WHEAT AND RICE IN DISEASE PREVENTION AND HEALTH

BENEFITS, RISKS AND MECHANISMS OF WHOLE GRAINS IN HEALTH PROMOTION

WHEAT AND RICE IN DISEASE PREVENTION AND HEALTH

BENEFITS, RISKS AND MECHANISMS OF WHOLE GRAINS IN HEALTH PROMOTION

Edited by

RONALD ROSS WATSON, BS PhD
*Mel and Enid Zuckerman College of Public Health, Health Promotion Sciences Division,
University of Arizona, Tucson, AZ, USA*

VICTOR R. PREEDY, BS PhD
*Department of Nutrition and Dietetics, Nutritional Sciences Division,
School of Biomedical & Health Sciences, King's College London, London, UK*

SHERMA ZIBADI, MD PhD
University of Arizona, Tucson, AZ, USA

AMSTERDAM • BOSTON • HEIDELBERG • LONDON
NEW YORK • OXFORD • PARIS • SAN DIEGO
SAN FRANCISCO • SINGAPORE • SYDNEY • TOKYO
Academic Press is an imprint of Elsevier

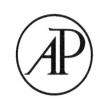

Academic Press is an imprint of Elsevier
32 Jamestown Road, London NW1 7BY, UK
225 Wyman Street, Waltham, MA 02451, USA
525 B Street, Suite 1800, San Diego, CA 92101-4495, USA

British Library Cataloguing-in-Publication Data
A catalogue record for this book is available from the British Library

Library of Congress Cataloging-in-Publication Data
A catalog record for this book is available from the Library of Congress

ISBN: 978-0-12-401716-0

For information on all Academic Press publications visit
our website at elsevierdirect.com

Typeset by TNQ Books and Journals
www.tnq.co.in

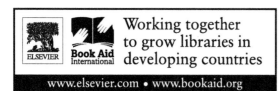

Contents

II

RICE AND OTHER WHOLE GRAINS IN HEALTH   279

Preface

Whole grains consist of the intact, ground, cracked or flaked kernel if it still has bran and the germ of the grain. Fiber intake in humans is alarmingly low, with long-term implications for risk of heart disease, hypertension, stroke, obesity, and diabetes, among other major public health problems. Eating wheat and rice as whole grains increases certain fibers known to prevent or reduce these chronic diseases. The bran and fiber enhance bowel regularity and gastrointestinal health, with improved weight loss and maintenance, and lower chronic heart disease. Currently less than 3% of American children and adults meet their appropriate fiber intakes, with consumption running at about 50% of the desired intake. Fiber is an under-consumed nutrient of public health concern, according to the 2010 Dietary Guidelines Advisory Committee. Several studies show that consuming 30 grams of whole grains daily reduces the likelihood of diabetes and heart diseases by about 30%.

In this book, bran from and on wheat and rice is reviewed by a number of experts. Part I, Wheat and Health, opens with a discussion of the role of whole wheat in pasta in health. Reviews of its fiber show vital modification of postprandial metabolic profile and health, digestive effects including childhood constipation, and reduction of prostate and colorectal cancer risk. Bran is shown to be important in providing antioxidants against antioxidant stress and as a source of cadmium, and there is an additional chapter on calcium, iron, and zinc for optimum health. Whole wheat plays an important role in gut function and nutrient utilization as well as growth and development of birds, described in chapters using poultry as a model for human health. Reviews show that whole grain affects phytate-degrading human bifidobacteria. Gluten from fiber is described in humans for its involvement with gut microbiota in health promotion. Finally, wheat fiber affects the sensory and health aspects when added to pasta.

In Part II, Rice and Other Whole Grains in Health, rice bran is described as a global public health opportunity.

Several authors document the role of whole rice in weight change, metabolic syndrome, and altering the glycemic index for diabetics. Oils in rice bran have benefits to health, and applications in the pharmaceutical industry. Genetically modified rice is suggested to have health benefits in reducing micronutrient malnutrition, and a potential impact via rice biofortification. Other authors describe extruded products from brown rice with unique physical and nutritional properties. Several chapters define the action of rice bran antioxidants in health and wellness. As with wheat, rice bran oil, fermented rice bran, and amino acid production from rice straw hydrolyzates are reviewed for health benefits.

Authors recognize that there are some risks connected with materials in whole grains. One author reviews adverse reactions to gluten and the exploitation of sourdough fermentation. Whole wheat has been documented as an occasional source of contaminants such as pesticides, which are then dissipated during their removal via processing. In developing countries, reviews show that whole rice and rice bran can be sources of arsenic for adults, and another chapter documents health risks in rice-based infant foods. Authors define the roles of rice bran, including arabinoxylan's immunomodulation as well as actions with anticancer agents. In addition, oryzanol is a developing bioactive component from rice bran. Exciting new developments in the use of enzyme-treated bran fiber from rice by-products produce novel functional foods for health promotion, using materials normally of limited nutritional value.

The book concludes with two reviews of bran and whole grains in health that are from neither wheat nor rice. Germinated barley foodstuffs reduce inflammatory bowel disease and show potential as a dietary therapy. Chickpeas are used to fortify wheat- and rice-based foods to increase fiber and phytochemical content. Overall, the uses of whole rice and wheat are varied, with substantial roles in health promotion and disease prevention.

Acknowledgements

The work of Dr Watson's editorial assistant, Bethany L. Stevens, in communicating with authors and working on the manuscripts was critical to the successful completion of the book and is very much appreciated. Support for Ms Stevens' and Dr Watson's work was graciously provided by Southwest Scientific Editing & Consulting LLD, and the Natural Health Research Institute (www.naturalhealthresearch.org). Finally, the work of Librarian of the Arizona Health Science Library, Mari Stoddard, was vital and very helpful in identifying key researchers who participated in the book.

Contributors

Anwaar Ahmed, BSc, MSc, PhD   Department of Food Technology, PMAS-Arid Agriculture University, Rawalpindi, Pakistan

Ahmed M. Amerah, PhD   Danisco Animal Nutrition, DuPont Industrial Biosciences, Marlborough, Wiltshire, UK

Akira Andoh, MD, PhD   Shiga University of Medical Science, Division of Mucosal Immunology, Graduate School of Medicine, Otsu, Shiga, Japan

Apostolis Angelis, PhD   University of Athens, Division of Pharmacognosy and Natural Products Chemistry, Department of Pharmacy, Athens, Greece

Paula Rossini Augusti, BSc, MSc, PhD   Federal University of Rio Grande do Sul, Department of Food Science, Institute of Food Science and Technology, Porto Alegre, Brazil

Mookambika Ramya Bai, MSc, MPhil   Madras Diabetes Research Foundation, Dr Mohan's Diabetes Specialties Centre, WHO Collaborating Centre for Non-Communicable Diseases, and International Diabetes Federation (IDF) Centre of Education, Gopalapuram, Chennai, India

Trust Beta, PhD   University of Manitoba, Richardson Centre for Functional Foods and Nutraceuticals, Smartpark, Winnipeg, Manitoba, Canada

Dieter Blancquaert, PhD   Ghent University, Department of Physiology, Laboratory of Functional Plant Biology, Ghent, Belgium

Erica C. Borresen, MPH   Colorado State University, Department of Environmental and Radiological Health Sciences, Fort Collins, Colorado, USA

Francisco Burló, PhD   Universidad Miguel Hernández, Departamento Tecnología Agroalimentaria, Grupo Calidad y Seguridad Alimentaria, Alicante, Spain

Alberto Caminero PhD   Universidad de León; Área de Microbiología, Facultad de Biología y Ciencias Ambientales, León, Spain; Universidad de León, Instituto de Biología Molecular, Genómica y Proteómica (INBIOMIC), León, Spain

Ángel A. Carbonell-Barrachina, PhD   Universidad Miguel Hernández, Departamento Tecnología Agroalimentaria, Grupo Calidad y Seguridad Alimentaria, Alicante, Spain

Claudia Cascio, PhD   De Montfort University, Faculty of Health and Life Sciences, Leicester, UK

Javier Casqueiro PhD   Universidad de León; Área de Microbiología, Facultad de Biología y Ciencias Ambientales, León, Spain; Universidad de León, Instituto de Biología Molecular, Genómica y Proteómica (INBIOMIC), León, Spain

Concha Castaño-Iglesias, PhD   Universidad Miguel Hernández, Departamento de Farmacología, Pediatría y Química Orgánica, Alicante, Spain

Un Jae Chang   Dongduk Women's University, Department of Food and Nutrition, Seoul, South Korea

Maria da Graça Kolinski Callegaro, PhD   Federal University of Santa Maria, Integrated Center for Laboratory Analysis Development (NIDAL), Department of Food Technology and Science, Center of Rural Sciences, Santa Maria, Brazil

Hans De Steur, PhD   Ghent University, Department of Agricultural Economics, Ghent, Belgium

Raffaella Di Cagno, PhD   University of Bari Aldo Moro, Department of Soil, Plant and Food Science, Bari, Italy

Mary R. Dicklin, PhD   Biofortis Clinical Research, Addison, Illinois, USA,

Silvina R. Drago, Dr   Universidad Nacional del Litoral, Instituto de Tecnología de Alimentos, Santa Fe, Argentina

Tatiana Emanuelli, PhD   Federal University of Santa Maria, Integrated Center for Laboratory Analysis Development (NIDAL), Department of Food Technology and Science, Center of Rural Sciences, Santa Maria, Brazil

Clara Fares   Consiglio per la Ricerca e la Sperimentazione in Agricoltura, Cereal Research Centre, Foggia, Italy

Christopher M. Fellows, BSc PhD   University of New England, School of Science and Technology, Armidale, New South Wales, Australia

Lynnette R. Ferguson DPhil, DSc   Discipline of Nutrition, Auckland, New Zealand

Xavier Gellynck, PhD   Ghent University, Department of Agricultural Economics, Ghent, Belgium

Mamdooh Helal Ghoneum, PhD   Charles Drew University of Medicine and Science, Department of Otolaryngology, Los Angeles, California, USA

Marco Gobbetti, PhD Professor   University of Bari Aldo Moro, Department of Soil, Plant and Food Science, Bari, Italy

Rolando J. González, Chemical Engineer   Universidad Nacional del Litoral, Instituto de Tecnología de Alimentos, Santa Fe, Argentina

Silvia Stanisçuaski Guterres, PhD   Department of Production and Control of Medicines, Faculty of Pharmacy, Federal University of Rio Grande do Sul, Porto Alegre, Brazil

Maria Halabalaki, PhD   University of Athens, Division of Pharmacognosy and Natural Products Chemistry, Department of Pharmacy, Athens, Greece

Gi Dong Han, PhD   Yeungnam University, Department of Food Science and Technology, College of Natural Resources, Gyeongsan, Republic of Korea

Parvez I. Haris, PhD   De Montfort University, Faculty of Health and Life Sciences, Leicester, UK

Monika Haros, PhD   Instituto de Agroquímica y Tecnología de Alimentos (IATA-CSIC), Paterna-Valencia, Spain

Philip J. Harris MA, PhD   University of Auckland, School of Biological Sciences, Auckland, New Zealand

Alexandra R. Herrán, MSc   Universidad de León; Área de Microbiología, Facultad de Biología y Ciencias Ambientales, León, Spain; Universidad de León, Instituto de Biología Molecular, Genómica y Proteómica (INBIOMIC), León, Spain

Masashi Higuchi, PhD   Meiji University, Organization for the Strategic Coordination of Research and Intellectual Property, Kawasaki, Kanagawa, Japan

Rhanissa Hirawan   University of Manitoba, Department of Food Science, Winnipeg, Manitoba, Canada

Yang Hee Hong   Korea University, Department of Food and Nutrition Seoul, South Korea

Masatoshi Hori, DVM, PhD   The University of Tokyo, Department of Veterinary Pharmacology, Graduate School of Agriculture and Life Sciences, Tokyo, Japan; The University of Tokyo, Development of Advanced Technology Laboratory Research Center for Food Safety, Tokyo, Japan

Takamitsu Hosoya, PhD   Tokyo Medical and Dental University, Institute of Biomaterials and Bioengineering, Graduate School of Biomedical Science, Tokyo, Japan

Md. Shafiqul Islam, DVM, MS, PhD   The University of Tokyo, Department of Veterinary Pharmacology, Graduate School of Agriculture and Life Sciences, Tokyo, Japan; Bangladesh Agricultural University, Department of Pharmacology, Mymensingh, Bangladesh

Muhammad Sameem Javed, BSc, MSc   National Institute of Food Science & Technology, University of Agriculture, Faisalabad, Pakistan

Eun Young Jung   Jeonju University, Department of Home Economic Education, Jeollabuk-do, South Korea

Osamu Kanauchi, PhD   Kirin Holdings Co., Ltd, Strategic Research and Development Department, Chuo-ku, Tokyo, Japan, and Shiga University of Medical Science, Otzu, Japan

Dongyeop Kim, PhD   Yeungnam University, Department of Food Science and Technology, College of Natural Resources, Gyeongsan, Republic of Korea; Hokkaido University, Division of Applied Bioscience, Graduate School of Agriculture, Sapporo, Japan

Dariusz Kokoszyński   University of Technology and Life Sciences, Faculty of Animal Breeding and Biology, Department of Poultry Breeding and Evaluation of Animal Products, Bydgoszcz, Poland

Willy Lambert, PhD   Ghent University, Department of Bioanalysis, Laboratory of Toxicology, Ghent University, Ghent, Belgium

Muriel Larauche, PhD   CURE: Digestive Diseases Research Center and Oppenheimer Family Center for Neurobiology of Stress, Digestive Diseases Division at the University of California Los Angeles, VA Greater Los Angeles Healthcare System, Los Angeles, California, USA

Christelle Lemus, PhD   University of Athens, Division of Pharmacognosy and Natural Products Chemistry, Department of Pharmacy, Athens, Greece

Helga Verena Leoni Maffei, MD, PhD   Full Professor of Pediatric Gastroenterology (retired), Professor Emeritus of São Paulo State University (UNESP), São Paulo, Brazil Past president of Pediatric Gastroenterology and Nutrition Societies: São Paulo (1986-8), and Latin-America (1987-9) São Paulo State University (UNESP), Department of Pediatrics – Botucatu Medical School, Botucatu, São Paulo, Brazil

Kevin C. Maki, PhD, FNLA   Biofortis Clinical Research, Addison, Illinois, USA

Eric V. Marietta, PhD   Mayo Clinic, College of Medicine, Division of Gastroenterology and Hepatology, Rochester, Minnesota, USA

Christian Matano, MSc   Bielefeld University, Faculty of Biology & CeBiTec, Bielefeld, Germany

Naoki Matsuki, DVM, PhD   The University of Tokyo, Department of Veterinary Clinical Pathobiology, Graduate School of Agriculture and Life Sciences, Tokyo, Japan

Tobias M. Meiswinkel, MSc   Bielefeld University, Faculty of Biology & CeBiTec, Bielefeld, Germany

Valeria Menga   Consiglio per la Ricerca e la Sperimentazione in Agricoltura, Cereal Research Centre, Foggia, Italy

Bruna Gressler Milbradt   Federal University of Santa Maria, Graduate Program in Food Science and Technology, Center of Rural Sciences, Santa Maria, Brazil

Keiichi Mitsuyama, MD, PhD   Kurume University School of Medicine, Inflammatory Bowel Disease Center, Division of Gastroenterology, Kurume, Japan

Tetsuya Mizoue, MD, PhD   Department of Epidemiology and Prevention, Center for Clinical Sciences, National Center for Global Health and Medicine, Tokyo, Japan

Joseph Birundu Mogendi, PhD   Ghent University, Department of Agricultural Economics, Ghent, Belgium, Mt Kenya University, Department of Nutrition and Dietetics, Thika, Kenya

Viswanathan Mohan, MD, FRCP, PhD, DSc, FNASc, FASc, FNA, FACP, FACE   Madras Diabetes Research Foundation, Dr Mohan's Diabetes Specialties Centre, WHO Collaborating Centre for Non-Communicable Diseases, and International Diabetes Federation (IDF) Centre of Education, Gopalapuram, Chennai, India

Sandra Munera-Picazo   Universidad Miguel Hernández, Departamento Tecnología Agroalimentaria, Grupo Calidad y Seguridad Alimentaria, Alicante, Spain

Joseph A. Murray, MD   Mayo Clinic, College of Medicine, Division of Gastroenterology and Hepatology, Rochester, Minnesota, USA

Reiko Nagasaka, PhD   Tokyo University of Marine Science and Technology, Department of Food Science and Technology, Tokyo, Japan

Ravi Naidu, PhD   University of South Australia, Center for Environmental Risk Assessment and Remediation (CERAR), Mawson Lakes, South Australia, Australia; and Cooperative Research Centre for Contamination Assessment and Remediation of the Environment (CRC-CARE), Salisbury South, South Australia, Australia

Akiko Nanri, PhD   Department of Epidemiology and Prevention, Center for Clinical Sciences, National Center for Global Health and Medicine, Tokyo, Japan

Vandana Nehra, MD   Mayo Clinic, College of Medicine, Division of Gastroenterology and Hepatology, Rochester, Minnesota, USA

Kristin M. Nieman, PhD   Biofortis Clinical Research, Addison, Illinois, USA

Katharina Nimptsch, PhD, MSc   Max Delbrück Center for Molecular Medicine (MDC), Molecular Epidemiology Research Group, Berlin, Germany

Esther Nistal PhD   Universidad de León; Área de Microbiología, Facultad de Biología y Ciencias Ambientales, León, Spain

Kazuyuki Ohara, PhD Tokyo University of Marine Science and Technology, Department of Food Science and Technology, Tokyo, Japan; The University of Tokyo, Laboratory of Marine Biochemistry, Graduate School of Agriculture and Life Sciences, Tokyo, Japan

Hiroshi Ozaki, DVM, PhD The University of Tokyo, Department of Veterinary Pharmacology, Graduate School of Agriculture and Life Sciences, Tokyo, Japan; The University of Tokyo, Development of Advanced Technology Laboratory Research Center for Food Safety, Tokyo, Japan

Elena Pastor-Cavada, Dr Instituto de la Grasa (CSIC), Sevilla, Spain

Jenifer Pérez-Andrés, MSc Universidad de León; Área de Microbiología, Facultad de Biología y Ciencias Ambientales, León, Spain; Universidad de León, Instituto de Biología Molecular, Genómica y Proteómica (INBIOMIC), León, Spain

Michelle Pietzak, MD University of Southern California Keck School of Medicine, Los Angeles County + University of Southern California Medical Center and Children's Hospital, Los Angeles, California, USA

Adriana Raffin Pohlmann, PhD Department of Organic Chemistry, Institute of Chemistry, Federal University of Rio Grande do Sul, Porto Alegre, Brazil

Mohammad Azizur Rahman, PhD University of Technology, Centre for Environmental Sustainability, Faculty of Science, Sydney, New South Wales, Australia

Mohammad Mahmudur Rahman, PhD University of South Australia, Center for Environmental Risk Assessment and Remediation (CERAR), Mawson Lakes, South Australia, Australia; and Cooperative Research Centre for Contamination Assessment and Remediation of the Environment (CRC-CARE), Salisbury South, South Australia, Australia

Tia M. Rains, PhD Biofortis Clinical Research, Addison, Illinois, USA

Amanda Ramírez-Gandolfo Universidad Miguel Hernández, Departamento Tecnología Agroalimentaria, Grupo Calidad y Seguridad Alimentaria, Alicante, Spain

Muhammad Atif Randhawa, BSc, MSc, PhD National Institute of Food Science & Technology, University of Agriculture, Faisalabad, Pakistan

Velmurugu Ravindran, BSc, MS, PhD Massey University, Institute of Veterinary, Animal and Biomedical Sciences, Palmerston North, New Zealand

Lucas Almeida Rigo, MSc Pharmaceutical Sciences Graduate Program, Faculty of Pharmacy, Federal University of Rio Grande do Sul, Porto Alegre, Brazil

Carlo Giuseppe Rizzello, PhD University of Bari Aldo Moro, Department of Soil, Plant and Food Science, Bari, Italy

Abdul Rohman MS., PhD., Apt Gadjah Mada University, Department of Pharmaceutical Chemistry, and Research Center of Halal Products, Yogyakarta, Indonesia; and Center of Research for Figh Science and Technology (Cirst) Universiti Teknologi Malaysia, Skudai, Malaysia

Nongluck Ruangwises, PhD Mahidol University, Department of Pharmaceutical Chemistry, Bangkok, Thailand

Suthep Ruangwises, PhD Chulalongkorn University, Department of Veterinary Public Health, Bangkok, Thailand

José María Ruíz de Morales, PhD Hospital de León, Departamento de Immunología, Altos de Nava, León, Spain; Universidad de León, Instituto de Biomedicina (IBIOMED), León, Spain

Ruy Carlos Ruver Beck, PhD Department of Production and Control of Medicines, Faculty of Pharmacy, Federal University of Rio Grande do Sul, Porto Alegre, Brazil

Elizabeth P. Ryan, PhD Colorado State University, Department of Environmental and Radiological Health Sciences, Fort Collins, Colorado, USA; Colorado School of Public Health, Fort Collins, Colorado, USA

Piyawat Saipan, PhD Khon Kaen University, Department of Veterinary Public Health, Khon Kaen, Thailand

Shengmin Sang, PhD North Carolina Agricultural and Technical State University, Center for Excellence in Post-Harvest Technologies, Kannapolis, North Carolina, USA

Juan Mario Sanz-Penella, PhD Instituto de Agroquímica y Tecnología de Alimentos (IATA-CSIC), Paterna-Valencia, Spain

Zumin Shi, MD, PhD University of Adelaide, Discipline of Medicine, Adelaide, South Australia, Australia

Antonio J. Signes-Pastor, PhD Universidad Miguel Hernández, Departamento Tecnología Agroalimentaria, Grupo Calidad y Seguridad Alimentaria, Alicante, Spain; and De Montfort University, Faculty of Health and Life Sciences, Leicester, UK

Mike J. Sissons, BAgSc, MAgSc, PhD NSW Department of Primary Industries, Tamworth Agricultural Institute, Calala, New South Wales, Australia

Alexios Leandros Skaltsounis, Prof University of Athens, Division of Pharmacognosy and Natural Products Chemistry, Department of Pharmacy, Athens, Greece

Khongsak Srikaeo, PhD Pibulsongkram Rajabhat University, Faculty of Food and Agricultural Technology, Muang Phitsanulok, Thailand

Hyung Joo Suh Korea University, Department of Food and Nutrition Seoul, South Korea

Birger Svihus, PhD Norwegian University of Life Sciences, Aas, Norway

Katarzyna Szarlej-Wcislo, MD, PhD Military Institute of Medicine, Department of Oncology, Warsaw, Poland

Yvette Taché, PhD CURE: Digestive Diseases Research Center and Oppenheimer Family Center for Neurobiology of Stress, Digestive Diseases Division at the University of California Los Angeles, VA Greater Los Angeles Healthcare System, Los Angeles, California, USA

Anne W. Taylor, PhD University of Adelaide, Discipline of Medicine, Adelaide, South Australia, Australia

Hideki Ushio, PhD The University of Tokyo, Development of Advanced Technology Laboratory Research Center for Food Safety, Tokyo, Japan; The University of Tokyo, Laboratory of Marine Biochemistry, Graduate School of Agriculture and Life Sciences, Tokyo, Japan

Ruchi Vaidya, MSc, PhD Madras Diabetes Research Foundation, Dr Mohan's Diabetes Specialties Centre, WHO Collaborating Centre for Non-Communicable Diseases, and International Diabetes Federation (IDF) Centre of Education, Gopalapuram, Chennai, India

Dominique Van Der Straeten, PhD Ghent University, Department of Physiology, Laboratory of Functional Plant Biology, Ghent, Belgium

Luis Vaquero, MD Hospital de León, Departamento de Gastroenterología, Altos de Nava, León, Spain

Sudha Vasudevan, MSc Madras Diabetes Research Foundation, Dr Mohan's Diabetes Specialties Centre, WHO Collaborating Centre for Non-Communicable Diseases, and International Diabetes Federation (IDF) Centre of Education, Gopalapuram, Chennai, India

Santiago Vivas, PhD Hospital de León, Departamento de Gastroenterología, Altos de Nava, León, Spain; Universidad de León, Instituto de Biomedicina (IBIOMED), León, Spain

Muhammad Wasim Sajid, BSc, MSc National Institute of Food Science & Technology, University of Agriculture, Faisalabad, Pakistan

Gabriel Wcislo, MD, PhD Military Institute of Medicine, Department of Oncology, Warsaw, Poland

Volker F. Wendisch, Prof. Dr. Bielefeld University, Faculty of Biology & CeBiTec, Bielefeld, Germany

Gary A. Wittert, MBBch, MD University of Adelaide, Discipline of Medicine, Adelaide, South Australia, Australia

Yingdong Zhu North Carolina Agricultural and Technical State University, Center for Excellence in Post-Harvest Technologies, Kannapolis, North Carolina, USA

WHEAT AND HEALTH

WHEAT COMPONENTS IN DISEASE PREVENTION: OVERVIEW

Whole Wheat Pasta and Health

Rhanissa Hirawan[*], *Trust Beta*[†]

[*]University of Manitoba, Department of Food Science, Winnipeg, Manitoba, Canada, [†]University of Manitoba, Richardson Centre for Functional Foods and Nutraceuticals, Smartpark, Winnipeg, Manitoba, Canada

CURRENT HEALTH CONDITION AND WHOLE GRAINS

Obesity

Statistics indicate that the rate of obesity has more than doubled since 1970, and Americans were still not meeting the United State Department of Agriculture (USDA) dietary recommendations in 2003 and 2005.[1] It has been shown that, after adjusted calculation for age and height, average body weights increased by almost 10% in the 20 years before the early 21st century, and that occurrence of clinical obesity has maintained its rapid increasing rate.[2] The increasing prevalence of the overweight trend is affecting not only developed countries, including the US and Canada, but also developing countries as they have experienced rapid economic growth.[3] There are currently more overweight than underweight people in the world,[4] where there is now widespread overconsumption of energy-dense, nutrient-poor foods resulting in diet-related chronic diseases. One of the well-known and well-repeated solutions is to decrease the consumption of refined grains by a significant amount; other recommendations include significantly reducing the intake of added fats, sugars, and sweeteners.

Whole Grain Foods and Health

Regular consumption of whole grain and whole wheat foods in place of refined grain provides a solution to the issue described above, for specific reasons. The discussion of whole grain in this chapter is focused on wheat as the major cereal produced, and one whose grain products are highly consumed worldwide.[5] According to the US Food and Drug Administration (FDA) Whole Grain Label Statement Draft Guidance written in 2006, "Cereal grains that consist of the intact, ground, cracked or flaked caryopsis, whose principal anatomical components – the

starchy endosperm, germ and bran – are present in the same relative properties as they exist in the intact caryopsis – should be considered a whole grain food".[6] The American Association of Cereal Chemists is currently (2012) updating their definition of whole grain as stated in their AACCI Standard Definitions.[7] Health Canada defines whole grain as products containing all three parts of the grain kernel, which are the bran, the endosperm, and the germ, while "Refined grains are whole grains that have had the germ and the bran removed".[8] In Canada, different types of flour are made by milling wheat, separating the different kernel parts and then recombining them to make specific types of flour, including whole wheat, whole grain, white cake and pastry, and all-purpose white flours. If all the parts are used in proportions similar to those of the original kernel, then the product is whole grain flour. Whole grain and whole wheat are different products. If 5% of the germ and bran is removed to reduce rancidity and prolong the shelf life of whole grain flour, it becomes whole wheat flour.[8] The definitions of whole grain and whole wheat name the parts of the grain kernel that must be included in order to be nominated whole grain or whole wheat. However, the amounts of these parts that must be present in the final product in order for it to be called a whole grain or whole wheat product are not specified. In order to achieve the health benefits that will be discussed in the next paragraph, and were summarized in a claim by General Mills, Inc. on March 10, 1999 as "Diets high in plant foods – i.e., fruits, vegetables, legumes, and whole grain cereals – are associated with a lower occurrence of coronary heart disease and cancers of the lung, colon, esophagus, and stomach", the definition of whole grain was further clarified as "foods that contain 51 percent or more whole grain ingredient(s) by weight per reference amount customarily consumed (RACC)".[9] In other words, the first ingredient on the ingredient listing must be a whole grain, such as whole wheat, oats, barley, rye, and millet.[10]

Whole grain possesses a specific food structure that provides increased satiety, and reduced transit time and glycemic response.[11] There are also health-promoting components that are concentrated in the bran and germ parts of the wheat kernel, including fiber, which provides improved fecal bulking, satiety, short-chain fatty acid production, and/or lowered glycemic response; magnesium, which improves glycemic homeostasis through increased insulin secretion; and bioactive compounds, including some minerals, vitamins, carotenoids, polyphenols, and alkylresorcinols, which have antioxidant and anticarcinogenic properties.[11,12] Health effects observed through large prospective population-based studies included lower risk of obesity and weight gain (especially abdominal fat accumulation) – effects also observed with a combination of high fruit and dairy intake and low white bread, processed meat, margarine, and soft drink intake[13–15] – a lower risk of cardiovascular diseases in regard to lower plasma cholesterol as well as LDL cholesterol levels,[16–19] and a lower risk of type 2 diabetes, including the effect of the particle size of whole grain in decreasing insulin response.[18,20,21] Removal of bran and germ in the production of refined grains eliminates these health benefits due to the removal of both these components and their synergistic effects.[22,23]

Despite the health benefits mentioned above, studies on whole grain consumption trends indicated a low level of less than one serving per day per person, which is well below the recommended level of three servings per day.[24,25] The socio-demographic group that consumes a greater amount of whole grain comprises the more health-conscious segment, which consists of women, older people, and more educated people.[25,26] Ratings for whole grain pasta when compared with their refined grain options regarding their relative pleasantness were equal, although there were also some inferior ratings.[27] Another issue with whole grain products is that the majority of the consumers perceive whole grain as providing a minor health benefit when compared with fruits and vegetables.[27] The pricing of whole grain products, especially pasta, is also a concern in efforts to promote the health benefits of these products. Whole grain product development should be focused on the types of foods that consumers appreciate and consider to be a major factor that can bring changes to their health conditions. The following summary of results from selected studies sheds some positive light on the promotion of whole grain intake. One study reported that staple foods such as bread and pasta were preferred to hedonistic foods such as biscuits and other snack products.[28] Whole grain intake that starts at an early age might remain a dietary habit for the long term when compared with a sudden and rapid change in dietary pattern at a later stage of life. Findings based on the eating habits of adolescents in Minneapolis/St Paul, MN, during the 2009–2010 academic year, regarding healthy foods including breakfast, fruit, vegetable, whole-grain, and low-fat dairy items, showed that adolescent friends share the same eating patterns.[29] This suggests that strategies designed by registered dietitians and health professionals to engage friends may enhance wholegrain intake in the everyday eating habits of adolescents. Another study found that dietary modeling involving substitution of a whole grain for a refined grain ingredient of foods commonly consumed by US children and teens, including breakfast cereals, popcorn, breads/rolls, other baked goods, pizza, rice/pasta, quick breads, and other grain-based savoury snacks, can increase the intake of whole grains.[30]

Current trends in scientific studies of whole grain versus refined grain are replete with results showing consistent health-benefiting properties, including lower body fat percentage in postmenopausal women, and in general, in relation to whole grain bread consumption,[19,31] and a lower BMI Z-score in schoolchildren (the BMI Z-score allows for a BMI comparison between a particular child and a group of children of the same age and sex).[32,33] Whole grain and also cereal fiber intake have been suggested to show correlations with the levels of the plasma alkylresorcinol and its urinary metabolites, 3,5-dihydroxybenzoic acid and 3-(3,5-dihydroxyphenyl)-1-propanoic acid.[34–36] This is because alkylresorcinols have been exclusively found in the whole grain and the bran of wheat, rye, and barley.[37] The very low trace amounts of intact alkylresorcinols that have been reported in refined grains are most likely due to bran contamination during milling.[38] These alkylresorcinol metabolites were also found to be highly associated with intake of cereal fiber, but not of fruit or vegetable fiber.[39] It was observed in one study that levels of plasma alkylresorcinols were inversely correlated with BMI scores in older adults.[40] However, the detection of these metabolites when there is a lower or no intake of alkylresorcinol-rich foods suggests other plant-based food sources[36] which are yet to be characterized. This suggests limitations to the use of alkylresorcinol metabolites as biomarkers for whole grain intake, and potentially the need for further processing of urine samples prior to quantification.[41] Other biomarkers are being used to measure whole grain intake in an attempt to correlate intake with the health condition of individuals. One group of researchers in Europe studied the combined effect of red meat and whole grain consumption using biomarkers that included C-reactive protein (CRP) for inflammation, gamma-glutamyltransferase (GGT) for oxidative stress, and GGT and alanine-aminotransferase (ALT) for hepatic fat accumulation.[42] The study concluded that levels of CRP, GGT, and ALT were inversely related to a high consumption of whole grain bread and directly related to a high consumption of red meat.[42]

USE OF WHOLE GRAIN IN PASTA PRODUCTS

Pasta Formulation

Many food products are made with a combination of whole grain and non-whole grain, for technical feasibility, shelf-life stability, taste, acceptance, and cost. Listed among such products are whole grain breakfast cereals (containing ≥ 25% of whole grain content), bread, hot cereals, and snacks, including crackers and muffins.[43] Several issues arise from this approach, where the relative proportions of whole and non-whole grain ingredients in the product are not clearly stated because information on the exact formulation is normally deemed proprietary to the food manufacturers.[43] However, pasta products may be exceptional, providing some solution to these issues in that the first ingredient of whole grain or whole wheat pasta, as found in regular grocery stores in North America, is durum wheat whole grain or whole durum wheat, and other ingredients that may be added include vitamins and minerals such as niacin, ferrous sulfate, thiamine mononitrate, riboflavin, and folic acid. In comparison to the manufacturing process of bread, for instance, pasta production does not require elaborate proving for its dough to rise to a certain volume. The latter therefore has the technical feasibility for using a large proportion of whole grain or whole wheat in the product. Shelf-life stability is also greatly enhanced through the drying process for pasta (<12% moisture content) compared to bread that is sold fresh after baking (<40% moisture content).

Pasta Glycemic Index and Glycemic Load

Durum wheat pasta made from regular refined semolina is commonly available as a good source of complex carbohydrates. In addition to its low fat levels, durum wheat pasta owes its low glycemic index and glycemic load to its high resistant starch content.[44–48] The glycemic index classifies foods which are high in carbohydrate content, based on the blood glucose level in the human body after a meal.[49] The blood glucose level is dictated by the nature of the carbohydrate, and type and extent of food processing.[49] The low glycemic index and glycemic load result in low glucose and insulin responses since the starch is not completely absorbed in the intestine, and thus the classification of pasta as a source of slow-release carbohydrates.[49–52] The gradual rate of release of sugars from pasta starch, which has been reported to be slower than other cereal products,[53] is due to the compact structure of pasta allowing for a very close protein network encapsulating starch granules that delays α-amylase attack[54–57] and the interaction with such components as dietary fiber.[58] The glycemic load

is a function of the carbohydrate intake and its glycemic index, as it estimates how much a food raises a person's blood glucose level following its consumption.[59] Studies found that a diet high in glycemic index and glycemic load increases the risk of selected cancers,[60] including digestive tract and prostate,[61] breast,[62] colorectal, and endometrial[63] cancers, although other reports do not support the direct relationship between glycemic index, glycemic load, and cancer risk.[64,65] The glycemic index of spaghetti (52) was found to be relatively low compared to higher values measured in white bread (100), barley (rich in amylose and β-glucans) (60), and vinegar (64).[66] Whole wheat durum pasta therefore combines the health benefits attributed to the low glycemic index of regular semolina and the phytochemicals of the bran and germ parts of durum wheat. The latter parts are removed during milling, since durum mills are designed to produce semolina predominantly from the endosperm fraction of the grain. Whole wheat durum pasta is made by incorporating the pulverized bran and germ back into the semolina.

Pasta Production

Pasta is traditionally made from hydrated semolina that is kneaded into dough and extruded into the desired shape. The semolina is transformed into homogenous dough during hydration and kneading. The use of whole wheat or whole grain durum, or the addition of non-traditional ingredients including whole wheat flour and wheat bran ingredients, changes the physical and chemical composition of uncooked and cooked pasta.[67,68] Whole wheat durum dough is generally weak and exhibits poor stability.[46] The main cause is the uneven distribution of the non-endosperm ingredients that leads to competitive hydration among the ingredients. Statements regarding the eating experience of pasta containing non-endosperm ingredients suggest that these products "can have a firm first bite but rapidly disintegrate in the mouth".[69] One study concluded that instrumental measurement of firmness, springiness, cohesiveness, and chewiness of these non-traditional pastas, including whole wheat durum spaghetti, needs to be combined with a sensory panel.[69] The probe type used in the instrumental measurement is dependent on the pasta shape, formulation, and cooking time, and level of discrimination desired. The firmness of cooked pasta made from commercial whole wheat durum flours ranged between 749 and 1020 N compared to the normal range of commercial durum wheat semolina pasta of 800–900 N as measured with an Instron instrument equipped with a Kramer cell.[70] Another study reported whole wheat durum spaghetti as having lower mechanical strength and cooked firmness, and greater cooking loss, than regular refined semolina spaghetti.[46,71]

A different investigation found that all spaghetti made with the addition of pulverized durum bran, ranging from 0% to 30% bran content in semolina, met both spaghetti quality cooking test standards of cooked firmness and cooking loss.[72] Similarly good performance was reported in durum semolina spaghetti samples containing 10%, 15%, and 20% added bran when tested against cooking resistance, cooking loss, and instrumental stickiness at the optimal cooking time and on overcooking.[73] The results were comparable to spaghetti samples without any added bran. In addition, the susceptibility to breakage during drying of the 15% and 20% bran-containing spaghetti decreased when compared with non-bran containing counterparts.[73] There is also the issue of physical appearance of whole wheat durum spaghetti. The surface of cooked whole wheat durum spaghetti was found to be rough with a reddish brown color when compared to the smooth and translucent yellow color of regular refined semolina spaghetti.

Sensory and Nutritional Properties

Sensory and nutritional aspects in one study found panelists preferring the flavor of 10% bran-containing spaghetti over non-bran-containing spaghetti, and a concomitant increase by 3.5 times in dietary fiber content, 40% in calcium content, and 150% in manganese content in the 10% bran spaghetti compared with 0% bran spaghetti.[72,73] The nutritional profiles of whole grain and refined pasta at the same portion of 100 g were reported by the National Institute for Health and Welfare in their Fineli database version 14 (www.fineli.fi) as follows: both had similar energy levels, protein, carbohydrate, iron, and folate contents, but different contents of fat (refined had 30% whole grain), fiber (refined had 50% whole grain), manganese (refined had 37% whole grain), and zinc (refined had 44% whole grain).[74] Single-screw extrusion of whole wheat flour to produce whole wheat spaghetti at 50 psi and 93°C resulted in a significant decrease of several essential amino acids, including 16% less lysine, 10% less threonine, 6% less leucine, and 5% less valine than the original whole wheat, even though the thermal processing was found to significantly increase protein digestibility.[75]

Color is an important pasta sensory quality that comprises (but is not limited to) the desirable yellow color that is the color of durum wheat endosperm. The less desirable brown color is likely an inherent brownness of the endosperm, but also a result of bran contamination. The less desirable reddish brown component is likely a result of some drying conditions. Melanoidins are the brown or reddish brown pigments formed through Maillard reactions during high-temperature drying of pasta, depending on the reducing sugar content of pasta and also the drying parameters.[76] Polyphenol oxidase

is highly concentrated in wheat bran including the tetraploid durum wheat bran.[77–79] This enzyme causes darkening and discoloration of wheat foods through its catalytic action in the reaction involving quinones producing brown and black pigmentation.[80]

Cost of Pasta

The difference in cost between whole grain and non-whole grain products was found to be small in bagel and bread products, with even lower prices for whole grain versus non-whole grain ready-to-eat and ready-to-cook cereals; however, the price of whole grain spaghetti macaroni was found to be more than two times higher than the price of their non-whole grain counterparts.[81] The average cost of whole grain spaghetti was $1.93 per pound in 1995 and $2.18 per pound in 1999, while the average price of non-whole grain spaghetti was $0.74 per pound in 1995 and $0.80 per pound in 1999.[81] Despite the higher charge per gram of whole grain spaghetti when compared with regular semolina pasta, whole grain spaghetti was included as one of the cheap health choices, at 23 cents per serving, among selected fruits, vegetables, pulses, etc., in a 2001 project to develop a healthy diabetes diet plan for the low-income population of South Alabama.[82] One serving of pasta is half a cup of cooked pasta, according to the Food Guide Pyramid of the Center for Nutrition Policy and Promotion, at a cost equal to $0.23 per 0.0625 pound or $3.68 per pound of spaghetti in 2001.[83] However, the availability of whole wheat spaghetti was very low according to market-based surveys conducted in 25 stores, including chain supermarkets (>20,000 square feet), small independent grocery stores (12,000–15,000 square feet), and supermarkets that sold bulk food items in Los Angeles and Sacramento.[84]

Factors Limiting Whole Grain Intake

Factors limiting whole grain consumption include consumers' lack of awareness of the health benefits of whole grain, inability to identify whole grain foods in the marketplace, association of whole grain products with lower sensory quality including taste and palatability, unfamiliarity with the preparation method of whole grain foods, and unwillingness to pay higher costs associated with whole grain foods.[81] Whole grain spaghetti, however, is among the whole grain foods that consumers can easily identify, in the same way as brown rice. It encompasses whole wheat and whole grain types, including the spaghetti types that are produced using buckwheat flour, bran, and brown rice. Whole grain spaghetti was among the whole grain foods that reached large-volume sales, along with oat bran ready-to-eat cereal, with the highest 5-year growth rate when compared with small-volume products, including whole wheat macaroni, fettuccine and rigatoni, spelt, millet and amaranth flour, graham flour, cracked wheat ready-to-cook cereal, and ready-to-eat cereals made with spelt and brown rice.[81] However, whole grain foods still make up a very small portion of total grain food sales. The abundance of studies on health benefits associated with consumption of whole grains also raises the question of the health effect of consuming refined grains. Total elimination of the consumption of refined grains, and especially of favorite foods such as white bread, white rice, or regular pasta, is likely unfeasible. Thus, Williams[85] collected literature with evidence that consumption of moderate levels of refined grain is not related to any health risks, including cardiovascular disease, diabetes, or overall mortality, as long as there is not overconsumption of refined grains, especially when combined with high levels of added fat, sugar, or sodium. However, reduced consumption of refined grains by one-third to one-half is all that is needed to achieve a diet that allows for the health benefits of whole grains to take effect.[85] This statement is further strengthened by another systematic review, where the summarized study results indicate how the proportion of macronutrients in a diet might not be a main factor in preventing obesity, although a diet abundant in whole grain and less refined grain was positively associated with lower weight gain and smaller waist circumference.[86]

BIOACTIVE COMPOUNDS OF WHOLE GRAIN FOUND IN PASTA

The health benefits of whole grain and its use in pasta as outlined above are very likely a result of synergistic effects of the many bioactive compounds in whole wheat grain.[74,87] Several bioactive phytochemical compounds have been studied in wheat. Those reported in pasta products include dietary fiber, oligosaccharides, phenolics (phenolic acids, alkylresorcinols, and flavonoids), lignans, and phytic acid.[43,74,88] Most of these compounds beneficial to health are highly concentrated in the bran and germ portions of whole grain.[43,89]

Dietary fiber is known to positively influence glucose and lipid metabolism.[44,45,90] The dietary fiber constituents along with other bran components that include alkylresorcinols, tocols, and sterols are key factors to be considered by plant breeders planning to develop varieties with health-promoting effects.[90] Studies on the role of fiber in human health have shown convincing inverse association between dietary fiber intake, through vegetable consumption and substitution of refined grains with whole grains, and total and specific mortality even in more recent findings on non-CVD, non-cancer inflammatory and respiratory diseases as well.[91] Total dietary fiber content was measured in regular refined wheat spaghetti and whole wheat spaghetti. Although dietary fiber could not be detected in regular spaghetti, it was found to be 10.36% in whole wheat spaghetti.[92]

Prebiotics generally include dietary fibers and indigestible oligosaccharides. Their indigestibility allows for better growth of bifidogenic and lactic acid bacteria in the human gastrointestinal tract.[93] The health benefits derived from regular intake of prebiotics include gut health maintenance, colitis prevention, cancer inhibition, immunopotentiation, cholesterol removal, reduced risk of cardiovascular disease, and prevention of obesity and constipation.[93] Some soluble dietary fibers from modern and old durum-type wheat varieties have been shown to have prebiotic effects when tested on *Lactobacillus* and *Bifidobacterium* strains.[94] Wheat bran is highly concentrated in arabinoxylans, hence enabling the production of arabinoxylooligosaccharides and xylooligosaccharides through enzymatic hydrolysis that occurs in the colon upon ingestion of arabinoxylans.[95,96] The degradation of arabinoxylan from the cell wall component of durum wheat bran in pasta into arabinoxylooligosaccharides and xylooligosaccharides is governed by certain factors, including the coarse particle size of pasta strands, the encapsulation of starch by gluten, and, in turn, the limited absorption of water by the starch.[97] These arabinoxylooligosaccharides and xylooligosaccharides from cereal-based food products were shown to have prebiotic effects in the colon of humans and animals through selective stimulation of beneficial intestinal microbiota.[96]

Phenolics, lignans, phytate, tocopherols, and tocotrienols are among the compounds acting as antioxidants in whole grain. Phenolics are compounds with one or more aromatic rings and one or more hydroxyl groups. They are the most studied bioactive compounds in whole grain. Phenolics exist in three forms: free, soluble-conjugated, and insoluble. The classes of phenolics include phenolic acids (hydroxycinnamic acid and hydroxybenzoic acid), alkyl- and alkenylresorcinols, and flavonoids (flavonols, flavones, isoflavones, flavanones, anthocyanidins, and flavanols). The flavanols include catechins, proanthocyanidins, and anthocyanins.

Phenolic acids are hydroxylated derivatives of benzoic and cinnamic acids, with hydroxycinnamic acids being more common than hydroxybenzoic acid. Hydroxycinnamic acids that are commonly measured in grains are *p*-coumaric, caffeic, sinapic, and ferulic acids, with ferulic acid normally found in the highest levels.[98–100] Analysis of flours from four wheat cultivars, using high performance liquid chromatography (HPLC), revealed that ferulic acid was the predominant phenolic acid in wheat grain (51.0%), followed by caffeic (22.8%) and *p*-coumaric (17.6%) acids.[101] The outer layers of grains contain most of the phenolic acids.[101,102] Three components of eight durum wheat grain samples comprising the starchy endosperm, aleurone layer, and pericarp were found to contain low levels of ferulic acid, a high content of *trans*-sinapic acid, and high levels of ferulic acid dehydrodimers, respectively.[103] Two studies on antioxidant activity in the outer layers of wheat obtained using a de-branning technique found that the first 5% pearled fraction contained the most pentosan, although it was lower in antioxidant activity; the next 5% pearled fraction had high levels of dietary fiber and antioxidant activity; and total dietary fiber and antioxidant activity decreased as amount of endosperm increased after removal of 10–20% pearlings.[104,105] Most phenolic acids are present in the bound form, and HPLC analysis showed that bound phenolics constituted 94.0% of total acids in four wheat cultivars.[101] These acids, predominantly ferulic acids, are esterified to arabinoxylans (ferulic acids as a molecular component of arabinoxylans are also known as pentosans) acting as cross-linking agents between these polysaccharides, or between the polysaccharides and lignins, playing a major role in the integrity of plant cell walls in the outer bran layers.[104,106,107] The bound ferulic acid of the bran layer is also considered to be a resistance factor against plant disease, especially *Fusarium* headblight.[108,109] Ferulic acid levels, along with their total phenolic contents, were measured in commercial spaghetti products (regular spaghetti, regular spaghetti with added inulin fiber, and whole wheat spaghetti).[110] Whole wheat spaghetti showed significantly higher ferulic acid and total phenolic contents than regular spaghetti; however, there was a 40% reduction in total phenolic content in regular and whole wheat spaghetti after cooking.[110] Regular spaghetti with added inulin fiber perceptibly behaved similarly to regular spaghetti in antioxidant properties, and these findings underscore the need to consume "whole" grains in order to fully benefit from the synergistic effects of the bioactive compounds in grains versus, for example, consumption of individual bioactive compounds in nutrient supplements.[110–112]

Alkyl- and alkenylresorcinols contain a long (normally 15–25 carbons) non-isoprenoid side chain attached to a hydroxybenzene ring.[98] Both types of resorcinols, present in significant amounts in cereals such as rye and wheat, have been shown to be bioactive compounds displaying antimicrobial action, cytotoxicity against cancerous cells, and protection of cellular lipid components from oxidation processes;[113] antioxidant properties (hydrogen donation and peroxyl radical-scavenging effects);[114] and potential prevention of coronary heart disease by increasing levels of γ-tocopherols.[115] Alkyl- and alkenylresorcinols are still present in significant enough amounts, even after grain processing, to impart potentially health-beneficial effects.[116–118] In a study on alkylresorcinol contents in durum wheat (*Triticum durum*) kernels and pasta products, pasta products containing 55% whole grain durum wheat flour and 45% refined durum wheat flour were shown to have approximately 50% of total alkylresorcinol contents when compared with whole grain durum wheat flour.[119]

In an investigation on alkylresorcinols as pasta product authentication markers, it was shown that even high drying temperatures did not influence the applicability of alkylresorcinols as markers.[118] Similar to other phenolics, alkyl- and alkenylresorcinols are also concentrated in the outer layer of grains.[114,116] Refined durum wheat flour was found to have trace amounts of alkylresorcinols, while whole grain durum wheat flour showed a high level of alkylresorcinol content.[119,120]

Flavonoids contains two aromatic rings that are linked by a three-carbon unit. Many types of flavonoids (flavonols, flavones, isoflavones, flavanones, anthocyanidins, and flavanols, which include catechins and proanthocyanidins, anthocyanins) are typically present in fruits, vegetables, and other plants.[99] C-glycosides of flavones are normally present in cereal grains including wheat,[121,122] while anthocyanins are present in colored cereal grains, with cyanidin being the most common form of anthocyanins.[123,124] Determination of phenolic compounds in durum wheat varieties using liquid chromatography coupled with time-of-flight mass spectrometry led to the identification of flavonoids including pelargonidin-3-glucoside, cyanidin3-glucoside, cyanidin chloride, apigenin, vitexin/isovitexin, apigenin-6/8-C-pentoside-8/6-C-hexoside, lucenin 1/3 (luteolin 6/8-C-xyloside-8/6-C-glucoside), more apigenin and luteolin derivatives, and other additional flavones.[125] Cyanidin-3-glucoside and peonidin-3-glucoside are commonly found in purple wheat and blue wheat.[124,126–128] One study reported the dose–response relationship as non-linear between intake levels of flavonoid monomers and polymers, indicating the need for further investigations to determine the health effects of flavonoids.[129] The potential health effects have been under active investigation, with quercetin, the most common flavonoid, not being detected after oral administration and its circulating metabolites showing low level of activity *in vitro*.[130] However, it was found that flavonoids undergo extensive metabolism through conjugation and deconjugation, producing free aglycones, which are the final effectors (for example, in blood vessels) as vasodilator and antihypertensive agents.[130] Flavonoid glycosides are present in some wheat grain products, for example in regular and whole wheat spaghetti, where they were identified as 6-C-glucosyl-8-C-arabinosyl apigenin and the sinapic acid ester of apigenin-C-diglycoside.[131] The contents were higher by 44% in whole wheat spaghetti than in regular spaghetti, providing further evidence that phenolic compounds along with dietary fiber are concentrated in the outer layers of grains and, that consumption of whole grain products is strongly recommended.[131]

Lignans consist of two phenylpropane units.[99] They are dietary phytoestrogens that are commonly found in plant foods such as flaxseeds and whole grains, including wheat, rye, corn, and oats.[132] The lignan group covers secoisolariciresinol, matairesinol, lariciresinol, pinoresinol, and syringaresinol.[132] Lignans are broken down into the metabolites enterodiol and enterolactone by mammalian intestinal microflora.[99] Lignans are found mainly in the bran layer of wheat grain.[133] Positive health effects of lignans have been observed in colon cancer[133–135] and breast cancer.[136,137] There are additional potential health effects of lignans in chronic diseases, including cardiovascular disease, prostate cancer, and intestinal cancer, and in menopausal symptoms and hepatotoxicity.[138] Lignans found in durum wheat and its products were 10- to 20-fold higher than the levels found in soft grain products, while 20–30% of the original content in durum wheat remained in semolina, with a slight reduction following processing into pasta.[139] Whole wheat spaghetti was found to contain 69% higher levels of secoisolariciresinol diglucosides than regular spaghetti.[131]

Another bioactive compound that has been found in spaghetti as the final product of durum wheat grain is phytic acid. In contrast to the negative implications regarding iron and zinc bioavailability, phytic acid was found to act as an antioxidant through formation of chelates with various metals, resulting in reduced levels of iron-catalyzed redox reactions and associated oxidative damage.[43,140] Phytic acid is concentrated in the wheat bran, as white flour contains no phytate.[140] Semolina pasta was found to contain 1.0 g/kg of dry matter of phytic acid, while levels in whole wheat spaghetti, to the best of our knowledge, have yet to be quantified.[141]

There is a need to emphasize that cereal grains are not consumed raw or unprocessed. For example, heat treatments are often involved in the form of high-temperature drying during pasta production, and cooking of dry pasta prior to consumption. Various observations have been made regarding the behavior of phenolic compounds in pasta products during processing and the

final cooking step. One investigation reported that the total phenolic acid content in rye and wheat flours was similar to that in the final bread and pasta products made from these flours.[98] Another study found a 50% decrease due to processing, but a 36–87% increase after cooking could have resulted from the release of esterified phenolic compounds from plant cell walls and also the formation of Maillard reaction products with considerable antioxidant activity during cooking.[142,143] A different observation was made when comparing cooked regular and whole wheat spaghetti, where cooking decreased total phenolic content of both products by 22–53%.[110]

NUTRIENTS IN WHOLE GRAIN PASTA

Bioactive phytochemicals continue to be actively investigated in terms of their molecular structures and structure–activity relationships in both *in vitro* and *in vivo* systems. Needless to say, bioactive compounds of durum wheat kernels coexist with traditional components that can be classified as major and minor nutrients. Whole wheat pasta retains most of the nutrients found in the durum wheat kernel. A nutrient profile of whole wheat pasta, on a limited number of observations (<10), is shown in Table 1.1. Major nutrients in macaroni (elbow) whole wheat dry pasta comprise carbohydrates (starch and non-starch polysaccharides), proteins, and lipids (Table 1.1). Whole wheat pasta is a good source of dietary fiber, providing 8 g per 100 g of macaroni. Major phenolic phytochemicals are associated with dietary fiber constituents of wheat. Chemical and gravimetric techniques are generally used to determine the proximate composition of carbohydrates, proteins, and fats. Individual amino acids are also listed in Table 1.1. Levels

TABLE 1.1 Nutrient Profile of Whole Wheat, Dry Pasta, Macaroni (Elbow)

Nutrient Name	Unit	Value per 100 g
PROXIMATES		
Moisture	g	7.34
Ash	g	1.6
Protein	g	14.63
Total fat	g	1.4
Carbohydrate	g	75.03
Alcohol	g	0
Energy (kcal)	kcal	348
Energy (kJ)	kJ	1456
Other carbohydrates		
Fiber, total dietary	g	8.3

(Continued)

TABLE 1.1 Nutrient Profile of Whole Wheat, Dry Pasta, Macaroni (Elbow)—cont'd

Nutrient Name	Unit	Value per 100 g
MINERALS		
Calcium, Ca	mg	40
Iron, Fe	mg	3.63
Magnesium, Mg	mg	143
Phosphorus, P	mg	258
Potassium, K	mg	215
Sodium, Na	mg	8
Zinc, Zn	mg	2.37
Copper, Cu	mg	0.454
Manganese, Mn	mg	3.055
VITAMINS		
Folacin, total	μg	57
Folate, naturally occurring	μg	57
Dietary folate equivalents, DFE	μg	57
Niacin	mg	5.13
Niacin equivalents	NE	8.263
Pantothenic acid	mg	0.984
Riboflavin	mg	0.143
Thiamin	mg	0.488
Vitamin B6	mg	0.223
Tocopherol, alpha	mg	0.78
AMINO ACIDS		
Tryptophan	g	0.188
Threonine	g	0.392
Isoleucine	g	0.57
Leucine	g	0.999
Lysine	g	0.324
Methionine	g	0.236
Cystine	g	0.306
Phenylalanine	g	0.728
Tyrosine	g	0.382
Valine	g	0.635
Arginine	g	0.517
Histidine	g	0.344
Alanine	g	0.457
Aspartic acid	g	0.66
Glutamic acid	g	5.073
Glycine	g	0.53
Proline	g	1.561
Serine	g	0.713

A. WHEAT COMPONENTS IN DISEASE PREVENTION: OVERVIEW

TABLE 1.1 Nutrient Profile of Whole Wheat, Dry Pasta, Macaroni (Elbow)—cont'd

Nutrient Name	Unit	Value per 100 g
LIPIDS		
Fatty acids, saturated, total	g	0.258
14:00	g	0.002
16:00	g	0.24
18:00	g	0.013
Fatty acids, monounsaturated, total	g	0.195
16:01	g	0.005
18:01	g	0.19
Fatty acids, polyunsaturated, total	g	0.556
18:02	g	0.529
18:03	g	0.027

Reference: Canada Nutrient File, 2010 (Food Code 4456).

of total polyunsaturated fatty acids (0.556 g) are twice as high as those of monounsaturated and saturated fatty acids for the limited number of observations (<10) for macaroni (elbow) whole wheat dry pasta. Minor nutrients include vitamins and minerals, with the latter usually being reported as total minerals if ash determination is conducted as part of the proximate analyses. Individual minerals are included, showing that macaroni (elbow) whole wheat dry pasta can serve as a source of phosphorus, potassium, and magnesium. Whole wheat pasta contains the B vitamin complex with pantothenic acid as one of the predominant vitamins.

References

1. Wells HF, Buzby JC. Dietary assessment of major trends in US food consumption, 1970–2005. USDA Economic Research Service, *Economic Information Bulletin Number 33*; March 2008:1–6.
2. Jeffery RW, Utter J. The changing environment and population obesity in the United States. *Obes Res* 2003;**11**:12S–22S.
3. Kearney J. Food consumption trends and drivers. *Phil Trans R Soc B* 2010;**365**:2793–807.
4. Popkin MB. Global nutrition dynamics: the world is shifting rapidly toward a diet linked with non-communicable dieases. *Am J Clin Nutr* 2009;**84**:289–98.
5. USDA. *Grain: World Markets and Trade [online]*. Available from: http://www.fas.usda.gov/grain_arc.asp; 2013 (accessed 2013 March 15).
6. Anderson S. *Whole Grain Label Statements. Draft Guidance*. College Park: Food and Drug Administration, US Department of Health and Human Services [online]. Available from: http://www.fda.gov/ohrms/dockets/98fr/06d-0066-gdl0001.pdf; 2006 (accessed 2013 March 15).
7. AACCI. *AACI Definitions [online]*. Available from: http://www.aaccnet.org/initiatives/definitions/Pages/default.aspx; (accessed 2013 March 15).
8. Canada H. *Whole grain – get the facts. [Online]*. Available from: http://www.hc-sc.gc.ca/fn-an/nutrition/whole-grain-entiers-eng.php; 2013 (accessed 2013 March 15).
9. Pape SM, Kracov DA, Spokes JJ, Boggs P. *Whole grain foods authoritative statement claim notification. Submitted on behalf of General Mills, Inc. to the Food and Drug Administration*; 1999.
10. Lang R, Jebb SA. Who consumes whole grains, and how much? *Pro Nutr Soc* 2003;**62**(01):123–7.
11. Fardet A. New hypotheses for the health-protective mechanisms of whole-grain cereals: what is beyond fibre? *Nutr Res Rev* 2010;**23**(01):65–134.
12. Okarter N, Liu RH. Health benefits of whole grain phytochemicals. *Crit Rev Food Sci Nutr* 2010;**50**:193–208.
13. Harland JI, Garton LE. Whole-grain intake as a marker of healthy body weight and adiposity. *Public Health Nutr* 2008;**11**(06):554–63.
14. McKeown NM, Troy LM, Jacques PF, Hoffmann U, O'Donnel CJ, Fox CS. Whole- and refined-grain intakes are differentially associated with abdominal visceral and subcutaneous adiposity in healthy adults: the Framingham Heart Study. *Am J Clin Nutr* 2010;**92**:1165–71.
15. Romaguera D, Angquist L, Du H, Jakobsen MU, Forouhi NG, Halkjaer J, et al. Food composition of the diet in relation to changes in waist circumference adjusted for body mass index. *PLoS ONE* 2011;**6**(8):e23384.
16. Seal CJaBI A. Whole grains and health, evidence from observational and intervention studies. *Cereal Chem* 2010;**87**(2):167–74.
17. Mellen PB, Walsh TF, Herrington DM. Whole grain intake and cardiovascular disease: a meta-analysis. *Nutr Metab Cardiovas* 2008;**18**:283–90.
18. Giacco R, Clemente G, Cipriano D, Luongo D, Viscovo D, Patti L, et al. Effect of the regular consumption of wholemeal wheat foods on cardiovascular risk factors in healthy people. *Nutr Metab Cardiovas* 2010;**20**:186–94.
19. Kristensen M, Toubro S, Jensen MG, Ross AB, Riboldi G, Petronio M, et al. Whole grain compared with refined wheat decreases the percentage of body fat following a 12-week, energy-restricted dietary intervention in postmenopausal women. *J Nutr* 2012;**142**:710–6.
20. de Munter JSL, Hu FB, Spiegelman D, Franz M, Van Dam RM. Whole grain, bran and germ intake and risk of type 2 diabetes: a prospective cohort study and systematic review. *PLOS Med* 2007;**4**(8):1386–95.
21. Heaton KW, Marcus SN, Emmett PM, Bolton CH. Particle size of wheat, maize, and oat test meals: effects on plasma glucose and insulin responses and on the rate of starch digestion *in vitro*. *Am J Clin Nutr* 1988;**47**:675–82.

22. Jacobs DR, Steffen LM. Nutrients, foods, and dietary patterns as exposures in research: a framework for food synergy. *Am J Clin Nutr* 2003;**78**:508S–13S.

23. Koh-Banerjee P, Franz M, Sampson L, Liu S, Jacobs DRJ, Spiegelman D, et al. Changes in whole-grain, bran, and cereal fiber consumption in relation to 8-y weight gain among men. *Am J Clin Nutr* 2004;**80**:1237–45.

24. Cleveland LE, Moshfegh AJ, Albertson AM, Goldman JD. Dietary intake of whole grains. *J Am Coll Nutr* 2000;**19**(3):331S–8S.

25. Lang R, Jebb SA. Who consumes whole grains, and how much? *P Nutr Soc* 2003;**62**(01):123–7.

26. Zunft HJF, Friebe D, Seppelt B, deGraaf C, Margetts B, Schmitt A, et al. Perceived benefits of heatlhy eating among a nationally-representative sample of adults in the European Union. *Eur J Clin Nutr* 1997;**51**:S41–6.

27. Arvola A, Lahteenmaki L, Dean M, Vassallo M, Winkelmann M, Claupein E, et al. Consumers' belief about whole and refined grain products in the UK, Italy and Finland. *J Cereal Sci* 2007;**46**:197–206.

28. Dean M, Shepherd R, Arvola A, Vassallo M, Winkelmann M, Claupein E, et al. Consumer perceptions of healthy cereal products and production methods. *J Cereal Sci* 2007;**46**:188–96.

29. Bruening M, Eisenberg M, MacLehose R, Nanney MS, Story M, Neumark-Sztainer D. Relationship between adolescents' and their friends' eating behaviours: breakfast, fruit, vegetable, whole-grain, and dairy intake. *J Acad Nutr Diet* 2012;**112**:1608–13.

30. Keast DR, Rosen RA, Arndt EA, Marquart LF. Dietary modeling shows that substitution of whole-grain for refined-grain ingredients of foods commonly consumed by US children and teens can increase intake of whole grains. *J Am Diet Assoc* 2011;**111**:1322–8.

31. Bautista-Castano I, Serra-Majem L. Relationship between bread consumption, body weight, and abdominal fat distribution: evidence from epidemiological studies. *Nutr Rev* 2012;**70**(4):218–33.

32. Choumenkovitch SF, McKeown NM, Tovar A, Hyatt RR, Kraak VI, Hastings AV, et al. Whole grain consumption is inversely associated with BMI Z-score in rural school-aged children. *Public Health Nutr* 2012:1–7.

33. Economos CD, Hyatt RR, Goldberg JP, Must A, Naumova EN, Collins JJ, Nelson ME. A community intervention reduces BMI z-score in children: Shape Up Somerville first year results. *Obesity* 2007;**15**:1325–36.

34. Aubertin-Leheudre M, Koskela A, Samaletdin A, Adlercreutz H. Plasma alkylresorcinol metabolites as potential biomarkers of whole-grain wheat and rye cereal fibre intakes in women. *Brit J Nutr* 2010;**103**(03):339–43.

35. Ross AB, Bourgeois A, Macharia HN, Kochhar S, Jebb SA, Brownlee IA, et al. Plasma alkylresorcinols as a biomarker of whole-grain food consumption in a large population: results from the WHOLEheart Intervention Study. *Am J Clin Nutr* 2012;**95**:204–11.

36. Landberg R, Townsend MK, Neelakantan N, Sun Q, Sampson L, Spiegelman D, et al. Alkylresorcinol metabolite concentrations in spot urine samples correlated with whole grain and cereal fiber intake but showed low to modest reproducibility over one to three years in US women. *J Nutr* 2012;**142**:872–7.

37. Landberg R, Kamal-Eldin A, Salmenkallio-Marttile M, Rouau X, Aman P. Localization of alkylresorcinols in wheat, rye and barley kernels. *J Cereal Sci* 2008;**48**:401–6.

38. Ross ABKS. Rapid and sensitive analysis of alkylresorcinols from cereal grains and products using HPLC-coularray-based electrochemical detecion. *J Agr Food Chem* 2009;**57**:5187–93.

39. Aubertin-Leheudre M, Koskela A, Marjamaa A, Adlercreutz H. Plasma alkylresorcinols and urinary alkylresorcinol metabolites as biomarkers of cereal fiber intake in Finnish women. Cancer Epidemiol. *Biomarkers Prev* 2008;**17**:2244–8.

40. Ma J, Ross AB, Shea KM, Bruce SJ, Jacques PF, Saltzman E, et al. Plasma alkylresorcinols, biomarkers of whole-grain intake, are related to lower BMI in older adults. *J Nutr* 2012;**142**:1859–64.

41. Marklund M, Landberg R, Andersson R, Aman P, Kamal-Eldin A. Alkylresorcinol metabolism in Swedish adults is affected by factors other than intake of whole-grain wheat and rye. *J Nutr* 2012;**142**:1479–86.

42. Montonen J, Boeing H, Fristche A, Schleicher E, Joost HG, Schulze MB, et al. Consumption of red meat and whole-grain bread in relation to biomarkers of obesity, inflammation, glucose metabolism and oxidative stress. Eur. *J. Nutr* 2012.

43. Jonnalagadda SS, Harnack L, H LR McKeown N, Seal C, Liu S, et al. Putting the whole grain puzzle together: health benefits associated with whole grains-summary of American Society for Nutrition 2010 Satellite Symposium. *J Nutr* 2011;**141**:1011S–22S.

44. Aravinda N, Sissonsa M, Egana N, Fellow C. Effect of insoluble dietary fibre addition on technological, sensory, and structural properties of durum wheat spaghetti. *Food Chem* 2012;**130**(2):299–309.

45. Modu S, Laila A, M ZA, P BB. Studies on the glycemic response of wheat at various level of processing fed to normal healthy rats. *Biokemistri* 2011;**23**(2):63–71.

46. Manthey FA, Schorno AL. Physical and cooking quality of spaghetti made from whole wheat durum. *Cereal Chem* 2002;**79**(4):504–10.

47. Bjorck I, Liljeberg H, Ostman E. Low glycaemic-index foods. *Br J Nutr* 2000;**83**(S1):149–55.

48. Kennedy ET, Bomwsn SA, Renee P. Dietary fat-intake in the US population. *J Am Coll Nutr* 1999;**18**(3):207–212.

49. Jenkins DJA, Wolever TMS, Taylor RH, Barker H, Fielden H, Baldwin JM, et al. Glycemic index of foods: a physiological basis for carbohydrate exchange. *Am J Clin Nutr* 1981;**34**:362–6.

50. Anderson IH, Levine AS, Levitt MD. Incomplete absorption of the carbohydrate in all-purpose wheat flour. New Engl. *J Med* 1981;**304**(15):891–2.

51. Levitt MD, Hirsch P, Fetzer CA. Sheehan Ma LAS. H2 excretion after ingestion of complex carboydrates. *Gastroenterol* 1987;**92**(2):383–9.

52. Bonomi F, D'Egidio MG, Iametti S, Marengo M, Marti A, Pagani MA, et al. Structure–quality relationship in commercial pasta: a molecular glimpse. *Food Chem* 2012;**135**:348–55.

53. Tudorica CM, Kuri V, Brennan CS. Nutritional and physicochemical characteristics of dietary fiber enriched pasta. *J Agric Food Chem* 2002;**50**:347–56.

54. Fardet A, Hoebler C, Baldwin PM, Bouchet B, Gallant DJ, Barry JL. Involvement of the protein network in the in vitro degradation of starch from spaghetti and lasagna: a microscopic and enzymic study. *J Cereal Sci* 1998;**27**:133–45.

55. Fardet A, Abecassis J, Hoebler C, Baldwin PM, Buleon A, Berot S, et al. Influence of technological modifications of the protein network from pasta on in vitro starch degradation. *J Cereal Sci* 1999;**30**:133–45.

56. Cunin C, Handshin S, Walther P, Escher F. Structural changes of starch during cooking of durum wheat pasta. *Lebensm.-Wiss.u.-Technol* 1995;**28**:323–8.

57. Dexter J, Dronzek BL, Matsuo RR. Scanning electron microscopy of cooked spaghetti. *Cereal Chem* 1978;**55**(1):23–30.

58. Esposito F, Arlotti G, Bonifati AM, Napolitano A, Vitale D, Fogliano V. Antioxidant activity and dietary fiber in durum wheat bran by-products. *Food Res Int* 2005;**38**:1167–73.

59. Foster-Powell K, Holt SHA, Brand-Miller JC. International table of glycemic index and glycemic load values: 2002. *Am J Clin Nutr* 2002;**76**:5–56.

60. Barclay AW, Petocz P, McMillan-Price J, Flood VM, Prvan T, Mitchell P, et al. Glycemic index, glycemic load, and chronic disease risk-a meta-analysis of observational studies. *Am J Clin Nutr* 2008;**87**:627–37.

61. Hu J, La Vecchia C, Augustin LS, Negri E, de Groh M, Morrison H, et al. Glycemic index, glycemic load and cancer risk. *Ann Oncol* 2012;**00**:1–7.

62. Dong JY, Qin LQ. Dietary glycemic index, glycemic load, and risk of breast cancer: meta-analysis of prospective cohort studies. *Breat Cancer Res Treat* 2011;**126**:287–94.

63. Gnagnarella P, Gandini S, La Vecchia C, Maisonneuve P. Glycemic index, glycemic load, and cancer risk: a meta-analysis. *Am J Clin Nutr* 2008;**87**:1783–801.

64. Mulholland HG, Murray LJ, Cardwell CR, Cantwell MM. Dietary glycaemic index, glycaemic load and breast cancer risk: a systematic review and meta-analysis. *Br J Cancer* 2008;**99**:1170–5.

65. George SM, Mayne ST, Leitzmann MF, Park Y, Schatzkin A, Flood A, et al. Dietary glycemic index, glycemic load, and risk of cancer: a prospective cohort study. *Am J Epidemiol* 2009;**169**:462–72.

66. Bjorck I, Elmstahl HL. The glycaemic index: importance of dietary fibre and other food properties. *P Nutr Soc* 2003;**62**(1):201–6.

67. Yalla SR, Manthey FR. Effect of semolina and absorption level on extrusion of spaghetti containing non-traditional ingredients. *J Sci Food Agric* 2006;**86**:841–8.

68. Dexter JE, Matsuo RR. Effect of semolina extraction rate on semolina characteristics and spaghetti quality. *Cereal Chem* 1978;**55**(6):841–52.

69. Manthey FA, Dick T. Assessment of probe type for measuring pasta texture. *Cereal Foods World* 2012;**57**(2):56–62.

70. Sahlstorm S, Mosleth E, Baevre AB. Influence of starch, gluten proteins and extraction rate on bread and pasta quality. *Carbohydr Polym* 1993;**21**:169–75.

71. Edwards NM, Bilideris CG, Dexter JE. Textural characteristics of wholewheat pasta and pasta containing non-starch polysaccharides. *J Food Sci* 1995;**60**(6):1321–4.

72. Kordonowy RK, Youngs VL. Utilization of durum bran and its effect on spaghetti. *Cereal Chem* 1985;**62**(4):301–8.

73. Chillo S, Laverse J, Falcone PM, Protopapa A, Del Nobile MA. Influence of the addition of buckwheat flour and durum wheat bran on spaghetti quality. *J Cereal Sci* 2008;**47**:144–52.

74. Poutanen K. Past and future of cereal grains as food for health. *Trends Food Sci Technol* 2012;**25**:58–62.

75. Arrage JM, Barbeau WE, Johnson JM. Protein quality of whole wheat as affected by drum-drying and single-screw extrusion. *J Agric Food Chem* 1992;**40**:1943–7.

76. Feillet P, Autran JC, Icard-Verniere C. Pasta brownness: an assessment. *J Cereal Sci* 2000;**32**:215–33.

77. Rani KU, Prasada Rao UJS, Leelavathi K, Haridas Rao P. Distribution of enzymes in wheat flour mill streams. *J Cereal Sci* 2001;**23**(3):233–42.

78. Jimenez M, Dubcovsky J. Chromosome location of genes affecting polyphenol oxidase activity in seeds of common and durum wheat. *Plant Breeding* 1999;**118**:395–8.

79. Lamkin WM, Milller BS, Nelson SW, Traylor DD, Lee MS. Polyphenol oxidase activities of hard red winter, soft red winter, hard red spring, white common, club and durum wheat cultivars. *Cereal Chem* 1981;**58**:27–31.

80. Anderson JV, Morris CF. An improved whole-seed assay for screening wheat germplasm for polyphenol oxidase activity. *Crop Sci* 2001;**41**:1697–705.

81. Kantor LS, Variyam JN, Allshouse JE, Putnam JJ, Lin BH. Choose a variety of grains daily, especially whole grains: a challenge for consumers. *J Nutr* 2001;**131** 473S–468S.

82. King A. *Rich eating on a poor income: can the poor afford to eat a healthy diabetes diet [Power Point Slides]*. Available from: http://aade2011.prod1.srdp.org/public/var/2/c/9/c/S23.pdf; 2001 (accessed 2013 March 15).

83. USDA Center for Nutrition Policy and Promotion. *Food Guide Pyramid. [Online]*. Available from: http://www.cnpp.usda.gov/FGP.htm; 2012 (accessed 2013 March 15).

84. Jetter KM, Cassady DL. The availability and cost of healthier food alternatives. *Am J Prev Med* 2006;**30**(1):38–44.

85. Williams PG. Evaluation of the evidence between consumption of refined grains and health outcomes. *Nutr Rev* 2012;**70**(2):80–99.

86. Fogelholm M, Anderssen S, Gunnarsdottir I, Lahti-Koski M. Dietary macronutrients and food consumption as determinants of long-term weight change in adult populations: a systematic literature review. *Food Nutr Res* 2012;**56**:1–45.

87. Liu RH. Potential synergy of phytochemicals in cancer prevention: mechanism of action. *J Nutr* 2004;**134** 3479S–3458S.

88. Okarter NaL RH. Health benefits of whole grain phytochemicals. *Crit Rev Food Sci Nutr* 2010;**50**(3):193–208.

89. Patel S. Cereal bran: the next super food with significant antioxidant and anticancer potential. *Mediterranian J Nutr Metabolism* 2012;**5**(2):91–104.

90. Andersson AAM, Andersson R, Piironen V, Lampi AM, Nystrom L, Boros D, et al. Contents of dietary fibre components and their relation to associated bioactive components in whole grain wheat samples from the HEALTHGRAIN diversity screen. *Food Chem* 2013;**136**:1243–8.

91. Landberg R. Dietary fiber and mortality: convincing observations that call for mechanistic investigations. *Am J Clin Nutr* 2012;**96**:3–4.

92. Anderson JW, Bridges SR. Dietary fiber content of selected foods. *Am J Clin Nutr* 1988;**47**:440–7.

93. Patel S, Goyal A. The current trends and future perspectives of prebiotics research: a review. *3 Biotech* 2012;**2**:115–25.

94. Marotti I, Bregola V, Aloisio I, Di Gioia D, Bosi S, Di Silvestro R, et al. Prebiotic effect of soluble fibres from modern and old durum-type wheat variaties on *Lactobacillus* and *Bifidobacterium* strains. *J Sci Food Agric* 2012;**92**:2133–40.

95. Delcour JA, Rouau X, Courtin CM, Poutanen K, Ranieri R. Technologies for enhanced exploitation of the health-promoting potential of cereals. *Trends Food Sci Tech* 2012;**25**:78–86.

96. Broekaert WF, Courtin CM, Verbeke K, Van De Wiele T, Verstraete W, Delcour JA. Prebiotic and other health-related effects of cereal-derived arabinoxylans, arabinoxylan-oligosaccharides and xylooligosaccharides. *Crit Rev Food Sci Nutr* 2011;**51**:178–94.

97. Colonna P, Barry JL, Cloarce D, Bornet F, Gouilloud S, Garmichle JP. Enzymic susceptibility of starch from pasta. *J Cereal Sci* 1990;**11**:59–70.

98. Mattila P, Pihlava JM, Hellstorm J. Contents of phenolic acids, alkyl- and alkenylresorcinols, and avenanthramides in commercial grain products. *J Agric Food Chem* 2005;**53**:8290–5.

99. Manach C, Scalbert A, Morand C, Remesy C, Jimenez L. Polyphenols: food sources and bioavailability. *Am J Clin Nutr* 2004;**79**:727–47.

100. Bravo L. Polyphenols: chemistry, dietary sources, metabolism, and nutritional significance. *Nutr Rev* 1998;**56**(11):317–33.

101. Wang L, Yao Y, He Z, Wang D, Liu A, Zhang Y. Determination of phenolic acid concentrations in wheat flours produced at difference extraction rates. *J Cereal Sci* 2012:1–6.

102. Rybka K, Sitarski J, Rchzynska-Bojanowska K. Ferulic acid in rye and wheat grain and grain dietary fiber. *Cereal Chem* 1993;**70**(1):55–9.

103. Peyron S, Surget A, Mabille F, Autran JC, Rouau X, Abecassis J. Evaluation of tissue dissociation of durum wheat grain (*Triticum durum* Desf.) generated by the milling process. *J Cereal Sci* 2002;**36**:199–208.

104. Sapirstein HD, Wang M, Beta T. Effects of debranning on the distribution of pentosans and relationships to phenolic content and antioxidant activity of wheat pearling fractions. *LWT Food Sci Technol* 2013;**50**:336–42.

105. Beta T, Nam S, Dexter JE, Sapistein HD. Phenolic content and antioxidant activty of pearled wheat and roller-milled fractions. *Cereal Chem* 2005;**82**(4):390–3.

A. WHEAT COMPONENTS IN DISEASE PREVENTION: OVERVIEW

106. Antoine C, Peyron S, Mabille F, Lapierre C, Brigitte B, Abecassis J, et al. Individual contribution of grain outer layers and their cell wall structure to the mechanical properties of wheat bran. *J Agric Food Chem* 2003;**51**:2026–33.

107. Peyron S, Abecassis J, Autran JC, Rouau X. Enzymatic oxidative treatments of wheat bran layers: effect on ferulic acid composition and mechanical properties. *J Agric Food Chem* 2001;**49**:4694–9.

108. Mckeehen JD, Busch RH. G FR. Evaluation of wheat (*Triticum aestivum* L.) phenolic acids during grain development and their contribution to Fusarium resistance. *J Agric Food Chem* 1999;**47**:1476–82.

109. Siranidou E, Kang Z, Buchenauer H. Studies on symptom development, phenolic compounds and morphological defence responses in wheat cultivars differing in resistance to Fusarium head blight. *J Phytopathology* 2002;**150**:200–8.

110. Hirawan R, Ser WY, Arntfield SD, T B. Antioxidant properties of commercial, regular- and whole-wheat spaghetti. *Food Chem* 2010;**119**:258–64.

111. Liu RH. Potential synergy of phytochemicals in cancer prevention: mechanism of action. *J Nutr* 2004;**134**:3479S–85S.

112. Jacobs DR, Tapsell LC, Temple NJ. Food synergy: the key to balancing the nutrition research effort. *Public Health Rev* 2012;**33**(2):507–29.

113. Kozubek A, Tyman JHP. Resorcinolic lipids, the natural non-isoprenoid phenolic amphiphiles and their biological activity. *Chemical Rev* 1999;**99**(1):1–25.

114. Kamal-Eldin A, Pouru A, Eliasson C, Aman P. Alkylresorcinols as antioxidants: hydrogen donation and peroxyl radical-scavenging effects. *J Sci Food Agric* 2000;**81**:353–6.

115. Ross AB, Chen Y, Frank J, Swanson JE, Parker RS, Kozubek A, et al. Cereal alkyresorcinols elevate gamma-tocophenol levels in rats and inhibit gamma-tocopherol metabolism *in vitro*. *J Nutr* 2004;**134**:506–10.

116. Ross AB, Shepherd MJ, Schuppaus M, Sinclair V, Alfaro B, Kamal-Eldin A, et al. Alkylresorcinols in cereals and cereal products. *J Agric Food Chem* 2003;**51**:4111–8.

117. Liukkonen KH, Katina K, Wilhelmsson A, Myllymaki O, Lampi AM, Kariluoto S, et al. Process-induced changes on bioactive compounds in whole grain rye. *Pro Nutr Society* 2003;**62**:117–22.

118. Knodler M, Most M, Schieber A, Carle R. A novel approach to authenticity control of whole grain durum wheat (*Triticum durum* Desf.) flour and pasta, based on analysis of alkylresorcinol composition. *Food Chem* 2010;**118**:177–81.

119. Landberg R, Kamal-Eldin A, Andersson R, Aman P. Alkylresorcinol content and homologue composition in durum wheat (*Triticum durum*) kernels and pasta products. *J Agric Food Chem* 2006;**54**:3012–4.

120. Menzel C, Kamal-Eldin A, Marklund M, Andersson A, Aman P, Landberg R. Alkylresorcinols in Swedish cereal food products. *J Food Composition Analysis* 2012;**28**:119–25.

121. King HG. Phenolic compounds of commercial wheat germ. *J Food Sci* 1962;**27**:446–54.

122. Asenstorfer RE, Wang Y, MD J. Chemical structure of flavonoid compounds in wheat (*Triticum aestivum* L.) flour that contribute to the yellow colour of Asian alkaline noodles. *J Cereal Sci* 2006;**43**:108–19.

123. Escribano-Bailon T, Santos-Buelga C, Rivas-Gonzalo JC. Anthocyanins in cereals. *J Chromatography A* 2004;**1054**:129–41.

124. Zofajova A, Psenakova I, Havrlentova M, Piliarova M. Accumulation of total anthocyanins in wheat grain. *Agric (Polnohospodarstvo)* 2012;**58**(2):50–6.

125. Dinelli G, Carretero AS, Di Silvestro R, Marotti I, Fu S, Benedettelli S, et al. Determination of phenolic compounds in modern and old varieties of durum wheat using liquid chromatography couple with time-of-flight mass spectrometry. *J Chromatography* 2009;**1216**:7229–40.

126. Zeven AC. Wheats with purple and blue grains: review. *Euphytica* 1991;**56**:243–58.

127. Abdel-Aal ES, Young C, Rabalski I. Anthocyanin composition in black, blue, pink, purple and red cereal grains. *J Agric Food Chem* 2006;**54**:4696–704.

128. Hosseinian FS, Li W, Beta T. Measurement of anthocyanins and other phytochemicals in purple wheat. *Food Chem* 2008;**109**:916–24.

129. Kay CD, Hooper L, Kroon PA, Rimm EB, Cassidy A. Relative impact of flavonoid composition, dose and structure on vascular function: a systematic revew of randomized controlled trials of flavonoid-rich foods. *Mol Nutr Food Res* 2012;**56**:1605–16.

130. Perez-Viscaino F, Duarte J, Santos-Buelga C. The flavonoid paradox: conjugation and deconjugation as key steps for the biological activity of flavonoids. *J Sci Food Agric* 2012;**92**:1822–5.

131. Hirawan R, Beta T. C-glycosylflavone and lignan diglucoside contents of commercial, regular, and whole-wheat spaghetti. *Cereal Chem* 2011;**88**(4):338–43.

132. Fardet A, Rock E, Remesy C. Is the *in vitro* antioxidant potential of whole grain cereals and cereal products well reflected *in vivo*? *J Cereal Sci* 2008;**48**:258–76.

133. Qu H, Madl RL, Takemoto DJ, Baybutt RC, Wang W. Lignans are involved in the antitumor activity of wheat bran in colon cancer SW480 cells. *J Nutr* 2005;**135**:598–602.

134. Kuijsten A, Arts IC, Hollman PC, van't Veer P, Kampman E. Plasma enterolignans are associated with lower colorectal adenoma risk. *Cancer Epidemiol Biomarkers* 2006;**15**:1132–6.

135. Johnsen NF, Olsen A, Thomsen BL, Christensen J, Egeberg R, Knudsen KE, et al. Plasma enterolactone and risk of colon and rectal cancer in a case-cohort study of Danish men and women. *Cancer Causes Control* 2010;**21**:153–62.

136. Touillaud MS, Thiebaut AC, Fournier A, Niravong M, Boutron-Ruault MC, Clavel-Chapelon F. Dietary lignan intake and postmenopausal breast cancer risk by estrogen and progesterone receptor status. *J Natl Cancer Inst* 2007;**99**:475–86.

137. Buck K, Zaineddin AK, Vrieling A, Linseisen J, Jenny CC. Meta-analyses of lignans and enterolignans in relation to breast cancer risk. *Am J Clin Nutr* 2010;**92**(1):141–53.

138. Landete J. Plant and mammalian lignans: a review of source, intake, metabolism, intestinal bacteria and health. *Food Res Int* 2012;**46**:410–24.

139. Granata OM, Russo G, Polito L, Traina A, Messina B, Carruba G. Sicilian durum wheat and its derivatives as a source of antitumoral compounds (lignans) in Mediterranean diet. *In 6th International Congress Flour-Bread*. 2011; *8th Croatian Congress of Cereal Technologists*. Opatjia, Croatia. p. 449–454.

140. Stevenson L, Phillips F, O'Sullivan K, Walton J. Wheat bran: its composition and benefits to heatlh, a European perspective. *Int J Food Sci Nutr* 2012 December;**63**(8):1001–13.

141. Torres A, Frias J, Granito M, Guerra M, Vidal-Varverde C. Chemical, biological and sensory evaluation of pasta products supplemented with alpha-galactoside-free lupin flours. *J Sci Food Agric* 2007;**87**:74–81.

142. Fares C, Platani C, Baiano A, Menga V. Effect of processing and cooking on phenolic acid profile and antioxidant capacity of durum wheat pasta enriched with debranning fractions of wheat. *Food Chem* 2010;**119**:1023–9.

143. Okarter N. *Whole grain consumption and health of the lower gastrointestinal tract: a focus on insoluble-bound phenolic compounds. [Online]*. Available from: http://cdn.intechweb.org/pdfs/29975.pdf; 2012 (accessed 2013 March 15).

Whole Grain and Phytate-Degrading Human Bifidobacteria

Juan Mario Sanz-Penella, Monika Haros

Instituto de Agroquímica y Tecnología de Alimentos (IATA-CSIC), Paterna-Valencia, Spain

LINES OF EVOLUTION IN CONSUMPTION OF WHOLE GRAINS

In recent decades, important socio-economic changes in the majority of the developed countries have substantially altered eating habits toward an increase in consumption of fat and proteins of animal origin, and have led to a decrease in the level of the population's physical activity. This trend is reflected in an increase in the incidence of diseases directly or indirectly related to an inadequate diet. In particular, the increase in the prevalence of diseases associated with metabolic syndrome has generated ongoing interest in the consumption of products made with whole grains, such as cereals and whole wheat flour or flour with bran, among others.[1] The rich composition of whole grains and their fractions, together with their high dietary fiber content, has motivated numerous nutritional interventions that have concentrated on highlighting their potential as a way of obtaining healthier, more nutritious foods.[2] According to various scientific studies, diets rich in whole grain foods and foods of plant origin and poor in lipids such as saturated fats and cholesterol can reduce the risk of suffering coronary diseases, certain types of cancer, and other chronic diseases. As a result, health claims began to be put forward for the consumption of whole grains in the United States in 1999, and in England and Sweden in 2002.[3] These claims established a direct relationship between consumption of whole grains and health. As research increasingly showed the benefits of whole grains, various countries and organizations throughout the world began to include them in their dietary recommendations. In 2003, The Australian Dietary Guidelines for Children and Adolescents proposed consumption of cereals such as bread, rice, pasta, and noodles, preferably made with whole grains. In 2004 the Ministry of Health

in Mexico announced its food health guidelines, declaring that "Consumption of cereals should be recommended, preferably whole cereals or foods derived from them. Moreover, their contribution of dietary fiber and energy should be highlighted." Subsequently, in 2007, Canada's Food Guide recommended consumption of at least three portions a day of whole grains such as barley, rice, oats, and even pseudocereals such as quinoa and amaranth. From 2008 onwards, European countries such as Denmark, Switzerland, Sweden, France, Germany, the Netherlands, and the United Kingdom declared their support for these recommendations.[4]

More than a decade after the first declaration regarding the health advantages of consuming whole grains, evidence for the benefits attributed to these products has become even stronger. One of the European Union's programs for reducing the risk of suffering diseases related to metabolic syndrome is HEALTHGRAIN, the aim of which is to increase intake of the bioactive compounds present in whole grains and in bran.[5,6] The activities connected with this project, which was created in 2005, are now being continued by the HEALTHGRAIN Forum, founded as an association in May 2010. Furthermore, the AACC International Report at The Second C&E Spring Meeting and Third International Whole Grain Global Summit in 2009 posed an important question: "Should we strive for getting 100% of the grain for 10% of the people or 90% of the grain for 90% of the people?"[7] This question suggests that an all-or-nothing strategy (whole wheat flour or refined flour) is not the most appropriate one. It has been shown that gradual and/or partial replacement of refined flour with ingredients obtained from whole grains in foods consumed by children of school age succeeds in increasing consumption of whole grain products.[8,9] Therefore, the manufacture of products formulated with a gradual increase in the outer layers of cereals might be a way of slowly adapting consumers to sensory changes in products made with whole grains. The Dietary Guidelines for Americans and the Healthy People 2020 program, which aim to promote healthy behavior in Americans during the next decade, recommend consumption of at least three portions of whole grains a day to reduce the risk of suffering cardiovascular diseases, type 2 diabetes, and certain types of cancer.[10,11]

THE ROLE OF CEREALS IN THE DIET

Cereals form one of the four basic food groups and are at the base of the healthy eating pyramid. Cereal-based products fit in perfectly with current dietary recommendations because they provide a feeling of fullness and avoid excessive consumption of calories; they contain little fat and it is unsaturated; they do not contain cholesterol; they are the best source of starch and fiber in our diet; and they have a low sugar content, with the exception of products with added sugar.[12] The United Nations Food and Agriculture Organization (FAO) has said that about 50% of diet energy should come from carbohydrates, cereals being the most representative group.

Wheat and rice are the most important cereals in the diet throughout the world, together with maize. Wheat accounts for most of the annual consumption of cereal grains in Europe, about half of the annual cereal consumption in Asia is rice, while maize is important primarily in Central and South America.[13] There are other less important cereals with a smaller production, such as barley, oats, and rye, which are mainly produced for human consumption, and sorghum and millet, which are used principally for animal consumption.[13]

Nutritional and Functional Importance of Outer Layers of Grains

One of the main contributions of whole grains is dietary fiber. Dietary fiber can play an important physiological role in maintaining general wellbeing and health, and the products that contain it are clear examples of functional foods.[14–16] Foods with dietary fiber improve gastrointestinal transit, help to reduce cholesterol levels, and are an excellent source of prebiotics, which help to strengthen the beneficial microbiota in our organism.[17] Products of this kind generally have a lower glycemic index than their fiber-free counterparts, maintaining better control of the blood sugar level.[18] Low consumption of dietary fiber has been associated with diseases such as atherosclerosis, dental caries, constipation, colon cancer, obesity, type 2 diabetes, and coronary disease, the latter two being preceded, in a large percentage of cases, by metabolic syndrome; whereas an increase in fiber content in the diet reduces the incidence of these diseases

and gastrointestinal disorders.[1,17,19] The quantity of dietary fiber consumed in a typical European diet is only 12–17 g/day, whereas the recommended daily intake, according to the European Food Safety Authority,[20] is 25 grams. In the United States, average consumption per person is similar, at 12–18 g/day, while recommendations for a suitable intake of dietary fiber are 38 g/day for men and 25 g/day for women.[21] With the aim of finding a solution to this problem, most countries in the world are developing programs aimed at promoting initiatives that will help to increase intake of dietary fiber in order to achieve the recommended values.

Apart from dietary fiber, the components of cereal grains that contribute to a healthier dietary profile are complex carbohydrates, minerals, vitamins, antioxidants, and other phytochemicals.[22] Most of these compounds are concentrated in the outer layers of the grain. The structure of all cereal grains is similar, consisting of three main parts: the pericarp, endosperm, and germ. The pericarp and germ are fractions that are removed in conventional milling of cereal grains, but they provide most of the biologically active compounds.[23] Specifically, they contain group B vitamins (thiamine, niacin, riboflavin, and pantothenic acid), vitamin E, minerals (calcium, magnesium, potassium, sodium, and iron), and essential amino acids (arginine and lysine), as well as other compounds such as phytic acid and polyphenols.[24] There is much research that suggests the inclusion of whole cereal flours, or mixtures of different grains or their fractions, to increase the nutritional value of products based on refined wheat flour.[3,7,25–32] However, despite the nutritional benefit that comes from the consumption of whole grains, whole wheat flours, and flours supplemented with bran, they contain substances whose activity inhibits the bioavailability of minerals, such as phytic acid (*myo*-inositol hexakisphosphate, $InsP_6$) or its salts, the phytates.[33,34]

PHYTIC ACID (MYO-INOSITOL HEXAKISPHOSPHATE, $I_{NS}P_6$)

Phytic acid is an organic acid widely found in natural systems, especially in plants, which has an important physiological function as a store of phosphorus and cations.[35] It consists of a cyclic polyalcohol of six carbon atoms called *myo*-inositol, in which each alcohol residue is phosphorylated. The phytic acid molecule has a total of 12 protons, 6 of them strongly dissociated [pK_a 2–3] and the others weakly dissociated [pK_a 5–9].[36,37] In accordance with this structure, at neutral pH and at the pH that foods normally present it is a negatively charged molecule with a great chelating capacity, so it is very able to form complexes with minerals or proteins (Fig. 2.1). The interaction of phytic acid with proteins is pH dependent, whereas interaction with metal cations

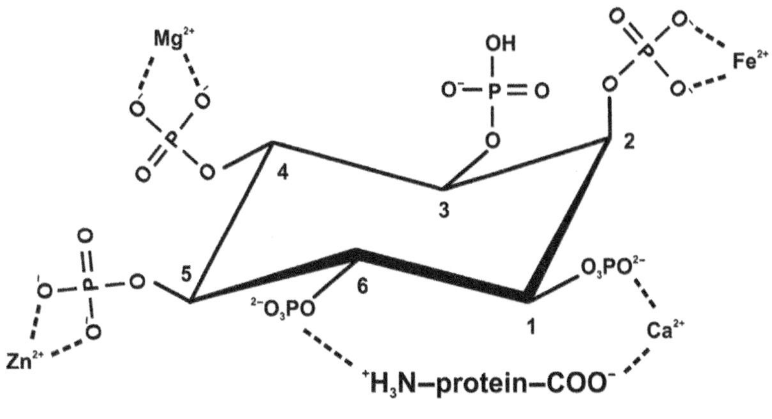

FIGURE 2.1 Suggested structure of $InsP_6$ complexed with proteins and/or divalent cations such as Ca^{2+}, Mg^{2+}, Fe^{2+}, and Zn^{2+}, at physiological pH.

is due exclusively to its numerous phosphate groups. Cations can bind to a single phosphate group, two phosphate groups of a single molecule, or phosphate groups of different molecules of phytic acid.[38]

In the context of human and animal nutrition, phytate has been considered an antinutritional factor because of the formation of complexes with proteins, affecting their solubility and digestibility; and with metal ions, strongly inhibiting their absorption.[39–41] However, beneficial health effects have also been attributed to it. Consumption of phytic acid can act positively against certain diseases, such as diabetes, atherosclerosis, kidney stones, and diseases connected with the heart.[42] Many of the mechanisms by which phytic acid acts have been attributed to its hydrolysis products, which have greater solubility and some of which have a conformation suitable for complexing intracellular metal cations. The special ability of some of these molecules to bind to metals can reduce the formation of hydroxyl radicals, acting as a natural secondary antioxidant in foods. This means that phytic acid is a precursor of molecules that provide protection against some kinds of cancer.[41,43,44] The metabolically active compounds derived from hydrolysis of phytic acid that could positively affect human health are extensively described in the literature.[45–49]

Distribution and Consumption

Phytates are found in all grains and seeds of cereals, oil-bearing plants, and legumes, and also in roots, tubers, fruits, nuts, and vegetables. The phytate content of cereals can vary between 0.1% and 2.2%, depending on the type of cereal.[50] Among all cereals, polished rice contains the lowest amounts of phytate (<0.25%), brown rice can reach values of 1%, while wild rice reaches values of 2.2%. On the other hand, the amount of phytate in different types of wheat (hard wheat, soft wheat, and durum wheat) ranges between 0.4% and 1.4%. The highest phytate content is found in some cereal milled fractions and protein products such as wheat bran (2.0–5.3%), rice bran (2.6–6.0%), wheat gluten (2.1%), and wheat protein concentrate (1.9–2.7%).[50]

Phytic acid is basically situated in the germ and in the bran fraction of cereals, mainly in the aleurone. The aleurone forms part of the endosperm, but it is very close to the outer coverings of the grain and therefore phytates are found in high quantities in products made from flour with a high degree of extraction.[35] Although there are studies on consumption of phytates in various countries, they are very sparse and not very recent. For the most part, diets in developed countries include cereals with a low degree of extraction, so phytate intake is moderate. Studies conducted between 1980 and 1990 reported that the mean phytate intake in Sweden was 180 mg/day,[51] whereas the British population consumed diets that were much richer in phytic acid, at between 504 and 848 mg/day.[52,53] On the other hand, in Italy there was a wider range in daily consumption of phytates, from 112 to 1367 mg/day, although the indicative average value was around 219–293 mg/day.[54,55] In Finland, average consumption of phytates was estimated at 370 mg/day.[56] Recent research conducted in the United Kingdom estimated phytate intakes for children, adolescents, adults, and the elderly population to be 496, 615, 809, and 629 mg/day, respectively – values that lie within the same range as those published in previous studies conducted in the same country.[57] In Spain, a recent study revealed an average phytate consumption of 422 mg/day, but this average increased to 672 mg/day when the diet included phytate-rich foods such as nuts, legumes, and whole cereals.[58] In developing countries, where whole grain cereals and other foods of plant origin make up a high proportion of the diet, it was observed that phytate intake is around 1–2 g/day, and in countries such as India, Nigeria, Malawi, Mexico, and Guatemala, consumption exceeds 2 g/day.[42,50]

Effect on Bioavailability of Minerals

As mentioned earlier, phytic acid is negatively charged at physiological pH, which gives it an extraordinary chelating power with an affinity for various components of foods such as proteins and minerals, as well

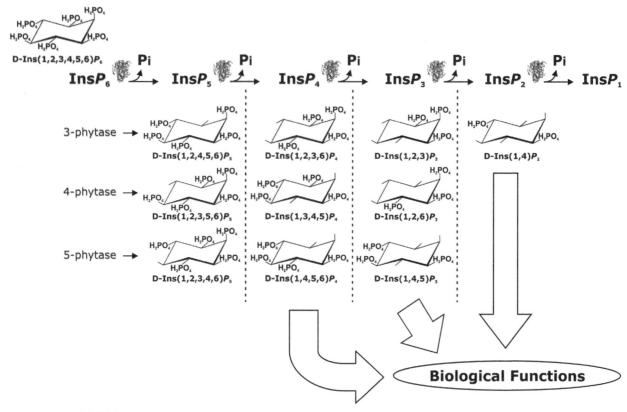

FIGURE 2.2   Sequence of phytic acid hydrolysis and generation of lower *myo*-inositol phosphate esters.

as starch and trace elements. Thus, phytic acid is capable of (1) affecting the enzyme activity, solubility, and digestibility of proteins;[41] (2) reducing the solubility of carbohydrates, affecting the digestibility and absorption of glucose;[41] and (3) reducing the bioavailability of minerals such as iron, zinc, calcium, magnesium, manganese, and copper,[39,40] forming complexes that are insoluble at physiological pH and impeding their absorption. Many studies have shown that a phytate-rich diet causes mineral deficiency,[40,59,60] particularly in unbalanced diets, in populations at risk, and in animal feed.[60,61]

Calcium is an essential nutrient for bone health and prevention of osteoporosis, which has become a global disease.[62] The calcium requirement depends on various factors, such as age, sex, physical activity, race, genetics, and several dietetic factors, including the phytates present in cereals and pulses, which reduce its absorption. After the process of gastric digestion, most of the calcium in the intestinal tract is bound to phytates and only a small percentage may be available for absorption. Although there are many factors that affect the bioavailability of this mineral,[39] the elimination of phytates improves its bioavailability.[63] Consequently, the bioavailability of calcium in foods of plant origin is generally deficient because of the presence of phytic acid.[62]

As for zinc, it is an essential mineral that is indispensable for the activity of many enzymes in our organism,

and it plays an important part in the proper functioning of the immune system. When the zinc contribution comes mainly from phytate-rich cereals, the processes that promote hydrolysis of phytates increase absorption of this mineral significantly.[64] Recent studies, both *in vitro* and *in vivo*, confirm the negative effect of phytic acid on the bioavailability of zinc,[65,66] the inhibiting effect being a process that is dependent on the $InsP_6$ concentration.[67]

Nutritional iron deficiency is the only deficiency with a significant prevalence in all developed countries, where the most vulnerable populations are women of child-bearing age, children, and adolescents. In earlier studies it was seen that iron in children' s cereals is less bioavailable because of the presence of phytates, whereas absorption increases significantly if they are eliminated.[68,69] In fortified foods, the bioavailability of iron was also affected by the presence of phytates, degradation of which also produced an increase in its absorption.[70] The study of the negative phytate effects on Fe bioavailability in whole grain products using the Caco-2 cell line, which approximates the biological response to the *in vivo* situation, has been well documented.[31,71–74] There are also studies in humans that show an increase in absorption of iron due to enzymatic hydrolysis of phytates in wheat rolls supplemented with wheat bran.[75]

Degradation of Phytic Acid

Phytase is a phosphomonoesterase capable of sequentially hydrolyzing phytic acid via pentakis-, tetrakis-, tri-, di-, and monophosphate of *myo*-inositol ($InsP_5$, $InsP_4$, $InsP_3$, $InsP_2$, $InsP_1$, respectively) and phosphate.[76] Hydrolysis of phytate has a two-fold benefit: (1) it improves absorption of minerals in the gastrointestinal tract, and (2) the *myo*-inositol phosphates with a lower degree of phosphorylation that are generated could have a positive effect on human health (Fig. 2.2). Three types of phytase are known, depending on the position on the inositol ring at which the initial attack of a phosphoester bond takes place: 3-phytase (EC 3.1.3.8) (phytate hydrolysis starts at the D3 position of the *myo*-inositol ring) or 1-phytase (name based on 1L-numbering system rather than 1D-numbering); 4-phytase (EC 3.1.3.26) (phytate hydrolysis starts at D4 position of the *myo*-inositol ring) or 6-phytase (name based on 1L-numbering system rather than 1D-numbering); and 5-phytase (EC 3.1.3.72) (phytate hydrolysis starts at D5 position of the *myo*-inositol ring). In general, depending on the type of phytase, the first hydrolyzed phosphate group of the *myo*-inositol ring can vary in position, which could generate different positional isomers of $InsP_5$. Subsequently, the hydrolysis will continue on another specific phosphate group of each enzyme, and so on, generating a particular hydrolytic profile for each enzyme.

The partially phosphorylated compounds that are generated may positively affect human health, because individual *myo*-inositol phosphate esters have been proposed to be metabolically active.[49] Several *myo*-inositol phosphates, including phytate, are present as intracellular molecules and the second messenger D-*myo*-inositol (1,4,5)-trisphosphate performs a range of cellular functions, including cell proliferation, by mobilizing intracellular Ca^{2+}.[47] This mobilization of intracellular calcium is modulated together with $Ins(1,3,4,5)P_4$, playing an important part in the internalization of calcium in the cell.[45,49]

An effect of extracellular phytate on the concentration of several intracellular *myo*-inositol phosphate esters has already been demonstrated in human erythroleukemia cells.[77] Furthermore, it has been reported that highly negatively charged *myo*-inositol polyphosphates can cross the plasma membrane and be internalized by cells.[78] *Myo*-inositol hexakisphosphate was shown to enter HeLa cells, followed by intracellular dephosphorylation to partially phosphorylated *myo*-inositol phosphates,[78] whereas turnover of *myo*-inositol (1,3,4,5,6)-pentakisphosphate was quite slow after internalization by SKOV-3 cells.[79] Myo-Ins$(1,4,5,6)P_4$ is also involved in epithelial response of the human intestine to infection by pathogenic microorganisms such as *Salmonella*.[47] Myo-Ins$(1,4)P_2$ has also been attributed with cell functions,

involved in replication of DNA by stimulation of DNA polymerase-α.[49] D-*myo*-inositol (1,2,6)-trisphosphate, for example, has been studied in connection with the prevention of diabetes complications and treatment of chronic inflammations as well as cardiovascular diseases.[46,80] With regard to the use of these compounds as possible pharmaceuticals, it has been seen that $Ins(1,2,6)P_3$ and myo-Ins$(1,4,5,6)P_4$ have anti-inflammatory activity, and the first of them is being evaluated as a possible analgesic in the treatment of chronic inflammations.[48] Because of its antiangiogenic and antitumor effects, *myo*-inositol (1,3,4,5,6)-pentakisphosphate was suggested as a promising compound for anticancer therapeutic strategies.[79]

Phytate breakdown products with 1,2,3-triphosphate grouping (equatorial–axial–equatorial) have a configuration that uniquely provides a specific interaction with iron which increases its solubility and inhibits its ability to catalyze hydroxyl radical formation.[81,82] Phytic acid also has the 1,2,3-triphosphate grouping, but when phosphates are removed from $InsP_6$ the lower isomers become more soluble.[83] The mineral-binding strength of inositol phosphates becomes progressively lower when phosphates are removed from the molecule, with the exception of the presence of the 1,2,3-triphosphate grouping. Myo-Ins$(1,2,3)P_3$ has been reported to be present at concentrations of $1-10\,\mu M$ in normal mammalian cells, where it was suggested to have a role in iron chelation as an intracellular iron transport agent and/or cellular antioxidant.[84–86] Furthermore, a study was made of the increase in absorption of calcium by means of $Ins(1,2,3,6)P_4$, which suggests that the compounds that contain the phosphate groups at positions 1,2,3 of the *myo*-inositol ring are potential candidates to increase the bioavailability of cations.[83]

Strategies for reducing or eliminating phytates include the addition of exogenous phytases (bacterial or fungal), the selection of varieties with high phytase activity or low phytate content, changes in agricultural conditions (optimization of fertilization), genetic engineering (overexpression of plant phytase), and changes in food production processes.[87] In the cereal malting, fermentation, steeping, and soaking stages, phytates could be sequentially hydrolyzed by the intrinsic phytase activity of the cereal,[88–90] whereas in the boiling stage (such as boiling of rice) the phytates are scarcely hydrolyzed or else they pass into the cooking water.[91] During germination of cereals, the level of phytase activity increased and reached its maximum value after 7 (16-fold), 6 (5-fold), 5 (7-fold), 7 (3-fold), and 8 (6-fold) days of germination for rice, maize, millet, sorghum, and wheat, respectively.[92] Significant reductions of phytates were seen in barley and rye germination processes.[93,94] Increase in phytase activity is always accompanied by a significant reduction in phytate content, releasing the phosphorus required for growth and development of the plant.[92]

Enzymatic degradation of phytates in cereal fermentation processes depends on many factors, such as time and temperature, pH, water activity, mineral salt concentration, additives, and process.[95] However, in whole products or products supplemented with bran the phytate content is maintained at high concentrations because of inefficient enzyme activity during the process.[89,90,93] Hydrolysis of InsP$_6$ in bakery products could be increased by strategies that involve lengthening process time,[96] increasing the quantity of phytase-producing yeast,[97,98] or increasing endogenous phytase activity by reducing pH, adding exogenous phytase, or both.[73,74,88–90,99–107] Tangkongchitr and colleagues[108] showed that degradation of InsP$_6$ in whole wheat bread after 300 minutes of fermentation was 23%. Faridi et al.[98] increased the quantity of yeast to reduce the InsP$_6$ content, while Harland and Harland[97] found that the InsP$_6$ content could be reduced both by increasing the fermentation stage and by increasing the concentration of added yeast. However, some studies indicated that increasing the yeast concentration did not increase, or only slightly increased, hydrolysis of InsP$_6$.[103,108–110] The addition of sourdough to a bread formulation also increases degradation of InsP$_6$ by activation of the endogenous phytase of cereals as a result of the decrease in pH.[99,100,104,111,112]

Commercial Phytases

Commercial phytases are currently available for administration in the preparation of monogastric animal feed. They are generally obtained by fermenting strains of genetically modified *Aspergillus* or by extraction of strains of *Aspergillus* not modified genetically from the culture medium.[113] Numerous studies have evaluated the effectiveness of commercial phytases on phytates in products for human consumption, but use of these enzymes remains in the experimental stage.[73,74,89,90,95,103–105,114–116] In the making of whole wheat bread, the addition of *Aspergillus niger* phytase resulted in a significant reduction of phytate, reaching 78%.[95] Subsequently, its use as an ingredient in the production of wheat rolls supplemented with wheat bran in order to increase absorption of iron in humans produced complete effective hydrolysis of phytates.[75] Porres and colleagues[114] used two fungal phytases (*A. niger* and *A. fumigatus*) and a bacterial phytase (*Escherichia coli*) in the preparation of whole wheat bread in order to maximize degradation of InsP$_6$, achieving hydrolysis percentages of over 75% after two and a half hours of fermentation. In later studies, Haros et al.[89,90] obtained hydrolysis percentages of up to 59% in whole wheat bread, and they achieved values close to 90% in the case of bread with bran by using *A. niger* phytase. There are few reports dealing with their applications in infant cereals containing different cereal flours (such as wheat, rice, corn, oat, barley, rye, sorghum, millet, etc.). In this food matrix, phytase treatment generally resulted in decreased phytate content and enhanced mineral bioavailability, as reflected by increased uptake of iron and zinc in intestinal epithelial (Caco-2) cell models.[115,116]

The use of commercial phytases could improve the bioavailability of minerals in cereal- or legume-based products by eliminating phytate during the manufacturing process.[73–75,103,105,114–116] The addition of phytases is a common practice in the preparation of animal feed. It consists in including a phytase that remains active during the process of preparing the feed, and subsequently in the digestive tract of monogastric animals. The use of phytases of microbial origin (*Schizosaccharomyces pombe*, *Penicillium funiculosum*, *Trichoderma reesei*, *A. niger*, and *A. oryzae*) is currently authorized in animal feed by European Commission Regulations.[117–121] However, these phytases are not yet of food grade and cannot be added to foods intended for human consumption or during their manufacture, even if they are deactivated during cooking.

Phytase-Producing Bifidobacteria

Increasing phytase activity seems to be the best strategy to reduce phytate content in cereal products. Haros et al.[122,123] found phytase activity in specific strains of the *Bifidobacterium* genus, suggesting their possible use in making bakery products in order to reduce phytate content significantly.

On the basis of previous studies on the production of phytase activity by various strains of bifidobacteria, the most productive ones were selected.[96,106,122,123] The strains under study were selected from a total of over 100 strains of the *Bifidobacterium* genus, isolated from a variety of ecosystems. A factor taken into account in the selection of phytase-producing strains was that the microorganisms were GRAS/QPS (Generally Regarded as Safe/Qualified Presumption of Safety), and mostly from human sources (Table 2.1). For the study of hydrolysis of phytates, the growth conditions for the selected strains were Garche's broth and MRS broth, both modified to replace inorganic phosphorus with sodium phytate and 3-[N-Morpholino]-propanesulfonic acid.[96,122] The strains were incubated at 37°C in anaerobic conditions until they reached the stationary phase, in accordance with Haros et al.[122] The cells were separated by centrifugation to determine biomass,[126] and the phytate and hydrolysis product contents in the supernatant were investigated by reverse-phase high-performance liquid chromatography.[122] The residual phytate content showed wide variability, depending on the strain used, but the strains of *B. pseudocatenulatum* and *B. longum* subsp. *infantis* achieved the greatest degradation of phytates, with the initial InsP$_6$ reduced to residual values of between 15% and 23% in modified Garche's broth (Table 2.2). From the phytase activity, residual

TABLE 2.1 Strains of the *Bifidobacterium* Genus Used in the Studies

Species	Strain	Source	Literature
B. longum subsp. *infantis*	ATCC 15697	Infant feces	Reuter[124]
B. pseudocatenulatum	ATCC 27919	Infant feces	Scardovi *et al.*[125]
B. breve	BIF27	Infant feces	Palacios *et al.*[106]
B. breve	BIF211	Infant feces	Palacios *et al.*[96]
B. longum	BIF307	Human adult feces	Palacios *et al.*[106]
B. longum	IG22	Chicken large intestine	Palacios *et al.*[96]
B. longum	ID23	Chicken small intestine	Palacios *et al.*[96]
B. animalis	KW1	–	Haros *et al.*[123]
B. bifidum	ATCC 29521	Infant feces	Haros *et al.*[123]
B. dentium	spp.	–	–

phytate, and biomass production results, it could be concluded that these strains or their enzyme preparations would be the best strategy for reducing InsP$_6$ contents in whole products or products with bran intended for human consumption (Table 2.2). Moreover, the phytases in these two strains show unique features with regard to the hydrolytic profile of InsP$_6$. The main InsP$_6$ degradation pathway by *B. pseudocatenulatum* by sequential removal of phosphate groups was mainly via (A) D/L-Ins(1,2,3,4,5)P_5 and D/L-Ins(1,2,3,4,6)P_5, (B) D/L-Ins(1,2,3,4)P_4, and (C) Ins(1,2,3)P_3/D/L-Ins(1,2,6)P_3 and D/L-Ins(1,2,4)P_3/D/L-Ins(1,3,4)P_3.[127] The first main step of InsP$_6$ degradation by the *B. pseudocatenulatum* phytate-degrading enzyme(s) was preferentially initiated at the L-6 (D-4) position of the *myo*-inositol ring, where the major *myo*-inositol pentakisphosphate generated has been identified as D/L-Ins(1,2,3,4,5)P_5. This is comparable to the enzymatic hydrolysis of seeds of higher plants such as rye, barley, spelt, oats, wheat, rice, and mung bean.[128] However, 6-phytase (EC 3.1.3.26) has not only been found in plants; *Escherichia coli* and *Paramecium* also initiate dephosphorylation of phytate at the L-6 position.[129] *B. pseudocatenulatum* also produced a relatively high concentration of D/L-Ins(1,2,3,4,6)P_5, which shows that the microorganism hydrolyzed the 5-position of the *myo*-inositol ring.[127] Both strains, *B. pseudocatenulatum* and *B. longum* subsp. *infantis*, generate isomers that contain phosphate groups at position (1,2,3), which might be involved in biological functions in the organism.[127] Furthermore, bifidobacteria are GRAS/QPS microorganisms, which would make them an especially suitable strategy for reducing InsP$_6$ contents in whole products intended for human consumption.

From a technological point of view, Palacios and colleagues[96,130] validated the use of strains of bifidobacteria of various origins in breadmaking, and they investigated the degradation of InsP$_6$ in whole wheat flour doughs fermented for long periods of time. The strains used in their study adapted to the fermentation process and acidified the dough, with a consequent decrease in the quantity of InsP$_6$. Subsequently, in breadmaking studies using *B. longum* subsp., the phytate content was reduced with respect to the control sample, basically by activation of endogenous phytase in the cereal as a result of reduction in pH.[106] However, the use of selected phytate-degrading *Bifidobacterium* strains (*B. pseudocatenulatum* and *B. longum* subsp. *infantis* from the ATCC) in the bread dough fermentation produced results with technological and sensorial quality similar to the controls, resulting in breads with significantly lower levels of InsP$_6$ and with residual amounts of *myo*-inositol triphosphates (InsP$_3$) after 1 hour of fermentation.[103] In that study, the degradation of InsP$_6$ content was up to 67%, whereas the InsP$_6$ + InsP$_5$ concentration was reduced by 32–60% with respect to the control levels (Fig. 2.3). The inclusion of commercial fungal phytase as a positive control in that investigation also significantly reduced the amount of InsP$_6$, but it also efficiently hydrolyzed the lower *myo*-inositol phosphates, which are considered to exert positive biological functions. In general, bread made with those strains of bifidobacteria did not show significant differences with respect to the control samples in terms of specific loaf volume, crumb structure, width/height ratio of the central slice, crust and crumb color, and crumb texture profile. The sensory characteristics of the product were similar to those of the control sample in the two formulations investigated (Fig. 2.4). The greatest differences were found between the formulations with different flours, mainly in the sensory perception of crumb softness and elasticity, largely due to the different bran content, with higher scores being obtained in the breads made with 50% whole wheat flour (Fig. 2.4).

Subsequently, the use of *B. pseudocatenulatum* in an indirect breadmaking process with sourdough made

TABLE 2.2 Hydrolysis of $InsP_6$ by Different Strains of Bifidobacteria in Semi-Synthetic Medium[a,b]

Strain	Medium	Biomass (%)	% InsP$_6$ Residual	InsP$_6$ (mM)	InsP$_5$ (mM)	InsP$_4$ (mM)	InsP$_3$ (mM)
B. infantis	Garche	18.7±0.7	22.5±0.3	1.5±0.9	1.3±0.6	1.2±0.3	3.0±0.5
ATCC 15697	MRS	20.8±0.2	20.4±0.4	1.5±0.5	0.9±0.2	1.4±0.1	3.1±0.3
B. pseudocatenulatum	Garche	10.9±0.0	14.6±0.3	1.0±0.3	1.7±0.5	3.1±0.5	2.2±0.3
ATCC 27919	MRS	2.4±0.1	90.7±0.7	6.7±0.8	2.0±0.2	0.3±0.0	0.0±0.0
*B. breve*BIF211	Garche	8.6±0.3	74.7±0.3	4.9±0.5	1.8±0.6	0.3±0.0	0.3±0.0
	MRS	15.2±0.2	100.2±0.7	7.2±0.1	2.2±0.1	0.4±0.1	0.2±0.1
*B. longum*IG22	Garche	9.2±0.6	95.8±1.2	6.3±0.1	2.3±0.2	0.3±0.0	0.3±0.1
	MRS	16.0±0.5	94.2±0.9	7.0±0.3	2.0±0.1	0.4±0.0	0.1±0.1
*B. longum*ID23	Garche	4.4±0.4	83.3±0.9	5.5±0.5	2.1±0.4	0.3±0.0	0.2±0.0
	MRS	13.4±0.8	68.2±0.2	5.1±0.4	1.5±0.4	0.3±0.1	0.1±0.1
*B. longum*BIF307	Garche	2.3±0.3	60.4±0.9	4.0±0.3	1.5±0.9	0.4±0.1	0.1±0.0
	MRS	6.8±0.1	76.1±0.5	5.7±0.1	1.9±0.3	0.3±0.0	0.0±0.0
*B. animalis*KW1	Garche	3.4±0.1	101.1±0.3	6.7±0.2	2.5±0.1	0.4±0.0	0.1±0.0
	MRS	7.1±0.3	78.9±0.8	5.9±0.3	1.8±0.1	0.3±0.0	0.0±0.0
B. bifidum ATCC 29521	Garche	0.7±0.1	62.2±0.6	4.1±0.2	1.7±0.1	0.4±0.0	0.1±0.0
	MRS	2.6±0.9	88.0±0.6	6.5±0.9	2.0±0.2	0.3±0.0	0.0±0.0
*B. breve*BIF27	Garche	9.3±0.9	63.1±0.5	4.2±0.2	1.7±0.8	0.4±0.2	0.2±0.0
	MRS	16.3±0.5	81.2±0.9	6.0±0.1	1.6±0.2	0.3±0.0	0.2±0.0
B. dentium spp.	Garche	6.9±0.8	94.1±0.4	6.2±0.5	2.3±0.1	0.3±0.0	0.2±0.0
	MRS	9.9±0.1	86.0±0.2	6.4±0.2	1.6±0.1	0.1±0.0	0.1±0.0
Control	Garche	—	100.0±0.4	7.0±0.5	2.1±0.3	0.3±0.0	0.0±0.0
	MRS	—	100.0±0.7	7.5±0.1	1.9±0.1	0.3±0.0	0.0±0.0

Culture conditions in Garche's broth and modified MRS, in which inorganic phosphate was replaced with sodium phytate and 3-[N-Morpholino]-propanesulfonic acid. Incubation until the start of the stationary phase ($\sim$14–18 hours) in anaerobiosis at 37 °C.

[a] *Mean $\pm$ SD*, n = 3.

[b] $InsP_6$, $InsP_5$, $InsP_4$, $InsP_3$; *hexakis-, pentakis-, tetra-, triphosphate of myo-inositol, respectively.*

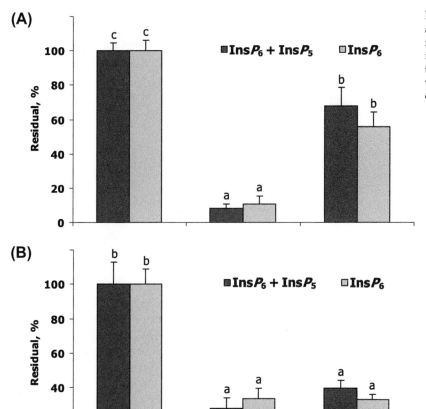

FIGURE 2.3 Relative residual amount of InsP$_6$ and InsP$_5$ in breads made with 100% of whole wheat flour (A) or 50% of whole wheat flour (B). InsP$_6$, *myo*-inositol hexakisphosphate; InsP$_5$, *myo*-inositol pentakisphosphate; d.m., dry matter. Mean ± SD, $n = 3$, bar values with same color and different letters are significantly different ($P < 0.05$).

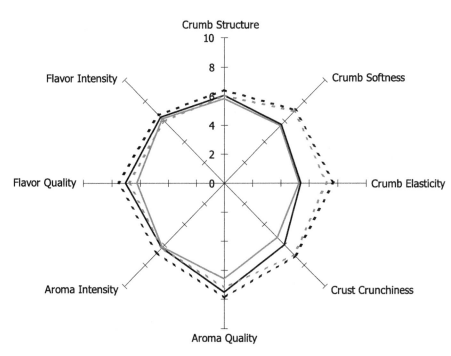

FIGURE 2.4 Sensory evaluation of breads with 100% of whole wheat flour (—) or 50% of whole wheat flour (---). Bread formulations: control bread (black), bread made with phytase-producing bifidobacteria (gray).

A. WHEAT COMPONENTS IN DISEASE PREVENTION: OVERVIEW

FIGURE 2.5   Relative residual amount of $InsP_6$ and $InsP_5$ in whole wheat bread with sourdough. Bread formulations with 0% (control), 5%, 10%, 15%, and 20% of sourdough inoculated with bifidobacteria. $InsP_6$, *myo*-inositol hexakisphosphate; $InsP_5$, *myo*-inositol pentakisphosphate; d.m., dry matter. Mean ± SD, $n = 3$, bar values with same color and different letters are significantly different ($P < 0.05$).

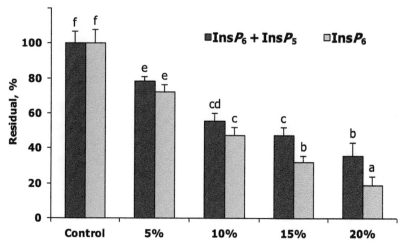

possible the formulation of whole wheat bread,[104] allowing an increase in phytate hydrolysis ranging from 28% to values over 80%, depending on the percentage of sourdough in the formulation (Fig. 2.5). The hydrolysis was largely due to the acidification of the dough, which produced a significant decrease in pH, close to the optimum pH of endogenous cereal phytase.[131] Furthermore, the study included investigation of an acid control, i.e., a formulation prepared with sourdough chemically acidified with a mixture of acetic and lactic acids to emulate the pH attained by the metabolism of bifidobacteria. The acid control showed a significant reduction of phytates in comparison with the sample made without sourdough, but significantly less than the sample made with phytase-producing bifidobacteria. These results suggested that the greater hydrolysis of $InsP_6$ observed in the samples with sourdough inoculated with bifidobacteria was due to the additional phytase activity contributed by the bacteria.[104] Furthermore, the quantity of *myo*-inositol phosphates with a lower degree of phosphorylation ($InsP_4$ and $InsP_3$) in the products made with sourdough supplemented with bifidobacteria remained at high concentrations with respect to the samples without sourdough, as also happened in direct application of bifidobacteria.[103] The use of bifidobacteria as a starter culture in sourdough formulations did not significantly affect bread performance, and increased its nutritional value. Only samples made with high replacement rates (15–20%) showed some differences in crumb hardness and specific loaf volume in comparison with the control, but the other parameters associated with technological quality remained without significant differences. Biochemical processes take place that affect carbohydrates and proteins during the sourdough production process, basically because of the metabolic activity of the microorganisms that proliferate during its preparation. The possible proteolytic activity associated with the bifidobacteria added and the lactobacilli present in the flour

might weaken the structure of the gluten network,[132] producing a slight decrease in specific loaf volume and consequently greater crumb firmness in the loaves with a high proportion of sourdough; however, these slight differences were not important in the sensory evaluation.[104] The lactic and acetic acids registered an increase with the addition of sourdough to the bread formula, and it is important to note that an increase in the amounts of these organic acids has been shown to lower the glycemic index of bread products.[133,134] The inclusion of phytase-producing bifidobacteria during the breadmaking process reduces phytates without affecting the technological and sensory quality of the product.[103,104]

Iron dialyzability and bioavailability from whole wheat breads made with phytase-producing bifidobacteria were also assessed.[73] Treatment with bifidobacteria increased the availability of iron in both processes (direct and indirect breadmaking); however, this was not reflected by an increase in iron uptake by Caco-2 cells. The authors suggested that the explanation for this behavior was that in the breads formulated with bifidobacteria the residual amount of $InsP_6$ was still higher than the threshold value of 0.135 µmol/g of bread at which inhibition begins in humans[75]; or that the phytate/Fe molar ratios were above critical values established as inhibitory of iron uptake, which should be lower than 1 and preferably lower than 0.4.[135] Although there was an effect on phytate reduction, it appeared to be still insufficient to improve iron bioavailability.[73]

Isolation and purification of bifidobacteria phytases and their inclusion in cereal fermentation processes might efficiently increase hydrolysis of phytates. Accordingly, first the location of the enzyme was investigated, and it was confirmed that the phytases were not extracellular. After cell disruption by treatment with lysozyme, subsequent sonication, and centrifugation and ultracentrifugation steps, phytase and phosphatase activity were measured in the three cell fractions obtained: cell wall, cell membrane, and cytoplasmic extract. The result obtained indicated that phytase activity was located mainly in the cell membrane fraction, because no activity was found in the cell-free supernatant, and only greater phosphatase activity in the cell wall extract. In order to release and solubilize the enzyme, the cell membrane fraction was resuspended in 20 mM Tris-HCl buffer at pH 6.15 in the presence of 1% Triton X100 or 15% glycerol. After the various treatments, phytase activity did not recover. This was basically because bifidobacteria phytases are associated with membrane, and therefore attempts to solubilize the enzyme always led to loss of activity or to inefficient solubilization, preventing its purification. Therefore it was decided to change strategy and use molecular biology techniques, permitting cloning and expression of the enzyme in another microorganism.[113] Accordingly, a search was made for possible phytases in genomes of producer strains (*B. pseudocatenulatum* ATCC 27919 and *B. longum* subsp. *infantis* ATCC 15697). The BLAST analysis and search for protein domains present in the Pfam database led to the identification of two gene loci that codify two proteins that have a histidine acid phosphatase domain.[136] This domain is present in a group of heterogeneous proteins that generally have phosphate ester hydrolysis activity, are active at acid pH, and have a histidine in the active center involved in catalysis.[113] The genes were amplified by PCR, excluding the sequences encoding the N-terminal signal peptides and the C-terminal hydrophobic domains, and cloned into the expression vector pQE80 for their purification as 6His-tagged proteins.[136] The enzymes were purified from *Escherichia coli* M15-induced cultures grown in LB by chromatography on Ni-nitrilotriacetic acid agarose columns.[136] These novel phytases are highly specific for hydrolysis of phytate, and render InsP$_3$ as the final hydrolysis product. They represent the first phytases characterized from this group of probiotic microorganisms, opening up possibilities for their use in the processing of high phytate-content foods. These purified bifidobacterial phytases were included in a food production process during infant cereal manufacture in two formulations (multicereal infant cereals containing rice, oats, barley, rye, maize, millet, sorghum, and wheat; and gluten-free infant cereals containing rice, maize, and tapioca).[105] This resulted in efficient phytate hydrolysis, up to almost 90%, which rendered lower *myo*-inositol phosphate products. The inclusion of phytases also significantly reduced the *myo*-inositol pentakisphosphate concentrations (up to 73%) as compared to control samples. Bifidobacterial phytase treatment increased zinc solubility by 25–30%, although calcium and iron solubility did not change, and mineral dialyzability also remained unchanged.

The effects of the inclusion of purified recombinant phytases from *B. pseudocatenulatum* ATCC 27919 and *B. longum* subsp. *infantis* ATCC 15697 on phytate levels of different bread formulations were also analyzed, compared to their counterparts without phytase (as negative control) and with commercial fungal phytase (as positive control).[137] Phytase inclusion did not affect final product quality, with the exception of a slight increase in loaf volume and a softening of the crumb. The addition of phytases from bifidobacteria contributed to the hydrolysis of phytate and significantly decreased its level in breads with more effectiveness than the commercial fungal phytase.[137]

Phytase Activity in the Gut

The phytase activity produced by intestinal microbiota can be considered of great importance from a nutritional point of view, because there is little endogenous activity.[138] Dietary phytic acid or wheat bran enhanced mucosal phytase activity in rat small intestine, but the increase was less pronounced in animals fed with wheat bran, probably because InsP$_6$ is less accessible to phytase.[139] It was suggested that a similar induction of phytase activity could also exist in humans or in the human gut microbiota. Phytase activity has been found in mucosal homogenates from the human small intestine at low levels; the activity, which may originate from gut microorganisms, was highest in the duodenum and lowest in the ileum.[140] It was reported that microbial activity in the intestine has only been associated with *Bacteroides* spp., *Clostridium* spp., and Gram-negative bacteria.[141] Irrespective of diet group (adults on conventional, vegetarian, or vegan diet, and breast-fed infants), the Gram-positive anaerobes and lactobacilli were characterized by the lowest ability to degrade phytate, whereas coliforms and proteobacteria-bacteroides cultures produced the highest amounts of intermediate *myo*-inositol phosphates.[142] However, a phytate-rich diet increases the potential of intestinal microbiota for phytate degradation and for bacteria to cooperate in this process.[142]

The phytate-degrading activity of bifidobacteria may contribute to phytic acid degradation during food processing, but also during gastrointestinal transit.[127] Potentially, the phytase-producing *Bifidobacterium* spp. could help in the development of a specific inositol phosphate isomer profile in fermented foods to improve their nutritional and health value, as well as *in vivo* in the gut. The *B. pseudocatenulatum* strain also showed a notable tolerance to bile, as well as a selective capacity of adhesion to human intestinal Caco-2.[127] Phytate-degrading activity is a novel metabolic trait which could contribute to the improvement of mineral absorption in the intestine as a nutritional probiotic feature with a potential trophic effect in the human gut.[127]

References

1. Aleixandre A, Miguel M. Dietary Fiber in the Prevention and Treatment of Metabolic Syndrome: A Review. *Crit Rev Food Sci* 2008;**48**:905–12.

2. Liu RH. Whole grain phytochemicals and health. *J Cereal Sci* 2007;**46**:207–19.

3. Marquart L, Asp NG, Richardson DP. Whole grain health claims in the United States, United Kingdom and Sweden. In: Van der Kamp JW, Asp NG, Jones JM, Schaafsma G, editors. *Dietary fibre – Bio-active carbohydrates for food and feed*. Wageningen: Wageningen Academic Publishers; 2004. p. 39–57.

4. Whole Grains Council. *Whole Grain Guidelines Worldwide*. Available at: http://www.wholegrainscouncil.org/whole-grains-101/whole-grain-guidelines-worldwide; 2011.

5. Poutanen K, Shepherd R, Shewry PR, Delcour JA, Björck IM, Van der Kamp JW. Beyond whole grain: the European HEALTHGRAIN project aims at healthier cereal foods. *Cereal Food World* 2008;**53**:32–5.

6. Poutanen K, Kervinen R, Van der Kamp JW, Poms R. *Enhancing health benefits of cereal foods*. Results, perspectives, challenges. Helsinki: Edita Prima Oy; 2010.

7. Miller Jones J. The Second C&E Spring Meeting and Third International Whole Grain Global Summit. *Cereal Food World* 2009;**54**:132–5.

8. Chu YL, Warre CA, Sceets CA, Murano P, Marquart L, Reicks M. Acceptance of two US Department of Agriculture commodity whole-grain products: a school-based study in Texas and Minnesota. *J Am Diet Assoc* 2011;**111**:1380–4.

9. Keast DR, Rosen R, Arndt EA, Marquart LF. Dietary modeling shows that substitution of whole-grain for refined-grain ingredients of foods commonly consumed by US children and teens can increase intake of whole grains. *J Am Diet Assoc* 2011;**111**:1322–8.

10. USDA. *US Department of Agriculture. Department of Health and Human Services*. Washington, DC: Nutrition and Your Health: Dietary Guidelines for Americans; 2005.

11. IOM (Institute of Medicine). Committee on Leading Health Indicators for Healthy People 2020. In: *Leading health indicators for healthy people 2020: Letter report*. Washington, DC: The National Academies Press; 2011.

12. Collar C. Panadería y salud. *Alimentación, nutrición y salud* 2007;**14**:33–46.

13. FAO. *Food and Agriculture Organization of the United Nations*. FAOSTAT. Available at: http://faostat.fao.org/; 2012.

14. Gamel TH, Linssen JP, Mesallam AS, Damir AA, Shekib LA. Seed treatments affect functional and antinutritional properties of amaranth flours. *J Sci Food Agric* 2006;**86**:1095–102.

15. Lamsal BP, Faubion JM. The beneficial use of cereal and cereal components in probiotic foods. *Food Rev Int* 2009;**25**:103–14.

16. Chandrasekara A, Shahidi F. Bioactivities and antiradical properties of millet grains and hulls. *J Agric Food Chem* 2011;**59**:9563–71.

17. ADA. Position of the American Dietetic Association: Health Implications of Dietary Fiber. *J Am Diet Assoc* 2008;**108**:1716–31.

18. Nilsson AC, Ostman EM, Hoist JJ, Bjorck IME. Including indigestible carbohydrates in the evening meal of healthy subjects improves glucose tolerance, lowers inflammatory markers, and increases satiety after a subsequent standardized breakfast. *J Nutr* 2008;**138**:732–9.

19. Escudero Alvarez E, Gonzalez Sanchez P. La fibra dietética. *Nutr Hosp* 2006;**21**:61–72.

20. EFSA Panel on Dietetic Products, Nutrition and Allergies (NDA). Scientific Opinion on Dietary Reference Values for carbohydrates and dietary fibre. *EFSA Journal* 2010;**8**:1462.

21. IOM (Institute of Medicine). *Food and Nutrition Board. Dietary Reference Intakes for Energy, Carbohydrate, Fiber, Fat, Fatty Acids, Cholesterol, Protein, and Amino Acids (Macronutrients)*. Washington, DC: The National Academies Press; 2005.

22. Slavin J. Whole grains and human health. *Nutr Res Rev* 2004;**17**:99–110.

23. Hemery Y, Chaurand M, Holopainen U, Lampi A-M, Lehtinen P, Piironen V, et al. Potential of dry fractionation of wheat bran for the development of food ingredients, Part I: Influence of ultra-fine grinding. *J Cereal Sci* 2010;**53**:1–8.

24. Miller G, Prakash A, Decker E. Whole-grain micronutrients. In: Marquart L, Slavin JL, Fulcher RG, editors. *Whole-Grain Foods in Health and Disease*. St Paul, MN: Eagan Press; 2002. p. 243–58.

25. Chavan JK, Kadan SS. Nutritional enrichment of bakery products by supplementation with nonwheat flours. *Crit Rev Food Sci* 1993;**33**:189–226.

26. Basman A, Koksel H. Effects of barley flour and wheat bran supplementation on the properties and composition of Turkish flat bread, yufka. *Eur Food Res Technol* 2001;**212**:198–202.

27. Tosi EA, Re ED, Masciarelli R, Sanchez H, Osella C. De la Torre MA. Whole and defatted hyperproteic amaranth flours tested as wheat flour supplementation in mold breads. *LWT-Food Sci Technol* 2002;**35**:472–5.

28. Sindhuja A, Sudha ML, Rahim A. Effect of incorporation of amaranth flour on the quality of cookies. *Eur Food Res Technol* 2005;**221**:597–601.

29. Dyner L, Drago SR, Piñeiro A, et al. Composition and potential contribution of iron, calcium and zinc of bread and pasta made with wheat and amaranth flours. *Arch Latinoam Nutr* 2007;**57**:69–78.

30. Bodroza-Solarov M, Filiocev B, Kevresan Z, Mandic A, Simurina O. Quality of bread supplemented with popped *Amaranthus cruentus* grain. *J Food Process Eng* 2008;**31**:602–18.

31. Sanz-Penella JM, Laparra JM, Sanz Y, Haros M. Bread supplemented with amaranth (*Amaranthus cruentus*): effect of phytates on *in vitro* iron absorption. *Plant Food Hum Nutr* 2012b;**67**:50–6.

32. Sanz-Penella JM, Wronkowska M, Soral-Śmietana M, Haros M. Effect of whole amaranth flour on bread properties and nutritive value. *LWT-Food Sci Technol* 2013;**50**:679–85.

33. Fretzdorff B, Brümmer JM. Reduction of phytic acid during breadmaking of whole-meal breads. *Cereal Chem* 1992;**69**:266–70.

34. Nielsen MM, Damstrup ML, Dal Thomsen A, Rasmussen SK, Hansen A. Phytase activity and degradation of phytic acid during rye bread making. *Eur Food Res Technol* 2007;**225**:173–81.

35. Reddy NR, Harland BF, Pierson MD. Accumulation and occurrence of phytate forms in dry beans. *Faseb J* 1989;**3** A759.

36. Barre R, Courtois JE, Wormser G. Étude de la structure de l' acide phytique au moyen de ses courbes de titration et de la conductivité de ses solutions. *Bull Soc Chim Biol* 1954;**36**:455–74.

37. Evans WJ, Pierce AG. Interaction of phytic acid with the metalions, copper (II), cobalt (II), iron (III), magnesium (II), and manganese (II). *J Food Sci* 1982;**47**:1014–5.

38. Weingartner KE, Erdman JW. Bioavailability of minerals in human soybean foods. *Illinois Res* 1978;**20**:4–5.

39. Lopez HW, Leenhardt F, Coudray C, Remesy C. Minerals and phytic acid interactions: is it a real problem for human nutrition? *Int J Food Sci Tech* 2002;**37**:727–39.

40. Konietzny U, Greiner R. Phytic acid: Properties and Determination. In: Caballero B, Trugo L, Finglas P, editors. *Encyclopaedia of Food Science and Nutrition*, 2nd ed. London: Elsevier; 2003. p. 4555–63.

41. Kumar V, Sinha AK, Makkar HPS, Becker K. Dietary roles of phytate and phytase in human nutrition: A review. *Food Chem* 2010;**120**:945–59.

42. Schlemmer U, Frolich W, Prieto RM, Grases F. Phytate in foods and significance for humans: Food sources, intake, processing, bioavailability, protective role and analysis. *Mol Nutr Food Res* 2009;**53**:S330–75.

43. Shamsuddin AM, Vucenik I. Mammary tumour inhibition by IP6: A review. *Anticancer Res* 1999;**19**:3671–4.

44. Shamsuddin AM. Anti-cancer function of phytic acid. *Int J Food Sci Tech* 2002;**37**:769–82.

45. Menniti FS, Bird GSJ, Glennon MC, Obie JF, Rossier MF, Putney Jr JW. Inositol polyphosphates and calcium signaling. *Mol Cell Neurosci* 1992;**3**:1–10.

46. Carrington AL, Calcutt NA, Ettlinger CB, Gustafsson T, Tomlinson DR. Effects of treatment with *myo*-inositol or its 1,2,6-triphosphate (PP56) on nerve conduction in streptozotocin-diabetes. *Eur J Pharmacol* 1993;**237**:257–63.

47. Shears SB. The versatility of inositol phosphates as cellular signals. *BBA-Mol Cell Biol L* 1998;**1436**:49–67.

48. Tarnow P, Cassuto J, Jonsson A, Rimback G, Hedman C. Postoperative analgesia by D-*myo*-inositol-1,2,6-triphosphate in patients undergoing cholecystectomy. *Anesth Analg* 1998;**86**:107–10.

49. Shi Y, Azab AN, Thompson MN, Greenberg ML. Inositol phosphates and phosphoinositides in health and disease. *Sub-Cell Biochem* 2006;**39**:265–92.

50. Reddy NR. Occurrence, distribution, content, and dietary intake of phytate. In: Reddy NR, Sathe SK, editors. *Food phytates*. Boca Raton, FL: CRC Press LLC; 2002. p. 25–51.

51. Torelm I, Bruce A. Phytic acid in foods. *Var Foeda* 1982;**34**:79–96.

52. Davies NT. Effects of phytic acid in mineral availability. In: Vahoung GV, Kritchevsky D, editors. *Dietary fiber in health and disease*. New York, NY: Plenum Press; 1982. p. 105–16.

53. Wise A, Lockie GM, Liddell J. Dietary intakes of phytate and its meal distribution pattern amongst staff and students in an institution of higher-education. *Br J Nutr* 1987;**58**:337–46.

54. Carnovale E, Lombardi-Boccia G, Lugaro E. Phytate and zinc content of Italian diets. *Hum Nutr Appl Nutr* 1987;**41A**:180–6.

55. Ruggeri S, De Santis N, Carnovale E. Intake and sources of phytic acid in Italian diets. In: Kozlowska H, Fornal J, Zdunczyk Z, editors. *Bioactive Substances in Food of Plant Origin*. Olsztyn: Proceedings of the International Conference Euro Food Tox IV. Centre for Agrotechnology and Veterinary Sciences; 1994. p. 355–9.

56. Plaami S, Kumpulainen J. Inositol phosphate content of some cereal-based foods. *J Food Compos Anal* 1995;**8**:324–35.

57. Amirabdollahian F, Ash R. An estimate of phytate intake and molar ratio of phytate to zinc in the diet of the people in the United Kingdom. *Public Health Nutr* 2010;**13**:1380–8.

58. Prieto RM, Fiol M, Perello J, et al. Effects of Mediterranean diets with low and high proportions of phytate-rich foods on the urinary phytate excretion. *Eur J Nutr* 2010;**49**:321–6.

59. Sandström B, Sandberg AS. Inhibitory effects of isolated inositol phosphates on zinc absorption in humans. *J Trace Elem Elect H* 1992;**6**:99–103.

60. Sandberg AS, Brune M, Carlsson NG, et al. Inositol phosphates with different numbers of phosphate groups influence iron absorption in humans. *Am J Clin Nutr* 1999;**70**:240–6.

61. Hurrell RF, Reddy MB, Juillerat MA, Cook JD. Degradation of phytic acid in cereal porridges improves iron absorption by human subjects. *Am J Clin Nutr* 2003;**77**:1213–9.

62. Dendougui F, Schwedt G. *In vitro* analysis of binding capacities of calcium to phytic acid in different food samples. *Eur Food Res Technol* 2004;**219**:409–15.

63. Kumagai H, Koizumi A, Suda A, et al. Enhanced calcium absorption in the small intestine by a phytate-removed deamidated soybean globulin preparation. *Biosci Biotech Bioch* 2004;**68**:1598–600.

64. Larsson M, Rossander-Hulthen L, Sandström B, Sandberg AS. Improved zinc and iron absorption from breakfast meals containing malted oats with reduced phytate content. *Br J Nutr* 1996;**76**:677–88.

65. Hunt JR, Beiseigel JM. Dietary calcium does not exacerbate phytate inhibition of zinc absorption by women from conventional diets. *Am J Clin Nutr* 2009;**89**:839–43.

66. Abd-El-Moneim MRA, El-Beltagi HS, Abd-El-Salam SM, Omran AA. Bioavailability of iron, zinc, phytate and phytase activity during soaking and germination of white sorghum varieties. *Adv Food Sci* 2011;**33**:133–40.

67. Fredlund K, Isaksson M, Rossander-Hulthen L, et al. Absorption of zinc and retention of calcium: Dose-dependent inhibition by phytate. *J Trace Elem Med Bio* 2006;**20**:49–57.

68. Hurrell RF, Juillerat MA, Reddy MB, et al. Soy protein, phytate, and iron absorption in humans. *Am J Clin Nutr* 1992;**56**:573–8.

69. Davidsson L, Galan P, Kastenmayer P, et al. Iron bioavailability studied in infants: the influence of phytic acid and ascorbic acid in infant formulas based on soy isolate. *Pediatr Res* 1994;**36**:816–22.

70. Layrisse M, Garcia-Casal MN, Solano L, et al. Iron bioavailability in humans from breakfasts enriched with iron bis-glycine chelate, phytates and polyphenols. *J Nutr* 2000;**130**:2195–9.

71. Haraldsson AK, Rimsten L, Alminger M, et al. Digestion of barley malt porridges in a gastrointestinal model: Iron dialysability, iron uptake by Caco-2 cells and degradation of *beta*-glucan. *J Cereal Sci* 2005;**42**:243–54.

72. Frontela C, Ros G, Martínez C. Phytic acid content and "in vitro" iron, calcium and zinc bioavailability in bakery products: the effect of processing. *J Cereal Sci* 2011;**54**:173–9.

73. Sanz-Penella JM, Laparra JM, Sanz Y, Haros M. Assessment of iron bioavailability in whole wheat bread by addition of phytase-producing bifidobacteria. *J Agric Food Chem* 2012c;**60**:3190–5.

74. Sanz-Penella JM, Laparra JM, Sanz Y, Haros M. Influence of added enzymes and bran particle size on bread quality and iron availability. *Cereal Chem* 2012d;**89**:223–9.

75. Sandberg AS, Hulthen LR, Türk M. Dietary *Aspergillus niger* phytase increases iron absorption in humans. *J Nutr* 1996;**126**:476–80.

76. Vohra A, Satyanarayana T. Phytases: Microbial sources, production, purification, and potential biotechnological applications. *Crit Rev Biotechnol* 2003;**23**:29–60.

77. Shamsuddin AM, Baten A, Lalwani ND. Effects of inositol hexaphosphate on growth and differentiation in K-562 erythroleukemia cell line. *Cancer Lett* 1992;**64**:195–202.

78. Ferry S, Matsuda M, Yoshida H, Hirata M. Inositol hexakisphosphate blocks tumor cell growth by activating apoptotic machinery as well as by inhibiting the Akt/NFkappaB-mediated cell survival pathway. *Carcinogenesis* 2002;**23**:2031–41.

79. Maffucci T, Piccolo E, Cumashi A, et al. Inhibition of the phosphatidylinositol 3-kinase/Akt pathway by inositol pentakisphosphate results in antiangiogenic and antitumor effects. *Cancer Res* 2005;**65**:8339–49.

80. Claxon A, Morris C, Blake D, et al. The anti-inflammatory effects of D-*myo*-inositol-1.2.6-trisphosphate (PP56) on animal models of inflammation. *Agents Actions* 1990;**29**:68–70.

81. Phillippy BQ, Graf E. Antioxidant functions of inositol 1,2,3-trisphosphate and inositol 1,2,3,6-tetrakisphosphate. *Free Radical Bio Med* 1997;**22**:939–46.

82. Dozol H, Blum-Held C, Guedat P, et al. Inframolecular acid-base studies of the tris and tetrakis myo-inositol phosphates including the 1,2,3-trisphosphate motif. *J Mol Struct* 2002;**643**:171–81.

83. Shen X, Weaver CM, Kempa-Steczko A, Martin BR, Phillippy BQ, Heaney RP. An inositol phosphate as a calcium absorption enhancer in rats. *J Nutr Biochem* 1998;**9**:298–301.

84. Hawkins PT, Poyner DR, Jackson TR, Letcher AJ, Lander DA, Irvine RF. Inhibition of iron-catalysed hydroxyl radical formation by inositol polyphosphates: a possible physiological function for *myo*-inositol hexakisphosphate. *Biochem J* 1993;**294**:929–34.

85. Barker CJ, French PJ, Moore AJ, et al. Inositol 1,2,3-triphosphate and inositol 1,2-biphosphate and/or 2,3-bisphosphate are normal constituents of mammalian-cells. *Biochem J* 1995;**306**:557–64.

86. Veiga N, Torres J, Mansell D, et al. "Chelatable iron pool": inositol 1,2,3-trisphosphate fulfils the conditions required to be a safe cellular iron ligand. *J Biol Inorg Chem* 2009;**14**:51–9.

87. Bohn L, Meyer AS, Rasmussen SK. Phytate: impact on environment and human nutrition. A challenge for molecular breeding. *J Zhejiang Univ Sci B* 2008;**9**:165–91.

88. Türk M, Carlsson NG, Sandberg AS. Reduction in the levels of phytate during wholemeal breadmaking; effect of yeast and wheat phytases. *J Cereal Sci* 1996;**23**:257–64.

89. Haros M, Rosell CM, Benedito C. Fungal phytase as a potential breadmaking additive. *Eur Food Res Technol* 2001;**213**:317–22.

90. Haros M, Rosell CM, Benedito C. Use of fungal phytase to improve breadmaking performance of whole wheat bread. *J Agr Food Chem* 2001;**49**:5450–4.

91. Toma RB, Tabekhia MM. Changes in mineral elements and phytic acid contents during cooking of 3 California rice varieties. *J Food Sci* 1979;**44**:619–21.

92. Azeke MA, Egielewa SJ, Eigbogbo MU, Ihimire IG. Effect of germination on the phytase activity, phytate and total phosphorus contents of rice (*Oryza sativa*), maize (*Zea mays*), millet (*Panicum miliaceum*), sorghum (*Sorghum bicolor*) and wheat (*Triticum aestivum*). *J Food Sci Tech* 2011;**48**:724–9.

93. Greiner R, Konietzny U, Jany KD. Purification and properties of a phytase from rye. *J Food Biochem* 1998;**22**:143–61.

94. Huebner F, O' Neil T, Cashman KD, Arendt EK. The influence of germination conditions on *beta*-glucan, dietary fibre and phytate during the germination of oats and barley. *Eur Food Res Technol* 2010;**231**:27–35.

95. Türk M, Sandberg AS. Phytate degradation during breadmaking – Effect of phytase addition. *J Cereal Sci* 1992;**15**:281–94.

96. Palacios MC, Haros M, Sanz Y, Rosell CM. Phytate degradation by *Bifidobacterium* on whole wheat fermentation. *Eur Food Res Technol* 2008;**226**:825–31.

97. Harland BF, Harland J. Fermentative reduction of phytate in rye, white, and whole wheat breads. *Cereal Chem* 1980;**57**:226–9.

98. Faridi HA, Finney GL, Rubenthaler GL. Iranian flat breads – relative bioavailability of zinc. *J Food Sci* 1983;**48**:1654–8.

99. Lopez HW, Ouvry A, Bervas E, et al. Strains of lactic acid bacteria isolated from sour doughs degrade phytic acid and improve calcium and magnesium solubility from whole wheat flour. *J Agr Food Chem* 2000;**48**:2281–5.

100. Lopez HW, Krespine V, Guy C, Messager A, Demigne C, Remesy C. Prolonged fermentation of whole wheat sourdough reduces phytate level and increases soluble magnesium. *J Agric Food Chem* 2001;**49**:2657–62.

101. Fernández A, Haros M, Rosell CM. Nutritional improvement of whole wheat bread though phytase activity during breadmaking. In: Courtin CM, Veraverbeke WS, Delcour JA, editors. *Recent Advances in Enzymes in Grain Processing, Part VI Applications Food.* Leuven: Katholieke Universiteit Leuven; 2003. p. 275–80.

102. Sanz-Penella JM, Collar C, Haros M. Effect of wheat bran and enzyme addition on dough rheological performance and phytic acid levels in bread. *J Cereal Sci* 2008;**48**:715–21.

103. Sanz-Penella JM, Tamayo Ramos JA, Sanz Y, Haros M. Phytate reduction in bran-enriched bread by phytase-producing bifidobacteria. *J Agric Food Chem* 2009;**57**:10239–44.

104. Sanz-Penella JM, Tamayo Ramos JA, Haros M. Application of bifidobacteria as starter culture in whole wheat sourdough breadmaking. *Food Bioprocess Tech* 2012a;**57**:10239–44.

105. Sanz-Penella JM, Frontela C, Ros G, Martinez C, Monedero V, Haros M. Application of bifidobacterial phytases in infant cereals: Effect on phytate contents and mineral dialyzability. *J Agric Food Chem* 2012e;**60**:11787–92.

106. Palacios MC, Haros M, Sanz Y, Rosell CM. Selection of phytate-degrading human bifidobacteria and application as starter cultures in whole-wheat dough fermentation. *Food Microbiol* 2008;**25**:169–76.

107. Rosell CM, Santos E, Sanz-Penella JM, Haros M. Wholemeal wheat bread: A comparison of different breadmaking processes and fungal phytase addition. *J Cereal Sci* 2009;**50**:272–7.

108. Tangkongchitr U, Seib PA, Hoseney RC. Phytic acid. 2. Its fate during breadmaking. *Cereal Chem* 1981;**58**:229–34.

109. Kadan RS, Phillippy BQ. Effects of yeast and bran on phytate degradation and minerals in rice bread. *J Food Sci* 2007;**72**:C208–11.

110. Harland BF, Frölich W. Effects of phytase from three yeasts on phytate reduction in Norwegian whole wheat-flour. *Cereal Chem* 1989;**66**:357–8.

111. Reale A, Konietzny U, Coppola R, Sorrentino E, Greiner R. The importance of lactic acid bacteria for phytate degradation during cereal dough fermentation. *J Agr Food Chem* 2007;**55**:2993–7.

112. Rizzello CG, Nionelli L, Coda R, De Angelis M, Gobbetti M. Effect of sourdough fermentation on stabilisation, and chemical and nutritional characteristics of wheat germ. *Food Chem* 2010;**119**:1079–89.

113. Haros M, Monedero V, Yebra MJ, Tamayo Ramos JA. Truncated phytases of bifidobacteria and uses thereof. Patent No.WO/2011/117452. PCT/ES2011/070198; 2011.

114. Porres JM, Etcheverry P, Miller DD, Lei XG. Phytase and citric acid supplementation in whole-wheat bread improves phytate-phosphorus release and iron dialyzability. *J Food Sci* 2001;**66**:614–9.

115. Frontela C, Haro JF, Ros G, Martinez C. Effect of dephytinization and follow-on formula addition on *in vitro* iron, calcium, and zinc availability from infant cereals. *J Agr Food Chem* 2008;**56**:3805–11.

116. Frontela C, Ros G, Martinez C. Iron and calcium availability from digestion of infant cereals by Caco-2 cells. *Eur Food Res Technol* 2009;**228**:789–97.

117. Commission Regulation (EC) No 785/2007 of 4 July 2007 concerning the authorisation of 6-phytase EC 3.1.3.26 (Phyzyme XP 5000G Phyzyme XP 5000L) as a feed additive.

118. Commission Regulation (EC) No 1141/2007 of 1 October 2007 concerning the authorisation of 3-phytase (ROVABIO PHY AP and ROVABIO PHY LC) as a feed additive.

119. Commission Regulation (EU) No 327/2010 of 21 April 2010 concerning the authorisation of a new use of 3-phytase as a feed additive for all minor avian species, other than ducks, and for ornamental birds (holder of authorisation BASF SE).

120. Commission Regulation (EU) No 891/2010 of 8 October 2010 concerning the authorisation of a new use of 6-phytase as a feed additive for turkeys (holder of authorisation Roal Oy).

121. Commission Regulation (EU) No 171/2011 of 23 February 2011 concerning the authorisation of 6-phytase (EC 3.1.3.26) produced by *Aspergillus oryzae* DSM 14223 as a feed additive for poultry and for porcine species and amending Regulation (EC) No 255/2005 (holder of authorisation DSM Nutritional Products Ltd represented by DSM Nutritional products Sp. z o.o).

122. Haros M, Bielecka M, Sanz Y. Phytase activity as a novel metabolic feature in *Bifidobacterium. FEMS Microbiol Lett* 2005;**247**:231–9.

123. Haros M, Bielecka M, Honke J, Sanz Y. *Myo*-inositol hexakisphosphate degradation by *Bifidobacterium infantis. Int J Food Microbiol* 2007;**117**:76–84.

124. Reuter G. Designation of type strains for *Bifidobacterium* species. *Intl J Syst Bacteriol* 1971;**21**:273–5.

125. Scardovi V, Tovatelli LD, Biavati B, Zani G. *Bifidobacterium cuniculi, Bifidobacterium choerinum, Bifidobacterium boum*, and *Bifidobacterium pseudocatenulatum*: four new species and their deoxyribonucleic acid homology relationships. *Intl J Syst Bacteriol* 1979;**29**:291–311.

126. Perrin S, Warchol M, Grill JP, Schneider F. Fermentations of fructo-oligosaccharides and their components by *Bifidobacterium infantis* ATCC 15697 on batch culture in semi-synthetic medium. *J Appl Microbiol* 2001;**90**:859–65.

127. Haros M, Carlsson NG, Almgren A, Larsson-Alminger M, Sandberg AS, Andlid T. Phytate degradation by human gut isolated *Bifidobacterium pseudocatenulatum* ATCC27919 and its probiotic potential. *Int J Food Microb* 2009;**135**:7–14.

128. Konietzny U, Greiner R. Molecular and catalytic properties of phytate-degrading enzymes (phytases). *Int J Food Sci Tech* 2002;**37** 791–12.

129. Van der Kaay J, Van Haastert PJM. Stereospecificity of inositol hexakisphosphate dephosphorylation by *Paramecium* phytase. *Biochem J* 1995;**312**:907–10.

130. Palacios MC, Sanz Y, Haros M, Rosell CM. Application of Bifidobacterium strains to the breadmaking process. *Process Biochem* 2006;**41**:2434–40.

131. Leenhardt F, Levrat-Verny MA, Chanliaud E, Remesy C. Moderate decrease of pH by sourdough fermentation is sufficient to reduce phytate content of whole wheat flour through endogenous phytase activity. *J Agr Food Chem* 2005;**53** 98–02.

132. Rollan G, De Angelis M, Gobbetti M, De Valdez GF. Proteolytic activity and reduction of gliadin-like fractions by sourdough lactobacilli. *J Appl Microbiol* 2005;**99** 1495–02.

133. Liljeberg H, Lönner C, Björck I. Sourdough fermentation or addition of organic acids or corresponding salts to bread improves nutritional properties of starch in healthy humans. *J Nutr* 1995;**125**:1503–11.

134. Liljeberg H, Björck I. Delayed gastric emptying rate may explain improved glycaemia in healthy subjects to a starchy meal with added vinegar. *Eur J Clin Nutr* 1998;**52**:368–71.

135. Hurrell RF. Phytic acid degradation as a means of improving iron absorption. *Int J Vitam Nutr Res* 2004;**74**:445–52.

136. Tamayo-Ramos JA, Sanz-Penella JM, Yebra MJ, Monedero V, Haros M. Novel phytases from *Bifidobacterium pseudocatenulatum* ATCC 27919 and *Bifidobacterium longum* subsp. *infantis* ATCC 15697. *Appl Environ Microbiol* 2012;**78**:5013–5.

137. García-Mantrana I, Monedero V, Haros M. Application of phytases from bifidobacteria in the development of cereal-based products with amaranth. *Eur Food Research Technol* 2013 submitted.

138. Sandberg AS, Andlid T. Phytogenic and microbial phytases in human nutrition. *Int J Food Sci Technol* 2002;**37**:823–33.

139. Lopez HW, Vallery F, Levrat-Verny MA, Coudray C, Demigne C, Remesy C. Dietary phytic acid and wheat bran enhance mucosal phytase activity in rat small intestine. *J Nutr* 2000;**130**:2020–5.

140. Iqbal TH, Lewis KO, Cooper BT. Phytase activity in the human and rat small-intestine. *Gut* 1994;**35**:1233–6.

141. Steer TE, Gibson GR. The microbiology of phytic acid metabolism by gut bacteria and relevance for bowel cancer. *Int J Food Sci Technol* 2002;**37**:783–90.

142. Markiewicz L, Honke J, Haros M, Świątecka D, Wróblewska B. Diet shapes the ability of human intestinal microbiota to degrade phytate - *in vitro* studies. *J Appl Microbiol* 2013;**115**:247–59.

A. WHEAT COMPONENTS IN DISEASE PREVENTION: OVERVIEW

WHEAT IN COMMERCIAL ANIMAL PRODUCTION

3

Effect of Whole Wheat Feeding on Gut Function and Nutrient Utilization in Poultry

Ahmed M. Amerah*, Velmurugu Ravindran†

*Danisco Animal Nutrition, DuPont Industrial Biosciences, Marlborough, Wiltshire, UK, †Massey University, Institute of Veterinary, Animal and Biomedical Sciences, Palmerston North, New Zealand

INTRODUCTION

Modern broilers are normally offered a complete balanced diet in pelleted form which requires the grains to be ground, mixed with other ingredients and subjected to thermal treatments before being pressed in a die. This process of pelleting the feed is known to improve weight gain, feed intake, and feed efficiency in broilers, irrespective of the grain source.[1] However, grinding and pelleting are relatively expensive and energy-consuming processes. It has been estimated that energy usage comprises between 25% and 30% of the manufacturing cost of broiler feed.[2] Taking into consideration that feed constitutes the greatest single expense in poultry production, at around 60% of the total cost, any reduction in energy consumption used for grinding and pelleting could significantly lower the cost of feed manufacture.

This need to reduce feed costs has led to renewed interest within the feed industry in whole grain feeding, which was a common practice in the early days of commercial poultry production.[3,4] In addition to feed cost savings, recent studies have shown that dietary whole wheat can improve gut health and digestive tract development (especially of the gizzard), and also improve nutrient digestibility.[5–8] Currently, adding whole wheat to broiler diets is a common practice in many European countries as well as Canada and Australasia. The major advantage of whole grain feeding comes from savings in the cost of grinding and pelleting. Thus the practical implication is that if birds fed whole grains perform at least as well as those fed a complete diet, then the economics will favor whole grain feeding. However, in the layer industry whole wheat feeding is not well established. The reason for this is not clear, but may be related to the well-developed gizzard in adult birds and that layers are usually fed mash diets based on coarsely ground grains. Studies examining the effect of whole wheat feeding on laying hens are limited. In general, these trials have shown similar or better performance with whole wheat feeding compared to those fed control mash diets.[9] The focus of this chapter will be on whole wheat feeding for broiler chickens, with a reference to laying hens where appropriate.

EFFECT OF MODERN PROCESSING TECHNOLOGY ON THE DEVELOPMENT OF THE DIGESTIVE TRACT

Development of the digestive tract in poultry, and especially of the gizzard, is known to be influenced by the degree of feed grinding. In nature, chickens are consumers of whole grain in addition to a range of protein-rich sources. The existence of the gizzard in the digestive system enables them to utilize whole grains efficiently. The gizzard is a muscular organ that reduces the particle size of ingested foods and mixes them with digestive enzymes.[10] The mechanical pressure applied in grinding by the gizzard may exceed 585 kg/cm².[11] However, when the grinding of grains is carried out by feed mills, this has negative effects on gizzard function. Under these conditions, the gizzard functions as a transit rather than a grinding organ.[12] The gizzard becomes relatively underdeveloped and the proventriculus becomes dilated when broilers are fed finely ground, processed diets.[8] This can negatively influence gut motility and gastric digestion. The resultant increase in undigested nutrients passing beyond the ileum may lead to increased growth and multiplication of pathogenic bacteria in the hindgut. Digestive organs other than the gizzard are usually less influenced by modern feed processing.[13–16]

METHODS OF WHOLE WHEAT FEEDING

Free Choice Feeding

The basic principle of choice feeding is that birds select freely from offered feed ingredients, and are able to compose their own diet according to their actual needs and production capacity. In this method, whole grain is offered along with either a balanced diet or a protein concentrate (components left when the grain is removed from the complete diet). Several studies have reported lower whole grain intake and inconsistent performance when broilers are offered the whole grain *ad libitum* with the protein concentrate.[17–19] This method is not commonly practiced in commercial poultry production systems, and it has been suggested that modern fast-growing broiler strains do not balance their energy intake, resulting in poor broiler performance.[17]

Mixed Feeding

Mixed feeding is the most commonly used method of whole grain feeding. In this method, whole grain is added either pre- or post-pelleting, replacing a portion of ground grains or diluting the complete balanced diet.

Whole Wheat Inclusion Post-Pelleting

In the post-pelleting method, whole wheat is added and mixed with a balancer diet either replacing part of the ground grain or diluting the complete pelleted balanced diet. This is the most widely used method because it does not involve changes in the existing feeding system and the inclusion rate can be easily manipulated. Commercially available computerized systems can be used to calculate and mix the whole wheat and the basal diet on the farm before the diet is fed through the normal feeding system. Guidelines to whole wheat inclusion rates are also suggested by the major broiler breeder companies.[20,21]

Whole Wheat Inclusion Pre-Pelleting

In the pre-pelleting method, whole wheat is added, replacing part of the ground wheat, and mixed with other ingredients before pelleting. However, concerns over pellet quality may limit the practical use of this method, especially at high inclusion levels of whole wheat. Reports from Norway, however, suggest that pellet quality is improved when whole cereals are included pre-pelleting.[22]

Sequential Feeding

Research into sequential feeding has been scant to date, and there has been no study directed towards developing a commercial feeding system. In broilers, however, studies have shown reduced weight gain with this type of feeding.[23–25] Recent studies with layers have shown improvements in feed efficiency using this feeding technique.[26,27]

EFFECT OF WHOLE WHEAT FEEDING ON GUT HEALTH

As noted previously, the current industry practice of feeding finely ground processed feed has negative effects on gizzard size and gut function in broiler chickens. Under these conditions the gizzard loses its grinding function and becomes relatively underdeveloped, and the proventriculus becomes enlarged.[8] Thus the gizzard becomes a transit rather than a grinding organ,[12] and the digesta is exposed to the low pH of the gizzard only for a short period of time. In contrast, dietary inclusion of whole wheat was found to restore gizzard function, increase gizzard size, and reduce proventricular dilation.[28]

Cumming[29] reported that an active normal gizzard, produced by the feeding of whole grains, plays some role in the resistance of chickens to coccidial infection. The effects of whole wheat feeding on coccidiosis are, however, inconclusive. Evans and colleagues[9] reported that layers fed diets with whole wheat had 2.5-fold lower oocyst output than those fed ground wheat diets. In contrast, Banfield and colleagues[30,31] found no effect of whole wheat inclusion in broiler diets on coccidial infection. Gabriel and colleagues[32,33] stated that although whole wheat feeding may have a small effect on coccidia development, it led to more deleterious effects on the birds during the acute phase of coccidiosis compared to the ground wheat diet. This adverse effect of whole wheat inclusion was attributed to higher gizzard activity leading to more coccidian sporocysts being mechanically liberated from the oocysts. These conflicting reports may be explained by differences in experimental methodology, such as the *Eimeria* species used, the challenge dose, type of basal diet, age of inoculation, age and strain of birds, age of introduction of whole grain, and quantity and type of whole grain fed.[32,33]

In general, studies have shown beneficial effects of whole wheat feeding on gut microflora (Table 3.1).[6,7,32] Whole wheat feeding has been reported to increase intestinal counts of some *Lactobacillus* species[6] and to reduce the number of *Clostridium perfringens* in the intestinal tract.[6,7] On the other hand, Gabriel and colleagues[33] reported no significant differences in the counts of *Lactobacillus* and *Escherichia coli* in the intestinal tract. Bjerrum and colleagues[7] challenged the birds with *Salmonella typhimurium* and found that birds fed whole wheat (100, 200 and 300 g/kg for 11–19, 20–27, and 28–41 days, respectively) had a lower number of salmonella-positive samples of gizzard contents and salmonella counts in ileal contents compared to those fed the pelleted ground wheat diet. Moen et al.[34] concluded that improvement in feed structure is a promising intervention strategy to reduce the zoonotic pathogen *Campylobacter jejuni* in poultry. The proposed mode of action of whole wheat feeding on pathogenic microflora is through the longer retention time at lower pH in the gizzard to process the whole grains (Table 3.1). This reduction in pH in the contents of the gizzard with whole wheat feeding may be related to the mechanical stimulation of the stomach, leading to an increased production of hydrochloric acid in the proventriculus. Therefore, a well developed gizzard may function as a barrier organ that prevents pathogenic bacteria from entering the distal digestive tract.[7] This effect of whole wheat on reducing the pH of gizzard contents may be similar to the effect of adding organic acids to poultry feeds. Samanta and colleagues[35] reported a reduction in gizzard pH from 3.23 to 2.61 when an organic acid blend was added at 2 kg/tonne of feed. An average reduction of gizzard pH from 3.61 to 2.83 was reported in three studies (Table 3.1). It is believed that the antibacterial effect of dietary organic acids in

chickens takes place in the crop and gizzard, where there is a limited possibility of changing the digesta pH.[36] This reduction in digesta pH in the upper digestive tract with organic acids will reduce the total microbial load entering the intestine, but will be particularly effective against *Escherichia coli*, *Campylobacter*, and *Salmonella*.[36] Another possible explanation for the lower numbers of pathogenic bacteria in birds fed whole wheat may relate to the better nutrient utilization and therefore lower concentration of undigested nutrients in the small intestine entering the hindgut.[13] It is known that higher concentrations of undigested protein in the distal gut will result in proliferation of proteolytic bacteria such as *Clostridium perfringens*.[37]

EFFECT OF WHOLE GRAIN INCLUSION ON NUTRIENT UTILIZATION

Whole wheat feeding usually results in a more developed gizzard, which may modulate the digestive process and improve the utilization of nutrients (Table 3.2).[5,14,38–40,45,48] Modulations of the digestive process include enhanced gizzard function, higher pancreatic and liver secretions, and increased gut motility.[40,41] In nature, refluxes are part of the normal digestive physiology of chickens. The purpose of these refluxes is to re-expose nutrients to digestive enzymes throughout the short digestive tract of poultry and improve nutrient utilization. A large, well-developed gizzard improves gut motility[42] due to increased cholecystokinin release in the pyloric region,[41] which in turn stimulates the secretion of pancreatic enzymes and gastro-duodenal refluxes.[43,44] Another possible reason for the improvement in nutrient digestibility with whole wheat feeding is the longer retention time

TABLE 3.1 Effect of Whole Wheat Inclusion on Gizzard pH and Ileal Microflora (Log10 cfu/g)

	Ground Wheat Diet	Whole Wheat	Reference
Gizzard pH	3.99[a]	3.31[b]	Gabriel et al.[32]
	3.34[a]	2.88[b]	Engberg et al.[6]
	3.50[a]	2.32[b]	Bjerrum et al.[7]
Clostridium perfringens	6.44	5.72	Engberg et al.[6]
	5.96[a]	3.78[b]	Bjerrum et al.[7]

[a,b] *Means in the same row with different superscripts differ significantly (P < 0.05).*

TABLE 3.2 Influence of Whole Wheat Inclusion on Nutrient Utilization and Apparent Metabolizable Energy (AME) Expressed as Percentage Changes Relative to Birds Fed the Control Diet

Basal Diet	Duration (days)	Inclusion Rate (g/kg)	Parameter	Reference
Wheat	14–42	333	3% in AME	Preston et al.[38]
Wheat	10–24	125	2% in ileal starch digestibility	Hetland et al.[5]
Wheat	25–38	300	3% in ileal starch digestibility	Hetland et al.[5]
Wheat	1–21	200	6% in AME	Wu et al.[14]
Wheat	1–20	375	3% in AME 5% in ileal starch digestibility	Svihus et al.[40]
Maize	1–21	200	4% in AME 2% in ileal lysine digestibility 3% in ileal methionine digestibility 10% in ileal cysteine digestibility	Biggs and Parsons[39]
Wheat	16–25	150	16% in AME 16% in ileal starch digestibility	Svihus et al.[48]
Wheat	7–21 22–35	100 200	1.5 in ileal N digestibility	Amerah et al.[45]

in the gizzard. When whole grains are fed to the chickens the feed stays longer in the gizzard – estimated to be 2 hours compared to 1 hour for a normal commercial diet[41] – which gives more time for mixing with digestive enzymes at low pH. This is expected to improve the gastric digestion and peptic digestion in the duodenum and, consequently, to reduce the bacterial load in the intestine. It should be noted that the gizzard development hypothesis, however, does not always explain the improvements in performance or apparent metabolizable energy observed with pre-pelleting[14] or post-pelleting[45] inclusion of whole wheat, suggesting the involvement of other factors.

Svihus[46] hypothesized that modern broiler strains overconsume pelleted feed, which results in overload of the digestive system and a reduction in nutrient digestibility. On the other hand, a well-developed gizzard functions as a regulator of feed intake and will improve nutrient digestibility. Svihus and Hetland[13] suggested that the gizzard may be the key site for the prevention of starch overload in the digestive tract. This thesis was supported by Amerah and colleagues,[47] who found that adding low levels of coarse insoluble fiber to poultry diets had beneficial effects on digestive tract development and starch digestibility, and consequently on feed efficiency of broilers.

The effect of whole wheat inclusion on the efficacy of exogenous enzymes is an interesting aspect since enzymes may stay longer in the gizzard at lower pH, which is, for example, the optimum condition for phytase. This may improve the efficacy of the phytase enzyme, leading to better phytate degradation and nutrient digestibility. Svihus and colleagues[48] reported higher phytate degradation when the retention time in the crop increases. However, no study to date has examined the interactions of phytase supplementation and whole wheat inclusion on poultry performance and nutrient utilization. For xylanase, Wu and Ravindran[15] concluded that substituting whole wheat for ground wheat in broiler diets is advantageous in terms of feed efficiency, and that this benefit can be further exploited with xylanase supplementation. On the other hand, different studies showed no interaction between xylanase and whole wheat inclusion, although whole wheat inclusion increased the relative weight of the gizzard.[6]

USE OF OTHER WHOLE GRAINS

Only limited studies have examined the effect of feeding whole grains other than wheat on poultry performance. The large grain size of corn may have limited its use for young broilers as a whole grain. However, a recent study has shown that broilers can utilize up to 25% of cracked corn from 0 to 41 days without a negative response on performance.[49] Olver and Jonker[50] reported no difference in weight gain and feed to gain of broilers from 21 to 56 days when fed whole corn or sorghum plus concentrate compared to a complete pelleted diet. These data suggest that cracked corn can be used for young broilers, and that older broilers are able to utilize the whole corn efficiently.

For barley, variable grain quality and higher viscosity effects compared to wheat may have limited its use as whole grain. Svihus et al.[51] found that broilers fed whole barley had higher feed to gain with no effect on weight gain compared to those fed rolled or ground barley in two experiments. In a third experiment, however, birds fed whole barley had higher weight gain with no effect on feed to gain. Bennet et al.[52] tested different levels of whole barley and reported that weight gain was decreased and feed to gain was higher with most inclusion levels of whole barley. Hidalgo et al.[53] concluded that whole seeds of pearl millet can be successfully included in broiler diets without adverse effects on broiler performance or carcass characteristics.

CONCLUSIONS

With the current situation of high feed and energy costs, there is renewed interest in whole grain feeding. Available data suggest that inclusion of whole wheat in broiler diets using a mixed feeding technique will have no adverse effect on broiler performance, but will have an economical advantage. Several studies have demonstrated the beneficial effects of whole wheat feeding on nutrient utilization, and this can be attributed to the positive effect of whole wheat on gizzard development. Higher gizzard functionality may also play a positive role in the control of bacterial populations in the gut. Systematic investigations on the relationship of whole wheat feeding with bird performance and gut health are warranted if feed efficiency is to be optimized.

References

1. Amerah AM, Ravindran V, Lentle RG, Thomas DG. Feed particle size: Implications on the digestion and performance of poultry. *Worlds Poult Sci J* 2007;**63**:439–51.
2. Dozier III WA. Reducing utility cost in the feed mill. *Watt Poult USA* 2002;**53**:40–4.
3. Carrick CW. The feeding of corn and its parts to mature cockerels in confinement. *Poult Sci* 1925;**4**:199–204.
4. Fritz JC. Effect of grinding on digestibility of argentine flint corn. *Poult Sci* 1934;**14**:267–72.
5. Hetland H, Svihus B, Olaisen V. Effect of feeding whole cereals on performance, starch digestibility and duodenal particle size distribution in broiler chickens. *Br Poult Sci* 2002;**43**:416–23.
6. Engberg RM, Hedemann MS, Steenfeldt S, Jensen BB. Influence of whole wheat and xylanase on broiler performance and microbial composition and activity in the digestive tract. *Poult Sci* 2004;**83**:925–38.

7. Bjerrum L, Pedersen K, Engberg RM. The influence of whole wheat feeding on salmonella infection and gut flora composition in broilers. *Avian Dis* 2005;**49**:9–15.

8. Taylor RD, Jones GP. The incorporation of whole grain into pelleted broiler chicken diets. II. Gastrointestinal and digesta characteristics. *Br Poult Sci* 2004;**45**:237–46.

9. Evans M, Singh DN, Trappet P, Nagle T. Investigations into the effect of feeding laying hens complete diets with wheat in whole or ground form and zeolite presented in powdered or grit form, on performance and oocyst output after being challenged with coccidiosis. *Proc 17th Aust Poult Sci Symp* 2005;**45**:187–90.

10. Duke GE. Alimentary canal: Anatomy, regulation of feeding and motility. In: Sturkie PD, editor. *Avian physiology.* New York, NY: Springer Verlag; 1986. p. 269–88.

11. Cabrera MR. *Effects of sorghum genotype and particle size on milling characteristics and performance of finishing pigs, broiler chicks, and laying hens.* Masters thesis. Kansas State University; 1994.

12. Cumming RB. *Opportunities for whole grain feeding.* Glasgow, UK: Proceedings of the 9th European Poultry Conference; 1994 219–222.

13. Svihus B, Hetland H. Ileal starch digestibility in growing broiler chickens fed on a wheat-based diet is improved by mash feeding, dilution with cellulose or whole wheat inclusion. *Br Poult Sci* 2001;**42**:633–7.

14. Wu YB, Ravindran V, Thomas DG, Birtles MJ, Hendriks WH. Influence of method of whole wheat inclusion and xylanase supplementation on the performance, apparent metabolisable energy, digestive tract measurements and gut morphology of broilers. *Br Poult Sci* 2004;**45**:385–94.

15. Wu YB, Ravindran V. Influence of whole wheat inclusion and xylanase supplementation on the performance, digestive tract measurements and carcass characteristics of broiler chickens. *Anim Feed Sci Technol* 2004;**116**:129–39.

16. Ravindran V, Wu YB, Thomas DG, Morel PCH. Influence of whole wheat feeding on the development of gastrointestinal tract and performance of broiler chickens. *Aust J Agric Res* 2006;**57**:21–6.

17. Amerah AM, Ravindran V. Influence of method of whole wheat feeding on the performance, digestive tract development and carcass traits of broiler chickens. *Anim Feed Sci Technol* 2008;**147**:326–39.

18. Rose SP, Burnett A, Elmajeed RA. Factors Affecting the Diet Selection of Choice-Fed Broilers. *Br Poult Sci* 1986;**27**:215–24.

19. Munt RHC, Dingle JG, Sumpa MG. Growth, Carcass Composition and Profitability of Meat Chickens Given Pellets, Mash or Free-Choice Diet. *Br Poult Sci* 1995;**36** 277–284.

20. Cobb Broiler Management Guide. Siloam Springs, AR: Cobb-Vantress Inc; 2008.

21. Ross Broiler Management Manual. Newbridge, UK: Aviagen Limited; 2009.

22. Svihus B. Norwegian poultry industry converts to whole grain pellets. *Feed Tech* 2001;**5**:22–3.

23. Forbes JM, Covasa M. Application of diet selection by poultry with particular reference to whole cereals. *Worlds Poult Sci J* 1995;**51**:149–65.

24. Erener G, Ocak N, Ozturk E, Ozdas A. Effect of different choice feeding methods based on whole wheat on performance of male broiler chickens. *Anim Feed Sci Technol* 2003;**106**:131–8.

25. Rose SP, Fielden M, Foote WR, Gardin P. Sequential Feeding of Whole Wheat to Growing Broiler-Chickens. *Br Poult Sci* 1995;**36**:97–111.

26. Umar Faruk M, Bouvarel I, Meme M, Rideau N, Roffidal L, Tukur HM, et al. Sequential feeding using whole wheat and a separate protein–mineral concentrate improved feed efficiency in laying hens. *Poult Sci* 2010;**89**:785–96.

27. Umar Faruk M, Bouvarel I, Mallet S, Ali MN, Tukur HM, Nys Y, et al. Is sequential feeding of whole wheat more efficient than ground wheat in laying hens? *Animal* 2011;**5**:230–8.

28. Jones GPD, Taylor RD. The incorporation of whole grain into pelleted broiler chicken diets: production and physiological responses. *Br Poult Sci* 2001;**42**:477–83.

29. Cumming RB. *The biological control of coccidiosis.* Amsterdam, The Netherlands: Proceedings of the 19th World Poultry Congress; 1992. p. 425–428.

30. Banfield MJ, Forbes JM. Effects of whole wheat dilution v. substitution on coccidiosis in broiler chickens. *Br J Nutr* 2001;**86**:89–95.

31. Banfield MJ, Kwakkel RP, Forbes JM. Effects of wheat structure and viscosity on coccidiosis in broiler chickens. *Anim Feed Sci Technol* 2002;**98**:37–48.

32. Gabriel I, Mallet S, Leconte M, Fort G, Naciri M. Effects of whole wheat feeding on the development of coccidial infection in broiler chickens. *Poult Sci* 2003;**82**:1668–76.

33. Gabriel I, Mallet S, Leconte M, Fort G, Naciri M. Effect of whole wheat feeding on the development of coccidial infection in broiler chickens until market-age. *Anim Feed Sci Technol* 2006;**129**:279–303.

34. Moen B, Rudi K, Svihus B, Skanseng B. Reduced spread of *Campylobacter jejuni* in broiler chickens by stimulating the bird's natural barriers. *J Appl Microbiol* 2012;**113**:1176–83.

35. Samanta M, Haldar S, Ghosh TK. Comparative efficacy of an organic acid blend and bacitracin methylene disalicylate as growth promoters in broiler chickens: effects on performance, gut histology, and small intestinal milieu. *Vet Med Int* 2010;**2010**:645150.

36. Dibner JJ, Buttin P. Use of organic acids as a model to study the impact of gut microflora on nutrition and metabolism. *J Appl Poult Res* 2002;**11**:453–63.

37. Drew MD, Syed NA, Goldade BG, Laarveld B, Van Kessel AG. Effects of dietary protein source and level on intestinal populations of *Clostridium perfringens* in broiler chickens. *Poult Sci* 2004;**83**:414–20.

38. Preston CM, McCracken KJ, McAllister A. Effect of diet form and enzyme supplementation on growth, efficiency and energy utilisation of wheat-based diets for broilers. *Brit Poult Sci* 2000;**41**:324–31.

39. Biggs P, Parsons CM. The effects of whole grains on nutrient digestibilities, growth performance, and cecal short chain fatty acid concentrations in young chicks fed ground corn soybean meal diets. *Poult Sci* 2009;**88**:1893–905.

40. Svihus B, Juvik E, Hetland H, Krogdahl A. Causes for improvement in nutritive value of broiler chicken diets with whole wheat instead of ground wheat. *Br Poult Sci* 2004;**45**:55–60.

41. Svihus B. The gizzard: function, influence of diet structure and effects on nutrient availability. *Worlds Poult Sci J* 2011;**67**:207–24.

42. Ferket P. Feeding whole grains to poultry improves gut health. *Feedstuffs (USA)* 2000;**4**:12–4.

43. Duke GE. Recent studies on regulation of gastric motility in turkeys. *Poult Sci* 1992;**81**:1–8.

44. Li Y, Owyang C. Vagal afferent pathway mediates physiological action of Cholecystokinin on pancreatic enzyme secretion. *J Clin Investig* 1993;**92**:418–24.

45. Amerah AM, Peron A, Zaefarian F, Ravindran V. Influence of whole wheat inclusion and a blend of essential oils on the performance, nutrient utilization, digestive tract development and ileal microbiota profile of broiler chickens. *Br Poult Sci* 2011;**52**:124–32.

46. Svihus B. The role of feed processing on gastrointestinal function and health in poultry. In: Perry GC, editor. *Avian gut function in health and disease.* Wallingford, Oxon: CAB International; 2006. p. 183–94.

47. Amerah AM, Ravindran V, Lentle RG, Thomas DG. Influence of insoluble fibre and whole wheat inclusion on the performance, digestive tract development and ileal microbiota profile of broiler chickens. *Br Poult Sci* 2009;**50**:366–75.

48. Svihus B, Sacranie A, Choct M. The effect of intermittent feeding and dietary whole wheat on performance and digestive adaptation in broiler chickens. *Poult Sci* 2010;**89**:2617–25.

49. Clark PM, Behnke KC, Fahrenholz AC. Effects of feeding cracked corn and concentrate protein pellets on broiler growth performance. *J Appl Poult Res* 2009;**18**:259–68.

50. Olver MD, Jonker A. Effect of choice feeding on the performance of broilers. *Br Poult Sci* 1997;**38**:571–6.

51. Svihus B, Herstad O, Newman CW, Newman RK. Comparison of performance and intestinal characteristics of broiler chickens fed on diets containing whole, rolled or ground barley. *Br Poult Sci* 1997;**38**:524–9.

52. Bennett CD, Classen HL, Riddell C. Feeding broiler chickens wheat and barley diets containing whole, ground and pelleted grain. *Poult Sci* 2002;**81**:995–1003.

53. Hidalgo MA, Davis AJ, Dale NM, Dozier III WA. Use of whole pearl millet in broiler diets. *J Appl Poult Res* 2004;**13**:229–34.

Whole Wheat in Commercial Poultry Production

Dariusz Kokoszyński

University of Technology and Life Sciences, Faculty of Animal Breeding and Biology, Department of Poultry Breeding and Evaluation of Animal Products, Bydgoszcz, Poland

WHEAT AS A FEED GRAIN

In addition to corn and rice, wheat (*Triticum* L.) is the most commonly cultivated cereal in the world. In 2011/2012, 695.7 million tonnes[1] of wheat was produced on 240 million hectares of arable land around the world. The largest wheat producers are China, at 18% (117.4 million tonnes) of world production, followed by India (13.3%), Russia (8.6%), and the USA (8.4%).[1,2]

Wheat grain is mainly processed into flour, which is used in the bread-making and confectionary industries, and for making pasta and culinary products. Other uses include production of starch, gluten, and bioethanol. Wheat processing by-products, such as bran, fodder flour, sprouts, gluten, and distillers grain, are fed to farm animals. Wheat grain is also an important component of most livestock diets. In Europe, about 45% of wheat grain is used as feed.[3,4]

Wheat is commonly used in diets of poultry, in particular broiler chickens, young broiler turkeys, and laying hens. This is the case in many countries which produce greater amounts of less expensive wheat grain compared to corn, or that have less favorable climatic and soil conditions to grow corn for grain, namely the United Kingdom,[5–8] Denmark,[9–11] Canada,[12–14] the Czech Republic,[15,16] Germany,[17–19] Poland,[20–23] Australia, and New Zealand.[24,25]

Until recently, corn was thought to be the best energy feed for poultry. The results of many studies with broiler chickens,[26,27] turkeys,[28] and laying hens[29–34] indicate that grain type (wheat vs corn) has no effect on the level of their production traits. It is now thought that wheat can be used in poultry diets as the sole grain. Its proportion in broiler and layer diets is unlimited, except that it is recommended that enzyme preparations be used in young

birds when wheat exceeds 40% of the diet.[35–37] Because no feed wheat cultivars are available, inferior grain, and even shriveled or sprouted grain, is used in diet manufacture. Feed wheat usually comes from the spring crop, which does not comply with the requirements for baking wheat.[3]

The considerable suitability of wheat grain in poultry nutrition is due to its high energy value (12.8–13.5 MJ ME/kg) resulting from high starch content, low amounts of crude fiber, and high nutrient digestibility.[38] However, the energy value of wheat is 8–10% lower than that of corn, mainly because wheat contains much less fat.[20,35] The major source of energy in wheat grain is nitrogen-free extracts (about 69%), including 60% of starch. However, the most concentrated energy source is fat, which accounts for about 1.7% of grain wheat. In poultry, the dietary energy level is considered to be decisive for nutrient intake. Where the amount of protein and the energy to protein ratio in the diet meet requirements, birds consume the feed only in amounts that meet their energy requirement.[39–42]

Wheat grain has the highest protein content of all cereals (9–18%), but levels vary widely according to the level of nitrogen fertilization, grain variety, soil richness, and environmental conditions. The most valuable batches of wheat that are high in protein are grown in continental and steppe climates, and originate from sites characterized by high temperature, high solar radiation, and long periods of precipitation deficiency during grain formation. When cultivated under such conditions, wheat grain may contain as much as 15–18% protein.[43] However, the overwhelming majority of wheat batches have inadequate protein concentrations for poultry and swine. This dietary protein deficiency has to be corrected with soybean, legume seeds, double-low rapeseed, or animal protein.

Wheat grain has low lysine, methionine, and threonine contents. Research showed lysine to be the first limiting amino acid that determines the biological value of wheat seed protein.[44–47] The second limiting amino acid in wheat is threonine[48–50] or methionine.[51,52] The relatively high phytase content of wheat may increase the utilization of phosphorus associated with phytic acid (about 60%).

The chemical composition and quality of different wheat batches may vary considerably, which has an effect on poultry performance. Wheat grain may provide up to 70% of energy, up to 35% of protein, and up to 25% of lysine in poultry diets.[21]

High proportions of wheat in poultry diets may lead to a deficiency of minerals and vitamins, which are less abundant in wheat than in other cereal species. Deficiencies of biotin (only <12% of which is available) should be expected, which may make birds excessively fat.[20]

Aside from nutrients, wheat grain contains small quantities of antinutritional factors, the most important of which are non-starch polysaccharides (NSP). Among these, water-soluble arabinoxylans (pentosans) and beta-glucans have strongest antinutritional effects. In birds, they increase gut viscosity and reduce nutrient availability by interfering with the secretion of digestive enzymes into the intestine.[4] Poultry have no non-starch polysaccharide-degrading enzymes in the small intestine. Supplementation of exogenous enzymes that contain xylanase, or xylanase and beta-glucanase, reduces their harmful effects. Good conditions for high activity of the supplemented exogenous enzymes are created by the crop environment due to the prevailing temperature and humidity, as well as pH conducive to NSP degradation. Supplementation of these enzymes reduces gut viscosity, enhances nutrient digestibility, increases body weight gains, and improves conversion of food and avian health. Particularly good results are obtained when supplementing these enzymes in young broilers.[10,53–65] In general, enzymes have little effect on improving the productivity of adult birds.[66,67]

Other antinutritional factors in wheat grain include inhibitors of digestive enzymes, mainly trypsin and chymotrypsin inhibitors, which reduce protein digestibility; the alpha-amylase inhibitor, which decreases starch digestibility; and alkylresorcinols, tannins, lectins, and phytins.[3]

Feed grains, including wheat, may contain mycotoxins produced by molds and fungi, which may infect grain before harvest, during harvest, or during storage. Fungi and molds that invade cereal grains may produce over 800 different mycotoxins.[68] The most common mycotoxins in cereals and compound feeds are deoxynivalenol (DON), nivalenol (NIV), T2 and HT2 toxins, diacetoxyscirpenol (DAS), moliniformin, and zearalenone (ZEA). These inhibit protein synthesis and have immunosuppressive

effects. They are responsible for depressed growth rate and reproductive problems. In large amounts, DON can also cause intestinal inflammation. Under favorable conditions, Aspergillus and Penicillum may appear during grain storage. They produce aflatoxins, ochratoxin A, citrinin, sterigmatocystin, and naphthoquinones. Aflatoxin B1, produced by Aspergillus flavus, is the most toxic.[21]

It is estimated that over 25% of the world's grain crops are infected with mycotoxins. In Europe, wheat is most often invaded with DON, NIV, and moliniformin, as well as ochratoxin A. Most often, mycotoxins in feeds occur in amounts that pose no real threat to animals. However, they are important for baking-wheat quality control. The presence of mycotoxins in cereals and feeds has been the subject of many analyses.[69–74] Numerous studies have also addressed the effect mycotoxins have on poultry performance.[75–79]

Wheat grain can also be infected with ergot, the sclerotial form of the fungus Claviceps purpurea containing toxic alkaloids, which poisons animals and cause them to die.[3,43]

In intensive poultry farming, wheat grain is predominantly used in ground form as a component of loose or pelleted feeds. It can also be used in the form of whole grains, which reduces the costs of crushing, pelleting, and transportation, as well as feeding costs. Another way of reducing feeding costs is to apply restricted feeding, whereby the amount of feed or a certain nutrient is limited. However, aside from reduced feeding costs, most experiments reported decreases in body weight, carcass weight, and meat weight.[80–85]

In commercial poultry production, whole wheat grain can be offered by several methods: (1) free choice, where whole grain and complete mixture are given *ad libitum* in separate feeders; (2) with part of the ground wheat found in the complete diet being replaced with whole grain and administered in one feeder; (3) with the feed mixture or protein/protein–mineral concentrate diluted with whole wheat grain – the so-called Danish system; and (4) alternately with the complete mixture (sequential feeding).

Observations to date[86] indicate that birds vary considerably in their ability to digest wheat grain. There are lines of broiler chickens with high (D+) or low (D−) wheat digestion capacity. Digestibility of fat, starch, and protein is significantly higher in the D+ line (77%, 94%, and 81%, respectively) compared to the D− line (62%, 91%, and 76%, respectively).

However, birds that digest wheat grain less efficiently have a larger proportion of breast muscle. This may suggest that meat content is unrelated to good digestion of feed.

Programs for feeding whole grain to poultry are applied mainly in Europe (especially in Scandinavia, The Netherlands, and the United Kingdom), Australia, New Zealand, Canada, and most recently in Turkey.[14,62,87–91]

WHOLE WHEAT GRAIN IN RELATION TO PRODUCTION LEVEL AND LIVABILITY AS AN INDICATOR OF HEALTH STATUS IN POULTRY

Over the past 50 years, the performance of broiler chickens, turkeys, ducks, and geese has been considerably improved, mainly as a result of breeding work – in particular, selection for improved feed conversion ratio and increased rate of growth. The rearing period of chickens has been shortened from 16 weeks in the 1950s to 5–6 weeks today. The considerable increase in body weight increased the incidence of birds with leg abnormalities, degeneration of hock joints, and deformed or fractured bones. An imbalance between the rate of body weight gain and the development of internal organs, especially the circulatory and respiratory systems, led to incidences of ascites and sudden death syndrome.[92,93]

Bennett and colleagues[13] showed that one way to reduce leg disorders could be to use whole wheat grain in poultry diets. Feeding broiler chickens of between 6 and 48 days of growth whole wheat grain (50–650 g/kg) supplemented with pelleted or mash diets caused a significant decrease in mortality due to leg problems up to 48 days of growth. The highest reduction in mortality due to skeletal and leg deformities (from 3.19% to 0.53%) was found in male broilers fed 50, 350, or 500 g/kg of whole grain until 6, 13, or 27 days of growth, respectively. Males receiving mash diets were lighter and more resistant.

In a study with Big 6 turkeys fed a diet containing whole wheat (108–405 g/kg of ration) from 4 to 22 weeks of age, flock health was considerably better (2.5% culling rate and mortality each) compared with turkeys receiving complete pelleted diets alone (7.5% culling rate and mortality each); this resulted from, among other things, their lower slaughter weight.[20]

Whole cereal grain, mostly wheat or barley, is primarily used in poultry nutrition to reduce feeding costs without adversely affecting profitability and production results. In a study with Cobb broiler chickens, replacing ground wheat with whole grain wheat at 100 g/kg or 200 g/kg of the diet increased body weight gains from 6 to 46 days of growth by 3.9% or 2.6%, and decreased feed consumption by 1.4% or 1.5%, respectively, which is of considerable relevance for breeders.[94]

However, when it is of poorer nutritive value and digestibility, whole grain used as a dietary component may carry the risk of slowing the growth rate of birds. Wheat given to birds should be of the highest possible quality. In Big 6 turkeys, replacing wheat in pelleted diet with low-protein (8.9–10.3%) whole wheat grain at 100–500 g/kg of wheat (Experiment I) from 4 to 15 weeks (females) or 22 weeks (males) reduced their slaughter weight by about 1000 g in relation to the control birds, which received a complete diet.[20]

Optimum economic results in young turkey nutrition were obtained when feeding protein concentrate (42.8% crude protein) supplemented with 400, 500, or 600 g/kg grain from 4, 7, and 9–10 weeks of rearing, respectively.[9] Dilution of the complete diets with a high level of whole wheat can negatively affect the growth and development of birds. Hybrid turkeys fed diets containing 150 g whole wheat from day 41, 350 g from day 62, and 500 g/kg from day 83 showed body weight reduction of 14.6% and breast muscle weight reduction of 7.3% compared to control birds receiving commercial mash. This feeding regimen also increased death losses in males compared to control birds.[14]

The beneficial effects of feeding whole wheat were also reported for table egg production. Bovans White layers receiving a diet containing 300 g/kg of whole wheat grain instead of the same amount of ground wheat, and supplemented with 150 g/t of the xylanase-containing enzyme preparation Ronozyme® WX produced 6.5% more eggs between 53 and 63 weeks of age compared to control birds, and 3.5% more eggs compared to layers fed whole grain and commercial mash, and consumed less feed for production of kg of eggs (by 7.0% or 7.5%, respectively). Hens receiving whole wheat grain, with or without supplemental xylanase, laid significantly heavier eggs.[95] Today it is necessary to use feed enzymes in the diets of poultry reared under intensive conditions. Diets high in wheat, triticale, or rye are supplemented with preparations containing arabinoxylanase, cellulase, beta-glucanase, and pectinase – i.e., enzymes that digest basic fiber components.[96]

Other studies[29,33,34] have shown cereal type (wheat vs corn) to have no effect on layer production traits, while substitution of corn with wheat,[31,32,97] and particle size of layer diets, had no effect on the quantity and quality of eggs laid.

A negative effect of using high wheat grain diets is the increased susceptibility of young broilers or layers to feather- and cannibalistic-pecking, as well as increased aggression.[98] These behaviors may intensify, especially when balanced rations (feed mixtures) are replaced with whole wheat grain. This decreases the intake of protein, minerals, vitamins, and other nutrients by the birds.

Effective results are obtained by feeding loose (less and less often), crumbled (young birds), or complete pelleted diets mixed with wheat grain, or protein concentrates and wheat grain from one or two different feeders. Simon and Delpech[99] found that broiler chickens adapt relatively easily to feed restrictions, which enables complete diets to be replaced with wheat grain. Research[100] showed that complete feed can be replaced with wheat grain at up to 300 g/kg of the diet without significantly affecting the body weight of slaughter-age chickens and feed conversion ratio. Feeding whole grain at up to 300 g/kg of the ration reduced feeding costs by 2.4–9.3%[89] in Hubbard chickens, and by 6.2–19.2% in Starbro chickens.[88] By replacing the control diet with increasing amounts of wheat grain (from 50–250 g/kg) as birds grew older, Dov and colleagues[101] obtained optimum production results in the form of reduced broiler production costs and considerable improvement in the economic result.

When comparing Cobb 500 broiler chickens receiving 100 g/kg of wheat grain from 6 to 21 days of age, and rolled wheat (control group) or 150, 250, 350, 450 and 610 g of whole wheat per kg feed from 21 to 42 days, it was found that the use of up to 450 g/kg of wheat grain had no negative effect on body weight and feed conversion, but significantly decreased the proportion of breast muscle in the carcass. Meanwhile, chickens receiving a diet containing 610 g/kg of whole grain had 3.4% lower body weight at the age of 6 weeks and 2.2% less efficient conversion of feed per kg of live weight gain. Dressing percentage was lower by 8.5%, and breast muscle content by 2.7 percentage points – i.e., by as much as 12.5% in relation to the control birds.[102] In another study,[103] replacing up to 450 g/kg of ground wheat with whole wheat grain compromised weight gains, increased individual variation, and increased fat levels in birds. In Avian chickens, there was a significant decrease in body weight gains and conversion of feed per kg of live weight gain when the diet contained 300 or 500 g/kg of whole or ground wheat.[91] According to Mazanowski,[37] the amount of grain used also depends on bird genotype. In Ross 308 broilers, wheat grain can be given from 20 days of age at up to 150 g/kg, followed by 200 g/kg, while in Cobb 500 chickens up to 450 g/kg of grain can be fed from 22 days of growth.

Other published studies concerning the effect of feeding whole wheat grain to broiler chickens on their performance have produced divergent results. Several experiments reported positive effects of feeding wheat grain to broilers,[104–106] while other researchers[107,108] found no benefits of giving whole wheat to broiler chickens.

The results of Danish studies indicated that adding 200 g/kg of whole wheat to the diet during the first weeks of life had no adverse effect on the amount of feed consumed until the fifth week of rearing, but reduced weight gains and increased feed conversion ratio.[109] Supplementation of a starter diet with low-protein wheat resulted in poorer weight gains, increased variation within the flock, and increased fat levels in chickens.[110]

Whole wheat grain as a supplement to complete diets or protein concentrates has been used for several dozen years in Denmark, The Netherlands, and the United Kingdom in intensive broiler production. Feeding the rations requires regular monitoring of body weight and ensuring the right energy to protein ratio to provide chickens with appropriate amounts of grain.[111]

In broiler chickens, whole wheat grain is added at 5% of the diet on days 7–9 of growth and gradually increased by five percentage points at 4-day intervals. From 31–32 days of age, broiler chickens receive a diet containing 350 g of grain per kg of feed until the end of rearing. This feeding system (the so-called Danish system) allows birds to consume nutrients of their choice while maintaining fixed proportions of grain and protein concentrate for the entire flock. The chicken feeding system with free choice of grain and concentrate containing 240 g protein/kg of feed was used in Denmark from the 1930s onwards, but was abandoned after the cage system and automatic feeders were introduced. It has again become significant now that computer scales (e.g., INDOOR or Big Dutchman) allow for accurate weighing and mixing of several feed ingredients.[21] The poultry feeding system based on free choice has been the subject of many studies involving broiler chickens.[90,112–129]

When broiler chickens and laying hens were fed by free choice, their nutrient requirements varied according to the time of day. This results, among other things, from changes in bird activity with time of day, and gave rise to the concept of sequential feeding. Sequentially fed Ross 308 broiler chickens given access to a standard diet for 18 hours of the day and whole wheat for the next 6 hours are characterized by 3.5% higher body weight at 42 days of age compared to birds receiving feed mixture and whole wheat grain (5–40 g of grain/kg mixture). However, sequentially fed birds were lighter than control chickens (by 3.8%) and those that had free choice between standard diet and whole wheat (by 6.9%). Sequentially fed chickens were characterized by poorer feed conversion compared to control birds (by 5.2%) and those fed free choice (by 0.2%), and were more efficient in feed conversion than birds fed a standard diet and whole wheat grain (by 8.4%).[89] The results of other studies indicate that sequential feeding had differential effects in laying hens. Leeson and Summers[130] and Robinson[131] reported lower egg production and egg weight, whereas Blair et al.[132] found increased feed consumption and no effect of this feeding system on the number and weight of eggs.

Whole wheat grain is also used in broiler breeder flocks. During the growth period (prior to the egg production period), most often from 6 weeks of age and during egg production, whole oat grain, whole wheat grain, or broken corn is added to the bedding. This makes the flock more active, enhances the condition of legs, increases egg fertility, improves flock survival, and also has a positive effect on bedding condition and indoor microclimate. Provided that purchase prices of broiler chickens after the egg production period are attractive, Hybro (a leading broiler breeding company) recommends that during the final dozen or so weeks of egg production the amount of feed be increased by offering whole wheat, barley, or oat grain at 15–30 g/day to improve the organoleptic properties of carcass and meat.[133]

Whole wheat grain or wheat and rye mixed at a 1:1 ratio and supplemented with essential vitamins and minerals may also be used as an alternative to restricted feeding. Feeding a low-protein whole wheat diet during the rearing period of broiler breeders resulted in decreased weight gains, increased carcass fat at 20 weeks of age, and poorer survivability. The use of wheat grain delayed the onset of sexual maturity by 5–8 days in relation to control birds receiving a mash diet.[134]

In duck feeding, it is best to use a mixture of different cereal species, in ground form, as a component of feed mixtures. The daily allowance of wheat grain for ducks should not exceed 50 g – i.e., about 20% of the feed consumed by an adult duck.[135] In an effort to reduce the cost of winter feeding (from October to the end of January in Europe), ostrich farmers abandon commercial diets offered by the feed industry and replace them with cereal grains.[136]

The renewed interest in feeding whole wheat grain results from intense competition between poultry producers who want to minimize production costs and market inexpensive products. Many countries, including members of the European Union, are abandoning intensive poultry farming systems, which is reflected in reduced stocking density of broiler chickens and hens and the introduction of enriched cages, under pressure from consumer and environmental groups. Moreover, feeding diets with whole grain to farmed birds is considered to be more natural and has a positive effect on bird health.[111]

In Poland, two feeding programs involving whole wheat have become available recently: Feed Mix Program (Broiler Wheat Mix and Turkey Wheat Mix) and Wheat Program. The former provides broiler chicken or broiler turkey producers with a pelleted diet containing about 20% of whole wheat grain. Under the latter program, producers receive a pelleted diet with a higher protein content than recommended for a given rearing period (concentrate) and have to administer whole wheat on their own from 11 days of rearing, according to a specific program. During the whole rearing period, wheat accounts for about 21% of feed consumed. Hama Plus (a poultry hatchery and distribution company) recommends adding good quality wheat (40 g/kg) when broilers are between 11 and 15 days old, and gradually increasing this amount by 20 g/kg every 3 days to reach a level of 160 g/kg.[137]

These broiler feeding programs enable the nutrient requirement of birds of different genotype to be optimally fulfilled while avoiding the periods of protein deficiency or excess. Birds exposed to protein deficiency increase their feed consumption and fatness. Excess protein is also unfavorable, as it increases the water and energy requirement of birds as well as the content of water and uric acid in excreted manure. Increasing the

content of water and nitrogen compounds in litter often increases the incidence of foot burns and breast blisters, which compromises the economic performance.[20,137] The use of imbalanced diets results in improper growth of birds, and in less efficient conversion of feed through the increase in metabolic heat production[7,8,138,139] A diet that does not meet the requirement may increase the risk of sudden death syndrome, fatty liver degeneration, and leg deformities.[12,140]

WHOLE WHEAT AS RELATED TO QUALITY OF POULTRY PRODUCTS AND HUMAN HEALTH

A large variety of poultry products (meat, eggs, feathers, goose fat, foie gras, and skin) is one of the factors contributing to the development of poultry production. Over the past several dozen years, global poultry meat production growth has been much higher compared to pork and beef. By way of example, during the period 1970–2006, poultry meat production increased by 461%, pork by 195%, and beef by 59%. Poultry meat production exceeded the volume of beef production in 2000, and is estimated to become higher than pork production within the next 6–10 years.[141,142] In 2010, poultry meat production was about 96 million tonnes. Worldwide egg production in 2010 was 64.1 million tonnes.[2]

The rapid increase in poultry meat and egg production was possible due to their low prices and high nutritional and dietetic value. The increase was also supported by a broad range of poultry products to suit the health, age, and wealth of customers; by the health of the products ensured by salmonellosis control programs and the health safety and quality assurance systems (HACCP, QAFP); by adjusting production conditions to meet customer expectations; and by the growing affluence of societies in developing countries. Recent years have seen increasing interest in functional food and products obtained from animals raised under semi-intensive or extensive conditions (Label Rouge, Free Farmed, etc.).[14]

Feeding systems that use whole wheat grain are considered more natural for birds, and thus have good development prospects. Data published on the effect of using whole wheat grain instead of ground wheat as a component of feed mixture offer no conclusive answer as to how this procedure affects dressing percentage (considered the most important trait for poultry slaughtering plants as it determines the quantity of the product intended for sale), as well as the characteristics desired by consumers: improved muscling (especially the breast part) and decreased carcass fatness (percentages of skin with subcutaneous fat and abdominal fat). The introduction of 100 g/kg (days 1–21) or 200 g/kg (days 22–35) whole wheat in place of ground wheat caused a slight deterioration in dressing percentage (percentage of eviscerated carcass in bird body prior to slaughter) and proportion of breast muscle, but also the percentage of abdominal fat, in Ross chickens.[24] Another study[94] found a significant decrease in abdominal fat content of Cobb chickens when 100 g/kg ground wheat was replaced with whole wheat grain. The use of whole wheat or cracked corn in the free-choice system caused a significant reduction in the proportion of breast muscle while increasing the proportion of abdominal fat.[87] In game pheasants, the substitution of complete feed with wheat grain during the final 7 weeks of rearing caused a significant reduction in body weight and weight of abdominal fat.[143] Reduction in carcass fatness, notably the amount of abdominal fat and subcutaneous fat, is a very important factor. High fatness of birds is associated with poorer feed conversion and increased production costs, and is not well received by consumers and processors. However, a certain amount of carcass fat is necessary as it positively affects the juiciness and flavor of meat.[144–149]

Excessive consumption of high-fat animal products encourages obesity and increases the risk of cardiovascular and heart diseases and the development of some neoplasms, especially colorectal cancer. Moreover, fat contains twice as much energy as protein or carbohydrates. According to FAO/WHO recommendations, the contribution of energy from fat in the average human diet should be decreased by 25–30%. The same experts also recommend reducing the proportion of energy from saturated fats (by one-third) and the consumption of cholesterol (by one-third), and increasing the proportion of energy from essential fatty acids (by one-half).[141]

A study[20] with Big 6 turkeys found differential effects of the date, amount, and mode of adding whole wheat on dressing percentage and carcass composition. Turkeys were fed, from 4–15 weeks (females) or 22 weeks (males), a pelleted diet (control group); a diet containing 108 g (weeks 4–6), 187 g (weeks 7–9), 292 g (weeks 10–12) and 405 g (weeks 13–15 or 22) wheat grain per kg of feed; or a pelleted diet and whole wheat (separate trough) in the free-choice system. Fifteen-week-old birds of both sexes, which also received wheat grain (Experiment I), had lower dressing percentage, proportion of breast and leg muscles, and proportions of abdominal fat, intestinal fat, and skin with subcutaneous fat compared to control birds and those fed by free choice. All feeding treatments, with or without whole wheat grain, ensured good post-slaughter results in 22-week-old turkey toms. Males fed pelleted diet and wheat grain (Experiment II) were characterized by slightly lower dressing percentage and significantly lower content of lower thigh muscles, and thigh and lower thigh muscles together, and significantly higher percentage of skin with subcutaneous fat, compared to the other groups of turkeys analyzed.

The feeding treatments of whole wheat had no negative impact on the basic chemical composition (content of dry matter, crude protein, crude fat, and crude ash) and physicochemical properties (water holding capacity, color, and pH_{48}) of breast muscle in 15-week-old birds of both sexes from all the groups receiving four or five feeds during the rearing period. Meat from males had significantly less crude protein and crude ash, and lighter color (higher L*) compared to females.[20]

The turkey feeding method had no effect on the sensory properties (tenderness, juiciness, aroma and flavor desirability and intensity) of muscles from 15- (male and female) and 22-week-old (male) birds. The introduction of whole wheat into turkey diets also had no significant effect on the fatty acid composition of breast muscle and liver (organ fats) as well as abdominal fat, intestinal fat, and subcutaneous fat (depot fats). Organ fats contained less unsaturated fatty acids (UFAs) than depot fats. Compared to turkey hens, 15-week-old turkey toms had a higher content of linoleic acid in organ and depot fats, which, according to some authors,[150,151] determines the value of fat.

Another study[152] found that laying hens fed a wheat- or triticale-based diet were characterized by higher weight gains, and laid more eggs that were heavier, compared to birds receiving a rye-based diet. Yolk cholesterol content in eggs from hens fed the wheat- or triticale-based diet was lower than for hens fed the rye-based diet. The yolk of eggs from hens fed the wheat- or rye-based diet had a lower content of linoleic acid and a greater oleic to linoleic acid ratio compared to eggs from hens receiving the triticale-based diet.

Feeding diets with wheat grain (300 g/kg) improved the flavor and aroma of boiled eggs from Isa Brown hens in relation to birds receiving a diet with rye.[21] Diets in which wheat was the sole cereal[153] contributed to improved flavor and a slight deterioration in the aroma of boiled eggs, compared to eggs from hens fed diets based on rye, triticale, awnless barley, or awned barley.

Ristic and colleagues[154] observed a slight deterioration in sensory properties, particularly the aroma of grilled breast and leg muscles from broilers, with an increasing supplement of whole wheat. The quality of abdominal fat also deteriorated. When the proportions of whole wheat were higher, the proportion of monounsaturated fatty acids increased at the cost of a reduction in polyunsaturated fatty acids. In another study,[155] breast muscle of Ross 208 chickens fed a diet with wheat grain had lower tenderness than when diets with ground corn were applied.

Replacing a complete pelleted diet with whole wheat (300 g/kg) for common pheasants between 5 and 16 weeks of age[156] increased dressing percentage and the proportion of breast and leg muscles in eviscerated carcass with neck from 16-week-old birds. Breast muscles of pheasants that also received wheat grain had significantly less myristic ($C_{14:0}$) and palmitoleic acids ($C_{16:1}$), and significantly more arachidonic acid ($C_{20:4}$) compared to the muscles of pheasants fed commercial diets alone. The decreased proportion of $C_{14:0}$ and increased $C_{20:4}$ are considered beneficial from a consumer perspective. The breast muscle of experimental pheasants (wheat grain) was characterized by significantly more polyunsaturated fatty acids (PUFAs) and a higher PUFA to SFA ratio.

Restricted feeding of common pheasants (whole wheat and feed mixture) contributed to a significant decrease in the calcium and zinc content of breast muscle. Lower proportions of sodium, zinc, magnesium, and iron were also found in the muscles of pheasants fed the mixture and wheat.[156] Compared to control pheasants receiving complete diets, 18-week-old birds (2 weeks older) fed a diet with wheat grain (300 g/kg) had lower proportion of meat and fat, and a higher proportion of bones, while 20-week-old birds had decreased proportions of breast muscle and abdominal fat, in the carcass.[157,158]

In another study,[159] feeding pheasants between 9 and 40 weeks of age a diet containing 800 g of commercial mixture and 200 g of whole corn and wheat mixture at a 1:1 ratio per kg of feed had a positive influence on the amino acid profile of breast muscles from farmed compared to wild pheasants. Feeding pheasants from 11 weeks of age wheat grain and corn as well as *ad libitum* forage (mixture of corn, sunflower, alfalfa, grass, and kale) had a favorable effect on the chemical composition of meat, especially the proportion of dry matter and crude protein, as well as the fatty acid profile of breast and leg muscles, in 40-week-old pheasants.[160]

Eggs from hens that were fed whole wheat and oyster shells and had pasture access had a more beneficial sensory profile compared to eggs from birds receiving a commercial layer diet with or without pasture access.[161] Research[162] also demonstrated that sequential feeding of Isa Brown hens (whole or pelleted wheat grain alternated with protein–mineral concentrate) significantly reduced hens' body weight (37 and 46 weeks) and proportion of abdominal fat (46 weeks). Experimental hens fed whole wheat grain from 19 to 46 weeks of age produced eggs with significantly greater albumen and shell weight and reduced yolk weight compared to control birds.

WHOLE WHEAT AS RELATED TO DIGESTIVE TRACT MORPHOLOGY, INTESTINAL MICROFLORA, ACTIVITY OF DIGESTIVE ENZYMES, AND HEALTH OF FARMED BIRDS

The avian digestive system is made up of the digestive tract and the glands arising from its epithelial wall (salivary, mucous and intestinal glands, liver, pancreas). The digestive tract of birds features five segments: oral cavity and beak, pharynx, esophagus, stomach, and intestine terminating in the cloaca. The tract is relatively short, between 2.0 and 2.5 m in length in an adult hen. The intestine to body-length ratio is 5–6:1 in hens and turkeys, and 4–5:1 in ducks and geese. In other monogastric farm animals of importance, such as pigs and horses, this ratio is much higher.[163]

The digestive tract develops very early in birds. In chicken embryos, the foregut is already beginning to develop early in the second day of incubation. In 1-day-old chicks it forms almost one-fourth of body weight, but this proportion decreases with hens' age. In 8-week-old broiler chickens, the digestive tract constitutes only around 5% of body weight. During the first week of life, development of the digestive tract is relatively more rapid compared to other internal organs, and even the body as a whole. During this period, intestinal villi almost double in length, while depth of crypts between the villi generally remains unchanged. In addition, activity of the digestive glands increases considerably.[164,165]

Development of the intestine is considerably influenced by the form and composition of the feed and the date of its administration post-hatching. Early feed access stimulates the growth of the digestive tract. Delayed access to feed slows intestinal development and negatively affects bird performance.[166]

Feeds given to chickens during the first 5–7 days, and to turkeys during the first 3–4 weeks, must be ideal in terms of quality, nutritive value, and form, because the intensive growth of birds in these periods is responsible for appropriate growth and development (high weight gains) during the rearing period. If cereal grains are added to the diets of birds too early, their gastrointestinal tract may become deformed, the rate of digesta passage may slow down, nutrient absorption may decrease, etc.[96,167,168] Therefore, it is recommended that whole wheat grain be fed to chickens not earlier than 5–7 days of age,[169] and to turkeys from 3–4 weeks of rearing.[7–9,20]

The physical form and structure of the feed have a considerable influence on its intake by poultry, as well as on development of the gastrointestinal tract, stomach and intestinal motility, secretion of digestive enzymes, and the amount and composition of intestinal microflora.[96] Grinding of feed (including wheat grain) by crushing increases grain surface area for the action of digestive juices, but is detrimental to intestinal motility. Excessively fine grinding accelerates the passage of digesta and makes it less digestible, sticks the beaks of farmed birds together and discourages them from eating, increases the amount of particulate matter in poultry houses, increases feed losses, and negatively affects production economics. Therefore, in production practice birds are fed diets in crumbled (first weeks of life) or pellet form. Pelleting of loose feeds reduces feed intake, improves body weight gains, and increases flock uniformity. In addition, it decreases the action of antinutritional factors, microbiological contamination, and particulate pollution inside poultry houses.[96]

The production results of young broiler chickens and turkeys encourage the use of diets containing whole or coarsely ground wheat grain. The addition of whole wheat to the diets of farmed birds contributes to proper gizzard development and function. The frequency and intensity of gizzard contractions also increases; when chickens are fed whole wheat grain the gizzard contracts three times per minute, and pressure inside ranges from 80 to 100 mmHg. The number of contractions and gizzard pressure decrease with decreasing feed consistency and hardness. The gizzard of hens ingesting watery feeds contracts twice per minute, with inside pressure of more than 10 mmHg.[170] More frequent and stronger contractions of the gizzard ensure feed is more thoroughly pounded. Also, gizzard weight increases, which is mainly due to better development of the body of the gizzard. The increased mechanical activity of the gizzard stops it from becoming slack and necrosed, and prevents the detachment of keratin epithelium lining the inside walls.[36] A large and well-developed gizzard contributes to improved intestinal peristalsis. This probably also increases the release of cholecystokinins, which stimulate the secretion of pancreatic enzymes and the gastroduodenal reflux.[171] Many research findings[10,94,102,118,124,125,172–176] support the beneficial effect of using whole grain on gizzard weight.

Gabriel and colleagues[177] found the relative weight of the gizzard in Ross PM3 cockerels to increase by 26% from 16 to 44 days of age when the amount of whole wheat was gradually increased from 200 g on day 8 to 400 g/kg diet on day 22 of growth. In another experiment,[178] in which the proportion of whole wheat fed to broiler chickens was gradually increased to 300 g/kg (trial 1), 400 g/kg (trial 2), or 500 g/kg (trial 3) diet, gizzard weight was higher by 50–90% at slaughter age compared to birds receiving pelleted commercial diets. After introducing 100 g/kg (days 7–21) or 200 g/kg (days 22–35) of whole wheat in the free-choice system, Amerah and Ravindran[25] obtained an approximately 200% higher gizzard weight. There is no straightforward relationship, then, between increase in gizzard weight and increasing the amount of grain. The different extents to which gizzard weight increased in different experiments is probably due to different degrees of grain hardness, bird genotypes, and nutritive values of feeds used in the control group.

Amerah and colleagues[179] found gizzard weight in chickens to be significantly higher when using hard compared to soft wheat, whereas in Bovans White laying hens Senkoylu et al.[95] observed that whole wheat supplemented with or without xylanase enzyme toward the end of the egg production period (53–63 weeks) had no significant effect on gizzard weight. Likewise, in a study involving common pheasants,[180] replacement of 300 g/kg complete pelleted diet with whole wheat grain from 5 to 16 weeks of rearing did not produce significant changes in the gizzard weight of these birds at 16 weeks of age.

Feeding birds with whole wheat is paralleled by a greater secretion of the hydrochloric acid and endogenous enzymes in the proventriculus, which precedes the gizzard. The lower pH of the gizzard prevents the development of pathogenic bacteria and is beneficial for bird health and survival. Moreover, it can help improve protein denaturation and hydrolysis.[177]

Frikha and colleagues[181] found that the form of diet and type of cereal fed to laying hens from days 1 to 45 had an effect on the weight and pH of gizzard in birds aged 120 days. Pullets fed pellets had relatively lower gizzard weight and higher pH of gizzard contents (day 120) compared to those fed mash until 45 days of age. In another experiment,[95] following the introduction of 300 g/kg whole wheat into the diets of Bovans White hens at the end of the egg production period, gizzard pH was observed to decline from 4.68 (control) to 4.35 (whole wheat) or 4.31 (whole wheat + xylanase).

Some studies[105,163] found increased weight of the proventriculus. In birds, the proventriculus is relatively small and tubular. Much less muscular than the gizzard, it is lined with mucosa that houses numerous digestive glands. These glands produce pepsinogen and hydrochloric acid. Hydrochloric acid denatures proteins, and pepsin breaks about 10% of pepsin bonds.[163] Other researchers[174,180] did not find a significant effect of feeding a diet with whole wheat grain on the development of avian proventriculus.

Engberg and colleagues[10] additionally obtained a significant increase in pancreas weight in 6-week-old Ross 208 chickens after adding whole wheat (100–300 g/kg depending on age) compared to control birds fed pellets. In addition, the activity of pancreatic lipase and chymotrypsin increased after adding Ronozyme® WX containing the enzyme xylanase. These enzymes have a positive effect on digestion of protein and fat in birds fed a wheat-based diet.[182,183] Apart from that, other experiments found significant increases in pancreas weight[62,163,173,184] and liver weight[180] as well as improved pancreatic and hepatic secretion[184,185] when whole wheat was fed to farmed birds.

Diet structure has differential effects on development of the intestine and its segments. Frikha et al.[181] found greater jejunal (by 8.0%) and ileal lengths (by 5.5%) in 120-day-old laying hens fed wheat mash or corn mash to 45 days of age compared to feeding pellets. Broiler chickens fed whole wheat and protein concentrate in separate feeders (free choice) had significant increases in jejunal and ileal weight and in small intestine weight compared to control birds receiving a ground wheat diet.[25]

Progressive increases in the proportion of whole wheat grain from 200 g/kg on day 8 to 400 g/kg on day 22 had no significant effect on relative weight and length of intestinal segments except for the jejunum, which was shorter.[177] Yasar *et al.*[91] found intestinal length to increase significantly in birds fed coarsely ground or whole wheat to the extent of 300–500 g/kg compared to birds receiving finely ground wheat.

A study with common pheasants[180] found different reactions of the birds of different sexes to dietary wheat grain. Males fed whole grain (300 g/kg) and commercial pelleted diet (700 g/kg) for 12 weeks of rearing (weeks 5–16) were characterized by a longer intestine and segments thereof compared to control birds that received commercial diets alone. However, an inverse reaction was found in females, which had a shorter intestine when fed whole wheat and the commercial diet.

Awad and colleagues[79] reported that 3-week feeding of wheat naturally contaminated with deoxynivalenol (DON) – a mycotoxin produced by the fungus *Fusarium graminearum* – at 5 mg DON/kg diet caused reductions in the absolute and relative weight of the small intestine (by 22.6% and 18.5%, respectively), and in the length (by 19.5%) and width (by 30.8%) of intestinal villi. However, the results of many experiments[10,24,62,95,104,163,173,174] have failed to confirm the modifying effect of adding whole wheat on the relative weight and length of intestinal segments. Studies also revealed the adjusting effect of using whole wheat grain on intestinal motility.[10,177]

Gradually increasing the amount of wheat grain from 200 g to 400 g/kg diet starting from day 8 of broiler chicken growth caused a significant increase in the villus to crypt length and surface ratios in the duodenum of 23-day-old chickens.[177] Meanwhile, Bovans White laying hens fed a diet containing 300 g/kg whole wheat with or without the enzyme xylanase had significantly greater crypt depth compared to those fed a commercial layer diet containing 300 g/kg ground wheat. The intestine of grain-fed hens is characterized by a lower villus height to crypt depth ratio, which is generally associated with poorer nutrient absorption, increased secretion of enzymes in the digestive tract, and lower disease resistance and poorer survivability.[163,186]

The digestive tract of birds is colonized by abundant microflora – a mixture of bacteria, yeast, molds, and protozoa, although bacteria are predominant. On the first day after chick hatching, 1 g of ileal contents has 10^8 colony forming units (CFUs), compared to 10^{10} CFU in 1 g of cecal contents. This population increases during the first 3 days to 10^9 (ileum) or 10^{11} (cecum), and becomes relatively stable for the next 30 days.[187] The most abundant populations of microorganisms inhabit the crop and the final section of the digestive tract, especially the ceca. In the proventriculus, gizzard, and small intestine,

microorganisms have less favorable colonization conditions (lower pH and/or slower gastrointestinal transit).

It is estimated that the small intestine of chickens is inhabited by about 640 different species of bacteria, and of these only 10% have been identified; 35% of the genera are known and the others are completely unknown.[187,188] Composition of the microflora varies according to the segment of the gastrointestinal tract. The small intestine is dominated by lactic fermentation bacteria (*Lactobacillus*), and in the ceca *Clostridium* and *Streptococcus* are equally as numerous as lactobacilli.[189]

The composition of gastrointestinal microflora is modified by many factors, including bird age, breed, diet composition, feed processing method, housing conditions, and the use of feed additives, in particular enzymes, coccidiostats, probiotics, and prebiotics.[169,188] In Europe, changes in microflora composition are also due to the withdrawal of in-feed antibiotics and slaughterhouse by-product meals as components of feed mixtures. To date, no substance/preparation has been found to act on Gram-positive bacteria, which form the majority of gastrointestinal microorganisms. The available preparations act on Gram-negative bacteria.[190]

It has also been established that the number of bacteria in the digestive tract of broiler chickens is increased by cereal-based diets, namely *Enterococcus* by corn- and sorghum-based diets, *Lactobacillus* by barley-based diets, *Escherichia coli* and *Lactobacillus* by oat-based diets, and *Streptococcus* by rye-based diets.[187]

Feeding broiler chickens with whole wheat grain (200–400 g/kg diet) significantly decreases the number of facultatively anaerobic bacteria in the ileum while slightly increasing the number of these bacteria in the jejunum and ceca. Supplementation of wheat grain slightly reduces the amount of *Lactobacillus* in the jejunum and ileum, and increases it in the ceca. In addition, the *E. coli* count was found to slightly decrease in all parts of the intestine in birds fed wheat grain compared to control birds.[177] A gradual increase in the proportion of wheat grain in the diet of Ross 208 chickens reduced the number of enterobacteria in the gizzard. There was also a tendency toward a gradual reduction in the number of *Clostridium perfringens* bacteria in the ileum and ceca of chickens fed a whole wheat diet.

Microflora composition and metabolism products have considerable effects on gastrointestinal health, the risk of intestinal diseases, and the course of the body's immune reactions. Maintaining the proper microbiological balance between different types of gastrointestinal microorganisms reduces the risk of health complications. When this balance is upset, harmful toxin-producing microorganisms proliferate, giving rise to diarrhea and body emaciation.[189]

In young growing birds, diarrhea may be induced by *E. coli*, *Campylobacter jejuni*, or *Salmonella* bacteria. Most often, however, diarrhea is caused by protozoa, especially *Eimeria* coccidia. Some viruses may also cause diarrhea.[189] Diarrhea in birds contributes to increased litter moisture and elevated amount of ammonia in the air, as well as skin ulcerations and breast blisters. Body weight loss and increased number of dirty eggs are also noted. The negative influence of gastrointestinal microflora results in dysbiosis and candidiasis in the upper section of the gastrointestinal tract, and in dysbiosis, necrosis, and subclinical and clinical coccidiosis in the middle and lower sections. Present in all acute diseases, intestinal dysbiosis is responsible for lack of appetite, meteorism, or diarrhea that occurs during infections. These symptoms usually subside after the acute phase of the disease is over.[190]

Following the withdrawal of antibiotic growth promoters in Europe there has been an increased risk of intestinal problems, especially those related to the presence of *Clostridium perfringens* bacteria, which cause necrotic enteritis. Today, the use of coccidiostats is regarded as the most important method for controlling necrotic enteritis. They are effective against not only *Eimeria* sp. protozoa, but also many intestinal bacteria, including *C. perfringens*. Another method for limiting the development of *Clostridium* bacteria is to use whole, crushed, or coarsely ground cereal grain. Branton et al.[191] found that death losses due to necrotic enteritis were more frequent when birds were fed finely ground (grain hammer mill) compared to coarsely ground feeds (roller mill). Engberg et al.[10] found wheat form (whole wheat or ground wheat in pellets) to influence the composition of intestinal microflora; birds fed a pelleted diet had larger populations *of C. perfringens* and *Lactobacillus*. Other studies[192,193] reported a reduction in the amount of *C. perfringens* in the intestine of broiler chickens fed a diet with whole wheat grain.

The use of whole wheat grain may assist in preventing coccidiosis, also known as bloody diarrhea. The symptoms may vary from slight irritation to intestinal hemorrhage, ichthyosis, and ulcerations. Birds consume less feed, which adversely affects their performance. Birds raised on litter under intensive conditions are particularly vulnerable to coccidiosis. To prevent the disease, coccidiostats are added to the diets of birds at risk, namely young chickens and turkeys. Birds that received whole wheat grain and balancer pellets under the free-choice system were found to excrete fewer oocysts compared to those fed pellets containing more protein.[124] This was probably due to physical destruction of oocysts by larger and more active gizzards of birds receiving the diet with whole wheat grain. However, this phenomenon is not always observed. Banfield et al.[194] found no significant reduction in fecal oocyst output of broiler chickens fed a diet supplemented with 200 g/kg of whole grain as compared to control birds that received finely ground feed. Likewise, Waldenstedt[195] observed no appreciable effect

of using wheat grain on oocyst counts in birds infected with *E. tunella* and *E. maxima*. In another study,[196] the introduction of 200 or 400 g/kg of whole wheat caused a significant increase in fecal oocyst counts paralleled by reduced performance of birds infected with *E. acervulina*. In turn, birds receiving whole wheat grain and infected with *E. maxima* had higher body weight gains than control birds on the standard diet.

Gabriel et al.[175] also reported differential effects of feeding whole wheat on the composition of intestinal flora following infection with different *Eimeria* species. Infection with *E. tunella* led to a greater number of *E. coli* in the intestine. *E. acervulina* and *E. maxima* infections did not cause significant changes in the composition of intestinal microflora. It should be noted, however, that *Escherichia coli* is unique in that it is found in the intestinal contents of healthy birds and has beneficial effects by producing the enzyme lactose and vitamin K. When intestinal bacterial balance is disturbed, increased pH (alkalization) causes autoinfection – *E. coli* proliferates and secretes the enzyme hyaluronidase, giving rise to unfavorable changes in the intestine and many deaths.

Feeding birds with whole wheat diets may also reduce the risk of ascites (abdominal dropsy), especially in fast-growing birds. Taylor and Jones[197] obtained a significant reduction in ascites mortality after supplementing the diet with whole wheat (200 g/kg) prior to pelleting. This could be associated with the lower oxygen requirement in slower-growing experimental (whole wheat) compared to control (standard feed) birds. Oxygen deficiency in fast-growing birds is considered one of the major causes of ascites.

Research findings[198] also confirm that *Salmonella typhimurium* can be significantly reduced in the stomach and ileum contents of infected chickens fed whole wheat compared to control birds. The use of whole wheat grain can also assist in preventing blackhead in turkeys. This disease is characterized by inflammation of the ceca and liver.[199]

The use of whole wheat in poultry nutrition also has a positive effect on hematological blood parameters. Higher red blood cell counts and higher hemoglobin levels were found in 15- and 22-week-old turkeys fed a whole wheat diet compared to control birds receiving a commercial mixture.[20] Much lower plasma levels of glucose and urea nitrogen were found in 42-day-old broiler chickens receiving 250 g/kg wheat grain compared to control birds.[200]

In summing up the results, it will be noted that using whole wheat grain in poultry diets is a centuries-old tradition and is now highly popular in extensive production systems. A renewed interest in feeding whole cereal grain under intensive production system is mainly due to efforts to minimize feeding costs, but also represents a move away from overly intensive poultry production systems in many countries and regions of the world. The use of whole wheat diets optimizes the amount of nutrients ingested with feed by individual birds according to their requirement while ensuring better development and operation of the digestive tract. This feeding system could be used in preventing gastrointestinal, vascular, and skeletal diseases, and in improving the indoor climate. However, the wheat grain used must be of high nutritive value and good quality to ensure high performance and good health in birds.

References

1. Cereals market – state and outlook. *IERIGŻ – PIB Warszawa*; 2012. 43: 5–6.
2. FAOSTAT. Top production. 2011:339.
3. Wężyk S, Krawczyk J. Wheat in poultry nutrition. *Polskie Drobiarstwo* 2005;**2**:2–5.
4. Lipiński K. Wheat grain in poultry nutrition. *Polskie Drobiarstwo* 2011;**12**:20–4.
5. Gilliat A. Broiler chicken and turkey nutrition in Poland, in accordance with the recommendations used in some EEC countries. *Drobiarstwo* 1992;**2**:32–4.
6. McNab J. Factors affecting the nutritive value of wheat for poultry. *Poultry Abstract* 1992;**18**:86.
7. Filmer D. A new system for livestock feeding. *Feeds Feeding* 1991;**7**(8):30–3.
8. Filmer D. Feeding whole wheat to poultry. *Feeds Feeding* 1992;**7**(8):39–40.
9. Høg C, Sorenson P. *Effect of whole wheat in the diet of broiler turkeys. Proceedings of 7 European Poultry Conference, Paris*; 1986. 1: 373–377.
10. Engberg RM, Hedemann MS, Steenfeldt S, Jensen BB. Influence of whole wheat and xylanase on broiler performance and microbial composition and activity in the digestive tract. *Poult Sci* 2004;**83**:925–38.
11. Horsted K, Hermansen JE. Whole wheat *versus* mixed layer diet as supplementary feed to layers foraging a sequence of different forage crops. *Animal* 2007;**1**:575–85.
12. Leeson S, Summers JD. Feeding wheat to broilers. *Poult Int* 1987;**26**:13–5.
13. Bennett CD, Classen HL, Riddell C. Feeding broiler chickens wheat and barley diets containing whole, ground and pelleted grain. *Poult Sci* 2002;**81**: 995–03.
14. Bennett CD, Classen HL. Effect of whole wheat dilution on performance and carcass characteristics of male turkeys. *J Appl Poult Res* 2003;**12**:468–75.
15. Horovský S, Koči S, Kociová Z. The effeciency of broilers fed the mixture containing whole wheat grains. *Živočisna Výroba* 1993;**38**:347–52.
16. Lichovníková M, Zeman L. Effect of housing system on the calcium requirement of laying hens and on eggshell quality. *Czech J Anim Sci* 2008;**53**:162–8.
17. Reiter K, Zerning F, Meyer H. Futterwahlverhalten bei Weizenbeifutterrung in der Putenmast. *Breicht Aus Karzfehn* 1994;**4**.
18. Tuller R. Zufütterung von Weizen Putenhännen. *Dtsch Geflügelwirtschaft und Schweinenproduction* 1988;**40**:708–16.
19. Tuller R. The addition of whole wheat grains to broiler grower feeds or supplement effect on performance and abdominal fat. Proceedings of XVIII World's Poultry Conference. Nagoya, 1988. 915–918.
20. Majewska T. Whole wheat grain in young slaughter turkey feeding. *Acta Academiae Agriculturae ac Technicae Olstenensis* 1995;**498**:1–65.
21. Smulikowska S. Nutritive value of rye, triticale and wheat for poultry. PAN, Instytut Fizjologii i Żywienia Zwierząt. *Jabłonna* 1998; pp. 156.
22. Kucharski K, Rutkowski A, Kochański A. The use of whole wheat and barley grain in the feeding of slaughter chickens. *Roczniki Naukowe Zootechniki* 2002;**29**:219–27.
23. Jankowski J, Mikulski D, Zduńczyk Z, Mikuska M, Juśkiewicz J. The effect of diluting diets with ground and pelleted or with whole wheat on the performance of growing turkeys. *J Anim Feed Sci* 2012;**21**:735–47.
24. Wu YB, Ravindran V. Influence of whole wheat inclusion and xylanase supplementation on the performance, digestive tract measurements and carcass characteristics of broiler chickens. *Anim Feed Sci Technol* 2004;**116**:129–39.
25. Amerah AM, Ravindran V. Influence of method of whole-wheat feeding on the performance, digestive tract development and carcass traits of broiler chickens. *Anim Feed Sci Technol* 2008;**147**:326–39.
26. Plaur K, Wójcik S. Suitability of wheat of different varieties as a component of broiler chicken diets. *Przegląd Naukowej Literatury Zootechnicznej* 1982;**1**:318–26.
27. Waldroup PW, Burnett WD, Hellwig HM. Performance of broiler chickens fed diets with different of corn, wheat and barley. *Poult Sci* 1985;**64**(suppl. 1):194.
28. Rous J. Comparison of the nutritional value of wheat and corn ground in compound feeds for slaughter chicken. *Živočina Výroba* 1972;**11**:833–4.
29. Lillie RJ, Denton CA. Evaluation of four cereal grain and three protein level combinations for layer performance. *Poult Sci* 1968;**47**:1000–4.
30. Quart MD, Marion JE, Harms RH. Influence of wheat particle size in diets of laying hens. *Poult Sci* 1986;**65**:1015–7.
31. Çiftci I, Yenice E, Eleroglu H. Use of triticale alone and in combination with wheat or maize. Effects of diet type and enzyme supplementation on hen performance, egg quality, organ weights, intestinal viscosity and digestive system characteristics. *Anim Feed Sci Technol* 2003;**105**:149–61.
32. Lázaro R, García M, Araníbar J, Mateos GG. Effect of enzyme addition to wheat-, barley- and rye-based diets on nutrient digestibility and performance of laying hens. *Br Poult Sci* 2003;**44**: 256–65.
33. Liebert F, Htoo JK, Sünder A. Performance and nutrient utilization of laying hens fed low-phosphorus corn-soybean diets supplemented with microbial phytase. *Poult Sci* 2005;**84**:1576–83.
34. Safaa HM, Jiménez-Moreno E, Valencia DG, Frikha M, Serrano MP, Mateos GG. Effect of main cereal of the diet and particle size of the cereal on productive performance and egg quality of brown egg-laying hens in early phase of production. *Poult Sci* 2009;**88**:608–14.
35. Bochenek M, Rutkowski A. Wheat grain in poultry nutrition. *Polskie Drobiarstwo* 2008;**12**:6–12.
36. Krystianiak S. Whole or ground wheat grain for poultry? *Hodowca Drobiu* 2011;**5**:12–5.
37. Mazanowski A. Modern broiler chicken production. Ed. Pro Agricola, Gerzwald, 2011. p. 246.
38. Sokół JL, Fabijańska M. Cereal grain. In: Animal nutrition and feed science. *Wydawnictwo Naukowe PWN, Warszawa* 2001: 209–32.
39. Richter G, Prinz M, Henning A. Studies on the requirements of turkeys in floor and the energy and crude protein content of the mixed-chuck. *Archiv für Tierenahr* 1980;**30**:373–80.
40. Emmersson DE, Denbow DM, Hulet RM. Selfselection of protein and energy by turkey breeder hens. *Poult Sci Symposium Ser* 1989;**21**:360–1.
41. Grabowski T. Effect of nutrition on carcass and poultry meat quality. *Biuletyn Informacyjny Drobiarstwa* 1990;**1**:5–11.

42. Jamroz D. Characteristics and possibility of using domestic feeds in concentrate mixtures and protein concentrates. *Przegląd Hodowlany* 1992;**4**:8–13.

43. Korbas M, Martyniuk S, Rozbicki J, Beale R. Take-all disease and other foot and root rot diseases of cereals. In: Fundacja Rozwój SGGW, Warszawa, editors; 2001.

44. Sell J, Hodgson GC, Shebeski JH. Triticale as a potential component of chick ration. *Can J Anim Sci* 1962;**42**:158–66.

45. Fernandez R, Lucas E, McGinnis J. Comparative nutritional value of different cereal grains as protein sources in modified chick bioassay. *Poult Sci* 1974;**53**:39–46.

46. Koreleski J, Ryś R, Kubicz M, Krasnodębska I. Cereal grain with elevated crude protein content in feeding trials with chickens and rats. *Roczniki Naukowe Zootechniki* 1985;**23**:183–99.

47. Šramková Z, Gregová E, Šturdík E. Chemical composition and nutritional quality of wheat grain. *Acta Chimica Slovaca* 2009;**2**:115–38.

48. Morey DD, Evans JJ. Amino acid composition of six grains and winter wheat forage. *Cereal Chemistry* 1983;**60**:461–4.

49. Horaczyński H. Evaluation of triticale grain protein with growing rats and chickens. *Roczniki Naukowe Zootechniki* 1985;**12** 195–03.

50. Surisdiarto Farrell DJ. High protein wheat in poultry diets. *Recent Adv Anim Nutr* 1989 285–04.

51. Ryś R, Koreleski J, Krasnodębska I, Kuchta M, Zegarek Z. Effect of nitrogen fertilization on feeding value of wheat grain in broiler chicken diets. *Roczniki Naukowe Zootechniki* 1977;**4**:183–95.

52. Rutkowski A. Nutritive value of grains for broiler chicken. *Roczniki AR Poznań* 1996;**267**:1–90.

53. Petterson D, Aman P. Effects of enzyme supplementation of diets based on wheat, rye or triticale on their productive value for broiler chicken. *Anim Feed Sci Technol* 1988;**20**:313–24.

54. Edney MJ, Campbell GL, Classen HL. The effect of beta-glucanase supplementation on nutrient digestibility and growth in broilers given diets containing barley, oat groats or wheat. *Anim Feed Sci Technol* 1989;**25** 193–200.

55. Cave NA, Wood PJ, Burrows VD. The nutritive value of naked oats for broiler chicks as affected by dietary additions of oat gum, enzyme, antibiotic, bile salt and fat-soluble vitamins. *Can J Anim Sci* 1990;**70**:623–33.

56. Friesen OD, Guenter B. The effect of enzyme supplementation on the apparent metabolizable energy and nutrient digestibilities of wheat, barley, oats and rye for the young broiler chick. *Poult Sci* 1992;**71**:1710–21.

57. Völker P, Tüller R. *Effect of Roxazyme G supplementation to wheat and wheat/barley based diets on the performance of growing turkey. Proceedings of 1st Symposium on Enzymes in Animal Nutrition.* Switzerland: Kartause Ittingen; 1993 141–143.

58. Richter G, Cyriaci G, Stölken B. Einsatz von Enzymgemischen in Broilerrationen mit Geerste, Roggenoder Triticale. *Arch Anim Nutr* 1994;**40**:823–30.

59. Veldman A, Vahl HA. Xylanase in broiler diets with differences in characteristics and content of wheat. *Br Poult Sci* 1994;**35**:537–50.

60. Cowan WD, Hastrup T. *Application of xylanases and beta-glucanases to the feed of turkey and ducks. Proceedings of the 10 European Symposium on Poultry Nutrition.* Turkey: Antalya; 1995 320–321.

61. Mikulski D, Jankowski J, Faruga A, Mikulska M. The effect of enzyme supplementation of triticale-barley feeds on fattening performance of turkeys. *J Anim Feed Sci* 1997;**6**:391–9.

62. Svihus B, Herstad O, Newman CW, Newman RK. Comparison of performance and intestinal characteristics of broiler chickens fed on diets containing whole, rolled or ground barley. *Br Poult Sci* 1997;**38**:524–9.

63. Svihus B, Gullord M. Effect of chemical content and physical characteristics on nutritional value of wheat, barley and oats for poultry. *Anim Feed Sci Technol* 2002;**102**:71–92.

64. Wu YB, Ravindran V, Thomas DG, Birtles MJ, Hendriks WH. Influence of method of whole wheat inclusion and xylanase supplementation on the performance, apparent metabolisable energy, digestive tract measurements and gut morphology of broilers. *Br Poult Sci* 2004;**45**:385–94.

65. Yang Y, Iji PA, Kocher A, Mikkelsen LL, Choct M. Effect of xylanase on growth and gut development of broiler chickens given a wheat-based diet. *Asian-Aus J Anim Sci* 2008;**11**:1659–64.

66. Vladimirova L, Surdjiska S. *Testing the effect of adding polyenzyme preparation in feeding layers. Proceedings of the 10th European Symposium on Poultry Nutrition.* Turkey: Antalya; 1995 330–331.

67. Polat C, Akyurek H, Konyali A, Senkölyu N. *Supplementation of an enzyme preparation to wheat and barley based diets fed to commercial Brown layers. Proceedings of the 10th European Symposium on Poultry Nutrition.* Turkey: Antalya; 1995 360–361.

68. Kleuskens H. *Hygiene of feed production, mold inhibitors – results of experiments. Proceedings IIIrd Symposium "Mycotoxins in food, raw materials and commercial feeds".* Poland: Bydgoszcz; 1996 71–73.

69. Wong LSL, Abramson D, Tekauz A, Leisle D, McKenzie RIH. Pathogenicity and mycotoxin production of *Fusarium* species causing head blight in wheat cultivars varying in resistance. *Can J Plant Sci* 1995;**75**:261–7.

70. Bata A. *Mycotoxin situation in Hungary. Proceedings IIIrd Symposium "Mycotoxins in food, raw materials and commercial feeds".* Poland: Bydgoszcz; 1996 41–47.

71. Tomczak M, Wiśniewska H. Stępień Ł, Kostecki M, Chełkowski J, Goliński P. Deoxynivalenol, nivalenol and moniliformin in wheat samples with head blight (scab) symptoms in Poland (1998–2000). *Eur J Plant Pathol* 2002;**108**:625–30.

72. Atalla MM, Hassanein NM, El-Beih AA, Youssef Y, A-G. Mycotoxin production in wheat grains by different *Aspergilli* in relation to different relative humidities and storage periods. *Nahrung* 2003;**47**:6–10.

73. Goswami RS, Kistler HC. Pathogenicity and in planta mycotoxin accumulation among members of the *Fusarium graminearum* species complex on wheat and rice. *Etiology* 2005;**95** 1397–04.

74. Nakagawa H, Ohmichi K, Sakamoto S, et al. Detection of a new Fusarium masked mycotoxin in wheat grain by high-resolution LC-Orbitrap™ MS. *Food Additives and Contaminants. Part A* 2011;**28**:1447–56.

75. Moran Jr ET, Hunter B, Ferket P, Young LG, McGirr LG. High tolerance of broilers to vomitoxin from corn infected with *Fusarium graminearum. Poult Sci* 1982;**61**:1828–31.

76. Harvey RB, Kubena LF, Rottinghaus GE, Turk JR, Casper HH, Buckley SA. Moniliformin from *Fusarium fujikuroi* culture material and deoxynivalenol from naturally contaminated wheat incorporated into diets of broiler chicks. *Avian Dis* 1997;**41**:957–63.

77. Swamy HVLN, Smith TK, Cotter PF, Boermans HJ, Seftons AE. Effects of feeding blends of grains naturally contaminated with *Fusarium* mycotoxins on production and metabolism in broilers. *Poult Sci* 2002;**81**:966–75.

78. Li YD, Verstegen MWA, Gerrits WJJ. 2003. The impact of low concentrations of aflatoxin, deoxynivalenol or fumonisin in diets on growing pigs and poultry. *Nutr Res Rev* 2003;**16**:223–39.

79. Awad WA, Böhm J, Razzazi-Fazeli E, Zentek J. Effects of feeding deoxynivalenol contaminated wheat on growth performance, organ weights and histological parameters on the intestine of broiler chickens. *J Anim Physiol Anim Nutr* 2006;**90**:32–7.

80. Cristofori C, Melluzi A, Giordani G, Sirri F. Early and late quantitative feed restriction of broilers: effect on productive traits and carcass fatness. *Archiv für Geflügelkunde* 1997;**61**:162–6.

81. Mazanowski A, Kokoszynski D, Korykowska H. Effect of restricted feeding on meat traits of broiler ducks. *Zeszyty Naukowe PTZ* 1998;**36**:211–8.

82. Mazanowski A, Kokoszyński D, Korytkowska H. Effect of restricted feeding on characteristics of meat ducks. Zeszyty Naukowe ATR Bydgoszcz. *Zootechnika* 1999;**30**:61–72.

83. Tůmová E, Skrivan M, Skrivanova V, Kacerovska L. Effect of early feed restriction on growth in broiler chickens, turkeys and rabbits. *Czech J Anim Sci* 2002;**47**:418–28.

84. Urdaneta-Rincon M, Leeson S. Quantitative and qualitative feed restriction on growth characteristics of male broiler chickens. *Poult Sci* 2002;**81**:679–88.

85. Camacho MA, Suarez ME, Herrera JG, Cuca JM, Garcia-Bojalil CM. Effect of age of feed restriction and microelement supplementation to control ascites on production and carcass characteristic of broilers. *Poult Sci* 2004;**83**:526–32.

86. Péron A, Gomez J, Mignon-Grasteau S, Sellier N, Besnard J, Derouet M, Juin H, Carré B. Effects of wheat quality on digestion differ between the D+ and D– chicken lines selected for divergent digestion capacity. *Poult Sci* 2006;**85**:462–9.

87. Leeson S, Caston LJ. Production and carcass yield of broilers using free-choice cereal feeding. *J App Poult Res* 1993;**2**:253–8.

88. Chołocińska A, Wężyk S. Effect of housing system on broiler chicken productivity. *Roczniki Naukowe Zootechniki* 1999;**26**:243–53.

89. Erener G, Ocak N, Ozturk E, Ozdas A. Effect of different choice feeding methods based on whole wheat on performance of male broiler chickens. *Anim Feed Sci Technol* 2003;**106**:131–8.

90. Krawczyk J, Cywa-Benko K, Wężyk S. The effect of using wheat grain in broiler chicken nutrition. *Roczniki Naukowe Zootechniki* 2002(supple. 16):229–34.

91. Yasar S. Performance, gut size and ileal digesta viscosity of broiler chickens fed with a whole wheat added diet and the diets with different wheat particle sizes. *Int J Poult Sci* 2003;**2**:75–82.

92. Kołacz R. Animal welfare and genetic progress. *Przegląd Hodowlany* 2006;**9**:8–11.

93. Schmidt CJ, Persia ME, Feierstein E, Kingham B, Saylor WW. Comparison of a modern line and a heritage line unselected since the 1950s. *Poult Sci* 2009;**88**:2610–9.

94. Plavnik I, Macovsky B, Sklan D. Effect of feeding whole wheat on performance of broiler chickens. *Anim Feed Sci Technol* 2002;**96**:229–36.

95. Senkoylu N, Samli HE, Akyurek H, Okur AA, Kanter M. Effects of whole wheat with or without xylanase supplementation on performance of layers and digestive organ development. *Ital J Anim Sci* 2009;**8**:155–63.

96. Mazanowski A. Goose breeding and raising. APRA sp. z o. o., Myślęcinek k. Bydgoszczy, Poland, 2012; pp. 402 (or 132, 146, 173).

97. Afsharmanesh M, Scott TA, Silversides FG. Effect of wheat type, grinding, heat treatment, and phytase supplementation on growth efficiency and nutrient utilization of wheat-based diets for broilers. *Can J Anim Sci* 2008;**88**:57–64.

98. Abrahamsson P, Tauson R, Elwinger K. Effects on production, health and egg quality of varying proportions of wheat and barley in diets for two hybrids of laying hens kept in different housing systems. *Acta Agric Scand A Anim Sci* 1996;**46**:173–82.

99. Simon J, Delpech P. Study of different methods of feeding for production of meat chickens of high quality. *Annales de Zootechnie* 1972;**21**(2):233–43.

100. Gill C, Viola S, Rand N, Noy Y, Dvorin A, Litman M, Gabai J, Yoselevitch Y, Mastbaum Y. *Effect of feeding programs and addition of whole grains on broiler performance. The Worlds Poultry Science Association*. Israel Branch, The 36th annual conversation; 1998. 20–22.

101. Dov C, Rimsky I, Dvorin A, Makovsky B, Gur N, Ptichi I. *Ben Shoshan A, Asaf Fishbein. The effect of feeding whole wheat. The Worlds Poultry Science Association*. Israel Branch, The 36th Annual Conversation; 1998. 16–17.

102. Rutkowski A, Wiąż M. The use of whole grain in broiler chicken nutrition. *Roczniki Naukowe Zootechniki* 2000(Suppl. 6):362–5.

103. Rutkowski A, Wiąz M. Application of wheat whole grain in broiler chicken nutrition. *Proceedings 12th European Symposium on Poultry Nutrition*. The Netherlands, Veldhoven 1999. p. 266.

104. Preston CM, McAllister A, McCracken KJ. Effect of diet form and enzyme supplementation on growth, efficiency and energy utilisation of wheat-based diets for broilers. *Br Poult Sci* 2000;**41**:324–31.

105. Nahas J, Lefrançois MR. Effects of feeding locally grown whole barley with or without enzyme addition and whole wheat on broiler performance and carcass traits. *Poult Sci* 2001;**80** 195–02.

106. Hetland HB, Svihus B, Olaisen V. Effect of feeding whole cereals on performance, starch digestibility and duodenal particle size distribution in broiler chickens. *Br Poult Sci* 2002;**43**:416–23.

107. Salah Uddin M, Rose SP, Hiscock TA, Bonnet S. A comparison of the energy availability for chickens of ground and whole grain samples of two wheat varieties. *Br Poult Sci* 1996;**37**:347–57.

108. Amerah AM, Ravindran V, Lentle RG. Influence of insoluble fibre and whole wheat inclusion on the performance, digestive tract development and ileal microbiota profile of broiler chickens. *Br Poult Sci* 2009;**50**:366–75.

109. Jensen JE. Choice feeding in practice. *Proceedings of the 9th European Poultry Conference*. UK: Glasgow; 1994; vol. II 223–226.

110. Belyavin CG. Nutritional management of broiler programmes. In: Garnsworthy PC, Cole DA, editors. *Recent Advances in Animal Nutrition*. Nottingham, UK: Nottingham University Press; 1995. p. 97–108.

111. Smulikowska S. Whole wheat grain in poultry nutrition – free-choice feeding system. *Polskie Drobiarstwo* 1994;**10**:11–3.

112. Cowan PJ, Michie W. Choice feeding of the turkey: use of a high-protein concentrate fed with either whole wheat, barley, oats or maize. *Zeitschrift für Tierphysiologie Tierernährung und Futtermittelkunde* 1997;**39**:124–30.

113. Cowan PJ, Mitchine W. Choice feeding of the male and female broiler. *Br Poult Sci* 1978;**19**:149–52.

114. Mastika LM, Cumming RB. Effect of nutrition and environmental variations on choice feeding of broilers. In: Farrell DJ, editor. *Recent Advances in Animal Nutrition in Australia*. Portland, ME: University of New England; 1985. p. 101–14.

115. Rose SP, Burnett A, Elmajeed RA. Factors affecting the diet selection of choice-fed broilers. *Br Poult Sci* 1986;**27**:215–24.

116. Sinurat AP, Balnave D. Free-choice feeding of broilers at high temperatures. *Br Poult Sci* 1986;**27** 587–84.

117. Munt RHC, Dingle JG, Sump MG. Growth, carcass composition and profitability of meat chickens given pellets, mash or free-choice diet. *Br Poult Sci* 1995;**36**:277–84.

118. Rose SP. The use of whole wheat in poultry diets. *World's Poult Sci J* 1996;**52**:59–60.

119. Olver M, Jonker A. Effect of choice feeding on the performance of broilers. *Br Poult Sci* 1997;**38**:571–6.

120. Yao J, Tian X, Xi H, Han J, Xu M, Wu X. Effect of choice feeding on performance, gastrointestinal development and feed utilization of broilers. *Asian-Aus J Anim Sci* 2006;**19**:91–6.

121. Graham JC. Individuality of pullets in balancing the ration. *Poult Sci* 1934;**13**:34–9.

122. Holcombe DJ, Roland DA, Harms RH. The ability of hens to adjust calcium intake when given a choice of diet containing two levels of calcium. *Poult Sci* 1975;**54**:552–61.

123. Emmans GC. The nutrient intake of laying hens given a choice of diets in relation to their production requirements. *Br Poult Sci* 1977;**18**:227–36.

124. Karunajeewa H. The performance of crossbred hens given free choice feeding of whole grains and a concentrate mixture and the influence of source of xanthophylls on yolk colour. *Br Poult Sci* 1978;**19** 699–08.

125. Forbes JM, Covasa M. Application of diet selection by poultry with particular reference to whole cereals. *World's Poult Sci J* 1995;**51**:149–65.

126. Olver MD, Malan DD. The effect of choice feeding from 7 weeks of age on the production characteristics of laying hens. *S Afr J Anim Sci* 2000;**30**:110–4.

127. Rose SP, Michie W. The food intake and growth of choice feed turkeys offered balancer mixture of different composition. *Br Poult Sci* 1982;**23**:547–54.

128. Erener G, Ocak N, Garipoglu V, Sahin A, Ozturk E. Feeding turkey poults with starter feed and whole wheat or maize in free choice feeding system: its effects on their performances. *Asian-Aus J Anim Sci* 2006;**19**:86–90.

129. Men BX, Ogle B, Lindberg JE. Effect of choice feeding on the nutrient intake and performance of broiler ducks. *Asian-Aus J Anim Sci* 2001;**14**:1728–33.

130. Leeson S, Summers JD. Voluntary food restriction by laying hens mediated through dietary self selection. *Br Poult Sci* 1978;**19**:417–24.

131. Robinson D. Performance of laying hens as affected by split time and split time composition dietary regimens using ground and unground cereals. *Br Poult Sci* 1985;**26** 299–09.

132. Blair R, Dewar WA, Downie JN. Egg production responses of hens given a complete mash or unground grain together with concentrate pellets. *Br Poult Sci* 1973;**14**:373–7.

133. Kolańczyk M. Raising broiler breeder flocks. Part 6. *Polskie Drobiarstwo* 2006;**12**:40–2.

134. Cave NA. The effect of whole wheat or whole rye plus wheat as grower rations on the growth and performance of broiler breeders. *Poult Sci* 1978;**57**:1609–15.

135. Mazanowski A. Ducks. Ed. PWRiL ü Warszawa, 1988. p. 348.

136. Horbańczuk J.O. Ostrich. Ed. IGHZ PAN Jastrzębiec, 2003. p. 302.

137. Majewska T. Whole wheat grain in broiler chicken nutrition. *Polskie Drobiarstwo* 1996;**12**:18–21.

138. Scott TA, Balnave D. Self-selection feeding for pullets. *Poult Int* 1989;**28**:36.

139. Summers JD, Bedford M, Sprott D. Sudden death syndrome: it is a metabolic disease. *Feedstuffs* 1987;**59**:20.

140. Olkowski AA, Wojnarowicz C, Nain S, Ling B, Alcorn JM, Laarveld B. A study on pathogenesis of sudden death syndrome in broiler chickens. *Reaserch Vet Sci* 2008;**85**:131–40.

141. Grabowski T, Kijowski J. Poultry meat and products – technology, hygiene, quality. *WNT Warszawa* 2003. p. 574.

142. Windhorst HW. The time-spatial dynamics of global poultry meat production between 1970 and 2006 and perspectives for 2016. *Zootecnika* 2008;**30**:16–31.

143. Sage RB, Putaala A, Woodburn MIA. Comparing growth and condition in post release juvenile common pheasants on different diets. *Poult Sci* 2002;**81** 1199–02.

144. Chizzolini R, Zanardi E, Dorigoni V, Ghidini S. Calorific value and cholesterol content of normal and low fat meat and meat products. *Trends Food Sci Technol* 1999;**10**:119–28.

145. Lippens M. *The influence of feed control on the growth pattern and production parameters of broiler chicken. Ph.D thesis*. Belgium: Gent University; 2003; pp. 203.

146. Zerhdaran S, Vereijken ALJ, Van Arendonk JAM, Van Der Waaij EH. Estimation of genetic parameters for fat deposition and carcass traits in broilers. *Poult Sci* 2004;**83**:521–5.

147. Zerhdaran S. *Genetic improvement for production and health in broilers. Ph.D thesis*. The Netherlands: Wageningen University; 2005; pp. 132.

148. Chartrin P, Méteau K, Juin H, et al. Effects of intermuscular fat levels on sensory characteristics of duck breast meat. *Poult Sci* 2006;**85**:914–22.

149. Kokoszyński D. Evaluation of meat traits in commercial crossbreds of pekin type ducks. Ed. UTP Bydgoszcz, Poland, 2011; pp. 113.

150. Kijowski J, Pikul J. Nutritive and dietetic value of turkey meat. *Drobiarstwo* 1980;**9**:4–5.

151. Kirchgeessner M, Ristić M, Kreuzer M, Roth FX. Einsatz von Feeten mit hohen Anteilen an freien Feetsären in der Broilermast. 2. Wochstum sowie Qualität von Schlachtkörper Fleich und Fett bei stufenweisem Auustausch von gesättigten durch ungesättigte Fettsäuren. *Archiv für Geflügelkunde* 1993;**57**:265–74.

152. Shafey TM, Dingle JG, McDonald MW. Comparison between wheat, triticale, rye, soyabean oil and strain of laying bird on the production, and cholesterol and fatty acid contents of eggs. *Br Poult Sci* 1992;**33**:339–46.

153. Śliwiński B, Rutkowski A. Possibility of using domestic grains in diets for layers producing consumption eggs. *Appl Sci Rep* 1997;**32**:167–75.

154. Ristic M, Kreuzer M, Roth FX, Kirchgessner M. Fattening performance, carcass value and meat quality of broiler at different supplementary feeding variations with grains of wheat. *Archiv für Geflügelkunde* 1994;**58**:8–17.

155. Komprda T, Zelenka J, Fajmonova E, Jarosova A, Kubis I. Meat quality of broilers fattened deliberately slow by cereal mixtures to higher age. 1. Growth and sensory quality. *Archiv für Geflügelkunde* 2000;**64**:167–74.

156. Kokoszyński D, Bernacki Z, Korytkowska H, Wilkanowska A. Effect of different feeding regimens for game pheasants on carcass composition, fatty acid profile and mineral content of meat. *Archiv für Geflügelkunde* 2014;**78** (in press).

157. Kokoszyński D, Korytkowska H. *The effects of wheat grain use on postslaughter traits in game pheasants. Proceedings of the XX International Poultry Symposium PB WPSA*. Poland: Bydgoszcz/Wenecja; 2008 111–112.

158. Kokoszyński D, Bernacki Z, Korytkowska H. The effect of adding whole wheat grain to feed mixture on slaughter yield and carcass composition in game pheasants. *J Cent Eur Agric* 2008;**9**:659–64.

159. Brudnicki A, Kułakowska A, Pietruszyńska D, Łożyca-Kapłon M, Wach J. Differences in the amino acid composition of the breast muscle of wild and farmed pheasants. *Czech J Food Sci* 2012;**30**:309–13.

160. Biesiada-Drzazga B, Socha S, Janocha A, Banaszkiewicz T, Koncerewicz A. Assessment of slaughter value and quality of meat in common 'Game' pheasants (*Phasianus colchicus*). *Food Sc Technol Qual* 2011;**74**:79–86.

161. Horsted K, Hammershøj M, Allesen-Holm BH. Effect of grass-clover forage and whole-wheat feeding on the sensory quality of eggs. *J Sci Food Agric* 2009;**90**:343–8.

162. Umar Faruk M, Bouvarel I, Mallet S, Ali MN, Tukur HM, Nys Y, Lescoat P. Is sequential feeding of whole wheat more efficient than ground wheat in laying hens? *Animal* 2011;**5**:230–8.

163. Langenfeld M.S. Anatomy of the chicken. Ed. PWN Warszawa-Kraków, 1992. p. 288.

164. Bugajak P. Causes of avian digestive disorders. *Polskie Drobiarstwo* 2002;**1**:11–3.

165. Konarkowski A. Digestive tract in turkey poults. *Polskie Drobiarstwo* 2005;**5**:18–9.

166. Geyra A, Uni Z, Sklan D. Enterocyte dynamics and mucosal development in the posthatch chick. *Poult Sci* 2001;**80**:776–82.

167. Antoniou TC, Marquardt RR, Cansfield PE. Isolation, partial characterization and antinutritional activity of a factor (pentosans) in rye grain. *Agric Food Chem* 1981;**59**:758–69.

168. Salih ME, Classen HL, Campbell GL. Response of chickens fed on hull-less barley to dietary β-glucanase at different ages. *Anim Feed Sci Technol* 1991;**33**:139–49.

169. Rutkowski A. Digestive tract structure and function. In *Poultry breeding and use*. Poland: PWRiL Warsaw; 2012. p. 83–5.

170. Bieguszewski H. Selected issues in avian physiology. In: Krzymowski T, editor. *Animal Physiology*. PWRiL Warsaw; 1983.

171. Duke GE. Recent studies on regulation of gastric motility in turkey. *Poult Sci* 1992;**71**:1–8.
172. Banfield MJ, Forbes JM. Effects of whole wheat dilution v. substitution on coccidiosis in broiler chickens. *Br Poult Sci* 2001;**86**:89–95.
173. Banfield MJ, Kwakkel RP, Forbes JM. Effects of wheat structure and viscosity on coccidiosis in broiler chickens. *Anim Feed Sci Technol* 2002;**98**:37–48.
174. Gabriel I, Mallet S, Leconte M. Differences in the digestive tract characteristics of broiler chickens fed on complete pelleted diet or on whole wheat added to pelleted protein concentrate. *Br Poult Sci* 2003;**44**:283–90.
175. Ravindran V, Wu B, Thomas DG, Morel PCH. Influence of whole wheat feeding on the development of gastrointestinal tract and performance of broiler chickens. *Aus J Agric Res* 2006;**57**:21–6.
176. Williams J, Mallet S, Leconte M, Lessire M, Gabriel I. The effects of fructo-oligosaccharides or whole wheat on the performance and digestive tract of broiler chickens. *Br Poult Sci* 2008;**49**:329–39.
177. Gabriel I, Mallet S, Leconte M, Travel A, Lalles JP. Effects of whole wheat feeding on the development of the digestive tract of broiler chickens. *Anim Feed Sci Technol* 2008;**142**:144–62.
178. Kiiskinen T. Feeding whole grain with pelleted diets to growing broiler chickens. *Agric Food Sci Finland* 1996;**5**:167–75.
179. Amerah AM, Ravindran V, Lentle RG, Thomas DG. Influence of feed particle size on the performance, energy utilization, digestive tract development, and digesta parameters of broiler starters fed wheat- and corn-based diets. *Poult Sci* 2008;**87**:2320–8.
180. Kokoszyński D, Bernacki Z, Cisowska A. *The effect of using whole wheat grain in the diet of game pheasants on their body weight, dimensions and development of some internal organs. Folia biologica (Kraków)*; 2010;**58**(1–2):101–6.
181. Frikha M, Safaa HM, Serrano MP, Arbe X, Mateos GG. Influence of the main cereal and feed form of the diet on performance and digestive tract traits of brown-egg laying pullets. *Poult Sci* 2009;**88** 994–02.
182. Dänicke S, Simon O, Jeroch H, et al. Effects of dietary fat type, pentosan level and xylanase supplementation on digestibility of nutrients and metabolizability of energy in male broilers. *Archiv für Tierernahr* 1999;**52**:245–61.
183. Hubener K, Vahjen W, Simon O. Bacterial responses to different cereal types and xylanase supplementation in the intestine of broiler chicken. *Arch Anim Nutr* 2002;**56**:167–87.
184. Svihus B, Juvik E, Hetland H, Krogdahl A. Causes for improvement in nutritive value of broiler chicken diets with whole wheat instead of ground wheat. *Br Poult Sci* 2004;**45**:55–60.
185. Wang C.C. Biochemistry and physiology of coccidian. In: The biology of the coccidian, P.L. Long (ed.), 1984, pp.167–228, Baltimore, MD, University Park Press.
186. Xu ZR, Hu CH, Xia MS, Zhan XA, Wang MQ. Effect of dietary fructooligosaccharide on digestive enzyme activities, intestinal microflora and morphology of male broilers. *Poult Sci* 2003;**82**:1030–6.
187. Apajalahti JHA, Kettunen A, Graham H. Characteristics of the gastro-intestinal microbial communities with special reference to the chicken. *World's Poult Sci J* 2004;**60**:223–32.
188. Lu J, Idris U, Harmon B, Hofacre C, Maurer JI, Lee MD. Diversity and succession of the intestinal bacterial community of the maturing broiler chicken. *Appl Environ Microbiol* 2003;**69**:6816–24.
189. Lerbier M, Leclercq B. Poultry nutrition. Ed. PWN Warsaw, 1995. p. 340.
190. Józefiak D, Kaczmarek S, Rutkowski A. Nutrient digestibility with regard to gastrointestinal microflora activity, part 2. *Polskie Drobiarstwo* 2006;**11**:10–3.
191. Branton SL, Lott BD, Deaton JW, Maslin WR, Austin FW, Pote LM, et al. The effect of added complex carbohydrates or added dietary fiber on necrotic enteritidis lesions in broiler chickens. *Poult Sci* 1997;**76**:24–8.
192. Engberg RM, Hedemann MS, Jensen BB. The influence of grinding and pelleting of feed on the microbial composition and activity in the digestive tract of broiler chickens. *Br Poult Sci* 2002;**43**:569–79.
193. Engberg RM, Hedemann MS, Steenfeldt S, Jensen BB. Influence of whole wheat and xylanase on broiler performance and microbial composition and activity in the digestive tract. *Poult Sci* 2004;**83**:925–38.
194. Banfield MJ, Doeschate Rahm Ten, Forbes JM. Effect of whole wheat and heat stress on a coccidial infection in broiler chickens. *Br Poult Sci* 1998;**39**:25–6.
195. Waldenstedt L, Elwinger K, Hooshmand-Rad P, Thebo P, Uggla A. Comparison between effects of standard feed and whole wheat supplemented diet on experimental *Eimeria tenella* and *Eimeria maxima* infections in broiler chickens. *Acta Vet Scand* 1998;**39**:461–71.
196. Banfield MJ, Kwakkel RP, Groenveld M, Doeschate Rahm Ten, Forbes JM. Effects of whole wheat substitution in broiler diets and viscosity on a coccidial infection in broilers. *Br Poult Sci* 1999;**40**:58–60.
197. Taylor RD, Jones GPD. The influence of whole grain inclusion in pelleted broiler diets on proventricular dilatation and ascites mortality. *Br Poult Sci* 2004;**45**:247–54.
198. Bjerrum L, Engberg RM, Pedersen K. The influence of whole wheat feeding on *Salmonella* infection and gut flora composition in broilers. *Avian Dis* 2005;**49**:9–15.
199. Majewska T. Turkeys are not chickens!. *Ogólnopolski Informator Drobiarski* 2000;**4**:46–9.
200. Çelik K, Uğur K, Uzatici A. Effect of supplementing broiler diets with organic acid and whole grain. *Asian J Anim Vet Adv* 2008;**3**:328–33.

WHEAT IN DIABETES AND HEART DISEASE PREVENTION

Wheat Fiber in Postprandial Metabolic Profile and Health

Kristin M. Nieman, Tia M. Rains, Mary R. Dicklin, Kevin C. Maki

Biofortis Clinical Research, Addison, Illinois, USA

INTRODUCTION

Observational studies suggest an inverse association between the intake of whole grain foods and chronic disease risk, including metabolic syndrome,[1,2] obesity,[3–5] type 2 diabetes mellitus,[6,7] cardiovascular disease (CVD),[7,8] and certain cancers.[9–13] Whole grains contain a number of constituents that may influence chronic disease risk, including fibers, vitamins, minerals, lignans, and phytochemicals. Increased consumption of total dietary fiber has also been inversely associated with risk for the development of chronic diseases.[14–17] The association was originally thought to be attributable to some soluble fibers which form viscous solutions in the gastrointestinal tract (e.g., oat bran, pectin, gums). When mixed with fluid in the gastrointestinal tract, such fibers produce a physical barrier to digestive enzymes through which simple sugars must travel to reach the intestinal brush border for absorption.[18–20] As such, postprandial glucose responses are attenuated when viscous fibers are consumed as part of carbohydrate-rich meals. However, results from recent prospective cohort and case–control studies have shown stronger inverse correlations between the consumption of non-viscous cereal fibers and disease risk, most notably for type 2 diabetes [6,16,21–23] and selected cancers.[24,25] The mechanisms by which cereal fibers might protect against disease are not well understood, but may involve increased intestinal transit time and improved insulin sensitivity.[26,27]

Wheat is the most highly consumed cereal grain in the United States.[28] It is comprised of approximately 11% insoluble fiber and 2% soluble fiber, most of which is localized to the bran and germ layers.[27,29] Wheat also contains a number of other compounds that may be relevant to human health, including antioxidants such as phenolic acids (e.g., ferulic acid), flavonoids, lignans, and carotenoids, in addition to vitamins (e.g., A, B, E, betaine, and choline) and minerals (e.g., magnesium and selenium).[27,30] This chapter will focus on the postprandial responses of wheat fiber intake and the potential mechanisms by which these responses may influence chronic disease risk (Fig. 5.1).

EFFECTS OF WHEAT ON POSTPRANDIAL INSULIN AND GLUCOSE RESPONSES

The influence of different dietary fibers on postprandial glucose and insulin responses has been an active area of investigation. In general, it is accepted that viscous dietary fibers reduce postprandial glucose and, consequently, the insulin response to a carbohydrate-containing meal, whereas non-viscous insoluble fibers impart little to no acute effect.[23] Wheat fiber is comprised of predominately insoluble fiber and is relatively low in viscosity compared to other grains (e.g., oats). However, several randomized controlled trials have demonstrated attenuated postprandial glucose and insulin responses in individuals with normal glucose tolerance following intake of whole wheat kernels or wheat bran (Table 5.1). In one of the earliest studies, consumption of 75 g of total carbohydrate as a wheat bran cereal, providing 18 g of total fiber, blunted the postprandial glucose and insulin response compared to an equivalent level of carbohydrate from glucose. Pinto beans, providing 2.8 g of total fiber, attenuated the postprandial rise in glucose and insulin to a similar degree, leading the authors to conclude that dietary fiber, in general, dampens glucose and insulin responses to a carbohydrate-containing meal.[31] Similar results have been shown in other studies following consumption of wheat-based cereals.[32,33] For example, Schenk and colleagues[32] reported a 55% decrease in the glucose area under the

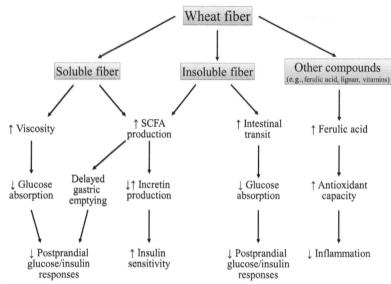

FIGURE 5.1   Potential postprandial effects of wheat fiber consumption *(modified from Fardet, 2010).*[27]

curve (AUC$_{0-180\ min}$) following intake of a wheat bran flake cereal (14 g fiber) versus a corn flake cereal. Wolever *et al.*[33] showed a smaller (−12%) but significant decrease in glucose AUC$_{0-120\ min}$ following intake of a whole grain wheat cereal (14 g fiber) versus a similar control.

Other investigators have shown similar results following consumption of intact wheat kernels, which contain the bran, endosperm, and germ components of the grain.[34-36] Wheat kernels hydrated with water to produce a porridge showed attenuated glucose (−7 to −28%) and insulin (−15 to −31%) responses relative to white bread controls.[34,36] Liljeberg *et al.*[35] showed similar results following consumption of a wheat bread prepared with intact whole grain wheat kernels (10.2 g fiber) compared to white wheat bread (3.2 g fiber). Postprandial glucose and insulin AUC responses over 120 minutes were reduced by 28% and 49%, respectively, in the wheat kernel bread versus control.

However, not all studies have shown similar results. In a small study of six subjects, Cara *et al.*[37] failed to show differences following a pasta meal containing added fiber from wheat (12.8 g) compared to a low-fiber pasta meal (2.8 g). Studies in which whole wheat was delivered as part of bread (6–13 g fiber) yielded similar results compared to white bread controls.[38,39]

Far fewer studies have evaluated postprandial responses after chronic (4–6 weeks) wheat consumption (Table 5.2).[40-42] In one of the largest studies, 28 overweight men consumed diets low in fiber (19 g/d) or high in fiber from wheat meal (32 g/d) for 4 weeks in a crossover design. There were no differences in fasting concentrations of glucose or insulin at the end of each treatment period, although 1-hour postprandial levels of glucose and insulin were 20% and 49% lower, respectively, for the high wheat-fiber diet versus low-fiber control.[42] However, two

smaller studies evaluating the effects of high wheat bran diets (11–26 g/d fiber) in healthy men failed to show differences in glucose or insulin AUC following a meal tolerance test at the end of each condition.[40,41] It has been suggested that both particle size and processing of the delivery vehicle may influence postprandial responses – a concept that is supported by the work of others on different fiber sources.[43-45] As such, it remains to be determined whether consumption of wheat bran or wheat bran bread, specifically, is effective at influencing the post-meal metabolic responses. Further research is needed to fully understand the relationships between wheat and wheat processing on postprandial glucose and insulin responses.

Arabinoxylans (AX) are one of the main constituents found in the cell wall of cereal grains. They are characterized by a xylose backbone with arabinose side chains. Within the bran and endosperm components of the wheat grain, AX comprises ~66% and ~88% of the non-starch polysaccharides, respectively.[46] AX are produced as a by-product of commercial processing of wheat endosperm into flour. They are of particular interest due to their viscosity and ability to act as a substrate for beneficial bacteria in the colon, increasing production of short-chain fatty acids (SCFAs), which promotes bowel health and, potentially, favorable metabolic outcomes.[47,48]

Several investigations have evaluated the post-meal metabolic responses to isolated AX from wheat. Lu *et al.*[49] showed that both 6 g and 12 g of AX consumed with a 75 g carbohydrate-containing mixed meal attenuated postprandial glucose concentrations by 20% and 41%, respectively, compared to no added AX in healthy individuals. Postprandial insulin concentrations also showed a dose–response effect (−17 and −33%, respectively for the 6 g and 12 g AX conditions). Similar responses were demonstrated in two longer-term

TABLE 5.1 Effects of Acute Wheat Fiber Intake on Postprandial Metabolic Outcomes

Reference	Study Design[a]	Treatments	Results[b]
Potter et al.[31,c]	• $n=9$ healthy men • Age (mean): 33.5 y	• Control: Liquid glucose/protein meal (75 g total CHO; 0 g fiber) • Wheat bran cereal (75 g total CHO; 8.2 g fiber)	• ↓ ~16% Glucose $Cmax_{0-180\,min}$ • ↓ ~38% Insulin $Cmax_{0-180\,min}$
Cara et al.[37]	• $n=6$ healthy and overweight men • Age (mean): 31.5 y	• Control: Low-fiber pasta meal (121 g total CHO; 2.8 g fiber) • Pasta meal with added wheat fiber (121 g total CHO; 12.8 g fiber)	• ↔ Glucose $AUC_{0-360\,min}$ • ↔ Insulin $AUC_{0-360\,min}$
Liljeberg et al.[35]	• $n=10$ healthy men and women • Age (mean): 38.0 y	• Control: White wheat bread (50 g available CHO; 2.1 g fiber) • Wheat bread with intact wheat kernels (50 g available CHO; 7.6 g fiber)	• ↓ 28% Glucose $AUC_{0-120\,min}$ • ↓ 49% Insulin $AUC_{0-120\,min}$
Granfeldt et al.[34]	• $n=9$ healthy men • Age (mean): 67.5 y	• Control: White wheat bread (50 g available CHO; 4.9 g fiber) • Wheat kernel porridge (50 g available CHO; 7.1 g fiber)	• ↓ 41% Glucose $AUC_{0-180\,min}$ • ↓ 31% Insulin $AUC_{0-180\,min}$
Lu et al.[49]	• $n=14$ healthy men and women • Age (mean): 32.0 y	• Mixed meal providing 75 g available CHO and one of the following: • 0 g AX (control) • 6.0 g AX • 12.0 g AX	• 6.0 g AX: ↓ 20% Glucose $AUC_{0-120\,min}$ • 12.0 g AX: ↓ 41% Glucose $AUC_{0-120\,min}$ • 6.0 g AX: ↓ 17% Insulin $AUC_{0-120\,min}$ • 12.0 g AX: ↓ 33% Insulin $AUC_{0-120\,min}$
Juntunen et al.[68]	• $n=20$ healthy men and women • Age (mean): 28.5 y	• Control: White wheat bread (50 g available CHO; 3.1 g fiber) • Whole-meal wheat pasta (50 g available CHO; 5.6 g fiber)	• ↓ 39% Glucose $Cmax_{0-180\,min}$ • ↓ 59% Insulin $Cmax_{0-180\,min}$ • ↓ 53% GIP $Cmax_{0-180\,min}$ • ↓ 37% GLP-1 $Cmax_{0-180\,min}$
Schenk et al.[32]	• $n=6$ healthy men • Age (mean): 27.8 y	• Control: Corn Flakes® (milled corn, 50 g available CHO; 1.7 g fiber) • All-Bran® cereal (wheat bran, 50 g available CHO; 38.5 g fiber)	• ↓ 55% Glucose $AUC_{0-180\,min}$ • ↔ Insulin $AUC_{0-180\,min}$
Wolever et al.[33]	• $n=77$ healthy and hyperinsulinemic men • Age (mean): 42.1 y	• Control: Corn Flakes® (milled corn, 25 g available CHO; 1.0 g fiber) • Fiber One® cereal (whole-grain wheat, 25 g available CHO; 14.0 g fiber)	• 12% ↓ Glucose $AUC_{0-120\,min}$ • ↔ Insulin $AUC_{0-120\,min}$
Weickert et al.[38]	• $n=14$ healthy women • Age (mean): 23.6 y	• Control: White bread (50 g available CHO; 2.9 g fiber) • Wheat fiber bread (50 g available CHO; 13.4 g fiber)	• ↔ Glucose $AUC_{0-180\,min}$ • ↔ Insulin $AUC_{0-180\,min}$ • ↔ GIP and GLP-1 $AUC_{0-300\,min}$
Najjar et al.[39]	• $n=10$ overweight or obese men • Age (mean): 59.0 y	• Control: White wheat bread (50 g available CHO; 1.5 g fiber) • Whole wheat bread (50 g available CHO; 6.3 g fiber)	• ↔ Glucose $AUC_{0-180\,min}$ • ↔ Insulin $AUC_{0-180\,min}$ • ↔ GIP and GLP-1 $AUC_{0-180\,min}$ • ↔ Insulin sensitivity[d,e]
Rosén et al.[36,c]	• $n=10$ healthy men and women • Age (mean): 26.0 y	• Control: White wheat bread (50 g available CHO; 4.4 g fiber) • Wheat kernel porridge (50 g available CHO; 19.8 g fiber)	• ↓ ~7% Glucose $AUC_{0-60\,min}$ • ↓ ~15% Insulin $AUC_{0-60\,min}$

Abbreviations: AUC, mean area under the curve; AX, arabinoxylan fiber; CHO, carbohydrate; Cmax, maximal response; GIP, glucose-dependent insulinotropic polypeptide; GLP-1, glucagon-like peptide-1.

[a] All references reported use of a randomized crossover study design.

[b] The most relevant study results are summarized as follows: increasing (↑), decreasing (↓), or no significant change (↔) in postprandial glucose, insulin, insulin sensitivity, and incretin hormone responses, compared to the control.

[c] Study results were estimated from a graphic representation of the data.

[d] Data not shown.

[e] As measured by Matsuda's insulin sensitivity index.[72]

C. WHEAT IN DIABETES AND HEART DISEASE PREVENTION

TABLE 5.2　Effects of Chronic Wheat Fiber Intake on Postprandial Metabolic Outcomes

Reference	Study Design[a]	Treatments	Results[b]
Munoz et al.[40]	• n = 15 healthy men • Age (mean): 36.5 y • Duration: 4 wk	• Control: Basal low-fiber diet (≤3.5 g/d fiber) • Hard red spring wheat bread (26.0 g/d fiber) • White wheat bran bread (26.0 g/d fiber)	• ↔ Glucose $AUC_{0-180\,min}$ • ↔ Insulin $AUC_{0-180\,min}$
Kestin et al.[41,c]	• n = 24 healthy men • Age (mean): 46.0 y • Duration: 4 wk	• Control: White wheat bread (low-fiber, 3.7 g/d fiber) • Wheat bran bread (10.9 g/d fiber)	• ↔ Glucose $AUC_{0-150\,min}$ • ↔ Insulin $AUC_{0-150\,min}$
Lu et al. 2004[50]	• n = 15 men and women with T2DM • Age (mean): 60.0 y • Duration: 5 wk	• Control: Bread and muffins (50% whole wheat flour; 50% white flour; 34.0 g/d fiber) • AX: Bread and muffins (50% whole wheat flour; 36% white flour; 14% AX fiber; 49.0 g/d fiber)	• ↓ 2 h Postprandial glucose • ↓ 2 h Postprandial insulin
McIntosh et al.[42]	• n = 28 overweight men • Age (mean): 52.5 y • Duration: 4 wk	• Control: Low-fiber diet (19.0 g/d fiber) • High-fiber whole-meal wheat diet (32.0 g/d fiber)	• ↓ 20% 1 h Postprandial glucose • ↓ 49% 1 h Postprandial insulin • ↔ FBG • ↔ FBI
Garcia et al.[51]	• n = 14 overweight or obese men and women with IGT and insulin resistance • Age (mean): 55.5 y • Duration: 6 wk	• Control: White flour rolls/powder (0 g/d AX) • White flour rolls/powder (15.0 g/d AX)	• ↓ 14% Glucose $AUC_{0-240\,min}$ • ↓ 10% Insulin $AUC_{0-240\,min}$

Abbreviations: AUC, mean area under the curve; AX, arabinoxylan fiber; FBG, fasting blood glucose; FBI, fasting blood insulin; IGT, impaired glucose tolerance; T2DM, type 2 diabetes mellitus.

[a] All references reported use of a randomized crossover study design.

[b] The most relevant study results are summarized as follows: increasing (↑), decreasing (↓), or no significant change (↔) in postprandial glucose and insulin responses, compared to the control or baseline condition, unless otherwise noted.

[c] Data not shown.

feeding studies.[50,51] Overweight subjects with impaired glucose tolerance and insulin sensitivity consumed bread and beverages with supplemental AX (15 g/d) or control (0 g/d) for 6 weeks, each in a crossover design. Postprandial glucose and insulin concentrations ($AUC_{0-240\,min}$) after a liquid meal tolerance test were 14% and 10% lower, respectively, after the AX treatment period.[51] Comparable results were shown in individuals with type 2 diabetes mellitus following 5 weeks of consuming breads and muffins prepared with AX.[50]

POTENTIAL MECHANISMS OF ACTION

The mechanisms whereby wheat attenuates postprandial glucose and insulin responses have not been clearly defined. One possibility is that insoluble fiber increases intestinal transit time, resulting in a decreased rate of absorption of nutrients, including carbohydrates.[23] However, it is likely that the mechanism is not limited to attenuations in nutrient absorption rates. The presence of indigestible fibers in the large intestine may lead to a cascade of processes that modulate glucose tolerance in the periphery. Resident colonic microbiota feed on indigestible material, producing SCFAs (acetate, butyrate, and propionate) as fermentative end products. Following absorption into the circulation, SCFAs have been shown to suppress the release of free fatty acids from adipose tissue and lower the total concentrations of free fatty acids in the circulation, which may improve insulin sensitivity.[52]

SCFAs may also increase production of glucagon-like peptide-1 (GLP-1), an incretin hormone secreted by enterocytes that stimulates secretion of insulin and may also increase insulin sensitivity (Table 5.3).[53–57] SCFAs stimulate GLP-1 secretion through a G-protein coupled cascade initiated by binding to free fatty acid receptors 2 and/or 3, also known as GPR43 and GPR41, respectively.[58,59] These receptors are expressed not only on the surfaces of GLP-1 secreting L cells of the colon, but also on leukocytes and adipocytes, where they are involved in the modulation of a variety of immune and metabolic functions that are only starting to be elucidated.[60–64] Cereal grains, and specifically wheat extracts, reportedly increase concentrations of fecal SCFAs and populations of fecal microbiota.[48,53,65,66] For example, a study in healthy subjects reported a 40% increase in fecal SCFA

TABLE 5.3 Potential Mechanisms for the Beneficial Effects of Chronic Wheat Fiber Consumption

Reference	Study Design[a]	Treatments	Results: Fecal Bacteria Content[b]	Results: Short-Chain Fatty Acid and Phenolic Acid Content[c]
Jenkins et al.[53]	• n = 24 healthy men and women • Age (mean) = 33.0 y • Duration: 2 wk	• Control: Low-fiber-supplemented diet (6 g/d fiber) • Wheat bran-supplemented diet (31 g/d fiber)	• NR	• Fecal total SCFA: 40% ↑ • Fecal acetic acid: 39% ↑ • Fecal butyric acid: 43% ↑ • Fecal propionic acid: 39% ↑ • Plasma total SCFA: ↔ • Plasma acetic acid: ↔ • Plasma butyric acid: 10% ↑ • Plasma propionic acid: ↔
McIntosh et al.[42]	• n = 28 overweight men • Age (mean): 52.5 y • Duration: 4 wk	• Control: Low-fiber diet (19.0 g/d fiber) • High-fiber whole-meal wheat diet (32.0 g/d fiber)	• NR	• Fecal total SCFA: ↔ • Fecal acetic acid: ↔ • Fecal butyric acid: ↔ • Fecal propionic acid: ↓ 12%
Costabile et al.[65]	• n = 31 healthy men and women • Age (mean): 25.0 y • Duration: 3 wk	• Control: Baseline restriction diet[d] • Wheat bran cereal (12.8 g/d fiber) • Whole-grain wheat cereal (13.0 g/d fiber)	• Bifidobacterium (wheat bran): ↔ • Bifidobacterium (whole-grain): 11% ↑ • Lactobacillus (wheat bran): ↔ • Lactobacillus (whole-grain): 7% ↑	• Plasma ferulic acid (wheat bran): 64% ↑ • Plasma ferulic acid (whole grain): 60% ↑
Freeland et al.[67]	• n = 14 hyperinsulinemic men and women • Randomized parallel • Age (mean): 29.1 y • Duration: 1 y	• Control: Rice Krispies® cereal (rice, 0.5 g/d fiber) • All-Bran® cereal (wheat bran fiber, 24.0 g/d fiber)	• NR	• Plasma acetic acid: 73% ↑ • Plasma butyric acid: 36% ↑ • Plasma propionic acid: ↔
Francois et al.[66]	• n = 63 healthy men and women • Age (mean): 42.0 y • Duration: 3 wk	• Control: 0 g/d AX supplement • AX supplement, 2.4 g/d • AX supplement, 8.0 g/d	• Bifidobacterium (2.4 g/d): ↔ • Bifidobacterium (8.0 g/d): 4% ↑ • Lactobacillus (2.4 g/d): ↔ • Lactobacillus (8.0 g/d): ↔	• Fecal total SCFA (2.4 g/d): ↔ • Fecal total SCFA (8.0 g/d): 8% ↑ • Fecal acetic acid (2.4 g/d): ↔ • Fecal acetic acid (8.0 g/d): 8% ↑ • Fecal butyric acid (2.4 g/d): ↔ • Fecal butyric acid (8.0 g/d): 5% ↑ • Fecal propionic acid (2.4 g/d): 3% ↑ • Fecal propionic acid (8.0 g/d): 8% ↑
Maki et al. [48,e]	• n = 65 healthy men and women • Age (mean) = 32.5 y • Duration: 3 wk	• Control: 0 g/d AX supplement • AX supplement, 2.2 g/d • AX supplement, 4.8 g/d	• Bifidobacterium (2.2 g): ↔ • Bifidobacterium (4.8 g): 17% ↑ • Lactobacillus (2.2 g): ↔ • Lactobacillus (4.8 g): ↔	• Plasma ferulic acid (2.2 g)[f]: 60% ↑ • Plasma ferulic acid (4.8 g)[f]: 65% ↑

Abbreviations: AX, arabinoxylan fiber, a by-product of wheat flour processing; NR, not reported; SCFA, short-chain fatty acids

[a] All references reported use of a randomized crossover study design unless otherwise noted.

[b] The most relevant study results are summarized as follows: increasing (↑), decreasing (↓), or no significant change (↔) in fecal bacterium count (log_{10} cells/g dry feces), as compared to the control or baseline condition, unless otherwise noted.

[c] Study results are summarized as follows: (↑), decreasing (↓), or no significant change (↔) in plasma phenolic acid concentration (μg/L) and fecal (μmol/g or mmol/d dry feces) or plasma (μmol/g or mmol/L plasma) short-chain fatty acid concentrations as compared to the control or baseline condition, unless otherwise noted.

[d] Actual fiber intake per day was not reported. Subjects were not allowed to consume high-bran or whole-grain breakfast cereal during the restriction diet period.

[e] Percent change was calculated from the difference in before and after treatment values for bacteria levels and after an acute meal test for ferulic acid concentrations.

[f] Actual values not reported. Percent change was calculated from a graphic representation of the data.

content after feeding a wheat bran-supplemented diet (31 g/d fiber) for 2 weeks, compared to a low-fiber diet (6 g/d fiber).[53] Freeland et al.[67] showed similar results; however, not all studies have demonstrated increases in SCFA content.[42]

Despite evidence that wheat fiber influences production of SCFA, data are discrepant with regard to the effects of wheat consumption on postprandial incretin response and may be influenced by the duration of exposure. Najjar et al.[39] reported no differences in postprandial GIP and GLP-1 concentrations following a meal tolerance test with whole wheat bread (6.3 g fiber) versus white wheat bread (1.5 g fiber; Table 5.1). Two other acute meal studies also failed to find differences in GIP or GLP-1 concentrations following intakes of wheat fiber or wheat germ test meals compared to controls.[37,38] However, Juntunen et al.[68] showed reduced levels of GIP and GLP-1, which paralleled the attenuated insulin response, following consumption of a whole meal wheat pasta test meal (7.9 g fiber) in comparison to the control meal (4.9 g fiber), in healthy individuals.

Chronic fiber intake may be necessary to appreciably raise SCFA levels in plasma. Wolever et al.[69] showed that 6–9 months of increased fiber intake were necessary to increase plasma acetate in subjects with diabetes, most likely due to proliferation of colonic acetate-producing bacteria over time. Chronic intake of wheat fiber (24 g/d) increased fasting plasma GLP-1 concentrations by 25% from baseline in hyperinsulinemic individuals after 12 months.[67] Whether similar results would be seen in subjects with normal glucose tolerance remains to be determined.

As previously mentioned, wheat fiber is rich in bioactive phytochemicals, which should also be considered as potential mechanisms for the beneficial effects of wheat fiber. Wheat phytochemicals may exert these beneficial effects through several physiologic mechanisms, including antioxidant activity and improved immune function, altered intestinal transit and absorption, and increased colonic SCFA production.[70,71] Several of the phytochemicals in whole grains provide antioxidant and anti-inflammatory effects, including phenolic compounds (Table 5.3).[27,55–57] Ferulic acid is the most abundant phenolic compound found in wheat, and its levels have been reported to be increased in the plasma of subjects following wheat fiber consumption.[48,65] However, the mechanisms linking wheat phytochemicals to beneficial effects on postprandial outcomes and chronic disease have yet to be clearly defined.[54]

CONCLUSIONS

Dietary fiber consumption, particularly cereal fibers, is associated with lower risk for chronic disease development, by mechanisms that have not been well defined at present. Cereal fibers, including wheat fiber, are mainly non-viscous (insoluble) and would not be expected to attenuate postprandial glucose and insulin responses to the same degree as viscous (soluble) fibers. However, several studies support a role of wheat, particularly whole wheat kernels, in decreasing post-meal glucose and insulin excursions. Differences in the processing of wheat and duration of consumption may influence the response. Whether this effect on post-meal metabolic responses is due to altered intestinal transit, colonic fermentation, stimulation of incretin release, or other mechanisms remains to be determined.

References

1. Sahyoun NR, Jacques PF, Zhang XL, Juan W, McKeown NM. Whole-grain intake is inversely associated with the metabolic syndrome and mortality in older adults. Am J Clin Nutr 2006;83(1):124–31.
2. Esmaillzadeh A, Mirmiran P, Azizi F. Whole-grain consumption and the metabolic syndrome: a favorable association in Tehranian adults. Eur J Clin Nutr 2005;59(3):353–62.
3. Giacco R, Della Pepa G, Luongo D, Riccardi G. Whole grain intake in relation to body weight: from epidemiological evidence to clinical trials. Nutr Metab Cardiovasc Dis 2011;21(12):901–8.
4. van de Vijver LP, van den Bosch LM, van den Brandt PA, Goldbohm RA. Whole-grain consumption, dietary fibre intake and body mass index in the Netherlands cohort study. Eur J Clin Nutr 2009;63(1):31–8.
5. Koh-Banerjee P, Rimm EB. Whole grain consumption and weight gain: a review of the epidemiological evidence, potential mechanisms and opportunities for future research. Proc Nutr Soc 2003;62(1):25–9.
6. de Munter JS, Hu FB, Spiegelman D, Franz M, van Dam RM. Whole grain, bran, and germ intake and risk of type 2 diabetes: a prospective cohort study and systematic review. PLoS Med 2007;4(8):e261.
7. McKeown NM, Meigs JB, Liu S, Wilson PW, Jacques PF. Whole-grain intake is favorably associated with metabolic risk factors for type 2 diabetes and cardiovascular disease in the Framingham Offspring Study. Am J Clin Nutr 2002;76(2):390–8.
8. Ye EQ, Chacko SA, Chou EL, Kugizaki M, Liu S. Greater whole-grain intake is associated with lower risk of type 2 diabetes, cardiovascular disease, and weight gain. J Nutr 2012;142(7):1304–13.
9. Larsson SC, Giovannucci E, Bergkvist L, Wolk A. Whole grain consumption and risk of colorectal cancer: a population-based cohort of 60,000 women. Br J Cancer 2005;92(9):1803–7.
10. Jacobs Jr DR, Marquart L, Slavin J, Kushi LH. Whole-grain intake and cancer: an expanded review and meta-analysis. Nutr Cancer 1998;30(2):85–96.
11. Chan JM, Wang F, Holly EA. Whole grains and risk of pancreatic cancer in a large population-based case-control study in the San Francisco Bay Area, California. Am J Epidemiol 2007;166(10):1174–85.
12. Aune D, Chan DS, Lau R, Vieira R, Greenwood DC, Kampman E, et al. Dietary fibre, whole grains, and risk of colorectal cancer: systematic review and dose-response meta-analysis of prospective studies. BMJ 2011;343 d6617.
13. Aune D, Chan DS, Greenwood DC, Vieira AR, Rosenblatt DA, Vieira R, et al. Dietary fiber and breast cancer risk: a systematic review and meta-analysis of prospective studies. Ann Oncol 2012;23(6):1394–402.
14. Park Y, Brinton LA, Subar AF, Hollenbeck A, Schatzkin A. Dietary fiber intake and risk of breast cancer in postmenopausal women: the National Institutes of Health-AARP Diet and Health Study. Am J Clin Nutr 2009;90(3):664–71.
15. Tucker LA, Thomas KS. Increasing total fiber intake reduces risk of weight and fat gains in women. J Nutr 2009;139(3):576–81.
16. Meyer KA, Kushi LH, Jacobs Jr DR, Slavin J, Sellers TA, Folsom AR. Carbohydrates, dietary fiber, and incident type 2 diabetes in older women. Am J Clin Nutr 2000;71(4):921–30.
17. Streppel MT, Ocke MC, Boshuizen HC, Kok FJ, Kromhout D. Dietary fiber intake in relation to coronary heart disease and all-cause mortality over 40 y: the Zutphen Study. Am J Clin Nutr 2008;88(4):1119–25.
18. Dikeman CL, Fahey GC. Viscosity as related to dietary fiber: a review. Crit Rev Food Sci Nutr 2006;46(8):649–63.
19. Wolever TM. Small intestinal effects of starchy foods. Can J Physiol Pharmacol 1991;69(1):93–9.
20. Jenkins DJ, Wolever TM, Leeds AR, et al. Dietary fibres, fibre analogues, and glucose tolerance: importance of viscosity. Br Med J 1978;1(6124):1392–4.

21. McKeown NM. Whole grain intake and insulin sensitivity: evidence from observational studies. *Nutr Rev* 2004;**62**(7 Pt 1):286–91.

22. Schulze MB, Schulz M, Heidemann C, Schienkiewitz A, Hoffmann K, Boeing H. Fiber and magnesium intake and incidence of type 2 diabetes: a prospective study and meta-analysis. *Arch Intern Med* 2007;**167**(9):956–65.

23. Weickert MO, Pfeiffer AF. Metabolic effects of dietary fiber consumption and prevention of diabetes. *J Nutr* 2008;**138**(3):439–42.

24. Hansen L, Skeie G, Landberg R, Lund E, Palmqvist R, Johansson I, et al. Intake of dietary fiber, especially from cereal foods, is associated with lower incidence of colon cancer in the HELGA cohort. *Int J Cancer* 2012;**131**(2):469–78.

25. Freudenheim JL, Graham S, Horvath PJ, Marshall JR, Haughey BP, Wilkinson G. Risks associated with source of fiber and fiber components in cancer of the colon and rectum. *Cancer Res* 1990; **50**(11):3295–300.

26. Anderson JW, Bryant CA. Dietary fiber: diabetes and obesity. *Am J Gastroenterol* 1986;**81**(10):898–906.

27. Fardet A. New hypotheses for the health-protective mechanisms of whole-grain cereals: what is beyond fibre? *Nutr Res Rev* 2010;**23**(1):65–134.

28. FAOSTAT. Food and Agriculture Organization of the United Nations, Rome. (retreived 6 December 2012). Available from: http://faostat.fao.org/; 2009.

29. Slavin JL, Martini MC, Jacobs Jr DR, Marquart L. Plausible mechanisms for the protectiveness of whole grains. *Am J Clin Nutr* 1999;**70**(Suppl. 3) 459S-63S.

30. Slavin J. Why whole grains are protective: biological mechanisms. *Proc Nutr Soc* 2003;**62**(1):129–34.

31. Potter JG, Coffman KP, Reid RL, Krall JM, Albrink MJ. Effect of test meals of varying dietary fiber content on plasma insulin and glucose response. *Am J Clin Nutr* 1981;**34**(3):328–34.

32. Schenk S, Davidson CJ, Zderic TW, Byerley LO, Coyle EF. Different glycemic indexes of breakfast cereals are not due to glucose entry into blood but to glucose removal by tissue. *Am J Clin Nutr* 2003;**78**(4):742–8.

33. Wolever TM, Campbell JE, Geleva D, Anderson GH. High-fiber cereal reduces postprandial insulin responses in hyperinsulinemic but not normoinsulinemic subjects. *Diabetes Care* 2004;**27**(6):1281–5.

34. Granfeldt Y, Hagander B, Bjorck I. Metabolic responses to starch in oat and wheat products. On the importance of food structure, incomplete gelatinization or presence of viscous dietary fibre. *Eur J Clin Nutr* 1995;**49**(3):189–99.

35. Liljeberg H, Granfeldt Y, Bjorck I. Metabolic responses to starch in bread containing intact kernels versus milled flour. *Eur J Clin Nutr* 1992;**46**(8):561–75.

36. Rosé LA, Ostman EM, Bjorck IM. Effects of cereal breakfasts on postprandial glucose, appetite regulation and voluntary energy intake at a subsequent standardized lunch; focusing on rye products. *Nutr J* 2011;**10**:7.

37. Cara L, Dubois C, Borel P, Armand M, Senft M, Portugal H, et al. Effects of oat bran, rice bran, wheat fiber, and wheat germ on postprandial lipemia in healthy adults. *Am J Clin Nutr* 1992;**55**(1):81–8.

38. Weickert MO, Mohlig M, Koebnick C, Holst JJ, Namsolleck P, Ristow M, et al. Impact of cereal fibre on glucose-regulating factors. *Diabetologia* 2005;**48**(11):2343–53.

39. Najjar AM, Parsons PM, Duncan AM, Robinson LE, Yada RY, Graham TE. The acute impact of ingestion of breads of varying composition on blood glucose, insulin and incretins following first and second meals. *Br J Nutr* 2009;**101**(3):391–8.

40. Munoz JM, Sandstead HH, Jacob RA. Effects of dietary fiber on glucose tolerance of normal men. *Diabetes* 1979;**28**(5):496–502.

41. Kestin M, Moss R, Clifton PM, Nestel PJ. Comparative effects of three cereal brans on plasma lipids, blood pressure, and glucose metabolism in mildly hypercholesterolemic men. *Am J Clin Nutr* 1990;**52**(4):661–6.

42. McIntosh GH, Noakes M, Royle PJ, Foster PR. Whole-grain rye and wheat foods and markers of bowel health in overweight middle-aged men. *Am J Clin Nutr* 2003;**77**(4):967–74.

43. Aston LM, Gambell JM, Lee DM, Bryant SP, Jebb SA. Determination of the glycaemic index of various staple carbohydrate-rich foods in the UK diet. *Eur J Clin Nutr* 2008;**62**(2):279–85.

44. Heaton KW, Marcus SN, Emmett PM, Bolton CH. Particle size of wheat, maize, and oat test meals: effects on plasma glucose and insulin responses and on the rate of starch digestion in vitro. *Am J Clin Nutr* 1988;**47**(4):675–82.

45. Jenkins DJ, Wesson V, Wolever TM, et al. Wholemeal versus wholegrain breads: proportion of whole or cracked grain and the glycaemic response. *BMJ* 1988;**297**(6654):958–60.

46. Ring SG, Selvendran RR. Isolation and analysis of cell wall material from beeswing wheat bran (Triticum aestivum). *Phytochemistry* 1980;**19**(8):1723–30.

47. Garcia AL, Steiniger J, Reich SC, Weickert MO, Harsch I, Machowetz A, et al. Arabinoxylan fibre consumption improved glucose metabolism, but did not affect serum adipokines in subjects with impaired glucose tolerance. *Horm Metab Res* 2006;**38**(11):761–6.

48. Maki KC, Gibson GR, Dickmann RS, Kendall CW, Chen CY, Costabile A, et al. Digestive and physiologic effects of a wheat bran extract, arabino-xylan-oligosaccharide, in breakfast cereal. *Nutrition* 2012;**28**(11–12):1115–21.

49. Lu ZX, Walker KZ, Muir JG, Mascara T, O'Dea K. Arabinoxylan fiber, a byproduct of wheat flour processing, reduces the postprandial glucose response in normoglycemic subjects. *Am J Clin Nutr* 2000;**71**(5):1123–8.

50. Lu ZX, Walker KZ, Muir JG, O'Dea K. Arabinoxylan fibre improves metabolic control in people with Type II diabetes. *Eur J Clin Nutr* 2004;**58**(4):621–8.

51. Garcia AL, Otto B, Reich SC, Weickert MO, Steiniger J, Machowetz A, et al. Arabinoxylan consumption decreases postprandial serum glucose, serum insulin and plasma total ghrelin response in subjects with impaired glucose tolerance. *Eur J Clin Nutr* 2007;**61**(3):334–41.

52. Tarini J, Wolever TM. The fermentable fibre inulin increases postprandial serum short-chain fatty acids and reduces free-fatty acids and ghrelin in healthy subjects. *Appl Physiol Nutr Metab* 2010;**35**(1):9–16.

53. Jenkins DJ, Vuksan V, Kendall CW, Wursch P, Jeffcoat R, Waring S, et al. Physiological effects of resistant starches on fecal bulk, short chain fatty acids, blood lipids and glycemic index. *J Am Coll Nutr* 1998;**17**(6):609–16.

54. Anson NM, van den Berg R, Havenaar R, Bast A, Haenen GR. Ferulic acid from aleurone determines the antioxidant potency of wheat grain (Triticum aestivum L.). *J Agric Food Chem* 2008;**56**(14): 5589–94.

55. Barone E, Calabrese V, Mancuso C. Ferulic acid and its therapeutic potential as a hormetin for age-related diseases. *Biogerontology* 2009;**10**(2):97–108.

56. Fardet A, Rock E, Rémésy C. Is the *in vitro* antioxidant potential of whole-grain cereals and cereal products well reflected *in vivo*? *J Cereal Sci* 2008;**48**(2):258–76.

57. Adom KK, Sorrells ME, Liu RH. Phytochemicals and antioxidant activity of milled fractions of different wheat varieties. *J Agric Food Chem* 2005;**53**(6):2297–306.

58. Tolhurst G, Heffron H, Lam YS, Parker HE, Habib AM, Diakogiannaki E, et al. Short-chain fatty acids stimulate glucagon-like peptide-1 secretion via the G-protein-coupled receptor FFAR2. *Diabetes* 2012;**61**(2):364–71.

59. Tazoe H, Otomo Y, Karaki S, et al. Expression of short-chain fatty acid receptor GPR41 in the human colon. *Biomed Res* 2009;**30**(3):149–56.

60. Xiong Y, Miyamoto N, Shibata K, Valasek MA, Motoike T, Kedzierski RM, et al. Short-chain fatty acids stimulate leptin production in adipocytes through the G protein-coupled receptor GPR41. *Proc Natl Acad Sci USA* 2004;**101**(4):1045–50.

61. Karaki S, Tazoe H, Hayashi H, Kashiwabara H, Tooyama K, Suzuki Y, et al. Expression of the short-chain fatty acid receptor, GPR43, in the human colon. *J Mol Hist* 2008;**39**(2):135–42.

62. Le Poul E, Loison C, Struyf S, Springael JY, Lannoy V, Decobecq ME, et al. Functional characterization of human receptors for short chain fatty acids and their role in polymorphonuclear cell activation. *J Biol Chem* 2003;**278**(28):25481–9.

63. Hong YH, Nishimura Y, Hishikawa D, Tsuzuki H, Miyahara H, Gotoh C, et al. Acetate and propionate short chain fatty acids stimulate adipogenesis via GPCR43. *Endocrinology* 2005;**146**(12):5092–9.

64. Al-Lahham S, Roelofsen H, Rezaee F, Weening D, Hoek A, Vonk R, et al. Propionic acid affects immune status and metabolism in adipose tissue from overweight subjects. *Eur J Clin Invest* 2012;**42**(4):357–64.

65. Costabile A, Klinder A, Fava F, Napolitano A, Fogliano V, Leonard C, et al. Whole-grain wheat breakfast cereal has a prebiotic effect on the human gut microbiota: a double-blind, placebo-controlled, crossover study. *Br J Nutr* 2008;**99**(1):110–20.

66. Francois IE, Lescroart O, Veraverbeke WS, Marzorati M, Possemiers S, Evenepoel P, et al. Effects of a wheat bran extract containing arabinoxylan oligosaccharides on gastrointestinal health parameters in healthy adult human volunteers: a double-blind, randomised, placebo-controlled, cross-over trial. *Br J Nutr* 2012;**108**(12):2229–42.

67. Freeland KR, Wilson C, Wolever TM. Adaptation of colonic fermentation and glucagon-like peptide-1 secretion with increased wheat fibre intake for 1 year in hyperinsulinaemic human subjects. *Br J Nutr* 2010;**103**(1):82–90.

68. Juntunen KS, Niskanen LK, Liukkonen KH, Poutanen KS, Holst JJ, Mykkanen HM. Postprandial glucose, insulin, and incretin responses to grain products in healthy subjects. *Am J Clin Nutr* 2002;**75**(2):254–62.

69. Wolever TM, Schrade KB, Vogt JA, Tsihlias EB, McBurney MI. Do colonic short-chain fatty acids contribute to the long-term adaptation of blood lipids in subjects with type 2 diabetes consuming a high-fiber diet? *Am J Clin Nutr* 2002;**75**(6):1023–30.

70. Lupton JR, Meacher MM. Radiographic analysis of the effect of dietary fibers on rat colonic transit time. *Am J Physiol* 1988;**255**(5 Pt 1):G633–9.

71. Gazzaniga JM, Lupton JR. Dilution effect of dietary fiber sources: An in vivo study in the rat. *Nutr Res* 1987;**7**(12):1261–8.

72. Matsuda M, DeFronzo RA. Insulin sensitivity indices obtained from oral glucose tolerance testing: comparison with the euglycemic insulin clamp. *Diabetes Care* 1999;**22**(9):1462–70.

6

Bioavailability of Calcium, Iron, and Zinc in Whole Wheat Flour

*Anwaar Ahmed**, *Muhammad Atif Randhawa*†, *Muhammad Wasim Sajid*†

*Department of Food Technology, PMAS-Arid Agriculture University, Rawalpindi, Pakistan, †National Institute of Food Science & Technology, University of Agriculture, Faisalabad, Pakistan

INTRODUCTION

Wheat (*Triticum aestivum* L.) is the world's second most cultivated cereal crop, after rice,[1] and is consumed as a staple food in many countries. Wheat is one of the major grains in the diet, and plays a significant role in the nutritional quality of the diet and in human health.[2] The nutrient composition of whole wheat grain flour is given in Table 6.1. However, despite adequate consumption, several nutritional problems related to micronutrient deficiencies have been reported in lower socioeconomic groups. This is because of phytate, present in cereal grains in relatively large quantities, which forms insoluble complexes with zinc, iron, and calcium in the human intestine and hinders their absorption by the body.[3] The formation of such insoluble phytate–mineral complexes leads to a decrease in mineral availability.[4–7]

Micronutrient deficiencies are referred to as "hidden hunger". Inadequacies in minute amount of vitamins and minerals have emerged as one of the most widespread and devastating nutritional deficiencies in the world. This "hidden hunger" has manifested itself in the development of several physiological–pathological conditions, such as anemia, growth and mental retardation, osteoporosis, and poor immunological responses.

Calcium deficiency may result in weak bones and teeth, and osteoporosis. Calcium also plays an important role in metabolic functions such as muscular function, nervous stimuli, enzymatic and hormonal activities, and transport of oxygen. It is necessary for blood clotting; cell membrane transport functions; release of neurotransmitters; synthesis and secretion of protein, hormones and intracellular enzymes; and regulation of heartbeat.[8] The widespread prevalence of osteoporosis due to inadequate calcium intake in the aged population is a real threat.[9]

Iron is required for various metabolic functions in the body, and its deficiency causes anemia, which reduces person's ability to perform physically demanding tasks and causes impaired productivity.[10] Iron deficiency anemia (IDA) is the most common micronutrient disorder in the world, negatively affecting both health and socioeconomic wellbeing.[11] Iron deficiency has been shown to reduce physical endurance, even in the absence of anemia,[12] and severe anemia has been associated with an increased risk of both maternal and child mortality.[13] IDA affects approximately 30% of the world population.[14]

Iron therapy in anemic adults is associated with a 5% increase in labor productivity (non-heavy labor work) and a 17% increase in productivity for heavy labor.[15] Iron deficiency anemia during pregnancy often leads to pre mature delivery.[16]

Zinc deficiency is responsible for many health complications, including impairment of physical growth, the immune system, and learning ability, combined with increased risk of infections, DNA damage, and development of cancer.[17–19] Zinc deficiency affects many aspects of metabolism,[20] including the activity of more than 300 enzymes, structure of many proteins, and control of genetic expression. Clinical signs of zinc deficiency include acrodermatitis, low immunity, diarrhea, poor healing, stunting, hypogonadism, fetal growth failure, teratology, other abnormalities of pregnancy, and neuropsychological abnormalities.[21] Nutritional zinc deficiency is particularly prevalent in developing countries[22,23] – 54.2% preschool children were reported to be zinc deficient in the North West Frontier Province (NWFP) in Pakistan.[24] Similarly, in a population based study in urban and rural Sindh, 54% of all pregnant women were observed to be zinc deficient.[25]

TABLE 6.1   Whole Wheat Grain Flour Nutrient Composition

Nutrient	Unit	Value per 100 g
PROXIMATES		
Water	g	10.74
Energy	kcal	340
Protein	g	13.21
Total lipid (fat)	g	2.50
Carbohydrate, by difference	g	71.97
Fiber, total dietary	g	10.7
Sugars, total	g	0.41
MINERALS		
Calcium, Ca	mg	34
Iron, Fe	mg	3.60
Magnesium, Mg	mg	137
Phosphorus, P	mg	357
Potassium, K	mg	363
Sodium, Na	mg	2
Zinc, Zn	mg	2.60

Nutrient values and weights are for edible portion.
Source: USDA Nutrient Database.

A comparable rate of subclinical zinc deficiency was seen among adolescent girls and boys in Sindh.[26] Approximately 61% of people in developing countries are at risk of low dietary zinc intake.[27]

MINERAL REQUIREMENTS AND CONSEQUENCES OF DEFICIENCY

Micronutrient malnutrition is a serious threat to the health and productivity of more than 2 billion people worldwide, even though it is preventable to a large extent.[28] Humans require at least 22 mineral elements for their wellbeing.[29–31] It is estimated that over 60% of the world's 6 billion people are iron deficient, over 30% are zinc deficient, 30% are iodine deficient, and 15% are selenium deficient, in addition to calcium, magnesium, and copper deficiencies.[32–36] These account for about 7.3% of the global burden of disease,[37] resulting in learning disabilities, reduced work capacity, serious illnesses, and even death.[38] Women and children are more vulnerable to micronutrient deficiencies because of their added requirements for reproduction and growth, respectively.[39] Malnutrition, related to calcium, iron, zinc, and copper, may lead to several physiological–pathological disorders.[40] In pregnant women, deficiencies of iron, zinc, and folic acid have been shown to increase risk of low birth weight, pregnancy complications, and birth defects.[41]

Calcium

Calcium serves as a second messenger in nearly every biological process, stabilizes many proteins, and when deficient is associated with a large number of diseases and disorders.[42] It is required for critical biological functions such as nerve conduction, muscle contraction, cell adhesiveness, mitosis, blood coagulation, glandular secretion, and structural support of the skeleton. An adequate intake of calcium reduces the risk of osteoporosis, hypertension, and, possibly, colon cancer. As a result of its expanding role in health, calcium has been designated as a "super nutrient".[43]

Calcium is the most abundant mineral in the body. Most (>99%) of the body's 1000–1200 g of calcium is located in the skeleton. Osteoporosis occurs due to calcium deficiency, resulting in brittle bones. Approximately 1.7 million hip fractures occur worldwide each year.[44] Osteoporosis is spreading due to inadequate calcium intake in the aged population.[9]

Calcium requirements are driven by high rates of bone mineral accretion throughout childhood and adolescence. The peak rate of bone mass accrual occurs at the age of 13 in girls and 14.5 in boys.[45] A cross-sectional study of 247 females aged between 11 and 32 years showed that approximately 90% of total body bone mineral content was achieved by 17.9, 95% by 19.3, and 99% by 22.1 years of age.[46] When men and women (mean age

71 years) were provided with 500 mg elemental calcium and 352 IU vitamin D, non-vertebral fracture rates were significantly reduced.[47] Moreover, subjects with a lower urinary sodium–potassium ratio but a higher calcium intake had the lowest supine blood pressure and prevalence of hypertension.[48] The calcium intake required by adults aged 19–50 years in order to achieve mean maximal retention or minimal loss was determined to be 1 g per day.[49] Rebecca and colleagues[50] recommended the intake of calcium to be 1.0–1.2 g/day for adults, with an upper tolerable limit of 2.5 g/day.

Iron

Iron deficiency affects 1.5–2.0 billion people globally,[14] most of whom live in developing countries.[51] In industrialized countries, approximately 15% of infants consume insufficient amounts of dietary iron.[52] Several studies have shown a prevalence of nutritional anemia of around 20–50% in developing countries, and between 2% and 28% in developed countries.[53,54]

Women and young children are especially at risk of iron deficiency. In women this results in poor pregnancy outcome, according to the United Nations (UN) estimates. Prevalence of anemia during pregnancy ranged from 18% in developed countries to 75% in South Asia,[55] and many severely anemic women have died during parturition.[10,56,57] IDA reduces a person's ability to perform physical tasks, with anemic laborers demonstrating impaired productivity, lower working capacity, and fatigue. In children, IDA results in lower growth rate, impaired cognitive scores, diminished ability to combat infection, reduced psychomotor and mental development, and decreased immune function and physical development.[58–62]

The National Nutrition Survey 2001–2012 has shown that 48.7% of mothers, and 29% of children under the age of 5 years, were iron deficient.[63] In a group of 100 children (aged 2–6 years) and 200 adult females (aged 17–35 years), hemoglobin levels below 11.5 g/dL were present in 47% children and 30% adult females.[64] In another survey, ferritin estimation was performed in 354 children to assess iron storage status.[65] Among these, 30% children were classified as normal and 70% anemic, according to WHO standards.[24] In a study on the nutritional status of male and female school children aged 6–12 years, it was found that a total of 36.1% children were stunted and 45.3% were underweight, while 25.2% were below standard weight for height.[66]

Iron deficiency was partly induced by vegetarian diets that contain low levels of poorly bioavailable iron.[67] Several researchers[68,69] described the nature of diet itself to be a major cause of reduced absorption of iron, suggesting that diets containing no meat and little ascorbic acid have very limited iron availability and can lead to iron deficiency.[70]

Zinc

Zinc was recognized in the 1960s as being essential for humans.[71] Zinc deficiency in humans was first observed in Middle Eastern dwarfs in 1963, and has since been documented worldwide.[72] Zinc deficiency is the fifth major cause of diseases and mortality in developing countries.[73,74]

In the world population, 2.7 billion people are estimated to be zinc deficient.[75] The percentage of national populations at risk for low zinc intake ranges from 1–13% in European and North American countries to 68–95% in South and South East Asia, Africa, and the Eastern Mediterranean regions. Globally, nearly half of the population is at risk for low zinc intake.[76] Approximately one-third of children in low-income countries had low height-for-age ratios with respect to international reference data, and Pakistan was no exception to this.[66]

Zinc has many diverse functions in the body. It is essential for growth and development, maintenance of appetite, testicular maturation, skin integrity, neurological function, wound healing, and immunocompetence. Zinc is essential for the activities of thymic, growth, and sex hormones, and for glucagon and insulin. In addition, it is recognized for its anti-infective and anticancer properties.[20,77] Zinc is a cofactor of superoxide dismutase enzymes, which play an important antioxidant role in detoxication of reactive oxygen species. It is also an important component of DNA, acting to stabilize phosphate groups and coordinate with bases.

The main clinical manifestations of severe zinc deficiency in humans are growth retardation, delay in sexual maturity, delay in skeletal maturation, development of orificial and acral dermatitis, diarrhea, alopecia, failure of appetite, appearance of behavioral changes, and increased susceptibility to infections due to development of a defective immune system. Symptoms of marginal or mild zinc deficiency are less obvious and often missed. They include reduced growth rate, impaired resistance to infection, delayed wound healing, and neurosensory defects such as taste abnormalities.[78–80] Zinc-deficient rats have been reported to have altered red and white blood cell counts, lower absolute reticulocyte numbers, changed leukocyte population, and lower plasma erythropoietin.[81–83]

Beneficial effects of zinc supplementation on vitamin A metabolism in malnourished children[84], preterm infants,[85] and adults with alcoholic cirrhosis[86] have been reported. Other studies showed no such effect of zinc on serum indicators of vitamin A metabolism.[87] Controlled trials of zinc supplementation in the prevention of infectious diseases have demonstrated reductions in the incidences of diarrhea, pneumonia, and malaria – the most common cause of death in children in developing countries.[88] Diabetes has an effect on zinc homeostasis. It might then lead to increased zinc excretion (hyperzincuria) and result in hypozincemia.

In men with low sperm counts, supplemental zinc for 4 months resulted in increased sperm counts.[89] The incidence of growth retardation of small babies significantly reduced when pregnant women were supplemented with 22.5 mg zinc daily.[90] Zinc supplementation could increase linear growth in stunted children.[91]

Zinc deficiency has been observed in 54.2% of preschool children.[24] Zinc supplementation decreased the incidence of infectious diseases such as diarrhea and acute lower respiratory tract infection and reduced child mortality in children over 1 year of age.[92] Plasma levels for retinol-binding protein and zinc among young infants presenting with diarrhea indicated that plasma zinc concentrations were significantly lower among those who were considered "small" at birth.[93] A meta-analysis of Zn supplementation trials with infants, preschoolers, and prepubertal children showed that Zn supplementation increased linear growth and weight gain.[92]

Zinc is often lacking, or present in only a poorly absorbable form, in the diets of poor families.[91] The food supply of nearly 50% of the global population is low in absorbable zinc because of limited availability of animal products.[76] Zinc is present in high concentrations in plants rich in phytates, which might inhibit its absorption.[94]

PHYTIC ACID: A POTENTIAL INHIBITOR OF MINERALS

The world food supply is dependent mainly on cereals, legumes, and oilseed crops. These foods are a good source of proteins, minerals, and vitamins, but unfortunately most of these foods may contain phytate as an antinutritional factor. This is an undesirable compound in foods because it may cause mineral deficiencies, especially in high-risk groups.[95]

Phytic acid (PA) is the hexaphosphoric ester of cyclohexane (inositol hexaphosphoric acid, IP6).[96] It is usually found as a complex with essential minerals and/or proteins.[97] Its biodegradation products are chelators of iron in particular, and of other divalent metals such as zinc, calcium, and manganese.

Phytic acid is widely distributed in foods, particularly cereal grains, legume seeds, and vegetables.[98] Wheat flour contains relatively high levels of phytic acid (6–10 mg/g), while in refined flour the concentration reduces to 2–4 mg/g. The concentration of PA is lower in commercially milled flours than in flours produced in a domestic environment.[99]

The role of PA is beneficial,[100] as well as having antinutritional effects.[101] Phytate works in a broad pH region as a highly negatively charged ion, and therefore its presence in the diet has a negative impact on the bioavailability of divalent and trivalent mineral ions such as Zn^{2+}, $Fe^{2+/3+}$, Ca^{2+}, Mg^{2+}, Mn^{2+}, and Cu^{2+}.[6,102,103] Phytic acid strongly inhibits the absorption of iron and other essential minerals.[3,69,97,104,105] It interferes with the functions of essential nutrients, so is considered a natural antinutrient substance.[106] The intake of PA relates negatively with the glycemic index of normal individuals.[107] In addition, the phosphorus in the phytate is not nutritionally available.[99]

Among the more promising approaches to reducing phytic acid content in cereals is to improve the bioabsorption of minerals through phytase treatment.[108] Enzymes with phytase-like activities are classified as histidine acid phosphatases (HAPs), purple acid phosphatases (PAPs), and b-propeller phosphatases;[109] and only HAPs and PAPs have been reported in plants, while the presence of PAP genes have been demonstrated in wheat grains.[110]

Reduction of PA can also be achieved by various food processes such as soaking, germination, fermentation,[18] milling, malting, and cooking.[111] Phytic acid was decreased considerably in whole grain flours by removing the hull.[112] It is common for the preparation of cereals to entail soaking and germination and/or fermentation.[113] These techniques are especially useful for preparing complementary foods and porridges.[114]

Milling has a major impact on both the phytate and mineral content of cereals and seeds. During processing of wheat, bran and germ are removed from the endosperm.[115] Bran, which forms about 14.5% of the grain, is a rich source of PA. Whole wheat flour contains over 800 mg phytate and 2–4 mg iron per 100 g, whereas unenriched white flour contains only 280 mg phytate and 1.2 mg iron per 100 g.[116] There is a sharp decrease in the phytic acid content in white patent flour and whole wheat flour.[117] Removal of phytate by modifying the process for producing soy protein was found to increase zinc absorption from 27% to 45%.[118]

Soaking under optimal conditions activated naturally occurring phytases in cereals and resulted in varying degrees of phytate hydrolysis, depending on the type of cereal.[119] During breadmaking, phytases are activated and may hydrolyze PA into IP5 and then into lower *myo*-inositol phosphate esters (IP4–IP1), which are less likely to bind minerals, and form weaker mineral complexes.[120,121] The reduction of PA content in different bread types may vary between 13% and 100%. The highest levels of PA remain in unleavened breads.[122]

Germination (malting) is a process in which whole grains are soaked and then germinated. Malting of wheat, barley, rye, and oats followed by soaking at pH 4.5–5 causes phytate degradation.[119]

Fermentation can hydrolyze most of the phytate in wheat so that iron absorption is improved.[123] Prolonged fermentation (48 hours at 23°C) of whole meal wheat bread reduces the total phytate content to the same level as that in low-phytate control rolls. It subsequently increases the absorption of iron seven-fold, to the same bioavailability as iron in the control bread, despite the five-fold higher total fiber content of whole meal flour.[4] It also improves the bioavailability of zinc[119] and presumably that of calcium and other minerals in cereals.[124] Similarly dephytinization of wheat flour increased the *in vitro* gastrointestinal bioavailability of minerals such as calcium, iron, zinc, and copper in different wheat varieties.[125]

Domestic cooking or industrial processing has also been reported to cause losses of phytic acid. Boiling or pressure-cooking of mung bean or black gram resulted in 5–15% phytic acid loss,[126] while losses in boiling maize, making popcorn, charcoal roasting, and cooking a chappatti caused 12%, 18%, 42%, and 53% losses, respectively.[127] Baking also resulted in a decrease in phytic acid content.[117] With the industrial process of extrusion cooking, losses of 10–30% were reported for rye,[128] rice, and millet,[129] although the decrease rose to 50% for cow peas.[130] Losses of up to 90% have been reported during canning of beans.[131] These phytate losses, reported during different cooking processes, could be attributed to a combination of heat and/or enzyme degradation.

Whole wheat bread is an important source of minerals but also contains considerable amounts of phytic acid, which is known to impair their absorption. Interaction of phytate with protein, vitamins, and minerals is an important factor that limits the nutritive value of wheat.[132] In the presence of phytate and calcium, absorption of other mineral is depressed due to formation of insoluble complexes.[133] For example, calcium-bound phytate shows greater affinity for zinc and forms co-precipitates, thereby reducing the reabsorption of endogenous zinc as well as affecting availability of dietary zinc.[134]

Levrat-Verny and colleagues[135] studied the absorption of minerals from diets based on whole wheat flour and white wheat flour in rats. The amounts of minerals absorbed were significantly enhanced (except for calcium) with the whole wheat flour diet. Moreover, plasma and tibial levels of magnesium, and plasma, liver, and tibial levels of iron, were significantly increased in rats fed on the whole wheat flour diet compared with those fed on the white flour diet.

Effects of increasing levels of phytate hydrolysis during breadmaking by the addition of varying amounts of rye sourdough and adjustment of pH with lactic acid were studied by Larsson and Sandberg.[136] Different pH values were used during bread preparation in order to study the influence of acidity in the dough. A decrease in phytate content was observed in bread containing rye bran, ranging from 66–97% of the initial phytate content in the raw materials. With a pH of between 4.4 and 5.4, more phytate was hydrolyzed in the scalded breads than in breads made with sourdough. Bread made with scalded oat flour with a sourdough content of 20% or 30% showed the most effective phytate decomposition in bread with oat flour or oat bran. Phytate content in unsoured bread with scalded oat bran was reduced to a maximum of 62% of the initial amount.

Phytate has an inhibitory effect on zinc absorption.[137] This notion is supported by Sandstrom *et al.*,[138] who made bread from wheat with different extraction rates. Direct evidence for a negative effect of phytate on zinc absorption was provided by a stable isotope study by Turnlund *et al.*,[139] and by adding phytate to milk formula in a radioisotope study on human volunteers.[140] Several single meal studies clearly showed a negative correlation between the presence of phytate or inositol phosphates and zinc absorption in humans.[141–143] Similarly, it was reported that in humans the absorption of zinc was significantly decreased, as compared to the test meal with no added phytate, when 50 mg of phytate P (269 mmol phytate) was added.[144]

Inhibition of zinc absorption is dependent on the dose of phytate.[99] Studies have involved adding sodium phytate in varying amounts. A significant negative effect of phytate on zinc absorption was found at levels of 50 mg of phytate phosphorus and above.[121] This effect of phytate on zinc absorption was in agreement with several previous studies on composite meals,[141,143] which also showed higher zinc absorption when phytate P was lower than 50 mg. For the high-phytate meals (100–280 mg phytate P), zinc absorption was very low, at 4–11%; for the low-phytate meals it was 21%.

The capacity of wheat bran to impair mineral absorption independent of its phytate content was studied by metabolic balance studies in humans.[144] Three breads were prepared, equivalent to white, brown, and whole meal, by adding bran in different quantities to white flour, and it was concluded that wheat bran is unlikely to exert a significant effect on mineral absorption in humans.

MICRONUTRIENT INTERACTIONS

Minerals such as calcium, iron, and zinc may interact with each other during absorption in the gut, insoluble complexes are formed, and hence their bioavailability is decreased. Previous multiple-meal studies on the effect of calcium on non-heme iron absorption also showed inconsistent and conflicting results. Healthy infants given iron-fortified formula with 1800 mg versus 465 mg of calcium showed no differences over 4 months in four measures of iron status.[145] Similarly, in preschool children, no difference of iron was observed in red blood cell incorporation after 5 weeks on a high-calcium diet (about 1000 mg per day) versus a low-calcium diet at about 500 mg per day.[146] Calcium supplementation as high as 1200 mg per day does not affect iron status in healthy premenopausal women.[147] In adolescent girls taking calcium supplementation of 1000 mg calcium per day (as calcium citrate malate) after breakfast and before bedtime for 4 years, no effect was observed on serum ferritin or red blood cell indexes.[148]

Calcium may interfere with the absorption of iron and zinc.[149,150] When non-heme iron absorption was measured for a 5-day period, 30% higher absorption was found for dairy calcium served at breakfast and dinner than for dairy calcium distributed more equally throughout the day.[151] In contrast, a 70% reduction in non-heme iron absorption was observed in a 1-day study in which subjects consumed supplemental calcium carbonate with the three main meals.[152] These results conflict with those obtained in a study by Reddy and Cook,[153] in which no difference in non-heme iron absorption between a low- and a high-calcium diet was found.

Interactions between trace elements like iron and zinc are primarily antagonistic. Thus, it was expected that when two chemically similar ions were present in the intestinal lumen, the one having molar excess would tend to exclude the other.[154,155] Preparations of nutrient supplements generally provide iron in much higher amounts than zinc; therefore, the interference of iron on zinc absorption was predominantly observed.[156,157]

Many studies showed that high concentrations of iron could have a negative effect on zinc absorption.[158,159] In another study, it was found that increasing the molar ratio of iron to zinc from 1:1 to 2.5:1 did not affect absorption of zinc from water.[160] An iron to zinc ratio of 25:1 decreased zinc absorption, but addition of the zinc ligand histidine decreased the inhibitory effect of this dose of iron, and zinc absorption increased from 34% to 47%. Sandstrom et al.[141] also observed no inhibitory effect on zinc absorption when iron and zinc were given with a meal of rice and meat sauce. The effect of calcium intake from a complete diet on non-heme iron absorption was examined. Calcium contents of the three diets averaged 280 mg, 684 mg, and 1281 mg per day, and the total iron contents were 10–11 mg per day for each diet. Iron absorption did not vary significantly across the calcium diets.[124]

In several other single-meal studies, calcium intake imparted a negative effect on both non-heme iron and heme iron absorption.[149,161–163] To counteract this putative effect, calcium supplements, dairy products rich in calcium, or calcium-fortified foods could be taken either with meals that were normally low in iron content or between meals. However, this might make it difficult for vulnerable groups to achieve the recommended daily calcium intake.[164]

The practical nutritional implications of the inhibitory effect of calcium are considerable because the addition of milk, a milkshake or cheese to common meals such as pizza or hamburger meals reduced iron absorption by 50–60%. It was recommended that the intake of dairy products be reduced in main meals providing most of the dietary iron.[165] Addition of extrinsic minerals to a diet high in phytate could result in significant impairments of growth and mineral utilization.[166]

Mendoza and colleagues[167] demonstrated that there was no significant effect of dietary calcium on iron absorption. Zinc absorption was not associated with the form of zinc consumed, but higher dietary calcium was marginally associated with lower zinc absorption. They concluded that a mixture of fortificants containing Na–Fe–EDTA, zinc sulfate or zinc methionine, ascorbic acid and citric acid, but without calcium, could improve iron and zinc absorption from food products.

The influence of a commercial cereal-based diet supplemented with bovine blood on iron, calcium, phosphorus, and magnesium metabolism in control and iron-deficient rats was studied by Pallares et al.[168] After feeding iron-deficient rats with a diet that contained 100 mg of iron per kg as elemental iron, the digestive and metabolic utilization of calcium, phosphorus, and magnesium decreased, whereas the sternum concentration of these minerals increased in comparison with control rats fed the same diet. Nevertheless, when cereal-based diet was supplemented with heme iron, no decrease in calcium or magnesium absorption was found in iron-deficient rats.

BIOAVAILABILITY STUDIES

Bioavailability refers to that fraction of nutrients which is utilized by the body out of the total undigested amount.[169] There is a consensus that in developing countries, poor dietary quality rather than quantity is the key determinant of impaired micronutrient status, including iron deficiency.[170–172] Populations with limited resources avoid hunger by consuming more cereals and tubers.[173] Phytic acid is found in high concentrations in cereals, reaching 3–6% of the weight of the grain.[99] The inhibitory effect of phytate on mineral availability is well known,[40,174] and phytic acid binds minerals such as zinc, iron, and calcium, making them unavailable for absorption.[175,176] The low bioavailability of iron in plant foods is caused by the presence of substances that inhibit iron absorption, such as phytate, etc.[177] The phytic acid to minerals ratio, referred to as mineral molar ratio, is important for determining the potential mineral bioavailability, which in general terms indicates higher mineral bioavailability when the molar ratio is low, and vice versa. Mineral molar ratios, therefore, have been suggested to be useful for assessing critical values for the availability of calcium.[178] Mineral bioavailability is complex, and phytate to mineral molar ratios ([phytate]: [mineral]) can be used as a simplified qualitative measure of their bioavailability in human food.[139,179–181] Owing to the high phytic acid (myo-inositol-1,2,3,4,5,6-hexakisphosphate: IP6) concentration of most cereal grains (1–4%), their mineral bioavailability is low.[182,183]

Less than 40% of the iron in meat, poultry, and fish[184] is in the heme form, which is more efficiently absorbed than the remaining non-heme iron present in these and all other foods. Heme iron is better absorbed (15–40%) than non-heme iron (1–15%).[185–188] Both forms are absorbed in inverse logarithmic proportion to body iron stores. However, this results in a greater range of efficiency for non-heme iron absorption compared with that for heme iron.[186–188] In contrast, because of apparent upregulation of non-heme iron absorption, non-heme iron contributes more than heme iron to the total amount of iron absorbed in people with low body iron stores.[186] Hence, the total iron content of a diet provides little information about its content of bioavailable iron, which is considerably influenced by the foods in the diet and could vary 10-fold from different meals of similar iron content.[70] Bioavailability of micronutrients, particularly zinc and iron, is low from plant foods. Bioavailability of iron is known to be influenced by various dietary components, which include both inhibitors and enhancers of absorption. Among inhibitors, phytic acid, tannins, dietary fiber, and calcium are the most potent, while organic acids are known to promote iron absorption.[189,190]

Several studies have been conducted on the bioavailability of iron in cereals. In a pilot field trial, 215 schoolchildren received hemoglobin-fortified biscuits (30 g) daily during two school periods, and their iron nutrition status was compared with that of children who received non-fortified biscuits (n = 212). Initially, both groups had comparably good iron nutrition. The fortified children presented higher mean ferritin values at the end of the first and second school periods. Good iron stores (serum ferritin greater than or equal to 20 μg/L) were present in 92% and 79% of the fortified and control subjects, respectively.[191]

Coudray and colleagues[192] compared the effect of ingestion of wheat flours on mineral status and bone characteristics in rats. White flour was tested either without further mineral supplementation, or with magnesium, iron, zinc, and copper supplementation. The rats fed on the white flour diet had the lowest feed intake, weight gain, fecal excretion, and intestinal fermentation. The magnesium and iron statuses were drastically lower in rats fed on the white flour diet than in those fed on whole wheat flour or control diets.

Fortification of lime-treated corn flour with reduced iron had no effect on iron bioavailability or utilization, probably due to the high phytate content.[193] In lime-treated corn flour, iron utilization by rats fed unfortified flour and flour fortified with reduced iron did not differ, but utilization was higher in rats fed corn flour fortified with iron sulfate, fumarate, and citrate than with reduced iron.

Ranhotra and colleagues[194] assessed iron in five types of Iranian flat bread and in the corresponding fermented doughs for its efficacy in promoting hemoglobin synthesis in hemoglobin-depleted rats. Bioavailability of iron in these breads differed significantly, ranging from 53% to 95%.

Hansen and colleague[195] evaluated the efficacy of intake of iron-fortified whole meal rye bread on the iron status of young women with low iron stores in a 5-month single-blind intervention study. Two parallel groups of women (20–38 y) were given 144 g of rye bread per day, either fortified with 6 mg iron as ferrous fumarate/100 g bread (i.e., 8.6 mg iron/d) (n = 21) or unfortified (n = 22), in addition to their normal diet. Blood samples were taken at 0, 2.5, and 5 months. There was no change in serum ferritin in subjects given iron-fortified bread. Hemoglobin was unchanged in the control group, at $124 \pm 8 \, g/L$. In the fortification group, there was a nonsignificant increase from 0 to 5 months: $124 \pm 6 \, g/L$ and $126 \pm 8 \, g/L$. Intake of fortified whole meal rye bread resulted in stabilization of iron stores of young women with poor iron status, which were otherwise reduced by intake of the unfortified control bread.

The bioavailability of zinc is also measured by radio-isotopic labeling techniques. The effect of iron on zinc absorption was measured by radio-isotopic labeling, followed by measurements of whole body retention of ^{65}Zn ($ZnCl_2$) by Valberg et al.[196] They found that zinc absorption was inhibited by inorganic and heme iron when the iron was given in water, but not by iron incorporated into a turkey meal.[197] No significant differences in zinc absorption were observed in adult males consuming iron-fortified weaning cereal, bread rolls, or infant formula when compared with those consuming the unfortified counterparts. Crofton et al.[198] also used radio-labeled iron and unlabeled iron in a single oral dose to measure plasma iron concentrations in healthy male volunteers. A significant reduction of plasma iron was observed with iron to zinc ratios of 1:1 and 1:2.5. A few years later, the effect of zinc on iron absorption in human subjects with use of a dual-radioisotope method (^{55}Fe and ^{59}Fe) was investigated by Rossander-Hulten et al.[159] The results suggested that, in water, a five-fold ratio of zinc to iron reduced iron absorption by 56%; however, fortification with zinc up to a ratio of 1:5 (iron to zinc) administered in a hamburger meal did not interfere with iron absorption. Studies in vitro have demonstrated an inhibitory effect of zinc on iron uptake.[199–202] There was a decrease in the uptake of 5 μM of iron in

Caco-2 cells, a human epithelial intestinal cell line, when incubated with graded doses of zinc (2.5–1000 µM), and a 50% inhibition in iron uptake was observed at a Zn:Fe molar ratio of 1.7:1.[203]

Iron and zinc appear to be highly bioavailable from foods made from fortified flour, but zinc sulfate co-fortification may have a detrimental effect on iron absorption. Iron absorption from the flour fortified with iron only was good (15.9 ± 6.8%), but, when corrections were made for hemoglobin concentrations, it was significantly lower from the flour co-fortified with zinc sulfate (11.5 ± 4.9%; $P < 0.05$) but not from the flour co-fortified with zinc oxide (14.0 ± 8.9%). Zinc absorption was not significantly different between the zinc oxide and zinc sulfate co-fortified flours (24.1 ± 8.2% compared with 23.7 ± 11.2%; $P = 0.87$).[204] Similarly, in a study when the Zn:Fe wt/wt ratio was kept constant it was observed that at higher doses of both minerals (11.71 mg of zinc and 10 mg of iron; Zn:Fe wt/wt ratio 1.17:1) iron bioavailability was inhibited by 56%, while no inhibitory effect was observed at lower doses (0.59 mg of zinc and 0.5 mg of iron; Zn:Fe wt/wt ratio 1.2:1). Zinc (11.71 mg) inhibited the absorption of 0.5 mg of iron when both minerals were given simultaneously; however, when zinc was given 30 or 60 minute before Fe, no inhibitory effect was observed.[205]

The bioavailability of Zn from vegetarian diets is also less than that in non-vegetarian diets. Plant foods rich in zinc, such as legumes, whole grains, nuts, and seeds, are also high in phytic acid, an inhibitor of zinc bioavailability.[206] Despite the high phytate content that lowered the fraction of zinc absorbed from unrefined foods, the higher zinc content of these foods might make these foods preferable to more refined products lower in zinc.[138] In a study, diets were supplied to young rats, with adequate quantities of iron (45 and 300 mg/kg diet) and zinc (14 and 45 mg/kg), for 2 months. A significant effect of iron supply, but not zinc, was evident on iron absorption; both iron and zinc diet concentrations had a significant influence on zinc absorption.[207]

Lopez de Romana and colleagues[182] measured zinc absorption from wheat products fortified with iron sulfate and either zinc sulfate or zinc oxide. Adult volunteers received either low-phytate bread ($n = 11$) or higher-phytate porridge ($n = 11$) once weekly on two or three occasions. The foods were fortified with one of the two zinc salts (60 mg elemental zinc/kg wheat flour) during week 1 and with the other during week 2, in random order. Zinc absorption from bread (13.8%; 95% CI: 11.8%, 16.2%) was significantly ($P < 0.001$) greater than from porridge (6.4%; 95% CI: 5.5%, 7.6%), presumably because of the greater phytate content of the porridge. With control for food type, there were no significant differences in zinc absorption from meals fortified with zinc sulfate or zinc oxide ($P = 0.24$). Indeed, most variation in

zinc bioavailability is well explained by zinc and phytate contents in the human diet. Therefore, the [phytate]:[zinc] ratio in food is considered to be a good indicator of zinc bioavailability.[76,181]

The bioavailability of zinc in bread and dough increases with the extraction rate of the flour used. A high relative zinc bioavailability (1.45) was found when a sangak bread-based diet with 80% flour extraction rate was used; in the corresponding dough, a low relative zinc bioavailability (0.95) was found. Femur zinc concentration in rats consuming bread-based diets increased significantly with the level of zinc fortification. It was concluded that zinc was more bioavailable when sangak bread was prepared using flour with an 80% extraction rate.[208]

Calcium also decreases bioavailability of iron and zinc during absorption. In a study, Gleerup et al.[209] investigated the duration of the inhibitory effect of calcium from milk and cheese (340 mg) in a breakfast meal on non-heme iron absorption from a hamburger meal eaten 2 or 4 hours after the breakfast. In another study, the effect of calcium fortification of bread on bone calcification in growing rats was investigated from breads prepared from flour fortified with calcium at 211 (US enrichment standard), 446, 924, and 1412 mg/100 g flour and fed to rats for 4 weeks.[210] Rats fed on highly fortified bread showed increased bone calcification. In a similar study conducted by Ranhotra et al.,[211] white pan breads were prepared with flour highly fortified with calcium, using calcium carbonate (38.8%) or a high-calcium whey powder (calcium 5.6%) as the calcium source. The bread was also prepared using calcium carbonate plus lactose. Calcium was added to flour at 924 mg/100 g of flour – a level 4.4-fold higher than that specified under the US enrichment standards. Breads were dried and finely ground to prepare test diets (Ca, 0.5%) which were then fed to growing rats for 4 weeks (growth phase) or 8 weeks (approaching maturity). At neither interval did femur ash content, femur calcium content, femur strength, or calcium absorption values differ significantly among groups fed breads fortified with calcium carbonate, calcium carbonate + lactose, or whey.

Calcium absorption from an extruded cereal prepared from intrinsically labeled wheat bran was compared with that from milk. Calcium absorption from the cereal (0.223 ± 0.046) was significantly less than from milk (0.375 ± 0.072). Sharla et al.[212] suggested that small children might benefit from calcium intakes similar to those recommended for older children without adverse effects on dietary iron utilization.

In a study, the apparent calcium absorption rate in rats fed diets containing 0.15% magnesium was significantly lower than that in rats fed diets containing 0.05% magnesium, and the calcium retention rate in rats fed diets containing 0.15% magnesium was significantly lower than that in rats fed diets containing 0.05% magnesium.[213]

It was reported that 10% and 20% beniseed flour substitution rates for wheat flour produced acceptable bread and cake, respectively, with significantly high mineral contents, particularly calcium.[214] It was also found that chicken eggshell powder contained high levels of calcium ($401 \pm 7 \, mg/g$), leading to the conclusion that it might be used as a calcium source in human nutrition.[215] Fortification of butter cake with eggshell at levels of 10% and 20% greatly increased its calcium content, with a noticeable increase in sodium, while it caused a reduction in phosphorus when compared with unfortified cake (100% wheat flour).[216] This led to an increase in the calcium to phosphorus ratio in the fortified cakes, which is in favor of the probable increase in calcium utilization in humans.[217]

Chicken bone extract powder (BEP) is another alternative inexpensive calcium source. It is rich in calcium ($30 \, g/100 \, g$) and has a calcium to phosphorus ratio of 2:1. Sittikulwitit et al.[218] determined calcium bioavailability of BEP and BEP-fortified products using an in vitro equilibrium dialysis method. BEP exhibited excellent calcium bioavailability, showing higher bioavailable calcium than milk and several calcium fortificants. Although phytate and dietary fiber had a negative effect on calcium bioavailability, BEP showed the lowest effect among all calcium sources.

Patwardhan and colleagues[219] evaluated the effect of extra calcium supplementation in the form of three different calcium salts (i.e., calcium carbonate (CaC), calcium lactate (CaL), and calcium phosphate (CaP), in a normocalcemic and a hypocalcemic status of the in vivo milieu. Male Wistar rats were divided into two groups: normocalcemic and hypocalcemic (induced by vitamin D deficiency). Both the groups were supplemented with extra 1.6% calcium in the form of either of these salts. It has been known for a long time that CaC supplementation shows hypercalcemic, hypomagnesemic and hypophosphatemic tendencies. CaL supplementation showed better results as compared with CaC supplementation.

Investigations regarding the effect of phytate hydrolysis were carried out through yeast fermentation, and of Maillard browning on calcium absorption by using leavened bread and underbaked and overbaked cookies, each made with intrinsically labeled wheat flour.[220] Calcium absorption from cookies was not affected by the extent of browning, and averaged 0.652 ± 0.087. However, calcium absorption from bread in the same women was higher (0.703 ± 0.108). It was reported in a study that meals containing 250 mg and 100 mg phytate-P (1344 and 538 mmol phytate) reduced calcium retention by about 65% and 30%, respectively, in humans, as compared to a meal with no added phytate.[102]

Phytate is the major form of phosphorus in plant seeds. Some hydrolysis products of phytate, including inositol pentakisphosphate (InsP$_5$), inositol tetrakisphosphate (InsP$_4$), and lower inositol phosphates (InsP$_3$ and InsP$_2$), are the result of phytate dephosphorylation by endogenous phytase, such as occurs in wheat bran.[221] It was reported in a study that a significant enhancing effect of Ins(1,2,3,6)P$_4$ on calcium absorption was found at the highest level studied (24.8 μmol or 16.8 mg; $P < 0.05$), which suggests that this compound may be a candidate for enhancing calcium absorption.[222]

CONCLUSION

It may be concluded from previous studies that deficiencies of Ca, Fe, and Zn in the diet result in several diseases. Unfortunately, wheat flour contains compounds such as phytate, which binds Ca, Fe, and Zn, forming insoluble complexes in humans and thus ultimately decreasing their bioavailability and making these minerals unavailable for absorption. These minerals also interact with one another and consequently their absorption is decreased. The bioavailability of micronutrients can be increased by reducing the phytate content of wheat flour (dephytinization) with endogenous or exogenous phytases.

References

1. Food Agric Organ 2012. Available at: www.faostat.fao.org.
2. Chaturvedi N, Sharma P, Shukla K, Singh R, Yadav S. Cereals Nutraceuticals, Health Ennoblement and Diseases Obviation: A Comprehensive Review. J Appl Pharm Sci 2011;1:06–12.
3. Nolan KB, Duffin PA. Effect of phytate on mineral bioavailability. In vitro studies on Mg++, Cu++, Ca++, Fe++ and Zn++ solubilities in the presence of phytate. J Sci Food Agri 1987;40:79–85.
4. Brune M, Rossander-Hulthén L, Hallberg L, Gleerup A, Sandberg AS. Iron absorption from bread in humans: Inhibiting effects of cereal fibre, phytate and inositol phosphates with different numbers of phosphate groups. J Nutr 1992;122:442–9.
5. Iqbal TH, Lewis KO, Cooper BT. Phytase activity in the human and rat small intestine. Gut 1994;35:1233–6.
6. Lopez HW, Leenhardt F, Coudray C, Remesy C. Minerals and phytic acid interactions: Is it a real problem for human nutrition? Int J Food Sci Technol 2002;37:727–39.
7. Konietzny U, Greiner R. Molecular and catalytic properties of phytatedegrading enzymes (phytases). Int J Food Sci Technol 2002;37:791–812.
8. Meschino J. Calcium: Requirements, Bioavailable Forms, Physiology and Clinical Aspects. Dynamic Chiropractic 2002: 20–18.
9. Abbasi W. Calcium deficiency widespread in country. The Nation 2002 7 February.
10. Basta SS, Soekirman MS, Karyadi D, Scrimshaw NS. Iron deficiency and the productivity of adult males in Indonesia. Am J Clin Nutr 1990;52:813–9.
11. Baltussen R, Knai C, Sharan M. Iron Fortification and Iron Supplementation are Cost-Effective Interventions to Reduce Iron Deficiency in Four Subregions of the World. J Nutr 2004;134: 2678–84.

12. Brownlie T, Utermohlen IV, Hinton PS, Giordano C, Haas JD. Marginal iron deficiency without anemia impairs aerobic adaptation among previously untrained women. *Am J Clin Nutr* 2002;**75**:734–42.

13. Brabin BJ, Hakimi A, Pelletier D. An analysis of anemia and pregnancy-related maternal mortality. *J Nutr* 2001;**131**:604–14.

14. Swanson CA. Iron intake and regulation: implications for iron deficiency and iron overload. *Alcohol* 2007;**30**:99–102.

15. Ross J, Horton S. *Economic consequences of iron deficiency*. Ottawa, Canada: The Micronutrient Initiative; 1998.

16. Scholl TO, Hediger ML, Fischer LR, Shearer JW. Anemia Vs Iron deficiency: Increased risk of pre-term delivery in a prospective study. *Am J Clin Nutr* 1992;**55**:985–8.

17. Hotz C, Brown KH. Assessment of the risk of zinc deficiency in populations and options for its control. *Food Nutr Bull* 2004;**25**:94–204.

18. Gibson RS. Zinc: the missing link in combating micronutrient malnutrition in developing countries. *Proc Nutr Soc* 2006;**65**:51–60.

19. Prasad AS. Zinc: Mechanisms of Host Defense. *J Nutr* 2007;**137**:1345–9.

20. Vallee BL, Falchuk KH. The biochemical basis of zinc physiology. *Physiol Rev* 1993;**73**:79–118.

21. Prasad AS. *Zinc in human nutrition*. Boca Raton, FL: CRC Press, Inc; 1979 33431.

22. Hess SY, Lonnerdal B, Hotz C, Rivera JA, Brown KH. Recent advances in knowledge of zinc nutrition and human health. *Food Nutr Bull* 2009;**30**:05–11.

23. Brown KH, Rivera JA, Bhutta Z, Gibson RS, King JC, Lonnerdal B. International Zinc Nutrition Consultative Group (IZiNCG) technical document #1. Assessment of the risk of zinc deficiency in populations and options for its control. *Food Nutr Bull* 2004;**25**:199–203.

24. Paracha PI, Jamil A. *Assessment of micronutrient (Iron, Vitamin A and Zinc) status in preschool children of NWFP, Pakistan*. Peshawar, Pakistan: Department of Human Nutrition NWFP Agricultural University; 2002.

25. Bhutta ZA. *The Sindh micronutrient survey in pregnancy; preliminary findings and outcomes*. Bhurban: Pakistan Pediatric Association Congress; 2001.

26. Wuehler S, Peerson J, Brown K. Estimation of the global prevalence of zinc deficiency using national food balance data. *FASEB J* 2000;**14**:510.

27. Brown KH, Wuehler SE. *Zinc and human health: results of recent trials and implications for program interventions and research*. Ottawa, Canada: The Micronutrient Initiative; 2000.

28. *Highlights of recent activities in the context of the World Declaration and Plan of Action for Nutrition*. Geneva, Switzerland: Nutrition Programme. World Health Organization; 1995.

29. Welch RM, Graham DR. Breeding crops for enhanced micronutrient content. *Plant Soil* 2004;**245**:205–14.

30. White PJ, Broadley MR. Biofortifying crops with essential mineral elements. *Trends Plant Sci* 2005;**10**:586–93.

31. Graham RD, Welch RM, Saunders DA. Nutritious subsistence food systems. *Adv Agronomy* 2007;**92**:1–74.

32. Frossard E, Bucher M, Mächler F, Mozafar A, Hurrell R. Potential for increasing the content and bioavailability of Fe, Zn and Ca in plants for human nutrition. *Journal of The Science of Food Agric* 2000;**80**:861–79.

33. Welch RM, Graham RD. Agriculture: the real nexus for enhancing bioavailable micronutrients in food crops. *J Trace Elem Med Biol* 2005;**18**:299–307.

34. Rude RK, Gruber HE. Magnesium deficiency and osteoporosis: animal and human observations. *J Nutr Biochem* 2004;**15**:710–6.

35. Grusak MA, Cakmak I. Methods to improve the crop-delivery of minerals to humans and livestock. In: Broadley MR, White PJ, editors. *Plant nutritional genomics*. Oxford, UK: Blackwell; 2005. p. 265–86.

36. Thacher TD, Fischer PR, Strand MA, Pettifor JM. Nutritional rickets around the world: causes and future directions. *Ann Trop Paediatr* 2006;**26**:1–16.

37. World Health Organization/United Nations University/UNICEF. *Iron deficiency anaemia, assessment, prevention and control: A guide for program managers*. Geneva, Switzerland: WHO; 2001 1–12.

38. Anonymous. *Code of Federal Regulation: Substances Generally Recognized as Safe*. Subpart F; Dietary Supplements. Washington, DC: US Govt Printing Office; 1994.

39. Calloway DH. *Human nutrition: Food and Micronutrient Relationships*. Agricultural Strategies for Micronutrients. Washington, DC: Working Paper 1: International Food Policy Research Institute; 1995.

40. Frontela C, Ros G, Martínez C. Phytic acid content "*in vitro*" iron, calcium and zinc bioavailability in bakery products: the effect of processing. *J Cereal Sci* 2011;**54**:173–9.

41. Seshadri S. Prevalence of micronutrient deficiency particularly of iron, zinc and folic acid in pregnant women in South East Asia. *Br J Nutr* 2001;**85**:87–92.

42. Weaver CM, Heaney RP, Nickel KP, Packard PI. Calcium Bioavailability from High Oxalate Vegetables: Chinese Vegetables, Sweet Potatoes and Rhubarb. *J Food Sci* 2006;**62**:524–5.

43. Miller GD, Anderson JJB. The role of calcium in prevention of chronic diseases. *J Am Coll Nutr* 1999;**18**:371–2.

44. Calcium: an emerging issue for developing countries. *Third report on the world nutrition situation*. Geneva: United Nations Sub-Committee on Nutrition ACC/SCN: World Health Organization; 1997. p. 44–6.

45. Martin AD, Baily DA, McKay HA, Whiting S. Bone mineral and calcium accretion during puberty. *The Am J Clin Nutr* 1997;**66**:611–5.

46. Teegarden D, Proulx WR, Martin BR, Xhao J, McCabe GP, Lyle RP, et al. Peak bone mass in young women. *J Bone Miner Res* 1995;**10**:711–5.

47. Dawson-Hughes B, Harris SS, Krall EA, Dallal GE. Effect of calcium and vitamin D supplementation in men and women age 65 and older. *The New England J Med* 1997;**337**:670–6.

48. Kwok TCY, Chan TYK, Woo J. Relationship of urinary sodium/potassium excretion and calcium intake to blood pressure and prevalence of hypertension among older Chinese vegetarians. *Eur J Clin Nutr* 2003;**57**:299–304.

49. Goulding A, Cannon R, Williams SM, Gold EJ, Taylor RW, Lewis-Barned NJ. Bone mineral density in girls with forearm fractures. *J Bone Miner Res* 1998;**13**:143–8.

50. Rebecca J, Bryant MS, Cadogan J, Weaver CM. The New Dietary Reference Intakes for Calcium:Implications for Osteoporosis. *J Am Coll Nutr* 1999;**18**:406–12.

51. Cook JD, Reusser M. Iron fortification: An update. *Am J Clin Nutr* 1983;**38**:648–59.

52. Yip R. Iron nutritional status defined. In: Filer Jr LJ, editor. *Dietary iron: birth to two years*. New York, NY: Raven Press; 1989. p. 19–36.

53. Arija V, Fernandez J, Salas J. Carencia de hierro y anemia ferropenica en la poblacion espanola. *Med Clín* 1997;**109**:425–30.

54. Van Moorsell L. Improving calcium and iron bioavailability through bioactive proteins. *International food ingredients* 1997;**4**:44–6.

55. Murphy JF, Riardon JO, Newcombe RG, Coles EC, Pearson JF. Relation of haemoglobin levels in first and second trimesters to outcome of pregnancy. *Lancetilla* 1986;**9**:92–4.

56. Llewelyn-Jones D. Severe anemia in pregnancy. *Aust N Z J Obstet Gynaecol* 1965;**5**:191–7.

57. Edgerton VR, Gardner GW, Ogiray KA, Ygunawadena Senewiratne B. Iron deficiency anemia and its effects on worker productivity pattern. *Br Med J* 1979;**2**:1546–9.

58. Lozoff B, Brittenham GM, Viteri FE, Wolf A, Urrutia JJ. 1982. The effect of short term oral iron therapy on developmental deficits in iron deficient anemic infants. *J Pediatr* 1992;**100**:351–7.

59. Ankett MA, Parks YA, Scott PA, Wharton BA. Treatment with iron increases weight gain and psychomotor development. *Archives of diseases in childhood* 1986;**61**:849–57.

60. Walter T, DeAndraca I, Chadud P, Perales CG. Iron deficiency anemia, adverse effects on infant psychomotor development. *Pediatrics* 1986;**84**:7–17.

61. Lotfi M, Mannar MGV, Merx RH, Naber-van den, Heuvel P. *Micronutrient fortification of foods: Current practices, research and opportunities. Ottawa, Canada: The Micronutrient Initiative and International Agriculture Centre.* Wageningen, The Netherlands: Wageningen University; 1996.

62. Walker AR. The remedying of iron deficiency: what priority should it have? *Br J Nutr* 1998;**79**:227–35.

63. Government of Pakistan. *Pakistan economic survey 2001–2, Economic Advisors Wing.* Islamabad, Pakistan: Finance Division; 2002.

64. Hamedani P, Hashmi KZ, Manji M. Iron depletion and anaemia: prevalence, consequences, diagnostic and therapeutic implications in a developing Pakistani population. *Curr Med Res Opin* 1987;**10**:480–5.

65. Molla A, Khurshid M, Molla AM. Prevalence of iron deficiency anaemia in children of the urban slums of Karachi. *J Pak Med Assoc* 1992;**42**:118–21.

66. Anwer I, Awan JA. Nutritional status comparison of rural with urban school children in Faisalabad District, Pakistan. *Rural Remote Health* 2003;**3**:130 (online). [accessed 2.02.13].

67. Chiplnkar SA, Tarwadi KV, Kavedia RB, Mengale SS, Paknikar KM, Agte VV. Fortification of vegetarian diets for increasing bio-available iron density using green leafy vegetables. *Food Res Int* 1999;**32**:169–74.

68. Cook JD, Finch CA. Iron Nutrition. *West J Med* 1975;**122**:474–81.

69. Hallberg L. Bioavailability of dietary iron in man. *Annu Rev Nutr* 1981;**1**:123–47.

70. Hallberg L, Hulthen L. Prediction of dietary iron absorption: an algorithm for calculating absorption and bioavailability of dietary iron. *The Am J Clin Nutr* 2000;**71**:1147–60.

71. Prasad AS, Halsted JA, Nadimi M. Syndrome of iron deficiency anemia, hepatosplenomegaly, hypogonadism, dwarfism and geophagia. *Am J Med* 1961;**31**:532–46.

72. Prasad AS, Miale A, Farid Z, Schulert A, Sandstead HH. Zinc metabolism in patients with the syndrome of iron deficiency anemia, hypogonadism, and dwarfism. *J Lab Clin Med* 1963;**61**:537–49.

73. White PJ, Broadley RM. Biofortification of crops with seven mineral elements often lacking in human diets-iron, zinc, copper, calcium, magnesium, selenium and iodine. *New Phytol* 2009;**182**:49–84.

74. *The World Health Report: reducing risks, promoting healthy life: overview.* Geneva: Switzerland; 2002.

75. Muller O, Krawinkle M. Malnutrition and health in developing countries. *Can Med Assoc J* 2005;**173**:279–86.

76. Brown KH, Wuehler SE, Peerson JM. The importance of zinc in human nutrition and estimation of the global prevalence of zinc deficiency. *Food Nutr Bull* 2001;**22**:113–25.

77. Walsh CT, Sandstead HH, Prasad AS. Zinc health effects and research priorities for the 1990s. *Environ Health Prospect* 1994;**102**:5–46.

78. Prasad AS. Clinical manifestations of zinc deficiency. *Ann Rev Nutr* 1985;**5**:341–63.

79. WHO. *Trace elements in Human nutrition and health.* Geneva, Switzerland: World Health Organization; 1996.

80. Gracey M. Nutritional effects and management of diarrhea in infancy. *Acta Paediar Suppl* 1999;**430**:110–26.

81. Paterson PG, Bettger WJ. Effect of dietary zinc intake on the hematological profile of the rat. *Comp Biochem Physiol* 1986;**83**:721–5.

82. El Hendy HA, Yousef MI, Abo El-Naga NI. Effect of dietary zinc deficiency on hematological and biochemical parameters and concentrations of zinc, copper, and iron in growing rats. *Toxicology* 2001;**167**:163–70.

83. Konomi A, Yokoi K. Zinc deficiency decreases plasma erythropoietin concen-tration in rats. *Biol Trace Elem Res* 2005;**107**:289–92.

84. Shingwekar AG, Mohanram M Reddy V. Effect of zinc supplementation on plasma levels of vitamin A and retinolbinding protein in malnourished children. *Act Clinica Chimica* 1997;**93**:97–100.

85. Hustead VA, Greger JL, Gutcher GR. Zinc supplementation and plasma concentration of vitamin A in preterm infants. *Am J Clin Nutr* 1988;**47**:1017–21.

86. Morrison SA, Russell RM, Carney EA, Oaks EV. Zinc deficiency: a cause of abnormal dark adaptation in cirrhotics. *Am J Clin Nutr* 1978;**31**:276–81.

87. Palin D, Underwood BA, Denning RC. The effect of oral zinc supplementation on plasma levels of vitamin A and retinol-binding protein in cystic fibrosis. *Am J Clin Nutr* 1979;**32**:1253–9.

88. Black RE. Zinc deficiency, immune function, and morbidity and mortality from infectious disease among children in developing countries. *Food Nutr Bull* 2001;**22**:155–62.

89. Tikkiwal M, Ajmera RL, Mathur NK. Effect of zinc administration on seminal zinc and fertility of oligospermic males. *Indian J Physiol Pharmacol* 1987;**31**:30–4.

90. Simmer K, Khanum S, Carlsson L, Thompson RPH. Nutritional rehabilitation in Bangladesh – the importance of zinc. *Am J Clin Nutr* 1988;**47**:1036–40.

91. Brown KH, Dewey K, Allen L. *Complementary feeding of young children in developing countries. A review of current scientific knowledge.* Geneva, Switzerland: World Health Organization; 1998.

92. Brown KH, Peerson JM, Baker SK, Hess SY. Preventive zinc supplementation among infants, preschoolers, and older prepubertal children. *Food Nutr Bull* 2009;**30**:12–40.

93. Bhutta ZA. Iron and zinc intake from complementary foods: some issues from Pakistan. *Pediatrics* 2000;**106**:1295–7.

94. Ferguson EL, Gibson RS, Thompson LU, Ounpuu S, Berry M. Phytate zinc and calcium contents of 30 East African foods and their calculated phytates: Zn, Ca:Phytate and Ca phytates Zn molar ratios. *J Food Composition Anal* 1988;**1**:316–25.

95. Davies NT. Anti-nutrient factors affecting mineral utilization. *Proc Nutr Soc* 1979;**38**:121.

96. Ravindran VG. Ravindran, Sivalogan S. Total and phytate phosphorous contents of various foods and foodstuffs of plant origin. *Food Chem* 1994;**50**:133–6.

97. Cheryan M. Phytic acid interactions in food systems. *Crit Rev Food Sci Nutr* 1980;**13**:297–335.

98. Zhou JR, Erdman JW. Phytic acid in health and disease. *Crit Rev Food Sci Nutr* 1995;**35**:495–508.

99. Febles CI, Arias A, Hardisson A, Rodrıguez-Alvarez C, Sierra A. Phytic acid level in wheat flours. *J Cereal Sci* 2002;**36**:19–23.

100. Feil B. Phytic acid. *J New Seeds* 2001;**3**:1–35.

101. Fredlund K. *Inhibition of calcium and zinc absorption by phytate in man. Methodological studies and hydrothermal processing of cereals to improve absorption.* PhD Thesis. Goteborg, Sweden: Chalmers University of Technology, Goteborg University; 2002.

102. Fredlund K, Isaksson M, Rossander-Hulthén L, Almgren A, Sandberg AS. Absorption of zinc and retention of calcium: Dose-dependent inhibition by phytate. *J Trace Elem Med Biol* 2006;**20**:49–57.

103. Lonnerdal B. 2002. Phytic acid-trace element (Zn, Cu, Mn) interactions. *Int J Food Sci Technol* 2002;**37**:749–58.

104. Navert B, Sandström B, Cederblad A. Reduction of the phytate content of bran by leavening in bread and its effect on zinc absorption in man. *Br J Nutr* 1985;**53**:47–53.

C. WHEAT IN DIABETES AND HEART DISEASE PREVENTION

105. Alabaster O, Tang Z, Shivapurkar N. Dietary fiber and the che-moreventive modelation of colon carcinogenesis. *Mutat Res* 1996;**350**:185–97.

106. Ko KM, Gold DV. Ferric ion-induced lipid peroxidation in eryth-rocyte membranes: effects of phytic acid and butylated hydroxy-toluene. *Mol Cell Biochem* 1990;**95**:125–8.

107. Yoon JH, Thompson LU, Jenkins DJA. The effect of phytic acid on *in vitro* rate of starch digestibility and blood glucose response. *Am J Clin Nutr* 1983;**1983**(38):835–42.

108. Wyss M, Pasamontes L, Friedlein A, Remy R, Tessier M, Kronen-berger A, et al. Biophysical characterization of fungal phytases (myo-inositol hexakisphosphate phospho-hydrolases): molecular size, glycosylation pattern, and engineering of proteo-lytic resis-tance. *Appl Environ Microbiol* 1999;**65**:359–66.

109. Lei XG, Porres JM, Mullaney EJ, Brinch-Pedersen H. Phytase: source, structure, and application. In J. of Polaina. In: MacCabe AP, editor. *Industial Enzymes: Structure, Function and Applications.* Dordrecht, The Netherlands: Springer; 2007. p. 505–30.

110. Dionisio G, Madsen VK, Holm PB, Welinder KG, Jorgensen M, Stoger E, et al. Cloning and characterization of purple acid phos-phatase phytases from wheat, barley, maize and rice. *Plant Physiol* 2011;**156** 1087–00.

111. Gibson RS, Yeundall F, Drost N, Mtitimuni B, Cullinan T. Dietary interventions to prevent zinc deficiency. *Am J Clin Nutr* 1998;**68**:484–7.

112. Reddy NR, Sathe SK, Salunkhe DK. Phytate in legumes and cere-als. *Adv Food Res* 1982;**28**:1–2.

113. Chavan JK, Kadam SS. Nutritional improvement of grains by fer-mentation. *Crit Rev Food Sci Nutr* 1980;**28**:349–400.

114. Svanberg U, Sandberg A. Improved iron availability in wean-ing foods through the use of germination and fermentation. In: Alnwick D, Moses S, Schmidt OG, editors. *Improving Young Child Feeding in Eastern and Southern Africa, Proceedings of a Workshop in Nairobi, Kenya.* Ottowa, Canada: IDRC 366; 1987.

115. INACG. *The effect of cereals and legumes on iron avialabity.* Washing-ton, DC: Nutrition Foundation; 1982.

116. Spiller G. *Dietary fiber in human nutrition.* Boca Raton, FL: CRC Press; 1993.

117. Tariq M. *Phytic Acid in Wheat as Influenced by Milling and Baking.* MSc Thesis. Faisalabad, Pakistan: Department of Food Technol-ogy, University of Agriculture; 1990.

118. Lonnerdal BJG, Bell AG, Hendrickx RA, Burns Keen CL. Effect of phytate removal on zinc absorption from soy formula. *Am J Clin Nutr* 1988;**48**:1301–6.

119. Sandberg AS. The effect of food processing on phytate hydro-lysis and availability of iron and zinc. *Adv Exp Med Biol* 1991;**289**:499–508.

120. Persson H, Turk M, Nyman M, Sandberg AS. Binding of Cu^{2+}, Zn^{2+}, and Cd^{2+} to inositol tri-, tetra-, penta-, hexaphosphates. *J Agric Food Chem* 1998;**46**:3194–200.

121. Sandberg AS, Brune M, Carlsson NG, Hallberg L, Skoglund E, Rossander-Hulthen L. Inositol phosphates with different num-bers of phosphate groups influence iron absorption in humans. *Am J Clin Nutr* 1999;**70**:240–6.

122. Reddy NR, Pierson MD. Reduction in antinutritional and toxic components in plant foods by fermentation. *Food Res Int* 1994;**27**:281–90.

123. El-Guindi M, Lynch SRJD. Cook. Iron absorption from fortified flat breads. *Br J Nutr* 1988;**59**:205–13.

124. Cook JD, Dassenko SA, Whittaker P. Calcium supplemen-tation:effect on iron absorption. *Am J Clin Nutr* 1999;**53**:106–11.

125. Akhter S, Saeed A, Irfan M, Malik KA. *In vitro* dephytinization and bioavailability of essential minerals in several wheat variet-ies. *J Cereal Sci* 2012;**56**:741–6.

126. Kataria A, Chauhan BM, Gandhi S. Effect of domestic process-ing and cooking on the antinutrients of black gram. *Food Chem* 1988;**30**:149–56.

127. Khan N, Zaman R, Elahi M. Effect of heat treatments on the phytic acid content of maize products. *J Sci Food Agric* 1991;**54**:153–6.

128. Fretzdorff B, Weipert D. Phytinsaure in Getreide und Getreideer-zeugnissen. Mitteilung 1. Phytinsaure und Phytase in Roggen und Roggenprodukt (Phytic Acid in Cereals and Cereal Products. Part 1. Phytic Acid and Phytase in Rye Products). *Zeitung für Leb-ensmittel Untersuchung und Forschung* 1986;**182**:287–93.

129. Dublish RK, Chanhan GS, Bains GS. Nutritional quality of extruded rice, ragi and defatted soy flour blends. *J Food Sci Technol* 1988;**25**:35–8.

130. Ummadi P, Chenoweth WL, Uebersax MA. The influence of extrusion processing on iron dialysability, phytates and tannins in legumes. *J Food Process Preservation* 1994;**19**:119–31.

131. Tabekhia MM, Luh BS. Effect of germination, cooking and can-ning on phosphorus and phytate retention in dry beans. *J Food Sci Technol* 1980;**45**:406–8.

132. Smith AK, Circle SJ. *Soybean Chemistry and Technology.* Westport, CT: Avi Publishing Company Inc; 1978.

133. Larson SR, Young KA, Cook A. Linkage mapping of two muta-tions that reduced phytic acid content of barley grain. *Theor Appl Genet* 1998;**97**:141–6.

134. Hardy RW. Phytate. *Aquaculture Mag* 1998;**11**:77–80.

135. Levrat-Verny MA, Coudray C, Bellanger J, Lopez HW, Demigne C, Rayssiguier Y, et al. Whole wheat flour ensures higher mineral absorption and bioavailability than white wheat flour in rats. *Br J Nutr* 1999;**82**:17–21.

136. Larsson M, Sandberg AS. Phytate reduction in bread containing oat flour, oat bran or rye bran. *J Cereal Sci* 1991;**14**:141–9.

137. Reinhold JG, Nasr K, Lahimgarzadeh A, Hedayati A. Effects of purified phytate and phytate-rich bread upon metabolism of zinc, calcium, phosphorus, and nitrogen in man. *Lancet* 1973;**1**:283–8.

138. Sandstrom B, Arvidsson B, Cederblad A, Bjorn-Rasmussen E. Zinc absorption from composite meals. I. The significance of wheat extraction rate, zinc, calcium, and protein content in meals based on bread. *Am J Clin Nutr* 1980;**33**:739–45.

139. Turnlund JR, King JC, Keyes WR, Gong B, Maynard CM. A stable isotope study of zinc absorption in young men: effects of phytate and a-cellulose. *Am J Clin Nutr* 1984;**40**:1071–7.

140. Lonnerdal BA, Cederblad L, Davidsson, Sandstrom B. The effect of individual components of soy formula and cows' milk formula on zinc bioavailability. *Am J Clin Nutr* 1984;**40**:1064–70.

141. Sandstrom B, Kivisto B, Cederblad A. Absorption of zinc from soy protein meals in humans. *J Nutr* 1987;**117**:321–7.

142. Kivisto B, Cederblad A, Davidsson L, Sandberg AS, Sandstrom B. Effect of meal composition and phytate content on zinc absorp-tion in humans from an extruded bran product. *J Cereral Sci* 1989;**10**:189–97.

143. Sandstrom B, Sandberg AS. Inhibitory effects of isolated phos-phates on zinc absorption in humans. *J Trace Elem Electrolytes Health Dis* 1992;**6**:99–103.

144. Andersson H, Navert B, Bingham SA, Englyst HN, Cummings JH. The effects of breads containing similar amounts of phytate but different amounts of wheat bran on calcium, zinc and iron balance in man. *Br J Nutr* 1983;**50**:503–10.

145. Dalton MA, Sargent JA, O'Connor GT, Olmstead EM, Klein RZ. Calcium and phosphorus supplementation of iron-fortified infant formula: no effect on iron status of healthy full-term infants. *Am J Clin Nutr* 1997;**65**:921–6.

146. Ames SK, Gorham BM, Abrams SA. Effects of high compared with low calcium intake on calcium absorption and incorpora-tion of iron by red blood cells in small children. *Am J Clin Nutr* 1999;**70**:44–8.

147. Bendich A. Calcium supplementation and iron status of females. *Nutrition* 2001;**17**:46–51.

148. Ilich-Ernst JZ, McKenna AA, Badenhop NE. Iron status, menarche and calcium supplementation in adolescent girls. *Am J Clin Nutr* 1998;**68**:880–7.

149. Hallberg L, Brune M, Erlandsson M, Sandberg AS, Rossander-Hulten L. Calcium: effect of different amounts on nonheme- and heme-iron absorption in humans. *Am J Clin Nutr* 1991;**53**:112–9.

150. Fordyce EJ, Forbes RM, Robbins KR, Erdman JWJ. Phytate, calcium/zinc molar ratios: are they predictive of zinc bioavailability? *J Food Sci* 1987;**52**:440–4.

151. Gleerup A, Rossander-Hulthen L, Gramatkovski E, Hallberg L. Iron absorption from the whole diet: comparison of the effect of two different distributions of daily calcium intake. *Am J Clin Nutr* 1995;**61**:97–104.

152. Minihane AM, Fairweather-Tait SJ. Effect of calcium supplementation on daily nonheme-iron absorption and long-term iron status. *Am J Clin Nutr* 1998;**68**:96–102.

153. Reddy MB, Cook JD. Effect of calcium intake on nonheme-iron absorption from a complete diet. *Am J Clin Nutr* 1997;**65**:1820–5.

154. Lonnerdal B. *Iron-zinc-copper interactions. In: Micronutrient interactions. Impact on child health and nutrition.* Washington, DC: USAID; 1996 3–10.

155. O'Dell B. Mineral interactions relevant to nutrient requirements. *J Nutr* 1989;**19**:1832–8.

156. Solomons N. Competitive interaction of iron and zinc inthe diet: consequences for human nutrition. *J Nutr* 1986;**116**:927–35.

157. Solomons NW, Ruz M. Zinc and iron interaction: concepts and perspectives in the developing world. *Nutr Res* 1974;**17**:177–85.

158. Whittaker P. Iron and zinc fortification in humans. *Am J Clin Nutr* 1998;**68**:442–6.

159. Rossander-Hulten L, Brune M, Sandstrom B, Lonnerdal B, Hallberg L. Competitive inhibition of iron absorption by manganese and zinc in humans. *Am J Clin Nutr* 1991;**54**:152–6.

160. Sandstrom B, Davidson L, Cederblad A, Lonnerdal B. Oral iron dietary ligands and zinc absorption. *J Nutr* 1985;**115**:411–4.

161. Deehr MS, Dallal GE, Smith KT, Taulbee JD, Dawson-Hughes B. Effects of different calcium sources on iron absorption in post-menopausal women. *Am JClin Nutr* 1990;**51**:95–9.

162. Hallberg L, Rossander-Hulthen L, Brune M, Gleerup A. Inhibition of haem-iron absorption in man by calcium. *Br J Nutr* 1993;**69**:533–40.

163. Monsen ER, Cook JD. Food iron absorption in human subjects. The effects of calcium and phosphate salts on the absorption of nonheme iron. *Am J Clin Nutr* 1976;**29**:1142–8.

164. Welch RM, Graham RD. Breeding for micronutrients in staple food crops from a human nutrition perspective. *J Exp Bot* 2002;**55**:353–64.

165. Hallberg L. Iron Balance in Pregnancy and Lactation. In: Fomon SF, Zlotkin S, editors. *Nestle Nutrition Workshop Series Vol. 20. Nutritional Anaemias.* New York, NY: Raven Press; 1992. p. 13–28.

166. Larsen T, Sandstrom B. Effect of calcium, copper, and zinc levels in a rapeseed meal diet on mineral and trace element utilization in the rat. *Biol Trace Elem Res* 1992;**35**:167–84.

167. Mendoza C, Peerson JM, Brown HK, Lönnerdal B. Effect of a micronutrient fortificant mixture and 2 amounts of calcium on iron and zinc absorption from a processed food supplement. *Am J Clin Nutr* 2004;**79**:244–50.

168. Pallares I, Campos MS, Lopez-Aliaga I, Barrionuevo M, Rodriguez-Matas MC, Gomez-Ayala AE, et al. Supplementation of a Cereal-Based Diet with Heme Iron:Interactions between Iron and Calcium, Phosphorus, and Magnesium in Rats. Magnesium in Rats. *J Agric Food Chem* 1996;**44**:1816–20.

169. Bilal R, Roohi S, Ahmad T, Trinidad TP. Iron fortification of wheat flour: bioavailability studies. *Food Nutr Bull* 2002;**23**(3):199–202.

170. Baker SJ, DeMaeyer EM. Nutritional anemia: its understanding and control with special reference to the work of the World Health Organization. *Am J Clin Nutr* 1971;**32**:368–417.

171. Allen. Marginal malnutrition and human function: The Nutrition CRSP. *Nutr Rev* 1993;**51**:255–67.

172. Enriching Lives. *Overcoming vitamin and mineral malnutrition in developing countries.* Washington, DC: World Bank; 1994.

173. Allen LH. An analytical approach for expanding the importance of dietary quality vs. quantity to the growth of Mexican children. *Food Nutr Bull* 1991;**13**:95–104.

174. Gargari BP, Mahboob S, Razavieh SV. Content of phytic acid and its mole ratio to zinc in floors and breads consumed in Tabriz, Iran. *Food Chem* 2007;**100**:1115–9.

175. Hallberg L, Rossander L, Skanberg AB. Phytates and the inhibitory effect of bran on iron absorption in man. *Am J Clin Nutr* 1987;**45**:988–96.

176. Gibson RS, Bailey KB, Gibbs M, Ferguson EL. A review of phytate, iron, zinc, and calcium concentrations in plant-based complementary foods used in low-income countries and implications for bioavailability. *Food Nutr Bull* 2010;**31**:S134–46.

177. Hurrell RF. Preventing iron deficiency through food fortification. *Nutr Rev* 1997;**55**(6):210–22.

178. Abebe YA, Bogale KM, Hambidge BJ, Stoecker K. Bailey, Gibson R S. Phytate, zinc, iron and calcium content of selected raw and prepared foods consumed in rural Sidama, Southern Ethiopia, and implications for bioavailability. *J Food Component Anal* 2007;**20**:161–8.

179. Hallberg L, Brune M, Rossander L. Iron absorption in man: ascorbic acid and dose-dependent inhibition by phy-tate. *Am J Clin Nutr* 1989;**49**:140–4.

180. Morris ER, Ellis R. Bioavailability of dietary calcium effect of phytate on adult men consuming non vegetarian diets. In: Kies C, editor. *American Chemical Society Symposium 275: nutritional bioavailability of calcium.* The Netherlands: American Chemical Society, Wagenington; 1985. p. 63.

181. Weaver CM, Kannan S. Phytate andmineral bioavailability. In: Reddy NR, Sathe SK, editors. *Food phytate.* Boca Raton, FL: CRC Press; 2002. p. 211–23.

182. Lopez-de-Romana D, Lonnerdal BK, Brown KH. Absorption of zinc from wheat products fortified with iron and either zinc sulfate or zinc oxide. *Am J Clin Nutr* 2003;**78**:279–83.

183. Palacios MC, Haros M, Sanz Y, Rosell CM. Phytate degradation by Bifidobacterium on whole wheat fermentation. *Eur Food Res Technol* 2008;**226**:825–31.

184. Sardar P, Randhawa HS, Abid M, Prabhakar SK. Effect of dietary microbial phytase supplementation on growth performance, nutrient utilization, body compositions and haematobiochemical profiles of *Cyprinus carpio* (L.) fingerlings fed soyprotein-based diet. *Aquaculture Nutr* 2007;**13**:444–56.

185. Lynch S, Skikne RBS, Cook JD. Food iron absorption in idiopathic hemochromatosis. *Blood* 1989;**74**:2187–93.

186. Cook JD. Adaptation in iron metabolism. *Am J Clin Nutr* 1990;**51**:301–8.

187. Taylor P, Martinez-Torres C, Leets I. Relationships among iron absorption, percent saturation of plasma transferrin and serum ferritin concentration in humans. *J Nutr* 1988;**118**:1110–5.

188. Hunt JR, Roughead ZK. Adaptation of iron absorption in men consuming diets with high or low iron bioavailability. *Am J Clin Nutr* 2000;**71**:94–102.

189. Gibson RS. Content and bioaccessibility of trace elements in vegetarian diets. *Am J Clin Nutr* 1994;**59**:1223S–32S.

190. Sandberg AS. Bioaccessibility of minerals in legumes. *Br J Nutr* 2002;**88**:281–5.

C. WHEAT IN DIABETES AND HEART DISEASE PREVENTION

191. Tallkvist J, Bowlus CL, Lonnerdal B. Functional and molecular responses of human intestinal Caco-2 cells to iron treatment. *Am J Clin Nutr* 2000;**72**:770–5.

192. Coudray C, Levrat-Verny MA, Tressol JC, Feillet-Coudray C, Horcajada-Molteni NM, Demigne C, et al. Mineral supplementation of white wheat flour is necessary to maintain adequate mineral status and bone characteristics in rats. *J Trace Elem Med Biol* 2001;**15**:131–7.

193. Hernandez M, Sousa V, Moreno A, Villapando S, Lopez-Alarcon M. Iron bioavailability and utilization in rats are lower from lime-treated corn flour than from wheat flour when they are fortified with different sources of iron. *J Nutr* 2003;**133**:154–9.

194. Ranhotra GS, Gelroth JA, Torrence JA, Bock MA, Winterringer GL, Faridi HA, et al. Iranian Flat Breads: Relative Bioavailability of Iron. *Cereal Chem* 1981;**58**:471.

195. Hansen M, Bæcha SB, Thomsenb AD, Tetensa I, Sandstrom B. Long-term intake of iron fortified wholemeal rye bread appears to benefit iron status of young women. *J Cereal Sci* 2005;**42**:165–71.

196. Valberg LS, Flanagan PR, Chamberlain MJ. Effects of iron, tin, and copper on zinc absorption in humans. *Am J Clin Nutr* 1984;**40**:536–41.

197. Davidsson L, Almgren A, Sandstrom B, Hurrell RF. Zinc absorption in adult humans: the effect of iron fortification. *Br J Nutr* 1995;**74**:417–25.

198. Crofton RW, Gvozdanovic D, Gvozdanovic S. Inorganic zinc and the intestinal absorption of ferrous iron. *Am J Clin Nutr* 1989;**50**:141–4.

199. Olivares M, Hertrampf E, Pizzarro F, Walter T, Cayazzo M, Llaguno S, et al. Hemoglobin-fortified biscuits: bioavailability and its effect on iron nutriture in school children. *Arch Latinoam Nutr* 1990;**4**:209–20.

200. Wien EM, Glahn RP, Van Campen DR. Ferrous iron uptake by rat duodenal brush border membrane vesicles: effects of dietary iron level and competing minerals (Zn^{+2}, Mn^{+2}, and Ca^{+2}). *J Nutr Biochem* 1994;**5**:571–7.

201. Arredondo M, Martı́nez R, Nunez MT, Ruz M, Olivares M. Inhibition of iron and copper uptake by iron, copper and zinc. *Biol Res* 2006;**39**:95–102.

202. Abd Rashed A. *In vitro* study to determine the effect of zinc on non-heme iron absorption. *Int J Collaborative Res Intern Med Public Health* 2011;**3**:354–68.

203. Roughead ZK, Hunt JR. Adaptation in iron absorption: iron supplementation reduces nonheme-iron but not heme-iron absorption from food. *Am J Clin Nutr* 2000;**72**:982–9.

204. Herman S, Griffin IJ, Suwarti S, Ernawati F, Permaesih D, Pambudi D, et al. Co-fortification of iron-fortified flour with zinc sulfate, but not zinc oxide, decreases iron absorption in Indonesian children. *Am J Clin Nutr* 2002;**76**:813–7.

205. Olivares M, Pizarro F, Ruz M. New insights about iron bioavailability inhibition by zinc. *J Nutr* 2007;**23**:292–5.

206. Harland BF, Oberleas D. Phytate in foods. *World Rev Nutr Diet* 1987;**52**:235–59.

207. Bougle D, Isfaoun A, Bureau F, Neuville D, Jauzac P, Arhan P. Long-term effects of iron: zinc interactions on growth in rats. *Biol Trace Elem Res* 1999;**67**:37–48.

208. Azar M. Bioavailability of zinc in sangak bread with different extraction rates of flour and in zinc fortified bread. *Dissertation Abstracts International, Thesis Publication* 1994;**54**:4458.

209. Gleerup A, Rossander-Hulten L, Hallberg L. Duration of the inhibitory effect of calcium on non-haem iron absorption in man. *Eur J Clin Nutr* 1993;**47**:875–9.

210. Ranhotra GS, Gelroth JA, Leinen SD. Increase in bone calcification in young rats fed bread highly fortified with calcium. *Cereal CheM* 1995;**67**:325–7.

211. Ranhotra GS, Gelroth AJ, Leinen SD. Utilization of Calcium in Breads Highly Fortified with Calcium as Calcium Carbonate or as Dairy Calcium. *Cereal Chem* 2000;**77**:293–6.

212. Sharla K, Ames BM, Gorham Abrams SA. Effects of high compared with low calcium intake on calcium absorption and incorporation of iron by red blood cells in small children. *Am J Clin Nutr* 1999;**70**:44–8.

213. Toba Y, Masuyama R, Katot K, Takadal Y, Aoet S, Suzuki K. Effects of dietary magnesium level on calcium absorption in growing male rats. *Nutr Res* 1999;**19**:783–93.

214. Emmanuel-Ikpeme C, Eneji C, Igile G. Nutritional and Organoleptic Properties of Wheat *(Triticum aestivum)* and Beniseed *(Sesame indicum)* Composite Flour Baked Foods. *J Food Res* 2012;**1**:84–91.

215. Schaafsma A, Pakan I, Hfstede G, Muskiet F, Van Der Veer E, Vries P. Mineral, amino acid and hormonal composition of chicken eggshell powder and evaluation of its use in human nutrition. *Poult Sci* 2002;**79**:1833–8.

216. Ibrahim SS, Abdalla SMA, Ramadan AH. Effect of Eggshell Powder Addition as a Source of Calcium Fortification on Butter Cake Quality. *J Agri Vet Sci Qassim Univ* 2012;**5**:109–18.

217. Makai F, Chudacek J. The treatment of osteoporosis with Biomin-H. *Arch Gerontol Geriatr* 1991;**2**:487–90.

218. Sittikulwitit S, Prapaisri PP, Sirichakwal P, Puwastien P, Chavasit V, Sungpuag P. *In vitro* bioavailability of calcium from chicken bone extract powder and its fortified products. *J Food Composition Anal* 2004;**17**:321–9.

219. Patwardhan UN, Pahuja DN, Samuel AM. Calcium bioavailability: an *in vivo* assessment. *J Nutr RE* 2001;**21**:667–75.

220. Weaver CM, Heaney RP, Nickel KP, Packard PI. Calcium Bioavailability from High Oxalate Vegetables: Chinese Vegetables, Sweet Potatoes and Rhubarb. *J Food Sci* 2006;**62**:524–5.

221. Peers FG. The phytase of wheat. *J Biochem* 1953;**53**:102–10.

222. Shen Y, Fan MZ, Ajakaiye A, Archbold T. True phosphorus digestibility and the endogenous phosphorus loss associated with corn for growing-finishing pigs are determined with the regression analysis technique. *J Nutr* 2002;**132**:1199–206.

7

Nutritive and Digestive Effects of Starch and Fiber in Whole Wheat

Birger Svihus

Norwegian University of Life Sciences, Aas, Norway

INTRODUCTION

On a global basis, wheat is among our most important food crops. Based on statistics from the FAO, it can be estimated that around 450 million tonnes of wheat are used for food every year, making it our most quantitatively important food cereal together with rice. Although wheat and other cereals are good sources of protein and several micronutrients, the quantitatively most important role of wheat is as a source of energy. On a global basis, cereals provide almost 50% of the food energy for the human population, according to the FAO. As with other cereals, the largest part of the wheat kernel is the endosperm fraction, the role of which is to be a nutrient source for the offspring (the germ) during sprouting. Starch dominates the endosperm, in the form of starch granules varying in size between 3 and 20 micrometers, embedded in a protein matrix. The germ contains the actual offspring from the mother plant, and is rich in protein, fat, and essential micronutrients such as minerals and vitamins. The outer part of the wheat kernel, the so-called bran, contains the various layers of tissue with roles such as protective function and as a reservoir for enzyme precursors used for nutrient mobilization during germination. This fraction contains a high fiber level, but is also a rich source of vitamins and minerals.

Due to significant associations found in epidemiological studies, whole wheat has been hypothesized to be protective against obesity, type 2 diabetes, and cardiovascular disease when compared to refined wheat products.[1,2] A number of components in whole wheat products, including starch and fiber, have been proposed to contribute to this effect, but few have been conclusively linked to these health benefits in controlled experiments.

As shown in Table 7.1,[3] nutrient composition varies considerably between the different parts of the wheat kernel, and, apart from its high energy content, the endosperm is the least nutrient-rich part of the kernel. Despite the fact that, from a nutritional point of view, flour made from the whole wheat kernel would constitute a much more nutritionally valuable source of nutrients, only the endosperm fraction of the wheat is usually used in human nutrition. While the whole wheat kernel was originally used for human consumption, a tradition emerged where the finer whiter parts of the ground wheat, which produced lighter bread, became more sought after. In Roman times, the whiteness of the bread became a token of social class, with the higher classes eating the white bread containing a high endosperm fraction and the lower classes eating the coarse and darker bread with more of the bran fraction. With the old stone-gristmills it was not possible to separate the different fractions in the grinding process, but sifting afterwards made removal of some of the bran fraction possible. In the 19th century, millers became more and more skilled at the art. However, the germ fraction was still part of the flour fraction, making the flour more colored, and, even worse, made the flour vulnerable to rancidity due to oxidation of the oil in the germ. With the invention of the roller mill system in the early 19th century, it was possible to produce the almost pure endosperm flour we know today as refined flour. In the roller-mill grinding system, the slightly soaked wheat is first cracked by a pair of rolls with a coarse surface such that the kernel is split into endosperm, germ, and bran. The endosperm is then further ground and purified through sifters, air classification systems, and further roller milling. This grinding system was introduced in the USA in the late 19th century, and quickly replaced the old stone mills. Today, this system of processing wheat into refined flour

TABLE 7.1 Composition of Different Wheat Fractions According to the USDA National Nutrient Database[3]

	Whole Wheat Flour	Refined Wheat Flour	Wheat Germ	Wheat Bran
Energy, kcal/100 g	340	364	360	216
Water,%	10.7	11.9	11.1	9.9
Protein,%	13.2	10.3	23.2	15.6
Fat,%	2.5	1	9.7	4.3
Starch,%	57.8	65	–	–
Dietary fiber,%	10.7	2.7	13.2	42.8
Iron, mg/100 g	3.6	1.2	6.3	10.6
Zinc, mg/100 g	2.6	0.7	12.3	7.3
Selenium, μg/100 g	61.8	33.9	79.2	77.6
Vitamin E, mg/100 g	0.71	0.06	16	1.49
Thiamin, mg/100 g	0.5	0.1	1.9	0.5
Folate, μg/100 g	44	26	281	79

is totally dominant worldwide. In Norway, close to 90% of the wheat used for human consumption is in the form of refined wheat flour, despite strong public promotion of whole wheat as a healthier alternative to refined wheat flour. It is therefore reasonable to assume that, on a global basis, at least 90% of the wheat products consumed are in the form of refined flour. In the US, in 2011, only 5% of the wheat flour consumed was whole wheat flour.[4]

STARCH

The starch content in whole wheat flour is around 58%, according to the USDA National Nutrient Database, which is only marginally lower than the 64% starch reported for refined flour. Pedersen and Eggum[5] found starch content as percentage of dry matter to increase from 70% to 81% when whole wheat was made into 80% extracted refined flour. Thus, starch is the quantitatively most important fraction of both whole wheat and refined flour. Due to the prominent role of wheat in many cultures, wheat starch will, in large parts of the world, be the most important source of energy in the diet. In Norway, for example, data from the Norwegian Health Directorate on average food consumption in 2011 indicate that wheat starch provided 16% of the total metabolizable energy intake, making it the largest single contributor to energy in the diet.

Two distinct populations of starch exist. Amylopectin consists of α1–4 glucose chains with frequent branches due to α1–6 bonds, while amylose is characterized by very few branches. Amylose has a molecular weight of around 500 kDa, but amylopectin has a much higher molecular weight in the order 50,000 kDa.[6] Amylose forms double helices or single helices in the native state,[6] and single helices give rise to a central cavity that can be filled with compounds such as iodine, alcohols, or fatty acids. Most starches contain between 200 and 250 g/kg amylose. In wheat, a range of 30–310 g/kg has been reported.[7–9] Starch is accumulated in granules in the endosperm, and the starch is deposited in layers with varying amylose and amylopectin content. Starch organization in the granule of cereals has been reviewed by Buléon et al.[6] and Donald,[10] and is only mentioned briefly here. The starch granule consists of alternating semicrystalline and amorphous layers. The semicrystalline layer is believed to consist of alternating 9-nm crystalline layers of double-helical α-glucans extending from intermittent branches of amylopectin, and the amorphous layers of amylopectin branch points. It has been hypothesized that one growth ring is laid down per day due to variation in photosynthetic activity and, thus, access to glucose.[11–12] Cornell et al.[13] found that the main peak for starch granule size was around 22 μm for wheat starch. A typical bimodal distribution in starch granule size has been reported in wheat, the large granules being between 16 and 26 μm in size and the small granules being between 2 and 10 μm in size.[8,14] The use of laser-scattering techniques has allowed finer separation of starch granules, and a trimodal distribution curve with peaks at 0.8, 4, and 22 μm has been found for wheat.[13,15]

Despite the extensive grinding process, starch granules are to a large extent intact in flour. Magnus et al.[16] reported that less than 5% of the starch granules were damaged. The extent to which starch granules in whole wheat flour are generally embedded in a protein matrix or surrounded by cell walls depends on the particle size of the flour. While refined flour is always ground to a particle size usually not exceeding 150 μm,[17] whole wheat flour may be ground on a stone mill to a much coarser particle size. However, whole wheat flour may also be produced by using a similar roller-mill grinding technique as for refined flour, where the endosperm and bran fraction of the wheat is combined with the flour in quantities equivalent to the original composition.[4] In this case, the starch fraction may have the same physical appearance in refined flour and whole wheat flour. Barros et al.[18] found that 99% of the particles of refined flour were smaller than 250 μm, 53–60% were smaller than 180 μm, and 23–33% were smaller than 75 μm. Kihlberg et al.[19] found 69–74% of the roller-milled whole wheat flour particles to be smaller than 250 μm, thus indicating that the difference in particle size from refined flour was mainly due to the particle size of reintroduced bran and germ particles. Likewise, Hallfrisch and Behall[20] found 100%, 90%, and 53% of the particles of finely ground whole wheat flour to be smaller than 150, 73, and 42 μm, respectively. In stone-milled whole wheat flour, only between 44% and 52% of the particles were smaller than 250 μm, indicating that this flour may have larger starch-rich particles.

In animal experiments, wheat starch has been shown to exhibit low digestibility in some cases.[21] However, wheat used in animal feeding differs from wheat used in human diets in that the former is of much coarser structure and is not heat treated to the same extent. Wheat used in human nutrition is almost invariably extensively heat treated, which destroys the starch granule structure and renders the starch much more available to digestion by the amylase secreted by the pancreas. Effects of processing on starch have been reviewed by Svihus et al.,[22] and will only be discussed briefly here. Changes in starch during processing have been extensively studied for human food applications. Most starches will gelatinize upon heating to above 80°C in excess water. Gelatinization markedly increases susceptibility for amylolytic degradation due to loss of crystalline structure.[23–26] In fact, Holm et al.[23] found a correlation of 0.96 between extent of gelatinization and digestion rate, indicating that the relationship is close to linear for pure starch. Donald[10] describes gelatinization as a swelling-driven process. Swelling occurs along the amorphous regions and, since the crystalline regions do not expand during swelling, stress increases at the interface between the crystalline and amorphous regions, where bonds exist between amylopectin in the crystalline regions and amylose in the amorphous regions. Thus, at a certain point in the swelling process the crystalline regions are rapidly and irreversibly broken and gelatinization is initiated. With excess water content, this onset of gelatinization usually occurs between 50°C and 70°C. Swelling causes nearly all amylose in the starch granule to leach out.[27] Viscosity increases during gelatinization, and is caused by swollen granules and gels consisting of solubilized amylose.[28]

Starch digestion generally occurs in the small intestine by the action of α-amylase, dextrinase, and glucoamylase. When measured on a total tract basis, starch digestibility appears to be almost complete for diets, independent of wheat bran content.[29] In comparative experiments with rats, even small-intestinal digestibility was 99% or higher. In an experiment with pigs, no difference in starch disappearance in the small intestine was found between refined flour and refined flour diluted with different bran fractions.[30] Steenfeldt et al.[31] found no differences in starch digestibility between flours made from whole wheat or the endosperm fraction in experiments with cockerels. Thus, despite surprisingly few studies on the starch digestibility of human subjects, starch appears to be more or less completely digested in the human digestive tract independent of the bran content. The rate at which starch is digested in humans can be indirectly measured through the blood glucose response after ingestion of a fixed amount of digestible carbohydrates. When refined flour products, which are known to result in a rather rapid increase in blood glucose levels, have been compared with whole wheat products, only small differences in the blood glucose response have been found.[17,32–33] This seems to corroborate the conclusion that wheat starch is rapidly digested independently of whether it is eaten as refined flour or whole wheat flour. How rapidly the starch from whole wheat flour is digested and absorbed will, however, be to some extent dependent on the particle size of the flour. Holt and Miller[33] showed that the glycemic index was significantly lower for cracked wheat (each grain cracked into approximately four pieces) than for finely ground whole wheat flour, but there was no difference in glycemic response between finely ground and coarsely ground whole wheat flour. Behall et al.[17] found that neither bread made from conventional whole wheat flour nor ultra-finely ground whole wheat flour gave a lower glycemic index than white bread made from refined flour. Similarly, Heaton et al.[34] found no differences in glycemic response or insulin response when subjects were fed baked products based on fine (78% smaller than 140 μm) as compared to coarse (16% smaller than 140 μm and 52% larger than 390 μm) whole wheat flour. Hallfrisch and Behall[20] found no differences in breath hydrogen between white bread, conventional and finely ground whole wheat bread, thus indicating small differences in fermentation independent of particle size.

FIBER

Wheat usually contains between 11% and 14% fiber, defined as non-starch polysaccharides plus lignin in the dietary fiber analysis.[35] A major fraction of the fiber comprises arabinoxylans, which usually constitute about half the fiber in wheat. The outer fractions of wheat, the pericarp and aleurone layers, have a higher fiber content than the endosperm. The pericarp, the aleurone layer, and the endosperm have been reported to contain 56%, 20%, and 3.5% dietary fiber, respectively.[30] The nature of the fiber fractions also varies between these different parts of the wheat kernel. The fibers of the pericarp are strongly lignified and contain around 30% cellulose.[30] The aleurone layer contains 22% cellulose, and is somewhat less lignified. The endosperm, in contrast, contains only 15% cellulose and very small amounts of lignin. Two-thirds of the fiber in wheat flour comprises arabinoxylans.[30] Since fiber content is highest in the aleurone layer and the outer layers of wheat, fiber content is strongly reduced in refined flour. The fiber content usually varies between 2.6% and 3.6%.[3,16] Due to the high content of cellulose and lignin, the fibers of the pericarp and aleurone layers are to some extent inert and will pass through the digestive tract without being altered and without affecting other nutrients. Le Gall et al.,[36] however, showed in experiments with pigs that fermentation was higher for whole grain flour than for refined flour diluted with cellulose, and thus indicated that some of the fibers in whole wheat flour may be fermentable. Hallfrisch and Behall,[20] on the contrary, did not find differences in fermentation, measured as breath hydrogen, between whole grain breads and refined flour bread.

NUTRITIONAL EFFECTS – WHOLE WHEAT FLOUR AND OBESITY

Obesity is a major nutrition-related health problem, and is caused by a net energy intake in excess of the energy used for basal metabolism and physical activity. From a nutritional point of view, it is thus the effect of a food on net energy intake which determines the contribution of a particular food to the problem of obesity. As already stated, wheat is the single most important contributor to energy intake in many cultures. In Norway, for example, data from the Norwegian Health Directorate for 2011 can be used to estimate that 22% of our metabolizable energy intake comes from wheat. In comparison, the other major sources of energy are milk, meat, and refined sugar, which contribute 17%, 13%, and 11% of our metabolizable energy intake, respectively. The main energy source in both refined and whole wheat flour is starch. Despite an earlier belief that the capacity of the human body to convert glucose into fat in so-called *de novo* lipogenesis was limited and of insignificant importance,[37–38] it is now clear that the capacity is in fact very large and thus that carbohydrates can contribute to obesity in a similar way to fat.[39–40] Pasquet et al.[41] studied a ritual fattening process among a tribe in Africa, where young lean men were overfed a starch-rich food (mainly sorghum with milk) for 2 months, and the difference between net fat deposition and fat intake indicated that *de novo* lipogenesis contributed at least 73 g body fat per day during the fattening period. This is also obvious and logical, since the capacity for storing glucose as glycogen is limited,[42] and the capacity for intake of digestible carbohydrate far exceeds the amount the body can use as an energy source. With a very high absorption capacity and no mechanisms for excretion of glucose, conversion into fat, mainly in the liver, is the only way the body can handle excess amounts.

Consumption of whole wheat products has been associated with decreased obesity when assessed in epidemiological studies.[1,2] The increased fiber content and decreased starch content will contribute to a lower energy concentration in whole wheat flour compared to refined flour. However, protein, and particularly fat content, is higher in whole wheat flour, and thus the energy concentration in whole wheat flour is only 7% lower than in refined flour.

In addition to energy concentration, the effect on satiety is another way foods may affect energy intake. Satiety results from a complex interplay between the brain, the digestive system, circulating fuels, and adipose tissue.[43] Different foods may affect satiety through subjective responses in the brain, or they may affect satiety through effects mediated via the digestive system or peripheral tissue such as adipose tissues. In experiments where products based on wheat have been compared with other foods, the satiating effect of wheat products has usually been relatively low. Holt et al.[44] found bread made from wheat flour generally to be less satiating than similar energy intakes of both fruits and other carbohydrate-rich foods, and protein-rich foods. The generally low satiating effect of bread and other products based on wheat flour may be explained by the low protein content, since it has been shown that protein gives a very high satiating effect.[45–48] In addition, it has been shown that high carbohydrate content contributes further to reduced satiety.[49] Bread made from whole wheat flour was reported to be more satiating than white bread.[44] Holt et al.[50] also observed a numerical but non-significant increase in the satiating effect of whole wheat bread compared to refined flour bread. Kristensen et al.[32] found whole grain bread to be more satiating than refined wheat flour bread, but did not observe any difference when pastas made from these two flour types were compared. Conversely, Hlebowicz et al.[51] did not observe differences in satiety when bread made from whole grain flour was compared with bread made from refined flour. The increased satiety sometimes observed with whole wheat flour could be due to increased fiber content, since fiber has been suggested to stimulate satiety.[52] However, the tendency for increased satiety could also be related to the increase in particle size, since Holt and Miller[33] showed that particle size was related to satiety. The differences in satiety response to whole wheat flour between experiments could therefore be due to the varying particle size of the whole wheat flour.

The moderate decrease in energy concentration and an inconsistent effect on satiety could explain the conflicting results of whole wheat intervention on weight loss. Kristensen et al.[53] carried out an intervention study where postmenopausal women were given a large part of an energy-reduced diet either as whole wheat products (minimum 50% whole wheat) or as refined wheat products. After 12 weeks there was no significant difference in weight loss, but total fat mass was significantly more reduced for the whole wheat group than the refined wheat group. Melanson et al.[54] compared diets with and without whole grain products in a weight-loss program for obese subjects, but found no difference in weight loss after 12 or 24 weeks between dietary interventions. Pereira et al.[55] also found no differences in weight between obese/overweight subjects after 6 weeks on a diet rich in either whole wheat products or refined wheat. Katcher et al.[56] reported a significantly greater weight loss in an experiment where participants were advised to consume whole grain products compared to a group advised against this food group.

The high starch and thus energy concentration in wheat and products based on wheat, and the rather low satiating effect of these products, means that wheat flour is a significant contributor to the high incidence of obesity in societies where large quantities of wheat are consumed. Replacing refined wheat flour with whole wheat flour may to some extent reduce this obesity-inducing effect of wheat products, but due to the marginal reduction in energy concentration and the variable effect on satiety, the effect will probably be modest at best.

WHOLE WHEAT FLOUR AND GLUCOSE METABOLISM

The starch in wheat is rapidly digested into glucose, which is absorbed in the small intestine. Thus, a high intake of wheat products will necessitate efficient handling of the large amounts of glucose entering the body. High amounts of glucose will trigger an insulin response, which will stimulate glucose uptake by the cells in the body, and thus results in a cascade of reactions such as a switch from fat oxidation to glucose oxidation, glycogen storage, and/or conversion of glucose into fat through de novo lipogenesis, dependent on the amount absorbed, activity level, and status of the body's glycogen stores. However, a growing proportion of the population has developed a reduced sensitivity to insulin and in some instances a reduced capacity to produce insulin, and thus has been diagnosed as having type 2 diabetes. The result is abnormally high blood glucose levels after ingestion of starch and other digestible carbohydrates. According to the International Diabetes Association, 366 million people worldwide suffer from diabetes. The highest prevalence is found in some of the Arab states, where it approaches 20% in a number of countries.[57] In China, prevalence increased from 2.6% to 9.7% during the period 2000–2010.[58]

Intake of nutrients which are converted to glucose is related to both the pathogenesis of type 2 diabetes[59] and the treatment of the condition.[60] Since wheat flour is quantitatively the most important source of glucose in many countries, this food group therefore obviously contributes both to the increasing prevalence of this disease and to the health problems associated with having developed the disease. A number of intervention trials have been carried out which demonstrate that reduction of starch and sugar intake through a reduced intake of wheat and other cereal products and sugar results in a regain of normal blood glucose levels in diabetic patients.[61–63] Replacement of wheat products based on refined wheat with whole grain products has been promoted as a way of reducing the problem of elevated blood glucose levels after ingestion of these products for persons with type 2 diabetes or impaired glucose tolerance. Indeed, Jenkins et al.[64] demonstrated that the glycemic index reduced proportionately with increased replacement of bread based on refined wheat flour with bread based on coarse whole wheat kernels. Several intervention trials carried out more recently, however, have indicated no large difference in blood glucose elevations between whole wheat and refined wheat products. Kristensen et al.[32] gave 20 subjects pasta or bread made from either whole wheat or refined wheat flour in a crossover experiment, and measured blood glucose levels regularly for 3 hours. Pasta consistently gave lower glycemic response values than bread, but no difference was observed between the flour types within the food groups. Similarly, Najjar et al.[65] found no difference in the blood glucose response in a similar experiment where bread based on refined wheat and whole wheat was compared in 11 overweight or obese men. Andersson et al.[66] did not find any differences in insulin sensitivity when overweight subjects were given whole grain or refined cereal products in a crossover study. In a similar study, however, Pereira et al.[55] found whole grain products to improve insulin sensitivity. As discussed above, it is possible that the coarse particle size in the experiment of Jenkins et al.[64] was the cause for the effect observed, and that the rather fine grinding commonly used in modern whole wheat products attenuates any effects on blood glucose response.

The high starch content in wheat and products based on wheat, which are rapidly and completely digested and absorbed as glucose, means that wheat flour is a significant contributor to type 2 diabetes and other health problems related to blood glucose regulation. Replacing refined wheat flour with whole wheat flour does not seem to alleviate this problem, except possibly when very coarsely ground whole wheat products are used.

References

1. Fardet A. New hypotheses for the health-protective mechanisms of whole-grain cereals: what is beyond fibre? *Nutr Res Rev* 2010;**23**: 65–134.

2. Bjorck I, Ostman E, Kristensen M, Anson NM, Price RK, Haenen GRMM, et al. Cereal grains for nutrition and health benefits: Overview of results from *in vitro*, animal and human studies in the HEALTHGRAIN project. *Trends Food Sci Technol* 2012;**25**:87–100.

3. USDA National Nutrient Database for Standard Reference. Available at: http://ndb.nal.usda.gov/index.html.

4. Doblado-Maldonado AF, Pike OA, Sweley JC, Rose DJ. Key issues and challenges in whole wheat flour milling and storage. *J Cereal Sci* 2012;**56**:119–26.

5. Pedersen B, Eggum BO. The influence of milling on the nutritive-value of flour from cereal-grains. 2. Wheat. *Qualitas Plantarum-Plant Foods Human Nutr* 1983;**33**:51–61.

6. Buléon A, Colonna P, Planchot V, Ball S. Starch granules: structure and biosynthesis. *Int J Biol Macromol* 1998;**23**:85–112.

7. Mohammadkhani A, Stoddard FL, Marshall DR. Survey of amylose content in Secale cereale, Triticum monococcum, T. turgidum and T. tauschii. *J Cereal Sci* 1998;**28**:273–80.

8. Peng M, Gao M, Abdel-Aal E-SM, Hucl P, Chibbar RN. Separation and characterization of A- and B-type starch granules in wheat endosperm. *Cereal Chem* 1999;**76**:375–9.

9. Abdel-Aal E-SM, Hucl P, Chibbar RN, Han HL, Demeke T. Physicochemical and structural characteristics of flours and starches from waxy and nonwaxy wheats. *Cereal Chem* 2002;**79**:458–64.

10. Donald AM. Review. Plasticization and self-assembly in the starch granule. *Cereal Chem* 2001;**78**:307–14.

11. Tester RF. Starch: the polysaccharide fractions. In: Frazier PJ, Donald AM, Richmond P, editors. *Starch: structure and functionality*. London, UK: The Royal Society of Chemistry; 1997. p. 163–71.

12. Smith AM. The biosynthesis of starch granules. *Biomacromol* 2001;**2**:335–41.

13. Cornell HJ, Hoveling AW, Chryss A, Rogers M. Particle size distribution in wheat starch and its importance in processing. *Starch* 1994;**46**:203–7.

14. Vasanthan T, Bhatty RS. Physicochemical properties of small- and large-granule starches of waxy, regular and high amylose barleys. *Cereal Chem* 1996;**73**:199–207.

15. Raeker MO, Gaines CS, Finney PL, Donelson T. Granule size distribution and chemical composition of starches from 12 soft wheat cultivars. *Cereal Chem* 1998;**75**:721–8.

16. Magnus EM, Brathen E, Sahlstrom S, Vogt G, Faergestad EM. Effects of flour composition, physical dough properties and baking process on hearth loaf properties studied by multivariate statistical methods. *J Cereal Sci* 2000;**32**:199–212.

17. Behall KM, Scholfield DJ, Hallfrisch J. The effect of particle size of whole-grain flour on plasma glucose, insulin, glucagon and thyroid-stimulating hormone in humans. *J Am Coll Nutr* 1999;**18**:591–7.

18. Barros F, Alviola JN, Rooney LW. Comparison of quality of refined and whole wheat tortillas. *J Cereal Sci* 2010;**51**:50–6.

19. Kihlberg I, Johansson L, Kohler A, Risvik E. Sensory qualities of whole wheat pan bread – influence of farming system, milling and baking technique. *J Cereal Sci* 2004;**39**:67–84.

20. Hallfrisch J, Behall KM. Breath hydrogen and methane responses of men and women to breads made with white flour or whole wheat flours of different particle sizes. *J Am Coll Nutr* 1999;**18**:296–302.

21. Svihus B. Research note: a consistent low starch digestibility observed in pelleted broiler chicken diets containing high levels of different wheat varieties. *Anim Feed Sci Technol* 2001;**92**:45–9.

22. Svihus B, Uhlen AK, Harstad OM. Effect of starch granule structure, associated components and processing on nutritive value of cereal starch: A review. *Anim Feed Sci Technol* 2005;**122**:303–20.

23. Holm J, Lundquist I, Bjorck I, Eliasson AC, Asp NG. Relationship between degree of gelatinisation, digestion rate *in vitro*, and metabolic response in rats. *Am J Clin Nutr* 1988;**47**:1010–6.

24. Bjorck I, Liljeberg H, Ostman E. Low glycaemic-index foods. *Br J Nutr* 2000;**83**:S149–55.

25. Kishida T, Nogami H, Himeno S, Ebihara K. Heat moisture treatment of high amylose cornstarch increases its resistant starch content but not its physiological effects in rats. *J Nutr* 2001;**131**:2716–21.

26. Perez H, Oliva-Teles A. Utilization of raw and gelatinized starch by European sea bass (Dicentrarchus labrax) juveniles. *Aquaculture* 2002;**205**:287–99.

27. Han X-Z, Hamaker BR. Amylopectin fine structure and rice starch paste breakdown. *J Cereal Sci* 2001;**34**:279–84.

28. Hermansson A-M, Kidman S. Starch – a phase-separated biopolymer system. In: Harding SE, Hill SE, Mitchell JR, editors. *Biopolymer mixtures*. Nottingham, UK: Nottingham University Press; 1995. p. 225–45.

29. Coles LT, Moughan PJ, Awati A, Darragh AJ, Zou ML. Predicted apparent digestion of energy-yielding nutrients differs between the upper and lower digestive tracts in rats and humans. *J Nutr* 2010;**140**:469–76.

30. Knudsen KEB, Hansen I. Gastrointestinal implications in pigs of wheat and oat fractions. *Br J Nutr* 1991;**65**:217–32.

31. Steenfeldt S, Knudsen KEB, Borsting CF, Eggum BO. The nutritive value of decorticated mill fractions of wheat. 2. Evaluation with raw and enzyme treated fractions using adult cockerels. *Anim Feed Sci technol* 1995;**54**:249–65.

32. Kristensen M, Jensen MG, Riboldi G, Petronio M, Bugel S, Toubro S, et al. Wholegrain vs refined wheat bread and pasta. Effect on postprandial glycemia, appetite, and subsequent *ad libitum* energy intake in young healthy adults. *Appetite* 2010;**54**:163–9.

33. Holt SHA, Miller JB. Particle size, satiety and the glycaemic response. *Eur J Clin Nutr* 1994;**48**:496–502.

34. Heaton KW, Marcus SN, Emmett PM, Bolton CH. Particle size of wheat, maize, and oat test meals: effects on plasma glucose and insulin responses and on the rate of starch digestion in vitro. *Am J Clin Nutr* 1988;**47**:675–82.

35. Svihus B, Gullord M. Effect of chemical content and physical characteristics on nutritional value of wheat, barley and oats for poultry. *Anim Feed Sci Technol* 2002;**102**:71–92.

36. Le Gall M, Serena A, Jorgensen H, Theil PK, Knudsen KEB. The role of whole-wheat grain and wheat and rye ingredients on the digestion and fermentation processes in the gut – a model experiment with pigs. *Br J Nutr* 2009;**102**:1590–600.

37. Acheson KJ, Schutz Y, Bessard T, Ravussin E, Jequier E, Flatt JP. Nutritional influences on lipogenesis and thermogenesis after a carbohydrate meal. *Am J Physiol* 1984;**246**:E62–70.

38. Schwarz J-M, Neese RA, Tumer S, Dare D, Hellerstein MK. Short-term alterations in carbohydrate energy intake in humans striking effects on hepatic glucose production, de novo lipogenesis, lipolysis, and whole-body fuel selection. *J Clin Invest* 1995;**96**:2735–43.

39. Acheson KJ, Schutz Y, Bessard T, Anantharaman K, Flail J-P, Jaquier E. Glycogen storage capacity and de novo lipogenesis during massive carbohydrate overfeeding in man. *Am J Clin Nutr* 1988;**48**:240–7.

40. Aarsland A, Chinkes D, Wolfe RR. Hepatic and whole-body fat synthesis in humans during carbohydrate overfeeding. *Am J Clin Nutr* 1997;**65**:1774–82.

41. Pasquet P, Brigant L, Froment A, Koppert GA, Bard D, de Garine I, et al. Massive overfeeding and energy balance in men: The Guru Walla model. *Am J Clin Nutr* 1992;**56**:483–90.

42. Acheson KJ, Flatt JP, Jequier E. Glycogen synthesis versus lipogenesis after a 500 gram carbohydrate meal in man. *Metabolism* 1982;**31**:1234–40.

43. Berthoud H-R, Sutton GM, Townsend RL, Patterson LM, Zheng H. Brainstem mechanisms integrating gut-derived satiety signals and descending forebrain information in the control of meal size. *Physiol Behav* 2006;**89**:517–24.

44. Holt SHA, Miller JCB, Petocz P, Farmakalidis E. A satiety index of common foods. *Eur J Clin Nutr* 1995;**49**:675–90.

45. Saris WHM, Tarnopolsky MA. Controlling food intake and energy balance: which macronutrient should we select? *Curr Opin Clin Nutr Metab Care* 2003;**6**:609–13.

46. Westerterp-Plantenga MS. The significance of protein in food intake and body weight regulation. *Curr Opin Clin Nutr Metab Care* 2003;**6**:635–8.

47. Halton TL, Hu FB. The effects of high protein diets on thermogenesis, satiety and weight loss: a critical review. *J Am Coll Nutr* 2004;**23**:373–85.

48. Veldhorst M, Smeets A, Soenen S, Hochstenbach-Waelen A, Hursel R, Diepvens K, et al. Protein-induced satiety: Effects and mechanisms of different proteins. *Physiol Behav* 2008;**94**:300–7.

49. Veldhorst MAB, Westerterp KR, van Vught AJAH, Westerterp-Plantenga MS. Presence or absence of carbohydrates and the proportion of fat in a high-protein diet affect appetite suppression but not energy expenditure in normal-weight human subjects fed in energy balance. *Br J Nutr* 2010;**104**:1395–405.

50. Holt SHA, Brand-Miller JC, Stitt PA. The effects of equal-energy portions of different breads on blood glucose levels, feelings of fullness and subsequent food intake. *J Am Diet Assoc* 2001;**101**:767–73.

51. Hlebowicz J, Lindstedt S, Bjorgell O, Hoglund P, Almér L-O, Darwiche G. The botanical integrity of wheat products influences the gastric distention and satiety in healthy subjects. *Nutr J* 2008;**7**:12.

52. Babio N, Balanza R, Basulto J, Bulló M, Salas-Salvadó J. Dietary fibre: influence on body weight, glycemic control and plasma cholesterol profile. *Nutr Hosp* 2010;**25**:327–40.

53. Kristensen M, Toubro S, Jensen MG, Ross AB, Riboldi G, Petronio M, et al. Whole grain compared with refined wheat decreases the percentage of body fat following a 12-week, energy-restricted dietary intervention in postmenopausal women. *J Nutr* 2012;**142**:710–6.

54. Melanson KJ, Angelopoulos TJ, Nguyen VT, Martini M, Zukley L, Lowndes J, et al. Consumption of whole-grain cereals during weight loss: Effects on dietary quality, dietary fiber, magnesium, vitamin B-6, and obesity. *J Am Diet Assoc* 2006;**106**:1380–8.

55. Pereira MA, Jacobs Jr DR, Pins JJ, Raatz SK, Gross MD, Slavin JL, et al. Effect of whole grains on insulin sensitivity in overweight hyperinsulinemic adults. *Am J Clin Nutr* 2002;**75**:848–55.

56. Katcher HI, Legro RS, Kunselman AR, Gillies PJ, Demers LM, Bagshaw DM, et al. The effects of a whole grain–enriched hypocaloric diet on cardiovascular disease risk factors in men and women with metabolic syndrome. *Am J Clin Nutr* 2008;**87**:79–90.

57. Alhyas L, McKay A, Majeed A. Prevalence of type 2 diabetes in the states of the co-operation council for the arab states of the gulf: A systematic review. *PLoS ONE* 2012;**7**:e40948.

58. Li H, Oldenburg B, Chamberlain C, O'Neil A, Xue B, Jolley D, et al. Diabetes prevalence and determinants in adults in China mainland from 2000 to 2010: A systematic review. *Diabetes Res Clin Pr* 2012;**98**:226–35.

59. Giaccari A, Sorice G, Muscogiuri G. Glucose toxicity: The leading actor in the pathogenesis and clinical history of type 2 diabetes – mechanisms and potentials for treatment. *Nutr Metab Cardiovas* 2009;**19**:365–77.

60. Wheeler ML, Dunbar SA, Jaacks LM, Karmally W, Mayer-Davis EJ, Wylie-Rosett J, et al. Macronutrients, food groups, and eating patterns in the management of diabetes. *Diabetes care* 2012;**35**:434–45.

61. Boden G, Sargrad K, Homko C, Mozzoli M, Stein TP. Effect of a low-carbohydrate diet on appetite, blood glucose levels, and insulin resistance in obese patients with type 2 diabetes. *Ann Intern Med* 2005;**142**:403–11.

62. Gannon MC, Nuttall FQ. Effect of a high-protein, low-carbohydrate diet on blood glucose control in people with type 2 diabetes. *Diabetes* 2004;**53**:2375–82.

63. Westman EC, Yancy Jr WS, Mavropoulos JC, Marquart M, McDuffie JR. The effect of a low-carbohydrate, ketogenic diet versus a low-glycemic index diet on glycemic control in type 2 diabetes mellitus. *Nutr Metab* 2008;**5**:36.

64. Jenkins DJA, Wesson V, Wolever TMS, Jenkins AL, Kalmusky J, Guidici S, et al. Wholemeal versus wholegrain breads: proportion of whole or cracked grain and the glycaemic response. *Br Med J* 1988;**297**:958–60.

65. Najjar AM, Parsons PM, Duncan AM, Robinson LE, Yada RY, Graham TE. The acute impact of ingestion of breads of varying composition on blood glucose, insulin and incretins following first and second meals. *Br J Nutr* 2009;**101**:391–8.

66. Andersson A, Tengblad S, Karlstrom B, Kamal-Eldin A, Landberg R, Basu S, et al. Whole-grain foods do not affect insulin sensitivity or markers of lipid peroxidation and inflammation in healthy, moderately overweight subjects. *J Nutr* 2007;**137**:1401–7.

WHEAT IN CANCER PREVENTION

Colorectal Cancer Prevention by Wheat Consumption: A Three-Valued Logic – True, False, or Otherwise?

Gabriel Wcislo, Katarzyna Szarlej-Wcislo

Military Institute of Medicine, Department of Oncology, Warsaw, Poland

INTRODUCTION

Modern science is permeated by any kind of analysis that relies on breaking something down into primary components. Thus, the method itself can be called "decomposable" in order to establish differences between entities.[1] More data concentrating on primary components would be helpful in achieving easier interpretation of investigated problems. This interpretation needs to be understood by using a language which is based upon primary logic and then mathematics. Looking through evidence from different medical investigations, it is not easy to infer a robust conclusion. "Simple" logic has been changing to a more sophisticated one that makes the interpretation more difficult to reach. The results from medical investigations very often cannot be interpreted with the use of bivalent logics such as classical sentential or Boolean logic, which provide only "true" and "false" alternatives. A three-valued logic appears to be a system in which there are three values indicating true, false, and an indeterminate third value.[2,3] More data are more difficult to interpret clearly, and therefore the answer should be positioned as one of the three-valued entities. We have this complicated situation in interpretation of collected data in the field of the preventive action of nutrients against malignant disease.

COLORECTAL CANCER: EPIDEMIOLOGY AND ETIOLOGY

Nutrients are substances in food that are primarily responsible for providing an energy source to run the system of a living organism independently of its structural organization. Humans are heterotrophs who must obtain their energy and nourishment from organic molecules manufactured by other organisms. Additional value in preserving health, in terms of preventing metabolic diseases and cancer, can be derived from eating "well-tailored" foods. Some nutrients in everyday foods, such as wheat, rye, and other grains, may be useful as strong preventive factors against disease, thus having clinical utility.

Another important part of the living system in the gut is the interaction between the intestinal microbiota and the central nervous system. Ingestion of *Lactobacillus ramnosus* is responsible for regulation of emotional behavior via changes of function in brain GABA (gamma-aminobutyric acid) receptor expression. GABA is the main central nervous system inhibitory neurotransmitter, and is significantly involved in regulating many physiological and psychological processes. Changes in GABA functions are implicated in the pathogenesis of anxiety and depression, which very often exist comorbidly with functional bowel disorders. Consumption of *Lactobacillus ramnosus* in experimental mice reduced the expression of GABA receptors (GABA $_{A\alpha2}$ at the level of mRNA) in the prefrontal cortex and amygdala with its increase in the hippocampus. The molecular events could be interpreted as important in reducing stress-induced corticosterone and anxiety- and depression-related behavior.[4] Moreover, accumulated experimental data have shown that colonization of the gut microbiota impacts mammalian brain development and subsequent adult behavior.[5] Bidirectional signaling between the gastrointestinal tract and the brain requires neural, hormonal, and immunological mechanisms. The gut–brain axis is a term coined to show how both systems are functionally responsible for maintaining the homeostasis of a living organism. Functional analysis of the gut microbiota in relation to the pathology of obesity, autism, and gastrointestinal diseases has been reported, and appears to have an increasing role in understanding many other abnormal conditions, hopefully including cancer.[6]

Colorectal cancer is the third most frequent cancer in men and the second in women. Male incidence rates appear greater than female rates for both proximal and distal cancers. Incidence rates declined by 2.9% per year during the period 1998–2001. This socially positive result comes from increased screening and polyp removal, which inhibits the progression of polyps to cancers. The mortality rate is similar in men and women, and is the fourth commonest cause of cancer death, which is the result of a better prognosis than more common cancers. Mortality rates from colorectal cancer have continued to decline in both men and women over the past 15 years at the level of 1.8% annually. Despite progress in screening, staging, and better treatments, over 35% of diagnosed patients with colorectal cancer die within 5 years. Only 40% of patients with colorectal cancer are diagnosed at a localized stage, when the rate of survival at 5 years is 90%.[7–10]

Management of colorectal cancer is based on surgery in most cases. For cancers that have not spread, surgical removal is often curative. A permanent colostomy is rarely needed for colon cancer, but a little more frequently required for rectal cancer. For rectal cancer, aside from surgery, chemotherapy alone or in combination with radiation therapy has been used successfully for many years. In colon cancer, other than surgery, chemotherapy used in an adjuvant setting or for palliation is considered as a mainstay in the treatment of such patients. In both cancers, rectal and colon, new treatment strategies have been approved since the beginning of the 21st century. Targeted therapy for colorectal cancer is available in clinical practice worldwide. There have been investigations regarding drugs that inhibit angiogenesis (the most developed strategy in the field of monoclonal antibodies and small molecules), with bevacizumab approved for the treatment of metastatic colorectal cancer, and EGFR (epidermal growth factor receptor) inhibitors such as cetuximab and panitumumab (both monoclonal antibodies) accepted for treating metastatic colorectal cancer with the expression of K-ras wild type.[11]

Colorectal cancer usually has a silent course without alarming signs and symptoms in its early stages. Therefore, a screening procedure should be helpful. For a clinically experienced physician, rectal bleeding, blood in the stool, a change in bowel habits, and cramping pain in the abdomen provide adequate signs and symptoms to suspect colorectal cancer. Risk factors are playing an increasing role in early detection of colorectal cancer. The primary risk factor for colorectal cancer is age, with more than 90% of cases diagnosed in patients older than 50 years. Risk is increased by a personal or family history of colorectal cancer and/or polyps, or a personal history of inflammatory bowel disease. Epidemiological investigations have revealed other risk factors to be smoking, alcohol consumption, physical inactivity, and a diet high in saturated fat and/or red meat with a low intake of fruits and vegetables. On the other hand, data have been reported focusing on the use of estrogen and non-steroidal anti-inflammatory drugs that may reduce colorectal cancer risk.[12]

Stools are a reservoir of many compounds, including indigestible parts of food, and many chemical substances, such as fecapentaenes, 3-ketosteroid, and heterocyclic amines, that are produced by the interaction of digestion and food products. It has been estimated that 10^{14} bacteria of hundreds of different species are colonized in the colon. Bacteria have indirect carcinogenic actions in the colon; they deconjugate and reduce bile acids, which further become active substances that promote cell proliferation and growth of adenomas.[13] Secondary bile acids (deoxycholic acid, lithocholic acid, 12-ketolithocholic acid) along with other fecal substances are responsible for the initiation of colorectal carcinogenesis. On the other hand, increased fiber intake in the form of wheat bran or cellulose may reduce the production and excretion of mutagens in stools.[14]

Fecapentaenes are characterized by highly potent mutagenic activity originating from intestinal bacterial production. High performance liquid chromatography (HPLC) analysis enables detection of at least eight forms of fecapentaene-like substances occurring in human stools. Two geometric isomers, fecapentaene-12 and fecapentaene-14, are present in paramount concentrations in the feces (21.7% of total), within fecalpentaene levels ranging from 5 µg to 6 mg/kg feces. Fecapentaenes are mutagens found in human feces that have direct genotoxic effects on colon epithelial cells. Fecapentaene-12 is considered a prototype substance that causes DNA single strand breaks, sister chromatid exchanges, and mutations in cultured human fibroblasts.[15–17]

Bile acids are associated with the digestion of fat. The presence of bile acids correlates with fat consumption, which is a known risk factor for colorectal cancer by activation of the AP-1 transcriptional factor associated with the promotion of malignant transformation in normal epithelial colon cells. Cholecystectomy is a surgical procedure that can result in high levels of bile acids in the cecum and ascending colon which might lead to increased frequency of right-sided colon cancer.[18,19]

Among the other significant etiologic factors, meat intake appears to have a critical role in the development of colorectal cancer. Cooking meats at high temperatures has long been considered a crucial factor in carcinogenesis, mainly regulated by heterocyclic amines. Thus it is thought that methods of red meat preparation and frequency of intake can be correlated with the prevalence not only of colorectal cancer but also of distal colorectal adenomas.[20,21]

It has been accepted that the human diet is too calorie-dense, with high animal fat, sugar (mostly refined carbohydrates) and alcohol contents. Despite divergent results of studies, in experimental studies positive results can be achieved, and in clinical trials results are very often inconclusive; current recommendations for decreasing the risk of colorectal cancer include dietary changes such as increased plant food intake with consumption of whole grains, vegetables, and fruits, and reduced intake of red meat.[22,23]

SCREENING FOR COLORECTAL CANCER

Cancer screening appears to have a crucial role in achieving clinical benefits at the social level. This goal is very practical, assuming detection of cancer at an early stage when it is treatable and curable. The screening procedure should lead to the early detection of asymptomatic or unrecognized malignant disease by the use of acceptable, inexpensive tests or examinations in a large number of individuals. The main aim of such a screening test is to reduce the morbidity and mortality from a particular cancer among the persons screened.[24] Several cancers are suitable for screening because of their substantial morbidity and mortality; their high prevalence in a preclinical state when detection is possible; the availability of a known treatment that can be applied in an early stage of cancer; and the availability of a good screening test characterized by accepted sensitivity and specificity, low cost, and little direct harm to a given subject. A short assessment of screening tests makes it easy to define cancers that could be suitable for intervention – namely, breast, cervix, colon and rectum, prostate, and other cancers important from the social standpoint.[25]

Patients diagnosed with localized colorectal cancer have a 90% 5-year survival rate.[26] Colorectal cancer mortality could be reduced both by early diagnosis and by cancer prevention using several methods, including polypectomy. Screening tests that can detect either cancer or adenomatous polyps are highly welcome.[27,28] The screening tests pursuing colorectal cancer can be divided in two broad categories: structural tests, and stool/fecal-based tests.[29]

A structural test is a tool for detection (e.g., radiologic imaging), or for detection and removal of adenomatous polyps by the use of an endoscopic instrument. An endoscopic examination may typically be a colonoscopy or a flexible sigmoidoscopy. Colonoscopy allows examination of the entire large bowel with removal of polyps in one session, but requires sedation of the patient. Therefore, this medical procedure is considered to be the current "gold standard" for the assessment of screening procedures. Polypectomy is also considered to be able to reduce colorectal cancer incidence by 50%.[30,31] Flexible sigmoidoscopy does not need sedation and careful bowel preparation, but it seldom crosses the boundary beyond 60 cm and is thus limited to examination of the end of the descending part of the colon tract. When examination by flexible sigmoidoscopy is positive in the form of multiple polyps larger than 1 cm, such patients should be referred for colonoscopy because of the higher propensity for adenomatous polyps to be located in the proximal part of the colon tract.[32] Virtual colonoscopy is an interesting diagnostic procedure that relies on computed tomographic colonography and has a radiation exposure dose of 10 mSv. This radiologic procedure may be useful for the detection of larger polyps measuring 10 mm or more. A positive finding with virtual colonoscopy requires a colonoscopy to remove the polyps.[33,34] A double-contrast barium enema has a marginal role in colorectal screening, and is typically used as an alternative for patients who cannot undergo colonoscopy.

Fecal tests are responsible for the detection of indications of cancer in stool samples, such as occult blood or changes in DNA from cancer cells. Currently, there are two fecal occult blood tests available; guaiac-based, and immunochemical. The guaiac-based tests have cancer detection rate of 37–79%. The range of detection is dependent on the size of the colon lesions (smaller lesions are less frequently detected) and non-human heme in food. The fecal immunochemical test directly detects human globin within hemoglobin, and does not require dietary restrictions. However, the sensitivity (25–72%) and specificity (59–97%) are also very wide.[35,36] A stool DNA test relies on detection of the presence of known DNA alterations that occur during colorectal carcinogenesis in tumor cells appearing in the stool. The first investigative attempt showed that K-ras mutation could be a marker of exfoliated tumor cells mixed in the stool.[37]

The incidence of colorectal cancer varies, and depends upon many factors due to both nature and nurture. The average risk of developing colorectal cancer emerges in humans at the age of 50 years and more, without a history of adenoma, colorectal cancer itself, inflammatory bowel disease, or family history predisposition. An increased risk of developing colorectal cancer embraces a personal history of adenomatous polyps, and factors defined above in the average risk group. Finally, high-risk syndromes are defined when a family history of Lynch syndrome or polyposis syndromes is precisely characterized. Table 8.1[38–48] shows representative results of large clinical studies screening individuals at an average risk of colorectal cancer development.

TABLE 8.1 Screening of Individuals at Average Risk of Colorectal Cancer: Representative Large Studies

Age at Entry	Number of Patients	Screening Method	Periodicity	Randomization (yes, no)	Outcome	Reference
I. STRUCTURAL SCREENING TEST						
50–90 years (mean 64 years)	2,412,077 patients	Complete colonoscopy	Not given	No	For every 1% increase in complete colonoscopy rate, the hazard of death from colorectal cancer decreased by 3%.	Rabeneck et al.[38]
60.3±8.7years	7882 patients	Colonoscopy	ND	No	Adenomatous polyps were detected in 23.5% of patients; hyperplastic lesions were detected in 21.4% of patients; advanced neoplasms were detected in 5.2% of patients; strong relationships between withdrawal times (less than 6 minutes vs 6 minutes and longer) and lesion-detection rates were observed.	Barclay et al.[39]
56.7±7.5 years	2436 patients	Screening colonoscopy at baseline and rescreening colonoscopy in those who had no neoplastic lesions in baseline colonoscopy	Rescreening after 5 years	No	Patients with no adenomas in screening were rescreened after 5 years; no cancer was found on rescreening colonoscopy; the risk of an advanced adenoma did not differ significantly between persons with no polyps at baseline and those with hyperplastic polyps at baseline (1.1% vs 2.0%), respectively; rescreening interval of 5 years or longer after a normal colonoscopic examination is sufficient.	Imperiale et al.[40]
45–91 years (mean 66 years)	261 patients	Rigid sigmoidoscopy	Sigmoidoscopy within 10 years before cancer diagnosis	No	Screening by sigmoidoscopy can reduce mortality from cancer of the rectum and distal colon (0.41 risk reduction [95% CI, 0.25–0.69]); screening once during 10 years can be efficacious as more frequent.	Selby et al.[41]
55–64 years	170,432 patients	Flexible sigmoidoscopy	Only once	Yes	Incidence of colorectal cancer in people attending screening was reduced by 33% (95% CI 0.67, 0.60–0.76) and mortality by 43% (95% CI 0.57, 0.45–0.72); the numbers that needed to be screened to prevent one colorectal cancer diagnosis or death were 191 (95% CI 145–277) and 489 (95% CI 343–852), respectively.	Atkins et al.[42]
Not given	4181 patients	CT colonography	Not given	No	CT colonography revealed, for large polyps (>1cm) per patient, average sensitivity 93% (95% CI: 73–98%) and specificity 97% (95% CI: 95–99%); sensitivity and specificity decreased to 86% (95% CI: 75–93%) and 86% (95% CI: 76–93%), respectively, when the threshold was lowered to include medium polyps (0.6–1cm). Data were inconclusive for small polyps (<0.6cm) due to heterogeneity. Of 150 cancers, 144 were detected (sensitivity 95.9%; 95% CI: 91.4–98.5%).	Halligan et al.[43]
Mean age of patients enrolled in included studies was 61.9 years	6393 patients	CT colonography		No	Sensitivity of CT colonography for detection of polyps <6mm was 48% (95% CI: 25–70%); for polyps 6–9mm, 70% (95% CI: 55–84%) and 85% (95% CI: 79–91%) for large polyps >9mm. Specificity was homogenous: 92% (95% CI: 89–96%, polyps <6mm), 93% (95% CI: 91–95%, polyps 6–9mm), and 97% (95% CI: 96–97%, for polyps >9mm).	Mulhall et al.[44]

Population / Age	Number of patients	Test / Method	Frequency		Results	Reference
Colonography group:57.0±7.2 years; Colonoscopy group:58.1±7.8 years	3120 patients (colonography group); 3163 patients (colonoscopy group)	CT colonography (CTC group); optical colonoscopy (OC group)	Once	No	Advanced neoplasia was confirmed in 100 of 3120 (3.2%) patients in CTC group and in 107 of 3163 (3.4%) in OC group (similar detection rates). 123 and 121 advanced neoplasms were found in CTC and OC groups, respectively. 14 cancers were found in CTC group and 4 cancers in OC group. The referral rate for OC in the primary CTC group was 7.9% (246 of 3120 patients). The total numbers of polyps removed in the CTC and OC groups were 561 and 2434, respectively.	Kim et al.[45]

II. STOOL/FECAL-BASED TEST

Population / Age	Number of patients	Test / Method	Frequency		Results	Reference
30.2% of patients were 50–59 years old; 39% of patients were 60–69 years old; 30.8% of patients were 70 or older	8104 study patients; 8065 were screened by Hemoccult II; 7904 were screened by Hemoccult II Sensa; 7493 were screened by HemeSelect; 7847 were screened by Hemoccult II Sensa and HemeSelect	Hemoccult II (detects the pseudoperoxidase activity of heme); Hemoccult II Sensa (detects the pseudoperoxidase activity of heme-more sensitive than Hemoccult II); HemeSelect (immunochemical test for human hemoglobin)	Once	No	The sensitivity for detecting carcinoma with Hemoccult II was 37.1% (95% CI: 19.7–54.6%), with combination Hemoccult II Sensa and HemeSelect was 65.6% (95% CI: 47.6–83.6%), with HemeSelect was 68.8% (95% CI: 51.1–86.4), and woтj Hemoccult II Sensa was 79.4% (95% CI: 64.3–94.5%). Specificity for detecting carcinoma was 86.7% with Hemoccult II Sensa, 94.4% with HemeSelect, 97.3% with combination test and 97.7% with Hemmoccult II.	Allison et al.[46]
50–74 years	15,011 patients	gFOBT-guaiac-based fecal occult blood test (arm 1); FIT-immunochemical FOBT(arm 2); FS – flexible igmoidoscopy(arm 3)	Once	Yes	gFOBT was positive in 2.8%, FIT in 4.8%, and FS in 10.2%. Detection rates for advanced neoplasia were: for FIT arm, 2.4%(OR 2.0 CI: 1.3–3.1); for FS arm, 8.0% (OR 7.0 CI: 4.6–10.7); for gFOBT arm, 1.1%. FS had a higher diagnostic yield of advanced neoplasia per 100 screened patients (2.4%) than gFOBT (0.6%) or FIT(1.5%).	Hol et al.[47]
50 years and older (mean 68.6 years)	4404 patients evaluated	Colonoscopy; Hemoccult II (detects the pseudoperoxidase activity of heme); the fecal DNA panel (21 mutations)	Once	648 patients were randomly selected for analysis from 1627 patients with minor polyps (tubular adenomas <1 cm and hyperplastic polyps); 1423 patients were randomly selected for analysis from 2318 patients with no polyps	Colonoscopy detected invasive adenocarcinoma in 31 patients. The fecal DNA panel detected 16 of 31 cancers (sensitivity 51.6%). Hemoccult II detected 4 of 31 cancers (sensitivity 12.9%) ($P=0.003$). Among 418 patients with advanced neoplasia (cancers plus large polyps), the DNA panel was positive in 76 (18.2%) whereas Hemoccult II was positive in 45 (10.8%) ($P=0.001$). As non-invasive test, the analysis of facal DNA detected a greater proportion of colorectal neoplasia than Hemoccult II test.	Imperiale et al.[48]

PREVENTION OF COLORECTAL CANCER

Prevention is defined as a medical activity that identifies significant various factors having important roles in carcinogenesis and that can be manipulated to alleviate their causal roles. Typically, prevention can be divided into two main categories: primary and secondary. Primary prevention of colorectal cancer includes a list of etiologic factors responsible for the development of this malignant disease. Among these are diet, energy intake, lifestyle and physical exercise, tobacco and alcohol use, parity, hormone use, and non-steroidal anti-inflammatory drug use. The list includes the prevalent factors regarding individuals with an average risk of colorectal cancer development. On the other hand, secondary prevention focuses on the identification of high-risk populations, embracing persons at increased risk of death from colorectal cancer in the presence of premalignant lesions or diagnosed early cancers. Secondary prevention strategies are used in, for example, the removal of adenomatous polyps by colonoscopic procedure, or even excision of the large bowel in famial adenomatous polyposis. Secondary prevention can therefore be used when a high-risk population of persons or patients has been characterized as needing accurate management to prevent colorectal cancer spreading. Table 8.2 presents factors important for primary and secondary prevention against colorectal cancer.

As indicated above, there are many factors of different categories that play important roles in colorectal carcinogenesis, and it is beyond the scope of this chapter to discuss them all. However, primary prevention of colorectal cancer by dietary modifications may be of critical value for all humans to be protected against colorectal cancer development, even if only partially. It seems that wheat, and especially wheat bran, consumption could be an important factor in providing health benefits in the sphere of colorectal cancer prevention.[49–51]

WHEAT CULTIVATION, CROPPING, AND BIOLOGY

Wheat is a well-known cereal grain that is grown on arable lands and is responsible for sustaining commercial food production worldwide. Wheat is the most important source of vegetable protein in human food and has the highest protein content in comparison with other cereals such as maize or rice. Wheat appears to be the most widely grown crop in the world. It represents a renewable resource for food, animal feed, and various kinds of industrial processes involving food. Wheat grows widely in various areas, but the best climate is found between latitudes 30–60 N and 27–40°S. It can be cultivated at elevations ranging from sea level to 3000 meters. Soil for wheat cultivation should be neutral to slightly acidic (pH 5.5–6.5), and the temperature approximately 25°C. All wheat species are annual plants. The most popular are spring wheat plants, which are planted in the spring, have a short growing season (less than 100 days), and are harvested in the fall. Conversely, winter wheat grains are planted in the fall and harvested in early summer. The average farm yield for wheat is approximately 3 tonnes per hectare, and the most productive farms are in The Netherlands and Belgium, where the yield is 8.9 tonnes per hectare. Wheat is a major staple crop worldwide, with consumption running at approximately 30% of dry matter and 60% of the daily calorie intake in some developing countries.[52,53]

Wheat (*Triticum* spp.) together with barley (*Hordeum* spp.) form the Poaceae, the largest family within the monocotyledonous plants, which constitute the most important cereal crops in the world. The genetics of wheat species is more complicated than in most other domesticated plants because some are diploid while others are stable polyploids, tetraploid, or even hexaploid. Einkorn wheat (*Triticum monococcum*) is diploid (AA), with two complements of seven chromosomes ($n = 7$) ($2n = 14$). Tetraploid ($4n = 28$) species with four sets of chromosomes include emmer wheat (*Triticum dicoccum*), which is less important in modern agriculture, and durum wheat (*Triticum durum*), which is widely cultivated by farmers worldwide. Common wheat, also known as bread wheat (*Triticum aestivum*),

TABLE 8.2 Factors Important for Primary Prevention or Secondary Prevention of Colorectal Cancer

Primary Prevention	Secondary Prevention
Age ≥ 50	Family history of colorectal cancer or polyps
Diet with low fiber and high animal fat (increased risk)	Familial polyposis syndromes (Peutz-Jeghers syndrome, Gardner syndrome, juvenile polyposis)
Alcohol and tobacco use (increased risk)	Hereditary non-polyposis colon cancer (Lynch syndromes I & II)
Energy intact resulting in overweight and obesity (increased risk)	Inherited colorectal cancer in Ashkenazi Jews
Sedentary lifestyle with low physical activity (increased risk)	Medial control of inflammatory bowel disease
Detection of inflammatory bowel disease and adenomatous polyps (jump in secondary prevention)	Bowel status after pelvic irradiation

is a hexaploid species ($6n = 42$) that is widely used throughout the world. Spelt wheat (*Triticum spelta*), which is cultivated in limited quantities, is also considered to be a subspecies of common wheat.[54] The presence of certain versions of wheat grains depends on the genetic variation, which has a great impact in higher protein content, better cultivation, and crop yields. Wheat is used as human food or for animal feed. On the other hand, farro is a food product composed of various species of wheat. Genetic selection has an interesting history, starting back in antiquity during domestication.

THE HISTORY OF WHEAT DOMESTICATION

Cereals were the first species that were domesticated by man, at almost the same time as dogs, sheep, and cattle. This process has been discovered independently on all continents. In the case of practical plants, domestication appears as the suite of morphological and anatomical changes that follow cultivation necessary for an altered human environment. Thus domestication is different from conscious cultivation, which in fact began with related wild species. Evolutionary botany is a natural discipline that uses molecular genetics tools and draws knowledge from archeological investigations and that may more precisely reconstruct the evolutionary scenarios of wheat domestication. Why farming became a turning point for the evolutionary progress of humankind will probably never be known. Some ethnologists claim that demographic expansion was the main cause for humans becoming farmers, in order to increase food resources due to an increase in human population; and the practice of primitive agriculture required more energy than hunting and gathering, so agriculture became a necessity rather than an adaptation to novel inhabited environments.[55,56]

Salt and silt are two important factors in the development of Mesopotamian agriculture. The semiarid climate with low soil permeability is responsible for dangerous accumulations of salt, which is harmful to crops and soil texture. This process is responsible for the progressive changes that contributed to the settlement and development of past civilizations regarding necessary plant cultivation and animal husbandry.[57] Wheat is one of the first cereals that were domesticated from the wild species, characterized by its ability to self-pollinate, which greatly facilitated the selection of more practical species. Archeological investigations suggest that wheat appeared in the Fertile Crescent and the Nile Delta.[58] Recent results have shown that einkorn wheat was domesticated at Nevali Cori in southern Turkey 9000 years ago. Domestication is considered to have

been a series of events, occurring at different places over many thousands of years, during which wheat persisted in cultivated fields. It has been suggested that domestication was a gradual process, being a result of the sedentary existence of our ancestors in the early villages of the Near East.[59] On the other hand, there have been results indicating that processing of wild cereal grains in the Upper Paleolithic (Ohalo II, Israel) was practiced at least 12,000 years before domestication in southwest Asia. The oldest evidence for processing of wild cereals as starch grains from barley and wheat was noted in grinding stones.[60]

One of the oldest mummies in the world, found in the Alps and better known by the popular humanizing nickname Ötzi, died at the age of 46 years approximately 5300 years ago. The corpse was perfectly preserved in ice for such a long time that meticulous investigations led to remarkable opportunities for extraordinary findings, including the contents of the colon, where the food residue had been preserved. Botanical assessment of the colon contents revealed bran and other remains of einkorn wheat and barley (45%), pollen (22%), and charcoal particles of coniferous wood (25%). Moreover, these studies revealed that Ötzi had been omnivorous, eating the meat of red deer and ibex.[61,62]

As indicated, domestication of plants and animals is the main factor responsible for changes in the development of human civilization. A pivotal position in the domestication of plants during early human agriculture development is held by einkorn wheat. For more than 50 years, the progress of molecular biology progress and its effective molecular techniques with appropriate scientific strategies have been playing a critical role in the determination of some wild species of plants that can be fully used as practical plants in modern agriculture. Phylogenetic analysis based on the allelic frequency of 288 amplified fragment length polymorphism marker loci, indicating a wild group of *Triticium monococcum boeticum* from the Karacadag mountains (southeast Turkey) that was likely the progenitor of cultivated einkorn wheat cereals. Moreover, archeological excavations of early agricultural settlements have supported this molecular conclusion.[63-65]

THE DEFINITION OF WHEAT BRAN AND DIETARY FIBER, AND A BRIEF CHEMISTRY

Industrialization and Westernization have led to the most prevalent ways of living in the modern world. Whether they always lead to a better and healthier life is highly debatable when taking into account new life-threats related to a disease associated with the progress of our civilization. Nearly 70 years after World War II ended, everyday living has been changing with an increase in wealth of entire societies – at least, this is a main goal of democratic governments. However, we know that an energy-dense, low-fiber diet, which is especially popular in economically developed parts of the world, plays a major role in the development of many diseases, such as obesity, cardiovascular disease, type 2 diabetes, and cancer.

The problem of eating the indigestible parts of plants in the context of pregnancy toxemia was described for the first time in 1953 by Eben Hipsley.[66] In the 1970s, Burkitt and Trowell shed some light on fiber, defined more than 20 years earlier, regarding its beneficial effects on cardiovascular disease, type 2 diabetes, and cancer.[67] It appeared that the intake of dietary fiber should have a major role in sustaining health in the sphere of some diseases that appear frequently in society. It is necessary, then, to define the term "dietary fiber". Initially, fiber was defined as insoluble fibrous plant material that was not digested in the upper intestinal tract, but this definition has changed with accumulated knowledge on the chemistry of dietary fiber. Dietary fiber is presently defined as carbohydrates consumed as food, which cannot be fully digested or absorbed in the upper intestinal tract. Carbohydrates are polymers with 10 or more monomeric units, which are not hydrolyzed by endogenous enzymes in the small intestine and belong to one of the following groups: (1) edible carbohydrate polymers that occur naturally in food as consumed; (2) carbohydrate polymers that have been obtained from raw material in food by physical, enzymatic, or chemical means, and have been shown, by generally accepted scientific evidence by competent authorities, to have beneficial physiological effects on health; (3) synthetic carbohydrate polymers that have been shown, by generally accepted scientific evidence by competent authorities, to have beneficial physiological effects on health. Thus, fiber compounds can be either soluble or insoluble in water. Soluble compounds behave like colloids; they are viscous and form gels, have the capacity to hold water, and can bind to or be adsorbed by bile acids and other organic molecules.[68,69] Wheat is a well-accepted source of protein, carbohydrates, minerals, B group vitamins, and dietary fiber, and is therefore considered to be an excellent health-building food.[70] Dietary fiber is mainly composed of starch and polysaccharides that occur naturally in plants. Table 8.3[71,72] lists chemical compounds that are present in dietary fiber, along with a brief description. There is also a group of various substances that are often associated with fiber but do not qualify to be included within the definition of dietary fiber, such as phenols, waxes, cutin, phytic acid, and phytosterols.[72]

BIOLOGICAL ACTIVITY OF WHEAT BRAN AND DIETARY FIBER COMPOUNDS IN COLORECTAL NORMAL AND CANCER CELLS

Accumulated evidence indicates that dietary fiber consumption may have a role in the prevention of development of colorectal cancer, closely associated with direct effects on stool bulk and bile acid output.[73–75] A number of mechanisms are postulated to play roles, as a result of fiber consumption, in the prevention of colorectal cancer development, including intestinal transit time, adsorption of metabolically active materials, intraluminal antioxidant activity, the chemical environment of the colon, and fecal flora and bacterial enzymatic activity. Dietary fiber is resistant to human intestinal enzymes, which may explain the greater fecal bulk seen with higher fiber intake. This leads to lower colonic exposure to carcinogens through a simple dilution effect due to fiber consumption.[76,77]

A body of accumulating animal evidence has shown that wheat bran plays a critical role in the prevention of development of a range of cancers, especially colorectal and breast. Wheat bran is a rich source of dietary fiber that includes many structures and chemical substances enabling protective activity against carcinogens. Dietary fiber makes up less than half of wheat bran; the rest consists of phytochemicals such as phytic acid, and various phenolic components (phenolic acid, lignans, and flavonoids).[78] The effects of wheat bran consumption at the macro level are mainly associated with the reduction in transit time, increased fecal bulking, and the dilution of potentially carcinogenic compounds. Fermentation of wheat bran by colonic bacteria produces short-chain fatty acids, including acetate, propionate, and butyrate, which are rapidly absorbed by the colonic mucosa. Butyrate is the main source of energy for epithelial cells lining the colon, and has a range of effects relevant to reducing colorectal cancer risk.[79] Conversely, when protein is fermented in the colon for a longer time, by-products such as ammonia and phenols (p-cresol and phenol) may be harmful in facilitating carcinogenesis. Supplementation of wheat bran consumption, especially directed against ammonia and phenol products, could be achieved by the use of resistant starch (i.e., undigested carbohydrate present in the colon lumen) which has physiologic characteristics such as increasing concentrations of short-chain fatty acids, a lower pH, and lower levels of ammonia, phenols, and secondary bile acids.[80] Many mechanisms have been reported that could explain, to a greater or lesser degree, the preventive activity of wheat bran, and in fact of its two main parts – i.e., dietary fiber and wheat bran oil (lipid fraction of wheat bran). Wheat bran fiber supplementation can inhibit cell proliferation of stimulated normal colon mucosa or colorectal cancer cell lines; moreover, inhibition of DNA synthesis has been detected.[81,82]

TABLE 8.3 Chemical Compounds of Dietary Fiber with Short Characterization[71,72]

Larger Structure	Chemical Group	Chemical Compound	Structural Description And Characteristics
Resistant and slowly-digested starch stored in plants as crystalline granules	–	Amylopectin	70–80% of edible starch as large branched molecules of more than 10,000 glucose monomers
		Amylose	20–30% of edible starch as fewer glucose monomers linked by α 1:4 glycosidic linkages
Non-starch polysaccharides	Glucans (insoluble or soluble state)	β-glucans	Consist of approximately 250,000 glucose monomers in form of thermo-reversible, worm-like and cylindrical molecules; can be viscous or soft gel (weight dependent)
		Cellulose	Stiff structure, unbranched crystalline β-glucans consisting of 2000–15,000 glucose monomers
	Hemi-celluloses (insoluble or soluble state)	Arabinoxylans	Structure of twisted ribbon consisting of 1500–5000 L-arabinose branches
		Xyloglucans	Bind to surface of cellulose microfibrils; occur in cell walls; have glucose backbone with xylose side chains
		Glucomannan	Consists of chains of repeating units of glucose and mannose bound by β 1:4 linkages with short side chains
	Beta-fructans (only soluble)	Inulins	Linear fructans consisting of 20–1000 β 2:1 linked fructose molecules; enzymatic hydrolysis yields 3—10 monomers
		Levans	Linear fructans made up of fructose molecules with β 2:1 and β 2:6 glycosidic links
		Graminans	Branched fructans consisting of β 2:1 and β 2:6 glycosidic-linked fructose molecules
	Galactans (only soluble)	Agar	Polymer of two classes of unbranched mixed α- and β-galactans: agarowe and agaropectin
		Corrageenans	Linear polymers of approximately 25,000 α-galactans
		Pectin	Complex, worm-like, flexible, acidic polysaccharides formed of partially methylated esters of α 1:4 D-galactose residues
	Mannans (only soluble)	–	Polymers of mannose complex structures
	Galacto-mannans (only soluble)	–	Consist of β 1:4 linked mannose backbone with α 1:6 D-galactose
	–	Xylan (only soluble)	Linear polysaccharide consisting of β 1:4 linked D-xylose (wood sugar)
Non-digestible oligosaccharides		Fructo-oligosaccharide	β 2:1 linear fructose polymer
		Galacto-oligosaccharide	Polymer of β-galactose molecules
		Raffinose-oligosaccharide	Trisaccharide consisting of galactose linked by α 1:6 linkage to sucrose
		Stachyose	Tetrasaccharide consisting of galactose and raffinose
		Verbascose	Pentasaccharide consisting of galactose and raffinose units

(Continued)

TABLE 8.3 Chemical Compounds of Dietary Fiber with Short Characterization[71,72]—cont'd

Larger Structure	Chemical Group	Chemical Compound	Structural Description And Characteristics
Sugar alcohols	Sorbitol, mannitol, erythriol, xylitol, isomalt, lactitol, maltitol	Erythriol	Absorber unchanged and oxidized partially to fructose
Non-digestible carbohydrate compounds bound to non-carbohydrate molecules	Glysocaminoglycan (bound to amino acids)	Chitin	Poly-glucosamino-glycan consisting of β-glucans linked by β 1:4 bonds to form acetyl-glucosamine
		Chitosan	Similar to chitin but less acetylated with lower molecular weight
		Hyaluronic acid (hyaluronian)	Non-sulfated polymer of glucoronic acid linked by glucosidic bonds to acetyl-glucosamine; viscous, slippery, and forms gel
	Glycoproteins (bound to proteins)	Psyllium	Combination of arabinoxylans, monosaccharides (arabinose, galactose, glucose, mannose, rhamnose, uronic acid, xylose); digested in upper intestinal tract, water-soluble, forms gels, holds water, binds organic molecules and is fermented in large bowel
		Gluten	Consists of gliadin, holdein, secalin, zein (avenin), and glutelin (protein) –all proteins responsible for immune reaction in celiac disease
		Heparan sulfate	Consists of two or three glucosaminoglycan chains of acetyl-glucosamine linked to glucuronic acid and iduronic acid
		Dermatan sulfate	Made up of cross-linked glucosamino-glycans, chains of acetyl-galactosamine and D-glucoronic or iduronic acid
		Chondroitin sulfate	Composed of glycosamino-glycan chain of more than 100 alternating acetyl-galactosamine and β-D-glucuronic acid
		Keratan sulfate	Large, highly hydrated glycoprotein composed of glycosamino-glycan of repeating units of acetyl-galactosamine and galactose
	Saccharides (bound to terpens and phenols)	Saponins	Group of complex linear or branched hydrophilic glycosides (glucose, galactose, xylose, glucoronic acid); insoluble in water, bind bile salts and organic material in intestine tract, make foam in water
		Lignins	Insoluble in water, not fermented in colon, complex phenolic macromolecule covalently linked in cellulose microfibrils in cell walls, filling spaces between cells, which is responsible for mechanical strength of plants

The results of such a broad biological activity of wheat bran rely on both the inhibition of cell proliferation in the case of cancer cells, and the development of aberrant crypt foci dispersed in normal colon mucosa.[83–85] Wheat bran oil has also strong colonic tumor inhibitory properties. The main mechanism leading to anticancer activity is probably associated with the alteration of iNOS (inducible nitric oxide synthase) and COX (cyclooxygenase)-1 and -2 enzyme activities. The anticancer action of wheat bran oil has been demonstrated in the Apc(Min/+) mouse model.[86,87] A mixture of chemical compounds present in wheat bran and whole grains has multidirectional pharmacological activities that could be responsible for a reduced risk of chronic disease and cancer. One of the most important mechanisms readily seen in anticancer action is antioxidant activity. Among the most active compounds that have such anticancer activity are phenols (ferulic acid) and other bound phytochemicals.[88]

Psyllium

Psyllium (ispaghula) is the common name for several plants belonging to the genus Plantago and whose seeds are primary used for the production of mucilage. Dietary fiber contains psyllium, which is a glycoprotein that is not absorbed by the small intestine. Structurally, psyllium is a complex chemical compound (see Table 8.3), being a soluble fiber with a mechanical action associated with its mucilaginous nature and reliance on the absorption of excess water while stimulating normal bowel elimination. Psyllium has both positive and negative effects; on the positive side, it is linked to normalization of higher levels of plasma cholesterol.[89]

Some experimental results have also shown that psyllium along with wheat bran can enhance inhibition of colon cancer, giving greater protective effects against azoxymethane-induced colonic tumors in Fischer-344 rats. Psyllium and wheat bran are active partners in maximum mammary tumor-inhibiting effects through decreased cecal β-D-glucuronidase activity due to the increased psyllium content. Unfortunately, no statistical significant differences in circulating estrogens or urinary estrogen excretion were observed.[90,91]

On the negative side, ingestion of a psyllium-containing cereal can lead to anaphylaxis that may end in death in sporadic cases.[92]

Fermented Wheat Germ Extract (FWGE, Avemar, Awge)

FWGE is defined as an extract of wheat germ derived from the germ of a wheat plant. It is available commercially as a dietary supplement, being the product of industrial fermentation of wheat germ and having a unique characteristic that is useful in anticancer management. Avemar pulvis is a powder consisting of an aqueous extract of fermented wheat germ with maltodextrin and silicon dioxide, standardized to contain circa $200\,\mu g/g$ of the natural constituent 2,6-dimethoxy-p-benzoquinone.[93,94]

The chemical composition of FWGE is complex because it is a multisubstance compound with two main biologically active entities: 2-methoxy benzoquinone and 2,6-dimethoxy benzoquinone. Biochemically, FWGE interferes with anaerobic glycolysis, the pentose cycle, and ribonucleotide reductase. Four mechanisms of action are postulated: a metabolic effect, an antiproliferative effect, an antimetastatic effect, and an immunological effect.

1. The metabolic effect of FWGE relies on inhibition of glucose uptake in cancer cells and interference with enzymes of anaerobic glycolysis – transkelotase, glucose-6-phosphate dehydrogenase, lactate dehydrogenase, and hexokinase. All the enzymes are necessary for the allocation of precursors for RNA and DNA synthesis.
2. An antiproliferative effect has been investigated in human tumor models *in vitro* and *in vivo*. Such experimental studies have shown potential antitumor activity in colon, testis, thyroid, ovary, lung, breast, gastric, head and neck, liver, glioblastoma, melanoma, cervical, and neuroblastoma human cancer cell lines. FWGE was found to reduce tumor growth in a dose-dependent manner.[95,96]
3. An antimetastatic effect has been observed alone or in combination with cytostatic drugs such as 5-fluorouracil or dacarbazine. Researchers used various tumor models, among them colon cancer cell lines, to demonstrate an antimetastatic effect of FWGE.[95,96]
4. An immunological effect was observed in preclinical studies when FWGE's action could not be attributed to its direct antiproliferative effect. *In vivo* experimental models have shown that FWGE is also effective by enhancing the activity of the immune system, for example, by stimulating NK cells (by reducing MHC I molecule expression), enhancing TNF secretion by macrophages, or increasing ICAM1 molecule expression on the vascular endothelial cells.[95,96]

FWGE appears to have an impact in reducing colon carcinogenesis induced by azoxymethane, as used in Fischer-344 rats. The antitumor activity of FWGE is mainly associated with previously described postulated mechanisms. A relatively new path that needs meticulous investigation is the inclusion of FWGE in combination with other well-accepted anticancer drugs, such as 5-fluorouracil, oxaliplatin or irinotecan, that have been clinically tested in the treatment of colorectal cancer patients. The most biologically active part of FWGE is benzoquinone, which itself has not been toxic in tested doses, but has anticarcinogenic action.[97–99] Aleurone is a protein that occurs in the form of minute granules, or in a special peripheral layer, in the endosperm of seeds. Fermentation of dietary fiber by microflora enhances the levels of effective metabolites to protect normal colon epithelium against malignant transformation. Wheat aleurone is a source of dietary fiber and has many biological activities, including regulation of cell growth, apoptosis, and differentiation. These processes could be responsible for the cancer-preventive action of fermented wheat aleurone in the colon.[100,101]

FWGE has mainly been tested in experimental models, but clinical trials have also been performed in patients with colon cancer and melanoma. In melanoma, a randomized pilot Phase II study was carried out in an adjuvant setting with the use of FWGE.[102] The open-label cohort trial was designed to compare anticancer treatments plus FWGE (dose of 9 g daily through 6 months) with anticancer treatments alone in colorectal cancer. The experimental group comprised 66 colorectal cancer patients, and the control group 104 colorectal cancer patients. End-point analysis revealed that progression-related events were significantly less frequent in the experimental group with FWGE treatment than in controls: new recurrences 3% vs 17.3%, $P < 0.01$; new metastases 7.6% vs 23.1%, $P < 0.01$; deaths 12.1% vs 31.7%, $P < 0.01$, respectively. Survival analysis showed significant improvements in progression-free survival ($P = 0.018$) and overall survival ($P = 0.027$) in patients given FWGE.[103]

Lignans

Lignans are chemical compounds, defined as phytoestrogens, found in plants. Plant lignans are polyphenols derived from phenylanaline (pinoresinol, lericiresinol, secoisolariciresinol, syringaresinol, or sesamin), and can be metabolized by intestinal bacteria to form mammalian lignans such as enerodiol and enterolactone. Lignans act as antioxidants and can bind to estrogen receptors in the breast tissue. The crucial role in the synthesis of mammalian lignins via the phenylpropanoid pathway is played by pinoresinol lariciresinol reductase.[104,105] Lignans (entroldiol and enterolactone) are involved in cytostatic activity against colon cancer cell lines. In spite of the lack of cytotoxicity, measured by proliferation capacity, DNA flow cytometry analysis revealed cell cycle arrest at the S phase with a readily seen decrease of cyclin A detected by Western blotting.[106]

Lignins

Lignins originating from wheat cereal may be responsible for protective activity against cancer.[107,108] Lignins are complex chemical compounds that fill the spaces in the cell walls between cellulose, hemicellulose, and xylem, forming tracheids and vessels in higher plants. Although lignins are indigestible by animal enzymes, they can be precursors of mammalian lignans.[109,110]

Tricin

Tricin is a flavonoid that was primarily found in rice bran, but can also be found in other grass species such as wheat, barley, and maize. Tricin can be prepared by chemical synthesis via the Baker–Venkata–Raman reaction between acetylsyringic acid and phloroacetophenone, or by separation by high performance liquid chromatography from an antioxidant product derived from bamboo leaves.[111] Tricin exhibits anti-growth activity in several human cancer cell lines via its well-expressed anti-inflammatory potential. Experimental results collected after determining tricin inhibitory activity against inflammation-related colon carcinogenesis in male Crj:CD-1 mice relied on decreased expression of TNF-α in the non-lesional crypts in the colon mucosa and the proliferation of adenocarcinomas.[112]

Phytic Acid

Phytic acid is a major fiber-associated component of wheat bran and legumes. The principal role of phytate in many plants is storage of phosphorus, especially in bran and seeds. Phytic acid, also known as hexaphosphorylated inositol (IP6), can be internalized by cells, and can therefore be responsible for changes in the biochemical functions of secondary messengers. Phytic acid targets cancer cells by modulation of cell signaling, alterations in the cell cycle, non-homologous end-joining DNA repair, or activation apoptosis.[113,114] Dietary fiber with endogenous phytic acid component, and pure exogenous phytic acid added to a low-fiber diet, can increase the rate of apoptosis and degree of differentiation in the distal colon.[115] One of the significant molecular targets for phytic acid appears to be nuclear factor-κB (NF-κB), a well-known member of the transcriptional factor family, which plays important roles in regulating the expression of genes involved in a number of cellular processes. Results of an experimental study performed on the colon cancer cell line Caco-2 showed that phytic acid primarily influences p65 (the NF-κB subunit) and IκBα gene expression by their stimulation, which is responsible for inhibition of cancer cell proliferation.[116]

Lunasin

Lunasin is a 43-amino acid peptide derived from the soybean 25 albumin seed protein that has both anticancer and anti-inflammatory activities. Although initially isolated in soybean, lunasin has recently also been isolated in barley and wheat. More recent experimental studies have demonstrated that lunasin can inhibit the growth of some cancer cells both in culture and in mouse *in vivo* models.[117–119] Lunasin is a unique peptide that contains, at its carboxyl end, nine asparagine residues, the RGD (arginine–glycin–asparagine) cell adhesion motif, and a predicted helix with structural homology to a conserved region of chromatin-binding proteins. The molecular and functional structure of lunasin has been confirmed in experiments showing arrest of mitosis, leading to apoptosis, when mammalian cells were transfected with the lunasin gene. This peptide binds to deacetylated histones and inhibits their acetylation. Therefore, when histones H3 and H4 are deacetylated, activities of histone acetyltransferase and phosphorylation of the Rb protein cannot be performed. The chemopreventative action of lunasin therefore seems to be a highly regulated acetylation-dependent process.[120,121] Lunasin has caused cytotoxicity to colon cancer cell lines and induced G2/M cell cycle arrest with a simultaneous increase in p21 expression. Apoptosis induced by lunasin has been stimulated by increased activity of caspase-9 and caspase-3. Effective cytotoxicity of lunasin against colon cancer cell lines has additionally been correlated with the expression of $\alpha_5\beta_1$ integrin.[122,123] Chemotherapeutics, especially oxaliplatin, play a pivotal role in colorectal cancer management. *In vitro* experimental results have demonstrated that lunasin potentiates the effect of oxaliplatin in preventing metastasis formation, by an $\alpha_5\beta_1$ integrin-dependent mechanism that suppresses FAK/ERK/NF-κB signaling.[124]

Apigenin

Apigenin is a natural flavone found in many plants. Natural flavones such as apigenin, naringenin, luteolin, tangeritin, and baicalein have many biological functions. Apigenin is abundantly present in common fruits and vegetables, including parsley, onions, oranges, tea, chamomile, and wheat sprouts, among others. It has been shown to possess significant anti-inflammatory, antioxidant, and anticarcinogenic properties.[125] In the carcinogenesis of colorectal tumors, it is accepted that aberrant crypts can be demonstrated (although not in all cases) and that this process depends mainly on the biological nature of the colon cancer. A diet containing apigenin was experimentally demonstrated to reduce by 57% ($P < 0.05$) more than four aberrant crypts/focus in azoxymethane-treated Sprague-Dawley rats.

On the other hand, naringenin lowered both the number of crypt foci by 51% ($P < 0.05$) and the proliferative index by 32% ($P < 0.05$). Both apigenin and naringenin increased apoptosis of luminal colon mucosa cells (78% and 97%, respectively; $P < 0.05$).[126] Apigenin along with TRAIL (human tumor necrosis factor-related apoptosis-inducing ligand) is responsible for induction of apoptosis by increased interaction of bcl-2 with caspase-8, -10, -9, and −3. These molecular events were detected only in colon cancer cell cells and other human cancer cell lines, and not in normal human peripheral blood mononuclear cells.[127] Various molecular mechanisms of the anticancer activity of apigenin have been reported. Both *in vitro* and *in vivo* studies have demonstrated that apigenin suppresses the growth of colorectal cancer cells via phosphorylation and upregulated expression of FADD (Fas-associated protein with death domain), and induction of proapoptotic proteins (NAG-1, p53) and the cell cycle inhibitor p21.[128,129] Metastasis formation in cancer progression is a turning point in the whole course of malignant disease. Therefore, there is a great need to find means of hampering or blocking metastasis formation. It seems that apigenin has a mechanism that could inhibit metastasis formation by CD26 molecule functions. CD26 is a multifunctional cell-surface protein that, through its associated dipeptidyl peptidase (DPPIV) and ectoadenosine deaminase (eADA) enzyme activities, can suppress pathways involved in tumor metastasis formation. Apigenin clearly upregulated cell-surface CD26 on human colorectal cancer cells (HT-29, HRT-18).[130]

Summary

Chemical compounds present in wheat bran are characterized by multifunctional activities, especially when assessed at the cellular and molecular levels. Some of the described substances are worth investigating in the context of supplementary helpers used during the arduous process of colorectal cancer treatment. The use of wheat bran-originating compounds along with anticancer drugs given alone or together with monoclonal antibodies, or with radiotherapy, which is especially important in patients with rectal cancer, appears to offer abundant future work for both laboratory scientists and physicians.

WHEAT BRAN CONSUMPTION, ADENOMATOUS POLYPS, AND COLORECTAL CANCER

The Irish surgeon and physician Dennis Burkitt is well known for his medical missionary work in Africa. In 1957, he and his co-workers identified the lymphoma that bears his name. His next success was firmly associated with observing disease patterns, and led to the nickname "fibreman". While working in Africa, Burkitt claimed that he had seen hardly any cases of many of the most common diseases in the United States and England. He hypothesized that these Western disorders had a single causative factor: deficiency of dietary fiber.[131] The medical problem of deficiency of dietary fiber is reflected throughout many fields of modern medicine, ranging from metabolic diseases and cardiac illnesses to cancer.[132]

Dennis Burkitt, as an astute clinician, drew his conclusions from meticulous surveys, but he did not have any knowledge of the biochemical and molecular background that represents dietary fiber/wheat bran deficiency in everyday eating. Food and feed represent an exceptional example of fast-growing market in which dietary supplements appear to have a critical role either in economic development by increasing profits, or in promotion of health. Therefore, it is necessary to have hard data regarding the role of many supplementary factors such as vitamins, minerals, and dietary fibers, reflecting the status of health among consumers. A variety of food chemical compounds used as ingredients of bread, whole grain cereals, and other snacks is frequently eaten by modern humans. Therefore, it is easy to hypothesize that food appears to be an important factor responsible for sustaining health, reflected by the longer lifespan among humans living in modern societies. Food has therefore probably had an exceptional role in the prevention of many diseases that naturally occurred in the past.[133–135]

The well-accepted fact that only 5–10% of all cancer cases are due to genetic defects leads to the conclusion that the remaining 90–95% are due to lifestyle factors such as diet, smoking, alcohol, physical activity, obesity, and sun exposure. The EPIC (European Prospective Investigation into Cancer and Nutrition) study was specifically designed to investigate the relationship between diet and cancer and other chronic diseases. The results showed the following associations in the gastrointestinal tract:

> Gastric cancer was inversely associated with high plasma vitamin C, some carotenoids, retinol, α-tocopherol, a high intake of cereal fiber, and high adherence to the Mediterranean diet, while red and processed meats were associated with increased risk. A high intake of dietary fiber, fish, calcium, and plasma vitamin D was associated with a decreased risk of colorectal cancer, while red and processed meat intake, alcohol intake, high body mass index (BMI), and abdominal obesity were associated with increased risk.[136]

Most of the present studies can be grouped as observational studies or intervention studies. Well-known limitations of observational studies embrace the collection and interpretation of dietary data, and therefore constrain conclusions from these studies. However, intervention studies testing the relationship between dietary fiber and colon cancer have focused on whether fiber supplementation or diet modification can affect the risk of adenomatous polyps, or even colorectal cancer, appearing. The blurred status of collected data evident at the interpretation stage, where final conclusions are hampered mainly by differences in dietary measurements, lack of standardization of supplemental sources, differences in metabolism among individual participants of the studies, and the retrospective nature of older studies. How these studies are designed and then performed is crucial to the level of evidence: level I evidence is derived from randomized, double-blind controlled clinical trials; level II evidence originates from well-designed controlled clinical trials or well-designed multicenter, prospective cohort, or case–control epidemiologic studies; and level III evidence comes from respected authorities with clinical experience, descriptive studies, or other clinical reports.[137–139]

Colorectal adenomatous polyps are defined as precursors to colorectal cancer. The relationship between diet and the appearance of polyps should help in identifying modifiable factors, with the paramount goal of decreasing the risk of colorectal cancer and reducing its incidence and mortality. It is accepted that adenomatous polyps are an informative endpoint for colorectal carcinogenesis. Several case–control studies[140–149] have shown inverse associations between fiber and colorectal adenoma. On the other hand, intervention studies have shown no protective association of a high-fiber diet or supplementary use of dietary fibers.[150–154]

In a randomized, partially double-blinded, placebo-controlled factorial trial, MacLennan et al.[155] showed that a modified diet with fat reduced to 25% of the total calories and daily supplementation with 25 g of wheat bran and a 20-mg capsule of β-carotene did not act preventively by significantly lowering the rate of new adenomas, but did reduce the risk of large adenomas (≥10 mm), although not in a statistically significant way. The American PLCO (Prostate, Lung, Colorectal, and Ovarian) Cancer Screening Trial was defined as a randomized controlled trial designed to investigate early detection of colon cancer and adenomas. Participants in the highest quintile of dietary fiber intake had a 27% (95% CI: 14–38, $P_{trend} = 0.002$) lower risk of adenoma than those in the lowest quintile. The range of total dietary fiber intake in the study population for the 10th to 90th percentiles was 12.6–36.4 g/day.[156] Despite the fact that evidence for an association between dietary fiber intake and colorectal polyps and cancer has been equivocal, there are some data showing a difference in response to fiber consumption between sexes. Results of the Wheat Bran

Trial and the Polyp Prevention Trial have shown that the adjusted odds ratio for adenoma recurrence in the intervention group was 0.91 (95% CI: 0.78–1.06), but for men the intervention was associated with statistically significant reduced odds of recurrence (0.81; 95% CI: 0.67–0.98) while for women no significant association was observed.[157] Diet modifications have also been assessed in interventional studies: in some studies dietary adherence to a low-fat, high-fiber diet was associated with a reduced risk of adenoma recurrence at the level of 35%, but in others no such result was found.[158,159]

Discrepancies in collected evidence are probably dependent on many other factors that have not been properly monitored or are even unknown, such as vitamins; active chemical compounds working co-carcinogenically or anti-carcinogenically and appearing during colonic fermentation; minerals – for instance, selenium, which has an inverse association with a decreased risk of colorectal cancer;[160] or other factors such as the inflammatory response in direct relation to functions of interleukins such as IL-1β, IL-8, IL-10, and IL-6.[161,162] The latter is considered to be a potential indicator for prevention of high-risk adenoma recurrence.

The link between dietary fiber intake and prevention of colorectal cancer was suggested more than 40 years ago. Clinical trials focusing on the role of wheat bran fiber supplementation in lower colorectal cancer risk have largely been performed safely, without significant gastrointestinal side effects and changes in body weight.[163] Many clinical trials establishing the association of dietary fiber intake with the risk of colorectal cancer have been performed, both as observational and as intervention studies. The results are conflicting, and it is impossible to draw final conclusions. A combination analysis of 13 case–control studies[164] and a meta-analysis of 16 case–control studies[165] presented an inverse association between fiber intake and risk of colorectal cancer incidence. In contrast to the above statement, 10 prospective studies avoiding the potential for recall and control selection bias have failed to support the association between beneficial dietary fiber intake and reduced risk of colorectal cancer.[166–175] However, the latest results seem predominantly to show a clinical benefit, by reduction of colorectal cancer risk, of consuming a 10-g daily dose of dietary fiber. Table 8.4[176–183] shows the results of clinical trials published since the year 2000.

Unfortunately, investigations regarding the relationship between wheat bran or dietary fiber intake and the reduced risk of colorectal cancer are not complete. There are many other problems, as indicated by the need to establish how dietary fiber should be mixed with other nutritional compounds. Which of the known sources of dietary fiber should be considered the best, taking into account the most frequently expressed beneficial results, indicating the clearest reduction in colorectal cancer risk? There is a question over the subject of how to maximize results by combining wheat bran or other sources of dietary fiber with NSAIDs (non-steroidal anti-inflammatory drugs), especially in patients with a propensity for colorectal polyps, or in the population of humans taking statins. Early results are encouraging, showing a reduced risk of colorectal cancer with 6-month interventions with atrovastin, sulindac, or ORAFTI® Synergy1 (a prebiotic fiber composed of oligofructose and polyfructose chains).[184]

Despite the real progress in medical management of colorectal cancer, it is still a huge challenge to achieve better results, because this malignant disease continues to constitute a significant proportion of the global burden of cancer morbidity and mortality. One million new cases of colorectal cancer are diagnosed each year and more than half a million people die from this disease – equivalent to approximately 8% of all cancer-related deaths worldwide.[185] More broadly defined needs for better results of preventive interventions must be supported by changes in lifestyle. This includes modification of the Western diet by increasing the consumption of plant foods and reducing red meat intake, along with maintenance of physical activity and appropriate body mass. Together, these activities should substantially reduce colorectal incidence and mortality.[186–188]

CONCLUSION

Colorectal cancer is still regarded as one of the most significant neoplasms, with a large number of cases diagnosed every year in industrialized societies. This form of cancer is responsible for a high rate of deaths among patients suffering from malignant disease. Many medical disciplines have made huge progress in the management of colorectal cancer: in diagnosis, gastroenterology offers modern techniques of visualizing the colonic mucosa and pathology gives a more precise diagnosis not only by assessment of cell morphology but by better molecular characterization; in surgery, modern surgical removal appears to be less invasive and patients recover faster than previously; and in oncology, chemotherapy has well-accepted significance either in the treatment of early colorectal cancer in an adjuvant setting, or in the advanced phase of the colorectal cancer in a palliative setting.

When knowledge shows clear causative relations among various factors, especially in cancers having tremendous importance in a society, it becomes necessary to use more active methods to change the action of harmful factors and hamper carcinogenesis. Colorectal cancer is considered to be one such important neoplasm, with a large number of cases worldwide, and an association with the Western lifestyle. It is a strong hope that both food and feed have important roles in tackling colorectal carcinogenesis. Accumulated evidence has shown

TABLE 8.4   The New Millennium Results of Clinical Trials on Dietary Consumption in Relation to Colorectal Cancer Risk

Study Design and Year of Report	Participants	Outcomes	Conclusions	References
Case–control (2001)	286 (174 males, 112 females) patients with histologically confirmed colon or rectal cancer vs 550 controls	OR: 0.55 for soluble non-cellulose polysaccharides; OR: 0.57 for total fibers; OR 58 for total insoluble fibers; OR 0.60 for vegetables; OR: 0.78 for fruit; OR: 0.74 for grain fibers	Significant inverse relationship of total dietary fiber intake with risk of colorectal cancer	Levi et al.[176]
Observational study – EPIC study (2003)	519,978	Adjusted RR: 0.75 (95% CI: 0.59–0.95) for highest vs lowest quintile of fiber intake; better protection for left side colon and for rectum Adjusted RR: 0.58 (0.41–0.85) highest vs lowest quintile of doubling fiber intake	Dietary fiber intake could reduce risk of colorectal cancer by 40%	Bingham et al.[177]
Prospective cohorts (2005)	76,947 women, 47,279 men	HR: 0.91 (95% CI: 0.87–0.95) for 5 g daily increase in fiber intake Adjusting for covariates used in EPIC study, HR: 0.99 (0.95–1.04)	Dietary fiber intake does not indicate important association with reduced colorectal cancer risk	Michels et al.[178]
13 Prospective cohort studies (2005)	725,628	Age adjusted RR: 0.84 (95% CI: 0.77–0.92)	Dietary fiber intake is inversely associated with risk of colorectal cancer in age-adjusted analysis; other dietary factors have no significant relationship	Park et al.[179]
Prospective nested case–control study (2010)	579 patients with histologically confirmed colorectal cancer vs 1996 controls	Multivariable-adjusted for colorectal cancer for highest vs. lowest quintile of fiber intake, OR: 0.66 (95% CI: 0.45–0.96, P_{trend} <0.012]	Dietary fiber intake is inversely associated with colorectal cancer risk	Dahm et al.[180]
Community-based case–control study (2010)	816 patients with histologically confirmed colorectal cancer vs 815 community controls	Soluble and insoluble dietary fibers are not associated with overall risk or subsite-specific risk of colorectal cancer	No protective association between dietary fiber intake and colorectal cancer risk	Uchida et al.[181]
25 prospective cohort and nested case–control studies (2011)	1.9 million participants in dietary fiber analysis and 14,400 cases of colorectal cancer	For 10 g daily of total dietary fiber (16 studies) RR: 0.90 (95% CI: 0.86–0.94, I^2=0%); for fruit fiber (9 studies) RR: 0.93 (0.82–1.05, I^2=23%); for vegetable fiber (9 studies) RR: 0.98 (0.91–1.06, I^2=0%); for legume fiber (4 studies) RR: 0.62 (0.27–1.42, I^2=58%); for cereal fiber (8 studies) RR: 0.90 (0.83–0.97, I^2=0%)	High intake of dietary fiber (cereal fiber) and whole grain are associated with reduced risk of colorectal cancer	Aune et al.[182]
Prospective Scandinavian HELGA cohort (2012)	108,081 cohort members with 1168 colorectal cancer patients (691 colon cancer and 477 rectal cancer)	For 10 g daily of total dietary fiber, IRR: 0.74 (95% CI: 0.64–0.86); for 2 g daily of total dietary fiber, IRR: 0.94 (0.91–0.98)	Dietary fiber has protective role against colon cancer but not rectal cancer	Hansen et al.[183]

Abbreviations: OR, odds ratio; RR, relative risk; IRR, incidence relative risk; HR, hazard ratio; CI, confidence interval; EPIC, European Prospective Investigation into Cancer and Nutrition; HELGA, Nordic Health – Whole Grain Food Project 070015.

heterogeneous results, with a slight bias in favor of a beneficial role of wheat bran/dietary fiber intake in the reduction of colorectal cancer risk. There is still the need, though, for more precise interpretation from planned controlled studies, showing how food consumption could modify the causative factors responsible for the pathogenesis of colorectal cancer. Therefore, a preventive action of food could offer more than even the most sophisticated methods of treatment of colorectal cancer, used at the disseminated phase of this malignant disease.

References

1. Beaney M. *Analysis. Stanford Encyclopedia of Philosophy.* Stanford, CA: Stanford Univerisity; 2009.

2. Prior AN. Three-valued logic and future contingents. *Philos Quart* 1953;**3**:317–26.

3. Malinowski G. Many-valued logic and its philosophy. In: Gabbay DM, Woods J, editors. *Handbook of the History of Logic,* vol. 8. Elsevier; 2007. p. 13–94.

4. Bravo JA, Forsythe P, Chew MV, Escaravage E, Savignac HM, Dinan TG, et al. Ingestion of *Lactobacillus* strain regulates emotional behavior and central GABA receptor expression in a mouse via vagus nerve. *Proc Natl Acad Sci* 2011;**108**:16050–5.

5. Heijtz RD, Wang S, Anuar F, Qian Y, Björkholm B, Samuelsson A, et al. Normal gut microbiota modulates brain development and behavior. *Proc Natl Acad Sci* 2011;**108**:3047–52.

6. Grenham S, Clarke G, Cryan JF, Dinan TG. Brain–gut-microbe communication in health and disease. *Front Physiol* 2011;**2**: 1–15.

7. Parkin DM, Pisani P, Ferlay J. Global cancer statistics. *CA Cancer J Clin* 1999;**49**:33–64.

8. Parkin DM, Pisani P, Ferlay J. Estinates of worldwide incidence of eighteen major cancers in 1985. *Int J Cancer* 1993;**54**:594–606.

9. Nelson RL, Dollear T, Freels SPV. The relation of age, race, and gender to the subsite location of colorectal carcinoma. *Cancer* 1997;**80**:193–7.

10. Siegel EM, Ulrich CM, Poole EM, Holmes RS, Jacobsen PB, Shibata D. The effects of obesity and obesity-related conditions on colorectal cancer prognosis. *Cancer Control* 2010;**17**:52–7.

11. Ortega J, Vigil CE, Chodkiewicz C. Current progress in targeted therapy for colorectal cancer. *Cancer Control* 2010;**17**:7–15.

12. Weitz J, Koch M, Debus J, Höhler T, Galle PR, Büchler MW. Colorectal cancer. *Lancet* 2005;**365**:153–65.

13. Parsonnet J. Bacterial infection as a cause of cancer. *Environ Health Perspect* 1995;**103**(suppl. 8):263–8.

14. Reddy B, Engle A, Katsifis S, Simi B, Bartram HP, Perrino P, et al. Biochemical epidemiology of colon cancer: effect of types of dietary fiber of fecal mutagens, acid and neutral sterols in healthy subjects. *Cancer Res* 1989;**49**:4629–35.

15. De Kok TM, ten Hoor F, Kleinjans JS. Identification and quantitive distribution of eight analogues of naturally occuring fecapentaenes in human feces by high-performance liquid chromatography. *Carcinogenesis* 1991;**12**:199–205.

16. Plummer SM, Grafstrom RC, Yang LL, Curren RD, Linnainmaa K, Harris CC. Fecapentaene-12 causes DNA damage and mutations in human cells. *Carcinogenesis* 1986;**7**:1607–9.

17. De Kok TM, van Faassen A, Bausch-Goldbohm RA, ten Hoor F, Kleinjans JC. Fecapentaene excretion and fecal mutagenicity in relation to nutrient intake and fecal parameters in humans on omnivorous and vegetarian diets. *Cancer Lett* 1992;**62**:11–21.

18. Glinghammar B, Holmberg K, Rafter J. Effects of colonic lumenal components on AP-1-dependent gene transcription in cultured human colon carcinoma cells. *Carcinogenesis* 1999;**20**:969–76.

19. Bernstein C, Bernstein H, Garewal H, Dinning P, Jabi R, Sampliner RE, et al. A bile acid-induced apoptosis assay for colon cancer risk and associated quality control studies. *Cancer Res* 1999;**59**:2353–7.

20. Thomas B. Heterocyclic amine levels in cooked meat and the implication for New Zealanders. *Eur J Cancer Prev* 1999;**8**:201–6.

21. Probst-Hensch NM, Sinha R, Longnecker MP, Witte JS, Ingles SA, Frankl HD, et al. Meat preparation and colorectal adenomas in a large sigmoidoscopy-based case-control study in California (United States). *Cancer Causes Control* 1997;**8**:175–83.

22. McIntosh GH. Colon cancer: dietary modifications required for a balanced protective diet. *Prev Med* 1993;**22**:767–74.

23. Campos FG, Logullo-Waitzberg AG, Kiss DR, Waitzberg DL, Habr-Gama A, Gama-Rodrigues J. Diet and colorectal cancer: current evidence for etiology and prevention. *Nutr Hosp* 2005;**20**:18–25.

24. Clark R. Principles of cancer screening. *Radiol Clin N Am* 2004;**42**:735–46.

25. Hulka BS. Screening for cancer: lessons learned. *J Occup Med* 1986;**28**:687–91.

26. Jemal A, Siegel R, Xu J, Ward E. Cancer statistics, 2010. *CA Cancer J Clin* 2010;**60**:277–300.

27. Levin B, Lieberman DA, McFarland B, Smith RA, Brooks D, Andrews KS, et al. Screening and surveillance for the early detection of colorectal cancer and adenomatous polyps, 2008: a joint guideline from the American Cancer Society, the US Multi-Society Task Force on Colorectal Cancer, and the American College of Radiology. *CA Cancer J Clin* 2008;**58**:130–60.

28. Rex DK, Johnson DA, Anderson JC, Schoenfeld PS, Burke CA, Inadomi JM, et al. American College of Gastroenetrology guidelines for colorectal cancer screening 2009. *Am J Gastroenetrol* 2009;**104**:739–50.

29. Burt RW. Colorectal cancer screening. *Curr Opin Gastroenetrol* 2010;**26**:466–70.

30. Citarda F, Tomaselli G, Capocaccia R, Barcherini S, Crespi M; Italian Multicentre Study Group. Efficacy in standard clinical practice of colonoscopic polypectomy in reducing colorectal cancer incidence. *Gut* 2001;**48**:812–5.

31. Winawer SJ, Zauber AG, Ho MN, O'Brien MJ, Gottlieb LS, Sternberg SS, et al. Prevention of colorectal cancer by colonoscopic polypectomy. The National Polyp Study Workgroup. *N Engl J Med* 1993;**329**:1977–81.

32. Weissfeld JL, Schoen RE, Pinsky PF, Bresalier RS, Church T, Yurgalevitch S, et al. Flexible sigmoidoscopy in the PLCO cancer screening trial: results from the baseline screening examination of a randomized trial. *J Natl Cancer Inst* 2005;**97**:989–97.

33. Kim DH, Pickhardt PJ, Taylor AJ, Menias CO. Imaging evaluation of complications at optical colonoscopy. *Curr Probl Diagn Radiol* 2008;**37**:165–77.

34. Hassan C, Laghi A, Pickhardt PJ, Kim DH, Zulo A, IaFrate F, et al. Projected impact of colorectal cancer screening with computerized tomographic colonography on current radiological capacity in Europe. *Aliment Pharmacol Ther* 2008;**27**:366–74.

35. Hewitson P, Glasziou P, Watson E, Towler B, Irwig L. Cochrane systematic review of colorectal cancer screening using the fecal occult blood test (hemocult): an update. *Am J Gastroenterol* 2008;**103**:1541–9.

36. Hundt S, Huang U, Brenner H. Comparative evaluation of immunochemical fecal occult blood tests for colorectal adenoma detection. *Ann Intern Med* 2009;**150**:162–9.

37. Sidransky D, Tokino T, Hamilton SR, Kinzler KW, Levin B, Frost P, et al. Identification of ras oncogene mutations in the stool of patients with curable colorectal tumors. *Science* 1992;**256**:102–5.

38. Rabeneck L, Paszat LF, Saskin R, et al. Association between colonoscopy rates and colorectal cancer mortality. *Am J Gastroenterol* 2010;**150**:1–8.

39. Barclay RL, Vicari JJ, Doughty AS, Johanson JF, Greenlaw RL. Colonoscopic withdrawal times and adenoma detection during screening colonoscopy. *N Engl J Med* 2006;**355**:2533–41.

40. Imperiale TF, Glowinski EA, Lin-Cooper C, Larkin GN, Rogge JD, Ransohoff DF. Five-year risk of colorectal neoplasia after negative screening colonoscopy. *N Engl J Med* 2008;**359**:1218–24.

41. Selby JV, Friedman GD, Quesenberry CP, Weiss NS. A case–control study of screening sigmoidoscopy and mortality from colorectal cancer. *N Engl J Med* 1992;**326**:653–7.

42. Atkin WS, Edwards R, Kralj-Hans I, Wooldrage K, Hart AR, Northover JM, et al. Once-only flexible sigmoidoscopy screening in prevention of colorectal cancer: a multicentre randomized controlled trial. *Lancet* 2010;**375**:1624–33.

43. Halligan S, Altman DG, Taylor SA, Mallett S, Deeks JJ, Bartram CI, et al. CT colonography in the detection of colorectal polyps and cancer: systematic review, meta-analysis, and proposed minimum data set for study level reporting. *Radiology* 2006;**237**:893–904.

44. Mulhall BP, Veerappan GR, Jackson JL. Meta-analysis: computed tomographic colonography. *Ann Intern Med* 2005;**142**:635–50.

45. Kim DH, Pickhardt PJ, Taylor AJ, et al. CT colonography versus colonoscopy for the detection of advanced neoplasia. *N Engl J Med* 2007;**357**:1403–12.

46. Allison JE, Tekawa IS, Ransom LJ, Adrain AL. A comparison of fecal occult-blood tests for colorectal-cancer screening. *N Engl J Med* 1996;**334**:155–9.

47. Hol L, van Leerdam ME, van Ballegooijen M, van Vuuren AJ, van Dekken H, Reijerink JC, et al. Screening for colorectal cancer: a randomised trial comparing guaiac-based and immunochemical faecal occult blood testing and flexible sigmoidoscopy. *Gut* 2010;**59**:62–8.

48. Imperiale TF, Ransohoff DF, Itzkovitz SH, Turnbull BA, Ross ME; Colorectal Cancer Study Group. Fecal DNA versus fecal occult blood for colorectal-cancer screening in an average-risk population. *N Engl J Med* 2004;**351**:2704–14.

49. Ferguson LR. Prospects for cancer prevention. *Mutat Res* 1999;**428**:329–38.

50. Vargas PA, Alberts DS. Primary prevention of colorectal cancer through dietary modification. *Cancer* 1992;**70**(5 suppl.):1229–35.

51. Schlormann W, Hiller B, Jahns B, Zöger R, Hennemeier I, Wilhelm A, et al. Chemopreventive effects of *in vitro* digested and fermented bread in human colon cancer. *Eur J Nutr* 2012;**51**:827–39.

52. Australian Government. Department of Health and Ageing Office of the Gene Technology Regulator. The biology of Triticum aestivum L. em Thell. (bread wheat). Version 2: February 2008. Available at: http://www.ogtr.gov.au.

53. Jaradat AA. Ecogeography, genetic diversity, and breeding value of wild emmer wheat (*Triticum dicoccoides* Korn ex Asch. & Graebn.) Thell. *Am J Crop Sci* 2011;**5**:1072–86.

54. Varshney RK, Langridge P, Graner A. Application of genomics to molecular breeding of wheat and barley. *Adv Genet* 2007;**58**:121–55.

55. Sramkova Z, Gregova E, Sturdik E. Genetic improvement of wheat – a review. *Nova Biotechnol* 2009;**9**:27–51.

56. Charmet G. Wheat domestication: lessons for the future. *CR Biologies* 2011;**334**:212–20.

57. Jacobsen T, Adams RM. Salt and silt in ancient Mesopotamian agriculture. *Science* 1958;**128**:1251–8.

58. Nesbitt M. Wheat evolution: integrating archeological and biological evidence. Pp. 37–59 in Wheat taxonomy: the legacy of John Percival. In: Caligari & PE Brandham PDS, editor. London: Linnean Society; 2001. Linnean Special Issue 3.

59. K-i Tanno. Willcox G: How fast was wild wheat domesticated? *Science* 2006;**311**:1886.

60. Piperno DR, Weiss E, Holst I, Nadel D. Processing of wild cereal grains in the Upper Paleotihic revealed by starch grain analysis. *Nature* 2004;**430**:670–3.

61. Dickson JH, Oeggl K, Handley LL. The iceman reconsidered. *Sci Am* 2003;**288**:70–9.

62. Dickson JH, Oeggl K, Holden TG, Handley LL, O'Connell TC, Preston T. The omnivorus Tyrolean Iceman: colon contents (meat, cereals, pollen, moss and whipworm) and stable isotope analyses. *Phil Trans R Soc Lond B* 2000;**355**:1843–9.

63. Peng J, Sun D, Nevo E. Wild emmer wheat, *Triticum dicoccoides*, occupies a pivotal position in wheat domestication process. *AJCS* 2011;**5**:1127–43.

64. Heun M, Schafer-Pregl R, Klawan D, Castagna R, Accerbi M, Borghi B, et al. Site of einkorn wheat domestication identified by DNA fingerprinting. *Science* 1997;**278**:1312–4.

65. Luo M-C, Yang Z-L, Kawahara T, Kawahara T, Waines JG, Dvorak J. The structure of wild and domesticated emmer wheat populations, gene flow between them, and the site of emmer domestication. *Theor Appl Genet* 2007;**114**:947–59.

66. Hipsley EH. Dietary fibre and pregnancy toxemia. *Br Med J* 1953;**2**:420–2.

67. Burkitt DP, Trowell HC. Dietary fibre and western diseases. *Irish Med J* 1977;**70**:272–7.

68. Cummings JH, Mann JI, Nishida C, Vorster HH. Dietary fibre: an agreement definition. *Lancet* 2009;**373**:365–6.

69. European Parliament Directive 2008/100/EC of the European Parliament. Official Journal. *L Series* 2008;**285**:9–12.

70. Kumar P, Yadava RK, Gollen B, Kumar S, Verma RK, Yadav S. Nutritional contents and medicinal properties of wheat: a review. Life Sciences and Medicine Research. *Volume* 2011. LSMR-22. Available at http://astonjournals.com/lsmr.

71. Sramkova Z, Gregova E, Sturdik E. Chemical composition and nutritional quality of wheat grain. *Acta Chim Slov* 2009;**2**:115–38.

72. Schultz E. *Dietary fibre*. E-book update; 2011. Available at http://www.effieschultz.com/files/pdf/dietary_fibre.pdf.

73. Ferguson LR, Harris PJ. Studies on he of specific dietary fibres in protection against colorectal cancer. *Mutat Res* 1996;**350**:173–84.

74. Kritchevsky D. Dietray fibre and cancer. *Eur J Cancer Prev* 1997;**6**:435–41.

75. Reddy BS. Role of dietary fibre in colon cancer: an overview. *Am J Med* 1999;**106**(1A):16S–9S discussion 50S-51S.

76. McPherson-Kay R. Fiber, stool bulk, and bile acid output: implications for colon cancer risk. *Prev Med* 1987;**16**:540–4.

77. Topping DL, Cobiac L. Dietary fibre. Potential role in etiology of disease. In: Caballero B, Allen L, Prentice D, editors. *Encyclopedia of human nutrition* 2nd ed. Elsevier; 2005. p. 578–85.

78. Ferguson LR, Harris PJ. Protection against cancer by wheat bran: role of dietary fibre and phytochemicals. *Eur J Cancer Prev* 1999;**8**:17–25.

79. Zoran DL, Turner ND, Taddeo SS, Chapkin RS, Lupton JR. Wheat bran diet reduces tumor incidence in a rat model of colon cancer independent of effects on distal luminal butyrate concentrations. *J Nutr* 1997;**127**:2217–25.

80. Muir JG, Yeow EGW, Keogh J, Pizzey C, Bird AR, Sharpe K, et al. Combining wheat bran with resistant starch has more beneficial effects on fecal indexes than does wheat bran alone. *Am J Clin Nutr* 2004;**79**:1020–8.

81. Alberts DS, Einspahr J, Rees-McGee S, Ramanujam P, Buller MK, Clark L, et al. Effects of dietary wheat bran fiber on rectal epithelial cell proliferation in patients with resection for colorectal cancers. *J Natl Cancer Inst* 1990;**82**:1280–5.

82. Zhu Y, Conklin DR, Chen W, Sang S. 5-alk(en)ylresorcinols as the major active components in wheat bran inhibit human colon cancer cell growth. *Bioorg Med Chem* 2011;**19**:3973–82.

83. Alabaster O, Tang Z, Shivapurkar N. Inhibition by wheat bran cereals of the development of aberrant crypt foci and colon tumours. *Food Chem Toxicol* 1997;**35**:517–22.

84. Earnest DL, Einspahr JG, Alberts DS. Protective role of wheat bran fiber: data marker trials. *Am J Med* 1999;**106**(1A):32S–7S.

85. Compher CW, Frankel WL, Tazelaar J, Lawson JA, McKinney S, Segall S, et al. Wheat bran decreases aberrant crypt foci, preserves normal proliferation, and increases intraluminal butyrate levels in experimental colon cancer. *J Parenter Enteral Nutr* 1999;**23**:269–77.

86. Reddy BS, Hirose Y, Cohen LA, Simi B, Cooma I, Rao CV. Preventive potential of wheat bran fractions against experimental colon carcinogenesis: implications for human colon cancer prevention. *Cancer Res* 2000;**60**:4792–7.

87. Sang S, Ju J, Lambert JD, Lin Y, Hong J, Bose M, et al. Wheat bran oil and its fractions inhibit human colon cancer cell growth and intestinal tumorigenesis in Apc (min/+) mice. *J Agric Food Chem* 2006;**54**:9792–7.

88. Adom KK, Liu RH. Antioxidant activity of grains. *J Agric Food Chem* 2002;**50**:6182–7.

89. Bell LP, Hectorn K, Reynolds H, Hunninghake DB. Cholesterol-lowering effects of soluble-fiber cereals as part of a pridentdiet for patientswith mild to moderate hypercholeterolemia. *Am J Clin Nutr* 1990;**52**:1020–6.

90. Alabaster O, Tang ZC, Frost A, Shivapurkar N. Potential synergism between wheat bran and psyllium: enhanced inhibition of colon cancer. *Cancer Lett* 1993;**75**:53–8.

91. Cohen LA, Zhao Z, Zang EA, Wynn TT, Simi B, Rivenson A. Wheat bran and psyllium diets: effects on N-methylnitrosourea-induced mammary tumorigenesis in F344 rats. *J Natl Cancer Inst* 1996;**88**:899–907.

92. Khalili B, Bardana EJ, Yunginger JW. Psyllium-associated anaphylaxis and death: a case report and review of the literature. *Ann Allergy Asthma Immunol* 2003;**91**:579–84.

93. Boros LG, Nichelatti M, Shoenfeld Y. Fermented wheat germ extract (Avemar) in the treatment of cancer and autoimmune diseases. *Ann NY Acad Sci* 2005;**1051**:529–42.

94. Heimbach JT, Sebestyen G, Semjen G, Kennepohl E. Safety studies regarding a standarized extract of fermented wheat germ. *Int J Toxicol* 2007;**26**:253–9.

95. Mueller T, Voigt W. Fermented wheat germ extract – nutritional supplement or anticancer drug? *Nutr J* 2011;**10**:89.

96. Telekes A, Hegedus M, Chae CH, Vékey K. Avemar (wheat germ extract) in cancer prevention and treatment. *Nutr Cancer* 2009;**61**:891–9.

97. Zalatnai A, Lapis K, Szende B, Rásó E, Telekes A, Resetár A, et al. Wheat germ extract inhibits experimental colon carcinogenesi in F-344 rats. *Carcinogenesis* 2001;**22**:1649–52.

98. Mueller T, Jordan K, Voigt W. Promising cytotoxicity activity profile of fermented wheat germ extract (Avemar) in human cancer cell lines. *J Exp Clin Res* 2011;**30**:42.

99. Hidvegi M, Raso E, Tomoskozi-Farkas R, Szende B, Paku S, Prónai L, et al. MSC, a new benzoquinone-containing natural product with antimetastatic effect. *Cancer Biother Radiopharm* 1999;**14**:277–89.

100. Stein K, Borowicki A, Scharlau D, Glei M. Fermented wheat aleurone induces enzymes involved in detoxification of carcinogens and in antioxidative defence in human colon cells. *Br J Nutr* 2010;**104**:1101–11.

101. Borowicki A, Michelmann A, Stein K, Scharlau D, Scheu K, Obst U, et al. Fermented wheat aleurone enriched with probiotic strains LGG and Bb12 modulates markers of tumor progression in human colon cells. *Nutr Cancer* 2011;**63**:151–60.

102. Demidov LV, Manziuk LV, Kharkevitch GY, Pirogova NA, Artamonova EV. Adjuvant fermented wheat germ extract (Avemar) nutraceutical improves survival of high-risk skin melanoma patients: a randomized, pilot, phase II clinical study with a 7-year follow-up. *Cancer Biother Radiopharm* 2008;**23**:477–82.

103. Jakab F, Shoenfeld Y, Balogh A, Nichelatti M, Hoffmann A, Kahán Z, et al. A medical nutriment has supportive value in the treatment of colorectal cancer. *Br J Cancer* 2003;**89**:465–9.

104. Velentzis LS, Woodside JV, Cantwell MM, Leathem AJ, Keshtgar MR, et al. Do phytoestrogens reduce the risk of breast cancer and breast cancer recurrence? What clinicians need to know. *Eur J Cancer* 2008;**44**:1799–806.

105. Ayella AK, Trick HN, Wang W. Enhancing lignan biosynthesis by overexpressing pinoresinol lariciresinolreductase in transgenic wheat. *Mol Nutr Food Res* 2007;**51**:1518–26.

106. Qu H, Madl RL, Takemoto DJ, Baybutt RC, Wang W. Lignans are involved in the antitumor activity of wheat bran in colon cancer SW480 cells. *J Nutr* 2005;**135**:598–602.

107. Harris PJ, Ferguson LR. Dietary fibres may protect or enhance carcinogenesis. *Mut Res* 1999;**443**:95–110.

108. Harris PJ, Ferguson LR. Dietary fibre: its composition and role in protection against colorectal cancer. *Mut Res* 1993;**290**:97–110.

109. Boerjan W, Ralph J, Baucher M. Lignin bios. *Ann Rev Plant Biol* 2003;**54**:519–49.

110. Begum AN, Nicolle C, Mila I, Lapierre C, Nagano K, Fukushima K, et al. Dietary lignins are precursors of mammalian lignans in rats. *J Nutr* 2004;**134**:120–7.

111. Jiao J, Zhang Y, Liu C, Liu J, Wu X, Zhang Y. Separation and purification of tricin from an antioxidant product derived from bamboo leaves. *J Agric Food Chem* 2007;**55**:10086–92.

112. Oyama T, Yasui Y, Sugie S, Koketsu M, Watanabe K, Tanaka T. Dietary tricin suppresses inflamation-related colon carcinogenesis in male Crj: CD-1 mice. *Cancer Prev Res (Phila)* 2009;**2**:1031–8.

113. Fox CH, Eberl M. Phytic acid (IP6), novel broad spectrum anti-neoplastic agent: a systemic review. *Complement Ther Med* 2002;**10**:229–34.

114. Jenab M, Thompson LU. The influence of phytic acid in wheat bran on early biomarkers of colon carcinogenesis. *Carcinogenesis* 1998;**19**:1087–92.

115. Jenab M, Thompson LU. Phytic acid in wheat bran affects colon morphology, cell differential and apoptosis. *Carcinogenesis* 2000;**21**:1547–52.

116. Kapral M, Parfiniewicz B, Strzałka-Mrozik B, Zachacz A, Weglarz L. Evaluation of the expression of transcriptional factor NF-kB induced by phytic acid in colon cancer cells. *Acta Polon Pharmac-Drug Res* 2008;**65**:697–702.

117. Hernandez-Ledesma B, de Lumen BO. Lunasin: a novel cancer preventive seed peptide. *Perspect Medicin Chem* 2008;**25**:75–80.

118. Hernandez-Ledesma B, Hsieh CC, de Lumen BO. Lunasin: a novel seed peptide for cancer prevention. *Peptides* 2009;**30**:426–30.

119. Seber LE, Barnett BW, McConnell EJ, Hume SD, Cai J, Boles K, et al. Scalable purification and characterization of the anticancer lunasin peptide from soybean. *PLoS ONE* 2012;**7** e35409.

120. Galvez AF, Chen N, Macasieb J, de Lumen BO. Chemopreventive property of a soybean peptide (lunasin) that binds to deacetylated histones and inhibits acetylation. *Cancer Res* 2001;**61**:7473–8.

121. Jeong JB, Jeong HJ, Park JH, Lee SH, Lee JR, Lee HK, et al. Cancer-preventive peptide lunasin from Solanum nigrum L. inhibits acetylation of core histones H3 and H4 and phosphorylation of retinoblastoma protein (Rb). *J Agric Food Chem* 2007;**55**:10707–1013.

122. Dia VP. Gonzalez-de Mejia E: Lunasin promotes apoptosis in human colon cancer cells by mitochondrial pathway activation and induction of nuclear clusterin expression. *Cancer Lett* 2010;**295**:44–53.

123. Dia VP. Gonzalez-de Mejia E: Lunasin induces apoptosis and modifies the expression of genes associated with extracellular matrix and cell adhesion in human metastatic colon cancer cells. *Mol Nutr Food Res* 2011;**55**:623–34.

124. Dia VP. Gonzalez-de Mejia E: Lunasin potentiates the effect of oxaliplatin preventing outgrowth of colon cancer metastasis, binds to $\alpha_5\beta_1$ integrin and suppresses FAK/ERK/NF-κB signaling. *Cancer Lett* 2011;**313**:176–80.

125. Patel D, Shukla S, Gupta S. Apigeninand cancer chemoprevention: progress, potential and promise (review). *Int J Oncol* 2007;**30**:233–45.

126. Leonardi T, Vanamala J, Taddeo SS, Davidson LA, Murphy ME, Patil BS, et al. Apigenin and naringenin suppress colon carcinogenesis through the aberrant crypt stage in azoxymethane-treated rats. *Exp Biol Med* 2010;**235**:710–7.

127. Horinaka M, Yoshida T, Shiraishi T, Nakata S, Wakada M, Sakai T. The dietary flavonoid apigenin sensitizes malignant tumor cells to tumor necrosis factor-related apoptosis-inducing ligand. *Mol Cancer Ther* 2006;**5**:945–51.

128. Wang QR, Yao XQ, Wen G, Fan Q, Li YJ, Fu XQ, et al. Apigenin suppresses the growth of colorectal cancer xenografts via phosphorylation and up-regulated FADD expression. *Oncol Lett* 2011;**2**:42–7.

129. Zhong Y, Krisanapun C, Lee S-H, Nualsanit T, Sams C, Peungvicha P, et al. Molecular targets of apigenin in colorctal cancer cells: involvment of p21, NAG-1 and p53. *Eur J Cancer* 2010;**46**:3365–74.

D. WHEAT IN CANCER PREVENTION

130. Lefort EC, Blay J. The dietary flavonoid apigenin enhances the activities of the anti-metastatic protein CD26 on human colon carcinoma. Clin Exp Metastasis 2011;28:337–49.

131. Burkitt DP. Epidemiology of cancer of the colon and rectum. Cancer 1971;28:8–13.

132. Coffin CS, Shaffer EA. The hot and cold facts of dietary fibre. Can J Gastroenterol 2006;20:255–6.

133. Kaczmarczyk MM, Miller MJ, Freund GG. The health benefits of dietary fiber: beyond the usual suspects of type 2 diabetes mellitus, cardiovascular disease and colon cancer. Metabol Clin Exp 2012;61:1058–66.

134. Gli A, Ortega RM, Maldonado J. Wholegrain cereals and bread: a duet of the Mediterranean diet for the prevention of chronic diseases. Public Health Nutr 2011;14:2316–22.

135. Pauwels EK. The protective effect of the Mediterranean diet: focus on cancer and cardiovascular risk. Med Princ Pract 2011;20:103–11.

136. Gonzalez CA, Riboli E. Diet and cancer prevention: contribution from the European Prospective Investigation into Cancer and Nutrition (EPIC) study. Eur J Cancer 2010;46:2555–62.

137. Rock CL. Primary dietary prvention: is the fiber story over? Recent Results Cancer Res 2007;174:171–7.

138. Duffy C, Perez K, Partridge A. Implications of phytoestrogen intake for breast cancer. CA Cancer J Clin 2007;57:260–77.

139. Ryan-Harshman M, Aldoori W. Diet and colorectal cancer. Review of the evidence. Can Fam Physician 2007;53:1913–20.

140. Hoff G, Moen LE, Trygg K, Frølich W, Sauar J, Vatn M, et al. Epidemiology of polyps in the rectum and sigmoid colon. Evaluation of nutritional factors. Scand J Gastroenterol 1986;21:199–204.

141. Macquart-Moulin G, Riboli E, Cornee J, Kaaks R, Berthezène P. Colorectal polyps and diet: a case-control study in Marseilles. Int J Cancer 1987;40:179–88.

142. Kune GA, Kune S, Read A, MacGowan K, Penfold C, Watson LF. Colorectal polyps, diet, alcohol, and family history of colorectal: a case-control study. Nutr Cancer 1991;16:25–30.

143. Little J, Logan RF, Hawtin PG, Hardcastle JD, Turner ID. Colorectal adenomas and diet: a case-control study of subjectsparticipating in the Nottingham faecal occult blood screening programme. Br J Cancer 1993;67:172–6.

144. Sandler RS, Lyles CM, Peipins LA, McAuliffe CA, Woosley JT, Kupper LL. Diet and risk of colorectal adenomas: macronutrients, cholesterol, and fiber. J Natl Cancer Inst 1993;85:884–91.

145. Neugut AI, Garbowski GC, Lee WC, Murray T, Nieves JW, Forde KA, et al. Dietary risk factors for the incidence and recurrence of colorectal adenomatous polyps: a case–control study. Ann Intern Med 1993;118:91–5.

146. Martinez ME, McPherson RS, Annegers JF, Levin B, et al. Association of diet and colorectal adenomatous polyps: dietary fiber, calcium, and total fat. Epidemiology 1996;7:264–8.

147. Haile RW, Witte JS, Longnecker MP, Probst-Hensch N, Chen MJ, Harper J, et al. A sigmoidoscopy-based case-control studyof polyps: macronutrients, fiber and meat consumption. Int J Cancer 1997;73:497–502.

148. Lubin F, Rozen P, Arieli B, Farbstein M, Knaani Y, Bat L, et al. Nutritional and lifestyle habits and water-fiber interaction in colorectal adenoma etiology. Cancer Epidemiol Biomarkers Prev 1997;6:79–85.

149. Breuer-Katschinski B, Nemes K, Marr A, Rump B, Leiendecker B, Breuer N, et al. Colorectal Adenoma Study Group. Colorectal adenomas and diet: a case-control study. Dig Dis Sci 2001;46:86–95.

150. Macrae F. Wheat bran fiber and development of adenomatous polyps: evidence from randomized, controlled clinical trials. Am J Med 1999;106:38S–42S.

151. Alberts DS, Einspahr J, Ritenbaugh C, Aickin M, Rees-McGee S, Atwood J, et al. The effect of wheat bran fiber and calcium supplementation on rectal mucosal proliferation rates in patients with resected adenomatous colorectal polyps. Cancer Epidemiol Biomarkers Prev 1997;6:161–9.

152. Alberts DS, Martinez ME, Roe DJ, Guillén-Rodríguez JM, Marshall JR, van Leeuwen JB, et al. Lack of effect of a high-fiber cereal supplement on the recurrence of colorectal adenomas. New Engl J Med 2000;342:1156–62.

153. Jacobs ET, Giuliano AR, Roe DJ, Guillén-Rodríguez JM, Alberts DS, Martínez ME. Baseline dietary fiber intake and colorectal adenoma recurrence in the wheat bran randomized trial. J Natl Cancer Inst 2002;94:1620–5.

154. Jacobs ET, Giuliano AR, Roe DJ, Guillén-Rodríguez JM, Hess LM, Alberts DS, et al. Intake of supplemental and total fiber and risk of colorectal adenoma recurrence in the wheat bran fiber. Cancer Epidemiol Biomarkers Prev 2002;11:906–14.

155. Lanza E, Yu B, Murphy G, Albert PS, Caan B, Marshall JR, et al. The Polyp Prevention Trial – Continued Follow-up Study: no effect of a low-fat, high-fiber, high-fruit, and vegetable diet on adenoma recurrence eight years after randomization. Cancer Epidemiol Biomarkers Prev 2007;16:1745–52.

156. Peters U, Sinha R, Chatterjee N, Subar AF, Ziegler RG, Kulldorff M, et al. Dietary fibre and colorectal adenoma in a colorectal cancer earlydetection programme. Lancet 2003;361:1491–5.

157. Jacobs ET, Lanza E, Alberts DS, Hsu CH, Jiang R, Schatzkin A, et al. Fiber, sex and colorectal adenoma: results of a pooled analysis. Am J Clin Nutr 2006;83:343–9.

158. Sansbury LB, Wanke K, Albert P, Kahle L, Schatzkin A, Lanza E, et al. The effect of strict adherence to a high-fiber, high-fruit and – vegetable, and low fat eating pattern on adenoma recurrence. Am J Epidemiol 2009;170:576–84.

159. MacLennan R, Macrae F, Bain C, Battistutta D, Chapuis P, Gratten H, et al. Randomized trial of intake of fat, fiber, and beta carotene to prevent colorectal adenomas. J Natl Cancer Inst 1995;87:1760–6.

160. Jacobs ET, Jiang R, Alberts DS, Greenberg ER, Gunter EW, Karagas MR, et al. Selenium and colorectal adenoma: results of a pooled analysis. J Natl Cancer Inst 2004;96:1669–75.

161. Bobe G, Murphy G, Albert PS, Sansbury LB, Young MR, Lanza E, et al. Do interleukin polymorphism play a role in the prevention of colorectal adenoma recurrence by dietary flavonols? Eur J Cancer Prev 2011;20:86–95.

162. Bobe G, Albert PS, Sansbury LB, Lanza E, Schatzkin A, Colburn NH, et al. Interleukin-6 as a potential indicator for prevention of high-risk adenoma recurrence by dietary flavonols in the Polyp Prevention Trial. Cancer Prev Res 2010;3:764–75.

163. Ho EE, Atwood JR, Benedict J, Ritenbaugh C, Sheehan ET, Abrams C, et al. A community-based feasibility study using wheat bran fiber supplementation to lower colon cancer risk. Prev Med 1991;20:213–25.

164. Howe GR, Benito F, Castelloto R, Cornée J, Estève J, Gallagher RP, et al. Dietary intake of fiber and decreased risk of cancers of the colon and rectum: evidence from the combined analysis of 13 case-control studies. J Nat Cancer Inst 1992;84:1887–96.

165. Trock B, Lanza E, Greenwald P. Dietary fiber, vegetables, and colon cancer critical review and meta-analyses of the epidemiologic evidence. J Natl Cancer Inst 1990;82:650–61.

166. Heilbrun LK, Nomura A, Hankin JH, Stemmermann GN, et al. Diet and colorectal cancer with special reference to fiber intake. Int J Cancer 1989;44:1–6.

167. Steinmetz KA, Kushi LH, Bostick RM, Folsom AR, Potter JD, et al. Vegetables, fruit, and colon cancer in the Iowa Womens' Health Study. Am J Epidemiol 1994;139:1–15.

168. Giovannucci E, Rimm EB, Stampfer MJ, Colditz GA, Ascherio A, Willett WC. Intake of fat, meat, and fiber in relation to risk of colon cancer in men. Cancer Res 1994;54:2390–7.

169. Kato I, Akhmedkhanov A, Koenig K, Toniolo PG, Shore RE, Riboli E. Prospective study of diet and female colorectal cancer: the New York University Womens' Health Study. *Nutr Cancer* 1997;**28**:276–81.

170. Sellers TA, Bazyk AE, Bostick RM, Kushi LH, Olson JE, Anderson KE, et al. Diet and risk of colon cancer in a large prospective study of older women: an analysis stratified on family history (Iowa, United States). *Cancer Causes Control* 1998;**9**:357–67.

171. Pietinen P, Malila N, Virtanen M, Hartman TJ, Tangrea JA, Albanes D, et al. Diet and the risk of colorectal cancer in a cohort of Finnish men. *Cancer Causes Control* 1999;**10**:387–96.

172. Fuchs CS, Giovannucci E, Colditz GA, Hunter DJ, Stampfer MJ, Rosner B, et al. Dietary fiber and the risk of colorectal cancer and adenoma in women. *N Engl J Med* 1999;**340**:169–76.

173. Terry P, Giovannucci E, Michels KB, Bergkvist L, Hansen H, Holmberg L, et al. Fruit, vegetable, dietary fiber, and risk of colorectal cancer. *J Natl Cancer Inst* 2001;**93**:525–33.

174. Mai V, Flood A, Peters U, Lacey Jr JV, Schairer C, Schatzkin A. Dietary fibre and risk of colorectal cancer in the Breast Cancer Detection Demonstration Project (BCDDP) follow-up cohort. *Int J Epidemiol* 2003;**32**:234–9.

175. McCullough ML, Robertson AS, Chao A, Jacobs EJ, Stampfer MJ, Jacobs DR, et al. A prospective study of whole grains, fruits, vegetables and colon cancer risk. *Cancer Causes Control* 2003;**14**:959–70.

176. Levi F, Pasche C, Lucchini F, La Vecchia C. Dietary fibre and the risk of colorectal cancer. *Eur J Cancer* 2001;**37**:2091–6.

177. Bingham SA, Day NE, Luben R, Ferrari P, Slimani N, Norat T, et al. Dietary fibre in food and protection against colorectal cancer in the European Prospective Investigation into Cancer and Nutrition (EPIC): an obseravtional study. *Lancet* 2003;**361**:1496–501.

178. Michels KB, Fuchs CS, Giovannucci E, Colditz GA, Hunter DJ, Stampfer MJ, et al. Fiber intake and incidence of colorectal cancer among 76,947 women and 47,279 men. *Cancer Epidemiol Biomarkers Prev* 2005;**14**:842–9.

179. Park Y, Hunter DJ, Spiegelman D, Bergkvist L, Berrino F, van den Brandt PA, et al. Dietary fiber intake and risk of colorectal cancer. A pooled analysis of prospective cohort studies. *J Am Med Assoc* 2005;**294**:2849–57.

180. Dahm CC, Keogh RH, Spencer EA, Greenwood DC, Key TJ, Fentiman IS, et al. Dietary fiber and colorectal cancer risk: a nested case-control study using food diaries. *J Natl Cancer Inst* 2010;**102**:614–26.

181. Uchida K, Kono S, Yin G, Toyomura K, Nagano J, Mizoue T, et al. Dietary fiber, source foods and colorectal cancer risk: the Fukuoka Colorectal Cancer Study. *Scand J Gastroenterol* 2010;**45**:1223–31.

182. Aune D, Chan DSM, Lu R, Vieira R, Greenwood DC, Kampman E, et al. Dietary fibre, whole grains, and risk of colorectal cancer: systematic review and dose-response meta-analysis of prospective studies. *Br Med J* 2011;**343** d6617.doi:10.1136/bmj.d6617.

183. Hansen L, Skeie G, Landberg R, Lund E, Palmqvist R, Johansson I, et al. Intake of dietary fiber, especially from cereal food, is associated with lower incidence of colon cancer in the HELGA cohort. *Int J Cancer* 2012;**131**:469–78.

184. Limburg PJ, Mahoney MR, Allen-Ziegler KL, Sontag SJ, Schoen RE, Benya R, et al. Randomized phase II trial of sulindac, atrovastin, and prebiotic dietary fiber for colorectal cancer chemoprevention. *Cancer Prev Res.* 2011;**4**:259–69.

185. Parkin DM, Bray F, Ferlay J, Pisani P. Global cancer statistics 2002. *CA Cancer J Clin* 2005;**55**:74–108.

186. Gingras D, Beliveau R. Colorectal cancer prevention through dietary and lifestyle modifications. *Cancer Microenvironment* 2011;**4**:133–9.

187. Caswell S, Anderson AS, Steele RJ. Bowel health to better health: a minimal contact lifestyle intervention for people at increased risk of colorectal cancer. *Br J Nutr* 2009;**102**:1541–6.

188. Franco A, Sikalidis AK, Solis-Herruzo JA. Colorectal cancer: influence of diet and lifestyle factors. *Rev Esp Enferm Dig (Madrid)* 2005;**97**:432–48.

D. WHEAT IN CANCER PREVENTION

Whole Grain and Dietary Fiber Intake and Risk of Prostate Cancer

Katharina Nimptsch

Max Delbrück Center for Molecular Medicine (MDC), Molecular Epidemiology Research Group, Berlin, Germany

INTRODUCTION

Prostate cancer is the second most frequent cancer among men worldwide, and the sixth most frequent cause of cancer death.[1] Screening by measurement of prostate-specific antigen (PSA) in blood became widely available in the 1990s, and since then the majority of prostate cancer cases have been initially detected by PSA screening in many industrialized countries. The wide availability of PSA tests has resulted in a shift in the mixture of diagnosed cases towards a growing number of early, localized prostate cancers, a proportion of which never become clinically significant during the lifetime,[2,3] while the proportion of advanced cancers at diagnosis has decreased. Compared to other types of cancer, prostate cancer has been shown to be affected to a great extent by genetic factors,[4] and the only established risk factors for prostate cancer are age, race/ethnicity, and family history of prostate cancer.[5] Nevertheless, the descriptive epidemiology of prostate cancer in the past 50–100 years supports a role for environmental factors, including diet, in prostate cancer etiology. First, the marked variation of prostate cancer incidence rates across the world, with lower rates in Africa and Asia and higher rates in industrialized areas such as Western Europe and the US,[1] suggests a potential role for environmental factors. This large difference in incidence rates across the world may partly be explained by the availability of screening practices, especially PSA screening. However, even before PSA screening became widely available, worldwide variation in incidence rates was apparent. Furthermore, prostate cancer mortality rates, which are less influenced by PSA screening rates, also vary substantially across countries worldwide.[1] The steady increase in prostate cancer incidence rates within the past 50 years, especially in industrialized countries, also suggests that prostate cancer may be influenced by lifestyle factors

that have changed over this same time period, such as diet. Again, this increase in incidence may be partly explained by increased use of PSA screening over time, but increases in incidence rates were already apparent before PSA screening became available, and increases in incidence rates are also observed in countries where PSA screening is not common, such as Japan and Eastern European countries.[6] Striking support for a role of environmental factors in the etiology of prostate cancer comes from migrant studies showing that men moving from countries with low prostate cancer incidence rates such as Japan to the US adapt to the host countries' incidence rates within one or two generations.[7,8]

The Western lifestyle is characterized by low physical activity; a positive energy balance; and a diet high in total and saturated fats, animal protein, and refined sugars, and low in dietary fiber. It has been proposed that the high prostate cancer incidence in Western countries and the increase in incidence rates over the past 50 years may be partly explained by the low content of fiber and whole grains in the Western diet. An estimated 95% of grains available for consumption in the US are refined.[9] During the industrial refining process, the outer bran layers as well as the germ are removed, and with them a variety of bioactive substances such as fiber, antioxidants, minerals, vitamins, phytoestrogens (lignans), and phenolic compounds.[10] According to a definition by Jacobs and colleagues, whole grain products comprise dark bread, brown rice, popcorn, wheat germ, bran, cooked oatmeal, bulgur, couscous, and breakfast cereals with a whole grain or bran content greater than 25% by weight.[11] Dietary fiber has been defined by the American Association of Cereal Chemists (AACC) as "the remnants of the edible part of plants and analogous carbohydrates that are resistant to digestion and absorption in the human small intestine with complete or partial fermentation in the human large intestine".[12] Whole grains are rich sources of dietary fiber, but fruit, vegetables, and legumes also provide considerable fiber in the human diet. The bioactive substances found in whole grain foods and foods high in dietary fiber may exert protective effects against prostate cancer through multiple and partially overlapping biological mechanisms.[10] While the consumption of whole grains is recommended worldwide because of the beneficial effects on obesity or weight gain, the reduced risk of cardiovascular diseases (including coronary heart disease, hypertension, and stroke), improved gut health, and lower risk of cancers of the upper gut and possibly colorectal cancer, and lower mortality rates,[13] it is less clear whether a diet with a high proportion of whole grains and a high fiber content may also be beneficial for prostate cancer prevention.

EXPERIMENTAL AND CLINICAL STUDIES SUGGESTING A PROSTATE CANCER-PROTECTIVE EFFECT OF WHOLE GRAINS

Animal studies have shown that whole grain rye and rye-based products have beneficial effects on prostate cancer progression, including delayed tumor growth and enhanced tumor cell apoptosis.[14,15] In a small human pilot study in men with prostate cancer, higher apoptosis rates were observed after 3 weeks of a rye bran bread diet compared to a refined wheat control diet.[16] In a small randomized controlled crossover trial in men with prostate cancer, a diet rich in whole grain and bran from rye compared with cellulose-supplemented refined wheat resulted in significantly lower plasma PSA concentrations, which can be considered a biomarker for prostate cancer progression.[17]

MECHANISMS SUGGESTED FOR DIETARY FIBER AND WHOLE GRAINS TO PLAY A ROLE IN PROSTATE CANCER ETIOLOGY

Gastrointestinal Response/Short-Chain Fatty Acid Production

In contrast to refined grains, whole grains are a rich source of fermentable carbohydrates such as dietary fiber, resistant starch, and oligosaccharides. During fermentation of insoluble fiber and undigested carbohydrates by the intestinal microflora, short-chain fatty acids, including butyrate, acetate, and propionate, are produced, of which butyrate is the preferred fuel of colonic mucosa cells.[10] Butyrate has also been shown to be a potent growth inhibitor, initiating cell differentiation and promoting apoptosis in several cancer cell lines, including

prostate cancer cells.[18] Thus, one potential mechanism through which dietary fiber and whole grains may lower risk of prostate cancer is the production of short-chain fatty acids in the gut microflora.

Hyperinsulinemia

Whole grain foods and foods rich in dietary fiber have been shown to slow digestion and delay absorption of carbohydrates. Blood glucose and insulin responses are affected by food structure –i.e., the more intact the physical or botanical structure of food ingredients, the lower and more delayed are postprandial blood glucose and insulin responses.[19] Breads made with a high proportion of whole cereal grains have been shown to reduce postprandial blood glucose profiles in diabetics more than white bread, but also more than "whole meal" bread, suggesting that the entity of whole grain ingredients is more effective in delaying digestion and absorption of carbohydrates than the mere dietary fiber content.[20]

Hyperinsulinemia and insulin resistance, i.e., reduced response of tissues to the physiological actions of insulin, have been proposed as one of the pathways through which diet and lifestyle factors may influence prostate cancer risk and progression.[21] The blood glucose and insulin response depends on the carbohydrate quality, which can be characterized by the content of dietary fiber or whole grains. A Western dietary pattern low in fiber and whole grains has been shown to be associated with insulin resistance.[22] Furthermore, in a randomized controlled trial, rye whole grain and bran product intake compared with refined wheat intake was associated with decreased fasting plasma insulin in men with prostate cancer.[17] Circulating insulin may influence prostate carcinogenesis either directly or indirectly through the potent mitogen insulin-like growth factor 1 (IGF-1).[23] Hyperinsulinemia enhances the bioactivity of IGF-1 by upregulating hepatic IGF-1 synthesis, or by reducing hepatic secretion of two IGF binding proteins (IGFBP-1 and IGFBP-2), resulting in higher free or bioactive IGF-1 levels.[23,24] The insulin and IGF responses are mediated by insulin receptors (IR) and IGF-1 receptors (IGF1R), both of which are widely expressed in normal tissues and are overexpressed in many cancer cell lines, including prostate cancer cells.[25] Binding of insulin or IGF-1 to their receptors is followed by a signal transduction cascade which may stimulate a number of cancerogenic phenotypes, including stimulation of cell proliferation, suppression of apoptosis, invasion, and metastasis, potentially enhancing promotion and progression.[26]

Blood concentrations of insulin and circulating C-peptide, which poses a more stable marker of insulin secretion, have been investigated in relation to prostate cancer in a number of epidemiological studies. In a Chinese case–control study, a 2.6-fold higher risk of prostate cancer was observed when comparing top and bottom tertiles of fasting plasma insulin.[27] While one Swedish cohort study found no association between insulin levels and risk of prostate cancer,[28] in another Swedish study circulating C-peptide tended to be positively associated with aggressive prostate cancer.[29] In the Physicians' Health Study, among men with prostate cancer, those with high prediagnostic C-peptide had a two-fold risk of dying from prostate cancer.[30] In a male Finnish cohort, elevated fasting serum insulin concentrations were associated with higher risk of prostate cancer.[31] Although not entirely consistent, these results support the hypothesis that high insulin may increase risk of prostate cancer, or at least prostate cancer progression and mortality.

The two most recent meta-analyses on circulating IGF-1 and prostate cancer risk consistently showed that high IGF-1 concentrations were moderately associated with higher risk of prostate cancer,[32,33] and one of them observed stronger associations with advanced than with localized prostate cancer.[33]

In summary, dietary intake of fiber and whole grains may influence prostate cancer risk through the insulin/IGF-1 axes. Fiber content and whole grains affect glucose and insulin responses. Hyperinsulinemia and insulin resistance have been plausibly linked to prostate carcinogenesis in a variety of experimental studies. Furthermore, serologic evidence supports the hypothesis that hyperinsulinemia and high circulating IGF-1 are associated with higher risk of prostate cancer, with slightly more consistent associations with advanced or aggressive prostate cancer.

Antioxidants

Oxidative stress denotes an imbalance between the production of reactive oxygen species and the antioxidant capacity of the target cell.[10] Oxidative stress induces DNA damage, thereby increasing the rate of cancer-initiating mutations.[34] Furthermore, oxidative stress promotes prostate cancer progression through triggering cell survival pathways, stimulation of growth signaling cascades that lead to more aggressive prostate cancer phenotypes, activation of inflammatory pathways, and development of hormone independence and castration resistance.[34]

Whole grains contain a variety of antioxidants, including vitamins such as vitamin E; minerals such as selenium, copper, zinc and manganese; phenolic acids; lignans; phytoestrogens; and phytic acid. All of these compounds are found in high concentrations in the outer layers of grains, and are thus mostly removed during the refining process. Therefore, the antioxidant potential of refined grains is close to zero whereas whole grains have a substantial antioxidant capacity that may lower the risk of prostate cancer.

Phytoestrogens

Phytoestrogens such as isoflavones, coumestans, and lignans are plant-derived compounds that exert estrogenic or anti-estrogenic effects due to their structural similarity to estrogen.[35] While isoflavones are abundant in soy, and coumestans originate from alfalfa sprouts and beans, lignans mainly originate from whole grain cereals, providing precursors for enterolactone and enterodiol, which are synthesized by the intestinal flora.[36] In vitro and in vivo studies have demonstrated preventive effects of lignans on prostate cancer development.[37] Proposed mechanisms include the modulation of steroid metabolism (reduction of serum 17β-estradiol and testosterone), as well as non-endocrine mechanisms such as inhibition of tumor formation and tumor cell growth, antioxidant activity, and inhibition of proteases, tyrosine kinases, and angiogenesis. Due to the lack of reliable data on content of lignans in various foods, direct assessments of dietary lignan intake in relation to risk of prostate cancer are scarce. Urinary lignan excretion in the form of enterolactone and enterodiol, as well as serum concentrations of these compounds, may serve as an indirect measure of lignans in the diet. However, so far neither urinary[38] nor blood concentrations[39,40] of enterolactone have been associated with risk of prostate cancer in nested case–control studies.

In summary, although there is evidence from in vitro and in vivo studies that whole grain-derived lignans may lower prostate cancer risk, this has not been supported by epidemiological studies investigating urinary or blood concentrations of enterolactone as an indirect measure of dietary lignan intake.

Dietary Fiber and Sex-Hormone-Binding Globulin

It has been suggested that dietary fiber influences prostate cancer risk through sex-hormone-binding globulin (SHBG), because dietary fiber has been shown to correlate with circulating SHBG in men[41] and higher serum SHBG concentrations have been associated with a modestly decreased prostate cancer risk.[42] However, because SHBG correlates inversely with insulin and IGF-1, it cannot be ruled out that the observed inverse association between SHBG and prostate cancer may be partly explained by the negative association between SHBG and the insulin/IGF axis, which itself is associated with higher risk of prostate cancer.

EPIDEMIOLOGICAL STUDIES RELATING HABITUAL INTAKE OF WHOLE GRAINS OR DIETARY FIBER TO RISK OF PROSTATE CANCER

Since 1992, epidemiological studies have been conducted with the aim of finding out whether the cancer-preventive effects of dietary fiber and whole grains that have been postulated and observed in experimental and clinical studies can also be seen at the population level (Table 9.1).

Case–Control Studies

In two early case–control studies conducted in the 1990s, no significant association between whole meal bread[43] or whole grain foods (essentially bread and pasta)[44] and risk of prostate cancer was observed. The first case–control study relating dietary fiber to risk of prostate cancer, which was published in 1995, found no association.[45] In 2004 a case–control study on the association between dietary fiber and risk of prostate cancer was published,[46] which had a more than four-fold number of cases compared to the case–control study from 1995.[45] In this study,[46] no association between total fiber intake and risk of prostate cancer was observed, but vegetable fiber was significantly inversely associated with risk of prostate cancer, whereas grain fiber was positively associated with prostate cancer risk.[46] In the first US-based case–control study on the association between dietary fiber and risk of prostate cancer,[47] dietary fiber intake was not associated with risk of prostate cancer, whereas a significant inverse association between dietary lignans and prostate cancer risk was observed. Four years later, a significant inverse association between fiber intake and prostate cancer risk was observed in another US-based case–control study.[48]

Cohort Studies

The first prospective investigation on the association between dietary fiber and risk of prostate cancer was conducted within the European Prospective Investigation into Cancer and Nutrition (EPIC).[49] Among 142,590 men, 2747 were diagnosed with prostate cancer during 8.7 years of follow-up. No association between total dietary fiber, cereal, fruit or vegetable fiber, and risk of prostate cancer was observed in this large study. When investigating subtypes of prostate cancer, no association was observed with advanced, localized, low-grade, or high-grade prostate cancer. In a large US cohort of 49,934 men of whom 5112 were diagnosed with prostate cancer between 1986 and 2007, no association between dietary fiber intake and risk of total or advanced/fatal prostate cancer was observed.[50] To the authors' surprise, in this study a significant positive association between whole grain intake and risk of prostate cancer was observed. The significant association, however, disappeared after restriction to PSA-screened participants. In a Danish cohort study comprising 26,691 men and 1081 prostate cancer cases diagnosed within 12 years of follow-up, no association between dietary fiber or consumption of whole grain products and prostate cancer risk was observed.[51] None of the specific whole grain products, such as whole grain rye, whole grain bread, or oatmeal, was individually associated with prostate cancer risk. In an Icelandic cohort study of 2268 elderly men of whom 347 were diagnosed with prostate cancer between 2002 and 2006, in line with previous cohort studies no association between whole grain rye bread, oatmeal, or whole wheat bread consumed in midlife was observed.[52] However, the aim of this study was to investigate whether consumption of whole grain products at different stages in life were associated with prostate cancer. It was observed that frequent rye bread consumption during adolescence was associated with lower risk of advanced prostate cancer and prostate-specific mortality.

While results of case–control studies were mixed, none of the three prospective cohort studies investigating the association between dietary fiber and risk of prostate cancer[49,50,53] observed that high fiber intake was statistically significantly associated with lower risk of prostate cancer. Similarly, none of the three cohort studies associating adult whole grain intake with risk of prostate cancer found a statistically significant association.[50–52] A significant inverse association between total fiber and risk of prostate cancer was observed in one case–control study,[48] and between vegetable fiber and risk of prostate cancer in another case–control study.[46] In general, findings from studies investigating the association between dietary intake and risk of disease in a case–control setting require cautious interpretation due to the possibility of systematic error. Thus, since the dietary exposure is assessed after the diagnosis, it is possible that, at the time of dietary assessment, cases had already changed their diet due to early disease symptoms. Furthermore, recall bias (i.e., the differential dietary reporting behavior in cases as compared to controls) may distort findings from case–control studies. Since in prospective cohort studies the dietary exposure is assessed before the diagnosis of disease, this type of bias is less of an issue. Both case–control and cohort studies have the limitation of measurement error in dietary assessment. The estimation of dietary fiber intake or whole grain intake by means of food frequency questionnaires or diet history is prone to error. Although the here reviewed prospective cohort studies used validated dietary assessment methods,[49–53] measurement error cannot be excluded. Since in prospective studies measurement error tends to be non-differential (i.e., not associated with the outcome)

TABLE 9.1 Epidemiological Studies Relating Whole Grains or Dietary Fiber Intake to Risk of Prostate Cancer

Reference	Study Type	Participants	Country	Dietary Assessment	Exposure	Intake Comparison	RR/OR (95% CI), p-trend	Adjustment Variables
Tabung et al.[54]	Case-only	930 African American men, 993 European American men with prostate cancer	USA	Diet history	Whole grains, dietary fiber	Highest versus lowest tertile	Whole grains with aggressive CaP 0.88 (0.63, 1.22), 0.15 Total fiber with aggressive CaP 0.61 (0.40, 0.93), 0.02	Age, race, energy intake, education, smoking status, physical activity, use of supplements, NSAIDs, PSA screening history, family history of prostate cancer, BMI
Drake et al.[53]	Prospective cohort	8128 men, 817 prostate cancer cases	Sweden	Diet history	Whole grains, dietary fiber	Highest versus lowest quintile	Whole grains Total CaP 1.00 (0.78, 1.28), 0.80 Low-risk 1.11 (0.82, 1.50), 0.61 High-risk 0.84 (0.55, 1.28), 0.71 Dietary fiber Total CaP 1.15 (0.89, 1.49), 0.13 Low-risk 1.24 (0.90, 1.70), 0.09 High-risk 0.97 (0.61, 1.52), 0.92	Year of study entry, season, energy, height, waist, physical activity, smoking, educational level, birth in Sweden, alcohol, calcium, selenium; competing risk by death from all causes was taken into account
Torfadottir et al.[52]	Prospective cohort	2268 men, 347 cases	Iceland	FFQ	Rye bread consumption in adolescence, midlife, and late life	Rye bread daily versus less than daily during adolescence Oat meal ≥5 versus ≤4 times/week during adolescence	Total CaP 0.76 (0.59, 0.98) Advanced CaP 0.47 (0.27–0.84) Total CaP 0.99 (0.77, 1.27) Advanced CaP 0.67 (0.37–1.20) Midlife and late life consumption of rye bread, oatmeal or whole wheat bread was not associated with CaP risk	Birth year, age, education, family history of prostate disease, going to a physician regularly, height, BMI, diabetes
Egeberg et al.[51]	Prospective cohort	26,691 men, 1081 prostate cancer cases	Denmark	FFQ	Whole grain products	Per 50 g/day (total whole grain products) or 25 g/day (whole grain rye bread, whole grain bread, oatmeal)	No association between whole grain products and prostate cancer risk, no association between specific whole grain products whole grain rye bread, whole grain bread, oatmeal and risk of prostate cancer, no risk associated with either stage or grade of disease	Age as time scale, adjusted for height, weight, school education, intake of red meat, processed meat, and dairy products, and smoking status
Nimptsch et al.[50]	Prospective cohort	49,934 men, 5112 cases	USA	FFQ	Whole grains, dietary fiber	Highest versus lowest quintile	Whole grains Total CaP 1.13 (1.03, 1.24), 0.001 Advanced/fatal CaP 1.11 (0.88, 1.40), 0.22 Dietary fiber Total CaP 1.01 (0.92, 1.12), 0.70 Advanced/fatal CaP 1.02 (0.80, 1.30), 0.81	Stratified by period and age, adjusted for BMI, height, diabetes, family history of CaP, race/ethnicity, smoking, vigorous physical activity, energy intake, alcohol, calcium, α-linolenic acid, and tomato sauce intake

(Continued)

TABLE 9.1 Epidemiological Studies Relating Whole Grains or Dietary Fiber Intake to Risk of Prostate Cancer—cont'd

Reference	Study Type	Participants	Country	Dietary Assessment	Exposure	Intake Comparison	RR/OR (95% CI), p-trend	Adjustment Variables
Lewis et al.[48]	Case–control	478 cases (373 incident, 105 prevalent), 382 controls	USA	FFQ	Dietary fiber	Highest versus lowest tertile	0.56 (0.35–0.89), <0.05	Age, education, BMI, smoking, family history of CaP, energy intake
Suzuki et al.[49]	Multicenter prospective cohort	2747 cases, 142,590 cohorts	10 European countries	FFQ	Dietary fiber	Per 10 g/day	Total CaP 0.97 (0.92, 1.3), 0.38; Localized stage 0.84 (0.70–1.01), 0.07; Advanced stage 1.01 (0.79–1.30), 0.94; Low grade 0.89 (0.73–1.09), 0.27; High grade 0.90 (0.71–1.15), 0.40; No association with fiber from cereal, fruits, or vegetables and risk of total, localized, advanced stage, low-grade or high-grade CaP	Stratified by study center, adjusted for age, energy intake, height, weight, smoking education, and marital status
McCann et al.[47]	Population-based case–control	443 cases, 538 controls	USA	FFQ	Dietary fiber	>38 g/day versus ≤23 g/day	0.79 (0.51–1.22), 0.25; 1.21 (0.73–2.01), 0.1	Age, education, BMI, smoking, total energy (first OR) + vegetables (second OR)
Pelucchi et al.[46]	Hospital-based multi-centre case–control	1294 cases, 1451 controls	Italy	FFQ	Dietary fiber	Highest versus lowest quintile	Total fiber 0.93 (0.71–1.22), ≥0.05; Vegetable fiber 0.62 (0.47–0.80), <0.05; Fruit fiber 0.82 (0.63–1.06), ≥0.05; Grain fiber 1.24 (0.94–1.62), ≥0.05	Age, study center, education, family history of prostate cancer, smoking, alcohol, total energy
Chatenoud et al.[44]	Hospital-based case–control	127 cases, 3220 controls	Italy	FFQ	Whole grain food (essentially bread or pasta)	High consumption (>3 days/week) versus low (no or rare) consumption	0.9 (0.4-1.7), 0.4	Age, education, smoking habits, alcohol intake, and BMI
Rohan et al.[45]	Case–control	207 cases, 207 controls	Canada	Diet history	Dietary fiber	Unspecified	No association	Age, energy, family history of PCa, BPH
Talamini et al.[43]	Hospital-based case–control	271 cases, 685 controls	Italy	FFQ	Whole meal bread	Unspecified	0.9, >0.05	Age, area of residence, education, BMI

Abbreviations: RR, relative risk; OR, odds ratio; CI, confidence interval; CaP, prostate cancer; PSA, prostate-specific antigen; BMI, body mass index; NSAIDs, non-steroid anti-inflammatory drugs.

and non-differential measurement error leads to a bias in estimates towards the null association, it cannot be excluded that an actual association between dietary fiber or whole grains and risk of prostate cancer has been missed due to inaccuracies in dietary assessment methods. Another potential source of bias in studies relating dietary fiber or whole grain intake to risk of prostate cancer is that high consumption of whole grains and fiber may be an indicator for a general healthy lifestyle. Thus, persons with high whole grain and fiber consumption may be more physically active, less often smokers, and less often obese than persons with low consumption. Furthermore, the health consciousness of persons with high whole grain and fiber intake may include more frequent participation in PSA screening, leading to detection bias – i.e., men with high whole grain or fiber intake may be more likely to be diagnosed with prostate cancer than men with low intake, who may also attend PSA screening less often. In such a scenario, a positive association between whole grain/fiber intake and risk of prostate cancer can be observed in the absence of a direct association between whole grain/fiber intake and prostate cancer. This seems to have been the case in the study within the Health Professionals Follow-up Study, where a significant positive association between whole grains and prostate cancer was observed, but no association after restriction of the study population to men who had participated in PSA screening.[50]

The so far mixed and null results regarding the association between whole grain or fiber intake and risk of prostate cancer from epidemiological studies argue against a strong cancer-protective effect of dietary fiber or whole grains on prostate cancer incidence. However, animal studies[14,15] and two small randomized trials in humans[16,17] have shown that whole grains particularly influence prostate cancer progression. While none of the prospective cohort studies observed an association between fiber[49–51] or whole grain[50,51,53] intake and risk of advanced prostate cancer, in a case-only study comprising 930 African Americans and 993 European Americans with prostate cancer, dietary intake of total fiber, insoluble fiber, and soluble fiber was significantly inversely associated with aggressive prostate cancer.[54] Whole grains, however, were not associated with aggressive disease in the same study.

CONCLUSION

While animal and clinical studies provide support for an effect of whole grains on prostate cancer progression, epidemiological evidence does not support the hypothesis that the risk of prostate cancer can be effectively reduced by high intake of whole grains or dietary fiber. There is some epidemiological support indicating that a high-fiber diet is inversely associated with prostate cancer aggressiveness, but this finding requires confirmation by future studies. While whole grains and fiber may have beneficial effects on metabolic diseases such as diabetes, cardiovascular diseases, or other types of cancer, given the currently available evidence a diet rich in dietary fiber and whole grains is unlikely to exert beneficial effects with respect to prostate cancer risk.

References

1. Ferlay J, Shin H, Bray F, Forman D, C. M, Parkin D. ea. GLOBOCAN 2008 v1.2, Cancer incidence and mortality worldwide. IARC CancerBase No. 10. Lyon, France: International Agency for Research on Cancer; 2010. Available from: http://globocan.iarc.fr.
2. Savage CJ, Lilja H, Cronin AM, Ulmert D, Vickers AJ. Empirical estimates of the lead time distribution for prostate cancer based on two independent representative cohorts of men not subject to prostate-specific antigen screening. Cancer Epidemiol Biomarkers Prev 2010;19(5):1201–7.
3. Savage CJ, Lilja H, Cronin AM, Ulmert D, Vickers AJ. Empirical estimates of the lead time distribution for prostate cancer based on two independent representative cohorts of men not subject to prostate-specific antigen screening. Cancer Epidemiol Biomarkers Prev 2010;19(5):1201–7.
4. Lichtenstein P, Holm NV, Verkasalo PK, Iliadou A, Kaprio J, Koskenvuo M, et al. Environmental and heritable factors in the causation of cancer–analyses of cohorts of twins from Sweden, Denmark, and Finland. N Eng J med 2000;343(2):78–85.
5. Hsing AW, Chokkalingam AP. Prostate cancer epidemiology. Front biosci 2006;11:1388–413.
6. Jemal A, Center MM, DeSantis C, Ward EM. Global patterns of cancer incidence and mortality rates and trends. Cancer Epidemiol Biomarkers Prev 2010;19(8):1893–907.
7. Shimizu H, Ross RK, Bernstein L, Yatani R, Henderson BE, Mack TM. Cancers of the prostate and breast among Japanese and white immigrants in Los Angeles County. Br J Cancer 1991;63(6):963–6.
8. Kolonel LN, Altshuler D, Henderson BE. The multiethnic cohort study: exploring genes, lifestyle and cancer risk. Nat rev 2004;4(7):519–27.
9. Pereira MA, Jacobs Jr DR, Pins JJ, Raatz SK, Gross MD, Slavin JL, et al. Effect of whole grains on insulin sensitivity in overweight hyperinsulinemic adults. Am J Clin Nutr 2002;75(5):848–55.
10. Slavin JL. Mechanisms for the impact of whole grain foods on cancer risk. J Am Coll Nutr 2000;19(Suppl. 3):300S–7S.
11. Jacobs Jr DR, Meyer KA, Kushi LH, Folsom AR. Whole-grain intake may reduce the risk of ischemic heart disease death in postmenopausal women: the Iowa Women's Health Study. Am J Clin Nutr 1998;68(2):248–57.
12. DeVries JW. On defining dietary fibre. Proc Nutr Soc 2003;62(1): 37–43.
13. Jones JM, Engleson J. Whole grains: benefits and challenges. Annu rev food sci technol 2010;1:19–40.
14. Bylund A, Zhang JX, Bergh A, Damber JE, Widmark A, Johansson A, et al. Rye bran and soy protein delay growth and increase apoptosis of human LNCaP prostate adenocarcinoma in nude mice. Prostate 2000;42(4):304–14.
15. Landstrom M, Zhang JX, Hallmans G, Aman P, Bergh A, Damber JE, et al. Inhibitory effects of soy and rye diets on the development of Dunning R3327 prostate adenocarcinoma in rats. Prostate 1998;36(3):151–61.
16. Bylund A, Lundin E, Zhang JX, Nordin A, Kaaks R, Stenman UH, et al. Randomised controlled short-term intervention pilot study on rye bran bread in prostate cancer. Eur J Cancer Prev 2003;12(5):407–15.

17. Landberg R, Andersson SO, Zhang JX, Johansson JE, Stenman UH, Adlercreutz H, et al. Rye whole grain and bran intake compared with refined wheat decreases urinary C-peptide, plasma insulin, and prostate specific antigen in men with prostate cancer. *J nutr* 2010;**140**(12):2180–6.

18. Tsubaki J, Hwa V, Twigg SM, Rosenfeld RG. Differential activation of the IGF binding protein-3 promoter by butyrate in prostate cancer cells. *Endocrinology* 2002;**143**(5):1778–88.

19. Bjorck I, Granfeldt Y, Liljeberg H, Tovar J, Asp NG. Food properties affecting the digestion and absorption of carbohydrates. *Am J Clin Nutr* 1994;**59**(Suppl. 3):699S–705S.

20. Jenkins DJ, Wesson V, Wolever TM, Jenkins AL, Kalmusky J, Guidici S, et al. Wholemeal versus wholegrain breads: proportion of whole or cracked grain and the glycaemic response, *Br Med J* 1988;**297**(6654):958–60.

21. Kaaks R. Nutrition, insulin, IGF-1 metabolism and cancer risk: a summary of epidemiological evidence. *Novartis Found Symp* 2004;**262**:247–60; discussion 60–68.

22. Giovannucci E, Rimm EB, Liu Y, Willett WC. Height, predictors of C-peptide and cancer risk in men. *Inter J Epidemiol* 2004;**33**(1):217–25.

23. Kaaks R, Lukanova A. Energy balance and cancer: the role of insulin and insulin-like growth factor-I. *Proc Nutr Soc* 2001;**60**(1):91–106.

24. Pollak M, Beamer W, Zhang JC. Insulin-like growth factors and prostate cancer. *Cancer Retastasis Rev* 1998;**17**(4):383–90.

25. Cox ME, Gleave ME, Zakikhani M, Bell RH, Piura E, Vickers E, et al. Insulin receptor expression by human prostate cancers. *Prostate* 2009;**69**(1):33–40.

26. Pollak M. Insulin and insulin-like growth factor signalling in neoplasia. *Nat Rev* 2008;**8**(12):915–28.

27. Hsing AW, Gao YT, Chua Jr S, Deng J, Stanczyk FZ. Insulin resistance and prostate cancer risk. *J Natl Cancer Inst* 2003;**95**(1):67–71.

28. Stattin P, Bylund A, Rinaldi S, Biessy C, Dechaud H, Stenman UH, et al. Plasma insulin-like growth factor-I, insulin-like growth factor-binding proteins, and prostate cancer risk: a prospective study. *J Natl Cancer Ins* 2000;**92**(23):1910–7.

29. Stocks T, Lukanova A, Rinaldi S, Biessy C, Dossus L, Lindahl B, et al. Insulin resistance is inversely related to prostate cancer: a prospective study in Northern Sweden. *Int J Cancer* 2007;**120**(12):2678–86.

30. Ma J, Li H, Giovannucci E, Mucci L, Qiu W, Nguyen PL, et al. Prediagnostic body-mass index, plasma C-peptide concentration, and prostate cancer-specific mortality in men with prostate cancer: a long-term survival analysis. *Lancet oncol* 2008;**9**(11):1039–47.

31. Albanes D, Weinstein SJ, Wright ME, Mannisto S, Limburg PJ, Snyder K, et al. Serum insulin, glucose, indices of insulin resistance, and risk of prostate cancer. *J Natl Cancer Ins* 2009;**101**(18):1272–9.

32. Roddam AW, Allen NE, Appleby P, Key TJ, Ferrucci L, Carter HB, et al. Insulin-like growth factors, their binding proteins, and prostate cancer risk: analysis of individual patient data from 12 prospective studies. *Ann Intern Med* 2008;**149**(7):461–71, W83-8.

33. Rowlands MA, Gunnell D, Harris R, Vatten LJ, Holly JM, Martin RM. Circulating insulin-like growth factor peptides and prostate cancer risk: a systematic review and meta-analysis. *Int J Cancer* 2009;**124**(10):2416–29.

34. Thapa D, Ghosh R. Antioxidants for prostate cancer chemoprevention: challenges and opportunities. *Biochem pharmacol* 2012;**83**(10):1319–30.

35. de Kleijn MJ, van der Schouw YT, Wilson PW, Adlercreutz H, Mazur W, Grobbee DE, et al. Intake of dietary phytoestrogens is low in postmenopausal women in the United States: the Framingham study(1–4). *J Nutr* 2001;**131**(6):1826–32.

36. Ganry O. Phytoestrogens and prostate cancer risk. *Prev med* 2005;**41**(1):1–6.

37. Webb AL, McCullough ML. Dietary lignans: potential role in cancer prevention. *Nutr Cancer* 2005;**51**(2):117–31.

38. Ward H, Chapelais G, Kuhnle GG, Luben R, Khaw KT, Bingham S. Lack of prospective associations between plasma and urinary phytoestrogens and risk of prostate or colorectal cancer in the European Prospective into Cancer – Norfolk study. *Cancer Epidemiol Biomarkers Prev* 2008;**17**(10):2891–4.

39. Stattin P, Adlercreutz H, Tenkanen L, Jellum E, Lumme S, Hallmans G, et al. Circulating enterolactone and prostate cancer risk: a Nordic nested case–control study. *Int J Cancer* 2002;**99**(1):124–9.

40. Travis RC, Spencer EA, Allen NE, Appleby PN, Roddam AW, Overvad K, et al. Plasma phyto-oestrogens and prostate cancer in the European Prospective Investigation into Cancer and Nutrition. *Br J Cancer* 2009;**100**(11):1817–23.

41. Longcope C, Feldman HA, McKinlay JB, Araujo AB. Diet and sex hormone-binding globulin. *J Clin Endocrinol Metab* 2000;**85**(1):293–6.

42. Roddam AW, Allen NE, Appleby P, Key TJ. Endogenous sex hormones and prostate cancer: a collaborative analysis of 18 prospective studies. *J Natl Cancer Inst* 2008;**100**(3):170–83.

43. Talamini R, Franceschi S, La Vecchia C, Serraino D, Barra S, Negri E. Diet and prostatic cancer: a case–control study in northern Italy. *Nutr cancer* 1992;**18**(3):277–86.

44. Chatenoud L, Tavani A, La Vecchia C, Jacobs Jr DR, Negri E, Levi F, et al. Whole grain food intake and cancer risk. *Inter J Cancer* 1998;**77**(1):24–8.

45. Rohan TE, Howe GR, Burch JD, Jain M. Dietary factors and risk of prostate cancer: a case–control study in Ontario, Canada. *Cancer Causes Control* 1995;**6**(2):145–54.

46. Pelucchi C, Talamini R, Galeone C, Negri E, Franceschi S, Dal Maso L, et al. Fibre intake and prostate cancer risk. *Int J cancer* 2004;**109**(2):278–80.

47. McCann SE, Ambrosone CB, Moysich KB, Brasure J, Marshall JR, Freudenheim JL, et al. Intakes of selected nutrients, foods, and phytochemicals and prostate cancer risk in western New York. *Nutr cancer* 2005;**53**(1):33–41.

48. Lewis JE, Soler-Vila H, Clark PE, Kresty LA, Allen GO, Hu JJ. Intake of plant foods and associated nutrients in prostate cancer risk. *Nutr cancer* 2009;**61**(2):216–24.

49. Suzuki R, Allen NE, Key TJ, Appleby PN, Tjonneland A, Johnsen NF, et al. A prospective analysis of the association between dietary fiber intake and prostate cancer risk in EPIC. *Int J Cancer* 2009;**124**(1):245–9.

50. Nimptsch K, Kenfield S, Jensen MK, Stampfer MJ, Franz M, Sampson L, et al. Dietary glycemic index, glycemic load, insulin index, fiber and whole-grain intake in relation to risk of prostate cancer. *Cancer Causes Control* 2011;**22**(1):51–61.

51. Egeberg R, Olsen A, Christensen J, Johnsen NF, Loft S, Overvad K, et al. Intake of whole-grain products and risk of prostate cancer among men in the Danish Diet, Cancer and Health cohort study. *Cancer Causes Control* 2011;**22**(8):1133–9.

52. Torfadottir JE, Valdimarsdottir UA, Mucci L, Stampfer M, Kasperzyk JL, Fall K, et al. Rye bread consumption in early life and reduced risk of advanced prostate cancer. *Cancer Causes Control* 2012;**23**(6):941–50.

53. Drake I, Sonestedt E, Gullberg B, Ahlgren G, Bjartell A, Wallstrom P, et al. Dietary intakes of carbohydrates in relation to prostate cancer risk: a prospective study in the Malmo Diet and Cancer cohort. *Am J Clin Nutr* 2012;**96**(6):1409–18.

54. Tabung F, Steck SE, Su LJ, Mohler JL, Fontham ET, Bensen JT, et al. Intake of grains and dietary fiber and prostate cancer aggressiveness by race. *Prostate cancer* 2012;**2012**:323296.

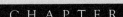

10

Bioactive Phytochemicals in Wheat Bran for Colon Cancer Prevention

Shengmin Sang, Yingdong Zhu

North Carolina Agricultural and Technical State University, Center for Excellence in Post-Harvest Technologies, Kannapolis, North Carolina, USA

INTRODUCTION

Colorectal cancer (CRC) is a leading cause of cancer deaths in the United States.[1] It ranks second only to lung cancer as the largest cause of cancer-related death in men and women combined. Epidemiological studies have suggested that dietary fiber plays an important role in the development of colon cancer.[2,3] For example, Burkitt's pioneering research pointed out that black Africans consuming high-fiber and low-fat foods had a lower mortality due to colon cancer than did white Africans on low-fiber, high-fat diets.[2] There was a lower incidence of colon cancer in the Finnish population than in the United States; despite the equally high consumption of fat by both populations, dietary fiber consumption by the Finnish population was twice that of the US population.[3] Case–control studies on the relationship between dietary fiber and colon cancer have provided more convincing results. Trock et al.[4] and Howe et al.[5] independently performed meta-analyses of several case–control studies conducted in populations with differing colon cancer rates and dietary practices. They found that relative risk decreased significantly as fiber intake increased. Freudenheim and colleagues[6] showed that colon cancer risk decreased with increased intake of grain fiber: insoluble grain fiber was more strongly associated with this risk reduction than the soluble fiber from vegetables and fruits. More recently, the European Prospective Investigation into Cancer and Nutrition Study showed that dietary fiber in foods was inversely related to incidence of large bowel cancer, the protective effect being greatest for the left side of the colon.[7] The American Prostate, Lung, Colorectal, and Ovarian Cancer Screening Trial also indicated that high intake of dietary fiber was associated with a lower risk of colorectal adenoma, after adjustment for potential dietary and non-dietary risk factors.[6] The inverse association was strongest for fiber from grains and cereals and from fruits.[8] Taken together, most of these studies support the hypothesis that dietary fiber, especially fiber from cereal sources, protects against colon cancer.[9–11]

WHEAT BRAN AND COLON CANCER

Human Intervention and Laboratory Animal Studies

Human intervention studies have shown mixed results on wheat bran (WB) consumption and the risk of colon cancer. A WB supplement was reported to inhibit epithelial cell proliferation within the rectal mucosal crypts of patients at high risk for recurrence of colorectal cancer,[12] but a later study did not confirm this.[13] A stronger support for the role of dietary WB in preventing the development of colorectal cancer comes from the Australian Polyp Prevention Project; a randomized study with a low-fat diet supplemented with WB (25 g/day) was found to significantly reduce the recurrence rate of large adenomas (defined as > 1 cm).[14] However, no association was found between WB consumption (13.5 g/day, which is about half of the dose used in the Australian Polyp Prevention Project) and adenoma recurrence in the WB fiber Randomized Trial in the United States.[15]

Human and animal studies indicated that not all fibers are equally efficacious. Intervention studies in humans consuming a high-fat/low-fiber diet demonstrated that adding WB to the diet favorably altered a number of biomarkers related to colon cancer risk, including fecal mutagenicity[16] and secondary bile acids.[17] In such studies, WB was more effective than corn bran or oat bran. Laboratory animal model studies have corroborated this concept.[18] WB is the only cereal bran that shows consistent protection against colon cancer in laboratory animal models.

Barbolt and Abraham[19] reported that a diet containing 20% WB decreased the incidence of 1,2-dimethylhydrazine(DMH)-induced colon tumors in rats. Male F344 rats fed WB and given azoxymethane (AOM)[20] or 3,2′-dimethyl-4-aminobiphenyl(DMAB)[21] had a lower incidence and multiplicity of small intestine and colon tumors than did those fed the control diet and treated with carcinogens. Dietary supplementation with WB also protected against the formation of colonic aberrant crypt foci (ACF) induced by 2-amino-3-methylimidazo[4,5-f]quinoline in the rat.[22] In the Apc(Min/+) mouse model, a diet containing 45% WB significantly decreased the tumor number in small intestine, and WB diets worked better than whole wheat diets.[23]

Role of Fiber

Although most of the human and animal studies show a correlation between WB consumption and reduction in the risk of colon cancer, the mechanism by which dietary WB protects against colon tumor development has not been fully explored. Most of the mechanisms are proposed based on the physiological function of fiber. A proposed mechanism for the action of WB is its fecal dilution effect.[24] Dietary intervention studies in humans indicated that WB supplementation increased fecal bulk, thereby diluting potential carcinogens and tumor promoters in the lumen of the colon.[16,17] Dietary fiber also decreased the formation of secondary bile acids, which increase colon cancer risk.[16,17] A second proposed mechanism for WB is its ability to accelerate the transit of fecal material through the colon, thus reducing access of luminal contents to the colonic epithelial cells.[24] In addition, butyric acid and orthophenolic acids, which are the fermentation products of WB fiber in the colon, have been proposed to be protective agents.[23,24] These proposed mechanisms are a subject of debate.[24] For instance, oat bran produced higher levels of luminal butyric acid than did WB, even though WB showed a protective effect on colon cancer and oat bran enhanced colon carcinogenesis.[25]

Role of Phytochemicals

Dr Reddy's group has previously compared the effects of specific WB fractions, including WB, dephytinized WB (WB-P), defatted WB (WB-F), dephytinized and defatted WB (WB-PF), and WB-PF fortified with 2% WB oil and/or with 0.4% phytate, on colon carcinogenesis in an AOM-induced rat tumor model.[26] They demonstrated for the first time that removal of lipids and lipid-soluble components from WB increased the multiplicity of colon tumors (35% increase, $P < 0.03$) and the tumor volume by about 43% compared with the WB control group. However, WB-PF fortified with excess WB oil (2%) alone or with 2% WB oil plus 0.4% phytate significantly suppressed the incidence (44–61% inhibition; $P < 0.02$ to $P < 0.001$), inhibited the multiplicity (45%–63% inhibition, $P < 0.0003$ to $P < 0.0001$), and reduced the volume (42–58% inhibition, $P < 0.03$ to $P < 0.01$) of adenocarcinomas of the colon as compared with WB, WB-P, WB-F, or WB-PF. Supplementation of WB-PF with phytate alone had no significant effect on colon tumorigenesis. These results indicate that the oil fraction of WB contains bioactive agents that inhibit colon carcinogenesis. Modulation of tumorigenesis by this oil fraction was associated with the alteration in inducible nitric oxide synthase (iNOS) and COX-2 activities. Feeding rats with the WB-PF fortified with excess bran oil significantly suppressed the activities of iNOS and COX-2 as well as the expression of these two enzymes in colon tumors compared with rats fed the WB diet or WB-PF diet.

The inhibitory effect of WB oil on tumorigenesis was also observed in our recent studies in the APC(Min+) mouse model.[27] Our results showed that the mice in the 2% WB oil-treated group had significantly fewer total tumors in small intestine than those in the control group ($P < 0.0001$), with 35.6% inhibition after adjustment of the experimental effect. A greater inhibition was found in the distal small intestine (40.6% inhibition, $P < 0.0001$) than in the middle or in the proximal small intestine. The 2% WB oil also significantly ($P < 0.0001$) inhibited the formation of tumors when analyzed by size, with the greatest inhibition on large tumors (>2 mm, 46.7%). All of these suggest that WB oil is the major active constituent of WB for the inhibition of colon tumorigenesis.

BIOACTIVE PHYTOCHEMICALS IN WHEAT BRAN

The nature of the chemical constituents of WB oil has not been fully delineated. It is known that bran oil consists mainly of triglycerides, as well as mono- and diglycerides, hydrocarbons, free fatty acids, and several lipid-soluble phytochemicals, including 5-alk(en)ylresorcinol, sphingolipids, free phytosterol, phytosterol ferulate, lignans, and phenolic acids.[28–30] The major fatty acids in the WB oil are oleic acid, palmitic acid, and linoleic acid.[29] Studies have shown no relationship between palmitic acid and colorectal cancer.[31] Most studies have indicated no relationship between oleic acid or linoleic acid and colon cancer, but some studies showed that consumption of these fatty acids increased the risk of colon cancer.[31] We and others have found that lipid-soluble phytochemicals are the active components in WB for colon cancer prevention.[27,29]

Alkylresorcinols

One of the major groups of phenolic compounds in whole grain wheat and rye comprises the 5-n-alkylresorcinols (ARs).[32] These are 1,3-dihydroxybenzene derivatives with an odd-numbered alkyl chain at position 5 of the benzene ring. ARs are only present in high amounts in wheat and rye, in which the length of the saturated alkyl tail varies between 15 and 27 carbons. They are generally not found in refined flour or in refined products from cereals. ARs exist in wheat and rye grains at levels of approximately 0.015–0.3% of whole kernel dry weight.[32] Therefore, ARs have been considered to be exposure markers to reflect whole grain wheat and rye consumption.[32]

In our effort to purify and identify the active components from WB oil, we fractionated WB oil through column chromatography into eight fractions.[33] Based on the MTT assay, fraction 7 (F7) had the highest growth inhibitory activity on HCT-116 human colon cancer cells.[33] Similar results were observed on HT-29 human colon cancer cells. Further LC/MS/UV analysis indicated that the major components in F7 are 5-alk(en)ylresorcinol analogues with compounds AR C19:0 and AR C21:0 as the most abundant components.

F7 was applied to a series of chromatographic steps to yield 14 alk(en)ylresorcinol-related analogues (Fig. 10.1).[33] The purified compounds include one new (10′Z,13′Z,16′Z)-5-(nonadeca-10′,13′,16′-trienyl)resorcinol (7), and 13 known alk(en)ylresorcinols (ARs) (1–6 and 8–14). Among the known compounds, (12′Z)-5-(nonadeca-12′-enyl)resorcinol (5), (10′Z,13′Z)-5-(nonadeca-10′,13′-dienyl)resorcinol (6), (16Z′)-5-(heneicos-16′-enyl)resorcinol (9), (12′Z)-5-(heneicos-12′-enyl)resorcinol (10), and 5-(2′-oxotricosyl)

resorcinol (13) were purified for the first time as individual compounds. Their structures were previously predicted from the mixture using mass spectrometry. The structure of compounds 1–4, 8, 11–12, and 14 was identified by comparison of their NMR and MS data with those reported in the literature.[28,34,35] They are 5-n-heptadecylresorcinol (1), (12′Z)-5-(heptadec-12′-enyl)resorcinol (2), 5-n-nonadecylresorcinol (3), (14′Z)-5-(nonadeca-14′-enyl)resorcinol (4), 5-n-heneicosylresorcinol (8), 5-(2′-oxoheneicosyl)resorcinol (11), 5-n-tricosylresorcinol (12), and 5-n-pentadecylresorcinol (14). The positions of the double bond in compounds 2 and 4 and the carbonyl group in 11 were established based on their key HMBC correlations.

All 14 analogues (1–14) except 10 were evaluated for growth-inhibitory activities against human colon cancer cells (HCT-116 and HT-29) using MTT assays.[33] Among the five dominant 5-alkylresorcinols, 5-n-heptadecylresorcinol (1, C17:0; IC$_{50}$ 18.94 μg/mL) had the strongest inhibitory effect on the growth of HCT-116 cells, followed by 5-n-nonadecylresorcinol (3, C19:0; IC$_{50}$ 36.19 μg/mL), whereas 5-n-heneicosenylresorcinol (8, C21:0), 5-n-tricosylresorcinol (12, C23:0), and 5-n-pentadecylresorcinol (14, C25:0) had almost no inhibitory effects, indicating that increasing the length of the side chain will diminish the observed inhibitory effects (ranged from C$_{17}$ to C$_{25}$). Similar results were observed on the HT-29 human colon cancer cells. We also observed that alk(en)ylresorcinols had better inhibitory effects than related alkylresorcinols especially on HCT-116 cells. Compounds 4–7, as members of the C$_{19}$ family owning unsaturated side chains, showed much stronger inhibitory effects than that of 5-n-nonadecylresorcinol (3, C19:0). Similarly, compound 9 (C21:1; IC$_{50}$ 22.28 μg/mL) had much better activity than that of heneicosenylresorcinol (8, C21:0). The presence of a carbonyl group in the alkyl chain enhanced the growth inhibitory effect of compound 11 (IC$_{50}$ 16.63 μg/mL), which had much better inhibitory effects than 8.

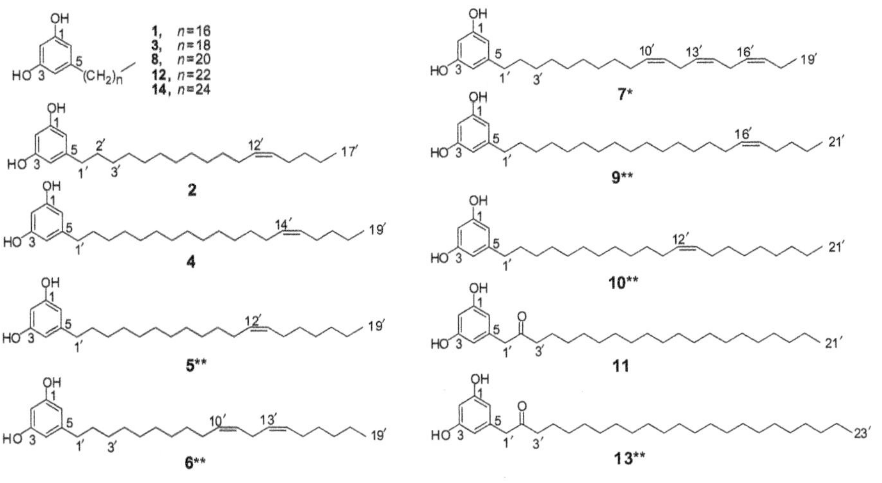

FIGURE 10.1 Structures of the major alkylresorcinols in wheat bran.

To further study the structure–activity relationships, we synthesized 15 ARs and their intermediates including AR C9:0–C15:0.[36] The synthetic AR analogues were evaluated for activities against the growth of human colon cancer cells HCT-116 and HT-29, and the chymotrypsin-like activity of the human 20S proteasome. Our results found that: (1) AR C13:0 and C15:0 had the greatest inhibitory effects in human colon cancer cells HCT-116 and HT-29, while decreasing or increasing the side-chain lengths diminished the activities; (2) two free meta-hydroxyl groups at C-1 and C-3 on the aromatic ring of the AR analogues greatly contributed to their antitumor activity; (3) the introduction of a third hydroxyl group at C-2 into the aromatic ring of the AR analogues yielded no significant enhancement in activity against HCT-116 cells and decimated the effects against HT-29 cells, but dramatically increased the activity against the chymotrypsin-like activity of the human 20S proteasome; and (4) AR C11:0 was found to have the greatest effect in a series of AR C9:0–C17:0 against the chymotrypsin-like activity of the human 20S proteasome.

Evidence on the anticancer effect of ARs is very limited, and most studies have been carried out using cancer cell lines. It has been reported that AR C15:0 could significantly inhibit the growth of BT-20 (IC_{50} 6.25 μg/mL), FM3A (IC_{50} 2.80 μM), and MCF-7 (IC_{50} 37.0 μM) breast cancer cells; NCI-H460 lung cancer cells (IC_{50} 34.2 μM); and HeLa epithelioid cervix carcinoma cells (IC_{50} 4.02 μg/mL).[32,37–39] Arisawa et al. compared the cytotoxicity of ARs with different lengths of side chain (C7:0 to C19:0) on KB cells.[38] They found that C13:0 was the most active AR, and that both increasing and decreasing the chain length would decrease the activity, indicating that the chain length played an important role on the cytotoxicity of ARs against KB cells. This is consistent with our observation on the effect of ARs against human colon cancer cells. Gasiorowski et al. attributed the anticancer effect of ARs to their ability to increase apoptosis in genotoxically damaged cells.[40] We are the first group to identify ARs as the major active components in wheat bran oil to inhibit the growth of human colon cancer cells. Our finding that one of the dominant ARs in wheat bran, 5-n-nonadecylresorcinol (3, C19:0), can inhibit the growth of human colon cancer cells is of significant importance. This indicates that ARs may play an important role in the observed in vivo efficacy of WB. Further studies on the in vivo efficacy of ARs could significantly contribute to our understanding of the colon cancer-preventive effect of WB.

Sphingolipids

Sphingolipids constitute a class of distinct compounds that are both endogenous to mammalian cells and available exogenously through dietary consumption. These unique lipids are composed of a sphingoid long-chain base, a fatty acid tethered to the amino group of the sphingosine, and a variable polar head-group. The sphingosine base and the fatty acid alone constitute ceramide and the linked head-groups can range from phosphocholine (sphingomyelin), to sugars (glycosphingolipids), to complex carbohydrates.[41] Mammalian cells usually contain sphingomyelin, a component not found in plants, and some neutral and acidic glycolipids as complementary constituents to phosphoglycerolipids and cholesterol in the plasma membrane structure.[42] Sphingolipids found in plant cells show more variety in their head-groups, positions of alkene double bonds on the structure, and location of the hydroxyl groups on the sphingoid base.[43] The predominant sphingolipids in plant extracts are glucosylceramide and inositolphosphorylceramide (IPC) derivatives.[44]

Given the complexity and great variety of sphingolipid structures, it is not surprising that these compounds exert a multitude of bioactivities. In addition to their contribution to membrane structure, a growing body of literature suggests that dietary sphingolipids have protective effects against colon cancer. Dietary sphingomyelin supplementation at 0.1% of the diet (wt/wt) reduced the number of aberrant crypt foci (ACF), an early marker of colon carcinogenesis, by ~ 70% in 1,2-dimethylhydrazine (DMH)-treated mice.[45] With longer feeding in the same model, sphingomyelin treatment suppresses the conversion of adenomas to adenocarcinomas.[46] Mazzei et al. found that dietary sphingomyelin suppressed intestinal inflammation and inflammation-driven colon cancer in dextran sodium sulfate- and azoxymethane-treated mice.[47] It has been reported that sphingadienes derived from soy and other natural sphingolipids are cytotoxic to colon cancer cells and reduce adenoma formation in APC(Min/+) mice.[48,49] Aida et al. observed that DMH-treated mice fed diets containing 0.1% or 0.5% maize cerebroside had greatly suppressed ACF formation, with about 60% less ACF than the control group.[50] The activity of sphingolipids from plant-derived sources is extended to other grains, including wheat, a major dietary source of these compounds.[51] For example, biological effects of sphingoid bases prepared from wheat flour were evaluated in DLD-1 human colorectal cancer cells and it was found that apoptosis was induced in a dose-dependent manner.[52]

Whether sphingolipids in WB contribute to its observed colon cancer-preventive effects is still unclear. Although there have been studies implicating ceramide mono-, di-, tri-, or tetrahexosides in wheat flour or wheat grain by FD-MS or GC-MS,[49,53,54] there is a dearth of information on the complete chemical profile of sphingolipids in WB as well as their anticancer activities. In our efforts to evaluate whether sphingolipids in WB contribute to the colon cancer-preventive properties displayed by this grain, we investigated the chemical profile of sphingolipids in WB and further determined the cytotoxic activities of these compounds against human colon cancer cells.

As an ongoing search for bioactive components against colon cancer in WB, the elaborate separation of a sphigolipids-enriched fraction (fraction 8) yielded 12 individual compounds, including 8 cerebrosides (1–8) and 4 ceramides (9–12) (Fig. 10.2).[55] Among them, sphingolipids 1, 6–9, 11, and 12 were reported for the first time as individual components from WB. The structures of sphingolipids 1 and 5–12 were identified using 1D and 2D NMR techniques, and confirmed by comparison of their NMR data with those already published. All 12 purified sphingolipids (1–12) were evaluated for growth-inhibitory effects against human colon cancer cells HCT-116 and HT-29, and showed weak but statistically significant activity at 200 μM in both cell lines. However, at low concentrations (25–50 μM), compounds 3 and 7 in HCT-116 cells and compounds 3 and 12 in HT-29 cells could promote cancer cell growth.

Dietary sphingolipids are enzymatically hydrolyzed to ceramides and free sphingoid bases, which have greater activity in this form, in the gastrointestinal tract.[56,57] Hence the sphingolipids observed in this study may show greater potency in vivo, thereby contributing to the chemopreventative properties associated with WB consumption. For instance, free sphingoid bases have been proven as inhibitors of colon carcinogenesis,[58] showing apoptosis-inducing effects in human colon cancer cells.[59,60] Studies also outline an effective chemopreventative strategy by which non-steroidal anti-inflammatory drugs are taken in tandem with foods rich

in sphingolipids and exert therapeutic activity through activation of lipid hydrolyzing enzymes, converting dietary sphingomyelin to its base ceramide.[61] Further study of the enzymatic metabolism of sphingolipids would be useful for simulating in vivo conditions in preclinical diagnostics.

Steroids

Cereals are one of the main dietary sources of natural phytosterols and their conjugates. Phytosterols and steryl ferulates are concentrated in the bran layers of wheat.[62] The steryl ferulates are accumulated in the intermediate layers, whereas the phytosterol composition varies within the wheat kernel.[62] Sitosterol (1 in Fig. 10.3A) and campestanyl ferulate are the major phytosterol and steryl ferulate in WB.[28,62] Many studies have shown that phytosterols have anticancer activities.[63–65] Epidemiological studies have shown positive correlations between increased dietary phytosterol intake and lower risk for colonic cancer.[66–68] Raicht et al. have shown that rats fed a diet containing 0.3% β-sitosterol had a significantly lower incidence of methylnitrosourea (MNU)-induced tumors than those receiving control diets.[69] Feeding dietary β-sitosterol at a level of 0.3% to MNU-induced rats also significantly decreases the rate of colonic epithelial cell proliferation and compresses the crypts' proliferous compartment.[70] Awad et al. found that dietary supplementation with 2% phytosterol (56% β-sitosterol, 28% campesterol, 10% stigmasterol, and 6% dihydrobrassicasterol) has a significant protective effect on cell proliferation in rat colonic mucosa.[63,71] They also

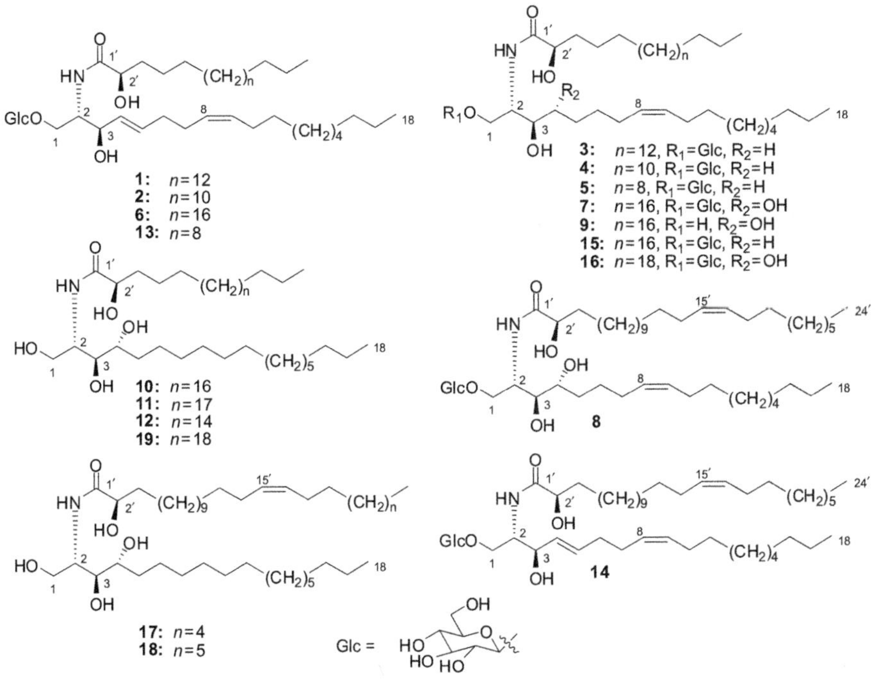

FIGURE 10.2 Structures of the major sphingolipids in wheat bran.

FIGURE 10.3 Structures of the major phytosterols and phytosterol ferulates (A), and lignans and phenolic acid (B), in wheat bran.

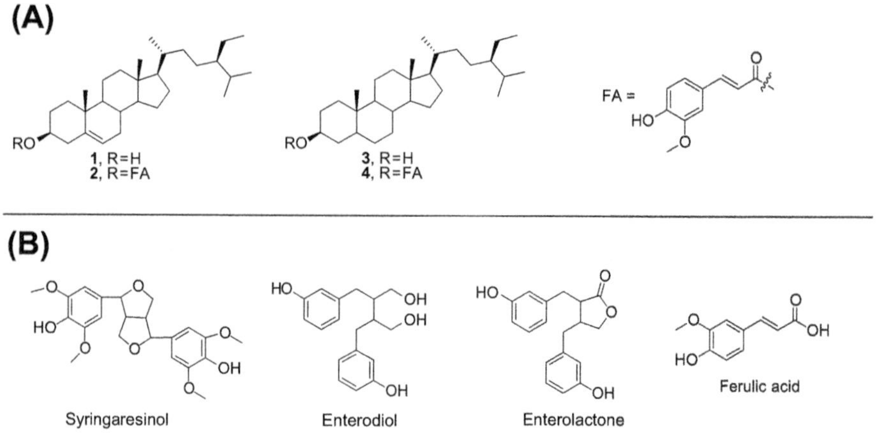

demonstrated that feeding diets supplemented with phytosterol for 22 days counteracted the hyperproliferative effect induced by bile acids in rat colon mucosa. Others reported similar results in mice.[72] It has been reported that β-sitosterol could significantly inhibit the growth of HT-29 human colon cancer cells.[73] Taken together, human, animal, and cell culture studies show that consumption of phytosterols can reduce the risk of colon cancer.

Lignans

Lignans form a group of phenolic compounds with a backbone of two phenylpropanoid (C6C3) units that are widely distributed in the plant kingdom, and includes various vegetables and cereals.[74] They present mainly in the bran part of cereal and are largely, in esterified forms, bound to the cereal matrix.[75] Syringaresinol, medioresinol, lariciresinol, pinoresinol, and secoisolariciresinal have been identified as the major lignans in WB, with syringaresinol being the most abundant one[75] (Fig. 10.3B). It has been reported that lignans can be converted by intestinal microflora to enterodiol and enterolactone (Fig. 10.3B).[76–79] The formation of lignans from WB in rats was reported by Nicolle and co-workers.[80] About 45 nmol/day enterodiol was excreted in urine after 2 weeks of a diet supplemented with 15% wheat bran. Treatment with enterodiol and enterolactone, alone or in combination, at 0–40 μM resulted in dose- and time-dependent inhibition of the growth of human colonic cancer SW480 cells.[81] DNA flow cytometric analysis indicated that the treatments induced cell cycle arrest at the S phase. Apoptosis analysis showed an increased percentage of apoptotic cells after enterodiol alone or combined treatments. In rats given the carcinogen azoxymethane, the lignin secoisolariciresinol diglycoside reduced the number of aberrant crypts foci in the distal colon compared with control rats given no lignan.[82,83] These results suggest that lignans may contribute to the colon cancer

prevention by WB. However, whether the amount of lignans in WB is high enough to reach the effective dose *in vivo* is still questionable.

Phenolic Acids

Phenols that possess a carboxylic acid are labeled phenolic acids. Phenolic acids have been reported to be in free, bound, or soluble-conjugated forms, and characterized from wholegrain, endosperm, bran, germ, flour, and gluten.[82,84,85] Wholegrain wheat flour was examined and the bran/germ layers accounted for 83% of the total phenolic acids measured.[86] Ferulic acid is the dominating phenolic acid in wheat, mainly found in the bound form, and is said to comprise 70–90% of the total phenolic acids present[82,85] (Fig. 10.3B). Wheat samples representing numerous strains and cultivars were screened for their *in vitro* ability to kill a human colon cancer cell, CaCo2.[87] Samples containing low, mid, and high *in vitro* protective ability were used to formulate balanced diets fed to Min mice. Wheat samples with a high ability to kill CaCo2 cells in culture had high levels of orthophenolic acids and produced elevated blood caffeic acid levels when used in diets. The antitumor activity of the wheat bran diets positively correlated with the levels of orthophenolic acids in the wheat samples. Specifically wheats, which elevated blood caffeic acid levels, had a strong antitumor effect.

CONCLUSIONS

In conclusion, many studies have found that phytochemicals, the non-fibrous components in WB, may be responsible for the observed anticancer effects. ARs, sphingolipids, phytosterols and their conjugates, and phenolic acids have been identified as the major phytochemicals in WB. Using human colon cancer cells as the guiding assay, we identified ARs as the major anticancer components in WB. However, the *in vivo* efficacy and the underlying molecular mechanisms of ARs are still unknown. In addition, the roles of microbiota in the generation of metabolites from WB phytochemicals and the impacts of WB phytochemicals on the bacterial entities have not been fully delineated. Understanding the impact of microbial-derived dietary metabolites has the potential to revolutionize interventions of various host pathologies, including cancer. Further studies on the cancer-preventive effects of phytochemicals in WB are important for understanding the relationship between WB consumption and the risk of colon cancer. In addition, there is no information regarding the metabolic profiles of the phytochemicals in WB. Using WB phytochemicals and their metabolites as the exposure markers for WB consumption is another topic for future research.

References

1. American Cancer Society. *Cancer Facts and Figures*. Available at: http://www.cancer.org/downloads/STT/CAFF2003PWSecured.pdf; 2003.
2. Burkitt DP. Epidemiology of cancer of the colon and the rectum. *Cancer* 1971;**28**:3–13.
3. Adlercreutz H. Western diet and western disease: some hormonal and biochemical mechanisms and associations. *Scand J Clin Lab Invest Suppl* 1990;**201**:3–23.
4. Trock B, Lanza E, Greenwald P. Dietary fiber, vegetables, and colon cancer: critical review and meta-analyses of the epidemiologic evidence. *J Natl Cancer Inst* 1990;**82**:650–61.
5. Howe GR, Benito E, Castelleto R, Esteve J, Gallagher RP, Iscovich JM, et al. Dietary intake of fiber and decreased risk of cancers of the colon and rectum: evidence from the combined analysis of 13 case–control studies. *J Natl Cancer Inst* 1992;**84**:1887–96.
6. Freudenheim JL, Graham S, Horvath PJ, Marshall JR, Haughey BP, Wilkinson G. Risks associated with source of fiber and fiber components in cancer of the colon and rectum. *Cancer Res* 1990;**50**:3295–300.
7. Bingham SA, Day NE, Luben R, Ferrari P, Slimani N, Norat T, et al. Dietary fibre in food and protection against colorectal cancer in the European Prospective Investigation into Cancer and Nutrition (EPIC): an observational study. *Lancet* 2003;**361**:1496–501.
8. Peters U, Sinha R, Chatterjee N, Subar AF, Ziegler RG, Kulldorff M, et al. Dietary fibre and colorectal adenoma in a colorectal cancer early detection programme. *Lancet* 2003;**361**:1491–5.
9. Reddy BS, Ekeland G, Bohe M, Engle A, Domellof L. Metabolic epidemiology of colon cancer: dietary pattern of fecal sterol concentrations of three populations. *Nutr Cancer* 1983;**5**:34–40.
10. McKeown-Eyssen GE, Bright-See E. Dietary factors in colon cancer: international relationships. *Nutr Cancer* 1984;**6**:160–70.
11. Jensen OM, MacLennan R, Wharendorf J. Diet, Bowel function, fecal characteristics and large bowel cancer in Denmark and Finland. *Nutr Cancer* 1982;**4**(4):5–19.
12. Alberts DS, Einspahr J, Rees-McGee S. Effects of dietary wheat bran fiber on rectal epithelial cell proliferation in patients with resection for colorectal cancers. *J Natl Cancer Inst* 1990;**82**:1280–5.
13. Alberts DS, Einspahr J, Ritenbaugh C. The effect of wheat bran fiber and calcium supplementation on rectal mucosal proliferation rates in patients with respected adenomatous colorectal polyps. *Cancer Epidemiol Biomarkers Prev* 1997;**6**:161–9.
14. MacLennan R, Macrae F, Bain C. Randomized trial of intake of fat, fiber, and beta carotene to prevent colorectal adenomas. The Australian polyp prevention project. *J Nat Cancer Inst* 1995;**87**:1760–6.
15. Jacobs ET, Giuliano AR, Roe DJ, Guillen-Rodriguez JM, Alberts DS, Martinez ME. Baseline Dietary Fiber Intake and Colorectal Adenoma Recurrence in the Wheat Bran Fiber Randomized Trial. *J Natl Cancer Inst* 2002;**94**:1620–5.
16. Reddy BS, Engle A, Katsifis S, Simi B, Bartram H-P, Perrino P, et al. Biochemical epidemiology of colon cancer: effect of types of dietary fiber on fecal mutagens, acid, and neutral sterols in healthy subjects. *Cancer Res* 1989;**49**:4629–53.
17. Reddy BS, Engle A, Simi B, Goldman M. Effect of dietary fiber on colonic bacterial enzymes and bile acids in relation to colon cancer. *Gastroenterology* 1992;**102**:1475–82.
18. Harris PJ, Ferguson LR. Dietary fibres may protect or enhance carcinogenesis. *Mutat Res* 1999;**443**:95–110.
19. Barbolt TA, Abraham R. The effect of bran on dimethylhydrazine-induced colon carcinogenesis in the rat. *Proc Soc Exp Biol Med* 1978;**157**:656–9.
20. Reddy BS, Mori H. Effect of dietary wheat bran and dehydrated citrus fiber on 3,2′-dimethyl-4-aminobiphenyl-induced intestinal carcinogenesis in male F344 rats. *Carcinogenesis* 1981;**12**:21–5.
21. Reddy BS, Mori H, Nicolais M. Effect of dietary wheat bran and dehydrated citrus fiber on azoxymethane-induced intestinal carcinogenesis in Fischer 344 rats. *J Natl Cancer Inst* 1981;**66**:553–7.
22. Ferguson LR, Harris PJ. Studies on the role of specific dietary fibres in protection against colorectal cancer. *Mut Res* 1996;**350**:173–84.
23. Drankhan K, Carter J, Madl R, Klopfenstein C, Padula F, Lu Y, et al. Antitumor activity of wheats with high orthophenolic content. *Nutri Cancer* 2003;**47**(2):188–94.
24. Lupton JR, Turner ND. Potential protective mechanisms of wheat bran fiber. *Am J Med* 1999;**106**:24S–7S.
25. Zoran DL, Turner ND, Taddeo SS. Wheat bran diet reduces tumor incidence in a rat model of colon cancer independent of effects on distal luminal butyric acid concentrations. *J Nutr* 1997;**127**:2217–25.
26. Reddy BS, Hirose Y, Cohen LA, Simi B, Cooma I, Rao CV. Preventive potential of wheat bran fractions against experimental colon carcinogenesis: Implication for human colon cancer prevention. *Cancer Res* 2000;**60**:4792–7.
27. Sang S, Ju J, Lambert JD, Lin Y, Hong J, Bose M, et al. Wheat bran oil and its fractions inhibit human colon cancer cell growth and intestinal tumorigenesis in Apc(min/+) mice. *J Agric Food Chem* 2006;**54**(26):9792–7.
28. Iwatsuki K, Akihisa T, Tokuda H, Ukiya M, Higashihara H, Mukainaka T, et al. Sterol ferulates, sterols, and 5-alk(en)ylresorcinols from wheat, rye, and corn bran oils and their inhibitory effects on Epstein-Barr virus activation. *J Agric Food Chem* 2003;**51**(23):6683–8.
29. Reddy BS, Hirose Y, Cohen LA, Simi B, Cooma I, Rao CV. Preventive potential of wheat bran fractions against experimental colon carcinogenesis: implications for human colon cancer prevention. *Cancer Res* 2000;**60**(17):4792–7.
30. Dinelli G, Segura-Carretero A, Di Silvestro R, Marotti I, Arraez-Roman D, Benedettelli S, et al. Profiles of phenolic compounds in modern and old common wheat varieties determined by liquid chromatography coupled with time-of-flight mass spectrometry. *J Chromatogr A* 2011;**1218**(42):7670–81.
31. Nkondjock A, Shatenstein B, Maisonneuve P, Ghadirian P. Specific fatty acids and human colorectal cancer: an overview. *Cancer Detect Prev* 2003;**27**(1):55–66.
32. Ross AB, Kamal-Eldin A, Aman P. Dietary alkylresorcinols: absorption, bioactivities, and possible use as biomarkers of whole-grain wheat- and rye-rich foods. *Nutr Rev* 2004;**62**(3):81–95.
33. Zhu Y, Conklin DR, Chen H, Wang L, Sang S. 5-alk(en)ylresorcinols as the major active components in wheat bran inhibit human colon cancer cell growth. *Bioorg med chem* 2011;**19**(13):3973–82.
34. Suzuki Y, Esumi Y, Kono Y, Sakurai A. Isolation of 5-(8′Z-heptadecenyl)resorcinol from etiolated rice seedlings as an antifungal agent. *Phytochemistry* 1996;**41**(6):1485–9.

35. Seki K, Haga K, Kaneko R. Phenols and a dioxotetrahydrodibenzo-furan from seeds of *Iris Pallasii*. *Phytochemistry* 1995;**38**(4):965–73.

36. Zhu Y, Soroka DN, Sang S. Synthesis and inhibitory activities against colon cancer cell growth and proteasome of alkylresorcin-ols. *J Agric Food Chem* 2012;**60**(35):8624–31.

37. Sumino M, Sekine T, Ruangrungsi N, Igarashi K, Ikegami F. Ardis-iphenols and other antioxidant principles from the fruits of Ardisia colorata. *Chem Pharm Bull (Tokyo)* 2002;**50**(11):1484–7.

38. Arisawa M, Ohmura K, Kobayashi A, Morita N. A cytotoxic con-stituent of Lysimachia japonica THUNB. (Primulaceae) and the structure–activity relationships of related compounds. *Chem Pharm Bull (Tokyo)* 1989;**37**(9):2431–4.

39. Chuang TH, Wu PL. Cytotoxic 5-alkylresorcinol metabolites from the leaves of Grevillea robusta. *J Nat Prod* 2007;**70**(2):319–23.

40. Barbini L, Lopez P, Ruffa J, Martino V, Ferraro G, Campos R, et al. Induction of apoptosis on human hepatocarcinoma cell lines by an alkyl resorcinol isolated from Lithraea molleoides. *World J Gastro-enterol* 2006;**12**(37):5959–63.

41. Duan RD. Physiological functions and clinical implications of sphingolipids in the gut. *J Dig Dis* 2011 Apr;**12**(2):60–70.

42. van Meer G, Hoetzl S. Sphingolipid topology and the dynam-ic organization and function of membrane proteins. *FEBS Lett* 2010;**584**(9):1800–5.

43. Sperling P, Heinz E. Plant sphingolipids: structural diversity, biosynthesis, first genes and functions. *Biochim Biophys Acta* 2003;**1632**(1-3):1–15.

44. Warnecke D, Heinz E. Recently discovered functions of glucosylce-ramides in plants and fungi. *Cell Mol Life Sci* 2003;**60**(5):919–41.

45. Reddy BS, Sharma C, Darby L, Laakso K, Wynder EL. Metabolic epidemiology of large bowel cancer. Fecal mutagens in high- and low-risk population for colon cancer. A preliminary report. *Mutat Res* 1980;**72**(3):511–22.

46. Reddy BS, Watanabe K, Sheinfil A. Effect of dietary wheat bran, alfalfa, pectin and carrageenan on plasma cholesterol and fecal bile acid and neutral sterol excretion in rats. *J Nutr* 1980;**110**(6):1247–54.

47. Sang S, Ju J, Lambert JD, Lin Y, Hong J, Bose M, et al. Wheat bran oil and its fractions inhibit human colon cancer cell growth and intestinal tumorigenesis in Apc(min/+) mice. *J Agric Food Chem* 2006;**54**(26):9792–7.

48. Zhu Y, Conklin DR, Chen H, Wang L, Sang S. 5-alk(en)ylresorcin-ols as the major active components in wheat bran inhibit human colon cancer cell growth. *Bioorg Med Chem* 2011;**19**(13):3973–82.

49. Fujino YO, M. Sphingolipids in wheat grain. *J Cereal Sci* 1983;**1**(2):159–68.

50. Aida K, Kinoshita M, Tanji M, Sugawara T. Prevention of aberrant crypt foci formation by dietary maize and yeast cerebrosides in 1,2-dimethylhydrazine-treated mice. *J Oleo sci* 2005;**54**(1):45–9.

51. Vesper H, Schmelz EM, Nikolova-Karakashian MN, Dillehay DL, Lynch DV, Merrill Jr AH. Sphingolipids in food and the emerging importance of sphingolipids to nutrition. *J Nutr* 1999;**129**(7):1239–50.

52. Sugawara T, Kinoshita M, Ohnishi M, Miyazawa T. Apoptosis in-duction by wheat-flour sphingoid bases in DLD-1 human colon cancer cells. *Biosci Biotechnol Biochem* 2002;**66**(10):2228–31.

53. Laine RA, Renkonen O. Ceramide di- and trihexosides of wheat flour. *Biochemistry* 1974;**13**(14):2837–43.

54. Fujino YO. M. Ito, S. Further studies on sphingolipids in wheat bran. *Lipids* 1985;**20**(6):337–42.

55. Zhu Y, Soroka DN, Sang S. Structure elucidation and chemi-cal profile of sphingolipids in wheat bran and their cytotoxic effects against human colon cancer cells. *J Agric Food Chem* 2013;**61**(4):866–74.

56. Schmelz EM, Roberts PC, Kustin EM, Lemonnier LA, Sullards MC, Dillehay DL, et al. Modulation of intracellular beta-catenin local-ization and intestinal tumorigenesis *in vivo* and *in vitro* by sphin-golipids. *Cancer Res* 2001;**61**(18):6723–9.

57. Sugawara T, Kinoshita M, Ohnishi M, Nagata J, Saito M. Digestion of maize sphingolipids in rats and uptake of sphingadienine by Caco-2 cells. *J Nutr* 2003;**133**(9):2777–82.

58. Schmelz EM, Bushnev AS, Dillehay DL, Liotta DC, Merrill Jr AH. Suppression of aberrant colonic crypt foci by synthetic sphingo-myelins with saturated or unsaturated sphingoid base backbones. *Nutr Cancer* 1997;**28**(1):81–5.

59. Aida KK, M, Sugawara T, Ono J, Miyazawa T, Ohnishi M. Apop-tosis inducement by plant and fungus sphingoid bases in human colon cancer cells. *J Oleo Sci* 2004;**53**(10):503–10.

60. Sugawara T, Kinoshita M, Ohnishi M, Miyazawa T. Apoptosis induction by wheat-flour sphingoid bases in DLD-1 human colon cancer cells. *Biosci Biotechnol Biochem* 2002;**66**(10):2228–31.

61. Chan TA, Morin PJ, Vogelstein B, Kinzler KW. Mechanisms un-derlying nonsteroidal antiinflammatory drug-mediated apoptosis. *Proc Natl Acad Sci USA* 1998;**95**(2):681–6.

62. Nurmi T, Lami AM, Nystrom L, Hemery Y, Rouau X, Piironen V. Distribution and composition of phtosterols and steryl ferulates in wheat grain and bran fractions. *J Cereal Sci* 2012;**56**:379–88.

63. Awad AB, Fink CS. Phytosterols as anticancer dietary components: evidence and mechanism of action. *J Nutr* 2000;**130**(9):2127–30.

64. Bradford PG, Awad AB. Phytosterols as anticancer compounds. *Mol Nutr Food Res* 2007;**51**(2):161–70.

65. Woyengo TA, Ramprasath VR, Jones PJ. Anticancer effects of phy-tosterols. *Eur J Clin Nutr* 2009;**63**(7):813–20.

66. Hirai K, Shimazu C, Takezoe R, Ozeki Y. Cholesterol, phytosterol and polyunsaturated fatty acid levels in 1982 and 1957 Japanese diets. *J Nutr Sci Vitaminol (Tokyo)* 1986;**32**(4):363–72.

67. Nair PP. Diet, nutrition intake, and metabolism in populations at high and low risk for colon cancer. Introduction: correlates of diet, nutrient intake, and metabolism in relation to colon cancer. *Am J Clin Nutr* 1984;**40**(Suppl. 4):880–6.

68. Nair PP, Turjman N, Kessie G, Calkins B, Goodman GT, Davidovitz H, et al. Diet, nutrition intake, and metabolism in pop-ulations at high and low risk for colon cancer. Dietary cholesterol, beta-sitosterol, and stigmasterol. *Am J Clin Nutr* 1984;**40**(Suppl. 4):927–30.

69. Raicht RF, Cohen BI, Fazzini EP, Sarwal AN, Takahashi M. Protec-tive effect of plant sterols against chemically induced colon tumors in rats. *Cancer Res* 1980;**40**(2):403–5.

70. Deschner EE, Cohen BI, Raicht RF. The kinetics of the protective effect of beta-sitosterol against MNU-induced colonic neoplasia. *J Cancer Res Clin Oncol* 1982;**103**(1):49–54.

71. Awad AB, Hernandez AY, Fink CS, Mendel SL. Effect of dietary phytosterols on cell proliferation and protein kinase C activity in rat colonic mucosa. *Nutr Cancer* 1997;**27**(2):210–5.

72. Janezic SA, Rao AV. Dose-dependent effects of dietary phytosterol on epithelial cell proliferation of the murine colon. *Food Chem Toxi-col* 1992;**30**(7):611–6.

73. Awad AB, Chen YC, Fink CS, Hennessey T. Beta-sitosterol inhibits HT-29 human colon cancer cell growth and alters membrane lip-ids. *Anticancer Res* 1996;**16**(5A):2797–804.

74. Adlercreutz H. Lignans and human health. *Crit Rev Clin Lab Sci* 2007;**44**(5-6):483–525.

75. Smeds AI, Jauhiainen L, Tuomola E, Peltonen-Sainio P. Char-acterization of variation in the lignan content and composition of winter rye, spring wheat, and spring oat. *J Agric Food Chem* 2009;**57**(13):5837–42.

76. Clavel T, Borrmann D, Braune A, Dore J, Blaut M. Occurrence and activity of human intestinal bacteria involved in the conversion of dietary lignans. *Anaerobe* 2006;**12**(3):140–7.

77. Clavel T, Henderson G, Alpert CA, Philippe C, Rigottier-Gois L, Dore J, et al. Intestinal bacterial communities that produce active estrogen-like compounds enterodiol and enterolactone in humans. *Appl Environ Microbiol* 2005;**71**(10):6077–85.

78. Clavel T, Henderson G, Engst W, Dore J, Blaut M. Phylogeny of human intestinal bacteria that activate the dietary lignan secoisolariciresinol diglucoside. *FEMS Microbiol Ecol* 2006;**55**(3):471–8.

79. Struijs K, Vincken JP, Gruppen H. Bacterial conversion of secoisolariciresinol and anhydrosecoisolariciresinol. *J Appl Microbiol* 2009;**107**(1):308–17.

80. Nicolle C, Manach C, Morand C, Mazur W, Adlercreutz H, Remesy C, et al. Mammalian lignan formation in rats fed a wheat bran diet. *J Agric Food Chem* 2002;**50**(21):6222–6.

81. Qu H, Madl RL, Takemoto DJ, Baybutt RC, Wang W. Lignans are involved in the antitumor activity of wheat bran in colon cancer SW480 cells. *J Nutr* 2005;**135**(3):598–602.

82. Ferguson LR, Harris PJ. Protection against cancer by wheat bran: role of dietary fibre and phytochemicals. *Eur J Cancer Prev* 1999;**8**(1):17–25.

83. Jenab M, Thompson LU. The influence of flaxseed and lignans on colon carcinogenesis and beta-glucuronidase activity. *Carcinogenesis* 1996;**17**(6):1343–8.

84. Adom KK, Sorrells ME, Liu RH. Phytochemicals and antioxidant activity of milled fractions of different wheat varieties. *J Agric Food Chem* 2005;**53**(6):2297–306.

85. Okarter N, Liu RH. Health benefits of whole grain phytochemicals. *Crit Rev Food Sci Nutr* 2010;**50**(3):193–208.

86. Stevenson L, Phillips F, O'Sullivan K, Walton J. Wheat bran: its composition and benefits to health, a European perspective. *Int J Food Sci Nutr* 2012;**63**(8):1001–13.

87. Drankhan K, Carter J, Madl R, Klopfenstein C, Padula F, Lu Y, et al. Antitumor activity of wheats with high orthophenolic content. *Nutr Cancer* 2003;**47**(2):188–94.

GLUTEN AND DISEASE

11

Immunologic Reactions to Wheat: Celiac Disease, Wheat Allergy and Gluten Sensitivity

Michelle Pietzak

University of Southern California Keck School of Medicine, Los Angeles County + University of Southern California Medical Center and Children's Hospital, Los Angeles, California, USA

BACKGROUND

Because of increases in celiac disease, wheat allergy, and gluten sensitivity, the gluten-free diet is no longer restricted to specialty food stores and small Internet distributors. In fact, products labeled as "gluten free" are now a 1 billion dollar business with exponential sales.[1] Today's gluten-free diet is perceived as "healthy" and "tasty", as opposed to dry and crumbling bread substitutes. The general public's recent embrace of the gluten-free lifestyle is also associated with a backlash, with the perception by many in the medical field that it is a "fad diet". When properly used, the gluten-free diet is medical nutritional therapy for celiac disease, dermatitis herpetiformis, and gluten-sensitive ataxia. Research is ongoing to see if the gluten-free lifestyle works for other conditions with gastrointestinal and neurologic symptoms, such as autism and irritable bowel syndrome. Some even propose that excluding gluten from the diet is healthier for everyone.

This review will differentiate between wheat allergy, celiac disease, and proposed "gluten-sensitive" syndromes. Some conditions, such as celiac disease, have decades of research showing the benefits of the gluten-free diet. Others, such as "gluten sensitivity", are evolving in definition, proposed pathophysiology, and treatment. The importance of celiac disease as the prototype for an autoimmune disorder which responds to gluten elimination will be highlighted. Important differentiators of celiac disease from these other conditions include its well-documented complications of nutritional deficiencies, co-morbid autoimmune conditions, and increased risk for a variety of malignancies. Wheat allergy will also be discussed, and how its symptoms and dietary treatment differ from those of celiac disease or gluten sensitivity. The concept of gluten sensitivity will be elaborated, with emphasis on the conditions known to respond to gluten elimination, and those that still require further definition and examination.

The gluten-free diet is challenging, and should not be taken lightly just because it is nutritional therapy and not a pharmacologic agent. United States food labeling presents many obstacles,[2,3] and unnecessary gluten restriction may impact a patient's ability to socialize, travel, and eat outside the home.[3] At present, additional studies on gluten-sensitive conditions are needed, using more rigorous scientific methods to further define the benefits of gluten elimination in those without true documented wheat allergy or celiac disease.

CELIAC DISEASE

Celiac disease is common, with a US prevalence estimated to be between 0.5% and 1% of the general population.[4,5] In addition to an increased awareness of the condition, the incidence of celiac disease is also thought to be rising in the US over the past several decades.[6] The condition, thought to be "autoimmune" by some researchers, is an immune-mediated reaction to gluten that occurs in genetically predisposed individuals. These specific patients react to dietary proteins, called prolamins, in certain grains, including wheat. All grain products, including rice, contain prolamins; however, the specific prolamins found in wheat (gliadin), rye (secalin), and barley (horedin) are the ones implicated in causing an immunologic reaction in celiac patients.[7] Oats, which contain avenin, will also cause a reaction in a small proportion of celiac patients.[8] The US has great potential for oats to be contaminated with wheat, as most oats are crop rotated and milled with wheat. Therefore, US oats are considered to have levels of contamination with wheat gluten high enough to make them unacceptable for the routine gluten-free diet.[9] In well controlled adults with celiac disease who have eliminated gluten strictly for many years, it may be possible that pure and uncontaminated oats can be incorporated safely into the diet. These oat products contain less than 20 mg of gluten per kg of oats.[10,11]

As with most studied autoimmune diseases, both a genetic predisposition and an environmental trigger are required to manifest the symptoms. In patients with celiac disease, the ingestion of gluten and a genetic predisposition with specific HLA (human leukocyte antigens) alleles are thought necessary. For example, infants who have not yet been exposed to gluten in the diet will not manifest the symptoms, even if they have the HLA alleles that put them at risk. Also, if an individual does not have the HLA alleles most found commonly in celiac disease, HLA DQ2 and HLA DQ8, they are at negligible risk of developing it. On the contrary, even though a significant proportion of the US population has these specific HLA alleles, the majority do not develop celiac disease.

Research in different patient populations implicates several modifying factors that may contribute to disease development in genetically at-risk individuals. An ESPGHAN (European Society for Pediatric Gastroenterology, Hepatology, and Nutrition) statement on complementary feeding recommends avoiding both early (less than 4 months of age) and late (greater than 7 months of age) introduction of gluten into the infant's diet. It is thought ideal to introduce gluten gradually, while the infant is still breastfeeding, to reduce the risk not only of celiac disease but also of type 1 diabetes mellitus and wheat allergy.[12] Cesarean delivery has also been associated with a higher incidence of celiac disease.[13] Boys and girls with celiac disease have been reported to have a different seasonality of month of birth.[14] Girls whose celiac disease was diagnosed prior to the age of 24 months had a different seasonality of month of birth from those who were diagnosed after age 24 months.[14] A higher risk for celiac disease has also been documented for those born during the summer months.[15] Infections during early childhood may appropriately activate the Th1 immune response, but may also lead to a presentation of celiac disease during the toddler years. This may explain why an increased risk for celiac disease has been found in children with repeated rotavirus infections as measured by antirotaviral antibody positivity.[16]

In addition to the HLA alleles, several additional genes have been reported to be associated with celiac disease susceptibility, including CCR3, IL12A, IL18RAP, RGS1, SH2B3, and TAGAP.[17] These genes are all implicated

in regulation of immune responses. The presence of autoimmune diseases in the patient or family (such as type 1 diabetes, autoimmune thyroid disease, rheumatoid arthritis, and autoimmune liver disease) also puts the patient at higher risk for celiac disease.[7] Patients with Down syndrome, Williams syndrome, Turner syndrome, and cystic fibrosis, for unclear reasons, are also at increased risk for celiac disease compared to the general population.[7,18,19] It is important to note, however, that elevated antigliadin antibodies (AGA) can be seen in Down syndrome and cystic fibrosis patients, perhaps due to increased intestinal permeability to these proteins.

In "classic" celiac disease, a child of toddler age, who has been ingesting gluten for several months, presents with diarrhea, weight loss, anorexia, vomiting, and abdominal distension. Unlike adults, who often see several healthcare practitioners before receiving the correct diagnosis, these children with protein-calorie malnutrition receive prompt medical attention. In the United States, "classic celiac disease" is a misnomer, as the majority of patients are now presenting in older age groups with symptoms outside of the gastrointestinal tract. Common misdiagnoses for these older patients include irritable bowel syndrome, lactose malabsorption, inflammatory bowel disease, and even "hypochondria".

Celiac disease can be confusing for the generalist to diagnose when it occurs outside of the "classic" gastrointestinal presentation. As an autoimmune condition, celiac disease symptoms can manifest in virtually every organ system. The next most common system affected in celiac disease is the musculoskeletal system, where arthritis, muscle pain, dental enamel defects, and osteopenia/osteoporosis are commonly seen. Short stature, delayed onset of puberty, and even idiopathic infertility can be seen in both men and women, prompting an endocrinology workup. In celiac women who are not diagnosed, or do not follow a gluten-free diet, there are higher rates of infertility, spontaneous abortions, fetal neural tube defects, and low birth-weight infants.[20,21] Trace vitamin and mineral deficiencies can include iron deficiency anemia, protein-calorie malnutrition, and low serum zinc, folic acid, selenium and vitamins B6, B12, D, E and K.[3,22] Neurologic complaints are common, and include headaches, seizures, anxiety, depression, schizophrenia, and peripheral neuropathy.[23,24] Improvement of long-standing neurologic symptoms is variable with the gluten-free diet and dietary supplements.[25]

Excellent serum antibodies are readily available to screen for celiac disease, and come in two types: those against gluten, and those against "self". The "antigluten" antibodies, antigliadin (AGA) IgG and antigliadin IgA, led to the first blood tests available on a mass scale to the general public. However, false positives can be seen in any condition in which the small bowel is more permeable to gluten. Therefore, using the anti-"self" antibodies is more accepted: anti-endomysial (EMA) IgA and anti-tissue transglutaminase (tTG) IgG and IgA. These last two antibodies have high sensitivity and specificity, and the likelihood of a false positive in an otherwise healthy individual is low. As young children will make food antibodies earlier than "self" antibodies, anti-endomysial IgA and antitissue transglutaminase IgG and IgA may not be as sensitive in younger children. Because of their lower sensitivity and specificity, antigliadin IgG and IgA are no longer routinely recommended as a first line screen for celiac disease in otherwise healthy adult patients. Recently developed IgG and IgA antibodies to deamidated gliadin peptide (DGP, a synthetic peptide derived from gamma gliadin of wheat) show improved sensitivity and specificity compared to AGA, and closely parallel the development of TTG IgA in developing celiac disease.[26,27] As IgA deficiency is more common in CD, and may yield falsely low AGA IgA, DGP IgA, EMA IgA, and tTG IgA titers, a total IgA level should also be measured. A tTG IgG can also be performed.[18]

In the United States, patients with symptoms and positive antibody testing require an endoscopic intestinal biopsy to confirm enteropathy prior to the initiation of a gluten-free diet.[18] These recommendations are changing as our European colleagues are using a combination of antibodies, genetic testing, and response to a gluten-free diet as criteria for diagnosis, possibly eliminating the need for pathology confirmation.

An interesting area of research involves exactly how gluten interacts with the gastrointestinal immune system. As opposed to ruminant animals (which chew their cud and pass wheat through a chambered stomach lined by bacteria), the human gastrointestinal tract incompletely digests gluten. Up to 50 different toxic gliadin fragments, which have the potential to stimulate an immune response, survive digestion and are absorbed (via a yet undiscovered mechanism) through the small-intestinal mucosa. The enzyme tTG, to which humans make a "self" antibody, is then thought to change the shape of gliadin into a conformation which has a strong affinity for HLA DQ2 (on antigen presenting cells). The antigen presenting cells then "present" gluten to the immune system as a foreign entity, stimulating the T helper 1 response, which leads to intestinal damage.[28] In contrast to wheat allergy and gluten sensitivity, these manifestations of celiac disease can cause permanent damage and result in nutritional deficiencies and higher rates of gastrointestinal malignancies.

WHEAT ALLERGY

In the United States, the top eight food allergens are milk, eggs, fish, crustacean shellfish, peanuts, tree nuts, soybeans, and wheat. Although approximately 5% of individuals in Westernized nations may have a true food allergy, only about 0.1% have a documented wheat allergy. However, most children with wheat allergies have reactions to the other common food allergens. As we have just seen in celiac disease, wheat allergy is an immune-mediated reaction to the proteins found in these food products. In contrast to celiac disease, wheat allergy is an IgE-mediated reaction to the water and salt-insoluble gliadins, particularly omega 5 gliadin.[29] Of interest, this protein fragment is also the major allergen of wheat-dependent exercised-induced anaphylaxis, commonly referred to as "Baker's asthma". Total serum IgE and specific IgE to wheat can be elevated in the blood. Skin prick tests using wheat protein extracts may show reactions on the back or forearm. It is important to differentiate celiac disease from wheat allergy, since those with the allergic response usually do not need to restrict other prolamin containing grains (rye, barley, and contaminated oats) from their diet. The wheat-free diet is therefore more liberal and less restricting, from a social standpoint (i.e., dining out at restaurants), than a strict gluten-free diet.

While symptoms of wheat allergy can occur in the gastrointestinal tract, they are more common in the skin and respiratory tract. Patients may complain of swelling, itching, and irritation in and around the lips, tongue, mouth, nose, eyes, and throat. Respiratory manifestations can include wheezing and shortness of breath, and, rarely, anaphylaxis. Hives and other simple pruritic rashes can be seen anywhere on the skin. In the gastrointestinal tract, the indicators of wheat allergy are very non-specific, and include nausea, vomiting, gas, cramps, bloating, diarrhea, and generalized abdominal pain. Unfortunately, the gastrointestinal manifestations of celiac disease, wheat allergy, and gluten sensitivity can be indistinguishable from each other. However, unlike celiac disease, wheat allergy does not cause permanent gastrointestinal or other organ damage once there has been resolution of the acute event.

Similar to celiac disease, the "classic" wheat allergy develops during the toddler years. However, unlike celiac disease (which is lifelong), wheat allergy is usually outgrown between the ages of 3 and 5 years. The allergenicity of wheat is hypothesized to be strengthened by activated tTG in these patients.[29] The gluten-free diet cannot be used to discriminate between celiac disease and wheat allergy, as both improve with elimination of wheat products from the diet. The best treatment of wheat allergy is avoidance. Antihistamines and corticosteroids may also be of benefit for severe reactions. As with peanut and shellfish allergies, wheat-allergic individuals should have epinephrine readily available in case of a life-threatening anaphylactic reaction. In celiac disease, while the immunologic reactions can be severe, with emesis, diarrhea, and dehydration, they do not cause anaphylactic reactions.

GLUTEN SENSITIVITY

By definition, gluten sensitivity exists when a patient has symptomatic improvement upon gluten withdrawal, and does not meet the criteria for celiac disease nor wheat allergy. A small bowel biopsy should be normal microscopically. There are no specific blood tests for gluten sensitivity, although some may have AGA IgG and/or IgA positivity, and some have reported a higher incidence of HLA DQ2. Gluten sensitivity is not thought to be immune related, in contrast to both celiac disease and wheat allergy. Unfortunately, the gastrointestinal complaints are non-specific, and it can be difficult to distinguish between these three conditions. Common in the gluten sensitive are dyspepsia, nausea, vomiting, borborygmi (intestinal rumbling noises), bloating, constipation, and overt diarrhea. Extra-intestinal symptoms commonly volunteered to improve when gluten-free include joint pain, bone pain, muscle cramps, fatigue, headaches, rashes, and swollen tongue. As in wheat allergy, and in contrast to celiac disease, the manifestations of gluten sensitivity are thought neither to cause permanent intestinal damage nor to result in nutritional deficiencies or higher rates of malignancies.

There are few published studies that try to elucidate the pathophysiologic mechanisms underlying gluten sensitivity. In one,[30] a 4-month supervised gluten challenge was given to subjects with biopsy-proven celiac disease, or with gluten sensitivity, or healthy controls (biopsied for dyspepsia). By definition, those labeled "gluten sensitive" were negative for EMA IgA, tTG IgA, and serum wheat IgE. However, about half had AGA IgG and/or AGA IgA, and HLA DQ2 and/or HLA DQ8. Those who were "gluten sensitive" experienced gas, diarrhea, weight loss, abdominal pain, glossitis, muscle cramps, leg numbness, bone and joint pain, osteoporosis, and unexplained anemia with the challenge. Immunologic markers in the "gluten-sensitive" group were also unique, in that they did not demonstrate elevations in either interleukin-6 or interleukin-21 (as seen in celiac disease). Biopsies of the "gluten sensitive" showed only a mild increase in intra-epithelial lymphocytes, and reduced expression of the T-regulatory cell molecules FOXP3 (forkhead box P3) and TGFB1 (transforming growth factor β_1). Interestingly, those who were "gluten sensitive" demonstrated increased expression of the gene CLDN4 (claudin 4, a tight junctional protein) and decreased intestinal permeability (as measured by urinary lactulose/mannitol), suggesting differences between this condition and celiac disease in regard to the function of the intestinal epithelial cell tight junctions. These results signified a decreased recruitment of T-regulatory cells to the small bowel in those "gluten sensitive" compared with subjects who were "gluten tolerant", and indicated a generalized more limited involvement for the adaptive immune system (as opposed to celiac disease). The innate immune system may play more of a role in those who are "gluten sensitive", as their biopsies showed higher expressions of toll-like receptors 1, 2, and 4 compared to healthy controls.[30]

Dermatitis herpetiformis and gluten-sensitive ataxia are two conditions that are often placed within the category of "gluten sensitivity". Some now consider these part of the "spectrum" of celiac disease. Autism, irritable bowel syndrome, and some other neurologic disorders have also been reported to show improvements on the gluten-free diet, indicating that perhaps these too are "gluten-sensitive" conditions.

Dermatitis Herpetiformis

The skin rash dermatitis herpetiformis (also known as Duhring's disease after the individual who first described it, in 1884) is thought by some to be pathognomonic for celiac disease. Due to its evolving appearance over time, the rash can be difficult to diagnose clinically without a biopsy. It particularly involves the extensor surfaces of the face, elbows, knees, and buttocks. In the beginning it presents as an erythematous macule (red and flat), then progresses to an urticarial papule (itchy and raised), and eventually manifests as a tense vesicle (fluid-filled hive). During the vesicular appearance, it is often mislabeled as chicken pox or varicella zoster. The condition may even mimic eczema or psoriasis, as patients will often unroof and scratch the lesions to the point where the chronic skin changes just appear scarred and inflamed. Distinguishing features of this skin rash are severe pruritus, and symmetrical distribution (i.e., both sides of face, both buttocks, both knees). While the majority of patients with dermatitis herpetiformis do not complain of noticeable gastrointestinal symptoms, the majority will demonstrate the classic villous atrophy on small bowel biopsy. The gold standard for diagnosis is a skin punch biopsy, which is an office procedure. This skin biopsy should be sent frozen for special granular IgA stains in the dermal papillae (which may be IgA reacting to tTG). Of note, the patient does not require endoscopy for small bowel biopsy if the skin biopsy confirms dermatitis herpetiformis. The medication of choice, in addition to diet, is dapsone, an anti-inflammatory antibiotic. This can alleviate severe pruritus but has several severe side effects, such as anemia, leukopenia (low white blood cells), and a flu-like syndrome. For this reason, close monitoring with blood tests is necessary for patients on this medication, although other medications are available. A strict gluten-free diet is recommended for those with dermatitis herpetiformis, to prevent flares and associated reported complications such as vitiligo, alopecia areata, sarcoidosis, autoimmune thyroid disease, type 1 diabetes, and systemic lupus erythematosis. Some patients are also sensitive to products containing latex and iodine.[31,32]

Ataxia and Other Neurologic Manifestations

"Gluten ataxia" was first described in 1998 in patients with progressive idiopathic ataxia (a lack of coordination of muscle movements) and elevated antigliadin IgG and IgA.[33] In this initial description, all had gait ataxia, some had limb ataxia, and most had peripheral neuropathy. Using MRI to study the brain, about 20% had evidence of cerebellar atrophy. On autopsy, two subjects demonstrated lymphocytic infiltration, similar to that seen in the small bowel in celiac disease, of the cerebellum, peripheral nerves, and posterior columns of the spinal cord. About a third, in fact, had distal duodenal biopsies consistent with celiac disease.[33] Several studies have since examined the higher prevalence of antigliadin IgG and IgA in patients with sporadic and familial ataxia.[25] As opposed to pure celiac disease, the 147 patients with gluten ataxia (followed over 12 years in one center) had an equal male : female ratio, and the mean age of onset of ataxia was 53 years. All were antigliadin IgG and/or IgA positive, 22% were EMA IgA positive, 56% were tTG IgA positive, and 70% were HLA DQ2+. Overall, 28% had biopsy-proven enteropathy and up to 60% had MRI evidence of cerebellar atrophy.[25]

As with the gut barrier, the mechanisms by which gluten interacts with the central nervous system have yet to be fully elucidated. *In vitro* research shows that there is an antibody cross-reactivity between gluten peptides and the Purkinje cells in the cerebellar cortex in human and rats.[34] Concomitantly, there is evidence for antibodies targeting Purkinje cell epitopes in the sera of patients with gluten ataxia.[34] TTG IgA deposits have been reported in both jejunal tissue and around the blood vessels of the brain (cerebellum, pons, and medulla) of gluten-sensitive patients.[35–37]. As with celiac disease, the gluten-free diet is the mainstay of treatment for gluten ataxia, although one uncontrolled trial reported improvement in four patients after intravenous immunoglobulin.[38]

Inflammatory myopathy has been reported to improve with a gluten-free diet with and without additional immunosuppression.[39] Similarly, sensory ganglioneuropathy has also been reported to respond to a gluten-free diet alone.[40] It is being debated in the literature whether or not multiple sclerosis, although reported to be associated with elevated antigliadin

IgG and IgA, should be part of the gluten-sensitivity spectrum (or whether these patients just have "occult" celiac disease).[41,42] Biopsy-proven celiac disease has also been associated with childhood partial epilepsy with occipital paroxysms.[43] A study of 75 biopsy-proven pediatric celiac disease patients showed many different neurologic manifestations, including ataxia, febrile seizures, single generalized seizures, muscular hypotonia with retarded motor development, and T2 hyperintensive white matter lesions on MRI (hypothesized to be from vasculitis or inflammatory demyelination).[44] Another study from 2004 controversially found that 75% of patients with untreated celiac disease exhibited at least one hypoperfused brain region as assessed by PET scan. These results were significantly different from healthy controls and celiac patients who maintained a gluten-free diet.[45] These perfusion defects, as reported in the superior and anterior areas of the frontal cortex and anterior cingulated cortex, have also been reported in depression, anorexia nervosa, and anxious-neurotic behaviors.[46–48] It is interesting to speculate whether these psychiatric disorders would also be "gluten-sensitive".

Irritable Bowel Syndrome

In blinded studies, some types of irritable bowel syndrome have shown symptomatic improvement with the gluten-free diet.[49] Recent publications indicate that irritable bowel syndrome is associated with small bowel bacterial overgrowth, as its symptoms are primarily pain, gas, bloating, and diarrhea, with or without constipation.[50] After 6 months of a gluten-free diet, the majority of those with diarrhea-predominant irritable bowel syndrome returned to normal stool frequency and gastrointestinal symptom score.[51] Favorable predictors of this clinical response included AGA IgG and TTG IgG positivity.[51] Irritable bowel syndrome is a common alternative diagnosis given to women with celiac disease, as they may also complain of gas, bloating, abdominal pain, and diarrhea alternating with constipation. It has also been reported that celiac disease and irritable bowel syndrome can co-exist in the same patient![52] Before finalizing the diagnosis of irritable bowel syndrome, most gastrointestinal experts and societies agree that it is cost-effective to first rule out celiac disease.

Some alternative practitioners suggest that the gastrointestinal symptoms, headache, and poor memory seen in irritable bowel syndrome may be attributed to intestinal overgrowth of the yeast *Candida albicans*. These patients are then subjected to a "*Candida* cleanse diet", eliminating sugar, white flour, yeast, and cheese. Many note symptomatic improvement on this diet, despite a lack of clinical trials showing efficacy. Perhaps these patients have another type of "gluten sensitivity", or perhaps the "cleanse" replaces processed foods with fresh ones, and white flour with whole grains, leading to a restitution of well-being.[53]

Autism and the Gluten-Free Casein-Free Diet

There are many hypotheses regarding the correct etiology and treatments for autism, one of which is the opioid hypothesis. This hypothesis suggests that autism results from excessive brain opioid activity during the neonatal period. Excessive opioid activity leads to inhibition of social motivation, resulting in aloofness and isolation. Arguments supporting this hypothesis include similar behaviors in animals after injections of exogenous opioids with decreased vocalization and increased aloofness; biochemical evidence of abnormal peripheral endogenous opioids in autistic patients; and case reports showing naltrexone (an opioid receptor blocking agent) to be therapeutic in autistic patients.[54,55] Reichelt theorized in 1991 that gluten and casein peptides, which have similar chemical structures, play a role in the pathogenesis of autism. A variety of disorders, including autism, schizophrenia, and postpartum psychosis, were thought to be due to an inability to process gluten and casein adequately.[56] These products of inadequate digestion, "gliadorphin" and "casomorphin", can be measured in the urine and cerebrospinal fluid of autistic patients. They theoretically cross both the gut and brain barriers, and then bind with endogenous opioid receptors, causing "interference of signal transmission". It has been proposed that "gliadorphin" and "casomorphin" have negative pharmacological effects on attention, learning, social interactions, and brain maturation.[57]

Complementary and alternative medicines are often used by the parents of children with autism spectrum disorders. These include high-dose dietary supplements, and many different types of restrictive diets. Supplements and diets are thought to be more acceptable and to have fewer issues with safety and side effects than prescribed pharmaceuticals for autism. However, even though diets and supplements are considered "food", there should still be equal concern to scrutinize the available evidence for their efficacy and effectiveness, as well as any associated risks. Cochrane Reviews published in 2004 and 2008, examined the evidence of the effect of diets on children, adolescents, and adults clinically diagnosed with autism spectrum disorder. Publications included trials in which gluten-free diet was compared to placebo (or no treatment); casein-free diet was compared to placebo (or no treatment), gluten-free casein-free diet was compared to placebo (or not treatment), and gluten-free diet was compared directly to casein-free diet. Measured outcomes included standardized autistic behavioral assessments, communication and linguistic

abilities, cognitive functioning, motor abilities, urine peptide concentrations, and disbenefits (harms, costs, and impact on quality of life).[58,59]

Between 1965 and 2007, 61 studies were identified; of these, only 3 were considered to be of a high enough quality to be included in the analysis.[57,60,61] The studies excluded had significant bias, or were not randomized or blinded and consisted mostly of case reports. The three publications consisted of two small trials: the first with 10 participants in each arm; the second with 15 participants in total. In the first trial, a gluten-free casein-free diet reduced the autistic traits of "social isolation" and "bizarre behavior" at only the age of 12 months. In the second trial, there was no significant difference in outcome measures between the diet group and the control group in regards to cognitive skills at 12 months, motor ability at 12 months, communication and language sampling at week 6 of the diet, or Childhood Autism Rating Scale at week 6 of the diet. Surprisingly, there were no reported adverse outcomes or potential disbenefits in regard to cost of the diet or further social isolation. The conclusion of these two meta-analyses was that this is an important area of investigation, and large-scale, good quality randomized control trials are needed.[58,59]

What might be an adverse outcome to using the gluten-free casein-free diet in autism? First, it costs significantly more than a standard diet to purchase gluten-free substitutes for bread, pasta, and other staples in the diet. Secondly, it involves extra effort in providing special meals for the child with autism and normal meals for the rest of the family. In autism, many children have well-established particular dietary preferences which are difficult to change with regard to texture and taste. It is also a challenge with the gluten-free diet to source food products that are guaranteed not to contain gluten or casein. While gluten is not an essential nutrient in the human diet, the loss of casein and its nutrients found in cow's milk products, such as calcium, protein, magnesium, potassium, and other vitamins and minerals, must be supplemented to the child in another way. Finally, the autistic patient is already perceived as "different", and further social restrictions via diet may place additional burdens on the family unit.[59]

WHY IS IT IMPORTANT TO KNOW THE DIFFERENCE BETWEEN CELIAC DISEASE, WHEAT ALLERGY, AND GLUTEN SENSITIVITY?

While treatment for celiac disease, wheat allergy, and gluten sensitivity is similar, it is important for patients, families, and healthcare practitioners to be able to differentiate between these disorders. A summary of the differences in antibodies, genes, and small bowel biopsy

TABLE 11.1 Antibody, Genetic and Biopsy Differences in Celiac Disease, Wheat Allergy, and Gluten Sensitivity

	AGA IgG	AGA IgA	TTG IgA	EMA IgA	Total IgA	Total IgE	Genes	Biopsy
Celiac disease	+	+	+	+	Normal	Normal	95% DQ2 5% DQ8 Others	Villous atrophy
Celiac disease IgA deficient	+	−	−	−	Low	Normal or low	95% DQ2 5% DQ8 Others	Villous atrophy
Wheat allergy	−	−	−	−	Normal	High	Family atopy	Eosinophilic inflammation
Gluten sensitivity	+/−	+/−	−	−	Normal	Normal	DQ2 common	Normal

findings is found in Table 11.1. For the following important reasons, celiac disease must be differentiated from other conditions, even if the patient states improvement on the gluten-free diet.

1. *Familial risk.* Relatives of patients with celiac disease are at much higher risk than the general population of developing celiac disease and also having other autoimmune disorders. Screening of first- and second-degree family members should be performed for celiac disease once the index case has been identified. Screening family members for wheat allergy or gluten sensitivity is not currently recommended, although atopic diseases (food allergy, asthma) may also run in families.
2. *Nutritional deficiencies.* Patients with celiac disease are at increased risk for malabsorption of protein, fat, iron, and the fat-soluble vitamins A, D, E, and K, leading to anemia and osteoporosis. Celiac patients often require iron and vitamin supplements and medical screens for nutritional deficiencies (i.e., anemia, vitamin levels, and bone density). As there is less intestinal damage with wheat allergy and gluten-sensitivity there is not the increased risk for these nutritional complications, and additional supplements, blood tests, and X-rays are not usually required.
3. *Degree of dietary restriction.* In celiac disease, a strict gluten-free diet, void of contamination, is required for symptomatic and histologic relief. In wheat allergy, only wheat restriction is needed, unless there are co-morbid food allergies. In gluten sensitivity, it is unclear whether such strict adherence, as with celiac disease, is required.
4. *Development of other autoimmune conditions.* Unfortunately, autoimmune conditions tend to travel together within the same patient and same family. Since celiac disease is an autoimmune condition, the patient is at risk for others, such as thyroid disease, type 1 diabetes, joint diseases, and liver diseases. Since wheat allergy and gluten sensitivity are not autoimmune conditions, these patients are not at an

increased risk of developing additional autoimmune conditions over that of the general population.
5. *Increased risk for malignancies.* Since celiac disease involves the activation of a particular type of white blood cell, the T lymphocyte, patients are at increased risk of developing T-cell enteropathy lymphoma.[62] Other gastrointestinal cancers, as well as skin cancer, have also been reported at higher rates in patients with celiac disease that is either untreated, or treated too late. Because food allergies and sensitivities do not involve this particular immune system pathway, and do not cause severe GI tract damage, these patients are not at increased risk for these particular cancers.
6. *Increased mortality.* Patients with celiac disease have a mortality rate two- to four-fold higher, at every age, than that of the general population. This is due to the above nutritional complications, co-morbid autoimmune conditions and higher rate of malignancies.[6,63] Patients with wheat allergy and gluten sensitivity do not have this increased risk of death due to these complications.

References

1. Gluten-Free Sector Still Hot in Tough Times. Available at: http://www.spins.com/news/03.31.09_Gluten_Free.php.
2. Pietzak M. Gluten-free food labeling in the United States. *J Pediatr Gastroenterol Nutr* 2005;**41**:567–8.
3. Pietzak MM. Follow-up of patients with celiac disease: achieving compliance with treatment. *Gastroenterology* 2005;**128**:S135–41.
4. Fasano A, Berti I, Gerarduzzi T, et al. Prevalence of celiac disease in at-risk and not at-risk groups in the United States: a large multicenter study. *Arch Intern Med* 2003;**163**:286–92.
5. Hoffenberg EJ, MacKenzie T, Barriga KJ, et al. A prospective study of the incidence of childhood celiac disease. *J Pediatr* 2003;**143**:308–14.
6. Rubio-Tapia A, Kyle RA, Kaplan EL, et al. Increased prevalence and mortality in undiagnosed celiac disease. *Gastroenterology* 2009;**137**:88–93.
7. Pietzak MM, Catassi C, Drago S, Fornaroli F, Fasano A. Celiac disease: going against the grains. *Nutr Clin Prac* 2001;**16**:335–44.
8. Arentz-Hansen H, Fleckenstein B, Molberg Ø, et al. The molecular basis for oat intolerance in celiac disease patients. *PLoS Med* 2004;**1**(1):e1.

9. Thompson T. Gluten contamination of commercial oat products in the United States. *N Engl J Med* 2004;**351**:2021–2.

10. Sey M, Parfitt J, Gregor J. Prospective study of clinical and histological safety of pure and uncontaminated Canadian oats in the management of celiac disease. *J Parenter Enteral Nutr* 2011;**35**:459–64.

11. Butzner JD. Pure oats and the gluten free diet: are they safe? *J Parenter Enteral Nutr* 2011;**35**:447–8.

12. ESPGHAN Committee on Nutrition. Complementary Feeding: A Commentary by the ESPGHAN Committee on Nutrition. *J Pediatr Gastroenterol Nutr* 2008;**46**:99–110.

13. Decker E, Engelmann G, Findeisen A, et al. Cesarean delivery is associated with celiac disease but not inflammatory bowel disease in children. *Pediatrics* 2010;**125**:e1433–1440.

14. Lewy H, Meirson H, Laron Z. Seasonality of birth month of children with celiac disease differs from that in the general population and between sexes and is linked to family history and environmental factors. *J Pediatr Gastroenterol Nutr* 2009;**48**:181–5.

15. Ivarrson A, Hernell O, Nystrom L, Persson LA. Children born in the summer have increased risk for coeliac disease. *J Epidemiol Community Health* 2003;**57**:36–9.

16. Stene LC, Honeyman MC, Hoffenberg EJ, et al. Rotavirus infection frequency and risk of celiac disease autoimmunity in early childhood: a longitudinal study. *Am J Gastroenterol* 2006;**101**:2333–40.

17. Hunt KA, Zhernakova A, Turner G, et al. Newly identified genetic risk variants for celiac disease related to the immune response. *Nat Genet* 2008;**40**:395–402.

18. National Institutes of Health Consensus Development Conference Statement on Celiac Disease, June 28–30, 2004. Gastroenterology. 2005;128:S1–S9.

19. Gravholt CH. Clinical practice in Turner syndrome (disease/disorder overview). *Nature Clin Pract Endocrinol Metab* 2005;**12**:41–52.

20. Bradley RJ, Rosen MP. Subfertility and gastrointestinal disease: "unexplained" is often undiagnosed. *Obstet Gynecol Surv* 2004;**59**:108–17.

21. O'Leary C, Wieneke P, Healy M, Cronin C, O'Regan P, Shanahan FL. Celiac disease and the transition from childhood to adulthood: a 28-year follow-up. *Gastroenterology* 2004;**99**:2437–41.

22. Harper JW, Holleran SF, Ramakrishnan R, Bhagat G, Green PH. Anemia in celiac disease is multifactorial in etiology. *Am J Hematol* 2007;**82**:996–1000.

23. Häuser W, Janke KH, Klump B, Gregor M, Hinz A. Anxiety and depression in adult patients with celiac disease on the gluten free diet. *World J Gastroenterol* 2010;**16**:2780–7.

24. Cascella NG, Kryszak D, Bhatti B, et al. Prevalence of celiac disease and gluten sensitivity in the United States clinical antipsychotic trials of intervention effectiveness study population. *Schizophr Bull* 2011;**37**:94–100.

25. Hadjivassiliou M, Sanders DS, Woodroofe N, Williamson C, Grunewald RA. Gluten ataxia. *Cerebellum* 2008;**7**:494–8.

26. Ankelo M, Kleimola V, Simell S, et al. Antibody responses to deamidated gliadin peptide show high specificity and parallel antibodies to tissue transglutaminase in developing coeliac disease. *Clin Exp Immunol* 2007;**150**:285–93.

27. Marietta EV, Rashtak S, Murray JA. Correlation analysis of celiac sprue tissue transglutaminase and deamidated gliadin IgG/IgA. *World J Gastroenterol* 2009;**15**:845–8.

28. Qiao SW, Bergseng E, Molberg O, et al. Antigen presentation to celiac lesion-derived T cells of a 33-mer gliadin peptide naturally formed by gastrointestinal digestion. *J Immunol* 2004;**173**:1757–62.

29. Inomata N. Wheat allergy. *Curr Opin Allergy Clin Immunol* 2009;**9**:238–43.

30. Sapone A, Lammers KM, Casolaro V, et al. Divergence of gut permeability and mucosal immune gene expression in two gluten-associated conditions: celiac disease and gluten sensitivity. *BMC Medicine* 2011;**9**:23.

31. Zone JJ. Skin manifestations of celiac disease. *Gastroenterology* 2005;**128**:S87–91.

32. Reunala T, Collin P. Diseases associated with dermatitis herpetiformis. *Br J Dermatol* 1997;**136**:315–8.

33. Hadjivassiliou M, Grunewald RA, Chattopadhyay AK, et al. Clinical, radiological, neurophysiological and neuropathological characteristics of gluten ataxia. *Lancet* 1998;**352**:1582–5.

34. Hadjivassiliou M, Boscolo S, Davies-Jones A, et al. The humoral response in the pathogenesis of gluten ataxia. *Neurology* 2002;**58**:1221–6.

35. Dieterich W, Ehnis T, Bauer M, et al. Identification of tissue transglutaminase as the autoantigen of celiac disease. *Nat Med* 1997;**7**:797–801.

36. Korponay-Szabo IR, Halttunen T, Szalai Z, et al. *In vivo* targeting of intestinal and extraintestinal transglutaminase 2 by coeliac autoantibodies. *Gut* 2004;**53**:641–8.

37. Hadjivassiliou M, Maki M, Sanders DS, et al. Autoantibody targeting of brain and intestinal transglutaminase in gluten ataxia. *Neurology* 2006;**66**:373–7.

38. Bürk K, Melms A, Schulz JB, Dichgans J. Effectiveness of intravenous immunoglobulin therapy in cerebellar ataxia associated with gluten sensitivity. *Ann Neurol* 2001;**50**:827–8.

39. Hadjivassiliou M, Chattopadhyay AK, Grünewald RA, et al. Myopathy associated with gluten sensitivity. *Muscle Nerve* 2007;**35**:443–50.

40. Hadjivassiliou M, Rao DG, Wharton SB, Sanders DS, Grunewald RA, Davies-Jones AG. Sensory ganglionopathy due to gluten sensitivity. *Neurology* 2010;**75**:1003–8.

41. Tengah CP, Lock RJ, Unsworth DJ, Wills AJ. Multiple sclerosis and occult gluten sensitivity. *Neurology* 2004;**62**:2326–7.

42. Hadjivassiliou M, Sander DS, Grünewald RA. Multiple sclerosis and occult gluten sensitivity. *Neurology* 2005;**64**:933–4.

43. Labate A, Gambardella A, Messina D, et al. Silent celiac disease in patients with childhood localization-related epilepsies. *Epilepsia* 2001;**42**:1153–5.

44. Kieslich M, Errázyruz G, Posselt HG, Moeller-Hartmann W, Zanella F, Boehles H. Brain white-matter lesions in celiac disease: a prospective study of 75 diet-treated patients. *Pediatrics* 2001;**108**(2)E21.

45. Addolorato G, Di Guida D, De Rossi G, et al. Regional cerebral hypoperfusion in patients with celiac disease. *Am J Med* 2004;**116**:312–7.

46. O'Connel RA. SPECT brain imaging in psychiatric disorders: current clinical status. In: Grünwald F, Kasper S, Biersack HJ, Möller HJ, editors. *Brain SPECT Imaging in Psychiatry*. Berlin, Germany: W. De Gruiter; 1995. p. 35–57.

47. Grasby PM, Bench C. Neuroimaging in mood disorders. *Curr Opin Psychiatry* 1997;**10**:73–8.

48. Davidson RJ, Abercrombie H, Nitschke JB, Putnam K. Regional brain function, emotion and disorders of emotion. *Curr Opin Neurobiol* 1999;**9**:228–34.

49. Biesiekierski JR, Newnham ED, Irving PM, et al. Gluten causes gastrointestinal symptoms in subjects without celiac disease: a double-blind randomized placebo-controlled trial. *Am J Gastroenterol* 2011;**106**:508–14.

50. Yamini D, Pimentel M. Irritable bowel syndrome and small intestinal bacterial overgrowth. *J Clin Gastroenterol* 2010;**44**:672–5.

51. Wahnschaffe U, Schulzke J-D, Zeitz M, Ullrich R. Predictors of clinical response to gluten-free diet in patients diagnosed with diarrhea-predominant irritable bowel syndrome. *Clin Gastroenterol Hepatol* 2007;**5**:844–50.

52. Häuser W, Musial F, Caspary WF, Stein J, Stallmach A. Predictors of irritable bowel-type symptoms and healthcare-seeking behavior among adults with celiac disease. *Psychosom Med* 2007;**69**:370–6.

53. Clinic Mayo. What is a candida cleanse diet and what does it do? Available at: http://www.mayoclinic.com/health/candida-cleanse/AN01679.

54. Panksepp J, Najam N, Soares F. Morphine reduces social cohesion in rats. *Pharmacol Biochem Behav* 1979;**11**:131–4.

55. Leboyer M, Bouvard MP, Launay JM, et al. Opiate hypothesis in infantile autism? Therapeutic trials with naltrexone. *Encephale* 1993;**19**:95–102.

56. Reichelt KL. Peptides in schizophrenia. *Biol Psychiatry* 1991;**29**:515–7.

57. Knivsberg AM, Reichelt KL, Høien T, Nodland M. A randomised, controlled study of dietary intervention in autistic syndromes. *Nutr Neurosci* 2002;**5**:251–61.

58. Millward C, Ferriter M, Calver S, Connell-Jones G. Gluten- and casein –free diets for autistic spectrum disorder. *Cochrane Database Syst Rev* 2004: CD003498. http://dx.doi.org/10.1002/14651858.CD003498.pub2.

59. Millward C, Ferriter M, Calver S, Connell-Jones G. Gluten- and casein –free diets for autistic spectrum disorder. *Cochrane Database Syst Rev* 2008: CD003498. http://dx.doi.org/10.1002/14651858.CD003498.pub3.

60. Knivsberg AM, Reichelt KL, Høien T, Nodland M. Effect of dietary intervention on autistic behavior. *Focus Autism Other Dev Disabl* 2003;**18**:247–56.

61. Elder JH, Shankar M, Shuster J, Theriague D, Burns S, Sherrill L. The gluten-free, casein-free diet in autism: results of a preliminary double blind clinical trial. *J Autism Dev Disord* 2006;**36**:413–20.

62. Smedby KE, Åkerman M, Hildebrand H, Glimelius B, Ekbom A, Askling J. Malignant lymphomas in coeliac disease: evident of increased risks for lymphoma types other than enteropathy-type T cell lymphoma. *Gut* 2005;**54**:54–9.

63. Corrao G, Corazza GR, Bagnardi V, et al. Mortality in patients with coeliac disease and their relatives: a cohort study. *Lancet* 2001;**358**:356–61.

E. GLUTEN AND DISEASE

12

Celiac Disease and its Therapy: Current Approaches and New Advances

Vandana Nehra, Eric V. Marietta, Joseph A. Murray

Mayo Clinic, College of Medicine, Division of Gastroenterology and Hepatology, Rochester, Minnesota, USA

Conflict of Interest

Both Dr Nehra and Dr Murray are investigators for Alvine, Inc. Dr Murray has served as an advisor to Alvine, Inc. and as a consultant to ImmunosanT, Inc. and Shire US Inc., and has received grant support from Alba Therapeutics.

INTRODUCTION

Celiac disease (CD) is an immune-mediated enteropathy that results from exposure to dietary gluten in genetically susceptible individuals. In 1940, Dr Willem-Karel Dicke, a Dutch pediatrician, reported the association of wheat protein with the symptoms of CD. With increasing awareness and rising prevalence, CD has been recognized as a disorder with both gastrointestinal and systemic manifestations including anemia, liver abnormalities, neurological disorders, and psychiatric diseases.[1] If unrecognized, there is a high risk of gastrointestinal tract malignancy,[2] enteropathy associated T cell lymphoma,[3] and other serious complications such as infertility, osteoporosis, and fractures. A gluten-free diet (GFD) remains the mainstay of treatment once diagnosis is confirmed; however, despite strict dietary adherence, some adults fail to achieve complete histologic recovery, which may have an impact on survival.[4] Recent advances in understanding the molecular mechanisms in CD have targeted pathogenic events in order to develop novel therapeutic strategies as an alternative to a GFD.

EPIDEMIOLOGY

The prevalence of CD varies across different countries. Based on serological testing and reported clinical diagnosis, the prevalence of CD in the United States has been calculated to be about 0.71% (1 in 141), with predominance among non-Hispanic Caucasians.[5] Compared to the United States, a higher prevalence of 1–1.5% has been reported from the United Kingdom and Ireland.[6] Overall, CD is underdiagnosed because of the silent and subclinical cases, and only 1 in 8 presenting with the classic symptoms.[7] Recent studies in the United States and Europe have reported a 2- to 4.5-fold increase in the prevalence of CD.[8,9] The reason for this trend is unclear, and cannot be solely explained on the basis of increased awareness and availability of serologic tests. Other explanations include the role of certain environmental triggers in genetically susceptible individuals, the worldwide increase in wheat consumption and enhanced gluten exposure, and, potentially, the role of changing industrial food processes, including breadmaking. The "hygiene hypothesis", based on the pattern of early childhood infections, may have an impact upon the changing epidemiology of this disease.[10]

CLINICAL PRESENTATION

Celiac disease may present with classical symptoms, atypical symptoms, or refractory disease. The classical presentation includes symptoms of diarrhea, weight loss, steatorrhea and failure to thrive, hypoalbuminemia, and deficiencies of micronutrients and fat-soluble vitamins. Presence of fever, anorexia, unexplained weight loss, gastrointestinal bleeding, or abdominal pain in patients with CD suggests the development of complications such as ulcerative jejunitis, small bowel adenocarcinoma, or enteropathy associated T cell lymphoma.

Atypical presentations may be associated with mild gastrointestinal symptoms or present with unexplained iron deficiency anemia,[11] metabolic bone disease,[12] neurological symptoms including idiopathic epilepsy and/or ataxia,[13] autoimmune thyroid disease,[14] infertility,[15] and cutaneous manifestations including dermatitis herpetiformis (DH).

The risk for association with other autoimmune disorders has been reported more frequently in patients with CD when compared to controls (14% vs 2.8%).[16] Prevalence of CD in patients with Diabetes mellitus type I has been estimated to range from 2–5% in adults and 3–8% in children.[17] Besides asymptomatic elevation of the liver transaminase levels,[14] CD may be associated with other chronic liver disorders such as autoimmune hepatitis,[18] primary biliary cirrhosis,[19] and cryptogenic liver disease.[20] Prevalence of CD is also increased in patients with Down syndrome (3–12%), and in Turner syndrome (2–10%).[17]

Non-Responsive Celiac Disease

This is characterized by a lack of response to a GFD once the diagnosis of CD has been confirmed, or the recurrence of clinical symptoms, and serological abnormalities while on a GFD, in a patient who had initially responded to dietary management.[21] Causes of non-responsive CD include non-compliance or inadvertent gluten contamination (36–51%), microscopic colitis, bacterial overgrowth, pancreatic insufficiency, lactose intolerance, and irritable bowel syndrome.[22]

Refractory Celiac Disease (RCD)

Refractory celiac disease (RCD) refers to persistent or recurrent gastrointestinal symptoms of diarrhea, weight loss, and malabsorption, with small bowel villous atrophy, despite adherence to a strict GFD for at least 12 months. Diagnosis of RCD can be made after exclusion of other causes of non-responsive CD or development of overt malignancy. Serologic tests for CD, including endomysial antibody (EMA) and tissue transglutaminase (TTG), are generally negative, but a positive serology may be present in 19–30% of patients despite being on a strict GFD,[23,24] hence a positive serology does not exclude the diagnosis of RCD. Therefore, RCD requires exclusion of other causes of non-responsive CD and villous atrophy. RCD has been classified as Type I or II. Type I is characterized by a normal intraepithelial lymphocyte phenotype and has a better prognosis than RCD type II. In RCD II, there is an abnormal phenotype of increased intraepithelial lymphocytes, characterized by the loss of CD3, CD4, and CD8 surface markers, but a preserved intracytoplasmic expression of CD3.[25] Detection of the abnormal lymphocyte clones is evaluated by flow cytometry or immunohistochemistry, and T-cell receptor rearrangement studies by PCR. Because of the aberrant intraepithelial population in RCD II, these patients are prone to frequent progression to enteropathy associated T-cell lymphoma, with 5-year survival rates of 40–58%.[9,23] Enteropathy associated T-cell lymphoma is rare in the general population,[26] reported occasionally in RCD I, and in 60–80% of patients with RCD II.[27,28] Although prognosis of RCD I is better than RCD II, the mortality and complication rates are still higher than that observed with uncomplicated CD.[24]

Dermatitis Herpetiformis

Dermatitis herpetiformis is a cutaneous condition that presents as clusters of intensely pruritic papulovesicular lesions on the extensor surface of the elbows, buttocks, scalp, and knees. Histologically, it is characterized by the deposition of IgA at the dermal–epidermal junction.[29] Like CD, there is a strong association with HLA DQ2 and DQ8.[30] All patients with DH have some manifestation of CD; 10–20% of such patients may present with classic gastrointestinal symptoms of diarrhea and malabsorption and 20% with atypical symptoms, while 60% of patients may have "silent" CD.[31] Both the skin condition and intestinal lesions respond to a gluten-free diet and recur with gluten exposure, though some patients may require treatment with a neutrophil inhibitor, such as dapsone, for treatment of DH.[32] Over the long term, by adherence to a strict gluten-free diet (GFD), 47% of patients with DH will be able to discontinue dapsone; however, about 15% will need ongoing treatment for control of dermatologic lesions.[33] The usual starting dose of dapsone is 100 mg/day, and side effects include hemolytic anemia, methemoglobinemia, and dapsone hypersensitivity syndrome.[34]

DIAGNOSIS

Serology

Serological testing is the initial test when there is a suspicion for CD or high-risk groups, such as first-degree relatives of patients with known CD. Available serologic tests for the detection of CD include deamidated antigliadin antibodies (IgA DGP , IgG DGP), endomysial antibodies (EMA), and tissue transglutaminase (TTG) antibodies (IgA TTG, IgG TTG).

In a systematic review of 34 studies, EMA and IgA TTG had specificities of >99% and >98%, respectively. Both EMA and IgA TTG had sensitivity of ~93% for diagnosis of CD.[35] Recombinant human IgA TTG demonstrated higher sensitivity, with comparable specificity when compared to EMA. Selective immunoglobulin A (IgA) deficiency has been reported in 2–2.6% of patients with CD and 0.2% of the general population,[36,37] hence it is advisable to measure the serum IgA level in order to avoid false negative results.

A finger stick-based TTG IgA test is available in some countries, and preliminary studies suggest good sensitivity and specificity, although additional studies are needed before recommending its widespread use.[38] Another point-of-care test based on the detection of antibodies against deamidated gliadin peptides reported high diagnostic accuracy, with sensitivity and specificity of 93.1% and 95%, respectively, and a negative predictive value of 99%, thus providing an efficient means of detecting CD in a primary care setting.[39] Although the deamidated gliadin peptide (DGP) antibody test is better than the gliadin antibody test, it is not better than the TTG IgA test. The pooled sensitivity of the DGP test was 87.8%, and of the TTG test was 93%. The pooled specificity for the TTG test was 96.5%, and for the DGP antibody test was 94.1%.[40] Hence, human recombinant IgA TTG is recommended as the test of choice for initial screening for CD.[41]

Though serologic tests are highly accurate for screening, they are not as useful in monitoring patients on a GFD, as normalization does not accurately predict a histologic recovery[42,43] or the assessment of strict adherence to a GFD.[22,44] It is expected that the serum titer will fall by 6 months and should normalize by 12 months.

Small Bowel Biopsy

Small bowel biopsy remains the gold standard for establishing the diagnosis of CD. Patients who are positive for IgA TTG should undergo esophagogastroduodenoscopy to obtain a small bowel biopsy in order to confirm the diagnosis of CD. The current recommendation is to obtain four to six biopsies from the second part of the duodenum and the mucosa of the bulb.[45–47] The histologic features are described using the Marsh–Oberhuber classification.[48] The spectrum ranges from Marsh 0, with no villous atrophy, to Marsh 4, which refers to total villous atrophy, increased intraepithelial lymphocytes, and crypt hypoplasia. In the presence of positive serology and characteristic histologic changes in the small bowel biopsy, the diagnosis of CD is confirmed.

In patients with high clinical suspicion for CD, and when diagnosis is unclear because of negative histology or serology, testing for HLA haplotypes associated with CD is helpful. HLA-DQ2 is present in 95% of patients with CD, and about 5–10% of patients with CD carry HLA-DQ8.

While all patients with CD have HLA DQ2 or DQ8, these markers are also present in 40% of the general population,[49] with CD developing in 2–5% of the gene carriers.[50] Hence, while carriage of the susceptibility genes is not at all sufficient for celiac disease to develop even in those with long exposure to gluten, the utility of this test is that diagnosis of CD is highly unlikely in the absence of these haplotypes.

TREATMENT

Once the diagnosis of CD is established, a strict GFD remains the mainstay of treatment. The term "gluten" refers to the storage proteins of wheat (gliadins and glutenin), barley (prolamines), and rye (hordeins). Grains that should be avoided include wheat, barley, rye, spelt, kamut, and triticale. Pasta, biscuits, bread, and cookies are obvious sources of gluten; however, seemingly "safe" foods may contain gluten. This will be the case if any of the ingredients are derived from wheat, barley, or rye – for example, thickening agents in soups. Also to be avoided are products that are processed in the same facility as wheat, barley, and rye, as are many rice- and corn-based cereals. Other ingredients that should be viewed with suspicion include malt or malt flavoring, hydrolyzed vegetable protein (HVP), modified food starch (and starch in foreign foods), natural flavorings, vegetable gum, and fat substitutes. Non-food items, such as medications and communion wafers, may also be unappreciated sources of gluten, as are food contaminants.

Although recent well-designed studies have demonstrated the safety of moderate amount of oats in the diet of patients with CD, the role of oats in CD remains controversial because of contamination by gluten during milling or processing. Additionally, a small number of patients may react directly to oats. Therefore, patients who intend to include oats in their GFD should be cautioned.

The amount of gluten acceptable in a GFD has been debatable, as is the exact amount of dietary gluten that can be tolerated by patients with CD without causing any symptoms or histological abnormalities in the small intestine. Consumption of 200 mg daily of gluten over a 4-week period by patients with CD was associated with the development of pathological changes in the small bowel mucosa.[51] In another study, 10–50 mg gluten daily over 3 months also resulted in intestinal histological abnormalities,[52] whereas in two other studies an average daily ingestion of 34–36 mg of gluten was well tolerated.[53,54] This suggests that the amount of daily gluten tolerated by different patients with CD is variable. However, gluten concentration of 20 ppm in foodstuffs, which would be equivalent to 6 mg of gluten daily, has a high likelihood of tolerance and is very unlikely to induce mucosal abnormalities.[55] This is in accordance with the *Codex Alimentarus* labeling guidelines for gluten-free foods to contain less than 20 ppm of gluten.[56]

A lifelong GFD is difficult to maintain, and compliance can be impacted because of expense, gluten contamination by cross-contact, and lack of availability, resulting in a decrease in quality of life. Even though patients adhere to a strict GFD, it is estimated that they may ingest 5–50 mg of gluten daily because of dietary contamination, cross-contact in the kitchen at home, or, perhaps most likely, in commercial kitchens.[52] Several efforts have been made to promote the provision of foods to patients requiring a GFD while reducing the danger of cross-contact in food-processing or commercial kitchens. In a survey conducted in the United Kingdom, 42% of patients with CD expressed dissatisfaction with their diet, and only 20% reported that a GFD was an acceptable treatment for their disease.[57] In general, adherence to a GFD has been reported to range from 42–91%,[58–60] as compared to a higher adherence (mean 80.4%) to treatment in other chronic gastrointestinal diseases.[61] Another issue is that greater than 50% of patients demonstrate persistent villous atrophy despite being on a strict GFD.[62–64] The risk of developing malignancy is higher in patients not adhering to a strict

GFD,[65] as well as those who do not respond to a GFD.[66] To prevent long-term complications, these patients may require alternative management therapies.[4]

Advances in understanding the molecular mechanisms in the pathophysiology of CD have led to the identification of pathogenic events that can be targeted with novel therapeutic strategies (Fig. 12.1). Wheat gluten is comprised of gliadin, low molecular weight glutenin (LMW-GS), and high molecular weight glutenin (HMW-GS). Gliadin is further subdivided into α, β, γ, and ω subunits. The α-gliadin is the most toxic fraction, though immunogenic T-cell stimulatory epitopes are also found in the γ-gliadins, and both the low molecular weight (LMW) and the high molecular weight glutenin.[67–69] Deamidation of the glutamine residues on α-gliadin subunits by TTG to glutamic acid enhances their immunogenicity. These peptides are then presented

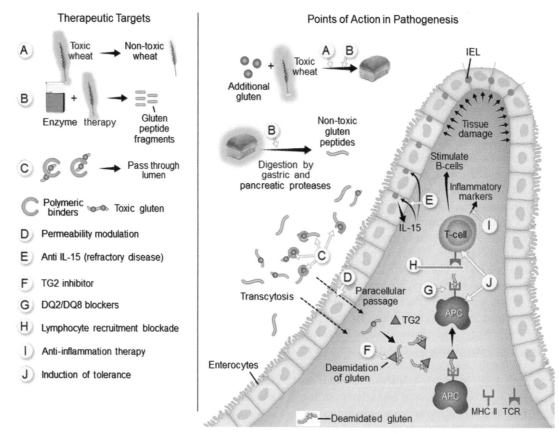

FIGURE 12.1 (A) Non-toxic wheat: generation of wheat species that lack the immunogenic gluten peptides. (B) Enzyme therapy: detoxification of the gluten peptides by enzymatic supplementation or treatment of the wheat flour with microbial proteases. (C) Polymeric binders: polymeric binders limit toxicity of gluten by preventing degradation and absorption. (D) Permeability modulation: zonulin antagonists (larazotide) inhibit gliadin-induced increased permeability by inhibition of zonulin release via receptor blockade. (E) Anti IL-15: gluten peptides evoke the innate immune response by inducing IL-15 expression and interaction between epithelial MIC and NKG2D receptor on surface of intraepithelial lymphocytes. This ligand–receptor interaction induces epithelial apoptosis by stimulation of the cytotoxic T lymphocytes. (F) TG2 inhibitors: gliadin peptides are deamidated by TG2 in the lamina propria. TG2 blockade can inhibit the adaptive immune response. (G) HLA blockade: Prevents binding of the gliadin peptides to HLA DQ2 or DQ8 on the surface of the antigen presenting cells. (H) Inhibition of T-lymphocyte recruitment blocks migration of immune cells to the intestinal tissues. (I) Anti-cytokine therapy: antibodies against IFN-γ and TNF-α produced in response to T-cell activation reduce mucosal injury in celiac disease. (J) Induction of immune tolerance: vaccine with immunogenic gluten peptides. Abbreviations: IL-15, interleukin; NKG2D, natural killer cell receptor D; MIC, major histocompatibility complex class I related chains; TG2, transglutaminase 2; IFN, interferon; TNF, tumor necrosis factor. See color plate at the back of the book.

to the T cells by HLA DQ2 or HLA-DQ8 molecules on the antigen presenting cells. The subsequent inflammation and pathogenic changes in the small bowel mucosa result from T-cell activation and the release of inflammatory cytokines. Novel therapeutic interventions have been developed to target different stages in the pathogenesis of CD, and some of these experimental therapies are currently in Phase I or II clinical trials.

Alteration of Wheat: Wheat Variants

An attractive alternative to a strict GFD would be the availability of modified wheat strains that lack the immunogenic gluten peptides but maintain the satisfactory baking qualities. This could be accomplished through genetic engineering by modifying or deleting the toxic gluten sequences.

The hexaploid wheat strain *Triticum aestivum* (AABBDD),which is currently used globally as bread wheat, has been derived from two ancient wheat strains: diploid *Triticum tauschii* (DD) and the tetraploid *Triticum turgidum* (AABB). *In vitro* studies reported that peptic–tryptic digests from the hexaploid wheat (bread) were more toxic to cultured small intestinal mucosal tissue from patients with CD as compared to digests from tetraploid (durum) wheat,[70] suggesting that durum wheat, if modified, may be less immunogenic in patients with CD. Genes encoding the gluten proteins are located on the A, B, or D genomes of wheat. HMW-GS and LMW-GS are encoded by loci on chromosome 1. Genes encoding for the α-gliadins are located within the Gli-2 locus on the short arm of chromosome 6D.[71] Deletion of the α-gliadin locus from the D genome on chromosome 6 in the hexaploid *Triticum aestivum* has been shown to reduce the number of T-cell stimulatory epitopes, but altered the baking properties. Alteration in the baking properties occurred because of decreased elasticity of the dough due to an altered ratio of the glutenin and gliadin proteins.[72] In contrast, deletion of the locus for ω- and γ-gliadins, along with that for low molecular weight glutenin (LMW-GS) on chromosome 1, decreased the expression of the T-cell stimulating epitopes, but retained desirable baking properties.[72] This approach for development of non-immunogenic wheat strains is still at the preclinical stages and remains under investigation.

Psyllium has been studied as a gluten replacement because of its minimal effect on odor and bread texture while retaining baking properties, and sensory analysis results reported high acceptance for bread prepared from psyllium dough among both celiac patients and healthy controls.[73] Sorghum, a grain related to maize has also been successfully utilized in baking gluten-free breads and other products. Preliminary *in vitro* and *in vivo* studies have been promising, but larger trials are needed before the feasibility of sorghum use in patients with CD is confirmed.[74]

Quinoa, which is a plant from the Andes that is rich in protein and other nutrients, has been considered a safe component for a GFD. To investigate the safety of using quinoa in celiac patients, 15 quinoa cultivars were tested *in vitro* for immunogenic celiac epitopes and immune reactivity, using monoclonal antibodies and cell proliferation assays. With the exception of two cultivars, quinoa seems generally safe for patients with CD.[75]

Gluten Detoxification

Pretreatment of Wheat Flour

Certain sourdough lactobacilli possess peptidases that can hydrolyze proline-rich gluten peptides in wheat flour, including the immunologically potent 33-mer peptide from the α2-gliadin, and thus decreasing their immunogenicity. Proteolysis of the wheat flour by sourdough lactic acid bacilli results in considerable, but not complete, hydrolysis of the wheat gliadins.[76] In a follow-up double-blind pilot study, 17 CD patients ingested two types of bread, each containing 2g gluten, and produced with baker's yeast or fermentation with sourdough lactobacillus. The sourdough bread was made from a mixture of wheat (30%) and flour from oats, millet, and buckwheat fermented with lactobacilli. The response was assessed by measurement of intestinal permeability, utilizing lactulose/l-rhamnose excretion. Of the 17 patients, 13 demonstrated increased intestinal permeability after ingestion of the baker's yeast bread, whereas the same 13 patients, when exposed to lactobacillus-treated bread, did not demonstrate any changes in intestinal permeability.[77]

Combination of sourdough lactobacilli with fungal proteases has been shown to result in complete hydrolyzation of the gluten, thus rendering it less toxic. Duodenal mucosal tissue from celiac patients, when treated with peptic tryptic digest from the hydrolyzed wheat after fermentation with sourdough lactobacilli and fungal proteases, demonstrated interferon-γ expression comparable to healthy controls.[78] Eight patients with known CD in remission ingested 200g daily of sweet baked goods (~10g of gluten) made from sourdough fermented wheat flour. No abnormality was reported in serology or intestinal permeability values after 60 days of challenge,[78] suggesting that gluten had been degraded. Probiotic preparation VSL#3 containing a mixture of lactic acid and bifido bacteria, when used as a starter for fermentation, decreased the immunogenicity of gluten by hydrolyzing the gliadin polypeptides.[79]

Another approach to decrease the immunogenicity of wheat gluten is incubation of wheat flour with microbial transglutaminase derived from *Streptomyces mobaraensis* and lysine methyl ester. Transamidation of the gliadin results in a loss of its affinity for the HLA-DQ2 molecules, and attenuates IFN-γ expression by T-cell lines from duodenal biopsies of adult celiac patients.[80] This approach of pretreatment of wheat flour utilizing sourdough lactobacilli, probiotics, and microbial proteases, though promising, has limited clinical trials, and further studies are required before non-immunogenic flours can be recommended. Potentially, this less immunogenic wheat flour could be consumed in conjunction with oral enzyme supplements or polymeric binders.

Oral Enzyme Therapy

Gliadin and other prolamines are partially resistant to degradation by the intestinal peptidases because of their high proline and glutamine content. Incomplete digestion of these proteins occurs because both the gastrointestinal peptidases, and the brush border dipeptidyl peptidase IV (DPPIV) and dipeptidyl carboxypeptidase I, have poor affinity for the peptide bonds adjacent to proline and glutamine, thus resulting in accumulation of the immunogenic 33-mer and the 26-mer long oligopeptide fragments.[81,82] Detoxification of gluten by oral administration of enzymes is an attractive alternative to GFD. Glutenases function as endopeptidases with the ability to effectively target the proline- and glutamine-rich peptide fragments, and rendering them non-immunogenic in susceptible individuals.

Prolyl endopeptidases (PEPs) expressed by certain bacteria and fungi, such as *Flavobacterium meningosepticum*, *Sphingomonas capsulate*, and *Myxococcus xanthum*, have demonstrated the ability to hydrolyze these proline and glutamine residues, but *Flavobacterium meningosepticum* and *Myxococcus xanthum* are susceptible to degradation by gastric acid and hence not optimal for oral administration.[83,84] Pretreatment of gluten with PEP derived from *Flavobacterium meningosepticum* destroyed its T-cell stimulatory properties.[85] In another double-blind randomized crossover study, 20 biopsy-proven asymptomatic CD patients in remission were exposed to gluten pretreated with *Flavobacterium meningosepticum* and did not develop fat or carbohydrate malabsorption in a majority of those who had developed symptoms after a 2-week gluten challenge.[86]

Aspergillopepsin from *Aspergillus Niger* and dipeptidyl peptidase IV (DPPIV) are two food-grade enzymes with the ability to detoxify gluten. Aspergillopepsin lacks specificity for the immunogenic gluten peptides, but has the ability to digest gluten into smaller peptides, thereby making them accessible to degradation by specific endopeptidases and exopeptidases. *In vitro* studies reported that, when used independently, neither Aspergillopepsin nor DDPIV can effectively cleave the immunotoxic gluten peptides. However, a combination of Aspergillopepsin and DDPIV was effective in detoxification of moderate amounts of gluten.[87]

A prolyl endopeptidase derived from *Aspergillus niger* can cleave the proline-rich peptides, is stable in the presence of gastric acid, and functions optimally at pH 4–5.[84] The ability of *Aspergillus niger* to cleave gluten peptides in bread was evaluated in a dynamic *in vitro* gastrointestinal model (TIM-1), and accelerated digestion of gluten in the gastric compartment[88] was reported with a small amount of gluten peptides entering the duodenum, thus limiting gluten toxicity in susceptible individuals and making *Aspergillus niger* a potential alternative treatment in CD. Based on these promising *in vitro* results, *Aspergillus niger* is undergoing further evaluation in a randomized double-blind control trial to assess the effect of *Aspergillus niger* supplementation with oral gluten on small bowel histology and serologic response in patients with CD (clinical trials.gov/show/NCT00810654). A randomized double-blind crossover study is investigating the impact of caloric density upon the efficacy of *Aspergillus niger* in gluten digestion (www.clinical trials.gov/NCT01335503).

Another therapeutic strategy has been to utilize a combination therapy for enhanced gluten degradation. EP-B2, a naturally occurring glutamine-specific cysteine endoprotease from barley (*Hordeum vulgare*), efficiently cleaves the 33-mer peptide, but is not able to completely hydrolyze the toxic QLPYPQP epitope. When used together, Aspergillopepsin and EP-B2 were effective in reducing the concentration of this toxic epitope. Co-administration of EP-B2 along with PEP from *Sphingomonas capsulate* in an *in vitro* study effectively detoxified gluten from whole wheat bread.[89] EP-B2 initiates the digestion of the gluten proteins, followed by SC PEP digesting the residual oligopeptides, thus minimizing gluten toxicity. ALV003 has been developed as an oral, fixed-dose 1:1 mixture of these two glutenases: EP-B2 (ALV001) and modified recombinant *Sphingomonas capsulate* (ALV002). The effect of ALV003 on symptoms and immune response was assessed in 20 known CD patients who were randomly assigned to ingest a large gluten meal pretreated with ALV003, or placebo. Although no difference in symptoms was noted between the two groups after gluten ingestion, the immune response to gluten was abolished in the ALV003 group, as evident by absence of gliadin or 33-mer specific T cells in the peripheral blood.[64] Safety and tolerability of ALV003 has been assessed in two Phase I clinical trials, which reported excellent tolerability without any adverse events.[90] In a randomized Phase IIA clinical trial in 41 patients with CD, ingestion of 2 g of gluten daily with ALV003 for 6 weeks attenuated the small bowel mucosal injury and serologic response to gluten, in contrast to the control subjects.[91] Currently, a Phase IIb clinical trial is underway with ALV003.

In a randomized double-blind placebo-controlled study, Stan-1, another combination of microbial food grade glutenases, was evaluated in 35 known celiac adolescents on a GFD with a persistent elevation of TTG. Ingestion of Stan-1 with 1 g gluten daily for 12 days did lead to reports of any difference between the two groups.[92]

Intraluminal Binding of Gluten by Polymeric Binders

The principle behind this approach is the ability to bind the ingested gluten by polymeric binders within the gastrointestinal lumen, thus limiting toxicity by preventing degradation and absorption. A high molecular weight polymeric binder, P (HEMA-co-SS), has the ability to selectively complex with α-gliadin, and thus counteracts the toxic effects of gluten on the small intestinal mucosa. In *in vitro* studies, PHEMA decreased the digestion of oral gluten, reduced gluten-induced paracellular intestinal permeability, and effectively attenuated the immune response to oral gluten in gluten-sensitized rodents.[93]

Permeability Modulation

Zonulin

Patients with active CD have been shown to have increased intestinal permeability, as measured by the lactulose/mannitol absorption test.[94] Zonulin is over-expressed in the intestinal epithelium of patients with CD. This molecule, identified as prehepatoglobin-2, is a modulator of intestinal permeability, and does this by regulating epithelial tight junctions. Interaction between gliadin peptides and intestinal mucosa induces the release of zonulin, which reduces electrical resistance at the epithelial tight junctions and facilitates paracellular diffusion of gluten peptides and other immunostimulatory substances across the mucosa, and is an early event in the cascade in the pathophysiology of CD.[94] A recent study reported that gliadin binds to the chemokine receptor CXCR3 on intestinal epithelial cells, and the released zonulin enhances permeability via the My-D88 pathway.[95] These observations led to the development of larazotide acetate (AT-1001), an octapeptide that inhibits the gliadin-induced increase in paracellular permeability by inhibition of zonulin release via receptor blockade.[96,97] In a Phase I double-blinded randomized placebo-controlled study, AT-1001 prevented gluten-induced permeability as measured by the lactulose–mannitol ratio, in 14 CD patients challenged with oral gluten. In this trial larazotide acetate was well tolerated when compared to placebo, and there were no adverse effects or gastrointestinal symptoms reported.[98] In a double-blind placebo-controlled randomized trial, patients with CD undergoing a gluten challenge were randomized to larazotide acetate or placebo. Although larazotide was well tolerated, no significant difference was observed in intestinal permeability when compared to placebo.[99] Gluten-induced symptoms and elevation of TTG IgA antibodies were prevented by the lower doses of larazotide acetate.[99]

R-Spondin 1

R-spondin protein is an epithelial mitogen that stimulates crypt cell growth in the large and small intestine. In a mouse model of drug-induced colitis, administration of R-spondin 1 decreased the severity of enterocolitis by inhibiting the production of proinflammatory cytokines, and enhancing regeneration of the mucosa by stimulating the growth of crypt cells.[100] These results suggest that R-spondin 1 may be useful in the treatment of gastrointestinal disorders with mucosal damage, such as inflammatory bowel disease, radiation-induced enterocolitis, and CD, by regeneration and restoration of mucosal architecture. It has not been tested in CD patients as yet.

Rho Kinase Inhibition

On gluten ingestion, patients with CD develop increased intestinal permeability triggered by interferon-γ produced by activated CD4T cells, and facilitated by Rho kinase (ROCK-1 and ROCK-2).[101,102] Rho A and Rho kinase regulate epithelial tight junctions and axon growth; hence they have been used in treatment of patients with spinal cord injury. Fasudil, a ROCK inhibitor, has been approved in Japan for treatment of cerebral vasospasm, and BA-210 is in Phase II trials in patients with spinal cord injury.[103] Though promising as a therapeutic option in CD by reversal of gluten-induced intestinal permeability through ROCK inhibition, more specific ROCK inhibitors need evaluation, as side effects of the currently available agent, fasudil, makes it undesirable for long-term use.

Blockade of Antigen Presentation

Inhibition of Tissue Transglutaminase

Deamidation of the gluten by TTG converts specific glutamine residues to glutamate, thereby unmasking the immunogenic T-cell epitopes that enhances their ability to bind to HLA DQ2 or DQ8 on the surface of the antigen presenting cells, resulting in an exaggerated T-cell response.[104] Thus, selective TTG inhibition seems to be an attractive non-dietary therapeutic option in management of CD. *In vitro* studies have shown that T-cell lines from intestinal biopsies of CD patients readily recognized deamidated gliadin epitopes following *in situ* treatment with TTG. However, inhibition of transglutaminase activity by an inhibitor abolished the T-cell response after gluten challenge.[105] TTG, a protein cross-linking enzyme, is ubiquitously expressed in mammalian tissues and supports the apoptosis program. Although deficiency of TTG function in TTG knockout mice is not associated with any physiological abnormalities,[106,107] they may develop autoimmunity and immune complex glomerulonephritis.[108] Selective inhibition of TTG can be accomplished with reversible or irreversible inhibitors.

Studies with imidazolium derivatives such as L682777 and R-283, as TTG inactivators, reported inactivation of factor XIIIa, thus making them unsuitable as a safe therapeutic option in CD.[109,110] Because of its ubiquitous expression, even selective inhibition of TTG has the potential for adverse effects. In animal models, selective inhibition of TTG by dihydroisoxazole compounds (e.g., KCC009) showed excellent oral bioavailability with few systemic adverse effects.[111,112] Currently, no clinical trials have been undertaken in humans because of the risk of adverse events.

Moreover, TTG blockade does not inhibit the innate immune response induced by the p31–43 non-immunodominant epitope of gliadin. This "innate" peptide induces expression of interleukin 15, resulting in an early inflammatory response that may lead to mucosal damage as well as increased permeability of the intestinal epithelium.[113] TTG inhibitors also do not inhibit the IgA-mediated transport of the toxic gliadin molecules to the lamina propria.[114] Hence the therapeutic role of even selective TTG inhibitors is limited, as, at best, this group of agents can only diminish the gliadin-induced adaptive immune response, without any impact on the innate immune response.

HLA DQ2/DQ8 Inhibitors

The role of HLA DQ2/DQ8 in the pathogenesis of CD makes them a target for therapeutic intervention. Binding of the deamidated gluten peptides to the HLADQ2/DQ8 molecules present on the surface of the antigen presenting cells leads to activation of the gluten-sensitized T cells. This interaction between gluten and the binding site on these HLA molecules can be inhibited by gluten analogues that may be developed by substituting the proline residues by azido prolines,[115] or using cyclic or dimeric peptides with enhanced affinity for the DQ2 binding sites.[116] However, the challenge remains to find an ideal blocking agent that has high oral bioavailability and does not interfere with the other Class 2 dependent responses. A gluten decapeptide (QQPQDAVQPF) derived from durum wheat has been shown in *in vitro* studies to inhibit activation of celiac peripheral blood lymphocytes on incubation with a peptic–tryptic digest of bread wheat gliadin and peptide 62–75 from α-gliadin.[117] These modified gluten peptides need further evaluation before being considered a therapeutic option in CD.

Blockade of Lymphocyte Recruitment

Alpha 4 Beta 7 and MAdCam-1

T lymphocytes express α4β7 , a principle mucosal homing receptor that interacts with mucosal addressin cell adhesion molecule 1 (MAdCam-1) on vascular endothelial cells, with subsequent entrance of the lymphocytes into the lamina propria.[118,119] MAdCam-1 and α4β7 are critical for lymphocyte homing to the gut, and both have a role in the pathogenesis of CD through lymphocyte recruitment. Patients with untreated CD had increased expression of MAdCam-1 in the duodenal mucosa and an associated depletion of α4β7-positive T cells in the peripheral blood.[120] This makes α4β7 both a mucosal addressing cell adhesion molecule-1 and an attractive target for therapy of CD. Trials with natalizumab, a monoclonal antibody against α4 integrin, in the treatment of Crohn's disease have been promising,[121] but no trials have yet been initiated in CD. The risk of side effects may not justify the use of such potent agents in CD.

CCR9 and CCL25

Chemokine receptor 9 (CCR9) is another receptor expressed on the surface of lymphocytes. Chemokine ligand 25 (CCL25), expressed by the intestinal epithelial cells, binds to CCR9 on the T lymphocyte and enables homing to the intestinal tissues. In a double-blind Phase II trial, CCX282-B, an oral CCR9 antagonist, was well tolerated and demonstrated a reduction in the Crohn's disease activity index (CDAI) in patients with active Crohn's disease.[122] This therapeutic approach in CD has been investigated in a Phase II clinical trial, although results have not been reported despite completion of the trial several years ago. CCX025, another oral CCR9 inhibitor, is also undergoing a Phase I clinical trial in CD.[50]

CXCL10 and CXCR3

CXCR3, a receptor expressed on the surface of the T lymphocytes, binds to CXCL10, a T-cell recruiting chemokine, and facilitates recruitment of T lymphocytes to the intestinal epithelium as an innate response to gliadin. Stimulation of human monocytes by gliadin has been shown to increase expression of multiple T-cell recruiting chemokines, including CXCL10.[123] The ability to block CXCL10 may represent a therapeutic target in CD, by blockade of T-cell recruitment.

Anti-CD3 Therapy

The CD3 protein complex is a co-receptor for the T-cell receptor. Anti-CD3 antibodies involves elimination of effector T cells and induction of regulatory T cells.[124] Monoclonal anti-CD3 antibodies are currently undergoing trials in type 1 diabetes and ulcerative colitis.[125–127] Although anti-CD3 therapy may have a potential role in CD, currently there are no trials underway.

Anti-CD 20 Therapy

Anti-CD 20 therapy has been shown to be beneficial in rheumatoid arthritis[128] and multiple sclerosis.[129] When gliadin links with TTG, the gliadin-specific CD4+ T helper cells interact with CD20+ B cells to assist them to differentiate into plasma cells and produce autoantibodies against TTG, thus amplifying the antigluten T-cell response.[130] Hence, anti-CD20 antibodies may have a role in the treatment of CD. A report that generation of mucosal IgA+ plasmablasts is not abrogated by anti-CD20 treatment suggests that if mucosally produced antibodies have a role in the pathogenesis of CD, then anti-CD20 therapy will be ineffective.[131] Rituximab, tositumomab, and ibritumomab are currently available anti-CD20 monoclonal antibodies approved for clinical use, but none has been evaluated in CD and they are unlikely to be used deliberately for the treatment of CD.[130]

Modulation of Inflammation

Anti-Interferon Gamma and TNF Alpha

Gluten peptides presented by their binding to the HLA Class II DQ2 and DQ8 molecules on the antigen presenting cells results in activation of the gluten-specific CD4 T helper cells. These activated CD4 T cells secrete proinflammatory cytokine interferon (IFN)-γ and tumor necrosis factor (TNF)-α, which stimulate macrophages to release proteolytic metalloproteinases (MMPs), which are responsible for the mucosal architectural remodeling[50] observed in CD.[132,133] Blockade of IFN-γ by an anti-IFN-γ gamma antibody prevented damage to the intestinal mucosa on exposure to gliadin-specific T cells, by inhibiting release of MMPs.[134] These IFN-γ antibodies also block the enhanced transepithelial gluten flux, without affecting the baseline gluten permeability in the absence of active inflammation;[135] however, there have been no clinical trials in CD. Monoclonal anti-TNF-α antibodies (infliximab and adalimumab) have been found to be beneficial in patients with inflammatory bowel disease. The beneficial role of these agents in RCD has been reported in case studies.[136,137]

Therapy Targeting IL-15

Secretion of IL-15 on gluten exposure by the antigen presenting cells in patients with CD induces expression of MIC on intestinal epithelial cells, which then binds to the NKG2D receptor on the surface of the intraepithelial lymphocytes.[138–141] This interaction results in proliferation of cytotoxic T lymphocytes that may have a role in the development of refractory sprue and malignant transformation.[142] Reversal of intestinal damage from autoimmune enteropathy in transgenic mice that overexpress IL-15 in the enterocyte has been demonstrated with the use of IL-15 blocking antibodies.[143] The IL-15 blocking antibodies induce apoptosis and reduce the number of intraepithelial lymphocytes in the intestinal epithelium of IL-15 transgenic models.[144] The role of IL-15 in the pathogenesis of CD, and in particular RCD, suggests that strategies blocking IL-15 or its signaling cascade may be an attractive therapeutic option, though trials are still awaited. IL-15 human monoclonal antibody has been evaluated in other autoimmune diseases, such as rheumatoid arthritis, with promising results.

Induction of Tolerance

Hookworm Infection

The observation that a high prevalence of autoimmune disorders occurs in developed countries led to a Phase II clinical trial to evaluate the role of hookworm infections upon the development of autoimmune diseases. In one study, the hookworm *Necator americanus* was used to determine whether a hookworm infection could modulate the gluten-induced immune responses in patients with known CD. In this double-blinded placebo-controlled study over 21 weeks, healthy celiac patients on a GFD had a cutaneous inoculation of the helminth larvae. No significant benefit was demonstrated on gluten-induced enteropathy;[145] however, there were some decreases in inflammatory immune responses after gluten challenge in hookworm-infected individuals.[146]

Immunotherapy

Patients with CD seeking alternatives to GFD preferred vaccination as an attractive option if they were unable consistently to maintain a GFD.[57] In the mouse model, repeated exposure by subcutaneous administration of the immunodominant gluten peptide was well tolerated and resulted in tolerant CD4 T lymphocytes.[147] Nexvax 2, a vaccine containing the commonly recognized immunodominant gluten peptides, has been developed to induce gluten tolerance in patients with CD. Nexvax was evaluated in a Phase I clinical trial in HLA DQ2 volunteers with CD. It was well tolerated, with activation of gluten-specific T cells in these patients (www.clinicaltrials.gov: NCT 00879749). Information regarding the long-term outcome of immunostimulation on the natural history of CD is awaited.

CONCLUSION

Advances in understanding of the pathophysiology of CD have led to the development of different therapeutic approaches that can be utilized as an alternative to a lifelong GFD. Many of these pharmacological agents are currently undergoing clinical trials to establish their safety and efficacy in maintaining clinical and histologic remission when used as an alternative to a GFD. The potential of novel therapies that may be used as an alternative to a GFD or as adjunctive therapy is promising, since lifelong adherence to a strict GFD is challenging, expensive, and may impact quality of life by restricting social activities.

References

1. Ludvigsson J, Rubio-Tapia A, van Dyke CT, Melton III LJ, Zinsmeister AR, Lahr BD, et al. Increasing incidence of Celiac Disease in North American Population. *Am J Gastroenterol* May 2013 (in press).

2. West J, Logan RF, Smith CJ, Hubbard RB, Card TR. Malignancy and mortality in people with coeliac disease: population based cohort study. *BMJ* 2004;329(7468):716–9.

3. Green PH, Fleischauer AT, Bhagat G, Goyal R, Jabri B, Neugut AI. Risk of malignancy in patients with celiac disease. *Am J Med* 2003;115(3):191–5.

4. Rubio-Tapia A, Rahim MW, See JA, Lahr BD, Wu TT, Murray JA. Mucosal recovery and mortality in adults with celiac disease after treatment with a gluten-free diet. *Am J Gastroenterol* 2010;105(6):1412–20.

5. Tack GJ, Verbeek WH, Schreurs MW, Mulder CJ. The spectrum of celiac disease: epidemiology, clinical aspects and treatment. *Nat Rev Gastroenterol Hepatol* 2010;7(4):204–13.

6. Dube C, Rostom A, Sy R, Cranney A, Saloojee N, Garritty C, et al. The prevalence of celiac disease in average-risk and at-risk Western European populations: a systematic review. *Gastroenterology* 2005;128(4 Suppl. 1):S57–67.

7. Cranney A, Rostom A, Sy R, Dube C, Saloogee N, Garritty C, et al. Consequences of testing for celiac disease. *Gastroenterology* 2005;128(4 Suppl. 1):S109–20.

8. Catassi C, Kryszak D, Bhatti B, Sturgeon C, Helzlsouer K, Clipp SL, et al. Natural history of celiac disease autoimmunity in a USA cohort followed since 1974. *Ann Med* 2010;42(7):530–8.

9. Rubio-Tapia A, Kyle RA, Kaplan EL, Johnson DR, Page W, Erdtmann F, et al. Increased prevalence and mortality in undiagnosed celiac disease. *Gastroenterology* 2009;137(1):88–93.

10. Scanlon SA, Murray JA. Update on celiac disease - etiology, differential diagnosis, drug targets, and management advances. *Clin Exp Gastroenterol* 2011;4:297–311.

11. Corazza GR, Valentini RA, Andreani ML, D'Anchino M, Leva MT, Ginaldi L, et al. Subclinical coeliac disease is a frequent cause of iron-deficiency anaemia. *Scand J Gastroenterol* 1995;30(2):153–6.

12. Stenson WF, Newberry R, Lorenz R, Baldus C, Civitelli R. Increased prevalence of celiac disease and need for routine screening among patients with osteoporosis. *Arch Intern Med* 2005;165(4):393–9.

13. Hadjivassiliou M, Rao DG, Wharton SB, Sanders DS, Grunewald RA, Davies-Jones AG. Sensory ganglionopathy due to gluten sensitivity. *Neurology* 2010;75(11):1003–8.

14. Volta U, Ravaglia G, Granito A, Forti P, Maioli F, Petrolini N, et al. Coeliac disease in patients with autoimmune thyroiditis. *Digestion* 2001;64(1):61–5.

15. Choi JM, Lebwohl B, Wang J, Lee SK, Murray JA, Sauer MV, et al. Increased prevalence of celiac disease in patients with unexplained infertility in the United States. *J Reprod Med* 2011;56(5-6):199–203.

16. Ventura A, Magazzu G, Greco L. Duration of exposure to gluten and risk for autoimmune disorders in patients with celiac disease. SIGEP Study Group for Autoimmune Disorders in Celiac Disease. *Gastroenterology* 1999;117(2):297–303.

17. Rostom A, Murray JA, Kagnoff MF. American Gastroenterological Association (AGA) Institute technical review on the diagnosis and management of celiac disease. *Gastroenterology* 2006;131(6):1981–2002.

18. Villalta D, Girolami D, Bidoli E, Bizzaro N, Tampoia M, Liguori M, et al. High prevalence of celiac disease in autoimmune hepatitis detected by anti-tissue tranglutaminase autoantibodies. *J Clin Lab Anal* 2005;19(1):6–10.

19. Volta U, Rodrigo L, Granito A, Petrolini N, Muratori P, Muratori L, et al. Celiac disease in autoimmune cholestatic liver disorders. *Am J Gastroenterol* 2002;97(10):2609–13.

20. Lindgren S, Sjoberg K, Eriksson S. Unsuspected coeliac disease in chronic 'cryptogenic' liver disease. *Scand J Gastroenterol* 1994;29(7):661–4.

21. Abdulkarim AS, Burgart LJ, See J, Murray JA. Etiology of nonresponsive celiac disease: results of a systematic approach. *Am J Gastroenterol* 2002;97(8):2016–21.

22. Leffler DA, Dennis M, Hyett B, Kelly E, Schuppan D, Kelly CP. Etiologies and predictors of diagnosis in nonresponsive celiac disease. *Clin Gastroenterol Hepatol* 2007;5(4):445–50.

23. Malamut G, Afchain P, Verkarre V, Lecomte T, Amiot A, Damotte D, et al. Presentation and long-term follow-up of refractory celiac disease: comparison of type I with type II. *Gastroenterology* 2009;136(1):81–90.

24. Rubio-Tapia A, Kelly DG, Lahr BD, Dogan A, Wu TT, Murray JA. Clinical staging and survival in refractory celiac disease: a single center experience. *Gastroenterology* 2009;136(1):99–107; quiz 352–3.

25. Ludvigsson JF, Leffler DA, Bai JC, Biagi F, Fasano A, Green PH, et al. The Oslo definitions for coeliac disease and related terms. *Gut* 2013;62(1):43–52.

26. Verbeek WH, Van De Water JM, Al-Toma A, Oudejans JJ, Mulder CJ, Coupe VM. Incidence of enteropathy–associated T-cell lymphoma: a nation-wide study of a population-based registry in The Netherlands. *Scand J Gastroenterol* 2008;43(11):1322–8.

27. Al-Toma A, Verbeek WH, Hadithi M, von Blomberg BM, Mulder CJ. Survival in refractory coeliac disease and enteropathy-associated T-cell lymphoma: retrospective evaluation of single-centre experience. *Gut* 2007;56(10):1373–8.

28. Daum S, Cellier C, Mulder CJ. Refractory coeliac disease. *Best Pract Res Clin Gastroenterol* 2005;19(3):413–24.

29. Zone JJ, Meyer LJ, Petersen MJ. Deposition of granular IgA relative to clinical lesions in dermatitis herpetiformis. *Arch Dermatol* 1996;132(8):912–8.

30. Collin P, Reunala T. Recognition and management of the cutaneous manifestations of celiac disease: a guide for dermatologists. *Am J Clin Dermatol* 2003;4(1):13–20.

31. Zone JJ. Skin manifestations of celiac disease. *Gastroenterology* 2005;128(4 Suppl. 1):S87–91.

32. Caproni M, Antiga E, Melani L, Fabbri P. Guidelines for the diagnosis and treatment of dermatitis herpetiformis. *J Eur Acad Dermatol Venereol* 2009;23(6):633–8.

33. Collin P, Pukkala E, Reunala T. Malignancy and survival in dermatitis herpetiformis: a comparison with coeliac disease. *Gut* 1996;38(4):528–30.

34. Sener O, Doganci L, Safali M, Besirbellioglu B, Bulucu F, Pahsa A. Severe dapsone hypersensitivity syndrome. *J Investig Allergol Clin Immunol* 2006;16(4):268–70.

35. Lewis NR, Scott BB. Systematic review: the use of serology to exclude or diagnose coeliac disease (a comparison of the endomysial and tissue transglutaminase antibody tests). *Aliment Pharmacol Ther* 2006;24(1):47–54.

36. Chow MA, Lebwohl B, Reilly NR, Green PH. Immunoglobulin A deficiency in celiac disease. *J Clin Gastroenterol* 2012;46(10):850–4.

37. Cataldo F, Marino V, Ventura A, Bottaro G, Corazza GR. Prevalence and clinical features of selective immunoglobulin A deficiency in coeliac disease: an Italian multicentre study. Italian Society of Paediatric Gastroenterology and Hepatology (SIGEP) and "Club del Tenue" Working Groups on Coeliac Disease. *Gut* 1998;42(3):362–5.

38. Raivio T, Korponay-Szabo I, Collin P, Laurila K, Huhtala H, Kaartinen T, et al. Performance of a new rapid whole blood coeliac test in adult patients with low prevalence of endomysial antibodies. *Dig Liver Dis* 2007;**39**(12):1057–63.

39. Bienvenu F, Besson Duvanel C, Seignovert C, Rouzaire P, Lachaux A, Bienvenu J. Evaluation of a point-of-care test based on deamidated gliadin peptides for celiac disease screening in a large pediatric population. *Eur J Gastroenterol Hepatol* 2012;**24**(12):1418–23.

40. Lewis NR, Scott BB. Meta-analysis: deamidated gliadin peptide antibody and tissue transglutaminase antibody compared as screening tests for coeliac disease. *Aliment Pharmacol Ther* 2010;**31**(1): 73–81.

41. Rashtak S, Ettore MW, Homburger HA, Murray JA. Comparative usefulness of deamidated gliadin antibodies in the diagnosis of celiac disease. *Clin Gastroenterol Hepatol* 2008;**6**(4):426–32; quiz 370.

42. Dickey W, Hughes DF, McMillan SA. Disappearance of endomysial antibodies in treated celiac disease does not indicate histological recovery. *Am J Gastroenterol* 2000;**95**(3):712–4.

43. Tursi A, Brandimarte G, Giorgetti GM. Lack of usefulness of anti-transglutaminase antibodies in assessing histologic recovery after gluten-free diet in celiac disease. *J Clin Gastroenterol* 2003;**37**(5):387–91.

44. Vahedi K, Mascart F, Mary JY, Laberenne JE, Bouhnik Y, Morin MC, et al. Reliability of antitransglutaminase antibodies as predictors of gluten-free diet compliance in adult celiac disease. *Am J Gastroenterol* 2003;**98**(5):1079–87.

45. Pais WP, Duerksen DR, Pettigrew NM, Bernstein CN. How many duodenal biopsy specimens are required to make a diagnosis of celiac disease? *Gastrointest Endosc* 2008;**67**(7):1082–7.

46. Hopper AD, Hadjivassiliou M, Hurlstone DP, Lobo AJ, McAlindon ME, Egner W, et al. What is the role of serologic testing in celiac disease? A prospective, biopsy-confirmed study with economic analysis. *Clin Gastroenterol Hepatol* 2008;**6**(3):314–20.

47. Bonamico M, Thanasi E, Mariani P, Nenna R, Luparia RP, Barbera C, et al. Duodenal bulb biopsies in celiac disease: a multicenter study. *J Pediatr Gastroenterol Nutr* 2008;**47**(5):618–22.

48. Oberhuber G, Granditsch G, Vogelsang H. The histopathology of coeliac disease: time for a standardized report scheme for pathologists. *Eur J Gastroenterol Hepatol* 1999;**11**(10):1185–94.

49. Hadithi M, von Blomberg BM, Crusius JB, Bloemena E, Kostense PJ, Meijer JW, et al. Accuracy of serologic tests and HLA-DQ typing for diagnosing celiac disease. *Ann Intern Med* 2007;**147**(5):294–302.

50. Schuppan D, Junker Y, Barisani D. Celiac disease: from pathogenesis to novel therapies. *Gastroenterology* 2009;**137**(6): 1912–33.

51. Catassi C, Rossini M, Ratsch IM, Bearzi I, Santinelli A, Castagnani R, et al. Dose dependent effects of protracted ingestion of small amounts of gliadin in coeliac disease children: a clinical and jejunal morphometric study. *Gut* 1993;**34**(11):1515–9.

52. Catassi C, Fabiani E, Iacono G, D'Agate C, Francavilla R, Biagi F, et al. A prospective, double-blind, placebo-controlled trial to establish a safe gluten threshold for patients with celiac disease. *Am J Clin Nutr* 2007;**85**(1):160–6.

53. Lohiniemi S, Maki M, Kaukinen K, Laippala P, Collin P. Gastrointestinal symptoms rating scale in coeliac disease patients on wheat starch-based gluten-free diets. *Scand J Gastroenterol* 2000;**35**(9):947–9.

54. Kaukinen K, Turjanmaa K, Maki M, Partanen J, Venalainen R, Reunala T, et al. Intolerance to cereals is not specific for coeliac disease. *Scand J Gastroenterol* 2000;**35**(9):942–6.

55. Akobeng AK, Thomas AG. Systematic review: tolerable amount of gluten for people with coeliac disease. *Aliment Pharmacol Ther* 2008;**27**(11):1044–52.

56. Fasano A, Catassi C. Clinical practice. Celiac disease. *N Engl J Med* 2012;**367**(25):2419–26.

57. Aziz I, Evans KE, Papageorgiou V, Sanders DS. Are patients with coeliac disease seeking alternative therapies to a gluten-free diet? *J Gastrointestin Liver Dis* 2011;**20**(1):27–31.

58. Hogberg L, Grodzinsky E, Stenhammar L. Better dietary compliance in patients with coeliac disease diagnosed in early childhood. *Scand J Gastroenterol* 2003;**38**(7):751–4.

59. Hall NJ, Rubin G, Charnock A. Systematic review: adherence to a gluten-free diet in adult patients with coeliac disease. *Aliment Pharmacol Ther* 2009;**30**(4):315–30.

60. Kemppainen T, Kroger H, Janatuinen E, Arnala I, Kosma VM, Pikkarainen P, et al. Osteoporosis in adult patients with celiac disease. *Bone* 1999;**24**(3):249–55.

61. DiMatteo MR. Variations in patients' adherence to medical recommendations: a quantitative review of 50 years of research. *Med Care* 2004;**42**(3):200–9.

62. Selby WS, Painter D, Collins A, Faulkner-Hogg KB, Loblay RH. Persistent mucosal abnormalities in coeliac disease are not related to the ingestion of trace amounts of gluten. *Scand J Gastroenterol* 1999;**34**(9):909–14.

63. Lanzini A, Lanzarotto F, Villanacci V, Mora A, Bertolazzi S, Turini D, et al. Complete recovery of intestinal mucosa occurs very rarely in adult coeliac patients despite adherence to gluten-free diet. *Aliment Pharmacol Ther* 2009;**29**(12):1299–308.

64. Tye-Din JA, Anderson RP, Ffrench RA, Brown GJ, Hodsman P, Siegel M, et al. The effects of ALV003 pre-digestion of gluten on immune response and symptoms in celiac disease *in vivo*. *Clin Immunol* 2010;**134**(3):289–95.

65. Holmes GK, Stokes PL, Sorahan TM, Prior P, Waterhouse JA, Cooke WT. Coeliac disease, gluten-free diet, and malignancy. *Gut* 1976;**17**(8):612–9.

66. Nielsen OH, Jacobsen O, Pedersen ER, Rasmussen SN, Petri M, Laulund S, et al. Non-tropical sprue. Malignant diseases and mortality rate. *Scand J Gastroenterol* 1985;**20**(1):13–8.

67. Sjostrom H, Lundin KE, Molberg O, Korner R, McAdam SN, Anthonsen D, et al. Identification of a gliadin T-cell epitope in coeliac disease: general importance of gliadin deamidation for intestinal T-cell recognition. *Scand J Immunol* 1998;**48**(2):111–5.

68. van de Wal Y, Kooy YM, van Veelen PA, Pena SA, Mearin LM, Molberg O, et al. Small intestinal T cells of celiac disease patients recognize a natural pepsin fragment of gliadin. *Proc Natl Acad Sci USA* 1998;**95**(17):10050–4.

69. van de Wal Y, Kooy YM, van Veelen P, Vader W, August SA, Drijfhout JW, et al. Glutenin is involved in the gluten-driven mucosal T cell response. *Eur J Immunol* 1999;**29**(10):3133–9.

70. Auricchio S, De Ritis G, De Vincenzi M, Occorsio P, Silano V. Effects of gliadin-derived peptides from bread and durum wheats on small intestine cultures from rat fetus and coeliac children. *Pediatr Res* 1982;**16**(12):1004–10.

71. Molberg O, Uhlen AK, Jensen T, Flaete NS, Fleckenstein B, Arentz-Hansen H, et al. Mapping of gluten T-cell epitopes in the bread wheat ancestors: implications for celiac disease. *Gastroenterology* 2005;**128**(2):393–401.

72. van den Broeck HC, van Herpen TW, Schuit C, Salentijn EM, Dekking L, Bosch D, et al. Removing celiac disease-related gluten proteins from bread wheat while retaining technological properties: a study with Chinese Spring deletion lines. *BMC Plant Biol* 2009;**9**:41.

73. Zandonadi RP, Botelho RB, Araujo WM. Psyllium as a substitute for gluten in bread. *J Am Diet Assoc* 2009;**109**(10):1781–4.

74. Ciacci C, Maiuri L, Caporaso N, Bucci C, Del Giudice L, Rita Massardo D, et al. Celiac disease: *in vitro* and *in vivo* safety and palatability of wheat-free sorghum food products. *Clin Nutr* 2007;**26**(6):799–805.

75. Zevallos VF, Ellis HJ, Suligoj T, Herencia LI, Ciclitira PJ. Variable activation of immune response by quinoa (*Chenopodium quinoa* Willd.) prolamins in celiac disease. *Am J Clin Nutr* 2012;**96**(2):337–44.

76. Di Cagno R, De Angelis M, Lavermicocca P, De Vincenzi M, Giovannini C, Faccia M, et al. Proteolysis by sourdough lactic acid bacteria: effects on wheat flour protein fractions and gliadin peptides involved in human cereal intolerance. *Appl Environ Microbiol* 2002;**68**(2):623–33.

77. Di Cagno R, De Angelis M, Auricchio S, Greco L, Clarke C, De Vincenzi M, et al. Sourdough bread made from wheat and nontoxic flours and started with selected lactobacilli is tolerated in celiac sprue patients. *Appl Environ Microbiol* 2004;**70**(2): 1088–96.

78. Di Cagno R, Barbato M, Di Camillo C, Rizzello CG, De Angelis M, Giuliani G, et al. Gluten-free sourdough wheat baked goods appear safe for young celiac patients: a pilot study. *J Pediatr Gastroenterol Nutr* 2010;**51**(6):777–83.

79. De Angelis M, Rizzello CG, Fasano A, Clemente MG, De Simone C, Silano M, et al. VSL#3 probiotic preparation has the capacity to hydrolyze gliadin polypeptides responsible for Celiac Sprue. *Biochim Biophys Acta* 2006;**1762**(1):80–93.

80. Gianfrani C, Siciliano RA, Facchiano AM, Camarca A, Mazzeo MF, Costantini S, et al. Transamidation of wheat flour inhibits the response to gliadin of intestinal T cells in celiac disease. *Gastroenterology* 2007;**133**(3):780–9.

81. Shan L, Molberg O, Parrot I, Hausch F, Filiz F, Gray GM, et al. Structural basis for gluten intolerance in celiac sprue. *Science* 2002;**297**(5590):2275–9.

82. Hausch F, Shan L, Santiago NA, Gray GM, Khosla C. Intestinal digestive resistance of immunodominant gliadin peptides. *Am J Physiol Gastrointest Liver Physiol* 2002;**283**(4):G996–1003.

83. Shan L, Marti T, Sollid LM, Gray GM, Khosla C. Comparative biochemical analysis of three bacterial prolyl endopeptidases: implications for coeliac sprue. *Biochem J* 2004;**383**(Pt 2):311–8.

84. Stepniak D, Spaenij-Dekking L, Mitea C, Moester M, de Ru A, Baak-Pablo R, et al. Highly efficient gluten degradation with a newly identified prolyl endoprotease: implications for celiac disease. *Am J Physiol Gastrointest Liver Physiol* 2006;**291**(4): G621–9.

85. Marti T, Molberg O, Li Q, Gray GM, Khosla C, Sollid LM. Prolyl endopeptidase-mediated destruction of T cell epitopes in whole gluten: chemical and immunological characterization. *J Pharmacol Exp Ther* 2005;**312**(1):19–26.

86. Pyle GG, Paaso B, Anderson BE, Allen DD, Marti T, Li Q, et al. Effect of pretreatment of food gluten with prolyl endopeptidase on gluten-induced malabsorption in celiac sprue. *Clin Gastroenterol Hepatol* 2005;**3**(7):687–94.

87. Ehren J, Moron B, Martin E, Bethune MT, Gray GM, Khosla C. A food-grade enzyme preparation with modest gluten detoxification properties. *PLoS One* 2009;**4**(7):e6313.

88. Mitea C, Havenaar R, Drijfhout JW, Edens L, Dekking L, Koning F. Efficient degradation of gluten by a prolyl endoprotease in a gastrointestinal model: implications for coeliac disease. *Gut* 2008;**57**(1):25–32.

89. Gass J, Bethune MT, Siegel M, Spencer A, Khosla C. Combination enzyme therapy for gastric digestion of dietary gluten in patients with celiac sprue. *Gastroenterology* 2007; **133**(2):472–80.

90. Siegel M, Garber ME, Spencer AG, Botwick W, Kumar P, Williams RN, et al. Safety, tolerability, and activity of ALV003: results from two phase 1 single, escalating-dose clinical trials. *Dig Dis Sci* 2012;**57**(2):440–50.

91. Lahdeaho ML, Maki M, Kaukinen K, et al. ALV003, a novel glutenase, attenuates gluten-induced small intestinal mucosal injury in celiac disease patients: a randomized controlled phase 2A clinical trial. *Gut* 2011;**60**:A12.

92. Korponay-Szabo IR, Tumpek J, Gyimesi J, Laurila K, Papp M, Maki M, et al. Food-grade gluten degrading enzymes to treat dietary transgressions in coeliac adolescents. *J Pediatr Gastroenterol Nutr* 2010;**50** E68–E6E.

93. Pinier M, Fuhrmann G, Galipeau HJ, Rivard N, Murray JA, David CS, et al. The copolymer P(HEMA-co-SS) binds gluten and reduces immune response in gluten-sensitized mice and human tissues. *Gastroenterology* 2012;**142**(2):316–25. e1–12.

94. van Elburg RM, Uil JJ, Mulder CJ, Heymans HS. Intestinal permeability in patients with coeliac disease and relatives of patients with coeliac disease. *Gut* 1993;**34**(3):354–7.

95. Lammers KM, Lu R, Brownley J, Lu B, Gerard C, Thomas K, et al. Gliadin induces an increase in intestinal permeability and zonulin release by binding to the chemokine receptor CXCR3. *Gastroenterology* 2008;**135**(1):194–204. e3.

96. Di Pierro M, Lu R, Uzzau S, Wang W, Margaretten K, Pazzani C, et al. Zonula occludens toxin structure-function analysis. Identification of the fragment biologically active on tight junctions and of the zonulin receptor binding domain. *J Biol Chem* 2001;**276**(22):19160–5.

97. Tripathi A, Lammers KM, Goldblum S, Shea-Donohue T, Netzel-Arnett S, Buzza MS, et al. Identification of human zonulin, a physiological modulator of tight junctions, as prehaptoglobin-2. *Proc Natl Acad Sci USA* 2009;**106**(39):16799–804.

98. Paterson BM, Lammers KM, Arrieta MC, Fasano A, Meddings JB. The safety, tolerance, pharmacokinetic and pharmacodynamic effects of single doses of AT-1001 in coeliac disease subjects: a proof of concept study. *Aliment Pharmacol Ther* 2007;**26**(5):757–66.

99. Kelly CP, Green PH, Murray JA, Dimarino A, Colatrella A, Leffler DA, et al. Larazotide acetate in patients with coeliac disease undergoing a gluten challenge: a randomised placebo-controlled study. *Aliment Pharmacol Ther* 2013;**37**(2):252–62.

100. Zhao J, de Vera J, Narushima S, Beck EX, Palencia S, Shinkawa P, et al. R-spondin1, a novel intestinotrophic mitogen, ameliorates experimental colitis in mice. *Gastroenterology* 2007;**132**(4):1331–43.

101. Beaurepaire C, Smyth D, McKay DM. Interferon-gamma regulation of intestinal epithelial permeability. *J Interferon Cytokine Res* 2009;**29**(3):133–44.

102. Utech M, Ivanov AI, Samarin SN, Bruewer M, Turner JR, Mrsny RJ, et al. Mechanism of IFN-gamma-induced endocytosis of tight junction proteins: myosin II-dependent vacuolarization of the apical plasma membrane. *Mol Biol Cell* 2005;**16**(10):5040–52.

103. Sollid LM, Khosla C. Novel therapies for coeliac disease. *J Intern Med* 2011;**269**(6):604–13.

104. Jabri B, Sollid LM. Mechanisms of disease: immunopathogenesis of celiac disease. *Nat Clin Pract Gastroenterol Hepatol* 2006;**3**(9):516–25.

105. Molberg O, McAdam S, Lundin KE, Kristiansen C, Arentz-Hansen H, Kett K, et al. T cells from celiac disease lesions recognize gliadin epitopes deamidated in situ by endogenous tissue transglutaminase. *Eur J Immunol* 2001;**31**(5):1317–23.

106. Nanda N, Iismaa SE, Owens WA, Husain A, Mackay F, Graham RM. Targeted inactivation of Gh/tissue transglutaminase II. *J Biol Chem* 2001;**276**(23):20673–8.

107. De Laurenzi V, Melino G. Gene disruption of tissue transglutaminase. *Mol Cell Biol* 2001;**21**(1):148–55.

108. Korponay-Szabo IR, Laurila K, Szondy Z, Halttunen T, Szalai Z, Dahlbom I, et al. Missing endomysial and reticulin binding of coeliac antibodies in transglutaminase 2 knockout tissues. *Gut* 2003;**52**(2):199–204.

109. Freund KF, Doshi KP, Gaul SL, Claremon DA, Remy DC, Baldwin JJ, et al. Transglutaminase inhibition by 2-[(2-oxopropyl) thio]imidazolium derivatives: mechanism of factor XIIIa inactivation. *Biochemistry* 1994;**33**(33):10109–19.

110. Maiuri L, Ciacci C, Ricciardelli I, Vacca L, Raia V, Rispo A, et al. Unexpected role of surface transglutaminase type II in celiac disease. *Gastroenterology* 2005;**129**(5):1400–13.

111. Choi K, Siegel M, Piper JL, Yuan L, Cho E, Strnad P, et al. Chemistry and biology of dihydroisoxazole derivatives: selective inhibitors of human transglutaminase 2. *Chem Biol* 2005;**12**(4):469–75.

112. Watts RE, Siegel M, Khosla C. Structure-activity relationship analysis of the selective inhibition of transglutaminase 2 by dihydroisoxazoles. *J Med Chem* 2006;**49**(25):7493–501.

113. Maiuri L, Ciacci C, Ricciardelli I, Vacca L, Raia V, Auricchio S, et al. Association between innate response to gliadin and activation of pathogenic T cells in coeliac disease. *Lancet* 2003;**362**(9377):30–7.

114. Matysiak-Budnik T, Moura IC, Arcos-Fajardo M, Lebreton C, Menard S, Candalh C, et al. Secretory IgA mediates retrotranscytosis of intact gliadin peptides via the transferrin receptor in celiac disease. *J Exp Med* 2008;**205**(1):143–54.

115. Kapoerchan VV, Wiesner M, Hillaert U, Drijfhout JW, Overhand M, Alard P, et al. Design, synthesis and evaluation of high-affinity binders for the celiac disease associated HLA-DQ2 molecule. *Mol Immunol* 2010;**47**(5):1091–7.

116. Xia J, Bergseng E, Fleckenstein B, Siegel M, Kim CY, Khosla C, et al. Cyclic and dimeric gluten peptide analogues inhibiting DQ2-mediated antigen presentation in celiac disease. *Bioorg Med Chem* 2007;**15**(20):6565–73.

117. Silano M, Di Benedetto R, Trecca A, Arrabito G, Leonardi F, De Vincenzi M. A decapeptide from durum wheat prevents celiac peripheral blood lymphocytes from activation by gliadin peptides. *Pediatr Res* 2007;**61**(1):67–71.

118. Salmi M, Jalkanen S. Molecules controlling lymphocyte migration to the gut. *Gut* 1999;**45**(1):148–53.

119. Berlin C, Berg EL, Briskin MJ, Andrew DP, Kilshaw PJ, Holzmann B, et al. Alpha 4 beta 7 integrin mediates lymphocyte binding to the mucosal vascular addressin MAdCAM-1. *Cell* 1993;**74**(1):185–95.

120. Di Sabatino A, Rovedatti L, Rosado MM, Carsetti R, Corazza GR, MacDonald TT. Increased expression of mucosal addressin cell adhesion molecule 1 in the duodenum of patients with active celiac disease is associated with depletion of integrin alpha4beta7-positive T cells in blood. *Hum Pathol* 2009;**40**(5):699–704.

121. Ghosh S, Goldin E, Gordon FH, Malchow HA, Rask-Madsen J, Rutgeerts P, et al. Natalizumab for active Crohn's disease. *N Engl J Med* 2003;**348**(1):24–32.

122. Keshav S, Vanasek T, Niv Y, Petryka R, Howaldt S, Bafutto M, et al. A Randomized Controlled Trial of the Efficacy and Safety of CCX282-B, an Orally-Administered Blocker of Chemokine Receptor CCR9, for Patients with Crohn's Disease. *PLoS One* 2013;**8**(3):e60094.

123. Rashtak S, Marietta E, Murray J. Gliadin Stimulation of Monocytes Leads to Increased Expression of Multiple T Cell Recruiting Chemokines: A Novel Innate Immune Response. *Clin Immunol* 2010;**135**:S47–S4S.

124. Chatenoud L. Immune therapy for type 1 diabetes mellitus – what is unique about anti-CD3 antibodies? *Nat Rev Endocrinol* 2010;**6**(3):149–57.

125. Herold C, Ganslmayer M, Ocker M, Zopf S, Gailer B, Hahn EG, et al. Inducibility of microsomal liver function may differentiate cirrhotic patients with maintained compared with severely compromised liver reserve. *J Gastroenterol Hepatol* 2003;**18**(4):445–9.

126. Wiczling P, Rosenzweig M, Vaickus L, Jusko WJ. Pharmacokinetics and pharmacodynamics of a chimeric/humanized anti-CD3 monoclonal antibody, otelixizumab (TRX4), in subjects with psoriasis and with type 1 diabetes mellitus. *J Clin Pharmacol* 2010;**50**(5):494–506.

127. Sandborn WJ, Colombel JF, Frankel M, Hommes D, Lowder JN, Mayer L, et al. Anti-CD3 antibody visilizumab is not effective in patients with intravenous corticosteroid-refractory ulcerative colitis. *Gut* 2010;**59**(11):1485–92.

128. Edwards JC, Szczepanski L, Szechinski J, Filipowicz-Sosnowska A, Emery P, Close DR, et al. Efficacy of B-cell-targeted therapy with rituximab in patients with rheumatoid arthritis. *N Engl J Med* 2004;**350**(25):2572–81.

129. Hauser SL, Waubant E, Arnold DL, Vollmer T, Antel J, Fox RJ, et al. B-cell depletion with rituximab in relapsing-remitting multiple sclerosis. *N Engl J Med* 2008;**358**(7):676–88.

130. Sollid LM, Molberg O, McAdam S, Lundin KE. Autoantibodies in coeliac disease: tissue transglutaminase – guilt by association? *Gut* 1997;**41**(6):851–2.

131. Mei HE, Frolich D, Giesecke C, Loddenkemper C, Reiter K, Schmidt S, et al. Steady-state generation of mucosal IgA+ plasmablasts is not abrogated by B-cell depletion therapy with rituximab. *Blood* 2010;**116**(24):5181–90.

132. Pender SL, Tickle SP, Docherty AJ, Howie D, Wathen NC, MacDonald TT. A major role for matrix metalloproteinases in T cell injury in the gut. *J Immunol* 1997;**158**(4):1582–90.

133. Ciccocioppo R, Di Sabatino A, Bauer M, Della Riccia DN, Bizzini F, Biagi F, et al. Matrix metalloproteinase pattern in celiac duodenal mucosa. *Lab Invest* 2005;**85**(3):397–407.

134. Przemioslo RT, Lundin KE, Sollid LM, Nelufer J, Ciclitira PJ. Histological changes in small bowel mucosa induced by gliadin sensitive T lymphocytes can be blocked by anti-interferon gamma antibody. *Gut* 1995;**36**(6):874–9.

135. Bethune MT, Siegel M, Howles-Banerji S, Khosla C. Interferon-gamma released by gluten-stimulated celiac disease-specific intestinal T cells enhances the transepithelial flux of gluten peptides. *J Pharmacol Exp Ther* 2009;**329**(2):657–68.

136. Gillett HR, Arnott ID, McIntyre M, Campbell S, Dahele A, Priest M, et al. Successful infliximab treatment for steroid-refractory celiac disease: a case report. *Gastroenterology* 2002;**122**(3):800–5.

137. Costantino G, della Torre A, Lo Presti MA, Caruso R, Mazzon E, Fries W. Treatment of life-threatening type I refractory coeliac disease with long-term infliximab. *Dig Liver Dis* 2008;**40**(1):74–7.

138. Hue S, Mention JJ, Monteiro RC, Zhang S, Cellier C, Schmitz J, et al. A direct role for NKG2D/MICA interaction in villous atrophy during celiac disease. *Immunity* 2004;**21**(3):367–77.

139. Maiuri L, Ciacci C, Auricchio S, Brown V, Quaratino S, Londei M. Interleukin 15 mediates epithelial changes in celiac disease. *Gastroenterology* 2000;**119**(4):996–1006.

140. Meresse B, Chen Z, Ciszewski C, Tretiakova M, Bhagat G, Krausz TN, et al. Coordinated induction by IL15 of a TCR-independent NKG2D signaling pathway converts CTL into lymphokine-activated killer cells in celiac disease. *Immunity* 2004; **21**(3):357–66.

141. Di Sabatino A, Ciccocioppo R, Cupelli F, Cinque B, Millimaggi D, Clarkson MM, et al. Epithelium derived interleukin 15 regulates intraepithelial lymphocyte Th1 cytokine production, cytotoxicity, and survival in coeliac disease. *Gut* 2006;**55**(4):469–77.

142. Mention JJ, Ben Ahmed M, Begue B, Barbe U, Verkarre V, Asnafi V, et al. Interleukin 15: a key to disrupted intraepithelial lymphocyte homeostasis and lymphomagenesis in celiac disease. *Gastroenterology* 2003;**125**(3):730–45.

143. Yokoyama S, Watanabe N, Sato N, Perera PY, Filkoski L, Tanaka T, et al. Antibody-mediated blockade of IL-15 reverses the autoimmune intestinal damage in transgenic mice that overexpress IL-15 in enterocytes. *Proc Natl Acad Sci USA* 2009;**106**(37):15849–54.

144. Malamut G, El Machhour R, Montcuquet N, Martin-Lanneree S, Dusanter-Fourt I, Verkarre V, et al. IL-15 triggers an antiapoptotic pathway in human intraepithelial lymphocytes that is a potential new target in celiac disease-associated inflammation and lymphomagenesis. *J Clin Invest* 2010;**120**(6):2131–43.

145. Daveson AJ, Jones DM, Gaze S, McSorley H, Clouston A, Pascoe A, et al. Effect of hookworm infection on wheat challenge in celiac disease – a randomised double-blinded placebo controlled trial. *PLoS One* 2011;**6**(3):e17366.

146. McSorley HJ, Gaze S, Daveson J, Jones D, Anderson RP, Clouston A, et al. Suppression of inflammatory immune responses in celiac disease by experimental hookworm infection. *PLoS One* 2011;**6**(9):e24092.

147. Keech CL, Dromey J, Chen ZJ, Anderson RP, McCluskey J. Immune Tolerance Induced By Peptide Immunotherapy in An HLA Dq2-Dependent Mouse Model of Gluten Immunity. *Gastroenterology* 2009;**136**(5):A57-A.

Gluten Metabolism in Humans: Involvement of the Gut Microbiota

Alberto Caminero[*,†], *Esther Nistal*[*], *Alexandra R. Herrán*[*,†],
Jenifer Pérez-Andrés[*,†], *Luis Vaquero*[**], *Santiago Vivas*[**,§],
José María Ruíz de Morales[‡,§], *Javier Casqueiro*[*,†]

[*]Universidad de León; Área de Microbiología, Facultad de Biología y Ciencias Ambientales, León, Spain, [†]Universidad de León, Instituto de Biología Molecular, Genómica y Proteómica (INBIOMIC), León, Spain, [**]Hospital de León, Departamento de Gastroenterología, Altos de Nava, León, Spain, [‡]Hospital de León, Departamento de Immunología, Altos de Nava, León, Spain, [§]Universidad de León, Instituto de Biomedicina (IBIOMED), León, Spain

INTRODUCTION

Wheat is a staple food for most of the world´s population.[1] At present, the cultivation of this cereal is widespread; it has become one of the most important crops in the world, together with maize and rice. Approximately 600 million metric ton are harvested annually, with cultivation extending over a vast geographical area.[1–3] The most important characteristics of wheat are the unique properties of wheat dough that allow it to be processed into a range of foodstuffs, notably bread, other baked products, and pastas. The properties of the dough are usually described as viscosity, elasticity, and cohesivity, and these properties are determined by the grain proteins, particularly the storage proteins that form a network in the dough called gluten.[2,4,5] Wheat gluten proteins are the major storage proteins that are deposited in the starchy endosperm cells of developing grain. These proteins form a continuous proteinaceous matrix in the cells of the mature dry grain and join together to form a continuous viscoelastic network when flour is mixed with water, forming dough. Therefore, the viscoelastic properties of gluten allow wheat to be used in bread and other processed foods, and thus gluten proteins are widely distributed throughout the food supply.[2,5,6] Despite the ubiquity of gluten in the diet, gluten proteins are the cause of the most common food-sensitive enteropathy in humans: celiac disease (CD).[7]

GLUTEN

Gluten is the rubbery mass that remains when wheat dough is washed to remove starch granules and water-soluble constituents. In practice, the term gluten refers to the fraction of water-insoluble protein, although lipids (up to 10%) and some water-insoluble starches are also present. Depending of the thoroughness of washing, the dry solid contains 75–85% of protein that plays a key role in determining the unique baking quality of wheat by conferring water absorption capacity, cohesivity, viscosity, and elasticity to the dough.[8] However, from a physiological viewpoint, gluten proteins appear in the endosperm of wheat grain, and their function is to store carbon, nitrogen, and sulfur to support seed germination and seedling growth. Gluten proteins have no other known biological role, and their viscoelastic properties in the dough appear to be a purely fortuitous consequence of their primary structure.[2,9] Furthermore, gluten proteins are capable of triggering one of the most common food-sensitive enteropathies in humans: celiac disease. Therefore, gluten is also the commonly used term for the complex of water-insoluble proteins that are harmful to patients with CD.[10]

Gluten proteins are among the most complex protein networks in nature because they have numerous different protein components, and they vary based on genotype, growing conditions, and technological processes.[8] Traditionally, gluten proteins have been divided into two groups according to their solubility in alcohol–water solutions (e.g., 60% ethanol): soluble gliadins and insoluble glutenins. The gliadin fraction consists of different highly homologue monomeric proteins (28–70 kDa) that are divided according to their electophoretic mobility into three families: α/β-, γ-, and ω-gliadins.[8,11,12] Hydrated gliadins contribute mainly to the viscosity and the extensibility of the dough system. In contrast, glutenins, the non alcohol-soluble fraction of gluten, are large aggregated proteins linked by interchain disulfide bonds. These large polymeric structures are responsible for the strength and elasticity of dough and are divided into low molecular (30–60 kDa) and high molecular weight (80–120 kDa) glutenins.[8,11,12] Therefore, gluten is a two-component glue in which gliadins can be understood as a plastizer or solvent for glutenins. Both fractions are prolamin proteins and are important contributors to the rheological properties of the dough, but their functions are different.[8] The name prolamin was originally based on the observation that these proteins have numerous repetitive sequences rich in proline and glutamine amino acids.[3] This characteristic primary structure has an important role in the physicochemical properties of gluten, and is responsible for the resistance of gluten proteins to human digestive proteases. Another important amino acid for the structure and function of gluten is cysteine. Although cysteine is not abundant within the amino acid sequences of gluten proteins, it is extremely important because it forms intrachain disulfide bonds within a protein, or interchain disulfide bonds between proteins.[8,13,14]

However, gluten is a common term not only limited to wheat proteins. Storage proteins with amino acid compositions similar to the wheat gliadin fraction have been identified in barley and rye (called hordeins and secalins, respectively). These cereals are evolutionarily related with wheat, belong to the *Triticeae* tribe, and possess common characteristics. Both hordein and secalin prolamins display properties that are similar to gliadin proteins and are frequently included in the broad term, gluten.[4,15] Moreover, different wheat varieties, such as kamut, emmer, or spelt, and hybrid cereals made from a cross of wheat and rye, such as triticale, have the same characteristics as their predecessor cereals. For this reason, the term gluten is used not only for wheat prolamins but also for barley, rye, kamut, durum, emmer, spelt and triticale proteins.[4,16,17] All of these proteins are capable of triggering the pathological process of CD. In contrast, other related cereals, such as oats, are under discussion: many experts consider them safe because most CD patients tolerate oats without any signs of intestinal inflammation, but others warn that this cereal may have a potentially toxic effect.[15,16,18] Recent studies have shown that the adverse effects of oats are closely linked to the variety.[19]

GLUTEN METABOLISM IN HEALTHY PEOPLE

Food is digested in the gastrointestinal tract into smaller components or nutrients that are more easily absorbed by the host. The nutritional requirements for amino acids in humans are met by dietary proteins that are assimilated in the small intestine. A typical Western diet usually contains approximately 100 g of protein per day; this amount of protein is metabolized through the gastrointestinal tract. The metabolic process involves the digestion of proteins to generate amino acids, dipeptides, or tripeptides that can be absorbed by the enterocytes.[20] However, not all the proteins are completely digested, and gluten prolamins are a good example of dietary proteins that are difficult for human digestive enzymes to digest. The great diversity of the human gut microbiota implies a vast catalogue of metabolic pathways and raises questions concerning the involvement of microorganisms in the metabolism of different nutrients, especially those that are recalcitrant to human digestive enzymes.

Gluten Metabolism in the Oral Cavity

The daily gluten consumption of the general population has been estimated at approximately 10–20 g, which is an extremely large amount.[21,22] Proteins ingested in the diet pass through the esophagus to the stomach, where the digestion of proteins begins in humans.[20] However, although the oral cavity is not considered to have a significant role in protein digestion, several studies have noted that the "port of entry" for the gastrointestinal tract may be where protein hydrolysis begins.[23–25]

Proline-rich proteins, also known as PRPs, are among the most abundant proteins in the saliva.[26] These proteins are rich in glutamine and proline residues, similar to gluten prolamins.[24] Helmerhorst and colleagues[23] identified glutamine endoproteasic activity while studying the digestome in the saliva. This activity is derived from dental plaque, suggesting a microbial origin. Glutamine endoprotease preferentially cleaves the basic PRPs in response to glutamine residue with a predominant specificity for the tripeptide Xaa–Pro–Gln. This proteolytic activity plays an important role in the degradation of salivary proteins and glutamine-containing dietary proteins.[23,24]

Wheat-derived gliadins and PRPs have several structural similarities (i.e., both are rich in glutamine and proline). Thus, both types of proteins may be substrates for oral microbial proteases. Indeed, a recent study from the same group described proteolytic activity toward gluten peptides in saliva. Helmerhorst *et al.*[24] have shown that oral proteolytic enzymes have the ability to cleave adjacent to tripeptides, which frequently occurs in gluten proteins. Moreover, highly immunogenic gluten-derived peptides resistant to human proteases, such as the 33-mer or 26-mer, were also completely degraded by the oral proteases. This proteolytic activity originates from the gluten-degrading bacteria naturally residing in the oral cavity.[24] The colonization of the oral cavity with microorganisms that produce proteases capable of hydrolyzing peptides with glutamine and proline residues may not be surprising, given that salivary PRPs as well as dietary wheat gluten proteins are prominent and abundant substrates in the oral cavity.[23,24]

The human mouth harbors one of the most diverse microbiomes in the human body, including viruses, fungi, protozoa, archaea, and bacteria. The bacterial community in the mouth is highly complex, with approximately 1000 species present; it is the second most complex community in the human body after the community in the colon.[27] Within the oral microbiota, the bacterial species with high activity toward gluten peptides in dental plaque have been identified as *Rothia mucilaginosa* and *Rothia aeria*. *Rothia* cells in suspension have been shown to degrade the initial amount of gliadin (250 μg/mL) by 50% in 30 minutes of incubation. Furthermore, these bacteria have the ability to hydrolyze gluten peptides that are resistant to human digestive proteases, even those that are highly immunogenic for CD patients. In addition, there are other microorganisms residing in the oral cavity that could be involved in the metabolism of gluten proteins, such as *Streptococcus mitis*, *Streptococcus penumoniae*, *Staphylococcus epidermidis*, *Bifidobacterium longum*, and *Bifidobacterium dentium*.[25]

The discovery of salivary microorganisms degrading dietary proteins *in vitro* prompts the question about the extent to which these microorganisms play a role in the metabolism of proteins. In the mastication process, foods are mixed with saliva, accelerating their breakdown by the digestive enzymes in the oral cavity. Oral microorganisms may survive in the swallowed food bolus and continue their digestive activity during or after gastric passage. *In vitro* studies with *R. aeria* have shown that its enzyme activities are not abolished at acidic pH values, and are optimally active under more basic pH conditions. Thus, it is possible that these enzymes resist the adverse conditions of the stomach and that enzymatic activity occurs in the small intestine.[25] Curiously, bacteria from the *Rothia* genus belong to the mucosa-associated microbiota of the proximal small intestine in both adults and children.[28,29] Therefore, it seems that oral microorganisms could play a role in the digestion of dietary gluten proteins in humans.[25]

Gluten Metabolism in the Stomach

Although proteolytic activity occurs in the oral cavity, it is generally accepted that significant protein digestion in the gastrointestinal tract begins in the stomach. The gastric phase of protein hydrolysis involves the proteolytic action of pepsin, which is secreted by the chief cells of the stomach as an inactive precursor called pepsinogen. This zymogene is activated by the acidic pH in the stomach lumen and by the autocatalytic hydrolysis of the active form of pepsin. Pepsin is an acid protease that is optimally active under acidic conditions. Therefore, pepsin remains active in the stomach lumen and initiates the digestion of dietary proteins. The end products of pepsin's action on proteins are large polypeptides.[20,30] However, details concerning gluten hydrolysis in the stomach are not known. Several works *in vitro* have shown that mammalian pepsin exerts only a partial proteolytic action on dietary gluten.[31–33]

On the other hand, there are no studies dealing with proteolytic microbiota in the human stomach. Although it seems unlikely that microorganisms residing in the stomach have an important role in gluten metabolism because of the low bacterial population, we think that the functional activity of this microbiota should be studied. The number of viable microbes that can be recovered from stomach contents is between 10^1–10^3 bacteria per gram, although higher counts can be obtained after a meal because of the transient increase in pH caused by the buffering action of food. This sparse population is a consequence of the low pH of the stomach and the relatively rapid transit of material through this organ (2–6 hours).[34,35] However, the microbiota of the stomach is perfectly adapted to live in this harsh habitat, and undigested dietary proteins, including gluten, could be used as nutrients. Thus, this microbiota could play an important role in protein digestion.

Nevertheless, *in vitro* studies have shown that gluten is only partially digested in the stomach, and high molecular weight gluten peptides arrive in the small intestine.[33,36]

Gluten Metabolism in the Small Intestine

The small intestine is the site at which major hydrolysis and food absorption occur in the digestive tract. The duodenum, also known as the proximal small intestine, is where proteins are mainly broken down. Protein and peptides from the stomach arrive in the duodenum, where they are converted to easily absorbed compounds, such as amino acids, dipeptides, and tripeptides. These compounds are transported by the enterocytes throughout the entire small intestine. The products of protein digestion enter into the bloodstream primarily as free amino acids, meeting the nutritional requirements for amino acids of the host.[20]

Digestion of Gluten Peptides by Human Proteases

The main proteolytic degradation of dietary proteins in the gastrointestinal tract appears to occur in the small intestine. When the stomach contents enter the small intestine, the presence of food and the acidic pH in the lumen stimulate endocrine cells, producing secretin and cholecystokinin hormones. Secretin acts on the pancreas and bile ducts to induce secretion of bicarbonate, which rapidly neutralizes the acid. Cholecystokinin induces the secretion of pancreatic fluid rich in digestive enzymes, and the secretion of bile by the gallbladder.[20] The main function of the pancreas is to produce digestive enzymes that are delivered to the small intestine for the hydrolysis of complex nutrients. Pancreatic secretions contain five enzymes that are known to be relevant to protein digestion at a neutral pH and show broad substrate specificity: trypsin, chymotrypsin, elastase, carboxypeptidase A, and carboxypeptidase B. All of these enzymes are secreted as inactive precursors. The first step in the activation of these zymogens is the activation of trypsin by the enteropeptidase associated with the brush border membrane of the intestinal epithelial cells. Trypsin then acts on the rest of the zymogens, generating the active forms.[37]

The polypeptides that enter the small intestine from the stomach are acted on by these pancreatic enzymes to generate smaller peptides consisting of six to eight amino acids.[20] However, gluten peptides are relatively resistant to proteolysis in the small intestine. Several studies have demonstrated that digestion of gliadins by pepsin and trypsin enzymes yields peptides of high molecular weight.[32,38,39] A recent *in vitro* study performed by Shan *et al.*[33] confirmed that gluten peptides

are unusually resistant to digestion by human digestive proteases. These authors have proposed that the high proline content of gluten peptides (15–25%) impairs their hydrolysis by pancreatic and brush border membrane proteases because these enzymes lack prolyl-endopeptidasic activity. As a result, gluten peptides are incompletely digested, and high molecular weight oligopeptides appear in the lumen of the small intestine.[33,40,41] In addition, bile is secreted in the small intestinal lumen by the gallbladder and could participate in the metabolism of some dietary proteins. Although bile secretion principally aids the digestion of lipids in the small intestine, conjugated bile acids also enhance the proteolysis of several dietary proteins, such as β-lactoglobulin and myoglobin. Nevertheless, the hydrolysis of other dietary proteins, such as chicken ovalbumin and gluten proteins, was not influenced by the presence of bile acids.[42]

Usually, peptides resulting from the digestion of proteins by pancreatic proteases are subjected to further hydrolysis by peptidases associated with the brush border membrane of the enterocytes. Although free amino acids are also generated, the hydrolysis products released into the intestinal lumen are mainly smaller peptides containing two or three amino acids[20] (Fig. 13.1). In the brush border, there are enzymes

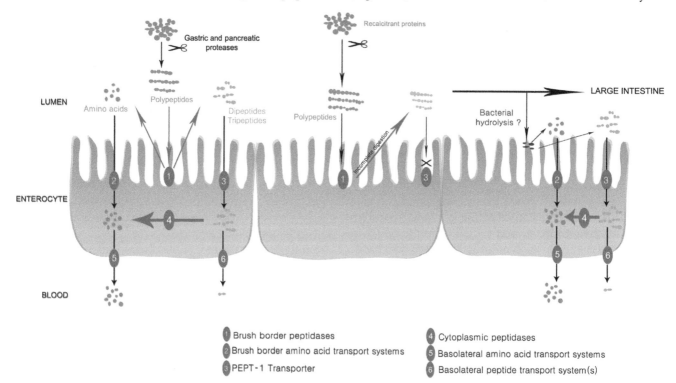

FIGURE 13.1 Model of protein digestion and absorption in the small intestine. Proteins are hydrolyzed to amino acids, dipeptides, and tripeptides by pancreatic and brush border membrane proteases. These products are transported into the enterocytes via specific transport systems in the brush border membrane. Once inside the cells, small peptides are subjected to hydrolysis by cytoplasmic peptidases to release free amino acids which are transported into the blood. The transport of small peptides across the basolateral membrane is a minor pathway. Recalcitrant proteins such as gluten prolamins are relatively resistant to proteolysis in the small intestine. As a result of the partial digestion, high molecular weight oligopeptides persist in the lumen of the small intestine because they are not transported by PEPT-1. These peptides could be hydrolyzed by bacterial proteases to easily absorbable compounds that would be used by the host. See color plate at the back of the book.

(e.g., dipeptidyl peptidase IV, aminopeptidase N, and dipeptidyl carboxypeptidase I) with the ability to break peptide bonds of proline residues. However, brush border enzymes exert only minimal proteolytic action on gluten peptides.[33,36,43,44] It has been shown that gluten peptides that are immunostimulatory for CD patients, such as peptides p57–68 or p62–75, are only partially degraded by brush border peptidases, but other peptides such as the 33-mer are totally resistant.[41,45,46] Like the pancreatic proteases, the brush border enzymes also lack prolyl-endopeptidasic activity, resulting in poor digestion of gluten peptides. Therefore, many high molecular weight oligopeptides (10 to ≥30 amino acid residues) persist in the lumen of the small intestine.[33]

Transport of Gluten Peptides across the Intestinal Epithelium

After the digestion process in the small intestinal lumen, the end products of highly digestible proteins are amino acids, dipeptides, and tripeptides. These compounds are absorbed differently in the small intestine. The transport of amino acids into the enterocytes is greater in the distal small intestine, and this process is mediated by a multitude of transport systems. Amino acids have different physicochemical properties, and thus a single transport system cannot handle all amino acids. Therefore, intestinal absorptive cells express several transport systems to absorb different groups of amino acids from the small intestinal lumen. In contrast, dipeptides and tripeptides are absorbed mainly in the proximal small intestine by a unique transporter. The protein responsible for intestinal peptide transport is PEPT-1, which only accepts small peptides with two or three amino acid residues.[47–50] Gluten digestion in the small intestine generates high molecular weight oligopeptides that are not transported by PEPT-1.[33] These large peptides remain in the intestinal lumen, where they could be substrates for bacterial metabolism.

Once inside the enterocyte, dipeptides and tripeptides are subjected to hydrolysis by cytoplasmic peptidases to release free amino acids. This characteristic is unique to protein assimilation because, in the case of carbohydrates, digestion in the intestinal lumen has to be complete before absorption into the enterocyte can occur.[20] The products of protein digestion enter the portal circulation mostly as free amino acids because of the efficient intracellular hydrolysis of peptides by cytoplasmic peptidases. Thus, intracellular peptidases in the enterocyte play a vital role in the terminal stages of protein assimilation.[20] The transport of amino acids from the cell into the blood occurs through multiple transport systems that are different from the amino acid transporters situated in the brush border membrane. Nevertheless, it is likely that some of the absorbed small peptides that are resistant to hydrolysis by cytoplasmic peptidases may be transported across the basolateral membrane intact (Fig. 13.1). In fact, there is evidence that small peptides containing proline and hydroxyproline appear in the blood after the ingestion of gelatin, and these peptides are known to be relatively resistant to hydrolysis by cellular peptidases.[51,52] Gluten prolamins also contain regions rich in proline; therefore, some of the gluten proteins ingested in the diet could enter into portal circulation as small peptides.

Is the Small Intestine Microbiota Involved in the Metabolism of Gluten Proteins?

Alimentary and endogenous proteins are mixed with the microbiota in the small intestinal lumen. The intestinal microbiota is metabolically active and plays a significant role in the host's physiology and metabolism. Although it has not been directly measured *in vivo* yet, there are several reasons to take the small intestinal microbiota into account when considering the metabolism of proteins in the small intestine.[53–55] As with bacteria in the large intestine, proteins and peptides from the diet are likely to provide amino acids for bacteria in the small intestine. These amino acids can be used for protein synthesis, generation of metabolic energy, and recycling of reduced cofactors.[53] Although several proteolytic bacteria have been described in the large intestine, there are no known bacteria capable of participating in protein digestion in the small intestine. The concentration and diversity of the bacteria in the small intestine are lower than in the large intestine. The duodenum, jejunum, and ileum are estimated to contain 10^4–10^5 cells/g, 10^6–10^7 cells/g and 10^7–10^8 cells/g, respectively.[56] However, the small intestine has a relatively high luminal concentration of peptides, which could allow the growth of proteolytic bacteria.[53] Furthermore, the metabolic compounds generated by microbial hydrolysis in the gut may be used by the host. For example, it seems that the microbiota is able to provide amino acids to the host for protein synthesis in the intestine. Thus, amino acid exchange between the intestinal bacteria and the host can proceed in both directions.[53,57–59] A recent study reported that the duodenal microbiota in adults is composed principally of bacteria belonging to the phyla *Firmicutes*, *Proteobacteria*, and *Bacteroidetes*. Moreover, the predominant genera were *Streptococcus* and *Prevotella*.[28] Some oral bacteria belonging to *Streptococcus* have been linked to gluten metabolism.[25] However, the role of these intestinal bacteria in the duodenal digestion of proteins is unknown.

Diet is the major environmental factor that influences the diversity and functionality of the gut microbiota.[60] The ubiquitous presence of gluten in the diet and the resistance of wheat prolamins to gastrointestinal digestion result in the presence of large amounts of high molecular weight oligopeptides in the lumen of the small intestine.[36] These gluten peptides are available for bacterial hydrolysis. Although the bacterial diversity in the small intestine is lower than in the large intestine, bacteria from this tract might participate in gluten metabolism. It has been shown that removing gluten from the diet can affect the bacterial population in the duodenum.[28] A recent study from our research group isolated bacteria from the duodenum with the ability to grow in media with gluten peptides as the sole nitrogen source (unpublished results). In this study, mostly Gram-positive bacteria were isolated, and some of them showed proteolytic activity toward gluten proteins. Previous research reported that bacterial proteases with the ability to hydrolyze gliadin were present in duodenum samples, although the results were restricted to the small intestine mucosa of CD patients.[61] Thus, small intestinal bacteria with the ability to hydrolyze gluten peptides seem to be part of the microbiota, at least in the duodenum. These data suggest that the small intestinal microbiota might participate in the metabolism of gluten and other dietary proteins. However, more studies are necessary to identify the role of these bacteria in the metabolism of gluten peptides.

Gluten Metabolism in the Large Intestine

The microbiota of the large intestine derives its energy from dietary compounds that escape digestion in the stomach and the small intestine. Thus, the human colonic microbiota works as an anaerobic digester that acts on material recalcitrant to digestion in the upper gut, using an array of metabolic pathways.[62] Because of the large amount of bacterial diversity in the large intestine, it is worth considering that the bacteria of the large intestine may participate in the metabolism of gluten proteins.

Digestion of Gluten Peptides in the Large Intestine

Alimentary protein digestion followed by amino acid and peptide absorption in the small intestinal epithelium is considered an efficient process. Nevertheless, unabsorbed dietary proteins enter the human large intestine as a complex mixture of protein and peptides.[53,63] The incomplete assimilation of some dietary proteins in the small intestine has been previously demonstrated, even with proteins that are known to be easily digested (e.g., egg protein).[64,65] The high proline content of wheat gluten and related proteins renders these proteins resistant to complete digestion in the small intestine. As a result, many high molecular weight gluten oligopeptides arrive in the lower gastrointestinal tract.[66] While gluten peptides

pass through the large intestine, proteolytic bacteria could participate in the hydrolysis of these peptides. A recent study from our group has shown that some of the gluten ingested in the diet is not completely digested while passing through the gastrointestinal tract, and is consequently eliminated in feces. Moreover, it has been shown that the amount of gluten peptides present in feces is proportional to the amount of gluten consumed in the diet. Therefore, several gluten peptides are resistant to both human and bacterial proteases in the gastrointestinal tract.[66,67]

The large intestine is the natural habitat for a large and dynamic bacterial community. Although the small intestine contains a significant density of living bacteria, the density in the large intestine is much higher. The large intestine has as many as 10^{11}–10^{12} cells per gram of luminal content that belong to thousands of bacterial taxa. Furthermore, the large intestinal microbiota is extremely complex and performs specific tasks that are beneficial to the host.[68–71] Among the important functions that the intestinal microbiota performs for the host are several metabolic functions.[72] In contrast to the rapid passage of dietetic components through the small intestine, the transit of the luminal material through the large intestine is considerably slower. The longer transit time in the large intestine has been associated with important bacterial metabolic activity.[53] Therefore, undigested food in the upper gut could be hydrolyzed by microbial metabolism in the large intestine, generating beneficial compounds for the host.

The composition and metabolism of intestinal microbiota is largely influenced by the diet.[60,73] Undigested dietetic compounds in the small intestine arrive in the large intestine, where they can be substrates for the metabolism of the large intestinal bacteria. Approximately 13 g of dietary proteins enter the colon daily; therefore, proteins and amino acids are available for bacterial fermentation in the colon.[62,72] However, the breakdown of proteins and peptides by colonic microbiota has been scarcely studied. Bacteria commonly utilize proteins as nitrogen, carbon, and energy sources.[53] The genetic diversity of the intestinal microbiota produces different enzymes and metabolic pathways that would not otherwise be present in the host, enabling the recovery of some of the energy ingested in the diet.[68,74] Thus, proteins that are resistant to human digestive proteases, such as gluten proteins, could be hydrolyzed by microbial proteases in the large intestine. The predominant proteolytic bacteria in fecal samples mostly belong to the genera *Bacteroides*, *Propionibacterium*, *Streptococcus*, *Lactobacillus*, *Fusobacterium*, *Clostridium*, *Bacillus*, and *Staphylococcus*.[74,75] As a consequence of bacterial metabolism in the colon, proteins and peptides are fermented to short-chain fatty acids (SCFAs) and branched-chain fatty acids (BCFAs), such as isobutyrate and isovalerate, as well as a range of nitrogenous compounds. Some of these metabolic products could have marked effects on the host.[62,76,77] It is well known that the substrates for bacterial production of SCFAs are mainly fiber and resistant starch. However, it is rarely noted that undigested proteins are another substrate for SCFA production. Indeed, several amino acids released from proteins in the large intestine are precursors of SCFAs and BCFAs.[53] A recent study by our group reported that a high consumption of gluten in the diet increases fecal SCFAs as well as the isobutyric acid. This result suggests that gluten ingested in the diet is capable of affecting microbial metabolism in the large intestine.[66]

The resistance of gluten peptides to pancreatic and brush border enzymes allows large amounts of high molecular weight peptides to enter the lower gastrointestinal tract. Therefore, gluten peptides are available for microbial metabolism in the large intestine and could be important to the composition of the intestinal microbiota. It has been shown that removing gluten from the diet affects the composition of the bacterial community in the large bowel.[78,79] De Palma et al.[78] observed that healthy subjects who followed a gluten-free diet for 1 month had reduced fecal populations of Lactobacillus and Bifidobacterium, but the population of Enterobacteriae such as E. coli appeared to increase. Similar results were obtained in studies with CD patients. Treated CD patients also showed a reduction in the diversity of Lactobacillus and Bifidobacterium species.[80,81] Therefore, it is possible that these bacterial groups are involved in intestinal gluten metabolism.

Caminero et al.[66] were the first to report the presence of enzymatic activity in human fecal samples ("fecal glutenasic activity") that has the ability to break down gluten proteins. Fecal glutenasic activity increases proportionally as gluten is incorporated into the diet. The authors hypothesized that glutenasic activity may originate in the microbial metabolism in the gut, suggesting that bacterial proteases play a role in the hydrolysis of gluten proteins.[66] Furthermore, unpublished results from our group showed the presence of prolyl-endopeptidasic and dipeptidyl-peptidasic IV (DPPIV) activities that hydrolyzed peptide bonds with proline residues in human fecal samples. These activities most likely have a bacterial origin as well. However, there are few studies that examine the bacteria in the large intestine with the ability to digest gluten proteins or derived peptides. Some interesting studies have been performed with bifidobacteria. Bifidobacterium strains isolated from feces, such as B. longum IATA-ES1, B. animalis IATA-A2, and B. bifidum IATA-ES2, are capable of digesting gliadin-derived peptides. The presence of these bifidobacterial strains during the simulation of intestinal digestion of gliadin proteins enables the generation of different gliadin peptide sequences, which could modify their toxic effects. Gliadin digestion inoculated with B. animalis and B. bifidum were cytotoxic for intestinal epithelial cells, whereas cytotoxicity was not observed in those inoculated with B. longum.[82] Furthermore, B. longum CECT 7347 was able to hydrolyze the immunogenic peptide 33-mer and modulate the immune response in CD patients.[82-84] This bacterium is commercially available in food as a probiotic bacterium for CD patients. Another large-intestinal bacterium with gliadin-hydrolyzing activity is Bacteroides fragilis. This bacterium was isolated from human feces and could also participate in the metabolism of gluten proteins.[85] In addition, some unpublished results from our group indicate the important role that some bacteria play in gluten metabolism. We have observed that mixed bacterial cultures from feces are capable of hydrolyzing the gluten proteins present in a culture medium. Moreover, some of these bacteria were isolated and can also completely hydrolyze gluten proteins. These proteolytic bacteria, which belong to Firmicutes and Actinobacteria phyla and reside in the large intestine, could play an important role in gluten metabolism.

Transport of the End Products of Digested Gluten in the Large Intestine

It is generally assumed that colonic luminal amino acids and small peptides are not significantly absorbed by the colonic epithelium except during a relatively short period of time after birth.[53] Although some studies have hypothesized that the colonic epithelial cells are capable of absorbing various amino acids[86-89] as well as small peptides,[90] it seems that they only serve a useful function in special situations such as the immediate postnatal period or in patients with ileostomies or chronic inflammation.[20,88,91,92] Data indicate that human PEPT-1 is not expressed in a healthy colon, and consequently small peptides are not transported in the large intestine.[91] Furthermore, amino acid transport studies in humans and mammalians yield no conclusive results.[57,58,93] Therefore, small peptides or amino acids generated in the large intestine by microbial proteolysis could not be transported into the colonocyte. Thus, even if gluten proteins were completely hydrolyzed in the large bowel by intestinal microbiota, the resulting compounds would not be available for the host. In contrast, amino acids are intensely metabolized by luminal bacteria; this is likely the primary fate for amino acids in the large intestine. Genomic and physiologic studies have shown that the intestinal microbiota possesses specialized enzymes for the utilization of amino acids. The amino acids generated in the large intestine that are not metabolized by the microbiota are excreted in feces and not used by the host.[53]

GLUTEN TOXICITY, CELIAC DISEASE AND GLUTEN METABOLISM

Gluten-Related Disorders

Gluten is often a component of processed food because its proteins confer extensibility and elasticity, which are important in food technology.[6] However, despite the ubiquity of gluten proteins in the diet, these proteins are not completely harmless for everyone. Gluten is the environmental trigger for celiac disesase, one of the most common food-sensitive enteropathies in humans. CD affects approximately 1 : 100 individuals in Western countries.[11] Gluten is not only injurious to CD patients. Recently, a new group of non-celiac patients has been identified who respond to the removal of gluten from the diet. These patients are considered to have "non-celiac gluten sensitivity" (NCGS), a new term in the spectrum of gluten intolerance.[10,94]

CD is a chronic small intestinal immune-mediated enteropathy precipitated by exposure to dietary gluten in genetically predisposed individuals.[10] The condition is characterized by chronic inflammation of the proximal small intestine with villous atrophy and malabsorption; it can manifest at any age and presents with a variety of clinical features.[95] Furthermore, CD is a unique autoimmune disorder because the environmental precipitant (gluten proteins) is known.[96] In CD patients, exposure to gluten results in varying degrees of intestinal damage that persist unless gluten is completely eliminated from the diet. A strict lifetime gluten-free diet is the only safe and efficient treatment currently available for CD patients.[97] However, although gluten proteins are the causative agent of CD, the metabolism of these proteins in patients with CD is not entirely known.

Recently, non-celiac gluten sensitivity (NCGS) has been identified as a new condition triggered by gluten. The term NCGS encompasses one or more of a variety of immunological, morphological, or symptomatic variations that are precipitated by the ingestion of gluten by people who do not have CD.[10] Unlike CD, the process by which gluten harms people with NCGS is unknown. The role of gluten proteins in CD is quite well known: the high molecular weight oligopeptides derived from the recalcitrance of gluten proteins to human digestive proteases are related to the immunological response. Nevertheless, it is unclear at this time which components of the grain trigger symptoms in people with NCGS. The only thing that has been proven is that these patients truly develop symptoms when they consume gluten in their diet.[10,94,98]

Gluten Metabolism in Celiac Disease Patients

Gluten proteins are poorly digested in the intestine in humans with or without CD because these proteins are relatively resistant to human proteolytic enzymes in the small intestine.[33] Incomplete digestion generates high molecular weight oligopeptides; some of them are capable of activating the immunological response associated with CD in genetically susceptible individuals.[33,40] Two types of gluten-derived peptides with deleterious effects for CD patients have been described: (1) immunogenic peptides, such as the 33-mer or the 26-mer peptides, which activate the adaptive immune response; and (2) toxic peptides, such as the 19-mer peptide, which activate the innate immune response. Thus, gluten has a dual effect on the bowel of CD patients, activating an innate and an adaptive immune response.[11,99] However, only a minority of genetically susceptible individuals develops CD. The metabolism of gluten proteins has not been extensively studied, and it is generally believed that the metabolism of gluten proteins is similar in CD patients and healthy people. Nevertheless, several studies have speculated that CD patients may demonstrate abnormal digestion of gluten proteins.[45,61,100,101]

Digestion of Gluten Proteins in CD Patients

Gluten proteins are resistant to complete digestion by human proteases in the small intestine.[33,40] Nonetheless, the relatively poor digestion of these proteins is not sufficient to cause CD, and there could be unknown differences in the ability to digest gluten proteins between healthy individuals and those susceptible to CD. The failure to digest these and other proteins might be exaggerated in the small intestine of individuals with active CD who have injuries to the epithelial cell brush border.[102] In fact, for a long time it was speculated that CD may be the result of an enzyme deficiency or abnormal digestion in CD patients. This theory was known as the "metabolic hypothesis" or the "missing enzyme hypothesis", and was supported by various studies.[100,101,103,104]

Some research groups in the 1980s showed that the intestinal mucosa in active CD patients was less efficient at hydrolyzing gliadin peptides.[101,103,104] Less efficient gliadin digestion was correlated with lower activity of several brush border membrane peptidases, including aminopeptidase N (AMP), DPPIV, glycyl-leucine dipeptidase, proline dipeptidase, and γ-glutamyl-transpeptidase, in biopsy homogenates of active CD patients. However, the products generated after digestion were the same in healthy individuals and in CD patients, and most of the brush border activities recovered in treated patients.[100] Thus, the pathogenic architecture of the duodenum in active CD patients could explain this defect because the recuperation of the duodenal architecture leads to the recovery of brush border enzyme activities. Although the metabolic hypothesis has been completely abandoned, a recent study using duodenal biopsies indicates that some immunogenic peptides, such as p57–68, are partially degraded by apical peptidases in non-CD subjects, whereas these peptides remain intact in patients with active CD.[45]

It has also been suggested that a primary defect in AMP and DPPIV could participate in the pathologic process of CD because some research has shown that the enzymatic activity of these enzymes decreases in CD patients treated with GFD.[43,100] DPPIV and AMP have the capacity to break down peptide bonds with proline residues. Furthermore, it has been shown that DPPIV has a significant role in the assimilation of peptides containing proline in rats.[43,44,105] Nevertheless, a genetic link between CD and the coding genes for DPPIV and AMP enzymes showed divergent results. An association with markers flanking the AMP region was reported in Irish and British patients with CD.[106,107] However, Italian patients showed no genetic link between CD and DPPIV or AMP coding genes.[108] Other studies reported that DPPIV and AMP may present altered or normal peptidase activity in CD patients on a gluten-free diet.[100,103,109,110] These divergent results might reflect the degree to which the villous epithelium has been restored, because brush border membrane enzyme activity parallels histological recovery.[43,111] Consequently, a deficiency in the activity of these enzymes is not clearly related to the etiology of CD. Therefore, although there are differences in the digestion of gluten proteins by human proteases between CD patients and healthy people, these differences seem to be a consequence of the disease, not the cause of it.

Is it Possible that the Microbial Digestion of Gluten Proteins is Different in the Bowel of CD Patients?

As mentioned above, the small intestinal microbiota may participate in the metabolism of gluten proteins. However, the role of the intestinal bacteria in the metabolism of proteins in humans is frequently underestimated. *In vitro* studies with human digestive proteases offer a good explanation for the appearance of undigested gluten peptides that interact with the human immune response system. However, a role for the small intestinal bacteria in the metabolism of gluten proteins should not be ruled out. The small intestinal microbiota could generate peptides that are more harmful than those generated by human digestive proteases. Indeed, Bernardo et al.[61] described a specific gliadinase pattern in duodenal samples from patients with CD that was absent in samples from non-CD patients. These authors have suggested that specific bacteria located in the mucosa of the small intestine of CD patients are responsible for producing proteolytic activities against gliadins. These bacteria would not appear in non-CD patients.[61] As a consequence, different immunogenic peptides capable of triggering CD in susceptible persons could be generated. *In vitro* studies showed that these

gliadinases release gliadin peptides that are immunogenic for monocyte-derived dendritic cells from both celiac and non-celiac subjects. If gliadin peptides also have immunogenic properties *in vivo* in the duodenum, they would provide a direct link between these activities and the disease by releasing immunogenic peptides that would remain masked in individuals lacking proteases (D. Bernardo, personal communication, 2013). Interestingly, the possible involvement of duodenal bacteria in the pathogenesis of CD has been described previously.[112]

Although there are no known small intestinal bacteria with the ability to participate in the metabolism of gluten proteins, several studies have indicated a role for the small intestinal microbiota in the pathophysiology of CD. Forsberg et al.[113] frequently found rod-shaped bacteria in the mucosa of CD patients that did not appear in non-CD control subjects, raising a question about the role of the small intestinal microbiota in CD.[113] The microbial communities that colonize the human gut influence many aspects of our health; indeed, various gastrointestinal pathologies are related to an alteration in the composition of gut microbiota.[60] In fact, numerous studies have shown differences in the composition of the intestinal microbiota between CD patients and non-CD volunteers.[80,81,114–118] It has been reported that CD patients frequently present altered intestinal bacterial groups such as *Bifidobacterium*, *Lactobacillus*, *Bacteroides*, *Prevotella Staphylococcus*, and *Escherichia*.[115–119] Within these groups there are some species with well-known proteolytic activity, as well as bacteria with the ability to cleavage gluten peptides. Fecal strains of the genera *Bacteroides* and *Bifidobacterium*, such as *Bacteroides fragilis* and *Bifidobacterium longum*, hydrolyze gliadin and gluten peptides.[75,82,85] Therefore, although there are no studies dealing with proteolytic bacteria in the small intestine, it is possible that the small intestinal dysbiosis in CD patients causes differences in the digestion of gluten proteins in the duodenum in relation to healthy people, and these differences may be involved in the development of CD.

Protein and peptides not digested in the small intestine arrive in the large intestine, where they serve as substrates for proteolytic bacteria. As a consequence of bacterial metabolism in the colon, undigested peptides are fermented to SCFAs, BCFAs, and nitrogenous compounds.[62] Although SCFAs are also produced from carbohydrates such as fiber and resistant starch, the exclusive precursors of BCFAs are proteins, which are thus good markers of protein metabolism in the large intestine.[53,76,120,121] It has been shown that high exogenous gluten intake in healthy volunteers increases the number of total SCFAs and BCFAs such as isobutyric acid.[66] This finding suggests that gluten proteins ingested in the diet arrive in the colon, where they are available for bacterial metabolism. Thus, SCFAs and especially BCFAs act as indirect indicators of the metabolism of proteins in the bowel. Several studies have shown that SCFAs and BCFAs appear altered in fecal samples from CD patients, indicating that there could be differences in the metabolic activity of the intestinal microbiota between healthy people and CD patients.[80,122,123] The explanation is generally associated with the presence of a characteristic microbiota in CD patients. However, could the imbalance of SCFAs and BCFAs in CD patients be caused by the metabolism of proteins? Tjellström et al.[122] reported a significantly higher concentration of acetic, isobutyric, and isovaleric acids, as well as total SCFAs, in fecal samples from children with CD, both at diagnosis and during treatment with a GFD, compared with healthy controls. The number of BCFAs in the feces of children with CD could indicate that protein digestion in the duodenum of CD patients is different from that in healthy people. Thus, a larger amount of protein would be arriving in the large intestine. Furthermore, this condition is independent of intestinal mucosa damage and gluten ingestion because the treated children also showed increased levels of BCFAs.[122] A recent study in a Spanish population showed that adults with CD also present different levels of SCFAs compared with healthy people. However, although BCFAs were increased in active CD patients, there was no significant difference in relation to healthy controls.[80]

Celiac Disease Therapies Related to Gluten Metabolism

CD is a widespread chronic disorder for which dietary adaptation is the only accepted form of therapy. Although GFD has proven to be a safe and effective therapy, it is not ideal. This type of diet is expensive, not readily available in many countries, and may have lower nutritional value, which can affect the patient's quality of life. Based on the current understanding of the pathogenesis of CD, several potential therapeutic targets are being explored. Some of these novel therapies are designed to modify the metabolism of gluten proteins in the human gut.[124]

Oral Proteases for Improving Gluten Hydrolysis

As mentioned above, gluten proteins are rich in glutamine and proline residues, and thus these proteins are highly resistant to degradation by gastric and pancreatic proteases.[125–129] This resistance results in the incomplete digestion of gluten proteins and the subsequent generation of long oligopeptides, such as the gliadin 33-mer and 26-mer peptides, which are well-known immunogenic peptides. These fragments can potently elicit an HLA-DQ2 or HLA-DQ8 restricted T-cell inflammatory response in patients with CD.[130,131]

Therapies that supplement oral protease focus on inactivating the immunogenic gluten epitopes using proteolytic hydrolysis. The most commonly studied enzymes with the ability to carry out this process are the proteases from the prolyl endopeptidase family (PEPs). These proteins are expressed in microorganisms and plants.[132,133] Shan et al.[33] first proposed the use of PEPs for the in vivo enzymatic detoxification of gluten. Some of these enzymes are able to cleave immunodominant proline-rich regions present in gluten proteins.[134] However, there are some concerns about the use of PEPs. These enzymes must not be inactivated by the acidic milieu of the stomach, and the majority of the epitope hydrolysis should occur in the stomach before the epitopes reach the small intestine.[133] In addition, PEP activity should be resistant to pepsin, pancreatic proteases, and intestinal brush border membrane peptidases. Different groups in both the United States and The Netherlands have demonstrated the efficacy of gluten protein digestion using different enzyme preparations.[126,128,129]

AN-PEP is a prolyl endopeptidase derived from Aspergillus niger that is being developed by an alimentary company (DSM).[135] In vitro studies have shown that AN-PEP is active at a pH between 2 and 8, with optimal activity at a pH ranging from 4 to 5. It resists digestion by pepsin and degrades all tested gluten peptides with a half-life ranging between 2.4 and 6.2 minutes.[128,129] AN-PEP accelerated the hydrolysis of gluten proteins in the stomach, degrading it into harmless fragments. Fewer toxic epitopes arrive in the duodenum, resulting in a reduction in the stimulation of T cells.[129] Based on these in vitro findings, a number of in vivo studies are underway. One of them is a randomized, double-blind, controlled trial investigating the efficacy of AN-PEP in detoxifying 8 g of gluten in a commercial food.[124,135,136] The study primarily focuses on the change in the small intestine histology, and other outcomes include the number of peripheral blood T cells and celiac antibodies. For this experiment, 14 patients consumed a special diet for three periods of 2 weeks each. For the first 2 weeks, the patients ate food prepared with gluten together with AN-PEP. Next, they were kept on a strict GFD for another 2 weeks. Finally, they were randomized to continue eating the same food containing gluten and AN-PEP, or gluten and a placebo. The safety profile was satisfactory, but there was no significant effect of AN-PEP on the prespecified outcomes, although a post hoc analysis showed a possible reduction in the intestinal deposits of anti-tTG IgA antibodies.[135,136] A new clinical trial for AN-PEP has also been announced, using 12 subjects to understand the extent of the degradation of gluten in the stomach (ClinicalTrials.gov identifier: NCT01335503).[136]

Another drug candidate, ALV003, is being developed as an orally administered mixture of two glutenases (ALV001 and ALV002).[127] ALV001 is a glutamine-specific cysteine endoprotease derived from germinating barley seeds (EP-B2). ALV002 is a prolyl endopeptidase from *Sphingomonas capsulate* (SC-PEP).[126,137] Both enzymes are active within the acidic environment of the stomach, and a 1:1 (w/w) formulation (ALV003) maximizes their glutenasic activity.[126] A Phase I clinical trial was conducted with 20 CD patients in remission who were randomized to receive a diet containing gluten (16 g a day for 3 days) after being pretreated with ALV003 (10 patients), or a diet containing gluten after being pretreated with a placebo (10 patients). The results showed that the immune response decreases, but ALV003 does not improve the clinical response.[125] A randomized controlled Phase IIa clinical trial has been performed in which CD patients received either ALV003 or a placebo daily for 6 weeks with 2 g of gluten. This study demonstrated that ALV003 can attenuate gluten-induced small intestinal mucosal injury in CD patients.[138] After this period of time, biopsies proved that small intestinal mucosal injuries were lower in patients treated with ALV003 than in placebo-treated patients, despite persistent intestinal inflammation in many patients on a strict GFD. Placebo-treated patients suffered more adverse events, such as distention, flatulence, eructation, abdominal pain, and diarrhea.[132,138]

In addition to these two company-sponsored clinical trials with proteases, a third protease mix was tested by an academic institution, Stanford University. The group led by Professor Khosla conducted a Phase II clinical trial with STAN1 (ClinicalTrials.gov identifier: NCT00962182). STAN1 is a cocktail of microbial enzymes commonly used in food supplements that shows modest gluten detoxification capacity.[139] A randomized, double-blind, placebo-controlled study was conducted with 35 CD patients who followed a GFD but had persistent seropositivity for tTG. The study evaluated the effect of STAN1 when the patients ingested 1 g of gluten per day for 12 weeks. No differences were found in serology between the placebo group and the patients treated with STAN1.[124,140]

The main problem with oral enzyme therapy is administering enough of the enzyme and allowing enough time for it to act on gluten proteins and peptides to complete the hydrolysis of the immunogenic gluten peptides with a daily gluten load (10–20 g). However, these enzymes may eliminate the detrimental side effects from lower gluten exposures, and as a result may improve the patient's response to low-level gluten exposure and reduce the incidence of refractory CD from inadvertent low-level gluten ingestion.[130]

CONCLUSIONS

Gluten is widespread in foods because of the properties of its proteins. Gluten is composed mainly of proteins that are ingested in the diet. Because of their high proline content, these proteins are only partially hydrolyzed by human digestive proteases in the small intestine, generating high molecular weight oligopeptides in the intestinal lumen. Oligopeptides and undigested proteins are good substrates for bacterial growth; however, the role of the intestinal bacteria in the metabolism of proteins is frequently underestimated. There is evidence that suggests that the human gut microbiota may be involved in the metabolism of gluten proteins. Diet is one of the major factors influencing the composition of gut bacteria, and removing gluten from the diet affects the bacterial population in the small and large intestines. Several studies have shown the presence of bacteria with the ability to hydrolyze gluten peptides in the oral cavity and in the large intestine. Nevertheless, knowledge about the role of the human gut microbiota in the metabolism of gluten proteins is scarce, and more studies are needed.

References

1. Shewry PR. Wheat. *J Exp Bot* 2009;**60**(6):1537–53.
2. Shewry PR, Halford NG, Belton PS, Tatham AS. The structure and properties of gluten: an elastic protein from wheat grain. *Philos Trans R Soc Lond B Biol Sci* 2002;**357**(1418):133–42.
3. Shewry PR, Halford NG. Cereal seed storage proteins: structures, properties and role in grain utilization. *J Exp Bot* 2002;**53**(370):947–58.
4. Shewry PR, Halford NG, Lafiandra D. Genetics of wheat gluten proteins. *Adv Genet* 2003;**49**:111–84.
5. Tosi P, Gritsch CS, He J, Shewry PR. Distribution of gluten proteins in bread wheat (*Triticum aestivum*) grain. *Ann Bot* 2011;**108**(1):23–35.
6. Belderok B. Developments in bread-making processes. *Plant Foods Hum Nutr* 2000;**55**(1):1–86.
7. Green P, Cellier C. Celiac disease. *N Engl J Med* 2007;**357**(17): 1731–43.
8. Wieser H. Chemistry of gluten proteins. *Food Microbiol* 2007; **24**(2):115–9.
9. Mills EN, Jenkins JA, Alcocer MJ, Shewry PR. Structural, biological, and evolutionary relationships of plant food allergens sensitizing via the gastrointestinal tract. *Crit Rev Food Sci Nutr* 2004;**44**(5):379–407.
10. Ludvigsson JF, Leffler DA, Bai JC, et al. The Oslo definitions for coeliac disease and related terms. *Gut* 2012.
11. Camarca A, Del Mastro A, Gianfrani C. Repertoire of gluten peptides active in celiac disease patients: perspectives for translational therapeutic applications. *Endocr Metab Immune Disord Drug Targets* 2012;**12**(2):207–19.
12. Wieser H. Relation between gliadin structure and coeliac toxicity. *Acta Paediatr Suppl* 1996;**412**:3–9.
13. Keck B, Köhler P, Wieser H. Disulfide bonds in wheat gluten: cystine peptides derived from gluten proteins following peptic and thermolytic digestion. *Z Lebensm Unters Forsch* 1995;**200**(6):432–9.
14. Köhler P, Belitz HD, Wieser H. Disulphide bonds in wheat gluten: isolation of a cystine peptide from glutenin. *Z Lebensm Unters Forsch* 1991;**192**(3):234–9.
15. Shewry PR, Tatham AS. The prolamin storage proteins of cereal seeds: structure and evolution. *Biochem J* 1990;**267**(1):1–12.
16. Hamer RJ. Coeliac Disease: background and biochemical aspects. *Biotechnol Adv* 2005;**23**(6):401–8.

17. Mamone G, Picariello G, Addeo F, Ferranti P. Proteomic analysis in allergy and intolerance to wheat products. *Expert Rev Proteomics* 2011;**8**(1):95–115.

18. Haboubi NY, Taylor S, Jones S. Coeliac disease and oats: a systematic review. *Postgrad Med J* 2006;**82**(972):672–8.

19. Comino I, Real A, de Lorenzo L, et al. Diversity in oat potential immunogenicity: basis for the selection of oat varieties with no toxicity in coeliac disease. *Gut* 2011;**60**(7):915–22.

20. Ganapathy V, Gupta N, Martindale RG. *Protein digestion and absorption*. 4th ed. San Diego, CA: Physiology of the gastrointestinal tract; 2006; 1667–1692.

21. van Overbeek FM, Uil-Dieterman IG, Mol IW, Köhler-Brands L, Heymans HS, Mulder CJ. The daily gluten intake in relatives of patients with coeliac disease compared with that of the general Dutch population. *Eur J Gastroenterol Hepatol* 1997;**9**(11):1097–9.

22. McAllister CS, Kagnoff MF. The immunopathogenesis of celiac disease reveals possible therapies beyond the gluten-free diet. *Semin Immunopathol* 2012;**34**(4):581–600.

23. Helmerhorst EJ, Sun X, Salih E, Oppenheim FG. Identification of Lys–Pro–Gln as a novel cleavage site specificity of saliva-associated proteases. *J Biol Chem* 2008;**283**(29):19957–66.

24. Helmerhorst EJ, Zamakhchari M, Schuppan D, Oppenheim FG. Discovery of a novel and rich source of gluten-degrading microbial enzymes in the oral cavity. *PLoS One* 2010;**5**(10):e13264.

25. Zamakhchari M, Wei G, Dewhirst F, et al. Identification of Rothia bacteria as gluten-degrading natural colonizers of the upper gastro-intestinal tract. *PLoS One* 2011;**6**(9):e24455.

26. Messana I, Cabras T, Pisano E, et al. Trafficking and postsecretory events responsible for the formation of secreted human salivary peptides: a proteomics approach. *Mol Cell Proteomics* 2008;**7**(5):911–26.

27. Wade WG. The oral microbiome in health and disease. *Pharmacol Res* 2012.

28. Nistal E, Caminero A, Herrán AR, et al. Differences of small intestinal bacteria populations in adults and children with/without celiac disease: effect of age, gluten diet, and disease. *Inflamm Bowel Dis* 2012;**18**(4):649–56.

29. Ou G, Hedberg M, Hörstedt P, et al. Proximal small intestinal microbiota and identification of rod-shaped bacteria associated with childhood celiac disease. *Am J Gastroenterol* 2009;**104**(12):3058–67.

30. Roberts NB. Review article: human pepsins - their multiplicity, function and role in reflux disease. *Aliment Pharmacol Ther* 2006;**24**(Suppl. 2):2–9.

31. Morón B, Cebolla A, Manyani H, et al. Sensitive detection of cereal fractions that are toxic to celiac disease patients by using monoclonal antibodies to a main immunogenic wheat peptide. *Am J Clin Nutr* 2008;**87**(2):405–14.

32. Frazer AC, Fletcher RF, Ross CA, Shaw B, Sammons HG, Schneider R. Gluten-induced enteropathy: the effect of partially digested gluten. *Lancet* 1959;**2**(7097):252–5.

33. Shan L, Molberg Ø, Parrot I, et al. Structural basis for gluten intolerance in celiac sprue. *Science* 2002;**297**(5590):2275–9.

34. Wilson M. *The gastrointestinal tract and its indigenous microbiota. Microbial inhabitants of human: their ecology and role in health and disease*. Cambridge, UK: Press syndicate of the University of Cambridge; 2005. p. 254–313.

35. Bik EM, Eckburg PB, Gill SR, et al. Molecular analysis of the bacterial microbiota in the human stomach. *Proc Natl Acad Sci USA* 2006;**103**(3):732–7.

36. Hausch F, Shan L, Santiago NA, Gray GM, Khosla C. Intestinal digestive resistance of immunodominant gliadin peptides. *Am J Physiol Gastrointest Liver Physiol* 2002;**283**(4):G996–1003.

37. Whitcomb DC, Lowe ME. Human pancreatic digestive enzymes. *Dig Dis Sci* 2007;**52**(1):1–17.

38. Pittman FE, Pollitt RJ. Studies of jejunal mucosal digestion of peptic-tryptic digests of wheat protein in coeliac disease. *Gut* 1966;**7**(4):368–71.

39. Kocna P, Fric P, Kocová-Holáková M, Slabý J, Kasafírek E, Hekkens WT. Isolation and analysis of peptidic fragments of alpha-gliadin using reversed-phase high-performance liquid chromatography. *J Chromatogr* 1988;**434**(2):429–38.

40. Shan L, Qiao SW, Arentz-Hansen H, et al. Identification and analysis of multivalent proteolytically resistant peptides from gluten: implications for celiac sprue. *J Proteome Res* 2005;**4**(5):1732–41.

41. Mamone G, Ferranti P, Rossi M, et al. Identification of a peptide from alpha-gliadin resistant to digestive enzymes: implications for celiac disease. *J Chromatogr B Analyt Technol Biomed Life Sci* 2007;**855**(2):236–41.

42. Gass J, Vora H, Hofmann AF, Gray GM, Khosla C. Enhancement of dietary protein digestion by conjugated bile acids. *Gastroenterology* 2007;**133**(1):16–23.

43. Heyman M, Abed J, Lebreton C, Cerf-Bensussan N. Intestinal permeability in coeliac disease: insight into mechanisms and relevance to pathogenesis. *Gut* 2012;**61**(9):1355–64.

44. Tiruppathi C, Miyamoto Y, Ganapathy V, Leibach FH. Genetic evidence for role of DPP IV in intestinal hydrolysis and assimilation of prolyl peptides. *Am J Physiol* 1993;**265**(1 Pt 1):G81–9.

45. Matysiak-Budnik T, Candalh C, Dugave C, et al. Alterations of the intestinal transport and processing of gliadin peptides in celiac disease. *Gastroenterology* 2003;**125**(3):696–707.

46. Matysiak-Budnik T, Candalh C, Cellier C, et al. Limited efficiency of prolyl-endopeptidase in the detoxification of gliadin peptides in celiac disease. *Gastroenterology* 2005;**129**(3):786–96.

47. Brandsch M. Transport of L-proline, L-proline-containing peptides and related drugs at mammalian epithelial cell membranes. *Amino Acids* 2006;**31**(2):119–36.

48. Ganapathy V, Miyamoto Y, Leibach FH. Driving force for peptide transport in mammalian intestine and kidney. *Beitr Infusionther Klin Ernahr* 1987;**17**:54–68.

49. Leibach FH, Ganapathy V. Peptide transporters in the intestine and the kidney. *Annu Rev Nutr* 1996;**16**:99–119.

50. Daniel H. Molecular and integrative physiology of intestinal peptide transport. *Annu Rev Physiol* 2004;**66**:361–84.

51. Prockop DJ, Keiser HR, Sjoerdsma A. Gastrointestinal absorption and renal excretion of hydroxyproline peptides. *Lancet* 1962;**2**(7255):527–8.

52. Bronstein HD, Haeffner LJ, Kowlessar OD. The significance of gelatin tolerance in malabsorptive states. *Gastroenterology* 1966;**50**(5):621–30.

53. Davila AM, Blachier F, Gotteland M, et al. Intestinal luminal nitrogen metabolism: Role of the gut microbiota and consequences for the host. *Pharmacol Res* 2012.

54. Bergen WG, Wu G. Intestinal nitrogen recycling and utilization in health and disease. *J Nutr* 2009;**139**(5):821–5.

55. Chen L, Li P, Wang J, et al. Catabolism of nutritionally essential amino acids in developing porcine enterocytes. *Amino Acids* 2009;**37**(1):143–52.

56. Cotter PD. Small intestine and microbiota. *Curr Opin Gastroenterol* 2011;**27**(2):99–105.

57. Metges CC. Contribution of microbial amino acids to amino acid homeostasis of the host. *J Nutr* 2000;**130**(7):1857S–64S.

58. Torrallardona D, Harris CI, Fuller MF. Microbial amino acid synthesis and utilization in rats: the role of coprophagy. *Br J Nutr* 1996;**76**(5):701–9.

59. Laparra JM, Sanz Y. Interactions of gut microbiota with functional food components and nutraceuticals. *Pharmacol Res* 2010;**61**(3):219–25.

60. Flint HJ, Scott KP, Louis P, Duncan SH. The role of the gut microbiota in nutrition and health. *Nat Rev Gastroenterol Hepatol* 2012;**9**(10):577–89.

61. Bernardo D, Garrote JA, Nadal I, et al. Is it true that coeliacs do not digest gliadin? Degradation pattern of gliadin in coeliac disease small intestinal mucosa. *Gut* 2009;**58**(6):886–7.

62. Tuohy KM, Hinton DJ, Davies SJ, Crabbe MJ, Gibson GR, Ames JM. Metabolism of Maillard reaction products by the human gut microbiota – implications for health. *Mol Nutr Food Res* 2006;**50**(9):847–57.

63. Bos C, Juillet B, Fouillet H, et al. Postprandial metabolic utilization of wheat protein in humans. *Am J Clin Nutr* 2005;**81**(1):87–94.

64. Evenepoel P, Geypens B, Rutgeerts P, Ghoos Y. Study of protein assimilation, using stable isotope techniques. *Rev Med Univ Navarra* 1998;**42**(2):104–8.

65. Evenepoel P, Claus D, Geypens B, et al. Amount and fate of egg protein escaping assimilation in the small intestine of humans. *Am J Physiol* 1999;**277**(5 Pt 1):G935–43.

66. Caminero A, Nistal E, Arias L, et al. A gluten metabolism study in healthy individuals shows the presence of faecal glutenasic activity. *Eur J Nutr* 2012;**51**(3):293–9.

67. Comino I, Real A, Vivas S, et al. Monitoring of gluten-free diet compliance in celiac patients by assessment of gliadin 33-mer equivalent epitopes in feces. *Am J Clin Nutr* 2012;**95**(3):670–7.

68. Guarner F, Malagelada JR. [Bacterial flora of the digestive tract]. *Gastroenterol Hepatol* 2003;**26**(Suppl. 1):1–5.

69. Neish AS. Microbes in gastrointestinal health and disease. *Gastroenterology* 2009;**136**(1):65–80.

70. Simrén M, Barbara G, Flint HJ, et al. Intestinal microbiota in functional bowel disorders: a Rome foundation report. *Gut* 2013;**62**(1):159–76.

71. Wylie KM, Truty RM, Sharpton TJ, et al. Novel bacterial taxa in the human microbiome. *PLoS One* 2012;**7**(6):e35294.

72. Cummings JH, Macfarlane GT. Role of intestinal bacteria in nutrient metabolism. *JPEN J Parenter Enteral Nutr* 1997;**21**(6):357–65.

73. Walker AW, Ince J, Duncan SH, et al. Dominant and diet-responsive groups of bacteria within the human colonic microbiota. *ISME J* 2011;**5**(2):220–30.

74. Macfarlane GT, Allison C, Gibson SA, Cummings JH. Contribution of the microflora to proteolysis in the human large intestine. *J Appl Bacteriol* 1988;**64**(1):37–46.

75. Macfarlane GT, Cummings JH, Allison C. Protein degradation by human intestinal bacteria. *J Gen Microbiol* 1986;**132**(6):1647–56.

76. Macfarlane S, Macfarlane GT. Regulation of short-chain fatty acid production. *Proc Nutr Soc* 2003;**62**(1):67–72.

77. Wong JM, de Souza R, Kendall CW, Emam A, Jenkins DJ. Colonic health: fermentation and short chain fatty acids. *J Clin Gastroenterol* 2006;**40**(3):235–43.

78. De Palma G, Nadal I, Collado MC, Sanz Y. Effects of a gluten-free diet on gut microbiota and immune function in healthy adult human subjects. *Br J Nutr* 2009;**102**(8):1154–60.

79. Kopecný J, Mrázek J, Fliegerová K, Kott T. Effect of gluten-free diet on microbes in the colon. *Folia Microbiol (Praha)* 2006;**51**(4):287–90.

80. Nistal E, Caminero A, Vivas S, et al. Differences in faecal bacteria populations and faecal bacteria metabolism in healthy adults and celiac disease patients. *Biochimie* 2012;**94**(8):1724–9.

81. Di Cagno R, Rizzello CG, Gagliardi F, et al. Different fecal microbiotas and volatile organic compounds in treated and untreated children with celiac disease. *Appl Environ Microbiol* 2009;**75**(12):3963–71.

82. Laparra JM, Sanz Y. Bifidobacteria inhibit the inflammatory response induced by gliadins in intestinal epithelial cells via modifications of toxic peptide generation during digestion. *J Cell Biochem* 2010;**109**(4):801–7.

83. Laparra JM, Olivares M, Gallina O, Sanz Y. Bifidobacterium longum CECT 7347 modulates immune responses in a gliadin-induced enteropathy animal model. *PLoS One* 2012;**7**(2):e30744.

84. Medina M, De Palma G, Ribes-Koninckx C, Calabuig M, Sanz Y. Bifidobacterium strains suppress *in vitro* the pro-inflammatory milieu triggered by the large intestinal microbiota of coeliac patients. *J Inflamm (Lond)* 2008;**5**:19.

85. Sánchez E, Laparra JM, Sanz Y. Discerning the role of *Bacteroides fragilis* in celiac disease pathogenesis. *Appl Environ Microbiol* 2012;**78**(18):6507–15.

86. Robinson JW, Luisier AL, Mirkovitch V. Transport of amino-acids and sugars by the dog colonic mucosa. *Pflugers Arch* 1973;**345**(4):317–26.

87. Lerner J, Sattelmeyer P, Rush R. Kinetics of methionine influx into various regions of chicken intestine. *Comp Biochem Physiol A Comp Physiol* 1975;**50**(1A):113–20.

88. Sepúlveda FV, Smith MW. Different mechanisms for neutral amino acid uptake by new-born pig colon. *J Physiol* 1979;**286**:479–90.

89. Ardawi MS. The transport of glutamine and alanine into rat colonocytes. *Biochem J* 1986;**238**(1):131–5.

90. Calonge ML, Ilundáin A, Bolufer J. Glycylsarcosine transport by epithelial cells isolated from chicken proximal cecum and rectum. *Am J Physiol* 1990;**258**(5 Pt 1):G660–4.

91. Merlin D, Si-Tahar M, Sitaraman SV, et al. Colonic epithelial hPepT1 expression occurs in inflammatory bowel disease: transport of bacterial peptides influences expression of MHC class 1 molecules. *Gastroenterology* 2001;**120**(7):1666–79.

92. Ziegler TR, Fernández-Estívariz C, Gu LH, et al. Distribution of the H+/peptide transporter PepT1 in human intestine: up-regulated expression in the colonic mucosa of patients with short-bowel syndrome. *Am J Clin Nutr* 2002;**75**(5):922–30.

93. Metges CC, Petzke KJ, El-Khoury AE, et al. Incorporation of urea and ammonia nitrogen into ileal and fecal microbial proteins and plasma free amino acids in normal men and ileostomates. *Am J Clin Nutr* 1999;**70**(6):1046–58.

94. Verdu EF, Armstrong D, Murray JA. Between celiac disease and irritable bowel syndrome: the "no man's land" of gluten sensitivity. *Am J Gastroenterol* 2009;**104**(6):1587–94.

95. Vivas S, Ruiz de Morales JM, Fernandez M, et al. Age-related clinical, serological, and histopathological features of celiac disease. *Am J Gastroenterol* 2008;**103**(9):2360–5, quiz 6.

96. Fasano A. Surprises from celiac disease. *Sci Am* 2009;**301**(2):54–61.

97. Setty M, Hormaza L, Guandalini S. Celiac disease: risk assessment, diagnosis, and monitoring. *Mol Diagn Ther* 2008;**12**(5):289–98.

98. Biesiekierski JR, Newnham ED, Irving PM, et al. Gluten causes gastrointestinal symptoms in subjects without celiac disease: a double-blind randomized placebo-controlled trial. *Am J Gastroenterol* 2011;**106**(3):508–14 quiz 15.

99. Arranz E, Garrote JA. [Immunology of celiac disease]. *Gastroenterol Hepatol* 2010;**33**(9):643–51.

100. Sjöström H, Norén O, Krasilnikoff PA, Gudmand-Høyer E. Intestinal peptidases and sucrase in coeliac disease. *Clin Chim Acta* 1981;**109**(1):53–8.

101. Carchon H, Serrus M, Eggermont E. Digestion of gliadin peptides by intestinal mucosa from control or coeliac children. *Digestion* 1979;**19**(1):1–5.

102. Kagnoff M. Celiac disease: pathogenesis of a model immunogenetic disease. *J Clin Invest* 2007;**117**(1):41–9.

103. Cornell HJ, Auricchio RS, De Ritis G, et al. Intestinal mucosa of celiacs in remission is unable to abolish toxicity of gliadin peptides on *in vitro* developing fetal rat intestine and cultured atrophic celiac mucosa. *Pediatr Res* 1988;**24**(2):233–7.

104. Cornell HJ. Mucosal digestion studies of whole gliadin fractions in coeliac disease. *Ann Clin Biochem* 1990;**27**(Pt 1):44–9.

105. Cunningham DF, O'Connor B. Proline specific peptidases. *Biochim Biophys Acta* 1997;**1343**(2):160–86.

106. Houlston RS, Tomlinson IP, Ford D, et al. Linkage analysis of candidate regions for coeliac disease genes. *Hum Mol Genet* 1997;**6**(8):1335–9.

107. Zhong F, McCombs CC, Olson JM, et al. An autosomal screen for genes that predispose to celiac disease in the western counties of Ireland. *Nat Genet* 1996;**14**(3):329–33.

108. Clot F, Babron MC, Percopo S, et al. Study of two ectopeptidases in the susceptibility to celiac disease: two newly identified polymorphisms of dipeptidylpeptidase IV. *J Pediatr Gastroenterol Nutr* 2000;**30**(4):464–6.

109. Bruce G, Woodley JF, Swan CH. Breakdown of gliadin peptides by intestinal brush borders from coeliac patients. *Gut* 1984;**25**(9):919–24.

110. Kreft D, Hauri H, Belli D, et al. The *in vitro* influence of gliadin peptides on the hydrolases of the duodenal brush border membrane in coeliac disease in remission. *Journal of Pediatric Gastroenterology and Nutrition* 1997;**24**(4).

111. Mercer J, Eagles ME, Talbot IC. Brush border enzymes in coeliac disease: histochemical evaluation. *J Clin Pathol* 1990;**43**(4):307–12.

112. Sanz Y, De Pama G, Laparra M. Unraveling the ties between celiac disease and intestinal microbiota. *Int Rev Immunol* 2011;**30**(4):207–18.

113. Forsberg G, Fahlgren A, Hörstedt P, Hammarström S, Hernell O, Hammarström ML. Presence of bacteria and innate immunity of intestinal epithelium in childhood celiac disease. *Am J Gastroenterol* 2004;**99**(5):894–904.

114. Collado MC, Calabuig M, Sanz Y. Differences between the fecal microbiota of coeliac infants and healthy controls. *Curr Issues Intest Microbiol* 2007;**8**(1):9–14.

115. Collado MC, Donat E, Ribes-Koninckx C, Calabuig M, Sanz Y. Imbalances in faecal and duodenal Bifidobacterium species composition in active and non-active coeliac disease. *BMC Microbiol* 2008;**8**:232.

116. De Palma G, Nadal I, Medina M, et al. Intestinal dysbiosis and reduced immunoglobulin-coated bacteria associated with coeliac disease in children. *BMC Microbiol* 2010;**10**:63.

117. Sanz Y, Sánchez E, Marzotto M, Calabuig M, Torriani S, Dellaglio F. Differences in faecal bacterial communities in coeliac and healthy children as detected by PCR and denaturing gradient gel electrophoresis. *FEMS Immunol Med Microbiol* 2007;**51**(3):562–8.

118. Sellitto M, Bai G, Serena G, et al. Proof of concept of microbiome-metabolome analysis and delayed gluten exposure on celiac disease autoimmunity in genetically at-risk infants. *PLoS One* 2012;**7**(3):e33387.

119. Iebba V, Aloi M, Civitelli F, Cucchiara S. Gut microbiota and pediatric disease. *Dig Dis* 2011;**29**(6):531–9.

120. Barker HA. Amino acid degradation by anaerobic bacteria. *Annu Rev Biochem* 1981;**50**:23–40.

121. Elsden SR, Hilton MG. Volatile acid production from threonine, valine, leucine and isoleucine by clostridia. *Arch Microbiol* 1978;**117**(2):165–72.

122. Tjellström B, Stenhammar L, Högberg L, et al. Gut microflora associated characteristics in children with celiac disease. *Am J Gastroenterol* 2005;**100**(12):2784–8.

123. Kopecný J, Mrázek J, Fliegerová K, Frühauf P, Tucková L. The intestinal microflora of childhood patients with indicated celiac disease. *Folia Microbiol (Praha)* 2008;**53**(3):214–6.

124. Stoven S, Murray JA, Marietta E. Celiac disease: advances in treatment via gluten modification. *Clin Gastroenterol Hepatol* 2012;**10**(8):859–62.

125. Tye-Din JA, Anderson RP, Ffrench RA, et al. The effects of ALV003 pre-digestion of gluten on immune response and symptoms in celiac disease. *in vivo. Clin Immunol* 2010;**134**(3):289–95.

126. Gass J, Bethune MT, Siegel M, Spencer A, Khosla C. Combination enzyme therapy for gastric digestion of dietary gluten in patients with celiac sprue. *Gastroenterology* 2007;**133**(2):472–80.

127. Siegel M, Garber ME, Spencer AG, et al. Safety, tolerability, and activity of ALV003: results from two phase I single, escalating-dose clinical trials. *Dig Dis Sci* 2012;**57**(2):440–50.

128. Stepniak D, Spaenij-Dekking L, Mitea C, et al. Highly efficient gluten degradation with a newly identified prolyl endoprotease: implications for celiac disease. *Am J Physiol Gastrointest Liver Physiol* 2006;**291**(4):G621–9.

129. Mitea C, Havenaar R, Drijfhout JW, Edens L, Dekking L, Koning F. Efficient degradation of gluten by a prolyl endoprotease in a gastrointestinal model: implications for coeliac disease. *Gut* 2008;**57**(1):25–32.

130. Mukherjee R, Kelly CP, Schuppan D. Nondietary therapies for celiac disease. *Gastrointest Endosc Clin N Am* 2012;**22**(4):811–31.

131. Caputo I, Lepretti M, Martucciello S, Esposito C. Enzymatic strategies to detoxify gluten: implications for celiac disease. *Enzyme Res* 2010;**2010**:174354.

132. Gujral N, Freeman HJ, Thomson AB. Celiac disease: prevalence, diagnosis, pathogenesis and treatment. *World J Gastroenterol* 2012;**18**(42):6036–59.

133. Tennyson CA, Lewis SK, Green PH. New and developing therapies for celiac disease. *Therap Adv Gastroenterol* 2009;**2**(5):303–9.

134. Gass J, Khosla C. Prolyl endopeptidases. *Cell Mol Life Sci* 2007;**64**(3):345–55.

135. Tack G, van de Water J, Kooy-Winkelaar E, et al. Can prolyl endoprotease enzyme treatment mitigate the toxic effect of gluten in coeliac patients? *Gastroenterology* 2010;**138**(5) S-54.

136. Crespo Pérez L, Castillejo de Villasante G, Cano Ruiz A, León F. Non-dietary therapeutic clinical trials in coeliac disease. *Eur J Intern Med* 2012;**23**(1):9–14.

137. Siegel M, Bethune MT, Gass J, et al. Rational design of combination enzyme therapy for celiac sprue. *Chem Biol* 2006;**13**(6):649–58.

138. Lahdeaho M, Maki M, Kaukinen K, et al. ALV003, a novel glutenase, attenuates gluten-induced small intestinal mucosal injury in celiac disease patients: a randomized controlled phase 2A clinical trial. *Gut* 2011;**60** A12.

139. Ehren J, Morón B, Martin E, Bethune MT, Gray GM, Khosla C. A food-grade enzyme preparation with modest gluten detoxification properties. *PLoS One* 2009;**4**(7):e6313.

140. Korponay-Szabo IR, Tumpek J, Gyimesi J, et al. Food-grade gluten degrading enzymes to treat dietary transgressions in coeliac adolescents. *J Pediatr Gastroenterol Nutr* 2010;**50** E68.

CHAPTER

14

Adverse Reactions to Gluten: Exploitation of Sourdough Fermentation

Raffaella Di Cagno, Carlo Giuseppe Rizzello, Marco Gobbetti

University of Bari Aldo Moro, Department of Soil, Plant and Food Science, Bari, Italy

INTRODUCTION

Celiac disease (CD), also known as celiac sprue and gluten-sensitive enteropathy, is a food hypersensitivity disorder caused by an inflammatory response to wheat gluten and similar proteins of barley and rye.[1] In recent years, the view of CD has undergone a profound revision. Nowadays, CD is considered, more than just a gluten-sensitive enteropathy, to be a systemic immune-mediated disorder elicited by gluten and related prolamines in genetically susceptible individuals. The common denominator for all subjects with CD is the presence of a variable combination of gluten-dependent clinical manifestations, specific autoantibodies (antitissue transglutaminase [TG]2 /anti-endomysium [EMA] antibodies), HLA-DQ2 and / or DQ8 haplotypes, and different degrees of enteropathy, ranging from lymphocytic infiltration of the epithelium to complete villous atrophy.[2] Reports of CD date back to the first century AD,[3] but it was not until 1888 that Samuel Gee gave the classical description of the disease,[4] and it was only in the 1930s that Dicke demonstrated that removal of wheat from the diet alleviated symptoms and signs of CD.[5] Nowadays, the prevalence of CD worldwide is increasing; it is estimated to be 0.5–2.0% in most of the European countries and the United States.[6] Such a rate establishes CD as one of the most common food intolerances.[7]

Gluten may also induce other pathological conditions, such as wheat allergy (WA),[8] which is an immunoglobulin (Ig)E-mediated disease also well characterized from the immunological and clinical point of view but completely unrelated to CD. More recently, attention was given to another entity, gluten sensitivity (GS), for which the limits and possible overlap with CD are still poorly defined.[9] GS subjects are unable to tolerate gluten and develop an adverse reaction when eating gluten that usually, and differently from CD, does not lead to damage in the small intestine. A number of morphological, functional, and immunological disorders have been considered under the umbrella of GS that miss one or more of the key CD criteria (enteropathy, associated HLA haplotypes, and presence of anti-TG2 antibodies), but respond to gluten exclusion.

Nowadays, the only effective treatment for CD consists of a lifelong gluten-free diet (GFD). The regression of symptoms in response to a GFD was also showed in WA and GS subjects. Nevertheless, gluten is a common, and in many countries unlabeled, ingredient in the human diet, presenting a big challenge for CD and WA patients, or GS subjects. There has therefore become an increasingly urgent need to develop safe and effective alternatives.

Beyond genetic predisposition, several environmental factors influence adverse reactions to gluten. Recent epidemiological studies show that the introduction of gluten-containing grains, which occurred about 10,000 years ago with the advent of agriculture, represented an evolutionary challenge that created the conditions for human diseases related to gluten exposure.[10] More recently, cereal food technology has changed dramatically by influencing the dietary habitudes of entire populations previously naïve to gluten exposure. Cereal baked goods are currently manufactured by a very accelerated process where long fermentations by sourdough, a cocktail of acidifying and proteolytic lactic acid bacteria with or without *Saccharomyces cerevisiae*, were almost totally replaced by the indiscriminate use of chemical and/or baker's yeast leavening agents. Under these technological circumstances, cereal components (e.g., proteins) are subjected to very mild or absent degradation during manufacture, resulting, probably, in less digestible foods compared to traditional and ancient sourdough baked goods.[11]

This chapter focuses on the biotechnologies that use selected sourdough lactic acid bacteria or probiotics to potentially counteract or decrease the adverse reactions to gluten (CD, WA, and GS) and the risk of gluten contamination.

SOURDOUGH AND CELIAC DISEASE

The Codex Alimentarius Commission of the World Health Organization and the FAO distinguishes gluten-free foods as those consisting of ingredients from wheat, rye, barley, oats, spelt, and their crossbred varieties with a gluten level of <20 ppm, or those that have been rendered GF with a gluten level of <200 ppm.[12] Recent advances have improved the understanding of the molecular basis of the CD disorder, and several targets have been developed for new treatments. Among the novel therapies for CD, the enzyme strategy to detoxify gluten is currently considered. It includes the oral administration of several bacterial endopeptidases, which have shown a different degree of tolerance to the gastrointestinal conditions.[13,14] During the past 10 years a biotechnological strategy has been developed that resembles the ancient tradition of using sourdough for breadmaking, in order to investigate its effect on CD. Primary and secondary proteolysis occurs during sourdough fermentation (Fig. 14.1). The primary activity of cereal proteases is promoted by acidification and the reduction of disulfide bonds of gluten by hetero-fermentative lactobacilli, which leads to the liberation of various sized polypeptides. Intracellular peptidases of sourdough lactic acid bacteria complete the proteolysis and liberate free amino acids, which in turn are subjected to various catabolic reactions by the same microorganisms.[15] When optimized and tailored, the degradation of cereal proteins may also have important repercussions on functional features of leavened baked goods. Preliminary studies on the hydrolysis of prolamins (>6000 ppm of gluten) from wheat and rye by using selected sourdough lactobacilli[16–20] created the required conditions for using these cereals in the GFD. An improved biotechnology protocol, which included a pool of 10 selected sourdough lactobacilli and fungal proteases, hydrolyzed gluten to less than 100 ppm during lengthy fermentation[21] (Fig. 14.2). Activity of fungal proteases was responsible for primary proteolysis, liberating various sized polypeptides. The large proportion of proline residues in the amino acid sequences characterizing the toxic peptides make them extremely resistant to further hydrolysis.[22–24] The specific cyclic structure of the proline imposes many restrictions on the structural aspects of peptides. To deal adequately with such peptides, a group of specific peptidases is necessary to hydrolyze peptide bonds. Prolyl endopeptidases (PEPs) of microbial origin are endoproteolytic enzymes that, in contrast to human gastrointestinal proteases, may readily cleave Pro-rich immune-stimulatory gluten peptides.[24] Through a complex system of ABC and ATP transporters, gluten peptides are moved across the cytoplasmic membrane of sourdough lactobacilli. Just a few minutes after entry, the concentration of polypeptides markedly decreases, being about 100 times lower than that in the environment.[25] A pool of intracellular peptidases of the selected sourdough lactobacilli was used to stimulate hydrolysis towards the 33-mer epitope (Fig. 14.1). The combined activity of peptidases was responsible for the complete degradation of the 33-mer or other synthetic immunogenic peptides, which occurred within 14 hours of incubation.[25] Lactic acid bacteria possess a very complex peptidase system,[26] although there is no unique strain that possesses the entire pattern of peptidases needed for hydrolyzing all the potential peptides where Pro is involved. Sweet baked goods were made using the complete hydrolyzed wheat flour. Two clinical challenges were carried out on celiac patients, who ingested the equivalent of approximately 8 or 10 g of native gluten per day for 60 days.[14,27] Hematology, serology, and intestinal permeability analyses showed complete tolerance by all celiac patients throughout the trial period; none of the CD patients suffered clinical complaints and none produced anti-TG2 antibodies or had modification of the small intestinal mucosa. No increase of CD3 and gamma delta cells was found, and the Marsh grade was unchanged after the challenge.

SOURDOUGH AND CEREAL ALLERGIES

Food allergies are of concern to both healthcare providers and the general population because of their markedly increased prevalence during the past few decades.[25] It is estimated that true food allergies affect up to 6–8% of children younger than 10 years of age, and 1–4% of the adult population.[28] Food allergies are immunologically mediated hypersensitivity responses to food antigens.[29] Typically, the immunological mechanism in food allergies is an immunoglobulin IgE-mediated Type I response, although recent advances reveal that food allergies may also involve Type II and Type IV components.[30] Expression of atopy (i.e., the atopic phenotype) is characterized by high serum total IgE concentration and by the presence of IgE antibodies specific to ordinarily harmless environmental antigens. IgE-mediated responses are characteristically divided in two phases: (1) the induction phase, during which the sensitization to an allergen occurs, and (ii) the effector phase, during which the clinical manifestations of allergy are triggered and expressed.

A list of identified allergens has been reported by International Union of Immunological Societies Allergen Nomenclature Subcommittee (www.allergome.org). Wheat flour (*Triticum aestivum* and *T. turgidum* var.

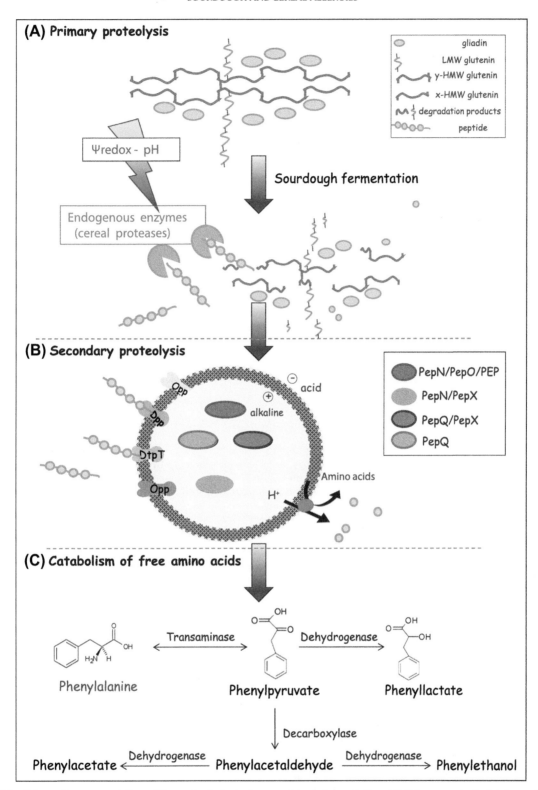

FIGURE 14.1 **Schematic representation of the proteolysis during sourdough fermentation.** (A) Primary proteolysis triggered by the acidification and reduction of disulfide bonds of gluten by hetero-fermentative lactobacilli, which in turn promote the primary activity of cereal proteases, which leads to the liberation of various sized polypeptides. (B) Secondary proteolysis by intracellular peptidases of sourdough lactic acid bacteria, which complete the proteolysis and liberate free amino acids. PepN, general aminopeptidase type N (EC3.4.11.11); PepO, endopeptidase (EC 3.4.23); PEP prolyl endopeptidyl peptidase (EC 3.4.21.26); PepX, X-prolyl dipeptidyl aminopeptidase (EC 3.4.14.5); PepQ, prolidase (EC 3.4.13.9). (C) Catabolism of free amino acids by sourdough lactic acid bacteria: example of catabolic reaction involving phenylalanine. *Figure adapted from Gobbetti et al.[45] See color plate at the back of the book.*

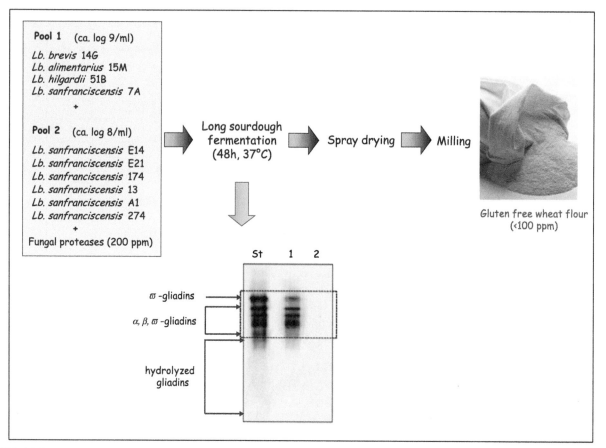

FIGURE 14.2 Schematic representation of the biotechnology protocol, which includes two pools (1 and 2) of 10 selected sourdough lactobacilli, fungal proteases (200 ppm), and long fermentation time (48 h, 37°C). The resulting wheat flour contains hydrolyzed gluten at less than 100 ppm, as shown by R5-Western blot gel. St, European gliadin standard; 1, chemically acidified dough; 2, dough fermented with selected lactobacilli and proteases. Lb, *Lactobacillus*. See color plate at the back of the book.

durum) constitutes one of the most frequent causes of food allergy. Depending on the route of exposure, cereal allergies may induce several clinical manifestations: classical food allergy affecting the skin, gut or respiratory tract; exercise-induced anaphylaxis; occupational rhinitis or asthma; and contact dermatitis. IgE antibodies play a fundamental role in all these clinical manifestations.[31,32] It was shown that gastrointestinal enzymes (pepsin, pancreatin, and trypsin) are not able to degrade cereal allergens, which reach the intestine unaltered, where they elicit the immune response.[33]

Identification of the wheat allergens was carried out by immunoblotting, preceded by electrophoresis of the proteins. In particular, immunoblotting methods were based on the use of sera from patients suffering from allergic symptoms after cereal ingestion.[25] Such analyses indicated that different protein components might contain IgE-reactive epitopes (e.g., low-Mr glutenin subunits and, especially, albumins, globulins, and gliadins in wheat).[25] Nineteen potential wheat allergens, such as α-amylase inhibitors, β-amylase, profilin, serpin, β-D-glucan exohydrolase, and 27K protein, were identified.[34] Through ELISA protocols, a comparison of IgE antibodies against wheat allergens in sera of allergic and healthy subjects was carried out.[34] IgA- and IgE-reactive antigens in wheat, using sera from patients with celiac disease and food allergy to wheat, were compared through two-dimensional electrophoresis (2-DE). IgA antibodies from celiac patients and IgE antibodies from allergenic patients recognized different profiles of wheat antigens.[35] Therefore, wheat contains antigens/epitopes that are preferentially recognized by celiac patients, whereas others elicit IgE-mediated food allergy.

After wheat, rye (*Secale cereale*) represents one of the most important cereals in the world economy. Most of the world rye harvest is used for breadmaking, especially in Central, Northern, and Eastern European countries. Rye flour was also considered a cause of food allergy. Rye secalins were shown to cross-react with ω-5 gliadin, one of the major allergens in wheat-dependent exercise-induced anaphylaxis, thus suggesting that they may also elicit symptoms in patients affected by cereal allergy.[36]

Processing of foods may influence the allergenicity of food proteins. The extent of the effects depends on several determinants, including the allergen and its biochemical and immunological properties, food matrix, processing conditions, thermodynamics of allergen–IgE interaction, and patient sensitivity (threshold, tolerance and permanency of allergenic reaction to a specific allergen).[37] Protein profiling through 2-DE and allergen detection by IgE have become powerful methods for analyzing changes of allergen content in complex matrixes during food processing and ipo-allergenic food production.[36,38,39]

Currently, the only treatment for food allergy is elimination of the offending food from the diet. Several proactive modalities, such as peptide immunotherapy, DNA immunization with immunostimulatory sequences, and anti-IgE therapy, are under investigation to provide an effective treatment for and prevention of food allergies in the near future.[36] However, enzymatic processing of raw materials may remove the allergenicity. Prerequisites are sufficient contact between the allergen, or epitope, and the enzyme, and sufficient control of undesired side effects that may affect sensory quality or processing properties. In some cases, proteolytic processing is insufficient to reduce allergenicity.[40] This may arise because of poor contact between proteases and allergens in the food matrix, or lack of specific proteases. However, the allergenicity of wheat flour prolamins may be decreased by treatment with the protease bromelain, which cleaves the prolamin IgE–epitope Gln–Gln–Gln–Pro–Pro near the proline residues, or by treatment with a non-food grade bacterial collagenase.[41]

Recently, it was demonstrated that selected high proteolytic lactic acid bacteria decreased the IgE-binding proteins from wheat and rye flours during sourdough fermentation.[36,38] In particular, hydrolysis of immunoreactive proteins was investigated after sourdough fermentation and after treatment of sourdough breads with enzymes (pepsin, trypsin, and pancreatin), mimicking the digestive process.[36] As shown by immunoblotting with sera from allergic patients, wheat sourdough fermentation caused the disappearance of some IgE-binding proteins (albumins/globulins and gliadins, mainly) with respect to the chemically acidified dough used as the control.[36] The IgE-binding protein profile of sourdough breads differed from those of baker's yeast breads. Moreover, the signals of the IgE-binding proteins contained in the sourdough breads disappeared after *in vitro* digestion with enzymes. The same effect by digestive enzymes was not found for baker's yeast breads, which showed persistent IgE-binding proteins. Thus, proteolytic activity by selected sourdough lactic acid bacteria may have a key role during food processing and might be employed to produce predigested products containing IgE-binding proteins degradable by digestive enzymes.[36] With the same approach, the capacity of the commercial probiotic preparation (VSL#3, VSL Pharmaceutical Inc., Gaithersburg, USA) to hydrolyze cereal allergens was studied.[38] When used as starters for breadmaking, probiotics determined a marked degradation of wheat proteins, including some IgE-binding proteins (e.g., the putative transcription factor APFI). Overall, hydrolysis of the immunoreactive proteins was achieved without a loss of functional performance, and with the hypoallergenic flour still being able to produce a muffin[41] or bread.[36,38]

SOURDOUGH AND GLUTEN SENSITIVITY

Beyond CD, the scientific community has recently defined GS as all those disorders attributed to gluten ingestion that do not meet the diagnostic criteria for celiac disease and that are probably involved in several pathologies, such as irritable bowel syndrome.[42] Reactions ascribed to GS do not involve allergic or autoimmune mechanisms. Intestinal (e.g., diarrhea, abdominal discomfort or pain, bloating) or extra-intestinal (headache, lethargy, attention-deficit/hyperactivity disorder, ataxia or recurrent oral ulceration) symptoms are often manifested during GS.[43] It is well established that GS symptoms decrease or disappear after gluten is withdrawn from the diet,[43] and very little is known about the quantity and the mechanisms that can trigger diseases and digestive problems.

It was hypothesized that daily consumption of wheat products with an intermediate content of gluten (significantly lower than the current one) may have a delaying effect on the susceptibility to GS, or even cause the absence of symptoms. Indeed, approaches targeting the uptake of toxic gluten peptides through enzyme breakdown, sequestering gluten, or restoring the epithelial barrier function were developed at the level of clinical trials. Thermal and enzyme treatments to obtain hypoallergenic or low-gluten wheat flour were proposed for making modified-gluten products, which are tolerated by susceptible individuals.[44]

With the aim of reducing, in part, the gluten concentration of wheat flour and increasing the proteolysis during food processing, the parameters of sourdough fermentation previously proposed for the complete gluten hydrolysis by Rizzello and colleagues[21] were modified, setting up a biotechnological process preserving the sensory acceptability and the technological properties of the flour. The degree of proteolysis, corresponding to a reduction of approximately 30% of the initial gluten (~ 58,000 ppm), was investigated by immunological, electrophoretic, and chromatographic analyses. The wheat flour with the intermediate content of gluten was used for breadmaking at pilot plant scale, and compared to a wheat flour bread control.[44] Chemical, structural, and sensory features were investigated, showing the technological suitability of the flour with the intermediate content of gluten and the good overall taste of the bread. The *in vitro* protein digestibility of the mild-gluten bread was higher than the control, as well as the nutritional quality, estimated by the calculation of different indexes (e.g., chemical and protein scores, essential amino acids index, protein efficiency ratio, biological value, and nutritional index).[44] All the improvements in the nutritional features of breads are related to the proteolysis carried out by lactic acid bacteria and fungal proteases during fermentation of flour. Nevertheless, *in vivo* studies are certainly needed to confirm this potentiality.

CONCLUDING REMARKS

The compliance with a gluten-free diet is an extremely challenging task, given the problems related to cross-contamination and lack of clear food labeling policies. Sourdough fermentation is a traditional process that has retained its importance in wheat baking because it improves bread quality by prolonging shelf life, increasing loaf volume, delaying staling, and improving bread flavor and nutritional properties.

Fermentation of wheat flours with selected sourdough lactic acid bacteria and fungal proteases following an ancient protocol which includes a long fermentation time has an effect on decreasing the gluten toxicity, as shown by several analytic techniques and several *in vitro*, *ex vivo*, and *in vivo* trials. Obviously, such wheat preparations with extended fermentation and completely degraded gluten need, likely the naturally gluten-free matrices, baking improvers to be used into gluten-free recipes. In response to the evolution of consumer demand, the protocol for obtaining flour with an intermediate content of gluten by sourdough fermentation may be also considered a useful tool for the manufacture of innovative and healthy foods.

References

1. Maki M, Mustalahti K, Korhonen J, Kulmala P, Haapalahti M, Karttunen T. Prevalence of celiac disease among children in Finland. *N Engl J Med* 2003;**348**:2517–24.
2. Di Sabatino A, Corazza GR. Coeliac disease. *Lancet* 2009;**373**:1480–93.
3. Adams F, translator. *On The Cœliac Affection. The extant works of Aretaeus, The Cappadocian*. London: Sydenham Society; 1856. p. 350–1.
4. Gee S. *On the celiac disease*. London: Saint Bartholomew's Hospital Reports; 1888;**24**:17–20.
5. Van Berge-Henegouwen GP, Mulder CJJ. Pioneer in the gluten free diet: Willem-Karel Dicke 1905-1962, over 50 years of gluten free diet. *Gut* 1993;**34**:1473–5.
6. Rewers M. Epidemiology of celiac disease: what are the prevalence, incidence, and progression of celiac disease? *Gastroenterology* 2005;**128**:47–51.
7. Fasano A, Catassi C. Current approaches to diagnosis and treatment of celiac disease: an evolving spectrum. *Gastroenterology* 2001;**120**:636–51.
8. Battais F, Richard C, Jacquenet S, Denery-Papini S, Moneret-Vautrin DA. Wheat grain allergies: an update on wheat allergens. *Eur Ann Allergy Clin Immunol* 2008;**40**:67–76.
9. Verdu EF, Armstrong D, Murray JA. Between celiac disease and irritable bowel syndrome: the "no man's land" of gluten sensitivity. *Am J Gastroenterol* 2009;**104**:1587–94.
10. Fasano A. *Prevalence and genetics, in AGA clinical Symposium-Celiac Disease Clinical Symposium, Program and abstracts of Digestive Disease Week*. New Orleans: Louisiana; 2004 May 15–20.
11. Gobbetti M. The sourdough microflora: interactions between lactic acid bacteria and yeast. *Trends Food Sci Technol* 1998;**9**:267–74.
12. Gallagher E, Gormley TR, Arendt EK. Recent advances in the formulation of gluten-free cereal-based products. *Trends Food Sci Technol* 2004;**15**:143–52.
13. Caputo I, Lepretti M, Martucciello S, Esposito C. Enzymatic strategies to detoxify gluten: implications for celiac disease. *Enzyme Res* 2010;**2010**:174354–64.
14. Di Cagno R, Barbato M, Di Camillo C, Rizzello CG, De Angelis M, Giuliani G, et al. Gluten-free sourdough wheat baked goods appear safe for young celiac patients: a pilot study. *Hepatol Nutr* 2010;**51**:777–83.
15. Gaenzle MG, Loponena J, Gobbetti M. Proteolysis in sourdough fermentations: mechanisms and potential for improved bread quality. *Trends Food Sci Technol* 2008;**19**:513–21.
16. Di Cagno R, De Angelis M, Lavermicocca P, De Vincenzi M, Giovannini C, Faccia M, et al. Proteolysis by sourdough lactic acid bacteria: effects on wheat flour protein fractions and gliadin peptides involved in human cereal intolerance. *Appl Environ Microbiol* 2002;**68**:623–33.
17. Di Cagno R, De Angelis M, Auricchio S, Greco L, Clarke C, De Vincenzi M, et al. Sourdough bread made from wheat and nontoxic flours and started with selected lactobacilli is tolerated in celiac sprue patients. *Appl Environ Microbiol* 2004;**70**:1088–96.
18. De Angelis M, Coda R, Silano M, Minervini F, Rizzello CG, Di Cagno R, et al. Fermentation by selected sourdough lactic acid bacteria to decrease coeliac intolerance to rye flour. *J Cereal Sci* 2006a;**43**:301–14.
19. De Angelis M, Rizzello CG, Fasano A, Clemente MG, De Simone C, De Vincenzi M, et al. VSL#3 probiotic preparation has the capacity to hydrolyze gliadin polypeptides responsible for celiac sprue. *Biochim Biophys Acta* 2006b;**1762**:80–93.
20. Gobbetti M, Rizzello CG, Di Cagno R, De Angelis M. Sourdough lactobacilli and celiac disease. *Food Microbiol* 2007;**24**:187–96.
21. Rizzello CG, De Angelis M, Di Cagno R, Camarca A, Silano M, Losito I, et al. Highly efficient gluten degradation by lactobacilli and fungal proteases during food processing: new perspectives for celiac disease. *Appl Environ Microbiol* 2007;**73**:4499–4407.
22. Auricchio S, Greco L, De Vizia B, Buonocore V. Dipeptidylaminopeptidase and carboxypeptidases activities of the brush border of rabbit small intestine. *Gastroenterol* 1978;**75**:1073–9.
23. Andria G, Cucchiara S, De Vizia B, De Ritis G, Mazzacca G, Auricchio S. Brush border and cytosol peptidase activities of human small intestine in normal subjects and celiac patients. *Pediatr Res* 1980;**14**:812–8.
24. Hausch F, Shan L, Santiago NA, Gray GM, Khosla C. Intestinal digestive resistance of immunodominant gliadin peptides. *Am J Physiol Gastrointest Liver Physiol* 2002;**283**:996–903.
25. De Angelis, Cassone A, Rizzello CG, Gagliardi F, Minervini F, Calasso M, et al. Mechanism of degradation of immunogenic gluten epitopes from *Triticum turgidum* L. var. *durum* by sourdough lactobacilli and fungal proteases. *Appl Environ Microbiol* 2010;**76**:508–18.
26. Kunji ERS, Mierau I, Hagting A, Poolman B, Konings WN. The proteolytic systems of lactic acid bacteria. *Ant Van Leeuwen* 1996;**70**:187–121.

27. Greco L, Gobbetti M, Auricchio R, Di Mase R, Landolfi F, Paparo F, et al. Safety for patients with celiac disease of baked goods made of wheat flour hydrolyzed during food processing. *Clin Gastroenterol Hepatol* 2011;**9**:24–9.

28. Kerbach S, Alldrick AJ, Crevel RWR, Dömötör L, DunnGalvin A, Mills ENC, et al. Managing food allergens in the food supply chain – viewed from different stakeholder perspectives. *Qual Assur Safety Crops Foods* 2009;**1**:50–60.

29. Johansson SGO, Hourihane JO, Bousquet J, et al. A revised nomenclature for allergy. An EAACI position statement from the EAACI nomenclature task force. *Allergy* 2001;**56**:813–24.

30. Johansson SG, Hourihane JO, Bousquet J, Bruijnzeel-Koomen C, Dreborg S, Haahtela T, et al. Revised nomenclature for allergy for global use: Report of the Nomenclature Review Committee of the World Allergy Organization. *J Allergy Clin Immunol* 2004;**113**:832–6.

31. Baldo BA, Wrigley CW. IgE antibodies to wheat flour components. Studies with sera from subjects with baker's asthma or celiac conditions. *Clin Allergy* 1978;**8**:109–24.

32. Ortolani C, Ispano M, Scibilia J, Pastorello EA. Introducing chemists to food allergy. *Allergy* 2001;**56**:5–8.

33. Astwood DJ, Leach JN, Fuchs RL. Stability of food allergens to digestion *in vitro*. *Nature Biotechnol* 1996;**14**:1269–73.

34. Sotkovský P, Hubálek M, Hernychová L, Novák P, Havranová M, Setinová I, et al. Proteomic analysis of wheat proteins recognized by IgE antibodies of allergic patients. *Proteomics* 2008;**8**:1677–91.

35. Costantin C, Huber WD, Granditsch G, Weghofer M, Valenta R. Different profiles of wheat antigens are recognised by patients suffering from coeliac disease and IgE-mediated food allergy. *Int Arch Allergy Immunol* 2005;**138**:257–66.

36. Rizzello CG, De Angelis M, Coda R, Gobbetti M. Use of selected sourdough lactic acid bacteria to hydrolyze wheat and rye proteins responsible for cereal allergy. *Eur Food Res Technol* 2006;**223**:405–11.

37. Shridhar KS, Girdhari MS. Effects of food processing on food allergens. *Mol Nutr Food Res* 2009;**53**:970–8.

38. De Angelis M, Rizzello CG, Scala E, De Simone C, Farris GA, Turrini F, et al. Probiotic preparation has the capacity to hydrolyze proteins responsible for wheat allergy. *J Food Prot* 2007;**70**:135–44.

39. Thomas K, Herouet-Guicheney C, Ladics G, Bannond G, Cockburn A, Crevel R, et al. Evaluating the effects of food processing on the potential human allergenicity of novel proteins: international workshop report. *Food Chem Toxicol* 2007;**45**:1116–22.

40. Malesi SJ. Food processing: effects on allergenicity. *Curr Opinion Allergy Clin Immunol* 2004;**4**:241–45.

41. Tanabe S, Arai S, Yanagihara Y, Mita H, Takahashi K, Watanabe M. A major wheat allergen has a Gln–Gln–Gln–Pro–Pro motif identified as an IgE-binding epitope. *Biochem Biophys Res Comm* 1996;**219**:290–3.

42. Troncone R, Jabri B. Coeliac disease and gluten sensitivity. *J Int Med* 2011;**269**:582–90.

43. Di Sabatino AD, Corazza GR. Non celiac gluten sensitive: sense or sensibility? *Annals Internal Med* 2012;**156**:309–11.

44. Rizzello CG, Curiel JA, Nionelli L, Vincentini O, Di Cagno R, Silano M, et al. Use of fungal proteases and selected sourdough lactic acid bacteria for making wheat bread with an intermediate content of gluten. *Food Microbiol* 2013 in press.

45. Gobbetti M, Rizzello CG, Di Cagno R, De Angelis M. How the sourdough may affect the functional features of leavened baked goods. *Food Microbiol* 2013 in press.

WHEAT FIBER

Antioxidant Properties of Wheat Bran against Oxidative Stress

Masashi Higuchi

Meiji University, Organization for the Strategic Coordination of Research and Intellectual Property, Kawasaki, Kanagawa, Japan

INTRODUCTION

The importance of wheat as a food component in humans has been mainly attributed to its ability to be ground into flour and semolina, which are the basic ingredients of bread (and other bakery products) and pasta, respectively.[1] Wheat bran, the hard outer layer of wheat grain, which includes part of the endosperm, is a by-product of wheat grain milling and grinding, and has also been used as a component of various animal feeds on a long-term basis. The physiological effects of wheat bran can be split into the following: nutritional effects from its constituent nutrients; mechanical effects in the gastrointestinal tract due to its fiber content; and antioxidant effects arising from its phytochemical constituents. Wheat bran has higher antioxidant activity than other milled fractions,[2] and contains various components such as phytic acid, polyphenols (including lignans and phenolic acids), vitamins, and minerals.[3] Moreover, components of wheat bran possess health benefits for humans, including preventative effects against cancer and type 2 diabetes.[4,5] Various studies have reported that these compounds exhibit significant antioxidant capabilities, including scavenging free radicals (e.g., reducing lipid oxidation), chelating metal ions, and activating antioxidant enzymes,[6–11] suggesting antioxidant properties of wheat bran. This chapter includes an overview of stress and oxidative stress and a discussion of the antioxidant properties of wheat bran.

WHAT IS STRESS?

Stress has been defined by abnormal alterations in physiological homeostasis such as bleeding, frigidity, exercise, hypoxia, and hypoglycemia.[12] In contrast, Selye defined stress as a condition characterized by systemic non-specific responses that are not due to a specific type of stimulus.[13] In reality, the body responds differently to different stimuli through specific and/or non-specific responses, and these can at times be difficult to quantify.[14] Nevertheless, these responses are generally and scientifically collectively referred to by the term "stress". Epidemiological research has identified stress as an exacerbating factor in many disorders – for example, an index combining stress and metabolic syndrome is used as an index of life expectancy.[15]

Stress factors are referred to as "stressors". As shown in Table 15.1, stressors are divided into two main classes, physiological and psychological. Recently analysis of biological alterations has demonstrated the presence of many factors involved in stress and biological regulation. Identifying the biological mechanism of stress and inhibiting the decline in biological function that it causes are important for maintaining good health in human and animals. The next section focuses on a specific type of stress, namely oxidative stress.

OXIDATIVE STRESS

Oxygen is an essential molecule for producing energy from foodstuffs in aerobic animals, whereas reactive oxygen, which is generated through the metabolism of oxygen, plays an important role in the maintenance of life in processes such as signal transduction and sterilization.[16,17] However, when reactive oxygen is produced in excess, it is associated with a great risk of toxicity in living organisms. Due to the existence of protective mechanisms for removing excess reactive oxygen, living

TABLE 15.1 Stressor as Cause of Stress

Case	Causal Factor
PHYSIOLOGICAL STIMULATION	
Physical stressor	Frigidity, noise, overwork, sleep deprivation, radioactivity
Chemical stressor	Oxygen, drug, food, cigarette
Biological stressor	Inflammation, infection, pollen
PSYCHOLOGICAL STIMULATION	
Psychological stressor	Anger, anxiety

TABLE 15.2 Respective Reactive Oxygen Species

Chemical Term	Molecular Formula	Half-Life (s)
RADICAL		
Superoxide anion radical	$O_2^{\bullet-}$	10^{-5}
Hydroxyl radical	$OH^{\bullet}$	10^{-9}
Peroxyl radical	$LOO^{\bullet}$	7
Alkoxyl radical	$LO^{\bullet}$	10^{-5}
NON-RADICAL		
Hydrogen peroxide	H_2O_2	Stable
Lipid hydroperoxide	LOOH	–
Hypochlorous acid	HClO	Stable
Ozon	O_3	Stable
Singlet oxygen	$^1O_2$	10^{-6}

organisms can cope effectively with this stress. However, tissue damage and failure arising from cancer, diabetes, and arteriosclerosis are caused by a disruption in the homeostatic balance between levels of reactive oxygen and the body's protective mechanisms,[16] referred to as oxidative stress.

Two types of reactive oxygen species (ROS) exist *in vivo*: (1) radicals with an unpaired electron, and (2) non-radicals with a paired electron, which can be subjected to the production of the radicals (Table 15.2). When oxygen is metabolized to water, superoxide anion radical ($O_2^{\bullet-}$) and hydrogen peroxide (H_2O_2) are produced, and hydroxyl radical ($OH^{\bullet}$) is generated in the presence of transition metal ions such as ferrous and cuprous ions. Therefore, during reaction with other radicals or molecules, new forms of free radicals or ROS are formed. Each ROS is characterized by different reactivities and half-life periods, and plays positive or negative roles. The following section describes the respective ROS and their transition metal ions.

Reactive Oxygen Species (ROS)

$O_2^{\bullet-}$ is produced under steady-state conditions by electron transport chains in mitochondria or chloroplasts, and by enzyme reactions in macrophages or neutrophils.[16,18] The amount of $O_2^{\bullet-}$ produced *in vivo* accounts for approximately 1–2% of oxygen molecules used in respiration. $O_2^{\bullet-}$ is produced by the addition of an electron to dioxygen, after which it becomes highly reactive (Eq. 1). However, $O_2^{\bullet-}$ itself does relatively little damage in the cell. Moreover, it is considered that the selective barrier does not allow $O_2^{\bullet-}$ to pass through. $O_2^{\bullet-}$ is metabolized by superoxide dismutase (SOD) enzyme under acidic conditions, leading to the formation of H_2O_2 (Eq. 2).

$$O_2 + e^- \rightarrow O_2^{\bullet-} \tag{1}$$

$$2O_2^{\bullet-} + 2H^+ \rightarrow H_2O_2 + O_2 \dots \tag{2}$$

H_2O_2 is widely generated by other enzymatic reactions in addition to its production via metabolism of $O_2^{\bullet-}$. Because H_2O_2 is not a free radical and does not contain unpaired electrons, it does not damage the cell due to its relatively low toxicity. However, once H_2O_2 has been produced it accumulates inside the cell for a long period due to its extended half-life, and diffuses through the plasma membrane; locally-generated H_2O_2 can cause cell injury.

Thy hydroxyl radical ($OH^{\bullet}$) is a neutral form of the hydroxide ion and has a high reactivity, making it a very dangerous radical with a very short *in vivo* half-life of approximately 10^{-9}s. Therefore, when produced *in vivo*, $OH^{\bullet}$ can react close to its site of formation. The production of ROS occurs through a series of chemical reaction (Eqs 3–5). The Haber–Weiss reaction generates $OH^{\bullet}$ from H_2O_2 and $O_2^{\bullet-}$ (Eq. 3) in a reaction catalyzed by transition metal ions, such as iron and copper, and is divided into two steps. The first step of the catalytic cycle involves reduction of the ferric ion to the ferrous ion (Eq. 4). The second step is the Fenton reaction, in which ferrous ion is oxidized by H_2O_2 to the ferric ion, $OH^{\bullet}$, and a hydroxyl anion (Eq. 5). In leukocytes, myeloperoxidase converts H_2O_2 to hypochlorous acid, one of the strongest physiological oxidants and a powerful antimicrobial agent.[19]

$$O_2^{\bullet-} + H_2O_2 \rightarrow O_2 + OH^{\bullet} + OH^- \dots \tag{3}$$

$$Fe^{3+} + O_2^{\bullet-} \rightarrow Fe^{2+} + O_2 \dots \tag{4}$$

$$Fe^{2+} + H_2O_2 \rightarrow Fe^{3+} + OH^{\bullet} + OH^- \dots \tag{5}$$

The schematic reaction of oxidative stress is summarized in Figure 15.1. The resulting $OH^{\bullet}$ can cause DNA strand breaks, inactivate enzymes, and initiate lipid peroxidation,[20–23] and is involved in tissue injury and the development of many diseases such as cancer, chronic

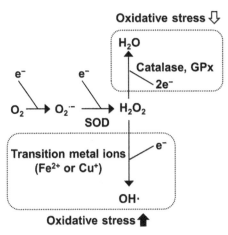

FIGURE 15.1 Schematic view of oxidative stress. The generation of reactive oxygen species, such as superoxide anion radical ($O_2^{\bullet-}$), hydrogen peroxide (H_2O_2), and hydroxyl radical (OH•), is promoted by a series of processes. $O_2^{\bullet-}$ is particularly important as the product of the one electron reduction of dioxygen (O_2). The superoxide dismutase (SOD) catalyzes the neutralization of superoxide followed by the production in H_2O_2. The generated H_2O_2 is decomposed in presences of antioxidant enzymes, such as catalase and glutathione peroxidase (GPx), to O_2 and hydrogen (H_2O). However, high active OH• is produced under a presence of transition metal ions, including iron or copper ions, leading to oxidative stress in the cell.

TABLE 15.3 Complications Caused by Iron Overload Disorder

Tissue	Complication
Liver	Cirrhosis, hepatocarcinoma
Heart	Cardiomyopathy
Pancreas	Diabetes
Pituitary	Hypogonadism
Thyroid	Hypothyroidism
Arthrosis	Arthralgia
Skin	Pigmentation

inflammation, atherosclerotic disease, diabetes, digestive tract disorder, and Alzheimer's and Parkinson's diseases.[16,24–26] Moreover, some reports have shown that continuous ROS induction may lead to premature embryogenesis and aging.[27,28] In summary, ROS generated in diverse tissues contribute to the development of diseases, and the regulation of their production is important to the survival of living organisms.

Iron as Respective Transient Metal Ion

Iron is an essential trace element for almost all organisms, and exists in two forms in the cell.[29] Functional irons are present in oxygen carriers, such as hemoglobin and myoglobin, and in the iron transporter transferrin. In addition, iron functions as a cofactor for redox enzymes, including catalase, aconitase, and succinate dehydrogenase. Therefore, iron is involved in various vital functions such as a resistance to infection, cognitive performance, physical capacity, work output, and, possibly, maintenance of body temperature.[30] Iron is normally stored bound with proteins, such as ferritin and hemosiderin, and is chemically stable. However, as described above, in the presence of an excess of stored iron, free ferrous ions are released more readily. Free iron can function as an electron donor, leading to the production of the most potent ROS, OH•, which in turn damages various cellular components such as membrane lipid, proteins, and nucleic acids through the Fenton reaction.[31,32] Recent study has demonstrated

the effect of diquat-induced oxidative stress on iron metabolism *in vivo*, indicating that high levels of hepatic free iron induce the production of highly reactive OH• through the Fenton reaction, causing subsequent oxidative injury in the liver.[33] Hemosiderosis, the pathological effect of iron accumulation in any given organ, is affected by iron in the form of ferritin and hemosiderin, and leads to tissue damage caused by iron overload disorder (Table 15.3).

Epidemiological studies have shown a relationship between body iron status and diseases in humans, including alcoholic cirrhosis, cancer, and type 2 diabetes.[34–37] Studies using experimental animals have also shown the involvement of iron in the development of atherosclerotic lesions, fulminant hepatitis, and liver cancer.[38,39] These results have demonstrated that iron chelators such as albumin, haptoglobin, lactoferrin, transferrin, and ferritin also have an important role in preventing oxidative stress-related diseases.[40] As described above, inhibiting the accumulation of excess iron and removal of ROS are important for preventing oxidative stress.

ANTIOXIDANT PROPERTIES OF WHEAT BRAN

Oxidation is a chemical reaction that transfers electrons or hydrogen from a substance to an oxidizing agent, leading to the generation of free radicals; antioxidants are molecules that inhibit the oxidation of other molecules. Chain reactions involving free radicals can cause damage or death to the cell. In contrast, antioxidants can terminate these chain reactions by removing free radical intermediates followed by inhibition of continuous oxidation reactions.[16,41] Two types of antioxidant exist: (1) intracellular or extracellular antioxidant enzymes, including catalase, SOD, and peroxidases (Table 15.4); and (2) non-enzymatic antioxidants, including various free radical quenchers such as vitamin C (ascorbic acid), vitamin E (α-tocopherol), vitamin A (carotenoids), flavonoids, thiols (including glutathione, lipoic acid, and ferritin),

TABLE 15.4 Cofactor, Localization, and Target of Antioxidant Enzymes

Antioxidant	Cofactor	Cellular Localization	Main target
Cu–Zn-SOD	Copper, zinc	Intracellular cytoplasmic space	$O_2^{\bullet-}$
Mn-SOD	Manganese	Mitochondrial space	$O_2^{\bullet-}$
EC-SOD	Copper, zinc	Extracellular space	$O_2^{\bullet-}$
Catalase	Iron	Peroxysome	H_2O_2
		Cytosol	
		Mitochondrion	
GPx	Selenium	Cytosol	H_2O_2
		Mitochondrion	LOOH

SOD, superoxide dismutase; GPx, glutathione peroxidase

TABLE 15.5 Antioxidant Properties of Non-enzymatic Antioxidants

Antioxidants	Antioxidant Properties
Vitamin C	Vitamin E regeneration
	GSH regeneration
Vitamin E	Scavenging free radical
	Membrane stabilization
Vitamin A	Scavenging free radical
Flavonoid	Metal ion chelation
	Activation of antioxidant enzyme
	Scavenging free radical
Glutathione	Substrate for GPx
(Reduced form)	Vitamins C and E regeneration
Lipoic acid	Scavenging free radical
	Vitamins C and E regeneration
	GSH regeneration
	Metal ion chelation
Ferritin	Iron chelation
Selenium	GPx cofactor
Lignan	Activation of antioxidant enzyme
	Scavenging free radical
Phytic acid	Metal ion chelation
Phenolic acid	Activation of antioxidant enzymes
	Scavenging free radical
	Metal ion chelation
	Cholesterol reduction

GSH, reduced glutathione; GPx, glutathione peroxidase

and micronutrients (selenium, iron, copper, zinc, and manganese), which act as enzymatic cofactors. Although selenium and other elements are commonly referred to as antioxidant nutrients, chemical elements have no antioxidant action *per se* but are required for the activity of some antioxidant enzymes. Under normal conditions, a balance between the activities and the intracellular levels of these antioxidants is essential for the health and survival of organisms. However, insufficient levels of antioxidants or inhibition of antioxidant enzymes cause oxidative stress and may damage or kill cells. Some compounds also contribute to antioxidant defense by chelating transition metals and preventing them from catalyzing the production of free radicals in the cell. Therefore, antioxidant capacity relies on the ability to scavenge radicals, activate antioxidant enzymes, and chelate transient metal ions.

Recently, antioxidants in grains, vegetables, and fruits have gained considerable attention for their potential in various applications, including improving the quality and safety of food products, preventing chronic diseases, and promoting general human health.[42] Wheat bran contains phytochemicals, such as phytic acid and phenolic acid (e.g., ferulic acid), in addition to antioxidants as described above, and can exert its effects by promoting scavenging of radicals, chelation of metal ions, and the activation of antioxidant enzymes (Table 15.5). The hydrophilic antioxidant activity of bran/germ fractions was shown to be nearly 30-fold higher than that of the respective endosperm fraction. In addition, lipophilic antioxidant activity is up to 90-fold higher in the bran/germ fractions, and the hydrophilic antioxidant activity was >80% of the total antioxidant activity,[6] indicating the characteristic antioxidant properties in wheat bran. Moreover, the ferrous ion chelating activity of bran samples ranges from 1 to 1.9 mg EDTA (a known reducing reagent) equivalent per gram of bran under the same

experimental conditions.[6] In addition to phytochemicals, some studies have reported that wheat bran plays a role in activating antioxidant enzymes, including SOD and GPx.[9–11] Therefore, wheat bran compounds exhibit significant capabilities in scavenging free radicals, chelating metal ion oxidants, and activating antioxidant enzymes.[6–11] Geographical factors influence the potential of wheat bran to serve as a dietary source of natural antioxidants, and its antioxidant ability is of considerable interest. The following section provides a detailed description of its representative antioxidants.

Antioxidant Enzymes

Superoxide Dismutase (SOD)

Cells are protected against oxidative stress by an interacting network of antioxidant enzymes. SOD is a rate-limiting enzyme that catalyzes dismutation, i.e., the breakdown of $O_2^{\bullet-}$ into oxygen and H_2O_2 (Eq. 6) at a rate $(2 \times 10^9 / M \bullet s)$, and decreases intracellular $O_2^{\bullet-}$ to levels of 100,000 parts or less.

$$2O_2^{\bullet-} + 2H^+ \rightarrow H_2O_2 + O_2 \cdots \qquad (6)$$

SODs are present in almost all aerobic cells and extracellular fluids, and are classified in terms of their metal ion cofactors, such as copper, zinc, manganese, or iron.[43-45] In human, SODs consist essentially of three isozymes: (1) the cytosolic copper/zinc SOD (Cu–Zn- SOD); (2) the mitochondrial manganese SOD (Mn-SOD);[44] and (3) the extracellular (EC) fluid form EC-SOD, which is particularly prominent in the vascular system, and which contains copper and zinc in its active sites.[46] Cu–Zn-SOD knockout mice are viable, but have numerous pathologies and a reduced lifespan. Although ovulation and pregnancy are normal in female Cu–Zn-SOD knockout mice, their offspring are born dead, resulting from a decline in their resistance to oxidative stress.[47] Mn-SOD appears to be the most biologically important of the three isozymes, and mice lacking this enzyme die soon after birth with problems such as decreased activities of succinate dehydrogenase and aconitase, dilated cardiomyopathy, accumulation of peroxide in liver and skeletal muscle, and metabolic acidosis.[48] Although EC-SOD knockout mice grow normally, they are sensitive to hyperoxia, resulting in a decreased survival rate caused by pulmonary edema.[49] Therefore, SOD plays an essential role in protection against oxidative stress *in vivo*. In addition to experiments in knockout animals, it has been reported that mutations in the Cu–Zn-SOD gene are associated with familial amyotrophic lateral sclerosis.[50] Alloxan-induced diabetic rats have decreased antioxidant enzyme capacities, and when fed wheat bran extracts containing sodium ferulate or feruloyl oligosaccarodes these mice are effectively protected against oxidative stress as a result of increased activity of SOD in the serum, liver, and testis.[9] Wheat bran may also act as a source of minerals, such as zinc and copper, which are known cofactors of SOD.

Catalase

Catalase, for which either iron or manganese are cofactors, functions as an antioxidant by catalyzing the conversion of H_2O_2 to water and oxygen (Eq. 7) and is localized to peroxisomes in most eukaryotic cells.[16,51] Catalase is effective in reducing high levels of H_2O_2. Although the effect of wheat bran on catalase is unclear, it may function to supplement levels of iron or manganese cofactors.

$$2H_2O_2 \rightarrow 2H_2O + O_2 \cdots \qquad (7)$$

Glutathione Peroxidase (GPx)

GPx, which contains selenium in its active center, is present in the cytosol and in mitochondria, and has a high degree of affinity for H_2O_2 compared with catalase.[16,52] GPx reduces and breaks down not only H_2O_2 but also lipid peroxide (LOOH) by catalyzing a redox reaction with reduced glutathione (GSH), which serves as an electron donor (Eqs 8, 9):

$$2GSH + H_2O_2 \rightarrow GSSG + 2H_2O \cdots \qquad (8)$$

$$2GSH + LOOH \rightarrow GSSG + LOH + H_2O \cdots \qquad (9)$$

During the GPx-catalyzed reaction, GSH is converted to its oxidized disulfide form (GSSG), which has a decreased ability to reduce peroxide. Once oxidized, GSH can be regenerated from GSSG by the enzyme glutathione reductase (GR), using reduced nicotinamide adenine dinucleotide phosphate (NADPH) as the electron donor and reducing equivalents. In the process, NADPH is oxidized to $NADP^+$, and NADPH is regenerated through the pentose phosphate pathway. Therefore, GPx-dependent redox cycle functions as a cellular antioxidant mechanism.[16] A previous study suggested that in GPx-deficient mice, impaired angiogenesis is associated with endothelial progenitor cell dysfunction.[53] Moreover, wheat bran can increase hepatic GPx activity *in vivo* in experimental animals by being involved in a selenium supplementation caused by wheat bran.[11] Selenium is also a key antioxidant component of wheat bran (see Selenium, below). In addition, the activity of GPx in the serum, liver, and testis of alloxan-treated rats, which are in an induced diabetic state, is elevated by feeding a diet containing sodium ferulate or feruloyl oligosaccharides (see Phenolic Acid, below).[9] Therefore, it is possible to protect against oxidative stress by harnessing the activity of GPx-dependent redox cycles more efficiently (Fig. 15.2), and this may be one of the essential functions of these cycles.

Non-Enzymatic Antioxidants

Ascorbic Acid (Vitamin C)

Ascorbic acid, a naturally occurring water-soluble organic compound (Fig. 15.3), is essential in the human diet because of its participation in many different biological processes. Many animals are able to produce ascorbic acid, because it is derived from glucose. In contrast, ascorbic acid is required as a dietary micronutrient in humans and other primates, such as the guinea pig, and is the most important antioxidant in extracellular fluids, while also being effective in the cytosol.[54] The antioxidant activity of vitamin C is primarily attributable to its ability to donate electrons and thereby function as a reducing agent, and this function has been studied extensively. In fluids, vitamin C has the ability to

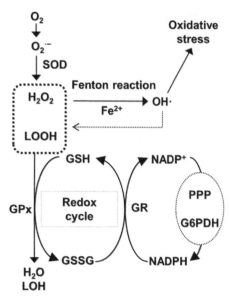

FIGURE 15.2 Glutathione redox cycle as antioxidant mechanism. Superoxide dismutase (SOD) has promoted the generation of hydrogen peroxide (H_2O_2), at least temporarily. However, catalase and glutathione peroxidase (GPx) can reduce free H_2O_2 into dioxygen (O_2) and hydrogen (H_2O) in the cell. GPx can break down not only H_2O_2 but also lipid hydroperoxide (LOOH) with reduced glutathione (GSH) as a substrate to their corresponding alcohols. In this process, GSH is converted to its oxidized glutathione (GSSG). Once oxidized, GSH can be reduced back by glutathione reductase (GR), using nicotinamide adenine dinucleotide phosphate (NADPH) as an electron donor. NADPH is supplied by the activation of glucose 6-phosphate dehydrogenase (G6PDH) in pentose phosphate pathway (PPP).

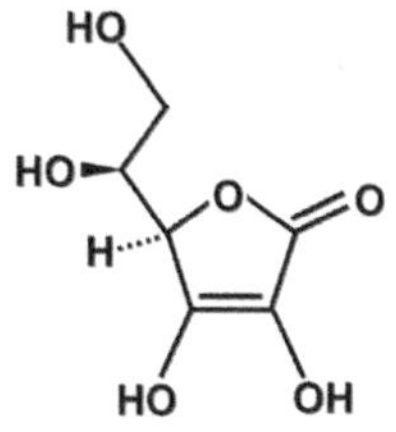

Ascorbic acid

FIGURE 15.3 Structure of ascorbic acid.

neutralize ROS (known as free radicals with an unpaired electron), such as $OH^{\bullet}$, $O_2^{\bullet-}$, peroxyl radical ($LOO^{\bullet}$), and alkoxyl radical ($LO^{\bullet}$), preventing cellular damage due to DNA fragmentation, enzyme inactivation, and lipid peroxidation. Inside cells, vitamin C supports the action of vitamin E and GSH by regenerating their active form after they have reacted with ROS.[55] Furthermore, vitamin C has been reported to have beneficial effects against cancer, cardiovascular disease, cataracts, cholesterol, lipid oxidation, hypertension, and aging,[56,57] and ascorbic acid supplementation has become popular for these conditions. Although vitamin C can play a role in the removal of radicals, it cannot account for antioxidant properties of wheat bran.

α-Tocopherol (Vitamin E)

Vitamin E is a fat-soluble vitamin, and consists of tocopherols and tocotrienols (Fig. 15.4). α-Tocopherol is the most active and abundant form of the tocopherols.[58] Compared with tocopherols, tocotrienols have a lower activity in vitamin E. Vitamin E has been called the most important chain-breaking antioxidant, due to its abundance in cells and mitochondrial membranes and its ability to act directly on ROS, preventing the propagation of free radicals.[59] In particular, vitamin E plays an important role in cell membranes by inhibiting lipid peroxidation. The molecular structure of vitamin E facilitates ROS inactivation in a lipid environment, particularly in the case of $LOO^{\bullet}$ radicals, which are generated by low density lipoprotein (LDL) oxidation in membranes or blood.[60,61] In addition, many different forms of tocopherols exist, including γ- and σ-tocopherols, whose scavenger function is lower than that of the alpha-type.[59] Furthermore, vitamin E interacts with numerous antioxidants, such as vitamin C, GSH, β-carotene, or lipoic acid, and these antioxidants have the capacity to regenerate vitamin E from its oxidized form. Vitamin E deficiency is rare and is rarely caused by a poor diet, but is rather attributable to three specific situations, namely (1) in persons who cannot absorb dietary fat; (2) in premature, very low birth weight infants; and (3) in individuals with rare disorders of fat metabolism.[62] Vitamin E deficiency can cause anemia due to oxidative damage to red blood cells and impairment of the immune response,[63,64] and epidemiological evidence suggests that high doses of vitamin E may reduce the risk of coronary heart disease.[65] Wheat bran can supply vitamin E through an ingestion pathway. However, a previous study has reported that the content of vitamin E is lower in Japanese wheat bran than in rice bran,[66] indicating that it may not be the main antioxidant in wheat bran, or that it may be removed during the wheat bran refining process.

Carotenoid

Carotenoids are organic pigments found in the chloroplasts and chromoplasts of plants and other photosynthetic organisms such as algae, bacteria, and fungi, and can be produced from fats and other basic organic metabolic building blocks by all these organisms. Carotenoids are divided into two classes, carotenes and xanthophylls.[67] Carotenes, including β-carotene and lycopen, are purely hydrocarbon. Xanthophylls, such as lutein and zeaxanthin, contain not only carbon and hydrogen, but also oxygen. In humans, four carotenoids – β-, α-, and γ-carotenes, and β-cryptoxanthin – have vitamin A activity. The structure of β-carotene is shown in Figure 15.5. One of the main mechanisms of the antioxidant action of carotenoids is the ability to quench singlet oxygen ($^1O_2$), which is the electronically excited

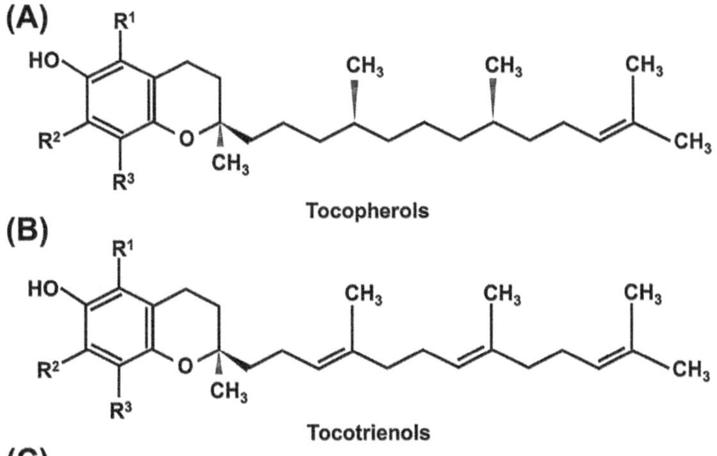

(A)

Tocopherols

(B)

Tocotrienols

FIGURE 15.4 **Structures of tocopherols and tocotrienols.** Two basic structures, which contain tocopherols (A) and tocotrienols (B), are shown. The corresponding –H or –H$_3$ in R$_1$–R$_3$ indicates the derivatives (C).

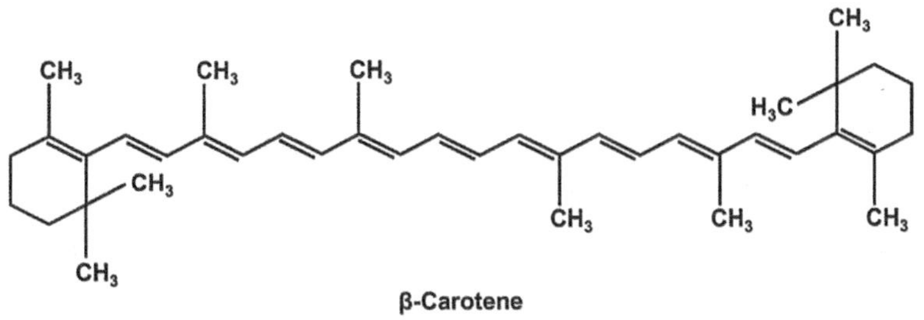

(C)

Derivative	R^1	R^2	R^3
α	CH$_3$	CH$_3$	CH$_3$
β	CH$_3$	H	CH$_3$
γ	H	CH$_3$	CH$_3$
δ	H	H	CH$_3$

FIGURE 15.5 Structure of β-carotene.

β-Carotene

form of oxygen and reacts with a number of biological molecules, including membrane lipids, to initiate peroxidation.[68] Reacted carotenoids can return to the ground state by releasing a small amount of heat and becoming more stable. In addition, β-carotene reacts with free radicals, such as LO• and LOO•, and is capable of transferring electrons (i.e., acting as an electron donor) and reducing free radicals to non-radical compounds, and in the process produces carotenoid radical cations.[68,69] A previous study also suggested that LDL-associated vitamin A can play a role in maintaining the antioxidant status of LDL during oxidative stress *in vivo*, and although they are less important than vitamin E in the antioxidant system, β-carotene and vitamin A act in tandem with vitamins C and E to protect cells against ROS.[70] Therefore, suboptimal intake of carotenoids may result in increased DNA damage and contribute to carcinogenesis through the reduced action of these antioxidants on $^1O_2$ and free radicals. Several investigations have demonstrated the antiproliferative effect of carotenoids on various cancer cell lines, and inhibition of cell cycle progression by lycopene has been shown in breast, lung, and prostate cell lines.[71–73] In human prostate cancer cell lines incubated with lycopene alone or with lycopene plus α-tocopherol, the combination of the two antioxidants strongly inhibited prostate cancer cell proliferation, whereas lycopene alone had very little effect.[72,74] Epidemiological studies have shown that people with a high β-carotene intake and high plasma levels of β-carotene have a significantly reduced risk of lung cancer.[75] However, no change in the relative risk of death by malignant neoplasms and cardiovascular disease was observed after supplementation with β-carotene.[76] Although wheat bran contains carotenoids such as β-carotene, zeaxanthin, lutein, and cryptoxanthin, it is inefficient compared with other antioxidants.[77]

Flavonoid

Flavonoids are phenolic substances formed in plants from amino acids including phenylalanine and tyrosine and malonate, with more than 4000 individual compounds known.[78] The basic flavonoid structure contains flavan nucleus, which consists of 15 carbon atoms arranged in three rings (C$_6$–C$_3$–C$_6$), and the various classes of flavonoids exist as flavones (e.g. apigenin and kaenpteral), flavanones (e.g. hesperetin and fisetin), catechins (e.g. catechin and epigallocatechin gallate), and anthocyanins (e.g. cyanidin and delphinidin). Each structure of flavonoid groups is shown in Figure 15.6. Because of the high reactivity of the hydroxyl group, flavonoids (Fl-OH) are able to reduce highly oxidizing free radicals with redox potentials by hydrogen atom donation, according to Eq. (10), where $R^{\bullet}$ represents superoxide anion, peroxyl, alkoxyl, and hydroxyl radicals.

$$Fl\text{-}OH + R^{\bullet} \rightarrow Fl\text{-}O^{\bullet} + RH \ldots \quad (10)$$

Previous in vitro work has indicated that flavonoids have the ability to chelate transition metal ions, such as free iron and copper, leading to decreased production of ROS, exemplified by the reduction of H_2O_2 and the generation of the highly reactive $OH^{\bullet}$ or by copper-mediated LDL oxidation.[79] In vitro, flavonoids have been shown to inhibit enzymes responsible for $O_2^{\bullet-}$ production (such as xanthine oxidase and protein kinase C) and others (such as glutathione s-transferase and NADPH oxidase) involved in ROS generation.[79,80] Flavonoids are important phytochemical components of wheat bran, and have been shown to be potent antioxidants with anticancer activity.[81,82] In addition, flavonoids have a role in the treatment of diabetes[83,84] by virtue of their ability to protect against hyperglycemic and alloxan-induced oxidative stress in experimental animal models.[85] In a large cohort of women, a clinical trial has shown that flavonoids are protective against type 2 diabetes.[86] Wheat bran contains low levels of flavonoids compared with wheat germ.[87]

Glutathione

Glutathione (L-γ-glutamyl-L-cysteinylglysin), the soluble and principal non-protein thiol-containing compound, is a tripeptide composed of cysteine, glutamic acid, and glycine. Its active group is represented by the thiol of cysteine residue. Glutathione is highly abundant in the cytosol (1–11 mM), nucleus (3–15 mM), and mitochondria (5–11 mM), and is produced in all organs, particularly in the liver. It consists of two types (Fig. 15.7), almost all of which (>98%) in the cell is GSH. Once oxidized, GSH is

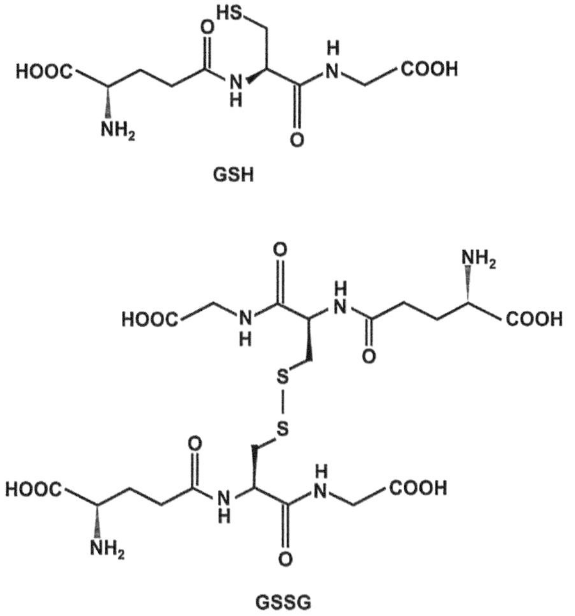

FIGURE 15.7　Structures of reduced and oxidized glutathione.

FIGURE 15.6　Structures of each groups of flavonoids. R_n indicates positions of hydroxyl groups, and these positions determine the antioxidant properties of flavonoids.

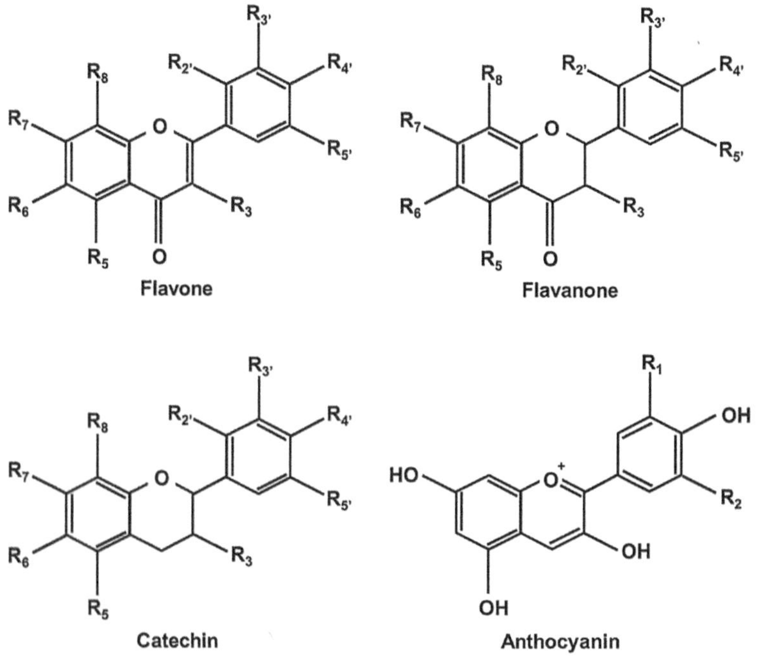

converted to GSSG, the oxidized form with decreased antioxidant properties. GSH is a multifunctional intracellular antioxidant and is considered to be the major thiol-disulfide redox buffer in the cell.[88] However, it not only protects cell membranes from oxidative stress[89] but can also prevent damage to important cellular components caused by ROS such as free radicals and peroxides. It can also act as a cofactor for several detoxifying enzymes, such as GPx (see Glutathione Peroxidase, above), participate in amino acid transport across the plasma membrane, and scavenge $OH^{\bullet}$ and $^{1}O_{2}$, which can theoretically be produced by neutrophils from the reaction of $H_{2}O_{2}$ with HClO, directly. GSH helps to maintain the sulf-hydryl groups of many proteins to ensure their normal function.[89] In addition, GSH regenerates important anti-oxidants, such as vitamins C and E, to their active forms. Moreover, glutathione can reduce the tocopherol radical of vitamin E either directly, or indirectly by reduction of monodehydroascorbate to ascorbate.[16,88,90] In addition, GSH deficiency has been linked to pulmonary diseases, such as chronic obstructive pulmonary disease (COPD), acute respiratory distress syndrome, neonatal lung damage, and asthma.[90] Many of the biological effects of anti-oxidants appear to be related to their ability to scavenge deleterious free radicals with modulation of cell-signaling pathways.[91] Both methionine and cysteine, as precursors of glutathione, contribute to the control of cell oxidative status, and are found in higher levels in wheat bran (0.6%).[92,93] However, a previous study reported no change in the hepatic GSH content of rats fed wheat bran.[11] Regardless of how GSH is generated, it protects against oxidative stress by activating the antioxidant mechanism in specific glutathione redox cycles, and this may be its essential function.

Lipoic Acid

Lipoic acid is both water- and fat-soluble, and is thus widely distributed in both cellular membranes and the cytosol of eukaryotic and prokaryotic cells. There are two forms of lipoic acid; α-lipoic acid (1,2-dithi-olane-3-pentanoic acid, 1,2-dithiolane-3-valeric acid or thioctic acid) and the reduced form dihydrolipoic acid (6,8-dimercaptoocatanoic acid or 6,8-thioctic acid) (Fig. 15.8). In addition to glutathione, lipoic acid is an important thiol antioxidant, and exerts its protective effects by scavenging free radicals, chelating metal ions, and recycling antioxidants. Moreover, it helps to reduce vitamins C and E from their oxidized forms and repairs protein damage due to oxidative stress either in the cytosol or in hydrophobic domains.[94] In particular, it is believed to play a pivotal role in protecting cells against lipid peroxidation. Both lipoic and dehydrolipoic acids eliminate $OH^{\bullet}$ generated by the Fenton reaction in the aqueous phase, whereas $O_{2}^{\bullet-}$ has been reported to be eliminated only by dihydrolipoic

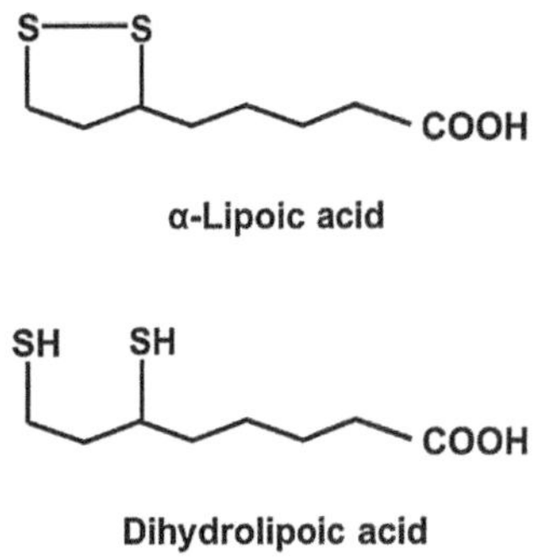

FIGURE 15.8 Structures of lipoic acids.

acid.[95,96] Moreover, dehydrolipoic acid plays a part in the non-enzymatic regeneration of GSH and ascorbic acid by reducing GSSG or dihydroascorbic acid (Eqs 11, 12), and recycles tocopherols.[94]

$$Dihydrolipoic\ acid + GSSG \rightarrow Lipoic\ acid + GSH \ldots (11)$$

$$Dihydrolipoic\ acid + Dehydroxyascorbic\ acid \rightarrow$$
$$Lipoic\ acid + Ascorbic\ acid \cdots \qquad (12)$$

In addition to its function as a radical scavenger, lipoic acid has chelating capability. Although lipoic acid does not chelate the ferric ion,[97] it has been shown to form a complex with the ferrous ion.[98] Moreover, a lipophilic complex of lipoic acid with the cupric ion has been invoked to explain protection against cupric ion-induced lipid peroxidation.[99] The chelating capacity of dihydrolipoic acid is more effective than that of lipoic acid, but a side effect is an increase in the formation of $OH^{\bullet}$ in vitro.[100] In fact, lipoic acid probably exerts it effects in diabetic rats by reducing lipid accumulation in adipose and non-adipose tissue.[101] However, it may not be a characteristic antioxidant in wheat bran.

Ferritin

Ferritin is an iron storage protein present in all living organisms and plays a central role in maintaining the delicate intracellular iron balance by regulating intracellular iron, an antioxidant.[102–104] Iron is required for normal cell growth and proliferation, and can have antioxidant effects as a cofactor of catalase. However, excess iron is potentially harmful due to production of the highly reactive $OH^{\bullet}$ by the Fenton reaction, as described previously (Eq. 5). Iron toxicity is minimized in cells because ferritin has the ability to store iron, accommodating up to 4500 iron atoms.[104,105] Furthermore, ferritin comprises 24 subunits of two functionally different types, termed H (heavy chain, heart-type) and L (light chain, liver type), in addition to a central cavity for iron storage.[106–108] The H subunit plays a crucial role in incorporating iron through its ferroxidase activity, and H ferritin gene knockout in the mouse is lethal.[109] In contrast, the L subunit lacks enzymatic activity but is involved in iron nucleation, allowing more iron to be sequestered. In addition, the expression of ferritin H and L mRNA is dependent on intracellular iron concentration and oxidative stress.[110,111] Therefore, ferritin can serve the dual function of storing and segregating iron in a bioavailable and non-toxic form, thereby contributing to the protective effect against oxidative stress. In normal animals without anemia, no effect of wheat bran feeding has been observed with respect to ferritin protein and stored iron levels in the liver – the main iron storage tissue[10] – indicating that ferritin synthesis is not affected by wheat bran and that the antioxidant effects of wheat bran are attributable to other factors.

Selenium

Selenium, which is present generally in nature, is an essential trace element in living organisms. Although excess levels of selenium are extremely toxic, trace amounts are necessary for cellular function in many organisms, including all animals. Selenium is a component of the unusual amino acids selenocysteine and selenomethionine.[112] In animals, selenium can function as cofactor for antioxidant enzymes such as GPx (see Glutathione Peroxidase, above) and certain forms of thioredoxin reductase found in animals and some plants. GPx, one of the selenium-dependent antioxidant enzymes, can catalyze certain reactions that remove ROS such as H_2O_2 and organic hydroperoxides, and functions in the protection of cells against oxidative stress. The activity of this enzyme in lung and liver is very low in selenium-deficient animals. Some studies have reported that dietary selenium deficiency decreases the activity of hepatic GPx, and renders rats and mice susceptible to diquat-induced oxidative stress or lethality.[113,114] Selenium deficiency, defined by low selenoenzyme activity levels in brain and endocrine tissues, occurs only when a low selenium status is linked with an additional stress, such as high exposure to mercury or as a result of increased oxidative stress due to vitamin E deficiency.[115] A previous study by our group demonstrated the selenium content of Japanese wheat bran to be 0.6 ppm, similar to other reported values (0.58 ppm), and that hepatic GPx activity is increased after wheat bran feeding.[11] Furthermore, the level of selenium in wheat bran is five-fold higher than that in okara and rice bran, both of which fail to protect against diquat-induced oxidative stress.[10] While the selenium content of wheat bran varies with soil, wheat bran can be used as a selenium supplement, leading to the increased GPx activity. Therefore, adding wheat bran to the diet may be an efficient way to remedy the selenium deficiency that frequently occurs in animals living in areas with low selenium content in the soil.[116]

Lignan

Lignans are a group of diphenolic compounds that are concentrated in the bran layer of cereal grain. The major lignan in wheat bran is secoisolariciresinol diglucoside,[117] which when consumed is converted by intestinal microflora to two lignan metabolites: enterodiol and enterolactone (Fig. 15.9). Lignan metabolites function as antioxidants and free radical scavengers, leading to decreased risk of cancer development.[118] A previous study has also found that enterolactone functions as an antioxidant against human LDL oxidation.[119] In addition, it has been shown to be capable of preventing colon cancer cell growth by inducing the phase 2 detoxification enzyme, NADPH:quinone reductase, in vitro. Lignans in wheat bran have been shown to have antitumor properties in mice and human cells that may be mediated by cytostatic and apoptotic mechanisms.[117] In addition, wheat bran inhibits the development of intestinal neoplasia, although the degree of inhibition differs significantly among the various wheat cultivars.[120] Further study is needed to verify the safety profile and effects of lignan.

Phytic Acid

Phytic acid, also known as inositol-6-phosphate or phytate in its salt form, is the principal storage form of phosphorus in many plant tissues (Fig. 15.10) and is localized mainly in the outer parts of the wheat kernel,

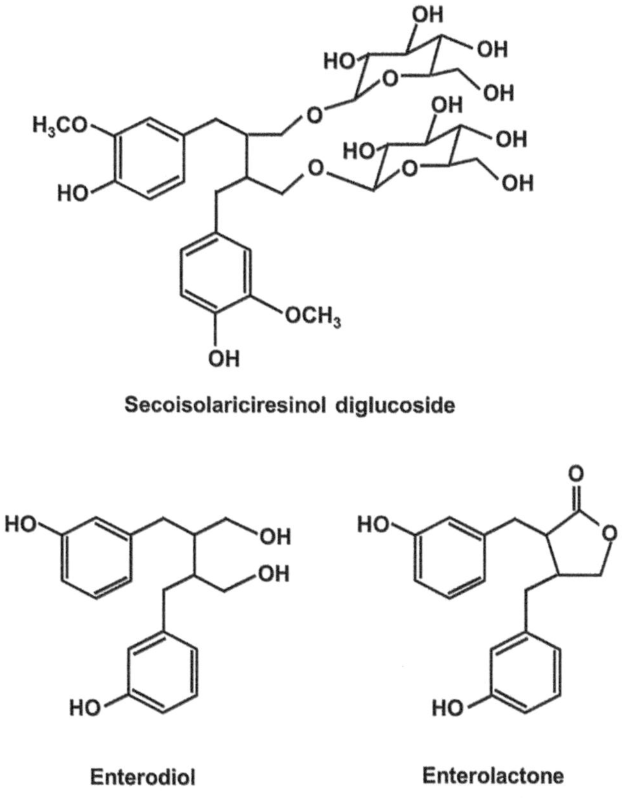

Secoisolariciresinol diglucoside

Enterodiol   **Enterolactone**

FIGURE 15.9   Structures of lignans.

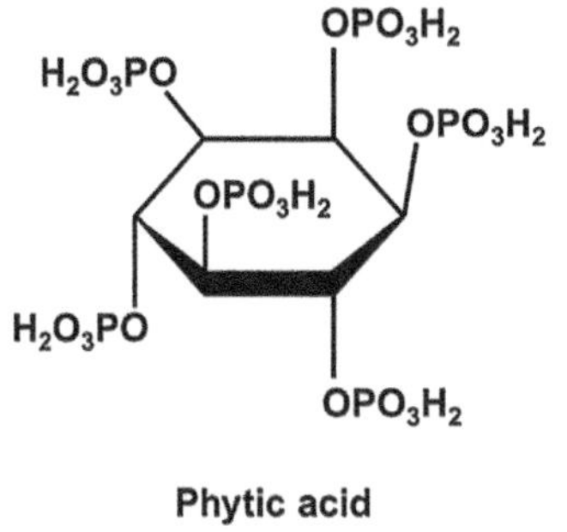

Phytic acid

FIGURE 15.10   Structure of phytic acid.

explaining its very high content in bran.[121] Phosphorus and inositol in phytate form are not generally bioavailable to non-ruminant animals because these animals lack the digestive enzyme phytase required to remove phosphate from the inositol in the phytate molecule. In contrast, ruminants readily digest phytate due to the phytase produced by rumen microorganisms. Phytate is not digestible by humans or non-ruminant animals, and thus is not a dietary source of either inositol or phosphate. Phytic acid may exert its greatest biologic effect through its antioxidant properties. It forms an iron chelate which inhibits iron-mediated oxidative reactions and limits site-specific DNA damage,[122,123] and can prevent tumor growth by suppressing the formation of the highly reactive $OH^\bullet$ and other ROS. Moreover, its antioxidant ability may aid in explaining the suppression of colon carcinogenesis by diets rich in phytic acid.[124] Therefore, tumor progression may also be limited by the chelating effect of other divalent cations such as magnesium and zinc because both are critical for tumor cell proliferation.[125] Indeed, in animal studies phytic acid has been shown to inhibit neoplastic growth in multiple types of cancer.[126,127] On the basis of the fact that phytic acid inhibits cell growth, generation of ROS, and cancer progression, there is no longer any doubt regarding its ability to chelate and inactivate pro-oxidant metals. At molar ratios of 0.25 phytate : iron and above, iron-promoted generation of $OH^\bullet$ is almost completely blocked by phytate. Its proposed mechanisms of action include an increase in natural killer cell activity, alteration in signal transduction, induction of genes involved in cell differentiation, and antioxidant activity.[128] One study has also correlated decreased osteoporosis risk with phytic acid consumption.[129] In contrast, phytic acid forms complexes with numerous cations, particularly zinc, calcium, and iron, generating insoluble salts unavailable for absorption through the intestinal tract.[130] Therefore, phytic acid is an antinutrient, despite its possible therapeutic effects, and the bioavailability of minerals in wheat bran is under debate due to the presence of phytic acid. However, other studies have observed no reducing effect of wheat bran feeding on stored iron in normal,

non-anemic rats,[10] indicating that wheat bran (possibly through the effect of phytic acid) may have an exclusive effect on excess free iron. Therefore, this process may contribute to mineral deficiencies in people whose diets rely on these foods for their mineral intake, such as those in developing countries. This point has indicated that natural wheat bran may be an appropriate food.

Phenolic Acid

Phenolic acids, a class of polyphenols, are ubiquitous in plant tissues. The majority of phenolic acids in wheat grain are insoluble and are bound by ester and ether linkages with polysaccharides, such as arabinoxylan and lignin, in the cell wall. Therefore, in wheat they are usually concentrated in the bran layer, and are an important factor in the antioxidant properties of wheat bran.[87] It has been noted that growing conditions and the interaction between environmental factors and genotype alter the antioxidant properties and phytochemical compositions of wheat bran.[8,131] Extracts of wheat bran with high concentrations of phenolic acids have been shown to have stronger antioxidant activity than other fractions of wheat.[132,133] The phenolic content of the bran/germ fraction is up to 18-fold higher than the corresponding endosperm samples.[6] Moreover, the content of bound phenolics is significantly higher than those of the free and esterified fractions, particularly in the case of wheat bran, leading to more potent scavenging capacity and chelating activity.[134,135] For example, phenolic acid has been reported to inhibit lipid peroxidation catalyzed by either iron or peroxyl radicals.[135] Moreover, a positive association exists between total phenolic content and ferrous ion,[134] suggesting that it has chelating capability. Low molecular weight phenolics encompass approximately 8000 naturally occurring compounds that possess a common structural feature, namely a phenol or an aromatic ring bearing at least one hydroxyl substituent.[136] Wheat bran extracts contain various phenolic acids, such as ferulic, vanillic, p-coumaric, caffeic, chlorogenic, gentisic, syringic, and p-hydroxybenzoic acids (Fig. 15.11).[132,135,137,138] Ferulic acid accounts for 59–60% of the total phenolic acid on a per weight basis, and, along with significant levels of syringic, p-hydroxybenzoic, vanillic, and coumaric acids at a concentration range of 4–33 µg/g bran in Trego wheat bran produced in Colorado,[6] it is the predominate phenolic acid.[135,138]

Ferulic acid (4-hydroxy-3-methoxycinnamic acid) is an abundant antioxidant and may be beneficial in the prevention and/or treatment of various disorders linked to oxidative stress, such as Alzheimer's disease, diabetes, cancer, cardiovascular disease, and atherosclerosis (as reviewed in Zhao and Moghadasian[139]). High levels of ferulic acid are found in both free and bound forms, and are concentrated in the bran of grains, the peel of fruits, and the roots and peel of vegetables. The content

FIGURE 15.11 Structures of various phenolic acids.

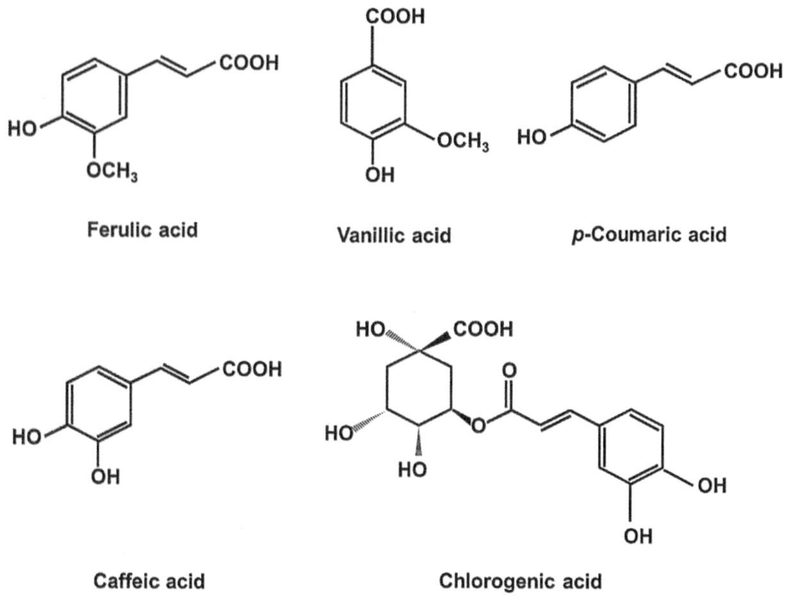

Ferulic acid

Vanillic acid

p-Coumaric acid

Caffeic acid

Chlorogenic acid

of ferulic acid is much higher in wheat bran than in other foods, and the levels of ferulic acid in a number of these foods are summarized in Table 15.6.[134,140–157]

The main mechanism of action of phenolic antioxidants is considered to be the scavenging of free radicals by donating the phenolic hydrogen atom,[158] and the characteristic antioxidant property of ferulic acid is its scavenging activity against peroxyl, hydroxyl, 2,2-diphenyl-1-picryhydraxyl radical (DPPH$^{•}$), 2,2-azino-di[3-ethylbenzthiazoline sulfonate] (ABTS$^{•+}$), $O_2^{•-}$, and OH$^{•}$, which is attributable to its phenolic nucleus and extended side chain.[159] Using electron spin resonance spectrometry[160,161] it has been estimated that at a concentration of 250 mg/L, ferulic acid scavenges 92.5% of OH$^{•}$ generated through the Fenton reaction. Compared with the well-known antioxidants vitamins E and C, wheat bran extract shows great DPPH$^{•}$ or $O_2^{•-}$ quenching capacity, although these differed in their relative activities.[7,77,162] Moreover, the cholesterol-lowering activity of ferulic acid has been confirmed, suggesting that it inhibits cholesterol synthesis by competitively inhibiting the activity of hydroxymethylglutaryl CoA reductase in the liver and increasing excretion of acidic sterol.[163] Ferulic acid has the potential to restore endothelial function in the aortas of spontaneously hypertensive rats, and to prevent trimethyltin-induced cognitive dysfunction in mice.[164,165] Furthermore, feruloyl oligosaccharide, which is released from wheat bran insoluble dietary fiber with xylanase from *Bacillus subtilis*, has scavenging activity against LOO$^{•}$, thereby inhibiting the peroxidation of erythrocytes *in vitro*.[166] The lipid peroxidation of erythrocytes is caused by 2,2′-azobis-2-amidinopropane dehydrochloride as an initiator of LOO$^{•}$. However, the presence of electron-donating groups on the benzene ring (3-methoxy, and, more importantly, 4-hydroxy)

of the ferulic acid moiety of feruloyl oligosaccharides gave the additional resonance structures of the resulting phenoxyl radical, contributing to the stability of this intermediate or even terminating free radical chain reactions.[166] Therefore, in the presence of feruloyl oligosaccharides (FH), the LOO$^{•}$ can be trapped and a new radical, F$^{•}$, produced (Eq. 13). Since the new radical F$^{•}$ is a stabilized radical, it can promote the rate-limiting hydrogen abstraction reaction (Eq. 13) and undergo a fast termination reaction (Eq. 14), and subsequently inhibit lipid peroxide.

$$LOO^{•} + FH \rightarrow LOOH + F^{•} \dots \qquad (13)$$

$$LOO^{•} + F^{•} \rightarrow LOOF \dots \qquad (14)$$

In addition, feeding feruloyl oligosaccharides significantly increases the activity of antioxidant enzymes, such as SOD and GPx, in the serum, liver, and testis of alloxan-induced diabetic rats, restoring them to almost normal levels or above.[9] Therefore, it is significant feature of the antioxidant properties of wheat bran against an oxidative injury.

CONCLUSION

This chapter has reviewed the antioxidant properties of wheat bran and its extracts. Wheat bran is relatively high in antioxidant activity compared with other foods, containing a balanced variety of antioxidants such as vitamins, minerals, lignans, phytic acid, and phenolic acids. *In vivo* and *in vitro* studies with wheat bran extracts have frequently reported that they are responsible for

TABLE 15.6 Levels of Ferulic Acid (FA) in Grains, Fruits, Vegetables, and Commercial Foods[a]

	FA Contents[b] (mg/100 g)	Serving Size (g)	mg/Serving	Reference(s)
GRAINS				
Refined corn bran	2610–3300	5	130–151	Saulnier and Thibault[140], Zhao et al.[141]
Barley extract	1358–2293	5	68–115	Madhujith and Shahidi[142]
Soft and hard wheat bran	1351–1456	5	68–73	Liyana-Pathirana and Shahidi[134]
Rice endosperm cell wall	910	5	45	Shibuya[143]
Fine wheat bran	530–540	5	26–27	Kroon and Williamson[144], Andreasen et al.[145]
Rye bran	280	5	14	Andreasen et al.[145], Mattila et al.[146]
Corn, dehulled kernels	174	30	52.2	Adom and Liu[147]
Whole wheat kernels	64–127	30	19–38	Adom and Liu[147], Nishizawa et al.[148]
Whole wheat flour	89	30	26.7	Mattila et al.[146]
Whole grain rye flour	86	30	25.8	Mattila et al.[146]
Whole brown rice	42	30	8.7–12.6	Adom and Liu[147], Nishizawa et al.[148]
Corn flour	38	30	11.4	Mattila et al.[146]
Whole oats	25	30	10.5	Mattila et al.[146], Adom and Liu[147]
Whole grain barley flour	35	30	7.5–10	Mattila et al.[146], Nishizawa et al.[148]
Oat bran	33			Mattila et al.[146]
FRUITS				
Grapefruit	10.7–11.6	125	13.4–14.6	Mattila et al.[149]
Orange	9.2–9.9	125	11.5–12.5	Mattila et al.[149]
Banana	5.4	125	6.75	Mattila et al.[149]
Berries	0.25–2.70	125	0.6–3.4	Mattila et al.[149]
Rhubarb	2	125	2.5	Mattila et al.[149]
Plum, dark	1.47	125	1.8	Mattila et al.[149]
Apple	0.27–0.85	125	0.3–1	Mattila et al.[149]
VEGETABLES				
Bamboo shoots	243.6	50	122	Nishizawa et al.[148]
Water dropwort	7.3–34	200	14.6–68	Sakakibara et al.[150]
Eggplant	7.3–35	200	14.6–70	Sakakibara et al.[150]
Red beet	25	100	25	Mattila and Hellström[151]
Burdock	7.3–19	100	7.3–19	Sakakibara et al.[150]
Soya bean	12	125	15	Mattila and Hellström[151]
Peanut	8.7	60	5.22	Mattila and Hellström[151]
Spinach/frozen	7.4	200	14.8	Mattila and Hellström[151]
Red cabbage	6.3–6.5	200	12.6–13	Mattila and Hellström[151]
Tomato	0.29–6	200	0.6–12	Mattila and Hellström[151], Bourne and Rice-Evans[152]
Radish	4.6	100	4.6	Mattila and Hellström[151]

(Continued)

F. WHEAT FIBER

TABLE 15.6 Levels of Ferulic Acid (FA) in Grains, Fruits, Vegetables, and Commercial Foods[a]—cont'd

	FA Contents[b] (mg/100 g)	Serving Size (g)	mg/Serving	Reference(s)
VEGETABLES				
Broccoli	4.1	200	8.2	Mattila and Hellström[151]
Carrot	1.2–2.8	100	1.2–2.8	Mattila and Hellström[151]
Parsnip	2.2	200	4.4	Mattila and Hellström[151]
Izuna	1.4–1.8	200	2.8–3.6	Sakakibara et al.[150]
Pot-grown basil	1.5	200	3	Mattila and Hellström[151]
Chinese cabbage	1.4	200	2.8	Mattila and Hellström[151]
Pot-grown lettuce	0.19–1.4	200	0.4–2.8	Mattila and Hellström[151]
Green bean/fresh	1.2	200	2.4	Mattila and Hellström[151]
Avocado	1.1	200	2.2	Mattila and Hellström[151]
COMMERCIAL FOODS AND BEVERAGES				
Sugar-beet pulp	800	10	80	Micard et al.[153]
Popcorn	313	60	187.8	Nishizawa et al.[148]
Whole grain rye bread	54	35	18.9	Mattila et al.[146]
Whole grain oat flakes	25–52	35	8.75–18	Mattila et al.[146], Nishizawa et al.[148]
Sweetcorn	42	60	24	Nishizawa et al.[148]
Pickled red beet	39	25	9.75	Mattila and Hellström[151]
Rice, brown, long-grain, parboiled	24	125	30	Mattila et al.[146]
Coffee	9.1–14.3	200	18.2–28.6	Mattila et al.[149], Nardini et al.[154]
Boiled spaghetti	13.6	100	13.6	Nishizawa et al.[148]
Pasta	12	100	12	Mattila et al.[146]
White wheat bread	8.2	35	2.87	Mattila et al.[146]
Orange juice	3–6.4	200	6–13.4	Mattila et al.[149], Rapisarda et al.[155]
Pickled red cabbage	1.5	50	0.5	Mattila and Hellström[151]
Bear	0.24–0.9	500	1–4.5	Mattila et al.[149], Bourne and Rice-Evans[152]

[a] Data are mean or a range of mean values reported. Data are total ferulic acid (FA) except for Sakakibara et al.,[150] which reported free FA. Total FA in the materials was detected by HPLC after absolute alkaline hydrolysis except for Madhujith and Shahidi[142] and Liyana-Pathirana and Shahidi,[134] which reported that total FA was detected by Folin-Ciocalteu's reagent. Free FA was detected by HPLC without hydrolysis.

[b] The contents were calculated using 100 g fresh edible part of foods, apart from Nishizawa et al.,[148] which was reported by 100 g dry matter.

Reprinted from Ref. 139: Zhao, Z. and Moghadasian, MH, Chemistry, natural sources, dietary intake and pharmacokinetic properties of ferulic acid: a review. Food Chemistry, 109(4), Table 1, 693–694, ©2008, with permission from Elsevier.

health benefits, as a result of their highly potent antioxidant properties. Phenolic acids, phytic acid, and lignans are characteristic and essential phytochemicals, and these components have been found to be concentrated in the wheat bran compared with other fractions in wheat or foods. Various solvent systems are used to prepare antioxidants of wheat bran, making it difficult to compare the antioxidant activities of wheat bran reported by different research groups. Other important factors are the area where the wheat bran was produced and the percentage of additives it contains, because bran samples of wheat from different sources may significantly differ in their antioxidant properties and phytochemical compositions.

Recently, the health benefits provided by food products have become critical marketing tools as a result of increasing consumer awareness of the role of food in health promotion and disease prevention. Epidemiological studies have been conducted on the consumption of wheat bran, and have shown that the risk of

TABLE 15.7 Studies on Prospective Protective Effects of Intake of Wheat Bran Against Oxidative Stress-Related Diseases

Disease	Reference(s)
Diabetes	Jensen et al.[172], de Munter et al.[177], Qi and Hu[178], Wang et al.[179]
Cardiovascular disease	Jensen et al.[172], Pereira et al.[173], Jacobs and Gallaher[180], Mozaffarian et al.[181]
Hypertension	Whelton et al.[175]
Cancer	Ferguson and Harris[4], Reddy et al.[174], Lupton and Turner[182], Freudenheim et al.[183], Sang et al.[184], Topping[185], Slavin[186]
Atherosclerosis	Venkatesan[187], Yu et al.[188]
Coronary heart disease	Craig[176], Pereira et al.[189]

cardiovascular disease can be reduced by consuming bran-based products.[167–171] These studies have shown that the addition of whole grain or bran reduces the risk of diabetes, cardiovascular disease, colon cancer, hypertension, and coronary heart disease.[172–176] Considering the above findings, eating whole wheat bran may be an extremely important and safe antioxidant. Furthermore, many studies encourage the hope that intake of wheat bran can prevent the onset or development of various oxidative stress-related diseases due to the various types of antioxidant it contains at moderate levels (Table 15.7).[172–189]

Organic wheat bran can easily be purchased in bulk from whole-food stores or organic markets, which is good news for people who prefer to make biscuits, pancakes, waffles, and cookies from scratch using healthier ingredients. However, these individuals should exercise caution when adding bran to foods, because it can induce diarrhea in individuals not accustomed to high-fiber foods. Wheat bran is also widely used as a major component in foods for livestock animals, such as cattle, American bison, goats, rabbits, guinea pigs, and horses. Identification of the biologically active phytochemicals of wheat bran has the potential to add value to this waste product in market segments including functional foods and nutraceuticals, or as a validated therapeutic pharmaceutical source.

References

1. Belderok B. Development in bread-making processes. *Plant Foods Hum Nutr* 2000;**55**:1–86.
2. Hemery Y, Rouau X, Lullien-Pellerin V, Barron C, Abecassis J. Dry processes to develop wheat fractions and products with enhanced nutritional quality. *J Cereal Sci* 2007;**46**:327–47.
3. Shewry PR. The Healthgrain programme opens new opportunities for improving wheat for nutrition and health. *Nutr Bull* 2009;**34**:225–31.
4. Ferguson LR, Harris PJ. Protection against cancer by wheat bran: role of dietary fibre and phytochemicals. *Eur J Cancer Prev* 1999;**8**:17–25.
5. Liu S, Manson JE, Stampfer MJ, Hu FB, Giovannucci E, Colditz GA. et al. A prospective study of whole-grain intake and risk of type 2 diabetes mellitus in US women. *Am J Public Health* 2000;**90**:1409–15.
6. Adom KK, Sorrells ME, Liu RH. Phytochemicals and antioxidant activity of milled fractions of different wheat varieties. *J Agric Food Chem* 2005;**53**:2297–306.
7. Yu L, Haley S, Perret J, Harris M, Wilson J, Qian M. Free radical scavenging properties of wheat extracts. *J Agric Food Chem* 2002;**50**:1619–24.
8. Zhou K, Yu L. Effects of extraction solvent on wheat bran antioxidant activity estimation. *Lebensm-Wiss u-Technol* 2004; **37**:717–21.
9. Ou SY, Jackson GM, Jiao X, Chen J, Wu JZ, Huang XS. Protection against oxidative stress in diabetic rats by wheat bran feruloyl oligosaccharides. *J Agric Food Chem* 2007;**55**:3191–5.
10. Higuchi M, Kobayashi S, Kawasaki N, et al. Protective effects of wheat bran against diquat toxicity in male Fischer-344 rats. *Biosci Biotechnol Biochem* 2007;**71**:1621–5.
11. Higuchi M, Oshida J, Orino K, Watanabe K. Wheat bran protects Fischer-344 rats from diquat-induced oxidative stress by activating antioxidant system: Selenium as an antioxidant. *Biosci Biotechnol Biochem* 2011a;**75**:496–9.
12. Cannon WB. Stresses and strains of homeostasis. *Am J Med Sci* 1935;**189**:1–14.
13. Selye H. A syndrome produced by diverse nocuous agents. *Nature* 1936;**138**:32.
14. Pacak K, Palkovits M, Yadid G, Kvetnansky R, Kopin IJ, Goldstein DS. Heterogeneous neurochemical responses to different stressors: a test of Selye's doctrine of nonspecificity. *Am J Physiol Regul Integr Comp Physiol* 1998;**275**:R1247–55.
15. Seeman TE, McEwen BS, Rowe JW, Singer BH. Allostatic load as a marker of cumulative biological risk: MacArthur studies of successful aging. *Proc Natl Acad Sci USA* 2001;**98**:4770–5.
16. Valko M, Leibfritz D, Moncol J, Cronin MTD, Mazur M, Telser J. Free radicals and antioxidants in normal physiological functions and human disease. *Int J Biochem Cell Biol* 2007;**39**:44–84.
17. Forman HJ, Torres M. Redox signaling in macrophages. *Mol Aspects Med* 2001;**22**:189–216.
18. Fleury C, Mignotte B, Vayssière JL. Mitochondrial reactive oxygen species in cell death signaling. *Biochimie* 2002;**84**:131–41.
19. Hampton MB, Kettle AJ, Winterbourn CC. Inside the neutrophil phagosome: oxidants, myeloperoxidase, and bacterial killing. *Blood* 1998;**27**:186–92.
20. Thomas CE, Aust SD. Reductive release of iron from ferritin by cation free radicals of paraquat and other bipyridyls. *J Biol Chem* 1986;**261**:13064–70.
21. Reif DW, Beales ILP, Thomas CE, Aust SD. Effect of diquat on the distribution of iron in rat liver. *Toxicol Appl Pharmacol* 1988;**93**:506–10.
22. McCord JM. Effects of positive iron status at a cellular level. *Nutr Rev* 1996;**54**:85–8.
23. Jones GM, Vale JA. Mechanisms of toxicity, clinical features, and management of diquat poisoning: A review. *Clin Toxicol* 2000;**38**:123–8.
24. Comporti M. Three models of free radical-induced cell injury. *Chem Biol Interactions* 1989;**72**:1–56.
25. Blau S, Kohen R, Bass P, Rubinstein A. Relation between colonic inflammation severity and total low-molecular-weight antioxidant profiles in experimental colitis. *Dig Dis Sci* 2000;**45**:1180–7.
26. Giasson BI, Ischiropoulos H, Lee VMY, Trojanowski JQ. The relationship between oxidative/nitrative stress and pathological inclusions in Alzheimer's and Parkinson's diseases. *Free Radic Biol Med* 2002;**32**:1264–75.

27. Lee HC, Wei YH. Mitochondrial alterations, cellular response to oxidative stress and defective degradation of proteins in aging. *Biogerontology* 2001;**2**:231–44.

28. Ornoy A. Embryonic oxidative stress as a mechanism of teratogenesis with special emphasis on diabetic embryopathy. *Reprod Toxicol* 2007;**24**:31–41.

29. Lieu PT, Heiskala M, Peterson PA, Yang Y. The roles of iron in health and disease. *Mol Aspect Med* 2001;**22**:1–87.

30. Crichton RR. Proteins of iron storage and transport. *Adv Prot Chem* 1990;**40**:281–363.

31. Harrison PM, Arosio P. The ferritins: molecular properties, iron storage function and cellular regulation. *Biochim Biophys Acta* 1996;**1275**:161–203.

32. Huang X. Iron overload and its association with cancer risk in humans: evidence for iron as a carcinogenic metal. *Mutat Res* 2003;**533**:153–71.

33. Higuchi M, Yoshikawa Y, Orino K, Watanabe K. Effects of diquat-induced oxidative stress on iron metabolism in male Fischer-344 rats. *Biometals* 2011b;**24**:1123–31.

34. Ganne-Carrié N, Christidis C, Chastang C, et al. Liver iron is predictive of death in alcoholic cirrhosis: a multivariate study of 229 consecutive patients with alcoholic and/or hepatitis C virus cirrhosis: a prospective follow up study. *Gut* 2000;**46**:277–82.

35. Stevens RG, Graubard BI, Micozzi MS, Neriishi K, Blumberg BS. Moderate elevation of body iron level and increased risk of cancer occurrence and death. *Int J Cancer* 1994;**56**:364–9.

36. Merk K, Mattsson B, Mattsson A, Holm G, Gullbring B, Bjorkholm M. The incidence of cancer among blood donors. *Int J Epidemiol* 1990;**19**:505–9.

37. Jiang R, Manson JE, Meigs JB, Ma J, Rifai N, Hu FB. Body iron stores in relation to risk of type 2 diabetes in apparently healthy women. *JAMA* 2004;**291**:711–7.

38. Lee TS, Shiao MS, Pan CC, Chau LY. Iron-deficient diet reduces atherosclerotic lesions in apo-E-deficient mice. *Circulation* 1999;**99**:1222–9.

39. Kato J, Kobune M, Kohgo Y, et al. Hepatic iron deprivation prevents spontaneous development of fulminant hepatitis and liver cancer in Long-Evans Cinnamon rats. *J Clin Invest* 1996;**98**:923–9.

40. Gutteridge JM. Lipid peroxidation and antioxidants as biomarkers of tissue damage. *Clin Chem* 1995;**1995**(41):1819–28.

41. Sies H. Oxidative stress: oxidants and antioxidants. *Exp Physiol* 1997;**82**:291–5.

42. Miller HE, Rigelhof F, Marquart L, Prakash A, Kanter M. Antioxidant content of whole grain breakfast cereals, fruits and vegetables. *J Am Coll Nutr* 2000;**19**:312S–9S.

43. Zelko IN, Mariani TJ, Folz RJ. Superoxide dismutase multigene family: a comparison of the CuZn-SOD (SOD1), Mn-SOD (SOD2), and EC-SOD (SOD3) gene structure, evolution, and expression. *Free Radic Biol Med* 2002;**33**:337–49.

44. Bannister JV, Bannister WH, Rotilio G. Aspects of the structure, function, and applications of superoxide dismutase. *CRC Crit Rev Biochem* 1987;**22**:111–80.

45. Johnson F, Giulivi C. Superoxide dismutases and their impact upon human death. *Mol Aspects Med* 2005;**26**:340–52.

46. Nozik-Grayck E, Suliman HB, Piantadosi CA. Extracellular superoxide dismutase. *Int J Biochem Cell Biol* 2005;**37**:2466–71.

47. Ho YS, Gargano M, Cao J, Bronson RT, Heimler I, Hutz RJ. Reduced fertility in female mice lacking copper-zinc superoxide dismutase. *J Biol Chem* 1998;**273**:7765–9.

48. Li Y, Huang TT, Carlson EJ, et al. Dilated cardiomyopathy and neonatal lethality in mutant mice lacking manganese superoxide dismutase. *Nature Genet* 1995;**11**:376–81.

49. Carlsson LM, Jonsson J, Edlund T, Marklund SL. Mice lacking extracellular superoxide dismutase are more sensitive to hyperoxia. *Proc Natl Acad Sci USA* 1995;**92**:6264–8.

50. Rosen DR, Siddique T, Patterson D, et al. Mutations in Cu/Zn superoxide dismutase gene are associated with familial amyotrophic lateral sclerosis. *Nature* 1993;**362**:59–62.

51. Lardinois OM. Reactions of bovine liver catalase with superoxide radicals and hydrogen peroxide. *Free Radic Res* 1995;**22**:251–74.

52. Sies H. Strategies of antioxidant defense. *Eur J Biochem* 1993;**215**:213–9.

53. Galasso G, Schiekofer S, Sato K, et al. Impaired angiogenesis in glutathione peroxidase-1-deficient mice is associated with endothelial progenitor cell dysfunction. *Circ Res* 2006;**98**:254–61.

54. Palmer FM, Nieman DC, Henson DA, et al. Influence of vitamin C supplementation on oxidative and salivary IgA changes following and ultramarathon. *Eur J Appl Physiol* 2003;**89**:100–7.

55. Evans WJ. Vitamin E, vitamin C, and exercise. *Am J Clin Nutr* 2000;**72**:647–52.

56. Gershoff SN. Vitamin C (ascorbic acid): new roles, new requirements? *Nutr Rev* 1993;**51**:313–26.

57. Meyers DG, Maloley PA, Weeks D. Safety of antioxidant vitamins. *Arch Intern Med* 1996;**156**:925–35.

58. Fuchs J, Weber S, Podda M, et al. HPLC analysis of vitamin E isoforms in human epidermis: correlation with minimal erythema dose and free radical scavenging activity. *Free Radic Biol Med* 2003;**34**:330–6.

59. Atkinson J, Epand RF, Epand RM. Tocopherols and tocotrienols in membranes: a critical review. *Free Radic Biol Med* 2008;**44**:739–64.

60. Vasankari TJ, Kujara UM, Vasankari TM, Vuorimaa T, Ahotupa M. Effects of acute prolonged exercise on serum and LDL oxidation and antioxidant defenses. *Free Radic Biol Med* 1997;**22**:509–13.

61. Liebler DC, Kling DS, Reed DJ. Antioxidant protection of phospholipid bilayers by α-tocopherol. *J Biol Chem* 1986;**261**:12114–9.

62. Traber MG, Sies H. Vitamin E in humans: demand and delivery. *Annu Rev Nutr* 1996;**16**:321–47.

63. Brigelius-Flohé R, Traber MG, Vitamin E. function and metabolism. *FASEB J* 1999;**13**:1145–55.

64. Kowdley KV, Mason JB, Meydani SN, Cornwall S, Grand RJ. Vitamin E deficiency and impaired cellular immunity related to intestinal fat malabsorption. *Gastroenterology* 1992;**102**:2139–42.

65. Stampfer MJ, Rimm EB. Epidemiologic evidence for vitamin E in prevention of cardiovascular disease. *Am J Clin Nutr* 1995;**62**:1365S–9S.

66. "Standard Tables of Feed Composition in Japan" [in Japanese]. Agriculture, Forestry and Fisheries Research Council Secretariat, Central Association of Livestock Industry. 1995; pp. 207–9.

67. Mortensen A, Skibsted LH. Importance of carotenoid structure in radical-scavenging reactions. *J Agric Food Chem* 1997;**45**:2970–7.

68. Krinsky NI. The biological properties of carotenoids. *Pure & Appl Chem* 1994;**66**:1003–10.

69. Burton GW, Ingold KU. β-Carotene: an unusual type of lipid antioxidant. *Science* 1984;**224**:569–73.

70. Livrea MA, Tesoriere L, Bongiorno A, Pintaudi AM, Ciaccio M, Riccio A. Contribution of vitamin A to the oxidation resistance of human low density lipoproteins. *Free Radic Biol Med* 1995;**18**:401–9.

71. Boileau TW, Liao Z, Kim S, Lemeshow S, Edman Jr JW, Clinton SK. Prostate carcinogenesis in N-methyl-N-nitrosourea (NMU)-testosterone-treated rats fed tomato powder, lycopene, or energy-restricted diets. *J Nutl Cancer Inst* 2003;**95**:1578–86.

72. Pastori M, Pfander H, Boscoboinik D, Azzi A. Lycopene in association with alpha-tocopherol inhibits at physiological concentrations proliferation of prostate carcinoma cells. *Biochem Biophys Res Commun* 1998;**250**:582–5.

73. Karas M, Amir H, Fishman D, et al. Lycopene interferes with cell cycle progression and insulin-like growth factor signaling in mammary cancer cells. *Nutr Cancer* 2000;**36**:101–11.

74. Sokoloski JA, Hodnick WF, Mayne ST, Cinquina C, Kim CS, Sartorelli AC. Induction of the differentiation of HL-60 promyelocytic leukemia cells by vitamin E and other antioxidants in combination with low levels of vitamin D3: possible relationship to NF-κB. *Leukemia* 1997;**11**:1546–53.

75. Omenn GS, Goodman DGE, Thornquist MD, et al. Effects of a combination of beta catotene and vitamin A on lung cancer and cardiovascular disease. *N Engl J Med* 1996;**334**:1150–5.

76. Hennekens CH, Buring JE, Manson JE, et al. Lack of effect of long-term supplementation with beta carotene on the incidence of malignant neoplasms and cardiovascular disease. *N Engl J Med* 1996;**334**:1145–9.

77. Zhou K, Su L, Yu LL. Phytochemicals and antioxidant properties in wheat bran. *J Agric Food Chem* 2004;**52**:6108–14.

78. Nijveldt RJ, van Nood E, van Hoorn DEC, Boelens PG, van Norren K, van Leeuwen PAM. Flavonoids: a review of probable mechanisms of action and potential applications. *Am J Clin Nutr* 2001;**74**:418–25.

79. Pietta PG. Flavonoids as antioxidants. *J Nat Prod* 2000;**63**:1035–42.

80. Brown JE, Khodr H, Hider RC, Rice-Evans CA. Structural dependence of flavonoid interactions with Cu^{2+} ions: implications for their antioxidant properties. *Biochem J* 1998;**330**:1173–8.

81. Braca A, Sortino C, Politi M, Morelli I, Mendez J. Antioxidant activity of flavonoids from *Licania licaniaeflora*. *J Ethnopharmacol* 2002;**79**:379–81.

82. Rice-Evans CA, Miller NJ, Paganga G. Structure–antioxidant activity relationships of flavonoids and phenolic acids. *Free Radic Biol Med* 1996;**20**:933–56.

83. Rahman K. Garlic and aging: new insights into an old remedy. *Aging Res Rev* 2003;**2**:39–56.

84. Rahimi R, Nikfar S, Larijani B, Abdollahi M. A review on the role of antioxidants in the management of diabetes and its complications. *Biomed Pharmacother* 2005;**59**:365–73.

85. Hedge PS, Rajasekaran NS, Chandra TS. Effects of the antioxidant properties od millet species on oxidative stress and glycemic status in alloxan-induced rats. *Nutr Res* 2005;**25**:1109–20.

86. Song Y, Manson JE, Buring JE, Sesso HD, Liu S. Associations of dietary flavonoids with risk of type 2 diabetes, and markers of insulin resistance and systemic inflammation in women: a prospective study and cross-sectional analysis. *J Am Coll Nutr* 2005;**24**:376–84.

87. Stevenson L, Phillips F. O'Sullivan, Walton J. Wheat bran: its composition and benefits to health, a European perspective. *Int J Food Sci Nutr* 2012;**63**:1001–13.

88. Masella R, Benedetto RD, Vari R, Filesi C. Giovannini. Novel mechanisms of natural antioxidant compounds in biological systems: involvement of glutathione and glutathione-related enzymes. *J Nutr Biochem* 2005;**16**:577–86.

89. Reed DJ, Fariss MW. Glutathione depletion and susceptibility. *Pharmacol Rev* 1984;**36**:23S–33S.

90. Pastore A, Federici G, Bertini E, Piemonte F. Analysis of glutathione: implication in redox and detoxification. *Clin Chim Acta* 2003;**333**:19–39.

91. Matés JM, Pérez-Gómez C, Núñez de Castro I. Antioxidant enzymes and human diseases. *Clin Biochem* 1999;**32**:595–603.

92. Fardet A. New hypotheses for the health protective mechanisms of whole-grain cereals: what is beyond fibre? *Nutr Res Rev* 2010;**23**:65–134.

93. Métayer S, Seiliez I, Collin A, et al. Mechanisms through which sulphur amino acids control metabolism and oxidative status. *J Nutr Biochem* 2008;**19**:207–15.

94. Navari-Izzo F, Quartacci MF, Sgherri C. Lipoic acid: a unique antioxidant in the detoxification of activated oxygen species. *Plant Physiol Biochem* 2002;**40**:463–70.

95. Suzuki YJ, Tsuchiya M, Packer L. Thioctic acid and dihydrolipoic acid are novel antioxidants which interact with reactive oxygen species. *Free Radic Res Commun* 1991;**15**:255–63.

96. Scott BC, Aruoma OI, Evans PEJ, et al. Lipoic and dihydrolipoic acid as antioxidants. A critical evaluation. *Free Rad Res* 1994;**20**:119–33.

97. Cornaro U, Cariati F, Bonomi F. Evidences for the formation of complexes of DL-dihydrolipoic acid (reduced lipoic acid) with Ni^{2+}, Co^{2+}, and Fe^{3+} salts. *Rev Port Quim* 1985;**27**:273–4.

98. Biewenga GP, Haenen GRMM, Bast A. The pharmacology of the antioxidant lipoic acid. *Gen Pharmacol* 1997;**29**:315–31.

99. Ou P, Tritschler HJ, Wolff SP. Thioctic (lipoic acid): a therapeutic metal-chelating antioxidant? *Biochem Pharmacol* 1995;**50**:123–6.

100. Scholich H, Murphy ME, Sies H. Antioxidant activity of dihydrolipoate against microsomal lipid peroxidation and its dependence on αα-tocopherol. *Biochim Biophys Acta* 1989;**1001**:256–61.

101. Song KH, Lee WJ, Koh JM, et al. alpha-Lipoic acid prevents diabetes mellitus in diabetes-prone obese rats. *Biochem Biophys Res Commun* 2005;**326**:197–202.

102. Andrews SC, Arosio P, Bottke W, et al. Structure, function, and evolution of ferritins. *J Inorg Biochem* 1992;**47**:161–74.

103. Harrison PM, Arosio P. The ferritins: molecular properties, iron storage function and cellular regulation. *Biochim Biophys Acta* 1996;**1275**:161–203.

104. Theil EC. Ferritin: Structure, gene regulation, and cellular function in animals, plants, and microorganisms. *Annu Rev Biochem* 1987;**56**:289–315.

105. Ford GC, Harrison PM, Rice DW, Smith JMA, Treffry A, White JL, Yariv J. Ferritin: design and formation of an iron-storage molecule. *Philos Trans R Soc Lond B Biol Sci* 1984;**304**:551–65.

106. Levi S, Luzzago A, Cesareni G, et al. Mechanism of ferritin iron uptake: activity of the H-chain and deletion mapping of the ferro-oxidase site A study of iron uptake and ferro-oxidase activity of human liver recombinant H-chain ferritin, and of two H-chain deletion mutants. *J Biol Chem* 1988;**263**:18086–92.

107. Levi S, Salfeld J, Franceshinelli F, Cozzi A, Dorner MH, Arosio P. Expression and Structural and functional properties of human ferritin L-chain from Escherichia coli. *Biochemistry* 1989;**28**:5179–84.

108. Orino K, Harada S, Natsuhori M, Takehara K, Watanabe K. Kinetic analysis of bovine spleen apoferritin and recombinant H and L chain homopolymers: iron uptake suggests early stage H chain ferroxidase activity and second stage L chain cooperation. *Biometals* 2004;**17**:129–34.

109. Ferreira C, Bucchini D, Martin ME, et al. Early embryonic lethality of H ferritin gene deletion in mice. *J Biol Chem* 2000;**275**:3021–4.

110. Tsuji Y, Ayaki H, Whitman SP, Morrow CS, Torti SV, Torti FM. Coordinate transcriptional and translational regulation of ferritin in response to oxidative stress. *Mol Cell Biol* 2000;**20**:5818–27.

111. Orino K, Watanabe K. Molecular, physiological and clinical aspects of the iron storage protein ferritin. *Vet J* 2008;**178**:191–201.

112. Stadtman TC. Selenocystein. *Annu Rev Biochem* 1996;**65**:83–100.

113. Burk RF, Lawrence RA, Lane JM. Liver necrosis and lipid peroxidation in the rat as the result of paraquat and diquat administration. Effect of selenium deficiency. *J Clin Invest* 1980;**65**:1024–31.

114. Fu Y, Cheng WH, Porres JM, Ross DA, Lei XG. Knockout of cellular glutathione peroxidase gene renders mice susceptible to diquat-induced oxidative stress. *Free Radic Biol Med* 1999;**27**:605–11.

115. Köhrle J, Jakob F, Contempre B, Dumont JE. Selenium, the thyroid, and the endocrine system. *Endocrine Rev* 2005;**26**:944–84.

116. Burk RF. Selenium in nutrition. *World Rev Nutr Diet* 1978;**30**:88–106.

117. Qu H, Madl RL, Takemoto DJ, Baybutt RC, Wang W. Lignans are involved in the antitumor activity of wheat bran in colon cancer SW480 cells. *J Nutr* 2005;**135**:598–602.

118. Davies MJ, Bowey EA, Adlercreutz H, Rowland IR, Rumsby PC. Effects of soy or rye supplementation of high-fat diets on colon tumor development in azoxymethane-treated rats. *Carcinogenesis* 1999;**20**:927–31.

119. Wang W, Goodman MT. Antioxidant properties of dietary phenolic agents in a human LDL-oxidation *ex vivo* model: interaction of protein binding activity. *Nutr Res* 1999;**19**:191–202.

120. Drankhan K, Carter J, Madl R, et al. Antitumor activity of wheats with high orthophenolic content. *Nutr Cancer* 2003;**47**:188–94.

121. O'Dell BL, de Boland AR, Koirtyohann SR. Distribution of phytate and nutritionally important elements among the morphological components of cereal grains. *J Agric Food Chem* 1972;**20**:718–21.

122. Graf E, Eaton JW. Antioxidant functions of phytic acid. *Free Radic Biol Med* 1990;**8**:61–9.

123. Midorikawa K, Murata M, Oikawa S, Hiraku Y, Kawanishi S. Protective effect of phytic acid on oxidative DNA damage with reference to cancer chemoprevention. *Biochem Biophys Res Commun* 2001;**288**:552–7.

124. Graf E, Eaton JW. Dietary suppression of colonic cancer. Fiber or phytate? *Cancer* 1985;**56**:717–8.

125. Urbano G, Lopez-Jurado M, Aranda P, Vidal-Valverde C, Tenorio E, Porres J. The role of phytic acid in legumes: antinutrient or beneficial function? *J Physiol Biochem* 2000;**56**:283–94.

126. Jenab M, Thompson LU. Phytic acid in wheat bran affects colon morphology, cell differentiation and apoptosis. *Carcinogenesis* 2000;**21**:1547–52.

127. Shamsuddin AM, Vucenik I. Mammary tumor inhibition by IP6: a review. *Anticancer Res* 1999;**19**:3671–4.

128. Fox CH, Eberl M. Phytic acid (IP6), novel broad spectrum antineoplastic agent: a systematic review. *Complement Ther Med* 2002;**10**:229–34.

129. Lopez-Gonzalez AA, Grases F, Roca O, Mari B, Vicente-Herrero MT, Costa-Bauza A. Phytate (myo-inositol hexaphosphate) and risk factors for osteoporosis. *J Med Food* 2008;**11**:747–52.

130. Maga JA. Phytate: its chemisty, occurrence, food interactions, nutritional significance, and methods of analysis. *J Agric Food Chem* 1982;**30**:1–9.

131. Yu L, Perret J, Harris M, Wilson J, Haley S. Antioxidant properties of bran extracts from "Akron" wheat grown at different locations. *J Agric Food Chem* 2003;**51**:1566–70.

132. Onyeneho SN, Hettiarachchy NS. Antioxidant activity of durum wheat bran. *J Agric Food Chem* 1992;**40**:1496–500.

133. Baublis AJ, Lu C, Clydesdale FM, Decker EA. Potential of wheat-based breakfast cereals as a source of dietary antioxidants. *J Am Coll Nutr* 2000;**19**:308S–11S.

134. Liyana-Pathirana CM, Shahidi F. Importance of insoluble-bound phenolics to antioxidant properties of wheat. *J Agric Food Chem* 2006;**54**:1256–64.

135. Baublis AJ, Decker EA, Clydesdale FM. Antioxidant effect of aqueous extracts from wheat based ready-to-eat breakfast cereals. *Food Chem* 2000;**68**:1–6.

136. Robbins RJ. Phenolic acids in foods: an overview of analytical methodology. *J Agric Food Chem* 2003;**51**:2866–87.

137. Kähkönen MP, Hopia AI, Vuorela HJ, et al. Antioxidant activity of plant extracts containing phenolic compounds. *J Agric Food Chem* 1999;**47**:3954–62.

138. Kim KH, Tsao R, Yang R, Cui SW. Phenolic acid profiles and antioxidant activities of wheat bran extracts and the effect of hydrolysis conditions. *Food Chem* 2006;**95**:466–73.

139. Zhao Z, Moghadasian MH. Chemistry, natural sources, dietary intake and pharmacokinetic properties of ferulic acid: a review. *Food Chem* 2008;**109**:691–702.

140. Saulnier L, Thibault JF. Ferulic acid and diferulic acids as components of sugar-beet pectins and maize bran heteroxylans. *J Sci Food Agric* 1999;**79**:396–402.

141. Zhao Z, Egashira Y, Sanada H. Phenolic antioxidants richly contained in corn bran are slightly bioavailable in rats. *J Agric Food Chem* 2005;**53**:5030–5.

142. Madhujith T, Shahidi F. Optimization of the extraction of antioxidative constituents of six barley cultivars and their antioxidant properties. *J Agric Food Chem* 2006;**54**:8048–57.

143. Shibuya N. Phenolic-acids and their carbohydrate esters in rice endosperm cell-walls. *Phytochemistry* 1984;**23**:2233–7.

144. Kroon PA, Williamson G. Hydroxycinnamates in plants and food: current and future perspectives. *J Sci Food Agric* 1999;**79**:355–61.

145. Andreasen MF, Kroon PA, Williamson G, Garcia-Conesa MT. Esterase activity able to hydrolyze dietary antioxidant hydroxycinnamates is distributed along the intestine of mammals. *J Agric Food Chem* 2001;**49**:5679–84.

146. Mattila P, Pihlava JM, Hellström J. Contents of phenolic acids, alkyl- and alkenylresorcinols, and avenanthramides in commercial grain products. *J Agric Food Chem* 2005;**53**:8290–5.

147. Adom KK, Liu RH. Antioxidant activity of grains. *J Agric Food Chem* 2002;**50**:6182–7.

148. Nishizawa C, Ohta T, Egashira Y, Sanada H. Ferulic acid contents in typical cereals [in Japanese, with abstract in English]. *Nippon Shokuhin Kagaku Kogaku Kaishi* 1998;**45**:499–503.

149. Mattila P, Hellström J, Törrönen R. Phenolic acids in berries, fruits, and bevarages. *J Agric Food Chem* 2006;**54**:7193–9.

150. Sakakibara H, Honda Y, Nakagawa S, Ashida H, Kanazawa K. Simultaneous determination of all polyphenols in vegetables, fruits, and teas. *J Agric Food Chem* 2003;**51**:571–81.

151. Mattila P, Hellström J. Phenolic acids in potatoes, vegetables, and some of their products. *J Food Compos Anal* 2007;**20**:152–60.

152. Bourne LC, Rice-Evans C. Bioavailability of ferulic acid. *Biochem Biophys Res Commun* 1998;**253**:222–7.

153. Micard V, Grabber JH, Ralph J, Renard CMGC, Thibault JF. Dehydrodiferulic acids from sugar-beet pulps. *Phytochemistry* 1997;**44**:1365–8.

154. Nardini M, Cirillo E, Netella F, Scaccini C. Absorption of phenolic acids in humans after coffee consumption. *J Agric Food Chem* 2002;**50**:5735–41.

155. Rapisarda P, Carollo G, Fallico B, Tomaselli F, Maccarone E. Hydroxycinnamic acids as markers of Italian blood orange juices. *J Agric Food Chem* 1998;**46**:464–70.

156. Clifford MN. Chlorogenic acids and other cinnamates – nature, occurrence and dietary burden. *J Sci Food Agric* 1999;**79**:362–72.

157. Herrmann K. Occurrence and content of hydroxycinnamic and hydroxybenzoic acid compounds in foods. *Crit Rev Food Sci Nutr* 1989;**28**:315–47.

158. Bakalbassis EG. Lithoxoidous AT and Vafiadis AP. Theoretical calculation of accurate absolute and relative gas- and liquid-phase O-H bond dissociation enthalpies of 2-mono-and 2,6-disubstituted phenols, using DFT/B3LYP. *J Phys Chem A* 2003;**107**:8594–606.

159. Graf E. Antioxidant potential of ferulic acid. *Free Radic Biol Med* 1992;**13**:435–48.

160. Ou S, Li Y, Gao K. A study on scavenging activity of wheat bran dietary fiber for free radical. *Acta Nutr Sin* 1999;**21**:191–4.

161. Ou S, Kwok KC. Ferulic acid: pharmaceutical functions, preparation and applications in foods. *J Sci Food Agric* 2004;**84**:1261–9.

162. Zhou K, Yin JJ, Yu LL. Phenolic acid, tocopherol and carotenoid compositions, and antioxidant functions of hard red winter wheat bran. *J Agric Food Chem* 2005;**53**:3916–22.

163. Kim HK, Jeong TS, Lee MK, Park YB, Choi MS. Lipid-lowering efficacy of hesperetin metabolites in high-cholesterol fed rats. *Clin Chim Acta* 2003;**327**:129–37.

164. Kim M, Choi J, Lim SJ, et al. Ferulic acid supplementation prevents trimethyltin-induced cognitive deficits in mice. *Biosci Biotechnol Biochem* 2007;**71**:1063–8.

165. Suzuki A, Yamamoto M, Jokura H, et al. Ferulic acid restores endothelium-dependent vasodilation in aortas of spontaneously hypertensive rats. *Am J Hypertens* 2007;**20**:508–13.

166. Yuan X, Wang J, Yao H. Antioxidant activity of feruloylated oligosaccharides from wheat bran. *Food Chem* 2005;**90**:759–64.

167. Halliwell B, Gutteridge JM, Cross CE. Free radicals, antioxidants, and human disease: where are we now? *J Lab Clin Med* 1992;**119**:598–620.
168. Gorinstein S, Bartnikowska E, Kulasek G, Zemser M, Trakhtenberg S. Dietary persimmon improves lipid metabolism in rats fed diets containing cholesterol. *J Nutr* 1998;**128**:2023–7.
169. Sabovic M, Lavre S, Keber I. Supplementation of wheat fiber can improve risk profile in patients with dysmetabolic cardiovascular syndrome. *Eur J Cardiovasc Prev Rehabil* 2004;**11**:144–8.
170. Willcox JK, Ash SL, Catignani GL. Antioxidants and prevention of chronic disease. *Crit Rev Food Sci Nutr* 2004;**44**:275–95.
171. Jensen MK, Koh-Banerjee P, Franz M, Sampson L, Gronbaek M, Rimm EB. Whole grains, bran, and germ in relation to homocysteine and markers of glycemic control, lipids, and inflammation. *Am J Clin Nutr* 2006;**83**:275–83.
172. Jensen MK, Koh-Banerjee P, Hu FB, et al. Intakes of whole grains, bran, and germ and the risk of coronary heart disease in men. *Am J Clin Nutr* 2004;**80**:1492–9.
173. Pereira MA, Jacobs Jr DR, Pins JJ, et al. Effect of whole grains on insulin sensitivity in overweight hyperinsulinemic adults. *Am J Clin Nutr* 2002;**75**:848–55.
174. Reddy BS, Hirose Y, Cohen LA, Simi B, Cooma I, Rao CV. Preventive potential of wheat bran fractions against experimental colon carcinogenesis: implications for human colon cancer prevention. *Cancer Res* 2000;**60**:4792–7.
175. Whelton PK, He J, Cutler JA, et al. Effects of oral potassium on blood pressure: meta-analysis of randomized controlled clinical trials. *J Am Med Assoc* 1997;**277**:1624–32.
176. Craig SAS. Betaine in human nutrition. *Am J Clin Nutr* 2004;**80**:539–49.
177. de Munter JS, Hu FB, Spiegelman D, Franz M, van Dam RM. Whole grain, bran and germ intake and risk of type 2 diabetes: a prospective cohort study and systematic review. *PLoS Med* 2007;**4**:e261.
178. Qi J, Hu FB. Dietary glycemic load, whole grains, and systemic inflammation in diabetes: the epidemiological evidence. *Curr Opin Lipidol* 2007;**18**:3–8.
179. Wang J, Sun B, Cao Y, Tian Y. Protein glycation inhibitory activity of wheat bran feruloyl oligosaccharides. *Food Chem* 2009;**112**:350–3.
180. Jacobs Jr DR, Gallaher DD. Whole grain intake and cardiovascular disease: a review. *Curr Atheroscler Rep* 2004;**6**:415–23.
181. Mozaffarian D, Kumanyika SK, Lemaitre RN, et al. Cereal, fruit, and vegetable fiber intake and the risk of cardiovascular disease in elderly individuals. *JAMA* 2003;**289**:1659–66.
182. Lupton JR, Turner ND. Potential protective mechanisms of wheat bran fiber. *Am J Med* 1999;**106**:24S–7S.
183. Freudenheim JL, Graham S, Horvath PJ, Marshall JR, Haughey BP, Wilkinson G. Risks associated with source of fiber and fiber components in cancer of the colon and rectum. *Cancer Res* 1990;**50**:3295–300.
184. Sang S, Ju J, Lambert JD, et al. Wheat bran oil and its fractions inhibit human colon cancer cell growth and intestinal tumorigenesis in Apc (min/+) mice. *J Agric Food Chem* 2006;**54**:9792–7.
185. Topping D. Cereal complex carbohydrates and their contribution to human health. *J Cereal Sci* 2007;**46**:220–9.
186. Slavin JL. Mechanisms for the impact of whole grain foods on cancer risk. *J Am Coll Nutr* 2000;**19**:300S–7S.
187. Venkatesan N, Devaraj SN, Devaraj H. A fibre cocktail of fenugreek, guar gum and wheat bran reduces oxidative modification of LDL induced by an atherogenic diet in rats. *Mol Cell Biochem* 2007;**294**:145–53.
188. Yu LL, Zhou K, Parry JW. Inhibitory effects of wheat bran extracts on human LDL oxidation and free radicals. *LWT* 2005;**38**:463–70.
189. Pereira MA, O'Reilly E, Augustsson K, et al. Dietary fiber and risk of coronary heart disease: a pooled analysis of cohort studies. *Arch Intern Med* 2004;**164**:370–6.

F. WHEAT FIBER

Wheat and Rice Dietary Fiber in Colorectal Cancer Prevention and the Maintenance of Health

Philip J. Harris, *Lynnette R. Ferguson*†

*University of Auckland, School of Biological Sciences, Auckland, New Zealand, †Discipline of Nutrition, Auckland, New Zealand

INTRODUCTION

Whole grain cereals, including wheat and rice, together with fruits and vegetables, are excellent sources of dietary fiber. However, the definition of dietary fiber and the methods of determining the dietary fiber content of foods have changed considerably since the term was first coined by Hipsley.[1] In this chapter we first outline the changes that have occurred in the definition of dietary fiber. We then indicate the range of chemical components included in each of these definitions, followed by the associated changes that have taken place in dietary fiber analysis. Finally, we comment on the implications of these changes for nutritional research and disease prevention.

CHANGES IN THE DEFINITION OF DIETARY FIBER

When the concept of dietary fiber was first coined, components of plant cell walls were the only components. In a footnote, Hipsley stated that the term "includes lignin, cellulose and the hemicelluloses". However, the first definition of dietary fiber which is usually quoted by nutritionalists is that of Trowell: "The skeletal remains of plant cells that are resistant to digestion by enzymes of man may be called dietary fiber (DF) to distinguish them from crude fiber (CF)".[2] In a further paper,[3] Trowell went on to emphasize that the term dietary fiber was introduced to distinguish it from the unsatisfactory term crude fiber, which had been internationally defined as "the portion of plant food resistant to hydrolysis by acid and subsequently by alkali". Trowell indicated that the concept of dietary fiber "provides a definition in terms of physiology as the remnants of plant cells resistant to hydrolysis by the alimentary enzymes of man, the group of substances that remain in the ileum but are partly hydrolyzed by bacteria in the colon." It was identified chemically as components of plant cell walls: cellulose, non-cellulosic polysaccharides (hemicelluloses and pectins), lignin, waxes, cutin, and suberin. This definition was extended to include indigestible dietary polysaccharides in addition to those in the plant cell wall.[4] These refer to non-starch polysaccharides obtained from plant cell walls and from sources other than plant cell walls.[5]

In the early 1990s, it became widely evident that two further components could potentially be added to the definition of dietary fiber: resistant starch, and non-digestible oligosaccharides (NDOs).[6] However, a fraction of dietary starch which escaped digestion in the mouth and small intestine had been discovered much earlier by Englyst and Cummings.[7] An international survey held in 1993 found that 80% of respondents were in favor of including resistant starch in the definition of dietary fiber and 65% were in favor of the inclusion of NDOs. Following this, the American Association of Cereal Chemists International consulted widely and proposed the following extended definition of dietary fiber:[8]

Dietary fiber is the edible parts of plants or analogous carbohydrates that are resistant to digestion and absorption in the human small intestine with complete or partial fermentation in the large intestine. Dietary fiber includes polysaccharides, oligosaccharides, lignin, and associated plant substances. Dietary fibers promote beneficial physiological effects, including laxation, and/or blood cholesterol attenuation, and/or blood glucose attenuation.

For the first time, this definition included physiological effects of dietary fiber. Physiological effects were also included in the first international agreed definition of dietary fiber that was finally adopted by the Codex Alimentarius Commission in 2009: [9]

Dietary fiber means carbohydrate polymers [1] with ten or more monomeric units [2] which are not hydrolysed by the endogenous enzymes in the small intestine of humans and belong to the following categories: edible carbohydrate polymers naturally occurring in the food as consumed; carbohydrate polymers, which have been obtained from food raw material by physiological, enzymic or chemical means and which have been shown to have a physiological effect of benefit to health as demonstrated by generally accepted scientific evidence to competent authorities; synthetic carbohydrate polymers which have been shown to have a physiological effect of benefit to health as demonstrated by generally accepted scientific evidence to competent authorities.

The two footnotes to the definition stated the following. Footnote [1]:

When derived from a plant origin, dietary fiber may include fractions of lignin and/or other compounds when associated with polysaccharides in the plant cell walls and if these compounds are quantified by the AOAC gravimetric analytical method for dietary fiber analysis. Fractions of lignin and the other compounds (proteic fractions, phenolic compounds, waxes, saponins, phytates, cutin, phytosterols, etc.) intimately "associated" with plant polysaccharides are often extracted with the polysaccharides in the AOAC 991.43 method. These substances are included in the definition of fiber insofar as they are actually associated with the poly- or oligosaccharidic fraction of fiber. However, when extracted or even reintroduced into a food containing non-digestible polysaccharides, they cannot be defined as dietary fiber. When combined with polysaccharides, these associated substances may provide additional beneficial effects (pending adoption of Section on methods of analysis and sampling).

Footnote [2]:

Decision on whether to include carbohydrates from 3 to 9 monomeric units should be left to national authorities.

We now discuss the wide variety of components currently included in the term "dietary fiber".

DIETARY FIBER COMPONENTS

Plant Cell Walls

Plant cell walls vary considerably in their compositions depending on plant species and cell types, but they all have a similar basic construction which comprises a fibrillar phase of cellulose microfibrils that is embedded in a matrix of non-cellulosic polysaccharides with a variety of structures.[10,11] In the cell walls of most fruits and vegetables these non-cellulosic polysaccharides are mainly pectic polysaccharides (pectins), with smaller proportions of xyloglucans. In contrast, in cereal grain cell walls these polysaccharides occur in only small proportions. Interestingly despite wheat and rice being major world cereals, much more has been published on the composition of the cell walls of wheat than of rice.

Botanically, the outer layers of the whole grain, which are removed during milling, are known as the bran layers, and comprise (from the outside in) the pericarp, seed coat (or testa), and aleurone.[12] In whole grains, a high percentage of the total non-starch polysaccharides (cell wall polysaccharides) in the grain is in these bran layers; in wheat, the proportion is 70%. The rest of the cell wall polysaccharides are in the thin cell walls of the starchy endosperm, the tissue in grains that contains the starch. In wheat and rice, the main cell wall polysaccharides, in both the bran layers and the starchy endosperm, are arabinoxylans, with much smaller proportions of $(1\rightarrow3)$ $(1\rightarrow4)$-β-glucans. In wheat, these arabinoxylans (Fig. 16.1) have been studied in considerable detail.[13,14] Their proportions and detailed structures vary among cultivars and with tissue type, more complex side chains being present in the pericarp walls. In the cell walls of the bran layers, particularly the aleurone, the arabinoxylans are esterified with ferulic acid and its dehydrodimers.[10–16] Much lower proportions of feruloylated arabinoxylans are present in the starchy endosperm cell walls of wheat. Ferulate and its dehydrodimers also occur in the cell walls of whole grain rice, although less is known about their distribution in the walls of different cell types than in wheat.[16,17]

In the cell walls of wheat aleurone and starchy endosperm, cellulose is present in only small proportions (2–4%), but in greater proportions (~30%) in the thick pericarp cell walls.[13,18] Similar proportions of cellulose have been reported in rice pericarp walls,[19] but higher proportions (~23%) in starchy endosperm walls. Rice is also unusual in that high proportions of glucomannans have been reported in their starchy endosperm cell walls.[13]

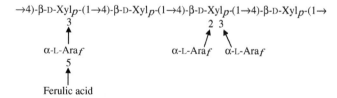

FIGURE 16.1 **The structure of the arabinoxylans found in wheat starchy endosperm cell walls.** The polysaccharide has a backbone of $(1\rightarrow4)$-linked β-Xyl*p* residues with single α-Ara*f* residues linked at *O*-3 or *O*-2 and *O*-3 of the Xyl*p* residues of the backbone. In the walls of the pericarp/seed coat layers, single α-D-glucuronic acid or α-D-4-*O*-methylglucuronic acid residues are joined at *O*-2 to some of the Xyl*p* residues and other, longer side chains may also be present.

In addition to polysaccharides, the walls of the outer (pericarp) bran layers of rice and wheat contain significant proportions of the phenolic polymer lignin, which confers hydrophobic properties to these walls.[16,19]

Non-Starch Polysaccharides Obtained from Plant Cell Walls and from Sources Other than Plant Cell Walls

Various polysaccharides extracted from plant cell walls are commonly used in the food industry and may be included in foods containing whole grain cereals.[5,20] They include soluble polysaccharides such as pectic polysaccharides (pectin), mostly from lemons, limes and apple pomace, as well as polysaccharides from the thick cell walls of various seeds. The latter include galactomannans from locust bean (carob) and guar seeds; xyloglucans from tamarind seeds; and a type of pectic polysaccharide (rhamnogalacturonan I) with mostly galactan side chains from several species of grain lupins such as *Lupinus angustifolius*. In addition, the insoluble cell-wall polysaccharide cellulose, obtained mostly from cotton linters or wood pulp, is used as a food additive. It is also used as the starting point for the production of a range of chemically modified celluloses that are water-soluble. These include sodium carboxymethyl cellulose, methyl cellulose, and hydroxypropylmethyl cellulose.

Other polysaccharides include non-starch polysaccharides from sources other than plant cell walls. These are mostly soluble polysaccharides and include polysaccharides exuded from plants (exudates gums), such as gum arabic, and mucilages produced by the outer layers of seeds, such as *Plantago ovata*, known as psyllium or ispaghula. They also include polysaccharides obtained from seaweed cell walls (carrageenans and agar) and those synthesized by some micro-organisms (e.g., gellan gum and xanthan gum).

Resistant Starches

For many years it was considered that all starch was fully digested by enzymes in the mouth and small intestine. However, the work of Hans Englyst and colleagues[21–23] showed that significant amounts of starch, referred to as resistant starch, are not digested. Resistant starch is defined as the sum of starch and the degradation products of starch that, on average, reaches the large intestine of healthy adult humans.[21,24] Four types of resistant starches, RS1–4, are now often recognized.[12,24–27]

RS1 is starch in the form of native (raw) granules entrapped in plant cells, and is physically inaccessible to α-amylases. This form of starch occurs in intact or coarsely milled cereal grains, including whole grain rice and wheat, and can be a significant source of dietary fiber in foods containing whole grain cereals. RS1 will also occur in other starch-rich seeds.

RS2 is starch in which the native (raw) starch granules are resistant to α-amylases because of their crystallinity. They include starch granules in potatoes, green banana fruit, and cultivars of plants with high-amylose starches. The latter include cereals, with cultivars of maize being the most well-known, although cultivars of wheat and rice, as well as barley, have been developed.[28–31] With the inclusion of resistant starch in the definition of dietary fiber, there is considerable interest in such cultivars as a way of increasing the dietary fiber content of foods. When starch granules swell (gelatinize) on being heated in water, this form of resistance is destroyed and the starch is digestible. The starch granules in potatoes and green banana fruit gelatinize at below 70°C, but the starch granules in the high-amylose maize cv. Hi-Maize® are fully gelatinized at 154–171°C – temperatures not usually reached during food processing.

RS3 is known as retrograded starch, and is formed when gelatinized starch is cooled. This form occurs in cooked foods that have been cooled. Amylose is particularly important in this process, as, on cooling, it retrogrades more quickly than amylopectin, so high-amylose starches are particularly good at producing this type of RS. RS4 consists of starches that are chemically modified in various ways, for example by being cross-linked, esterified or etherized, and are often used in processed foods. These different forms of resistant starch are likely to produce different physiological effects in the colon, and may occur together in foods.

Non-Digestible Oligosaccharides

Soon after resistant starch was discovered, non-digestible oligosaccharides were also recognized as being potential dietary fibers. These are water-soluble oligosaccharides that are resistant to digestion in the human small intestine but are degraded by bacteria in the colon. Some NDOs occur naturally in food plants, whereas others are synthetic or semisynthetic. Those that occur naturally in food plants include fructans, comprising inulin and fructo-oligosaccharides (FOS), which are commercially extracted for the food industry from chicory roots and Jerusalem artichoke tubers.[32] However, they also occur in cereal grains such as wheat, but only in small amounts in the mature grain (1.3–2.5%[13]), with much higher amounts occurring during grain filling.[33–35] Experimental bread has been made incorporating meal from immature wheat grains to increase the FOS content.[36] Another group of NDOs, the α-galactosides, are best known to occur in the seeds of leguminous plants,[37] but small amounts of raffinose and stachyose occur particularly in the embryo (germ) of mature grains.[34,38] Semisynthetic NDOs include the β-galacto-oligosaccharides, which are produced from lactose by the transglycosylating activity of microbial β-galactosidases.[35] They also include resistant maltodextrins, for example Fibersol-2, which are produced by heating maize starch under low moisture conditions with HCl, then treating with α-amylase to remove the digestible portion.[39] Polydextrose is a synthetic NDO made by vacuum thermal polymerization of glucose.[40]

CHANGES IN ANALYTICAL METHODS FOR DETERMINING DIETARY FIBER

The earliest method of determining the dietary fiber content of human and animal foods was the Weende method, developed in Germany in the 19th century.[41] This method involves treatment of the food with hot acid and alkali, and the residue, known as crude fiber is then quantified. This severely underestimates the cell wall content, and the residue contains mostly cellulose, as well as a variable proportion of non-cellulosic polysaccharides and lignin; it is better regarded as a fraction defined by the method itself.[41,42] The introduction of detergent fiber methods by van Soest in the 1960s was an important step forwards.[43–46] Neutral detergent fiber (NDF) and acid detergent fiber (ADF) are the residues left after extraction with hot neutral and acid detergent solutions, respectively. These methods were initially developed for forages, but later applied to human foods. NDF residues contain most of the cell wall components except for pectic polysaccharides, and may also contain heat-damaged proteins. ADF residues contain cellulose, lignin, and variable proportions of other cell wall polysaccharides.[42,45]

The growing interest in dietary fiber in foods in the 1970s and early 1980s led to the development of a number of dietary fiber methods in which digestible components, such as starch and proteins, were usually removed by enzyme preparations.[47–49] Further development of enzymatic methods in the USA resulted in the Prosky method.[6,50–53] (AOAC Official Method of Analysis 985.29), and further development of the Southgate method in the UK resulted in the Englyst method.[22,54–56] The Prosky method, in various forms, has been used extensively in the USA and other countries, including EC countries other than the UK. This is an enzymatic–gravimetric method which involves first the enzymatic degradation of starch and then protein, followed by the addition of ethanol to a final concentration of ~80% v/v, and the insoluble material is then dried and weighed. In contrast to the Prosky method, the Englyst method is an enzymatic–chemical method, which also involves a similar enzymatic degradation and precipitation with ethanol, but the insoluble residue is analyzed chemically for non-starch polysaccharides (NSPs) calculated by summing the individual neutral monosaccharides and uronic acids obtained by

acid hydrolysis. Unlike the Prosky method, in the Englyst method[22] a pretreatment with DMSO together with the α-amylase treatment ensures that starch is totally removed. Dietary fiber estimated by the Englyst method also does not include lignin, suberin, or cutin, so the values are lower than those obtained by the Prosky method. The Prosky value divided by 1.33 gives an approximation to the Englyst value, but this difference varies considerably with different foods.[56,57] Until 1999, when it was replaced by the Prosky method, the Englyst method was the recommended UK method for dietary fiber.

Following the international survey in 1993 regarding the possible inclusion of NDOs and resistant starch in dietary fiber and their subsequent inclusion in definitions, methods were developed to determine resistant starch and a range of specific NDOs.[6] For example, AOAC Official Methods were approved for resistant starch, fructans, galacto-oligosaccharides, and resistant maltodextrins.[6] This resulted in total dietary fiber values being calculated by adding these individual components to the Prosky total dietary fiber value. However, as McCleary[6] points out, some of the NDOs are partly quantified by the Prosky method. For example, this applies to the fructans, polydextrose, and fibersol-2 (a resistant maltodextrin). This also applies to resistant starch, where the residue quantified in the Prosky method includes some resistant starch, particularly RS3. These additions resulted in some double counting. To solve these problems, McCleary[6,58,59] devised a new method for total dietary fiber, which fits with the Codex Alimentarius Commission (2009) definition of dietary fiber. The method is similar in principle to the Prosky method and uses an extended digestion of starch at 37°C as described in a method for quantifying resistant starch (AOAC Official Method 2002.02).[60] After addition of ethanol, the soluble, low molecular weight component is analyzed for NDOs by HPLC. The method for measuring total dietary fiber[59] has been adopted as AOAC Official Method 2009.01, and a version of the method which gives soluble and insoluble dietary fiber has been adopted as AOAC Official Method 2011.25. Results using these new methods have already been applied to cereal products.[61] Potentially, the method could also be adapted for research purposes to give values for many of the components of dietary fiber, including resistant starch and specific NDOs.

IMPLICATIONS OF CHANGING DEFINITIONS OF DIETARY FIBER FOR THE PREVENTION OF COLORECTAL CANCER BY WHOLE GRAIN WHEAT AND RICE DIETARY FIBER

In the 1970s, Trowell, together with Burkitt, Painter, and Walker, put forward a series of hypotheses known as "dietary fiber hypotheses" in which they postulated that many diseases common in the modern Western world were, at least in part, caused by an insufficient intake of dietary fiber.[2–4,62,63] As well as colorectal cancer, these diseases included appendicitis, diverticular disease, ischemic heart disease, gallbladder disease, obesity, and diabetes mellitus. Burkitt brought dietary fiber and these hypotheses to the attention of the public in his popular book, *Don't Forget Fiber in your Diet*.[64] This, together with the results of increasing research activity on this topic, led government organizations around the world to recommend minimum intakes of dietary fiber. However, the original concept of dietary fiber as envisaged by Hipsley has now changed to encompass components other than plant cell walls.

Resistant starch is now a component of dietary fiber, and whole grain wheat and rice may contain RS1, RS2, and, when cooked and cooled, RS3. There have also been strenuous efforts to publicize the beneficial properties of resistant starch,[30,31] and so breeding efforts have been addressed towards developing high-amylose cultivars to increase the resistant starch content of grains. High-amylose rice appears to have a superior ability, compared with the parent rice, in decreasing body weight gain, while increasing fecal mass, fecal moisture, and short-chain fatty acids. All these properties may be beneficial in protecting against obesity, diabetes, and other risk factors for the metabolic syndrome.[65–67] High-amylose wheat appears to have similar health benefits.[68] However, current evidence (see below) indicates that resistant starch may not be the most beneficial type of dietary fiber in relation to prevention of colorectal cancer.

As was envisaged in the 1970s, the plant cell wall component of the dietary fibers of whole wheat and rice grains may play the major role in preventing colorectal cancer. Most of the cell walls in these grains are in the bran layers, and many of these cell walls are compositionally different from those in the rest of the grain, although much more is known about the composition of wheat than rice cell walls. The walls of the outer bran layers (pericarp) contain the phenolic polymer lignin, which covalently links to the non-starch polysaccharides and reduces the digestibility of these polysaccharides by hydrolytic enzymes produced by bacteria in the colon. This resistance of lignified cell walls to digestion and fermentation means that they may be largely intact in fecal deposits, and may be more likely to enhance fecal bulk and reduce transit times compared with non-starch polysaccharides alone.[69,70] Lignin also makes the cell walls hydrophobic. This property may be beneficial in that it increases the abilities of the cell walls to adsorb carcinogens.[71,72]

In both wheat and rice, the major non-starch polysaccharides in the cell walls of the bran layers as well as the starchy endosperm are arabinoxylans. To these polysaccharides are esterified varying amounts of the hydroxycinnamic ferulic acid (Fig. 16.1). Interestingly, the amount of ferulate is much greater on the arabinoxylans in the bran layers than in the starchy endosperm. At least some of this ferulate can be released into the colon by esterases produced by bacteria in this location, although the presence of lignin in some of these walls may well inhibit this process. Ferulic acid and related hydroxycinnamic acids have antioxidant, antimutagenic, and anti-inflammatory effects, and may be involved in cell–cell signaling and gene regulation.[73–77]

We have also extended our work on the cell walls of wheat bran layers by comparing the chemical composition and potential anticancer properties of two fractions, one pericarp-rich and one aleurone-rich, obtained by a special milling process. Interestingly, both fractions have different properties that may relate to cancer prevention through different mechanisms.[70,78]

The original dietary fiber hypotheses suggested that plant cell walls, largely in the form of non-starch polysaccharides, protected against colorectal cancer.[69] However, it is increasingly realized that other cell wall components, especially phenolic components, have important physiological effects on humans. Thus, it appears that the phenolic compounds rather than the non-starch polysaccharides in the cell walls of the bran layers are more likely to protect against colorectal cancer. However, much of the traditional database on foods has focused on non-starch polysaccharides, which are readily analyzed and quantified by the Englyst method.

COHORT STUDIES ON DIETARY FIBER INTAKE AND COLORECTAL CANCER RISK

The most comprehensive analysis of cohort studies is provided by the WCRF/AICR continuous update, published in 2010.[79] This review summarized a total of 22 prospective studies, published before December 2009. The authors performed a meta-analysis of the overall dataset, including a sub-analysis on cancer subsite (colon and rectal cancer). They also separated data for men and women, to conclude that the data for each of these groups were statistically significant, and released a press statement to this effect, which was widely dispersed. Frustratingly, with few exceptions, the method of assessment of non-starch polysaccharides or dietary fiber has not been described in detail in most of the studies, and it is usually impossible to pull apart data on wheat or rice from those of other dietary fiber sources. The Nurses' Health Study and the Health Professional Follow-up Study assessed dietary fiber intake using two methods: the Prosky and the Englyst.[80] The UK branch of the EPIC study also used two methods: the Englyst and the earlier Southgate method.[81] However, all of these methods detect a range of materials.

Dahm et al.[82] set up a prospective case–control study, using data from seven different UK-based cohort studies – two EPIC studies (Norfolk and Oxford), the Guernsey Study, the MRC National Survey of Health and Development, the Oxford Vegetarian Study, the UK Woman's Cohort Study and the Whitehall II study – to consider the impact of increased dietary fiber intake on colorectal cancer risk for 579 cases and 1996 matched controls. Although data were not consistent among studies, there was a general trend towards decreased colorectal cancer risk with increased DF intake. Similar data were available from The Pooling Project of Prospective Studies of Diet and Cancer.[83] None of these studies, however, distinguished the sources or nature of dietary fiber on colorectal cancer risk.

For the association between cereal dietary fiber intake and risk of colorectal cancer, a 10% decreased risk was observed in the age-adjusted model comparing the highest quintile to the lowest quintile; however, the association was attenuated when potential colorectal cancer risk factors were accounted for.[83]

DIETARY INTERVENTION STUDIES

The most definitive data, and those that allow discrimination of specific dietary fiber sources, are from dietary intervention studies. A collation of dietary intervention studies that purport to consider dietary fiber protection against colorectal cancer is provided in Table 16.1.[84–90]

The two studies cited as showing either weak or no effect of wheat bran protection against colorectal cancer are worth considering in some detail. The first of these was published by DeCosse and colleagues.[90] They considered a high-risk colorectal cancer population – subjects with familial adenomatous polyposis (FAP). Over a 4-year period, 58 FAP patients were supplemented with 4 g of ascorbic acid (vitamin C)/day plus 400 mg of α-tocopherol (vitamin E)/day alone or with a wheat bran-derived grain dietary fiber supplement (22.5 g/day), supplied by Kelloggs, or a similar-appearing placebo that was low in dietary fiber. This was a randomized, double-blind, placebo-controlled study, whose endpoint was rectal polyps in these patients. The strongest benefit was shown by those patients supplementing with the high dietary fiber supplement during the middle 2 years of the trial. These data are considered to provide evidence for inhibition of early stages of colorectal cancer by a wheat bran fiber supplement, fed in excess of 11 g/day.

Alberts and colleagues[87] considered dietary supplementation with a wheat bran fiber in a randomized trial that questioned whether this could reduce the recurrence of colorectal adenomas. Their population group comprised 1429 men and women, between 40 and 80 years of age, who had had at least one colorectal adenoma removed up to 3 months before the study. Their diet was supplemented with either 13.5 g or 2 g per day of what the authors described as "wheat bran fiber". No statistically significant differences between the groups were found.

At first sight, the trial by Schatzkin et al.[88] may appear to support the work of Alberts et al.,[87] but contradict the earlier work by DeCosse and colleagues.[90] Their hypothesis was similar: that regular consumption of a high dietary fiber diet protected against recurrence of rectal polyps. Their population, however, was different from that of DeCosse et al., whereby these were not FAP patients but rather members of the population whose polyps had been detected in screening programs. The study, however, was quite sizable, recruiting 2079 men and women aged 35 years or older who had had at least one colorectal adenoma removed within the previous 6 months. Subjects were randomly assigned to one of two groups who received high or low levels of dietary counseling. At the end of the trial period, there were no significant differences in colonic dysplasia or adenoma recurrence between the two groups. Similar negative results were obtained by McKeown-Eyssen et al.[89] in the Toronto polyp prevention trial.

THE CAPP TRIALS

The most comprehensive evidence of a dietary fiber protecting or not against colorectal cancer must come from the CAPP1 and CAPP2 trials.[84,85] These are both very comprehensive and well-designed studies, which decisively tested the ability of resistant starches to protect against the development of colorectal cancer. The rationale for both studies was similar. Plant breeders are creating high-amylose wheat and rice cultivars, on the assumption that the resistant starch will have good physiological effects. While some potentially useful physiological effects have indeed been seen in some studies,[30,31] the evidence from the CAPP trials definitively proves that they do not protect against colorectal cancer.

The CAPP1 trial[84] established a large randomized, placebo-controlled trial of 600 mg/d aspirin and/or 30 g/d of resistant starch or placebo, administered to 206 young FAP patients for a minimum of 1 year ranging to a maximum to 12 years. The resistant starch was administered in two sachets per day, each containing a 1:1 mix of potato starch and Hylon® VII (a high-amylose maize starch). Both of these starches are RS2. The study design was exceptionally rigorous, with the primary endpoint being polyp number after the intervention, and the

TABLE 16.1 Dietary Fibers which have been Subjected to Clinical Trial

Study Name	Type of Study	Nature of Dietary Fiber	Endpoint of Study	Odds Ratio or Other Measure of Risk	Reference
CAPP1	Clinical trial (FAP patients)	1:1 raw potato starch and high amylose maize starch (Hylon® VII)	Adenoma	Odds ratio of 1.05 (95% CI, 0.73–1.49, P=non-significant	Burn et al.[84]
CAPP2	Clinical trial (FAP patients)	1:1 Novelose® 240 and Novelose® 330	Colorectal cancer	Incidence rate ratio of 1.15 (95% CI 0.66–2.00, P=non-significant)	Mathers et al.[85]
European Cancer Prevention Organisation Study Group	Clinical trial (normal individuals)	3.5 g/day ispaghula husk	Adenoma	Odds ratio of 1.67 (95% CI 1.01–2.76, P=0.042)	Bonithon-Kopp et al.[86]
Phoenix Colon Cancer Prevention Physician's Network	Clinical trial (normal individuals)	13.5g/day "Wheat bran fiber", "shredded cereal" and/or "high dietary fiber bar"	Adenoma	Relative risk of 0.99 (95% CI 0.71–1.36, P=0.93)	Alberts et al.[87]
Polyp Prevention Trial	Observation study with counseling	18g dietary fiber/1000 kcal diet	Adenoma	Relative risk of 1.00 (95% CI, 0.90–1.12, P=non-significant)	Schatzkin et al.[88]
Toronto Polyp Prevention Group	Observation study with counseling	50g/day dietary fiber	Adenoma	Relative risk of 1.2 (95% CI 0.6–2.2, P=non-significant)	McKeown-Eyssen et al.[89]
Wheat bran Fiber Intervention Study	Clinical trial (FAP patients)	22.5g/day wheat bran dietary fiber	Adenoma	Relative risk of 0.65±1.38, P=non-significant	DeCosse et al.[90]

F. WHEAT FIBER

secondary endpoint being polyp size. While this clinical trial showed significant effects in those subjects taking 600 mg of aspirin daily, resistant starch supplementation had no significant effect on adenoma recurrence. The CAPP2 study[82] had a somewhat similar trial design. However, this study used Novelose 240 and Novelose 330, which are resistant starches produced by National Starch and Chemical Co. Bridgewater NJ (USA). Both are produced from high-amylose maize cultivars: Novelose 240 is a RS2 in which the starch granules are thermally modified, and Novelose 330 is a highly retrograded RS3. Again, however, the results for the resistant starch trial arm were negative.

Although these trials are cited in some circles as disproving the dietary fiber hypothesis, we would contend that this is not the case. Indeed, the trial results may justify excluding resistant starches from the current dietary fiber definition. Other components of wheat and rice dietary fiber, apart from the resistant starches, are likely to protect against colorectal cancer.

References

1. Hipsley EH. Dietary "fiber" and pregnancy toxaemia. *Br Med J* 1953;**2**:420–2.
2. Trowell H. Crude fiber, dietary fiber and atherosclerosis. *Atherosclerosis* 1972;**16**:138–40.
3. Trowell H. Definition of fiber. *Lancet* 1974:503.
4. Trowell H, Southgate DAT, Wolever TMS, Leeds AR, Gassull MA, Jenkins DJA. Dietary fiber redefined. *Lancet* 1976:967.
5. Harris PJ, Ferguson LR. Dietary fiber: its composition and role in protection against colorectal cancer. *Mutat Res* 1993;**290**:97–110.
6. McCleary BV. Development of an integrated total dietary fiber method consistent with the Codex Alimentarius definition. *Cereal Foods World* 2010;**55**:24–8.
7. Englyst HN, Cummings JH. Digestion of the polysaccharides of some cereal foods in the human small intestine. *Am J Clin Nutr* 1985;**42**:778–87.
8. Anon. The definition of dietary fiber. *Cereal Foods World* 2001;**46**:112–26.
9. Phillips GO, Cui SW. An introduction: Evolution and finalisation of the regulatory definition of dietary fiber. *Food Hydrocolloids* 2011;**25**:139–43.
10. Harris PJ. Diversity in plant cell walls. In: Henry RJ, editor. *Plant diversity and evolution: genotypic and phenotypic variation in higher plants*. Wallingford, UK: CAB International Publishing; 2005. p. 201–27.
11. Harris PJ, Stone BA. Chemistry and molecular organization of plant cell walls. In: Himmel ME, editor. *Biomass recalcitrance: deconstructing the plant cell wall for bioenergy*. Oxford: Blackwell Publishing; 2008. p. 61–93.
12. Ferguson LR, Harris PJ. Dietary fiber carbohydrates and their fermentation products. In: Knasmüller S, DeMarini DM, Johnson I, Gerhäuser C, editors. *Chemoprevention of cancer and DNA damage by dietary factors*. Weinheim: Wiley-VCH Verlag; 2009. p. 721–9.
13. Fincher GB, Stone BA. Chemistry of nonstarch polysaccharides. In: Wrigley C, Corke H, Walker CE, editors. *Encyclopedia of grain science*. Oxford, UK: Elsevier; 2004. p. 206–23.
14. Saulnier L, Sado P-E, Branlard G, Charmet G. Guillon, F. Wheat arabinoxylans: Exploiting variation in amount and composition to develop enhanced varieties. *J Cereal Sci* 2007;**46**:261–81.
15. Bunzel M, Ralph J, Brüning P, Steinhart H. Structural identification of dehydrotriferulic and dehydrotetraferulic acids isolated from insoluble maize bran fiber. *J Agric Food Chem* 2006;**54**:6409–18.
16. Bunzel M, Ralph J, Lu F, Hatfield RD, Steinhart H. Lignins and ferulate-coniferyl alcohol cross-coupling products in cereal grains. *J Agric Food Chem* 2004;**52**:6496–502.
17. Bunzel M, Ralph J, Marita J, Hatfield RD, Steinhart H. Diferulates as structural components in soluble and insoluble cereal dietary fibre. *J Sci Food Agric* 2001;**81**:653–60.
18. Fincher GB, Stone BA. Cell walls and their components in cereal grain technology. *Advances in Cereal Science and Technology* 1986;**8**:207–95.
19. Shibuya N, Nakane R, Yasui A, Tanaka K, Iwasaki T. Comparative studies on cell wall preparations from rice bran, germ, and endosperm. *Cereal Chem* 1985;**62**:252–58.
20. Harris PJ, Smith BG. Plant cell walls and cell-wall polysaccharides: structures, properties and uses in food products. *Int J Food Sci Technol* 2006;**41**:129–43.
21. Englyst HN, Kingman SM, Cummings JH. Classification and measurement of nutritionally important starch fractions. *Eur J Clin Nutr* 1992;**46**(Suppl. 2):S33–50.
22. Englyst HN, Quigley ME, Hudson GJ. Determination of dietary fiber as non-starch polysaccharides with gas-liquid chromatographic, high performance liquid chromatographic or spectrophotometric measurement of constituent sugars. *Analyst* 1994;**119**:1497–509.
23. Englyst KN, Englyst HN. Carbohydrate bioavailability. *Br J Nutr* 2005;**94**:1–11.
24. Asp N- G. Resistant starch. *Eur J Clin Nutr* 1992;**46**(Suppl. 2):S1.
25. Fuentes-Zaragoza E, Riquelme-Navarrete MJ, Sánchez-Zapata E, Pérez-Álvarez JA. Resistant starch as functional ingredient: A review. *Food Res Int* 2010;**43**:931–42.
26. Alsaffar AA. Effect of food processing on the resistant starch content of cereals and cereal products – a review. *Int J Food Sci Technol* 2011;**46**:455–62.
27. Landon S, Colyer CGB, Salman H. The resistant starch report: an Australian update on health benefits, measurement and dietary intakes. *Food Aus Suppl* 2012:1–18.
28. Morell MK, Konik-Rose C, Ahmed R, Li Z, Rahman S. Synthesis of resistant starches in plants. *J AOAC Int* 2004;**87**:740–8.
29. Jane J, Ao Z, Duvick SA, Wiklund M, Yoo S-H, Weng K- S. Structures of amylopectin and starch granules: how are they synthesized? *J Appl Glycoscience* 2003;**50**:167–72.
30. Bird AR, Flory C, Davies DA, Usher S, Topping DL. A novel barley cultivar (*Himalaya 292*) with a specific gene mutation in starch synthase IIa raises large bowel starch and short-chain fatty acids in rats. *J Nutr* 2004;**134**:831–5.
31. Bird AR, Vuaran MS, King RA, Noakes M, Keogh J, Morell MK, et al. Wholegrain foods made from a novel high-amylose barley variety (*Himalaya 292*) improve indices of bowel health in human subjects. *Br J Nutr* 2008;**99**:1032–40.
32. Flamm G, Glinsmann W, Kritchevsky D, Prosky L, Roberfroid M. Inulin and oligofructose as dietary fiber: a review of the evidence. *Crit Rev Food Sci Nutr* 2001;**41**:353–62.
33. Pollock CJ, Cairns AJ. Fructan metabolism in grasses and cereals. *Annu Rev Plant Biol* 1991;**42**:77–101.
34. Biesiekierski JR, Rosella O, Rose R, Liels K, Barrett JS, Shepherd SJ, et al. Quantification of fructans, galacto-oligosaccharides and other short-chain carbohydrates in processed grains and cereals. *J Hum Nutr Diet* 2011;**24**:154–76.
35. Gosling A, Stevens GW, Barber AR, Kentish SE, Gras SL. Recent advances refining galactooligosaccharide production from lactose. *Food Chem* 2010;**121**:307–18.
36. Mujoo R, Ng PKW. Physicochemical properties of bread baked from flour blended with immature wheat meal rich in fructooligosaccharides. *J Food Sci* 2003;**68**:2448–52.

37. Martinez-Villaluenga C, Frias J, Vidal-Valverde C. Alpha-galactosides: antinutritional factors or functional ingredients? *Crit Rev Food Sci Nutr* 2008;**48**:301–16.

38. Black M, Corbineau F, Gee H, Côme D. Water content, raffinose, and dehydrins in the induction of desiccation tolerance in immature wheat embryos. *Plant Physiol* 1999;**120**:463–71.

39. Ohkuma K, Wakabayashi S. Fibersol-2: a soluble, non-digestible, starch-derived dietary fibre. In: McCleary BV, Prosky L, editors. *Advanced dietary fibre technology*. Oxford: Blackwell Science; 2001. p. 509–23.

40. Craig SAS, Holden JF, Troup JP, Auerbach MH, Frier HI. Polydextrose as soluble fiber: physiological and analytical aspects. *Cereal Foods World* 1998;**43**:370–6.

41. Southgate DAT. *Determination of food carbohydrates*. London: Applied Science Publishers Ltd.; 1976.

42. Jung H- JG. Analysis of forage fiber and cell walls in ruminant nutrition. *J Nutr* 1997;**127**:810S–3S.

43. Van Soest PJ. Use of detergents in the analysis of fibrous feeds. 1. Preparation of fiber residues of low nitrogen content. *J Assoc Official Agric Chemists* 1963;**46**:825–8f29.

44. Van Soest PJ. Use of detergents in the analysis of fibrous feeds. 2. A rapid method for the determination of fiber and lignin. *J Assoc Official Agric Chemists* 1963;**48**:829–35.

45. Van Soest PJ, Robertson JB, Lewis BA. Symposium: carbohydrate methodology, metabolism, and nutritional implications in dairy cattle. Methods for dietary fiber, neutral detergent fiber, and non-starch polysaccharides in relation to animal nutrition. *J Dairy Sci* 1991;**74**:3583–97.

46. Van Soest PJ, Wine RH. Use of detergents in the analysis of fibrous feeds. IV. Determination of plant cell-wall constituents. *J Assoc Official Agric Chemists* 1967;**50**:50–5.

47. Southgate DAT. Determination of carbohydrates in foods. 2. Unavailable carbohydrates. *J Sci Food Agric* 1969;**20**:331–5.

48. Schweizer TF, Würsch P. Analysis of dietary fiber. *J Sci Food Agric* 1979;**30**:613–9.

49. Asp N-G, Johannson CG, Hallmer H, Siljestrom M. Rapid enzymatic assay of insoluble and soluble dietary fiber. *J Agric Food Chem* 1983;**31**:476–82.

50. Prosky L, Asp N-G, Furda I, DeVries JW, Schweizer TF, Harland BF. Determination of total dietary fiber in foods and food products and total diets: interlaboratory study. *J Assoc Official Anal Chemists* 1984;**67**:1044–53.

51. Prosky L, Asp N-G, Furda I, DeVries JW, Schweizer TF, Harland BF. Determination of total dietary fiber in foods and food products: collaborative study. *J Assoc Official Anal Chemists* 1985;**68**:677–9.

52. DeVries JW, Prosky L, Li B, Cho S. A historical persective on defining dietary fiber. *Cereal Foods World* 1999;**44**:367–9.

53. Prosky L. What is fiber? Current controversies. *Trends Food Sci Technol* 1999;**10**:271–5.

54. Englyst H, Wiggins HS, Cummings JH. Determination of the non-starch polysaccharides in plant foods by gas-liquid chromatography of constituent sugars as alditol acetates. *Analyst* 1982;**107**:307–18.

55. Englyst HN, Cummings JH. Improved method for measurement of dietary fiber as non-starch polysaccharides in plant foods. *J AOAC* 1988;**71**:808–14.

56. Englyst HN, Quigley ME, Englyst KN, Bravo L, Hudson GJ. Dietary fiber. Measurement by the Englyst NSP procedure, measurement by the AOAC procedure. Explanation of the differences. *J Assoc Public Anal* 1996;**32**:1–52.

57. Buttriss JL, Stokes CS. Dietary fiber and health: an overview. *Br Nutr Found Nutr Bull* 2008;**33**:186–200.

58. McCleary BV. An integrated procedure for the measurement of total dietary fiber (including resistant starch), non-digestible oligosaccharides and available carbohydrates. *Anal Bioanal Chem* 2007 Sep;**389**(1):291–308.

59. McCleary BV, DeVries JW, Rader JI, Cohen G, Prosky L, Mugford DC, et al. Determination of total dietary fiber (CODEX definition) by enzymatic–gravimetric method and liquid chromatography: collaborative study. *J AOAC Int* 2010;**93**:221–33.

60. McCleary BV, McNally M, Rossiter P. Measurement of resistant starch by enzymic digestion in starch samples and selected plant materials: collaborative Study. *J AOAC Int* 2002;**85**:1103–11.

61. Hollmann J, Themeier H, Neese U, Lindhauer MG. Dietary fiber fractions in cereal foods measured by a new integrated AOAC method. *Food Chem* 2013;**140**:586–9.

62. Burkitt DP, Walker AR, Painter NS. Effect of dietary fibre on stools and the transit-times, and its role in the causation of disease. *Lancet* 1972;**2**:1408–12.

63. Burkitt, DP. Epidemiology of large bowel disease: the role of fibre. *Proceedings of the Nutrition Society* 1973;**32**:145–9.

64. Burkitt D. *Don't forget fiber in your diet: to help avoid many of our commonest diseases*. London, UK: Martin Dunitz Ltd; 1979.

65. Wu F, Yang N, Toure A, Jin Z, Xu X. Germinated brown rice and its role in human health. *Crit Rev Food Sci Nutr* 2013;**53**:451–63.

66. Zhu L, Gu M, Meng X, Cheung SC, Yu H, Huang J, et al. High-amylose rice improves indices of animal health in normal and diabetic rats. *Plant Biotechnol J* 2012;**10**:353–62.

67. Yang R, Sun C, Bai J, Luo Z, Shi B, Zhang J, et al. A putative gene sbe3-rs for resistant starch mutated from SBE3 for starch branching enzyme in rice (*Oryza sativa* L.). *PLoS ONE* 2012;**7**:e43026.

68. Hallstrom E, Sestili F, Lafiandra D, Bjorck I, Ostman E. A novel wheat variety with elevated content of amylose increases resistant starch formation and may beneficially influence glycaemia in healthy subjects. *Food Nutr Res* 2011:55–61.

69. Ferguson LR, Chavan RR, Harris PJ. Changing concepts of dietary fiber: implications for carcinogenesis. *Nutr Cancer* 2001;**39**:155–69.

70. Harris PJ, Chavan RR, Ferguson LR. Production and characterisation of two wheat-bran fractions: an aleurone-rich and a pericarp-rich fraction. *Mol Nutr Food Res* 2005;**49**:536–45.

71. Ferguson LR, Roberton AM, Watson ME, Triggs CM, Harris PJ. The effects of a soluble-fiber polysaccharide on the adsorption of carcinogens to insoluble dietary fibers. *Chem-Biol Interact* 1995;**95**:245–55.

72. Funk C, Weber P, Thilker J, Grabber JH, Steinhart H, Bunzel M. Influence of lignification and feruloylation of maize cell walls on the adsorption of heterocyclic aromatic amines. *J Agric Food Chem* 2006;**54**:1860–7.

73. Ferguson LR, Zhu S-T, Harris PJ. Antioxidant and antigenotoxic effects of plant cell wall hydroxycinnamic acids in cultured HT-29 cells. *Mol Nutr Food Res* 2005;**49**:585–93.

74. Harris PJ, Ferguson LR. Dietary Fibres and Human Health. *Mol Nutr Food Res* 2005;**49**:517–8.

75. Srinivasan M, Sudheer AR, Menon VP. Ferulic Acid: therapeutic potential through its antioxidant property. *J Clin Biochem Nutr* 2007;**40**:92–100.

76. Fardet A. New hypotheses for the health-protective mechanisms of whole-grain cereals: what is beyond fiber? *Nutr Res Rev* 2010;**23**:65–134.

77. Lee S, Monnappa AK, Mitchell RJ. Biological activities of lignin hydrolysate-related compounds. *BMB Rep* 2012;**45**:265–74.

78. Ferguson LR, Harris PJ, Kestell P, Zhu ST, Munday R, Munday CM. Comparative effects in rats on protection against the mutagenicity of 2-amino-3-methylimidazo[4,5-*f*]quinoline by intact wheat bran and two wheat bran fractions. *Mutat Res* 2011;**716**:59–65.

79. WCRF/AICR. *Continuous update report. The Associations between Food, Nutrition and Physical Activity and the Risk of Colorectal Cancer*. WCRF/AICR; 2010.

80. Michels KB, Fuchs CS, Giovannucci E, Colditz GA, Hunter DJ, Stampfer MJ, et al. Fiber intake and incidence of colorectal cancer among 76,947 women and 47,279 men. Cancer Epidemiol. *Biomarkers Prev* 2005;**14**:842–9.

81. Bingham SA, Day NE, Luben R, Ferrari P, Slimani N, Norat T, et al. Dietary fibre in food and protection against colorectal cancer in the European Prospective Investigation into Cancer and Nutrition (EPIC): an observational study. *Lancet* 2003;**361**:1496–501.

82. Dahm CC, Keogh RH, Spencer EA, Greenwood DC, Key TJ, Fentiman IS, et al. Dietary fiber and colorectal cancer risk: a nested case-control study using food diaries. *J Natl Cancer Inst* 2010;**102**:614–26.

83. Park Y, Hunter DJ, Spiegelman D, Bergkvist L, Berrino F, van den Brandt PA. Dietary fiber intake and risk of colorectal cancer: a pooled analysis of prospective cohort studies. *JAMA* 2005;**294**:2849–57.

84. Burn J, Bishop DT, Chapman PD, Elliott F, Bertario L, Dunlop MG, et al. A randomized placebo-controlled prevention trial of aspirin and/or resistant starch in young people with familial adenomatous polyposis. *Cancer Prev Res* 2011;**4**:655–65.

85. Mathers JC, Movahedi M, Macrae F, Mecklin JP, Moeslein G, Olschwang S, et al. Long-term effect of resistant starch on cancer risk in carriers of hereditary colorectal cancer: an analysis from the CAPP2 randomised controlled trial. *Lancet Oncol* 2012;**13**:1242–9.

86. Bonithon-Kopp C, Kronborg O, Giacosa A, Räth U, Faivre J. Calcium and fiber supplementation in prevention of colorectal adenoma recurrence: a randomised intervention trial. European Cancer Prevention Organisation Study Group. *Lancet* 2000;**356**:1300–6.

87. Alberts DS, Martinez ME, Roe DJ, Guillen-Rodriguez JM, Marshall JR, van Leeuwen JB, et al. Lack of effect of a high-fiber cereal supplement on the recurrence of colorectal adenomas. Phoenix Colon Cancer Prevention Physicians' Network. *N Engl J Med* 2000;**342**:1156–62.

88. Schatzkin A, Lanza E, Corle D, Lance P, Iber F, Caan B, et al. Lack of effect of a low-fat, high-fiber diet on the recurrence of colorectal adenomas. Polyp Prevention Trial Study Group. *N Engl J Med* 2000;**342**:1149–55.

89. McKeown-Eyssen GE, Bright-See E, Bruce WR, Jazmaji V, Cohen LB, Pappas SC, et al. A randomized trial of a low fat high fiber diet in the recurrence of colorectal polyps. Toronto Polyp Prevention Group. *J Clin Epidemiol* 1994;**47**:525–36.

90. DeCosse JJ, Miller HH, Lesser ML. Effect of wheat fiber and vitamins C and E on rectal polyps in patients with familial adenomatous polyposis. *J Natl Cancer Inst* 1989;**81**:1290–7.

Sensory, Technological, and Health Aspects of Adding Fiber to Wheat-Based Pasta

Mike J. Sissons[*], *Christopher M. Fellows*[†]

[*]NSW Department of Primary Industries, Tamworth Agricultural Institute, Calala, New South Wales, Australia,
[†]University of New England, School of Science and Technology, Armidale, New South Wales, Australia

INTRODUCTION

Dietary fiber is that fraction of polysaccharides resistant to digestion in the human small intestine which is fermented in the large intestine. This category includes cellulose, hemicellulose, arabinoxylans, arabinogalactans, polyfructose, oligosaccharides (inulin, gums, pectins and mucilages), material bound to cell walls (lignin, waxes, cutin, phytates, saponins, tannins, and suberin), and resistant starch. Some of these products are used in the food industry as stabilizers in small amounts (<1%), but higher levels are needed to achieve nutritional and health benefits.

Dietary fiber consumption has been shown to reduce glycemic and insulinemic responses to ingestion of carbohydrates, reduce the risk of colorectal cancers, reduce serum concentrations of cholesterol and triglycerides, enhance vitamin and mineral absorption, and encourage the formation of short-chain fatty acids (SCFAs) with probiotic effects in the large intestine, while the capacity of fiber to increase satiety has a documented effect in combating obesity. However, consumer acceptance of high-fiber foods is low: our instinctive preference is for low-fiber foods, and the trajectory of culinary history has been to more refined foods with reduced fiber content. Thus, improving methods by which dietary fiber can be effectively "disguised" in foods is necessary for the health benefits of fiber consumption to be realized.

Pasta is a uniquely suitable substrate for fortification with dietary fiber. As a staple food, it provides the opportunity to supplement the diet with a large amount of fiber, so is more suitable for supplementation than biscuits or similar snack foods. In addition, the texture of pasta is much less sensitive to the incorporation of additional ingredients than bread, where complex and easily disrupted interactions between surface-active proteins and entrained gases give rise to the preferred light textures.[1] Accordingly, when bread and pasta are enriched with fiber to a similar degree the pasta has been reported to be more acceptable to sensory panels than the bread. In comparison to bread, pasta is also much less perishable, making it unnecessary to prepare as a fortified foodstuff locally, and making its distribution an economic proposition at a much lower rate of consumer uptake. Furthermore, cases have been reported where the beneficial effects of equivalent amounts of supplementation are greater for pasta than for breads – for example, a greater reduction of serum cholesterol has been reported on substitution with oat (rich in β-glucan) added to pasta than for bread.[2]

Many dietary fibers have been added to pasta and the technological, sensory, and nutritional properties of the products investigated. The majority of this work has involved fortification of semolina or flour with whole flours from high-fiber sources, such as barley and buckwheat flour, and the subsequent manufacture of pasta (usually dried). There have also been numerous reports on pasta enriched with resistant starches, soluble fibers (e.g., inulin) and insoluble fibers (e.g., bran, chitosan).

The main barrier to consumer acceptance of pasta enriched with dietary fiber is the negative impact of dietary fiber on the sensory/textural properties of the pasta. These effects on pasta properties that can be measured semiquantitatively by sensorial analysis are amenable to quantitative measurement using standard technological/rheological tests, and throughout this review these technological measurements will be used as proxies to supplement the relatively small number of reports on the sensory analysis of fiber-enriched pasta. Properties such as firmness, stickiness, etc., measured instrumentally, have been shown to correlate strongly with the perceptions of sensory panels.[3]

The water absorption and retention capacity of dietary fibers differs depending on the botanical source, how the fibers are processed, and the actual particle size of the fiber used in the food.[4] Fiber incorporation can impair desirable pasta properties in several ways. Particles of fiber are usually significantly larger than starch granules and cannot be mixed with complete homogeneity, causing disruption/dilution of the starch–protein matrix present in unsubstituted pasta and giving a weaker, softer product. Fibers frequently hydrate more rapidly than starch, with the same results: at optimal cooking time (OCT) starch granules contain less moisture than in the unsubstituted product, while the swollen fiber makes the overall structure weak and soft. This hydrophilicity of fibers can also lead to greater adhesiveness in substituted pasta, especially if demixing leads to a concentration of fiber material at the surface of the pasta. Phase separation and the impact of the fiber on the flow properties of the dough may also lead to esthetically unappealing surface textures. All these effects can alter the formation of the pasta structure. If pasta structure is altered, product texture and other properties will also change. For single fiber additions into food matrices, generally as more of the fiber is added then the greater will be the effect on the food structure. While some fiber sources are colorless and flavorless, this is not true of most of the natural fibers of nutritional interest, and the invariably darker colors imparted to the pasta are a barrier to consumer acceptance, as are any changes in the expected pasta flavor. Conversely, a "whole grain" color may serve as a marker that the pasta is fiber-enriched and encourage the acceptance of the product by health-minded consumers. The main bioactive components and effect of fiber sources used in pasta formulations are summarized in Table 17.1. While some display specific health benefits, it is in all cases unclear whether these have a chemical basis or arise purely through the impact of these sparingly digestible molecules on the nature of the digesta. Figure 17.1 illustrates the references in this table to fiber sources from different parts of the cereal seed.

This chapter will discuss the documented impacts of fiber supplementation of conventional durum pastas on nutritional, sensory, and technological properties, avoiding the related area of pastas based entirely on higher-fiber non-durum sources, or substitution of pasta with ingredients intended primarily to improve protein content, protein value, or mineral and vitamin content.

Minimizing the negative impact of dietary fiber incorporation is a major focus of research, and this review discusses the relative impacts of different fibers on the technological/sensory properties of pasta.

TABLE 17.1 A Selection of Bioactive Compounds in Fibers

Bioactive Compound	Wheat Kernel Location/Other Source	Biological Effects
β-glucan (barley and oat)	Starchy endosperm and aleurone layer	Hypocholesterolemic, hypoglycemic
Cellulose, lignan, hemicellulose	Bran, pericarp, aleurone layer	Laxation, fecal bulking, hypocholesterolemic, hypoglycemic, reduction of risk of cardiovascular disease and cancer
Resistant starch	Endosperm	Fecal bulk, prebiotic, fermentation in colon to produce SCFAs, hypoglycemic
Xanthan gum	Soluble bacterial gums manufactured by fermentation	Increases digesta viscosity, produces SCFAs in large intestine, hypoglycemic
Inulin	Immature grain, artichoke	Prebiotic, SCFA production, enhances calcium absorption, hypoglycemic
Guar gum	Indian cluster bean (*Cyamopsis tetragonoloba*)	Fermented by colonic bacteria, lowers lipids, hypoglycemic
Locust bean gum	Locust bean (*Ceratonia siliqua*)	Increases digesta viscosity
Arabinoxylan	Pericarp	Hypocholesterolemic

HEALTH EFFECTS OF PASTA SUPPLEMENTATION WITH FIBER

Supplementation of Pasta with Whole Flours

Cereal, pseudo-cereal, and legume flours have been extensively investigated as ingredients in pasta formulations. These serve not only as fiber sources, but in many cases also have possible additional health benefits, such as increasing protein content or incorporating antioxidants.

Barley (*Hordeum vulgare*) and Oats (*Avena sativa*)

Flours made from barley and oats contain levels of β-glucans (2–20% barley; 4–6% oats) much higher than in wheat flour (0.5–2.3%),[5,6] so replacement of semolina with barley or oat flour is one way to increase the amount of fiber in pasta with a relatively small impact on properties. Yokoyama *et al.* have verified that 40% substitution of semolina with barley flour gives a marked reduction in postprandial plasma glucose and plasma insulin levels in human test subjects, with the rise in postprandial insulin on barley-enriched pasta consumption being approximately half the rise seen for conventional pasta.[7]

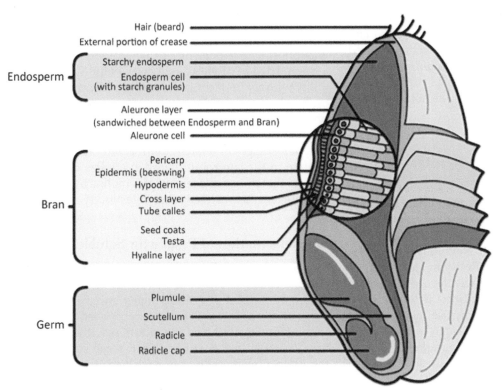

FIGURE 17.1 Structure of a wheat grain. http://www.grainchain.com/14-to-16/technology/images/seed.gif. See color plate at the back of the book.

Endosperm
- Hair (beard)
- External portion of crease
- Starchy endosperm
- Endosperm cell (with starch granules)
- Aleurone layer (sandwiched between Endosperm and Bran)
- Aleurone cell

Bran
- Pericarp
- Epidermis (beeswing)
- Hypodermis
- Cross layer
- Tube calles
- Seed coats
- Testa
- Hyaline layer

Germ
- Plumule
- Scutellum
- Radicle
- Radicle cap

Buckwheat (*Fagopyrum esculentum*)

The high content of protein, fiber, and antioxidants in pseudo-cereal species has made them of increasing interest as functional foods in recent decades, and considerable work has been carried out on the supplementation of durum pasta with buckwheat, quinoa, and amaranth flour. Buckwheat, though producing a cereal-like grain, is not a grass. It has a high protein content with a balanced amino acid composition and significant amounts of antioxidants (phenols and rutin), and, due to its short growing season, has historically been an important crop in northern Eurasia.[8] Boiled buckwheat has a high content of resistant starch, a useful functional ingredient.

Legumes

Unprocessed legume starches are digested with more difficulty than unprocessed cereal starches. This has been attributed both to the presence of a higher proportion of resistant starch in legumes and to high amounts of dietary fiber in the cell walls giving a greater physical barrier to digestion.[9,10] In addition, the high protein content of legumes, and the fact that they contain significant amounts of lysine and threonine in which durum pasta is deficient, has made them favored targets as sources for pasta supplementation.[11]

In vitro glucose release over 20 minutes was reduced on supplementation of pasta with faba bean (*Vicia faba*) or green pea (*Pisum sativum*) flour, with no significant difference seen between the legumes or between high and low drying temperatures.[11] Substitution of pasta with 15–45% common bean flour (*Phaseolus vulgaris*) had a lower fraction of digestible starch the greater the amount of bean flour added (as determined by the resistant starch assay of Goñi *et al.*),[12] though no apparent effect on the rate of *in vitro* digestion was observed.[13,14]

Chickpea (*Cicer arietinum*) has a similar protein content and amino acid profile to soybean, and is produced in large volumes on the Indian subcontinent.[15] Chickpea seeds have been considered a suitable source of dietary protein, due to the good balance of amino acids, the high protein bioavailability, and relatively low levels of antinutritional factors.[16] Chickpea flour also increases the mineral and fat content of pasta,[17] and is high in dietary fiber.[18]

Osorio-Diaz *et al.* investigated the substitution of pasta noodles with 20% and 40% chickpea flour. Relative to control pasta, the 20% substituted pasta exhibited a $13.8 \pm 1.1\%$ decrease of *in vitro* starch digestibility over 180 minutes, while the 40% substituted pasta exhibited a $26.5 \pm 2.8\%$ decrease.[19]

Foods containing soybean (*Glycine max*) have been shown to reduce risks of heart disease,[20] and there is some evidence that they can reduce the risks of certain cancers which are related to steroid hormones, such as breast and prostate cancer.[21] Addition of 10% soybean or lentil flour in durum spaghetti gave no significant changes to *in vitro* digestion relative to control pasta.[22]

Marinangeli et al. prepared pasta containing 30% yellow pea (Lathyrus aphaca) flour.[23] The integrated in vivo glycemic response over 150 minutes showed a reduced response from the yellow pea flour containing pasta in comparison to a whole meal wheat pasta (161 ± 19 compared with $179 \pm 20\,mM/min$) which was not deemed to be significant.

Supplementation of Pasta with Resistant Starch

There are a number of ways in which starches resistant to digestion in the small intestine may arise. Resistant starch 1 (RS1) is physically inaccessible starch occurring in partly milled grains, seeds, legumes, and tubers, which is only digested when the solid mass containing the starch granules is disrupted. Resistant starch 2 (RS2) is semicrystalline native starch where the accessibility of digestive enzymes before gelatinization is limited; raw potato, green banana, and high-amylose maize are the main RS2 sources. Resistant starch 3 (RS3) is semicrystalline starch formed in situ through retrogradation of amylose on cooling of gelatinized starch. Resistant starch 4 (RS4) is starch that has been chemically modified to reduce its digestibility, such as acetylated or hydroxypropylated starch; finally, starch–lipid complexes formed in the preparation of starch-based foods have been defined as Resistant starch 5 (RS5).

There are inconsistencies in the data reported thus far on the extent to which RS substitution can impact digestibility, with some studies suggesting it is purely a substitution effect[24] while others appear to suggest a broader effect of RS on generating a more indigestible structure.[25]

Resistant Starch 1

While no work has been done setting out explicitly to reduce the glycemic index of pasta by incorporating RS1, it is possible that the observed effects of adding non-durum flours in reducing in vitro or in vivo digestibility (see above) are partially attributable in some cases to incorporation of more coarsely ground material.

Resistant Starch 2 and 3

Two commercial RS2 sources from maize (Hi-Maize® 260 and Hi-Maize® 1043) at 10–20% substitution of a pasta dried at 35–40°C (low temperature drying) reduced the in vitro starch digestibility of pasta compared to a durum wheat pasta control.[26] Incorporation at 2.5–10% of Hi-Maize 260 pasta dried at 30–40°C also reduced the in vitro starch digestibility.[25] Aravind et al. found that in vitro digestibility was reduced to a degree consistent with the replacement of starch with RS2 and RS3, with no evident synergistic effects.[24]

Resistant Starch 4

It has been reported that a wheat starch cross-linked with phosphate (Fibersym® 70), when added at 10–20% to a pasta dried at 35–40°C, reduced in vitro starch digestibility without impacting on sensory properties.[26] Novelose® 480, a high-amylose maize starch cross-linked with phosphate, at substitution levels of 2.5–10% in pasta dried at 30–40°C,[25] was found to significantly decrease the percentage of starch hydrolyzed at 90 minutes relative to the control in digestion studies in vitro, suggesting that mere replacement of semolina by RS was not a significant factor in reducing digestibility.

Supplementation of Pasta with Soluble Fibers

Incorporation of whole flours can have negative effects through dilution of the durum semolina, which can be minimized by adding highly enriched fiber fractions. There is clearly a continuum between substitution with a whole flour and substitution with an isolated fiber, as most flours will have had some component of the grain preferentially removed, and it is not usually possible to rigorously purify an extract from natural sources so that all non-fiber components are removed. We have followed the common practice of classifying fibers into "soluble" and "insoluble", but it should be noted that again there is a continuum: most naturally occurring fiber sources will have both soluble and insoluble components under a given set of conditions, and the range of possible conditions used in pasta preparation means that the same fiber may be effectively soluble in one formulation and insoluble in another.

β-Glucans

Naturally occurring (1→3) (1→4) β-glucans have both soluble and insoluble components, with only 30–43% of β-glucan in oat brans reported to be soluble in water at 38°C,[27] but will be considered here as soluble fibers. Aravind et al. prepared pasta containing up to 20% Barley Balance® (5% β-glucan) and found a reduction in total reducing sugar release of 17% for the highest degree of substitution.[28] Brennan and Tudorica found that substitution of semolina with Hi-Sol (a flour containing approximately 12% β-glucan) in fresh pasta reduced in vitro starch hydrolysis over 300 minutes by up to 50% at an estimated total β-glucan content of 10%.[29]

The effectiveness of β-glucan in lowering serum cholesterol has been linked to molar mass, with some evidence that lower molar mass fractions are ineffective.[5] In a similar way, the effectiveness of a low molar mass commercial β-glucan source (Glucagel™, approx 150 kDa) in reducing postprandial serum glucose levels was much less than that of a higher molar mass (Barley Balance™, approx 700 kDa) commercial β-glucan (Table 17.2).[30]

TABLE 17.2 Decrease in Incremental Area under Curve of Excess Serum Glucose (%) or Reducing Sugar Released (%) (*in vitro*) of Substituted Pastas Relative to Control Pasta[32]

% Substitution with Glucagel	Glucagel (Approx 75% β-Glucan, 150 kDa)		% Substitution with Barley Balance	Barley Balance (Approx 25% β-Glucan, 650–700 kDa)	
	In Vivo	*In Vitro*		*In Vivo*	*In Vitro*
2.5	−8.6 ± 1.5	−6.3 ± 10.6	7.5	19.3 ± 4.0	12.7 ± 8.7
4.7	4.6 ± 0.8	12.6 ± 8.7	14.3	25.7 ± 5.3	26.3 ± 7.4
6.9	32.8 ± 7.0	12.6 ± 8.7	21.1	31.9 ± 6.8	30.3 ± 7.0
7.2	3.5 ± 0.6	8.6 ± 9.1	27.1	42.6 ± 8.4	42.5 ± 5.7
11.2	29.5 ± 5.4	13.8 ± 8.6	32.8	51.5 ± 11.2	42.2 ± 5.8

Raw data for determining *in vitro* AUC provided by S. Chillo, personal communication.

As the effectiveness of fiber in promoting health outcomes has been linked to increased viscosity of intestinal digesta,[31] and molar mass and viscosity are highly correlated, these findings are not surprising. This cannot be the whole story, however, considering that low amounts of incorporation of Glucagel were observed to increase the glycemic index, and that Chillo *et al.* report that on *in vitro* digestion there was no observable difference in viscosity of the digested pastas prepared from the two β-glucan sources.[32]

Decreased *in vitro* starch digestion of pasta was observed by Cleary and Brennan for pastas at low levels (~10%) of β-glucan incorporation.[33] This may again be related to differences in scale, and β-glucan may conceivably both increase the local viscosity and/or restrict enzyme access (reducing GI) and disrupt the formation of the starch–protein matrix (increasing GI) while having no effect on the global viscosity of a partially digested pasta suspension.[34]

As endogenous β-glucanases can lower the molar mass of β-glucan during processing, the nature of the foodstuff and its processing history may be vital in ensuring that beneficial health properties are retained: it has been reported that fresh pasta contained low molar mass β-glucan while conventional macaroni (dried at high temperature) prepared from the same raw material had a higher molar mass β-glucan, probably because the endogenous heat-labile β-glucanases were destroyed on pasta drying.[34]

Inulin

Inulin is a polydisperse fructan with a degree of polymerization (DP) of 2 to 60 consisting mainly of D-fructose joined by β-(2→1) linkages with a terminal D-glucose residue.[35] A soluble fiber with a neutral taste, inulin resists digestion and is fermented in the colon to produce large amounts of short-chain fatty acids (SCFAs).[36] These play a vital role in maintenance of colonic integrity and metabolism. They are produced

when dietary fiber is fermented by colonic bacteria. SCFAs are avidly absorbed in the colon, at the same time as sodium and water absorption and bicarbonate secretion. Once absorbed, SCFAs are used preferentially as fuel for colonic epithelial cells and have trophic effects on the epithelium. SCFAs may be the effector of the beneficial role of fiber in prevention of colon cancer.

In vitro digestion studies have shown an effect of inulin addition proportional to the amount of inulin added; no significant reduction in projected GI was found for 2.5% substitution, while a 15% reduction was found at 10% substitution.[37] Brennan *et al.* hypothesized that inulin acts either by competing for available water with the starch or by forming a protective matrix around the starch granules limiting water movement, gelatinization, and accessibility to starch-degrading enzymes.[38] In subsequent work, Brennan and Tudorica used the same source of inulin and reported no significant change in projected GI at up to 10% substitution.[37] As there are no obvious differences in the pasta preparation methods described in the two papers, it is unclear why.

Aravind *et al.* found that a higher DP inulin (12–13) decreased *in vitro* hydrolysis at up to 5% substitution, but a lower DP inulin (6–7) was ineffective.[39] At higher substitution levels of the higher DP inulin, *in vitro* hydrolysis returned to levels comparable with the control. This non-intuitive result may be rationalized by a competition between a protective effect of the inulin reducing accessibility of the starch to amylases (reducing GI) and a disruptive effect of the inulin reducing the cohesiveness of the starch–protein matrix (increasing GI). Both of these effects would be expected to be less pronounced at lower DP.

Guar Gum

Guar gum is a galactomannan derived from the Indian Cluster Bean (*Cyamopsis tetra-gonoloba*), consisting of a β-1,4-mannose backbone partially substituted with α-1,6 galactose side chains. As far back as 1974 guar gum was seen as a strong possibility for preparing functional pasta, with the patenting of a low calorie pasta containing up to 50% guar.[40] Gatti et al. provided evidence that guar galactomannan considerably reduces GI and lowers serum cholesterol at a level of 20% substitution.[41] Although Gatti et al. state that the pasta was found to be of acceptable quality in a clinical setting, since then there has been surprisingly little work done on this system.

Brennan and Tudorica found a significant effect of guar gum in reducing in vitro hydrolysis of fresh pasta, with about half the total reducing sugar release over 300 minutes with 10% guar gum substitution compared to the control.[37] Aravind et al. only reported a reduction of 24% in reducing sugar release over 300 minutes for 20% guar gum (G4129, intrinsic viscosity 900 mL/g) substitution of pasta dried at 65°C.[42] This difference may be due to the different drying protocols employed, or differences in the molar mass and/or side-chain distribution of the guar gums employed.

Locust Bean Gum

The locust bean, Ceratonia siliqua, produces a gum which, like guar gum, consists of a β-1,4-mannose backbone partially substituted with α-1,6 galactose side chains, but has a lower degree of side-chain substitution. Pasta with 2.5–10% locust bean gum has been found to have a very similar impact to guar and xanthan gum on in vitro digestion, reducing it by about 60% over 300 minutes.[37]

Xanthan Gum

The bacterial polysaccharide xanthan gum is a β-1,4-glucose backbone with regular side chains consisting of two mannose residues and a glucuronate residue, where one of the mannoses may be acetylated and one may be pyruvylated. On addition to pasta at 2.5–10% substitution, it was found to have the most significant effect on reduction of in vitro digestion (by approximately 70% over 300 minutes) of any of the eight fibers investigated in a study by Brennan and Tudorica.[37]

Carboxymethylcellulose

Carboxymethylcellulose (CMC) is a cellulose derivative with carboxymethyl groups bound to some of the hydroxyl groups of the glucopyranose monomers which make up the cellulose backbone, with food-grade CMC, which is usually used as the sodium salt, having a degree of substitution in the range 0.65–0.95 and a molar mass significantly lower than most cellulose sources.[43] Over 300 minutes, Aravind et al. found a decrease of 18% in starch hydrolysis in pastas dried at 65°C with 1.5% CMC.[42]

Supplementation of Pasta with Insoluble Fibers

The common mental image of "fiber" is, of course, indigestible fibers comprising celluloses and hemicelluloses that impart a distinctive texture to foods – a texture associated with things that are good for you, rather than

pleasant to eat. A significant amount of research has been carried out on pasta incorporating such fibers, primarily derived from bran or vegetable by-products.

Brans

One concern with consumption of large amounts of brans are antinutritional effects from phytic acid, which strongly complexes divalent minerals to reduce the bioavailability of species such as Ca^{2+} and Fe^{2+}, in which many consumers even in developed countries are deficient.[44] Upon cooking, however, phytic acid is degraded and no longer acts as an antinutrient.

When substituted with 28.6% oat bran, fettucini dried at 90°C gave a glycemic response over 120 min of 64 ± 13 mM/min and insulinemic response of 15.6 ± 1.4 μM/min compared to 77 ± 12 mM/min and 20.1 ± 2.5 μM/min, respectively, for a control sample.[45] Bustos et al. made pasta from bread wheat dried at 45°C, and found in vitro hydrolysis gave a significantly reduced predicted GI at 2.5–7.5% oat bran substitution (GI: 71.5 ± 0.9 compared with 83.4 ± 0.3 control).[25] However, this value increased to that of the control at 10% substitution, which may be related to the effect of oat bran on the overall cohesiveness of the pasta matrix; at 10% (but not 7.5%) substitution, significant increases in the amount of amylose and protein present in the cooking water were found.[25] It is likely that a large part of the observed benefits of oat bran are due to the increased β-glucan content of oat flour, as discussed above.

Vegetable Fibers

A number of vegetable by-products have been used to supplement pasta, including amaranth leaves,[46] mango peel,[47] pea fibers,[37] and carrot fibers.[48] Brennan and Tudorica investigated the effect of 2.5–10% pea fiber and bamboo fiber on the technological properties[29] and in vitro digestion[37] of fresh pasta. A pea fiber product (Exafine®, Cosucra, Belgium) had relatively little impact on in vitro digestion over 300 minutes, while a bamboo fiber product (Qualicel® 41B, CFF, Germany), had a more pronounced impact on in vitro digestion, reducing it by about 30% over 300 minutes.

SENSORY AND TECHNOLOGICAL IMPACTS

Supplementation of Semolina with Whole Flours

The traditional and best raw material for the manufacture of pasta is semolina, and partial substitution of semolina with non-gluten fibers can potentially interfere with the formation of the protein network in the pasta that prevents the dissolution of starch from the pasta during cooking. These ingredients can also modify the rheological properties of the dough or alter the sensory acceptability and cooking quality of the pasta. Therefore, balanced formulations and suitable processing technologies must be used to produce acceptable pasta as close as possible to the durum-only pasta. Therefore, the amount of the ingredient that can be used to substitute for semolina represents a balance between nutritional improvement and achievement of satisfactory sensory and functional properties of the pasta.

Barley (*Hordeum vulgare*) Flour

Barley is a good source of fiber (13–28% dry mass),[49] with the main fibers being β-glucan (2–20% dry mass) and arabinoxylan (3.4–8% dry mass)[50] with variation due to differences between different types and varieties of barleys. Very high degrees of substitution with barley flour have been reported to give acceptable pasta; in fact, pasta has been prepared from 100% barley flour that was acceptable to a sensory panel in all respects except for color.[51] Berglund *et al.* reported reduced scores for sensory textural attributes for pasta comprising 75% barley flour.[52] At incorporation levels of 20% and 40%, Basinskiene and Schoenlechner demonstrated that barley flour had a less deleterious effect on cooking loss, water absorption, and noodle hardness than equivalent amounts of oat, amaranth, buckwheat, or quinoa flours: of the additives investigated; it was the only one reported to decrease rather than increase cooking loss.[53] Marconi *et al.* (2000) added barley-pearling fractions to semolina at 50% substitution (45% durum semolina, 5% gluten), obtaining a pasta which was darker in color but gave acceptable textural quality on cooking.[54]

Oat (*Avena sativa*) Flour

Oat contains 2–7% β-glucan by total dry weight of the kernel, of a higher molecular weight than barley β-glucan.[55] Oat also contains arabinoxylans (2.2–4.1% dry weight).[50] Few publications have appeared on the supplementation of durum-based pasta with oat flour. Osipova and Volchkov have reported that the use of 40–60% whole grain oat flour in pasta formulations significantly increased the viscosity and firmness of the formulation, impairing extrusion.[56,57]

Buckwheat (*Fagopyrum esculentum*) Flour

Buckwheat is used in significant quantities on its own in East Asia to produce noodles, so buckwheat flour is an obvious choice for supplementation of durum pasta. Pasta fortified with 5–30% buckwheat flour has been reported to have acceptable rheological and sensory properties.[3,58] Due to the innate color of the buckwheat flour, such pastas are typically a chocolate-brown color. While water absorption was found to be slightly greater on average on incorporation of buckwheat flour, no impact on cooking time was observed for pastas dried at 30–40°C.[3] Cooking loss increased with degree of substitution, from 6.5–7.2% at 5% substitution to 7.2–8.0% at 25% substitution. Firmness (measured as the work required to cut through two pasta strands) also decreased with degree of substitution, from 4.5–4.8 to $2.9–3.6 \times 10^{-4}$ Nm, respectively. Both these effects were more pronounced for pastas produced from dark buckwheat flour than light buckwheat flour. The dark buckwheat flour was of similar overall composition, with slightly higher lipid content, but was reported to give a grittier feel to the pasta in sensory analysis.[3] This suggests that, although particle size was not measured, the dark buckwheat flour was a coarser material than the light flour, which may have been partially responsible for the differences in behavior in the pasta.

Rayas-Duarte *et al.* carried out an extensive sensory analysis of pastas substituted with buckwheat flour, and found that overall acceptability remained high although there were significant differences in sensory perception scores.[3] Consistent with instrumental measurements, substituted pastas were assessed as less firm, with this effect greater at higher degrees of substitution and for the dark rather than light buckwheat flour. The pasta prepared with the dark buckwheat flour was judged to be significantly stickier and grittier than control pasta at all degrees of substitution.

At 20% incorporation, Yalla and Manthey found little impact of buckwheat bran flour on water absorption, in contrast to a significant decrease in absorption with incorporation of flaxseed flour (~5%) and an increase in absorption with incorporation of wheat bran (~10%).[59] Buckwheat bran flour generally had little impact on DDT, and durum semolina doughs prepared with buckwheat bran flour were significantly stickier at the high moisture content range of formulations than conventional semolina, consistent with a reduced degree of water uptake into starch granules.

It was observed by Yalla and Manthey that the non-traditional ingredients they investigated had a coarser particle size than semolina.[59] It is unclear to what extent simple physical differences such as these may underpin many of the changes in textural and sensory properties reported on incorporation of fibers in pasta.

Legume Flours

A range of legume flours has been investigated for supplementation of pasta, and in general they display similar properties, regardless of the legume flour used. Undesirable odors and flavors can arise from oxidation of lipid-rich legumes, so thermal deactivation of lipoxygenases may be necessary.[60]

Pasta supplemented with up to 30% broad bean (*Vicia faba*) flour was prepared by Gimenez *et al.*[61] All levels of incorporation of bean flour had detrimental effects on dough quality, with 10% substitution giving a fall in

Farinograph stability and an increase in water absorption. The substituted pasta displayed a greater cooking loss and reduced OCT, but marginally lower water absorption. While cooking loss was proportional to the amount of bean flour incorporated, water absorption was independent, suggesting that the former is due to the loss of soluble bean flour components and the latter is due to the effect of bean flour on the overall matrix structure. The reduced water absorption was mirrored in sensory analysis, where panel respondents scored the substituted pastas higher on firmness upon overcooking (OCT + 10 extra minutes of cooking).[61]

Petitot et al. prepared durum pasta substituted with 35% faba bean or green pea flours.[11,62] Pastas were firmer both in sensory and instrumental tests. The only significant differences between the faba bean results and the green pea results was that sensory panels found the surface of the green pea flour substituted pastas to be considerably rougher.[62]

Drying temperature was found to be vastly more significant in determining sensory and rheological properties of the pasta than the nature of the legume flour, despite differences in protein and fiber content, and particle size distribution, of the flours. Though higher drying temperature reduced many of the negative effects of legume flour incorporation, it also gave a more rubbery product than the control pasta and significantly higher amounts of Maillard products imparting colors and flavors that could impact negatively on consumer acceptance.[62] Microscopic investigation of the pastas showed a disruption of the protein network in the legume-substituted pastas, but conversely birefringence showed a reduced degree of starch gelatinization, suggesting a lower degree of hydration.[11,62]

Petitot et al. suggested that differences in the hydration properties of the substituted pastas could arise largely from differences in particle size distribution, and proposed that this be known and uniform in these types of studies. They provide particle size distributions for the flours used – a practice necessary if the contribution of different variables to pasta properties on incorporation of different ingredients is ever to be clarified (Fig. 17.2).[62]

With increasing substitution of semolina with common bean (Phaseolus vulgaris) flour, Gallegos-Infante et al. found increased cooking loss, decreased water absorption and OCT. The amount of resistant starch increased in the substituted pastas to a greater degree than would be expected from simple addition of the resistant starch component of the bean flour, suggesting that additional resistant starch is formed on processing.[13,14]

Substitution of pasta with 5–25% bean flour derived from roasted or unroasted navy or pinto beans (Phaseolus vulgaris) was found to increase dough water absorption

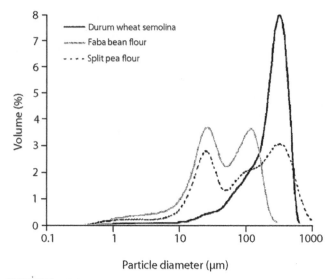

FIGURE 17.2   Particle size distributions of semolina and flours used in preparation of legume-fortified pasta.[64] *Reproduced with permission from Petitot et al.[62]*

and have little effect on dough development time (DDT) but increased dough stability and decreased the mechanical tolerance index, with greater effects seen at higher degrees of legume flour incorporation.[63] Despite the greater water absorption of the dough, the formed pasta had lower water absorption. In sensory evaluations, mouthfeel, color, appearance, and acceptability were ranked well down from the control pasta in all cases.[63]

Durum wheat flour can carry 5–10% of chickpea flour and still meet the specification of pasta products in terms of firmness, cooking quality, and sensory evaluation.[64] Wood investigated pasta containing up to 30% chickpea flour and found decreased cooking loss and stickiness with increasing levels of substitution, while instrumental measurements showed a steady decrease in firmness and resilience.[65] In sensory analysis, overall acceptability of pasta substituted with up to 30% chickpea flour was not inferior to control durum pasta, but the most substituted pasta was rated as firmer than the control by sensory panelists, in contradiction to the instrumental results. Sabanis et al. prepared lasagne from chickpea flour and durum wheat blends and reported that though consumers preferred spaghetti without legume additives, they liked ones supplemented with 20% chickpea.[64] Lasagne with up to 50% chickpea flour was investigated and significant increases in water absorption and DDT were observed, while dough strength significantly declined. On cooking, the water uptake of the lasagne supplemented with chickpea was significantly less, with equivalent amounts of 50% chickpea pasta absorbing half as much water, leading to unacceptable textural properties for 10% substitution or greater, giving lasagne that was less firm and more easily broken. Flavor, color, and overall acceptability were rated well by a sensory panel at 5% and 10% substitution, but pastas prepared at higher degrees of substitution were rated poorly.

Zhao *et al.* produced pasta substituted with 5–30% of a range of legume flours. Of the legumes investigated, chickpea had the greatest trypsin inhibiting activity, and some of this activity remained in the cooked pasta with the higher chickpea-flour contents.[66] Optimal cooking times for the substituted pastas were similar to the control, while cooking loss and firmness increased and cooked weight decreased with increasing legume incorporation. In sensory tests, firmness and stickiness increased with increasing chickpea flour substitution, and elasticity decreased.[66] While a trained sensory panel rated the chickpea fortified pasta most highly in terms of overall quality of the four legume-fortified pastas investigated (green pea, yellow pea, lentil, and chickpea), it was rated the lowest in a consumer acceptance study (though the differences between the four legume-fortified pastas in this study were not significant). The pastas substituted with yellow pea flour were rated second in quality by the sensory panel. Pasta substituted with 5–30% whole green pea flour had increased OCT, cooking loss, and firmness. Sensory tests confirmed the increase in firmness and noted a marked decrease in elasticity; stickiness was dependent on the cultivar used, with *Toledo* green peas giving less sticky pasta than the control, and *Majorette* green peas giving a stickier product. Indicative of the range of variation within and between legume species, the *Toledo* cultivar also gave the highest overall cooking loss for all the legume flours investigated, while the *Majorette* cultivar gave the least.[66] Pastas substituted with 5–30% lentil (*Lens culinaris*) flour had the lowest overall acceptability and the highest stickiness when assessed by the trained sensory panel, but the highest value in consumer acceptance tests. At all levels of substitution, lentil flour gave firmer and less elastic pasta in both technological and sensory tests.

Chillo *et al.* investigated the impact of incorporation of 10% of a number of legume flours (mung bean, soybean, lentil, and chickpea) on technological properties and *in vitro* digestion of pasta.[22] For chickpea flour, no change in water absorption or cooking loss was observed. Hardness increased approximately 25%, which was attributed to the higher protein content. No significant differences were seen in water absorption, while OCT increased slightly (5.0 to 6.0 minutes) and adhesiveness and hardness both increased (190±20 compared with 290±40 mN to break three strands). It was the only legume flour investigated for which cooking loss increased (from 7.8±0.3 to 8.9±0.2), but this difference was not considered to be of practical significance. Addition of 10% soybean flour in durum spaghetti slightly reduced cooking loss and water absorption.[22] The modified pasta was found to be harder than the control

(285±48 compared with 193±16 mN) and, while more adhesive than the control pasta, was the least adhesive of the four legume-modified pastas. This is possibly attributable to the higher lipid content of the soybean compared to the other legumes used. With 10% lentil flour incorporation, Chillo *et al.* found a small increase in OCT and decrease in cooking loss, as well as an increase in hardness and in stickiness.[22] The increase in hardness was less than that observed in the same study for chick pea, mung bean, and soybean flours, while the increase in adhesiveness was greater.

In sensory analysis of spaghetti prepared with up to 35% of commercial defatted heat-treated soy flour dried at 40°C, Shogren *et al.* found no significant differences from control spaghetti in texture.[67] This is in contrast to the previous work of Buck *et al.* (flour dried at 25°C), where soybean flour gave pasta that was markedly firmer than the control at 10% and 20% incorporation.[68] Similarly, the work of Taha *et al.* found increasing firmness on supplementation with soy flour of pastas also containing maize flour.[69] However, Shogren *et al.* found pastas with 25–50% defatted soy flour gave increased intensity for the "starchy mouthcoating" response on sensory analysis, and pasta with 35% or greater soy meal was perceived as "grainy", with higher values of bitter and "beany" flavors reported by panelists for pasta incorporating 50% soybean flour.[67]

Nasehi *et al.* carried out a multivariate analysis of more than 20 pasta formulations containing durum wheat flour and 9–39% soy flour.[70] They found that firmness and stickiness were not affected, and while soy flour impacted negatively on color, no beany flavor was noted in sensory analysis except at the very highest levels of substitution. Sensory analysis of pasta fortified with 30% yellow pea flour found it to be not significantly different from the control by panelists except in terms of odor, which was judged to be inferior.[23]

Pasta prepared with lentil flour at degrees of substitution between 5% and 25% were ranked well down from a control pasta in all cases for mouthfeel, color, appearance, and acceptability.[63] In Farinograph studies, dough stability increased and mechanical tolerance index decreased at all substitution levels, with a more pronounced effect at higher degrees of substitution; DDT was not significantly different from the control for the roasted lentil flour but shorter (2.5 vs 3.5 minutes at all substitution levels) for the unroasted lentil flour.[63]

Pasta prepared with 5–12% fermented pigeon pea (*Cajanus cajan*) flour and dried at 50°C for 2 hours showed a markedly greater cooking loss than control pasta (6–8% compared with 3%), as well as an increased OCT and greater water absorption (217–224% compared with 152%, independent of the amount of pigeon pea flour incorporated). At all levels of incorporation the overall acceptability of the pasta in sensorial analysis was reduced, but it was judged that the reduction in sensory quality at up to 10% incorporation was acceptable.[71]

No impact on average water absorption or OCT was observed in pastas produced with 5–30% lupin (*Lupinus albus*) flour and dried at 30–40°C.[3] Cooking loss increased at all levels of substitution, to a degree proportional to the level of substitution, while a small increase in firmness unrelated to level of substitution was observed. In sensory evaluations, this same increase in firmness unrelated to substitution level was reported, with increasing stickiness and grittiness values proportional to the level of substitution.[3]

In conclusion, while the nutritional effect of incorporating non-wheat flours in pasta can be beneficial, the negative impact of diluting the semolina is apparent with all ingredients at substitution levels high enough to be of substantial health benefit. In the case of ingredients where the non-fiber components are not significantly different in their nutritional effects from wheat, it may be more advisable to use an extracted fiber (see Supplementation of Pastas with Soluble Fibers, below). Where there are substantial other benefits from, for example, essential amino acids absent in wheat and antioxidants, as in the case of legume-substituted pasta, the negative effects on textural and sensory properties may be acceptable. The results of Petitot *et al.* suggest that processing has a greater effect on textural properties than the type of legume used in the formulation.[62]

Supplementation of Pasta with Resistant Starch

Resistant Starch 2

Two commercial RS2 sources from maize (Hi-Maize 260 and Hi-Maize 1043) at 10% to 20% substitution of a pasta dried at 35–40°C had no impact on sensory properties compared to a durum wheat pasta control.[26] Hi-Maize 260 was also investigated by Bustos *et al.*, who found that incorporation at 2.5–10% in pasta dried at 30–40°C also had minimal impact on sensory quality.[25] Hi-Maize 260 incorporation reduced cooking loss and water absorption and produced a pasta with equivalent or superior textural properties compared to the control.[25]

Vernaza *et al.* investigated Hi-Maize 260, preparing formulations containing up to 25% Hi-Maize 260 together with up to 0.70% of a lipid (Dimodan B-727, a monoglyceride produced from palm oil).[72] For pasta dried at 60–85°C they found significant reductions in OCT and water absorption, and increases in cooking loss, all of which scaled with the amount of RS2 added. Increased firmness was observed for pastas incorporating RS2, with the firmest being the pasta with 12% Hi-Maize 260 and no added lipid. Stickiness was also generally reduced with greater RS2 incorporation.[72] Substitution of pasta dried at 65°C with 10–50% Hi-Maize 1043 was investigated by Aravind *et al.*[24] They observed a significant increase

in Farinograph water absorption and decrease in DDT, but saw significant increases in cooking time only at 50% substitution. Water absorption decreased with the amount of RS2 substitution, and there was no impact on stickiness. Pasta with 10% Hi-Maize 1043 was firmer than control pasta, while pasta with 50% Hi-Maize 1043 was less firm. No adverse impact of the RS2 on flavor or odor was detected in sensory analysis, and no significant differences were found in textural attributes (firmness, slippery, rubbery, chewy, floury mouthfeel, rubbery or mouthdrying) between the control and pastas with 10% or 20% Hi-Maize 1043 substitution.

Besides high-amylose corn starch, pasta has been prepared with sweet potato (*Ipomea batatas*)[73,74] and banana (*Musa paradisiaca*)[75,76] starches. Agama-Acevedo *et al.* substituted durum semolina with 15–45% banana flour in preparing pasta dried at 45°C.[76] These levels of banana flour gave pastas of reduced diameter compared to the control, but did not negatively impact technological properties of the pastas to any great extent; the products were slightly firmer, stickier, and more elastic, while water absorption increased somewhat at low levels of banana starch substitution and decreased at higher levels. Despite these variations, sensory analysis of the pastas by a sample of 200 consumers found no difference between the control and all levels of banana flour substitution; all were perceived as equally inferior to commercial durum pasta. Hernandez-Nava prepared pasta with 5–20% banana starch, and found small decreases in diameter and firmness and small increases in cooking loss with increasing banana starch content.[75] In sensory analysis, the substituted pastas with 5–15% banana starch were rated significantly better overall than the control by an untrained panel of 40 testers.

Resistant Starch 3

Sozer and colleagues found that 10% substitution of durum pasta with an RS3 (unspecified) had minimal impact on sensory quality and textural properties, giving a product that was much more acceptable than one with an equivalent amount of bran substitution.[77] Water absorption was only slightly greater for the RS3-substituted pasta, while cooking loss was less than the control at short cooking times and greater at cooking times longer than 10 minutes.[77] Aravind *et al.* found a slightly more pronounced effect of substitution on the properties of pasta dried at 65°C with 10–20% of an RS3 (Novelose 330) than equivalent amounts of an RS2 (Hi-Maize 1043).[24] Farinograph water absorption increased and dough development time decreased to a similar extent with the two resistant starches, but cooking loss was higher for RS3 than RS2 at the same level of substitution and cooking time was reduced to a greater extent. As with pasta prepared with RS2, Aravind *et al.* found that pastas with 10% RS3 substitution were somewhat firmer than the control, while the firmness at 20% substitution was equivalent to the control; this is probably attributable to the reduced water absorption of the RS competing with the effect of the substituent on diluting the gluten and/or disrupting the starch/protein matrix, with the former effect dominating at lower levels and the latter at higher levels of substitution. Sensory evaluation found no significant differences in textural or flavor attributes between the substituted pastas and the control.

Resistant Starch 4

Novelose 480 was used at substitution levels of 2.5–10% in pasta dried at 30–40°C.[25] It was found to reduce water absorption and increased the hardness and stickiness of the pasta, though the product obtained was still of acceptable quality in sensory evaluations.[25]

In summary, incorporation of resistant starch appears to be a facile way to introduce large quantities of fiber into pasta without imparting undesirable properties.

Supplementation of Pasta with Soluble Fibers

β-Glucan

Cleary and Brennan fortified pasta with a β-glucan enriched fraction extracted from barley containing approximately 70% β-glucan, and found a significant drop in hardness (measured in terms of the force required to sever a pasta strand) and increase in water absorption even at the lowest level of fortification (2.5%).[33] They observed that hardness did not decrease further on increasing the proportion of the β-glucan enriched fraction to 10%, while water absorption only increased slightly. These results suggest the effect of β-glucan incorporation arises primarily from the disruptive effect of the fiber on the starch–protein matrix. [33] On the other hand, the decrease in the *in vitro* starch digestion observed by Cleary and Brennan (see β-Glucans, above) was approximately linear with the amount of β-glucan incorporation, suggesting that this effect is not strongly coupled with the gross changes to structure impacting hardness and water absorption. Cleary and Brennan suggested the barley β-glucan extract both restricted starch gelatinization and modified the starch–gluten matrix, reducing the rates of sugar release, but these effects would have to operate on a smaller size scale than that responsible for the overall changes in pasta properties.

At levels of substitution of up to 10% β-glucan, Chillo *et al.* found no significant impact on hardness, color, or optimal cooking time for pasta dried at 25°C, but greater cooking loss and stickiness and some deterioration in color values at all levels of substitution.[32]

Aravind *et al.* prepared pasta containing up to 20% Barley Balance™.[28] As semolina water absorption was affected by the presence of the β-glucan source, water content was adjusted to give similar Farinograph behavior; the pasta was dried at 65°C. All pastas had lower cooking loss, swelling index, and pasta water absorption than the control. Substituted pastas were firmer than the control, and only had significantly greater stickiness at 20% substitution. Pasta substituted with 7.5% Barley Balance™ was found to have sensory properties similar to pasta made from only durum semolina, while at substitution levels of 15% and higher panelists noted a bran aftertaste and described the pasta as increasingly rubbery and chewy.

Inulin

Brennan and colleagues prepared fresh pasta substituted with inulin (Frutafit® HD, DP 12–14) at 2.5–10% and found a decrease in water absorption, elasticity, and firmness, all of which scaled with the amount of inulin present.[29,38] They observed no significant differences in cooking loss or adhesiveness across the range of inulin levels investigated.[38]

Sensory analysis of pastas prepared with inulin (Fibruline XL, DP >20) substituted for 5–15% of semolina assessed the textural properties of pasta at 5% substitution as equivalent to the control, at 10% substitution the pasta was judged distinctly inferior in terms of hardness, stickiness, and appearance.[78] Flavor was judged inferior at all inulin incorporation levels above 2%.

Aravind *et al.* investigated two different inulins of different DP, Frutafit® HD (DP 12–13) and TIC LV-100 (DP 6–7).[39] These were used to prepare pastas (dried at 65°C) at up to 10% substitution (LV-100) and 20% substitution (Frutafit HD). Farinograph measurements showed a decrease in water absorption with increased inulin addition, and a much longer mixing time requirement. Small clumps in the mixture were observed, suggesting uneven moisture distribution through preferential absorption of water by inulin. Cooking time decreased and cooking loss increased with increasing inulin incorporation, and the cooking time effect was more pronounced for the lower DP inulin. Reduction in firmness was seen only at 20% substitution for the higher DP inulin, whereas substitution with the lower DP inulin gave reduced firmness at levels of 7.5%. There were no significant changes in pasta stickiness and cooked pasta diameter with addition of either inulin. Aravind *et al.* carried out sensory analysis on the pastas produced with the lower DP inulin, which had the more significant effect in technological measurements (12 panelists), and the pasta prepared at 7.5% substitution could not be distinguished from the control by the testers. Firmness, rubberiness, and chewiness were all reported by the sensory panel as reduced at the highest level of substitution.

Guar Gum

Aravind *et al.* found that addition of up to 20% guar gum increased stickiness (from 21.2 to 42.1 mN) and had a smaller effect in increasing cooking loss and water absorption.[42] In sensory tests the pastas were assessed as being comparable to the control at up to 10% guar gum incorporation, with the pasta containing 15% guar gum being assessed well for overall quality but having significantly reduced scores for firmness, chewiness, and rubberiness. Brennan and Tudorica likewise reported only small decreases in firmness and elasticity measured instrumentally for up to 10% guar gum, with a small increase in stickiness that was independent of the amount of guar gum present.

Locust Bean Gum

Pasta with 2.5–10% locust bean gum had decreased cooking loss and increased firmness at all levels of substitution, and, like guar gum, gave a small increase in stickiness that was independent of the amount of gum present.[29]

Xanthan Gum

Xanthan gum was used by Edwards et al. to substitute semolina in durum pasta, and found to enhance firmness without impairing other qualities at 1% and 2% substitution.[79] Enhancement of firmness and elasticity at low levels of xanthan gum incorporation (2.5%) was found by Brennan et al., with only a small increase in stickiness, with values for all properties dropping to levels similar to the control by 10% substitution.[29]

Carboxymethylcellulose (CMC)

Komlenić and colleagues added up to 0.75% CMC to pasta dried at 35°C, and in sensory tests found a small reduction in stickiness and no impact on taste or firmness, giving overall acceptability scores slightly above or equivalent to that of the control at all levels of substitution.[80] Cooking loss increased somewhat with increasing levels of CMC substitution (from 6.1–6.5% in the control to 8.6–9.8% with 0.75% CMC).

Aravind et al. found that 1.5% substitution of pasta with CMC had no significant impact on sensory properties, instrumentally measured firmness, stickiness, or cooking loss, but increased water absorption to a small extent.[42]

In summary, significant nutritional effects can be seen at low levels of certain high-viscosity soluble fibers, such as guar gum and carboxymethylcellulose, without any impact on technological and sensory properties; however, the nutritional effects do not appear to scale linearly, and different soluble fibers can exhibit very different behaviors. In addition, marked differences attributable to molar mass exist between pasta produced with different sources of nominally the same fiber, such as β-glucan and inulin.

Supplementation of Pasta with Insoluble Fibers

Brans

Kaur and colleagues prepared a series of substituted pastas (dried at 45–50°C) with up to 25% bran derived from a variety of sources, and sensory tests suggested that acceptable product could be produced with up to 10% of all brans investigated, with some brans giving acceptable product at much higher substitution levels (Fig. 17.3).[81] The water absorption values reported by Kaur et al. increase with bran content in a very similar way across all brans investigated.[81]

FIGURE 17.3 Sensory analysis acceptability scores for different insoluble fibers. *Adapted from Kaur et al.[81]*

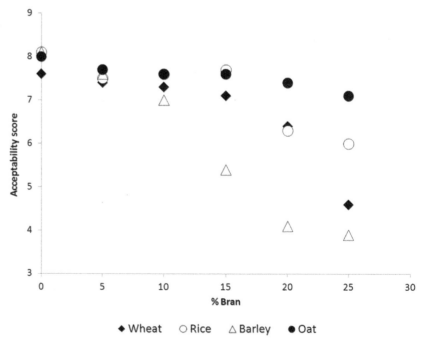

OAT BRAN

Bustos and colleagues found that incorporating up to 10% oat bran in pasta reduced hardness, elasticity, and chewiness, in both instrumental and sensory tests, with sensory analysis giving a much lower overall acceptability score for pasta substituted with 10% oat bran than 10% resistant starch.[25]

WHEAT BRAN

Kordonowy and Youngs found that incorporation of 10–30% durum wheat bran in spaghetti reduced the degree of protein loss on cooking and the extent of checking (minute cracks on the pasta surface that can lead to strand breakage), but otherwise had deleterious effects.[82] They reported mean bran particle sizes in the range of 0.15–0.17mm, measured by laser diffraction. Dough development time increased steadily with degree of bran addition, firmness decreased, cooking loss increased, and the weight of the cooked pasta decreased. All pastas incorporating bran scored significantly inferior in sensory evaluations of texture, flavor, and color. Kordonowy and Youngs employed a total of 51 people in carrying out sensory analysis, and collected information on their bread consumption preferences; the overall rating of the pasta attractiveness was strongly related to bread preferences, with respondents preferring brown bread rating the flavor and texture of the substituted pasta less unfavorably. Only those panelists with the strongest brown bread preference rated any feature of the bran substituted pasta on a par with the unsubstituted pasta, however, with the 10% bran pasta rated marginally above the control pasta for flavor by this group.[82]

Pasta containing 40–50% wheat bran dried at 80°C was prepared by Sudha et al.[83] Reductions in firmness from 156 to 113mN were seen on going from a control pasta to a 50% bran pasta made with untreated bran, but bran that had been steam heat-treated before addition gave a considerably firmer product (130.5mN at 50% substitution). Dry heat-treated bran gave products only marginally firmer than the pastas substituted with raw bran. Cooking loss was much greater in the non-heated bran substituted pastas than the control, but this was reduced significantly (although still greater than the control) using heat-treated bran.

Aravind et al. prepared durum pasta with 10% to 30% of bran substitution.[84] Bran substitution resulted in increased cooking loss, decreased water absorption, firmness, and stickiness. In sensory testing, all substituted pastas showed a profile distinctly different from the control, approaching but not as extreme as the results reported for a commercial whole meal pasta.

BARLEY BRAN

Comparing various bran sources from wheat, rice, barley, and oats in the preparation of fiber-enriched pasta, barley bran had to be used at a lower dosage than the other bran sources because of its lower overall acceptability score (sensory) (Fig. 17.3).[81]

Vegetable Fibers

Yaseen and colleagues produced durum pasta substituted with 10% to 20% fiber from potato peels and derived by removing juice from carrot and orange.[48] Fibers were milled to a fine powder before addition and 1% gum arabic was added as a binder to the pasta formulations, which were dried at 70°C. Dough stability was reduced and DDT increased to similar degrees in Farinograph measurements for the three fibers, and all fibers had greater water absorption, though to very different extents. Cooking loss and water absorption of pasta increased significantly for all fibers. Appearance, color, flavor, cohesiveness, and stickiness were rated significantly worse by sensory panelists than the control for all pastas made with potato or carrot fiber, but equivalent values to the control were obtained for all pastas made with orange fiber.

Mango-peel fiber sieved through a 150-micron sieve was used by Ajila et al. to supplement durum pasta (dried at 85°C) at 2.5–7.5% substitution.[47] Cooking loss increased at higher levels of substitution, as did firmness (73.5 ± 1.2mN for 7.5% compared with 44.0 ± 1.7mN for control). Overall quality in sensory analysis was rated significantly below the control for 5% and 7.5% mango-peel fiber substituted pasta, but the adverse reaction was primarily to taste rather than to texture.

Brennan and Tudorica investigated the effect of 2.5–10% pea fiber and bamboo fiber on the technological properties[29] of fresh pasta. Pea fiber (Exafine, Cosucra. Belgium) and bamboo fiber (Qualicel 41B, CFF, Germany) reduced firmness at all levels of substitution, and had relatively little impact on elasticity or stickiness.

DISCUSSION

It is clear that the addition of a large range of fibers to pasta formulations can have very diverse impacts on pasta technological, sensory, and nutritional properties, and that these can often be counterintuitive. While a fiber may reduce GI without impairing technological properties at low levels of substitution, at higher levels of substitution it may impair the textural properties of the pasta without having any nutritional benefit through its negative effect on the cohesion of the material. This suggests that the effect of a fiber on the micro scale (e.g., in forming an impermeable matrix on the surface of starch granules to restrict access by amylases, a mechanism for reducing GI) must be carefully distinguished from its effect on the macro scale (e.g., in mixing poorly and encouraging the pasta strand to disintegrate more rapidly during cooking).

In this summary we have seen marked differences in results not only between different fibers but also for different sources of the same fiber, and very rarely has significant characterization of the fiber been carried out to explain these differences. This is especially true with the soluble fibers, where differences in molar mass and structure can lead to profoundly different outcomes.

In the same way, particle size appears to play a major role in the success of supplementation of durum pasta with whole flours, and it is often unclear whether differences seen between different flours reflect chemical differences or differences in milling; however, particle size and particle size distributions have very rarely been characterized. The importance of particle size as a variable was explicitly raised by Li and Walker, who highlighted it as a significant part of their future investigations.[85]

It is important to note that the physical properties of pasta are very dependent on the drying protocols employed, which have been alluded to rather than described in detail here, and differences in drying procedure complicate considerably the task of comparing different reports on a particular fiber, or comparing the impact of different fibers. While drying at higher temperatures usually improves textural properties, Holm *et al.* saw very little difference in *in vitro* digestion behavior of pasta dried at low and high temperatures,[45] suggesting that this may be a way to improve the properties of substituted pastas that appear to be unacceptable from reports made on fresh pasta. Conversely, in several systems summarized here, on comparison of different reports a smaller impact of the substituting fiber is seen for pastas dried at higher temperatures – understandable, if what we surmise about the role of the starch/protein matrix in reducing GI is correct.

Besides raising the pasta drying temperature, there is scope for improving the technological and sensory properties of substituted pastas by adding additional protein or a viscous hydrocolloid. Both these strategies are commonly employed in making pasta from non-durum sources, and have been illustrated in this summary in the discussion of a pasta made primarily from sweet potatoes.[86] Gluten addition is one obvious strategy, referred to explicitly by Manno,[87] and legume protein extracts have also been used in pasta supplementation.[88] Small quantities of carboxymethylcellulose or xanthan gum, for example, can have dramatic effects on textural properties.[89,90]

A further strategy for improving the properties of substituted pasta is to increase the degree of cross-linking in the diluted semolina-derived protein through addition of transglutaminase.[91–93] Furthermore, much of the research has focused on using single fibers in pasta formulations. Possibly the use of multiple fibers and/or other components can be used more effectively which could affect product structure, satiety, gut health, and more controlled regulation of the GI of foods.

References

1. Cubadda RE, Marconi E. Developing functional foods enriched with natural barley β-glucans: a review. *Ingredienti Alimentari* 2008;**7**(1):6–13.
2. Frank J, Sundberg B, Kamal-Eldin A, Vessby B, Åman P. Yeast-leavened oat beads with high or low molecular weight beta-glucan do not differ in their effects on blood concentrations of lipids, insulin, or glucose in humans. *J Nutr* 2004;**134**:1384–8.
3. Rayas-Duarte P, Mock CM, Satterlee LD. Quality of spaghetti containing buckwheat, amaranth, and lupine flours. *Cereal Chem* 1996;**73**(3):381–7.
4. Guillon F, Champ M. Structural and physical properties of dietary fibers, and consequences of processing on human physiology. *Food Res Int* 2000;**33**:233–45.
5. Andersson AAH, Åman P. Functional barley products. In: Hamaker BR, editor. *Technology of Functional Cereal Products*. Cambridge, UK: Woodhead Publishing; 2008. p. 261–80.
6. Lim HS, White PJ, Frey KJ. Genotypic effects on beta-glucan content of oat lines grown in two consecutive years. *Cereal Chem* 1992;**69**:262–5.
7. Yokoyama WH, Hudson CA, Knuckles BE, Chiu M-C, Sayre RN, Turnlund JR, et al. Effect of barley beta-glucan in durum wheat pasta on human glycemic response. *Cereal Chem* 1997;**74**:293–6.
8. Nikolic N, Sakac M, Mastilovic J. Effect of buckwheat flour addition to wheat flour on acylglycerols and fatty acids composition and rheology properties. *LWT-Food Sci Technol* 2010;**44**(3):650–5.
9. Tovar J, Björck IM, Asp NG. Incomplete digestion of legume starches in rats: A study of precooked flours containing retrograde and physically inaccessible starch fraction. *J Nutr* 1992;**122**:1500–7.
10. Tovar J, Granfeldt Y, Björck IM. Effect of processing on blood glucose and insulin responses to starch in legumes. *J Agr Food Chem* 1992;**40**:1846–51.
11. Petitot M, Barron C, Morel M- H. Impact of legume flour addition on pasta structure: consequences on its *in vitro* starch digestibility. *Food Biophys* 2010;**5**:284–9.
12. Goñi I, Garcia-Diaz L, Mañas E, Saura-Calixto F. Analysis of resistant starch: A method for food and food products. *Food Chem* 1996;**56**:445–9.
13. Gallegos-Infante JA, Rocha-Guzman NE, Gonzalez-Laredo RF, Ochoa-Martinez LA, Corzo N, Bello-Perez LA, et al. Quality of spaghetti pasta containing Mexican common bean flour (*Phaseolus vulgaris* L.). *Food Chem* 2009;**119**(4):1544–9.
14. Gallegos-Infante J-A, Bello-Perez LA, Rocha-Guzman NE, Gonzalez-Laredo RF, Avila-Ontiveros M. Effect of the addition of common bean (*Phaseolus vulgaris* L.) flour on the *in vitro* digestibility of starch and undigestible carbohydrates in spaghetti. *J Food Sci* 2010;**75**(5):H151–6.
15. Friedman M. Nutritional value of proteins from different food sources. *J Agric Food Chem* 1996;**44**(1):6–29.
16. Cordoso-Sandiago AR, Moreira-Araujo RSR, Pinto e Silva MEM, Area GAJ. The potential of extruded chickpea corn and bovine lung for malnutrition programs. *Innov Food Sci Emerg* 2001;**2**:203–9.
17. Goñi I, Valentin-Camazo C. Chickpea flour ingredient slows glycemic response to pasta in healthy volunteers. *Food Chem* 2003;**81**:511–5.
18. Dalgetty DD, Byung-Kee B. Isolation and characterization of cotyledon fibers from peas, lentils, and chickpeas. *Cereal Chem* 2003;**80**:310–5.
19. Osorio-Diaz P, Agama-Acevedo E, Mendoza-Vinalay M, Tovar J, Bello-Perez LA. Pasta added with chickpea flour: chemical composition, *in vitro* starch digestibility and predicted glycemic index. *Ciencia Tecnol Alime* 2008;**6**(1):6–12.
20. Messina M. Soyfoods and disease prevention: Part 1: Coronary heart disease. *Agro Food Ind Hi-Tec* 2003;**14**:7–10.

21. Wietrzyk J, Grynkiewicz G, Opolski A. Phytoestrogens in cancer prevention and therapy - mechanism of their biological activity. *Anticancer Res* 2005;**25**:2357–66.

22. Chillo S, Monro JA, Mishra S, Henry CJ. Effect of incorporating legume flour into semolina spaghetti on its cooking quality and glycemic impact measured *in vitro*. *Int J Food Sci Nutr* 2010;**61**(2):149–60.

23. Marinangeli CPF, Kassis AN, Jones PJH. Glycemic responses and sensory characteristics of whole yellow pea flour added to novel functional foods. *J Food Sci* 2009;**74**(9):S385–9.

24. Aravind N, Sissons MJ, Fellows CM, Blazek J, Gilbert EP. Optimization of resistant starch II and III levels in durum wheat pasta to reduce *in vitro* digestibility while maintaining processing and sensory characteristics. *Food Chem* 2013;**36**:1100–9.

25. Bustos MC, Perez GT, Leon AE. Sensory and nutritional attributes of fiber-enriched pasta. *LWT-Food Sci Technol* 2011;**44**(6):1429–34.

26. Gelencsér T, Gál V, Hódsagi M, Salgó A. Evaluation of quality and digestibility characteristics of resistant starch-enriched pasta. *Food Bioprocess Technol* 2008;**1**:171–9.

27. Luhaloo M, Mårtennson A-C, Andersson R, Åman P. Compositional analysis and viscosity measurements of commercial oat bran. *J Sci Food Agric* 1998;**76**:142–8.

28. Aravind N, Sissons M, Egan N, Fellows CM, Blazek J, Gilbert EP. Effect of β-glucan on technological, sensory, and structural properties of durum wheat pasta. *Cereal Chem* 2012;**89**(2):84–93.

29. Brennan CS, Tudorica CM. Fresh pasta quality as affected by enrichment of nonstarch polysaccharides. *J Food Sci* 2007;**72**(9):S659–65.

30. Chillo S, Ranawana DV, Pratt M, Henry CJK. Glycemic response and glycemic index of semolina spaghetti enriched with barley β-glucan. *Nutrition* 2011;**27**(6):653–8.

31. Schkoda PM. Barley beta glucans application in obesity. *Agro Food Ind Hi-Tec* 2008;**19**(Suppl. 5):14–5.

32. Chillo S, Ranawana DV, Henry CJK. Effect of two barley β-glucan concentrates on *in vitro* glycemic impact and cooking quality of spaghetti. *LWT-Food Sci Technol* 2011;**44**(4):940–8.

33. Cleary L, Brennan C. The influence of a (1→3)(1→4)-β-D-glucan rich fraction from barley on the physico-chemical properties and *in vitro* reducing sugars release of durum wheat pasta. *Int J Food Sci Technol* 2006;**41**(8):910–8.

34. Åman P, Rimsten L, Andersson R. Molecular weight distribution of beta-glucan in oat-based foods. *Cereal Chem* 2004;**81**:356–60.

35. Waterhouse AL, Chatterton NJ, editors. *Glossary of Fructan Terms. Science and Technology of Fructans*. Boca Raton, FL: CRC; 1993.

36. Roberfroid MB. Dietary fiber, inulin, and oligofructose – a review comparing their physiological effects. *Critical Rev Food Sci* 1993;**33**:103–48.

37. Brennan CS, Tudorica CM. Evaluation of potential mechanisms by which dietary fiber additions reduce the predicted glycemic index of fresh pastas. *Int J Food Sci Technol* 2008;**43**:2151–62.

38. Brennan CS, Kuri V, Tudorica CM. Inulin-enriched pasta: effects on textural properties and starch degradation. *Food Chem* 2004;**86**(2):189–93.

39. Aravind N, Sissons MJ, Fellows CM, Blazek J, Gilbert EP. Effect of inulin soluble dietary fiber addition on technological, sensory, and structural properties of durum wheat spaghetti. *Food Chem* 2012;**132**(2):993–1002.

40. Wren MA, Mullen JD, inventors; General Mills, Inc., assignee. Low calorie pasta. Application: US, US patent 1972-314657, 3843818. 1974 19721213.

41. Gatti E, Catenazzo G, Camisasca E, Torri A, Denegri E, Sirtori CR. Effects of guar-enriched pasta in the treatment of diabetes and hyperlipidemia. *Ann Nutr Metab* 1984;**28**:1–10.

42. Aravind N, Sissons M, Fellows CM. Effect of soluble fiber (guar gum and carboxymethylcellulose) addition on technological, sensory and structural properties of durum wheat spaghetti. *Food Chem* 2012;**131**(3):893–900.

43. BeMiller JN. Hydrocolloids. In: Arendt EK, Dal Bello F, editors. *Gluten-Free Cereal Products and Beverages*. New York, NY: Elsevier; 2008. p. 203–15.

44. Ekholm P, Virkki L, Ylinen M, Johansson L. The effect of phytic acid and some natural chelating agents on the solubility of mineral elements in oat bran. *Food Chem* 2003;**80**(2):165–70.

45. Holm J, Koellreutter B, Würsch P. Influence of sterilization, drying and oat bran enrichment of pasta on glucose and insulin responses in healthy subjects and on the rate and extent of *in vitro* starch digestion. *Eur J Clin Nutr* 1992;**46**:629–40.

46. Borneo R, Aguirre A. Chemical composition, cooking quality, and consumer acceptance of pasta made with dried amaranth leaves flour. *LWT-Food Sci Technol* 2008;**41**(10):1748–51.

47. Ajila CM, Aalami M, Leelavathi K. Prasada Rao UJS. Mango peel powder: A potential source of antioxidant and dietary fiber in macaroni preparations. *Innov Food Sci Emerg* 2010;**11**(1):219–24.

48. Yaseen AAE, Shouk AA. High dietary fiber pasta: processing and evaluation. *Egypt J Food Sci* 2007;**35**:47–58.

49. Åman P, Hesselman K, Tilly A- C. The Variation in Chemical Composition of Swedish Barleys. *J Cereal Sci* 1985;**3**:73–7.

50. Collins HM, Burton RA, Topping DL, Liao M-Y, Bacic A, Fincher GB. Variability in fine structures of noncellulose cell wall polysaccharides from cereal grain: Potential importance in human health. *Cereal Chem* 2010;**87**(4):272–82.

51. Melland R, Newman RK, McGuire CF, Eslick RF. The effects of bleach treatment on pasta made from a series of barley genotypes. *Cereal Res Commun* 1984;**12**:201–7.

52. Berglund PT, Fastnaught CE, Holm ET. Food uses of waxy hull-less barley. *Cereal Food World* 1992;**37**:707–14.

53. Basinskiene L, Schoenlechner R. The influence of alternative cereals on noodle quality. *Chemine Technologija (Kaunas, Lithuania)* 2007;**1**:74–9.

54. Marconi E, Graziano M, Cubadda RE. Composition and utilization of barley pearling by-products for making functional pastas rich in dietary fiber and beta-glucans. *Cereal Chem* 2000;**77**:133–9.

55. Beer MU, Wood PJ, Weisz J, Fillion N. Effect of cooking and storage on the amount and molecular weight of (1–3)(1–4)-β-glucan extracted from oat products by an *in vitro* digestion system. *Cereal Chem* 1997;**74**:705–9.

56. Osipova GA, inventor Orlovskii Gosudarstvennyi Tekhnicheskii Universitet, assignee. Pasta production method. Application: RU patent 2008-103888.2358453. 2009 20080201.

57. Osipova G, Volchkov A. New recipe component for pasta. *Khlebo-produkty* 2008;**7**:51–2.

58. Manthey FA, Yalla SR, Dick TJ, Badaruddin M. Extrusion properties and cooking quality of spaghetti containing buckwheat bran flour. *Cereal Chem* 2004;**81**:232–6.

59. Yalla SR, Manthey FA. Effect of semolina and absorption level on extrusion of spaghetti containing non-traditional ingredients. *J Sci Food Agric* 2006;**86**(5):841–8.

60. Alasino M, Andrich O, Sabbag N, Costa S, Torres M, Sánchez H. Baking with pea flour previously subjected to enzyme inactivation. *Arch Latinoam Nutr* 2008;**58**(4):397–402.

61. Gimenez MA, Drago SR, De Greef D, Gonzalez RJ, Lobo MO, Samman NC. Rheological, functional and nutritional properties of wheat/broad bean (*Vicia faba*) flour blends for pasta formulation. *Food Chem* 2012;**134**(1):200–6.

62. Petitot M, Boyer L, Minier C, Micard V. Fortification of pasta with split pea and faba bean flours: Pasta processing and quality evaluation. *Food Res Int* 2010;**43**(2):634–41.

63. Bahnassey Y, Khan K, Harrold R. Fortification of spaghetti with edible legumes. II. Rheological, processing, and quality evaluation studies. *Cereal Chem* 1986;**63**(3):216–9.

64. Sabanis D, Makri E, Doxastakis G. Effect of durum flour enrichment with chickpea flour on the characteristics of dough and lasagne. *J Sci Food Agric* 2006;**86**:1938–44.

65. Wood JA. Texture, processing, and organoleptic properties of chickpea-fortified spaghetti with insights to the underlying mechanisms of traditional durum pasta quality. *J Cereal Sci* 2009;**49**(1): 128–33.

66. Zhao YH, Manthey FA, Chang SKC, Hou H-J, Yuan SH. Quality characteristics of spaghetti as affected by green and yellow pea, lentil, and chickpea flours. *J Food Sci* 2005;**70**(6):371–6.

67. Shogren RL, Hareland GA, Wu YV. Sensory evaluation and composition of spaghetti fortified with soy flour. *J Food Sci* 2006;**71**(6): S428–32.

68. Buck JS, Walker CE, Watson KS. Incorporation of corn gluten meal and soy into various cereal-based foods and resulting product functional, sensory, and protein quality. *Cereal Chem* 1987;**64**(4): 264–9.

69. Taha SA, Kovacs Z, Sagi F. Evaluation of Economical Pasta Products Prepared from Durum SemolinalYellow Corn Flour/Soy Flour Mixtures. 2. Cooking Behavior, Firmness and Organoleptic Properties. *Acta Aliment Hung* 1992;**21**:163–70.

70. Nasehi B, Mortazavi SA, Razavi SM, Tehrani MM, Karim R. Effects of processing variables and full fat soy flour on nutritional and sensory properties of spaghetti using a mixture design approach. *Int J Food Sci Nutr* 2009;**60**(Suppl. 1):112–25.

71. Torres A, Frias J, Granito M, Vidal-Valverde C. Fermented Pigeon Pea (*Cajanus cajan*) Ingredients in Pasta Products. *J Agric Food Chem* 2006;**54**(18):6685–91.

72. Vernaza MG, Biasutti E, Schmiele M, Jaekel LZ, Bannwart A, Chang YK. Effect of supplementation of wheat flour with resistant starch and monoglycerides in pasta dried at high temperatures. *Int J Food Sci Technol* 2012;**47**(6):1302–12.

73. Gopalakrishnan J, Menon R, Padmaja G, Sajeev MS, Moorthy SN. Nutritional and functional characteristics of protein-fortified pasta from sweet potato. *Food Nutr Sci* 2012;**2**(9):944–55.

74. Krishnan JG, Menon R, Padmaja G, Sajeev MS, Moorthy SN. Evaluation of nutritional and physico-mechanical characteristics of dietary fiber-enriched sweet potato pasta. *Eur Food Res Technol* 2012;**234**(3):467–76.

75. Hernandez-Nava RG, Berrios JdJ, Pan J, Osorio-Diaz P, Bello-Perez LA. Development and characterization of spaghetti with high resistant starch content supplemented with banana starch. *Food Sci Technol Int* 2009;**15**(1):73–8.

76. Agama-Acevedo E, Islas-Hernandez JJ, Osorio-Diaz P, Rendon-Villalobos R, Utrilla-Coello RG, Angulo O, et al. Pasta with unripe banana flour: physical, texture, and preference study. *J Food Sci* 2009;**74**(6):S263–7.

77. Sozer N, Dalgic AC, Kaya A. Thermal, textural and cooking properties of spaghetti enriched with resistant starch. *J Food Eng* 2007;**81**:476–84.

78. Negro C, Tommasi L, De Bellis L, Miceli A, D'Oria F. Development of improved pasta enriched with inulin. *Ingredienti Alimentari* 2007;**6**(5):23–6.

79. Edwards NM, Biliaderis CG, Dexter JE. Textural characteristics of whole wheat pasta and pasta containing non-starch polysaccharides. *J Food Sci* 1995;**60**(6):1321–4.

80. Komlenić DK. Ugarĉić-Hardi Ž, Jukić M. Sensory Properties of Hydrocolloid-enriched Pasta from Two Flour Types of *Triticum aestivum* Wheat. *Deut Lebensm Rundsch* 2006;**102**(8):368–72.

81. Kaur G, Sharma S, Nagi HPS, Dar BN. Functional properties of pasta enriched with variable cereal brans. *J Food Sci Technol* 2012;**49**(4):467–74.

82. Kordonowy RK, Youngs VL. Utilization of durum bran and its effect on spaghetti. *Cereal Chem* 1985;**62**:301–8.

83. Sudha ML, Ramasarma PR, Rao GV. Wheat bran stabilization and its use in the preparation of high-fiber pasta. *Food Sci Technol Int* 2011;**17**(1):47–53.

84. Aravind N, Sissons M, Egan N, Fellows C. Effect of insoluble dietary fiber addition on technological, sensory, and structural properties of durum wheat spaghetti. *Food Chem* 2011;**130**(2):299–309.

85. Li J, Walker CE. Effect of water absorption and mung bean middlings content on mung bean - durum semolina composite pasta quality. *Getreidetechnologie* 2009;**63**(4):26–36.

86. Gopalakrishnan J, Menon R, Padmaja G, Sajeev MS, Moorthy SN. Nutritional and functional characteristics of protein-fortified pasta from sweet potato. *Food Nutr Sci* 2011;**2**(9):944–55.

87. Manno D, Filippo E, Serra A, Negro C, De Bellis L, Miceli A. The influence of inulin addition on the morphological and structural properties of durum wheat pasta. *Int J Food Sci Technol* 2009;**44**:2218–24.

88. Doxastakis G, Papageorgiou M, Mandalou D, Irakli M, Papalamprou E, D'Agostina A, et al. Technological properties and non-enzymatic browning of white lupin protein enriched spaghetti. *Food Chem* 2006;**101**(1):57–64.

89. Barcenas ME, de la O-Keller J, Rosell CM. Influence of different hydrocolloids on major wheat dough components (gluten and starch). *J Food Eng* 2009;**94**(3-4):241–7.

90. Chillo S, Civica V, Iannetti M, Suriano N, Mastromatteo M, Del Nobile MA. Properties of quinoa and oat spaghetti loaded with carboxymethylcellulose sodium salt and pregelatinized starch as structuring agents. *Carbohyd Polym* 2009;**78**(4):932–7.

91. Sissons M, Aravind N, Fellows CM. Quality of fiber-enriched spaghetti containing microbial transglutaminase. *Cereal Chem* 2010;**87**(1):57–64.

92. Basman A, Koksel H, Atli A. Effects of increasing levels of transglutaminase on cooking quality of bran supplemented spaghetti. *Eur Food Res Technol* 2006;**223**(4):547–51.

93. Kovacs ET. Use of enzyme transglutaminase for developing pasta products with high quality. 3rd International Congress "Flour-Bread 05" and 5th Croatian Congress of Cereal Technologists. *Opatija, Croatia*; 2005. p. 258–63.

18

Dietary Fiber and Wheat Bran in Childhood Constipation and Health

Helga Verena Leoni Maffei

São Paulo State University (UNESP), Department of Pediatrics – Botucatu Medical School, Botucatu, São Paulo, Brazil

INTRODUCTION

It is now over 40 years since Burkitt and colleagues described softer/bulkier stools and shorter transit time in populations with unrefined diets than in populations with refined diets.[1] Much has been published since then about the role of dietary fiber (DF) in the gastrointestinal tract of healthy people, but great gaps in our knowledge about the relation of DF with childhood constipation still prevail. Chronic childhood functional constipation (CFC) is highly prevalent worldwide,[2] leads to a great economical burden, is often associated with behavior problems, and has an important impact on quality of life.[3] It can therefore be considered a public health problem. Also, recurrence rates are very high,[4–5] and thus it can be inferred that long-term follow-up and maintenance of a dietary fiber-rich diet for lifetime are very important.

A great proportion of CFC begins in the first months of life, after weaning and before toilet training.[6–9] It is crucial, therefore, that preventive measures begin at weaning.

PREVENTION OF CHILDHOOD FUNCTIONAL CONSTIPATION

In theory, to prevent CFC one should avoid the multiple intermingled factors considered to be involved in its physiopathology:

- Constitutional predisposing factors[10] cannot be avoided, but have been looked for,[11] and some are potentially treatable.
- Absence of human milk during infancy[12] and/ or low DF intake leads to hard stools.[13] Anorexia (accompanying infectious episodes or other causes) can also result in low DF intake.
- Dermatitis and fissures in the perianal region can both occur during diarrhea; however, fissures often appear after elimination of hard stools. Cow's milk allergy also leads to anal dermatitis and can cause constipation.[14]
- Retentive behavior is usually caused by the attempt to avoid painful evacuation due to hard stools and/ or to dermatitis/fissures. In fact, painful defecation was the event most often reported by mothers as causing the constipation in their children.[15] In addition, inadequate school toilet conditions, bullying, and other stressful life events may trigger retentive behavior and constipation;[16] stressful events, however, can also diminish appetite, thus acting through the low dietary/DF intake mechanism. Retentive behavior has also been attributed to forceful/precocious toilet training; however, constipation has been shown to be present before toilet training.[17]

Besides weaning, other precipitators of CFC (infectious diarrhea, cow's milk allergy) occur mainly during the first year of life and explain its frequent early onset.[6–9] Whatever the causes of hard stools, of dermatitis/ fissures, and of retentive behavior, these factors cause a vicious circle that maintains and aggravates CFC. Therefore, whenever present, the treatment of these causes should not be postponed.

The Role of Breastfeeding in Prevention: Weaning and DF Recommendations

Exclusively breastfed infants produce more and softer stools than those on cow's milk formulas.[12] Human milk protects against constipation, and during transition to formula or cow's milk stool frequency decreases and the proportion of hard stools increases.[18–20] The risk of constipation increases 4.5-fold in infants up to 6 months of age without breast milk, when compared to predominantly breastfed infants, and 2.1-fold in infants with breast *plus* cow's milk/formula feeding and/or complementary food.[8] The protective effect of human milk is still evident in 6- to 24-month-old children when complementary food is added, but not when cow's milk is also added.[21] The protective effect of breast milk has been ascribed, among other factors, to its high content of non-absorbable oligosaccharides: being prebiotic substances, these behave like soluble fiber. Formulas with added prebiotics have, therefore, the potential to keep stool characteristics closer to those of breastfed infants.[20,22] However, although promising, it has not been shown that these formulas prevent constipation; in fact, constipation has been exceptionally evaluated in these studies.[23] Regardless, although several prebiotic supplemented formulas have been commercialized over the last decade, according to the ESPGHAN, independent non-company funded trials are still needed before its routine use can be recommended.[24] Moreover, when studying stool characteristics it should be reported which formulas infants received, to allow better analysis of constipation frequencies.[18,25]

According to World Health Organization (WHO) recommendations, the ideal would be exclusive breastfeeding for 6 months, and partial breastfeeding up to 2 years or beyond while receiving adequate complementary foods.[26] In Europe it is recommended that infants begin complementary foods at 4–6 months, switching to cow's milk at the end of the first year of age.[27] However, compliance with the weaning guidelines is poor, since a high proportion of infants in various countries had received solid food before the age of 4 months.[7,28–32] Also breastfeeding is clearly far from desirable, since a great proportion of infants receive human milk substitutes before the age of 6 months.[33,34] However, WHO and European guidelines do not give specific advice for non-breastfed infants under the age of 6 months; in Brazil and the UK, formula is recommended as the sole food for these younger than 6-month-old infants who present to the pediatrician already without breastmilk.[35,36] Moreover, although not recommended, infants of economically underprivileged families are often fed cow's milk, since it is less expensive than formulas. Relactation should be tried for these infants as a first step, and, if not successful, formulas should be advised (if affordable). However, this is a vulnerable period, since constipation often begins in the absence of human milk's protective factors.[6–9] In fact, constipation (and also colic/excessive crying, which could be secondary to it) is a frequent reason alleged by mothers for introducing solid foods before the recommended age, or changing formulas.[33,37] Therefore, the question arises whether complementary food containing DF should be "officially"

anticipated for these infants. They are capable of accepting it, as is supported by the mentioned surveys.[28–32] The author's personal recommendation is to introduce easily mashed/pressed fruit and then progressively gluten-free non-refined cereals and vegetables, with good results: adequate growth and no constipation. However, the possible role of DF during this vulnerable period has to be proven with well-designed studies, since so far it is based on empirical observations and on indirect evidence.[6–9] One could worry about early introduction of solid food and future allergies,[38] but this association has not been shown to occur.[39] However, more studies are needed to confirm these data, since sensitization might occur.[40] Regardless, only poorly sensitizing foods should be advised for these infants less than 4 months old, as described.

When weaning occurs after the age of 4–6 months, complementary foods should be introduced according to the guidelines of each country/region, if available. In general, fruit (not juices), vegetables, and whole grain bread, pasta, and rice are recommended.[35,41–44] Additionally, the author lays emphasis on the peel/bagasse of fruit and the grain of pulses in addition to its broth. However, although foods containing DF are recommended when complementary food is introduced, to our knowledge there is only one recommendation, from Italy, regarding the amount of DF to be given: 6 g per day for 9- to 10-month-old infants.[41] Other widely followed recommendations begin at 1,[45] 2,[46] or 3 years of age.[47] The lack of recommendations for infants weaned off breast milk before the age of 12 months might induce some restraint regarding introduction of the necessary amount of DF. This is seemingly due to the fear that DF in infants may lead to faltering growth and mineral imbalance. However, this was found not to occur after 6 months of a DF-rich diet, at least not in older children; in fact, serum ferritin even increased.[48]

The most widely used recommendation is easy to apply and very practical: age (years) +5–10 g per day (American Health Foundation).[47] The American Academy of Pediatrics recommends 0.5 g/kg per day; this recommendation has the disadvantage that obese children often exceed what seems a reasonable amount, or even the proposed higher limit of 35 g/day for 18-year-old boys. The recommendation of the Institute of Medicine (IOM) is based on adult data: 14 g DF/1000 kcal;[45] moreover, it has the inconvenience that functional fiber (synthetically produced fibers with known physiological benefits that are added to foods) is included in the total recommended amount, but this is not listed in food or nutrient databases or on food labels. The average intake of functional fiber in adults is estimated at approximately 5 g per day – a relatively small amount.[49] The Food Guide Pyramid[46] (now substituted by MyPlate) is very practical and illustrative; both these guides recommend portions of different food sources (including those which contain DF), but not exact amounts of DF.

DF versus Constipation: Does DF Prevent Constipation? Possible Confounding Factors

Studies evaluating whether DF intake prevents childhood constipation are based on comparisons between constipated versus non-constipated children, and results are controversial. Most studies detected an inverse relation between DF intake and constipation. Thus, a significantly greater intake of DF or DF-containing foods[13,50–54] (A. Vicentini and H. Maffei, personal communication) – or a non-significantly greater intake[55] – has been documented in control than in constipated children. Furthermore, constipated schoolchildren in Turkey had a lower consumption rate of fruit and vegetables and a higher consumption rate of milk-group foods, biscuits, and macaroni than non-constipated children.[56] Other studies have not detected a lower DF intake in constipated children,[57] particularly those in pediatric age extremes: 6-month to 2-year-old infants[8] and adolescents.[58,59] Interestingly, a significantly lower DF intake in constipated infants aged 6 months–2 years than in control children was observed in another study (A. Vicentini and H. Maffei, personal communication).

Many factors can contribute to the cited discrepancies and will be discussed: the definition of CFC, the dietary assessment method, the number of food sources inquired about, the food table with the DF content, the soluble/insoluble DF ratio, the "fiber paradox", the possible associated ontogenetic lactase deficiency, etc.

1. *Definitions of CFC.* Definitions of CFC must be broad enough to detect a range from mild disturbances in the bowel habit of otherwise healthy children to severe alterations in children attended in specialty clinics.[60] If the definition is somewhat restrictive, like the globally accepted Rome III criteria,[61,62] a child with mild constipation (hard stools every second day with straining, without the other symptoms of the definition) might be erroneously included in the control group, mainly in community surveys during which a rectal exam is not performed. Thus, constipated and "control" children are not clearly separated and this will influence DF intake results. The reverse of the "Boston Working Group" definition[63] is an option, since it will include in the control group those children with adequate bowel habits: soft stools (mushy or cylindrical without cracks), passed without pain or straining; absence of large stools that may clog the toilet periodically; absence of recurrent abdominal pain, enuresis, non-structural urinary tract infections, fecal soiling, and of a feeling of incomplete elimination; three or more stools per week, unless the child is breastfed. Also, asking about frequent episodes of "want but can't" can avoid inclusion of children with "occult" constipation in the control group.[7]

2. *Dietary assessment method/food sources.* The preferred assessment method to evaluate an individual's usual food intake depends on several aspects, including the aim of the study. No single method is optimal under all conditions.[64] Food records have been considered good methods, but are difficult to apply in everyday practice. According to Kranz et al.,[65] "only a composite diet quality index can begin to capture the multidimensional nature of what people eat". Regardless, when choosing a method to assess DF intake, one has to consider that children often have limited fruit, vegetable, and whole grain intake and thus there is a large day-to-day variation. Therefore, a single dietary 24-hour recall (24-hR), although practical and widely used, might underestimate the intake if the child eats these food groups once or twice per week, but not in the last 24 h; in contrast, it might lead to overestimation if the only weekly intake occurred in the last 24 h. Furthermore, the "usual day method" might be impossible to apply to children eating fruit and vegetables every second day, for instance. A recent study has shown that the quantitative food frequency questionnaire for the previous month seems more suitable to detect the described daily variations in DF intake than a single 24-hR (A. Vicentini and H. Maffei, personal communication), but more studies are necessary to unravel this issue. To better discriminate between study groups, the greatest possible number of representatives for each food source (foods, food preparations, and industrialized products) should be included, detailing cereals (whole grain, wheat bran/other DF-containing supplements), vegetables, and whether fruit is consumed with peel and seeds, and citrus fruit with bagasse. Removing the peel was found to reduce the fiber content in apples by 6–11% and in pears by 34%.[66] In fact, studying 2- to 12-year-old children, those of the control group had a significantly greater DF intake than constipated children (median 18.0 g/d vs 15.3 g/d) and the only significant differences for the food groups were a greater intake of fruit with peel/bagasse in controls than in children with constipation (5.1% vs 1.8% of total DF), and less refined grains (42.5% vs 47.0%). For peeled fruit the intake was similar, although somewhat greater in the control group (13.3% vs 10.1%).[67]

3. *Food tables and insoluble/soluble fiber ratio.* The widely used food tables from UK, USA, and Australia[68–70] do not present insoluble (IF) and soluble (SF) fiber separately, and thus the IF/SF ratio has rarely been used.[71,72] Taking into account that these components have different physiological effects, and that on

theoretical grounds IF is better for laxation than SF,[73,74] knowing this ratio makes a difference. Refined cereals, fruit without peel/bagasse, and the pulp of pulses can result in a reasonable amount of DF intake, but since this constitutes mainly SF, the desired bowel habit may not be achieved. One Brazilian Table presents soluble and insoluble fiber,[75] but it overestimates SF;[76] since rice and beans are staple foods in Brazil, beans being rich in SF and non-absorbable oligosaccharides, this might falsely inflate SF and total DF data and has to be considered when analyzing the results.[77] Moreover, the usually employed food tables are somewhat incomplete and often do not contain foods commonly consumed in countries other than those from which the food table originated. Thus, it might be necessary to use data from several tables to ensure that as few as possible foods of the population's eating habits are excluded (A. Vicentini and H. Maffei, personal communication). The UK and the USA tables are based on similar analytical DF methods,[68,69] but, should different methods be involved, they have to be stated.

4. *The fiber paradox.* Conflicting results in the literature could in part be explained by the so-called dietary fiber paradox.[78] Heaton states that "constipated patients will almost certainly have increased their DF intake in an effort to help themselves, and so may have normalized what was originally a low intake". This statement was again emphasized in the Constipation Guidelines of the American Gastroenterological Association: "the studies do not take into account the number of persons who increased their fiber intake as treatment for constipation".[79] Were dietary measures to occur without an adequate bowel washout, constipation would usually not subside, leading to a false impression that DF was unhelpful.

5. *Ontogenetic lactase deficiency.* The possible associated ontogenetic lactase deficiency might help in keeping a normal bowel habit in children older than 2 years of age, in spite of a low DF intake. Therefore, along with the dietary assessment, one should ask about milk intolerance and/or other possible (albeit rarer) sugar intolerances.

All the above factors should be considered before stating that DF does not protect against constipation.

POPULATION SURVEYS OF DF INTAKE

Several population surveys (mainly from North America, and also from Europe, with hundreds and mostly thousands of children) have detected that DF intake in general is far below what is recommended by the American Health Foundation.[49,80–88] Thus, only 45% of 4- to 6-year-olds and 32% of 7- to 10-year-olds consumed adequate fiber to meet the age + 5 rule.[89] Figure 18.1, containing data from the literature,[49,80–88] clearly depicts that DF intake worsens with increasing age. However, since the data represent mean intake for approximate mean age groups, a great proportion of younger children with less than the minimum recommended intake (<age (y)+5g/d) is not shown in Figure 18.1A. Thus, 55.3% of children aged 2–5 years consumed less than age+5g/d, and this proportion had increased to 60.2% 10 years later.[81] At the other extreme, 17.1% of 2- to 5-year-old children consumed more than age (y)+10g/d, 32.7% of whom consumed more than age+15g/d (a little bit less after 10 years). Moreover, a proportion (although smaller) of older children and adolescents had a DF intake above age+10g/d.[81] Mean data from Spain are also above the proposed upper limit (Fig. 18.1B); nevertheless, the authors draw attention to the fact that "Spanish children's eating habits are reasonably

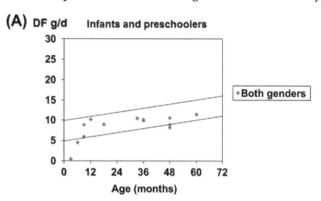

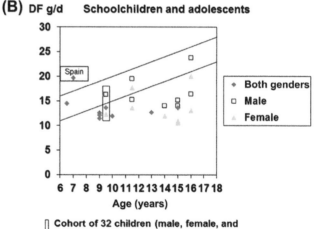

Cohort of 32 children (male, female, and both genders), followed for 2 years

FIGURE 18.1 Mean dietary fiber intake according to mean age groups: (A) infants and preschoolers; (B) school children and adolescents. Means of age groups are approximate, since mean ages are not available from the literature; for instance, the calculated mean for age group 2–5 years is 48 months. Oblique lines represent the limits of the recommended DF intake according to the American Health Foundation: age (years)+5–10g/day.[47] Please see color plate at the back of the book. *Information from a compilation of literature data.[49,81–88]* See color plate at the back of the book.

in line with the American food pyramid guidelines, but consumptions of cereals and fruit should be improved".[83] Also, 2- to 3-year-old children and 4- to 5-year-old children in the upper quartile of DF intake had a mean intake above age + 10 g/d, at 16.4 g/d and 18.24 g/d, respectively.[49] In fact, in this study[49] the high amount of DF intake better conforms to dietary reference intakes (DRI) and the Food Guide Pyramid or MyPlate recommendations.[45,46,90] However, only a few children met the DRI recommendation of 14 g DF/1000 kcal of energy consumed, even after considering a hypothetical estimated average of 5 g per day functional fiber.[49] Similarly, the few studies approaching specifically whole grain intake have in general shown low intakes when confronted with the recommendation to consume at least 50% of all grains as whole grains. This was recently reviewed by Stewart,[91] and will not be detailed further in this chapter.

These data might explain high constipation prevalence. One cannot be sure, however, that children with constipation have not been included in the surveyed general population. Some surveys are decades old, with data from 1976 –1988,[80,81] but in fact data are similar to those collected more recently.[49,82–84,86,87] Indeed, it is unfortunate that dietary guidelines do not seem able to induce better dietary habits.[92] Nevertheless, recommendations are far from settled, and still need to be validated.

THE ROLE OF DIETARY FIBER IN THE TREATMENT OF CHILDHOOD FUNCTIONAL CONSTIPATION

Treatment of CFC involves four partially intermingled steps:

1. Education – very important, mainly in childhood
2. Colorectal disimpaction, *per os* or *rectum* (this step should be fully accomplished to avoid the "fiber paradox")
3. Treatment of anal fissures, and sphincter reconditioning
4. Maintenance treatment with laxatives and diet.

Education includes explanations about the need of disimpaction and how it will be implemented, the technique for sphincter reconditioning, and the importance of a DF-rich diet. The DF amount and the possible food choices according to the child's preferences should be discussed in detail; the new MyPlate[90] and the older Food Guide Pyramid[46] are both illustrative and helpful, the latter somewhat more so.

When constipation is detected in its initial stage, sphincter reconditioning and maintenance treatment should suffice. However, when detected later on, treatment may have become a complex issue, since secondary changes ensue along with constipation's progression: (1)

long-standing distension of the rectal ampulla leads to altered expulsion dynamics and so-called "obstructed defecation", accompanied by fecal soiling and/or enuresis and the emotional disturbances (poor self-esteem, social withdrawal) secondary to it;[93] and (2) colonic transit time progressively increases, leading to slow-transit constipation (STC), often considered an almost irreversible condition. Since STC probably is due to chronic rectosigmoid stasis,[94] one could ask whether these changes might have been prevented, had effective treatment started early, and had recurrences been avoided. In fact, 85% of adults without such changes responded to DF treatment, but only 37% and 20%, respectively, when such changes were present.[95]

It is unfortunate that often only little emphasis is placed on the use of DF for treating constipation. Other treatment modalities are much more discussed.[10,96] In fact, besides the vague statements that "increase in DF intake is widely recommended as a first treatment step for childhood constipation" or "a balanced diet that includes whole grain, fruits and vegetables is recommended", rarely is further discussion dedicated to DF treatment in the guidelines.[63,97,98] Conversely, it is stated that "the effectiveness of fiber treatments is currently too weak to support a definitive recommendation for fiber supplementation in the treatment of constipation".[97,98] Laxatives have been used instead, but should not be used for life, whereas a DF-rich diet can be lifelong.

Dietary Treatment of Constipation

Due to lack of details about DF intake in CFC guidelines, the author's dietary advice is based on theoretical knowledge about the effects of DF on bowel habits,[73,74] other literature data,[1,12,13,41,46–48,78,79,99–102] and clinical experience.[7,67] Thus, the recommended diet is that according to the Food Guide Pyramid/MyPlate for all food groups,[46,90] with an emphasis on fruits with peel/bagasse, and on pulses, vegetables, seeds, and nuts. At least five daily portions of fruits/vegetables, one of non-sifted pulses and of seeds/nuts, are recommended. A written leaflet listing the DF-dense foods within each food group is provided, while those with almost no DF, such as melon, watermelon, and cucumber without skin, are also indicated. Non-refined cereals are included in the advice, but, apart from corn, these are relatively expensive in Brazil. Therefore, taking into account that whole grain foods like bread, pasta, and rice are not part of the usual Brazilian diet, plain wheat bran is recommended in approximate amounts: 5–10 g per day for age <1 year, 10–20 g per day for ages 1–2 years, and 20 g per day for older children. Wheat bran is cheap and tested by governmental entities for food security in Brazil, and it has the best weight/weight ratio among foods (g food intake/g increase in fecal weight).[73] It can be used – in the proportion 2 parts of refined flour to 1 part of bran – to prepare bread, desserts, cakes, pancakes, and "farofa" (manioc flour roasted with varied ingredients, which is very popular in the country). Otherwise, it can be slightly roasted and added to a humid (but solid) food constituent. Bran is usually not well accepted in fluids such as soups and beverages. Adequate fluid intake has to be ensured, but this is not usually a problem. Fruit juice is allowed, as long as it contains the whole fruit, is non-sifted, and has no added sugar. Suggestions for "good" snacks (between meals) and for "good" sweets (after meals) are given: olives, popcorn, mixed nuts, dried fruits, coconut-filled chocolate, pumpkin compote, passion fruit mousse with seeds, and so forth. Gaseous beverages and junk food are discouraged. A decrease in protein intake is advised whenever excess is reported.[103] A prospective evaluation throughout 24 months confirmed that this recommendation is a feasible, cheap, and effective tool for treating constipated children (along with the other treatment tools) in everyday clinical attendance.[103]

Evaluating Dietary Treatment of Constipation

Studies in Adults

A recent review on the effects of DF on the management of adult constipation[104] considered six eligible randomized controlled trials: four used SF (one with an inulin/maltodextrose mixture, three with psyllium), with a favorable outcome; only two used IF, and the results were conflicting.[102,105] In one of the IF trials,[105] women consumed either fiber-rich rye bread (37 g/d DF derived from it) or low-fiber toast (6.6 g/d DF from it). Transit time, fecal frequency and consistency, and straining were significantly improved with rye bread. However, it is not clear how much DF from other food sources was consumed. The other IF trial had a cross-over double-blind design, with a basal period followed by 4-week periods of either placebo–bran or bran–placebo sequences.[102]

This trial has been cited as having no effect of bran supplementation on constipation; however, this conclusion deserves a more detailed analysis. In the placebo–bran sequence, oro-anal transit time and stool frequency improved significantly with bran, but no difference was noted in the bran–placebo sequence. According to the authors, "the lack of any significant difference in the latter sequence should not be regarded as evidence of no benefit of 20 g of bran added to the diet containing 15 g/day of DF, but rather as the result of the carry-over effect of the previous bran treatment". Other aspects can be pointed out in this study, as follows: During the first placebo period, 3/12 patients (25%) needed bowel washout rescue therapy (due to having passed no stools for 8 days), while no patient in the first bran period needed it;

The proportions of patients at the end of the first treatment period (without the carry-over effect) not straining to pass stools in relation to those with the symptoms at baseline were 28.6% (2/7) for placebo and 55.6% (5/9) for bran. The proportions were almost twice as high after bran intake, although not significantly, perhaps due to the small number of patients with straining in the basal period (only 16); The weekly fecal weight, obtained by multiplying the means of daily stool weight and stool frequency, was >50% heavier in both bran periods (838.4 g) than in both placebo periods (550.8 g). Together, these data could be indicative of possible benefits of bran.[100,101]

Older studies not cited in the review[104] also seem to indicate a beneficial effect of wheat bran.[100,101]

Studies in Children

Few studies have approached the effect of treating constipated children with DF-rich diets and/or DF supplements. An attempt to increase DF in regular food without an additional DF supplement led to a significant DF increase.[106] However, only about 25% of children attained DF intake above the minimum recommended age + 5 g rule; constipation relief could be in part attributed to bowel cleanout and to the laxative still used by most children at the end of the study.

Supplementation with SF (glucomannan,[107] DF mixture with mainly SF,[108,109] guar gum[110]) has been used with favorable results. In these studies, DF supplements were used like laxatives, without an attempt to improve the DF amount in the diet. If children do not improve their diet, constipation will possibly recur after discontinuing the supplement. Long-term studies, after discontinuance of these supplements, are needed, since only 4- to 8-week interventions have been published so far. Most common side effects of SF are colonic fermentation and increased satiety. Thus, these SF supplements are a plausible choice for constipated obese children.[111,112] Also, neurologically impaired children may benefit from DF supplementation, either as soluble[113] or insoluble fiber.[114]

The studies in which the supplements were mainly IF are listed in Table 18.1.[48,99,103,114–117] Notwithstanding the different criteria used and the methodological fragilities, an overview of the table indicates a good response to the treatment schedules used. The duration of most studies was longer than the usual 4–8 weeks with SF. In six of the seven studies the supplemented IF was wheat bran, and in four of these an additional effort was made to implement an otherwise high-fiber diet. The only controlled, randomized, double-blind study was the one supplemented with cocoa husk.[116] This probably reflects the difficulty of "blinding" wheat bran intake in children. The other problem is the alleged bad acceptance of wheat bran, in contrast to cocoa husk which seems

TABLE 18.1 Treatment of Chronic Childhood Functional Constipation (CFC) with Insoluble Fiber (IF) Supplements

Reference (Year)	Age, n	Inclusion Criteria Washout	Study Design Duration	Planned Intervention	Baseline Data[a] Food Table (FT)l	Outcome[a]	Observations
Zoppi et al.[115] (1982)	6–16 months n=6	Mild constipation Washout ?	No control, 3-day basal diet 1 month	Wheat (w.) bran[b], 15 g/d (age <12 months); 30 g/d (age >12 months)	DF 0.32 g/kg per day Stool/d 0.5, small, dry Food table?	DF 1.39 g/kg per day Stools/d 1.5, soft	NS blood biochemical decrease. Fecal biliary salt/cholesterol increase
Olness and Tobin[99] (1982)	2–12 years, n=60	CC[c], soiling or both Washout (≥1 enema)	Retrospective clinical experience 6 weeks + 24 months follow-up	High-fiber diet with w. bran Exclusion/reintroduction of "constipating" foods	Previous treatment failures in 68.3%[d] Soiling in 30.0%	After 4.3 weeks: soft stools every 24–48 h; 11.7% soiling (6 w); 10.0% recurrence[e]	Emphasis on patient responsibility was considered additional factor of success
McClung et al.[48] (1993)	4–12 years, n=16	Soiling >3 months, >1 treatment failure Washout (1–3 weeks)	Prospective DF supplement; mineral oil at start 6 months	High-fiber diet plus 0.25 g/kg per day DF from w. bran, Metamucil®, and/or other product	Age	DF (FT[118]) 4–5y	0.71 g/kg per day 6–12y	0.31 g/kg per day Stool weight 71 g/d	75% no soiling[f] 0.71; 0.71 g/kg per day; 0.61; 0.37 g/kg/day[g] Stool weight 224 g/d	No anthropometric/biochemical alterations Ferritin and stool water increased
Tse et al.[114] (2000)	3–17 years, n=20	Developmental disabilities, oral feeds, >1 laxative/week No washout	Prospective laxative (lax) need/week (w) 72 days	All Bran® two-stage increase: (A) 20d, no bran 10d; (B) 42d. Lax after 2 d no stools	FT from Hong Kong DF 2 g/d Lax 1.22/w	(A) (B) DF 17 g/d 21 g/d Lax 0.90/ 0.71/w w p<0.05 <0.01	Amount consumed per child was not measured
Castillejo et al.[116] (2007)	3–10 years, n=48	Adult Rome II, no washout 7d/DF treatment 2 weeks Washout (1 enema)	Controlled, randomized, double-blind 4 weeks	Cocoa husk + β-fructosan DF 5.3 g/d (age 3–6 years), 10.6 g/d (age 7–10 years) plus toilet training	<3 stools/w 33.9% Hard stools 95.8% FT? Cocoa Placebo DFg/d 12.3 13.4	Cocoa Placebo Hard 41.7% 75.0% ISC[h] 58.3% 25.0% CTT[i] decreased	No blood biochemical differences. No weight alteration

(Continued)

F. WHEAT FIBER

TABLE 18.1 Treatment of Chronic Childhood Functional Constipation (CFC) with Insoluble Fiber (IF) Supplements—cont'd

Reference (Year)	Age, n	Inclusion Criteria Washout	Study Design Duration	Planned Intervention	Baseline Data[a] Food Table (FT)/	Outcome[a]	Observations
Chao et al.[117] (2008)	3–14 years, n=422	<3 stools/ week, over >2 months Washout?	Prospective diet program; CC severity score 12 weeks (every 2 weeks)	High-fiber diet with wheat bran; bran intake was not detailed	Score: severe 43.6% Age · DF 5.8 years · 6.0g/d 10.2 years · 9.8g/d FT from Taiwan	Score: severe, 17.3%; mild, 33.6%; any, 49.1% Higher DF intake in patients with <versus >60% symptoms (P<0.001)	DF cutoff for CC relief Age · DF 3–7 years · 10.0g/d 8–14 years · 14.5g/d
Maffei and Vicentini[103] (2011)	3 months–15.6 years, n=28	≥2 items of "Boston criteria"[63] Washout (3–10 enemas)	Prospective clinical and dietary evaluation 2–4 follow-up visits (80 visits); 4–14 months (n=14) 4–24 months (n=14)	High-fiber diet[j] with wheat bran: 5–10g/d (age <12 months); 10–20g/d (age 12–24 months); 20g/d (age ≥2 years)	Soil 44%, RAP 39%, Enuresis/UTI[k] 21% <3 stools/week 32% DF: · 60.7% <age+5; · 17.9% >age+10 FTs: · UK,USA,Australia, Brazil	DF/bran associated to REC[l] (P<0.03) Last visit: 75% REC DF: · 17.9% <age+5; · 60.7% >age+10 Bran: · 7.9g/d[m] (n=18)	DF good acceptance and REC were already occurring at first follow-up visit (0.5–3.5 months), and were maintained at subsequent visits[n]

[a] *Data are presented as mean, unless otherwise stated.*
[b] *Commercial wheat bran, composition obtained from Milupa/Germany*
[c] *CC=Chronic constipation, 41.7% from birth or >5 years.*
[d] *There was no rigorous dietary approach in previous treatments; therefore, the authors considered these children as their own controls.*
[e] *With subsequent amelioration.*
[f] *25% reduced soiling.*
[g] *Increased and then decreased to basal value.*
[h] *ISC=subjective improvement in stool consistency, NS increase in stool frequency.*
[i] *CTT=colonic transit time: in children with basal CTT >50th percentile, the total and right colonic transit time (TT) decreased significantly (rectal TT p 0.051) after cocoa husk.*
[j] *According to the Food Guide Pyramid[46].*
[k] *Soil=soiling (retentive functional incontinence), RAP=recurrent abdominal pain, UTI=urinary tract infection*
[l] *REC=Bowel habit recovery: asymptomatic (71.4%) or improved, no CC complications (3.6%).*
[m] *Median bran intake by 18 children at the last visit.*
[n] *Median data were kept steady after initial amelioration, but individual fluctuations occurred. See Table 18.2 for further details.*

easy to accept.[116] However, the high pentose content of wheat bran's highly predominant IF is better for laxation than cellulose, the main insoluble component of cocoa husk.[73] In fact, the study with cocoa husk barely indicated its benefit, when compared to the control group receiving only toilet training procedures. The studies with wheat bran, being not controlled, do not prove its benefit, but prove it is acceptable to children and is not harmful. In addition, it is very difficult to attain the necessary amount of DF to treat CFC only with the usual food sources.[106] Wheat bran contains around 40% of mainly IF, and therefore greatly contributes to achieving a good DF intake.[103]

No major difficulties with bran acceptance have been referred to in most studies shown in Table 18.1.[99,115,117] However, in everyday practice increasing DF intake by constipated children can be bound by difficulties,[50,103] and intervention studies describing techniques trying to overcome these problems have been published.[119–122] Goal-setting has been used for adolescents, but the reported success could be due to other simultaneously used interventions.[119] Emphasis on patient's responsibility seems helpful.[99] An interesting point rating scheme to increase DF intake was reported in a small number of boys with retentive fecal incontinence.[120] However, children who received verbal and written advice on how to increase their DF intake and those with an additional point rating scheme showed similar results after 6 months; thus, 71.4% and 75% of the children, respectively without or with point rating, accepted ≥age+5g/d DF.[121] An advantage in point rating occurred only after 3 months. Curiously, after 12 months the proportion of children meeting the age+5g/d target was significantly higher in the control group without point rating.[121] These results indicate that a good and detailed orientation could suffice for most children. In fact, groups of children receiving either physician's dietary advice or an additional dietitian's advice both achieved a significant increase in DF intake, somewhat better with the additional advice.[122] However, these children were followed for only 1 month,[122] and, in the author's own experience, ongoing support is necessary. Thus, after the initial extensive personal and written dietary advice mentioned previously, children received dietary reinforcement from a physician at each follow-up visit and from a dietitian at some visits. Whenever the desired DF intake was not achieved, children and families were directed to a bimonthly session with a dietitian; there they received explanations and recipes, tasted foods containing wheat bran, and prepared a very tasty mixture of powdered milk, bran and sugar (2:1:1 proportions) *plus* water to give it a puréed consistency. The results of this approach, for 28 children followed prospectively over 4–24 months, are summarized in Table 18.2.[103]

The four children without bran acceptance at any visit presented the same proportion of bowel habit recovery; they accepted an otherwise very DF-dense diet, despite this being much more expensive and difficult to achieve, since the median proportion of DF due to bran was 26.9%.[103] DF intake above the maximum recommended, at 57.5% of the follow-up visits in this study, could raise concerns about micronutrient bioavailability and children's growth. It was, however, in accordance with the Food Guide Pyramid[46] and with the recommendation of the Institute of Medicine.[45] Moreover, anthropometric data of the children did not indicate a negative influence of the high DF/bran amounts; instead, there was a slight increase in height/age score after intervals with bran.[123] This is supported by other studies.[48,124] One must also consider that DF intake recommendations for children are based on an estimate for healthy children, and constipated children might require more DF, at least for some time after starting treatment.

Possible adverse effects of excessive DF/bran intake, mainly when a large quantity of SF is ingested, include bloating, abdominal distension/cramping, and loose stools. These symptoms can, however, also be consequent upon constipation. A careful clinical history should be able to distinguish both situations. In the author's experience, these symptoms are not present when the bowel habit has recovered, notwithstanding the high DF intake.[103] It is possible, however, that they occur when the bowel washout is not effective.

Recurrence rates are high[4,5] and should be carefully avoided. Therefore, after recovery from constipation children should not be immediately discharged from the outpatient unit but return for a visit after some months to ensure that they are symptom-free and maintaining the DF-rich diet. The DF-rich diet should be kept for life and a rescue plan should be taught, to be used whenever constipation symptoms reappear: laxatives for some days, and reinforcement of DF intake. Should symptoms not subside, or reappear, new medical advice should be sought before complications develop.

FINAL REMARKS

In population surveys, DF consumption is below the recommended amount in a great proportion of children, and this proportion increases among schoolchildren and adolescents. Children with functional constipation have, according to most studies, a lower DF intake than children without constipation signs. Many confounding factors can contribute to the existing controversial results, which occur mainly in infants below the age of 2 years and in adolescents. Thus, current knowledge seems to indicate that adequate DF intake may prevent constipation. However, the beneficial effect of a DF-rich diet

TABLE 18.2   Data from 28 Children[a] with CFC, at 108 Visits over 24 Months[104]

DF intake > age + 10 g/d	23 children, at 57.5% of 80 follow-up visits
Wheat bran acceptance	24 children, at 70% of 80 follow-up visits; 13 continuous, 7 intermittent, 4 rarely. Median intake 20 g/day. Median intakes: REC[b] 15.5 g/day, BAD BH[c] 3.0 g/day Median proportion of DF due to bran: 26.9%
Significant associations	Bran acceptance vs > age + 10 g/day DF Higher DF intake and higher bran intake each, vs BH REC during intervals between visits
Bowel habit at last visit, n = number of children	*21 REC*: 20 asymptomatic, 1 improved, 18 off laxatives; 12 with continuous REC at all follow-up visits, 8 with intermittent REC, 1 only at last visit *7 BAD BH*: 5 with REC at some/all previous visits, in 4 of them BAD BH recurred after bran discontinuance; 2, with only 2 follow-up visits, never had REC

[a] *Median age (range) 7.25 years (0.25–5.6).*

[b] *BH REC: Bowel habit recovery; improved BH, no complications of constipation.*

[c] *BAD BH: Worse/unaltered BH relative to first visit, or improved but still complications. See Table 18.1 for further details.*

still has to be proven with carefully designed studies. This diet probably has to be lifelong, since it also has the potential to help prevent obesity, diabetes, cardiovascular diseases, and colonic/rectal cancer,[125–127] and to decrease mortality from several other causes.[128] While waiting for these studies, more proactive strategies trying to improve dietary habits could be implemented. In a controlled community (mainly elderly people) intervention trial, the consumption of whole grain bread increased and laxative sales decreased.[129] This is a good example of what can be done.

Treatment of childhood constipation should be as vigorous as possible in trying to be effective, to avoid the undesirable evolution to non-responsive constipation and to surgical interventions[10,130] in an originally functional disorder. One important step in the treatment of constipation, after adequate bowel washout procedures, is a DF-rich diet, with or without DF supplements. However, although again there are many clinical indications that this could be effective, conclusive well-designed studies are still necessary. It is the author's opinion that it is necessary to change the paradigm: the focus must lie on prevention beginning at weaning, lifelong adequate DF intake, and prompt treatment at the earliest signs of constipation. In the author's clinical experience a DF-rich diet, with wheat bran supplementation, is very helpful and should not be neglected.

References

1. Burkitt DP, Walker ARP, Painter NS. Effect of dietary fibre on stools and transit time, and its role in the causation of disease. *Lancet* 1972;2:1408–12.
2. Mugie SM, Benninga MA, Di Lorenzo C. Epidemiology of constipation in children and adults: a systematic review. *Best Pract Res Clin Gastroenterol* 2011;25:3–18.
3. Wald A, Sigurdsson L. Quality of life in children and adults with constipation. *Best Pract Res Clin Gastroenterol* 2011;**25**:19–27.
4. van den Berg MM, van Rossum CH, de Lorijn F, Reitsma JB, Di Lorenzo C, Benninga MA. Functional constipation in infants: a follow-up study. *J Pediatr* 2005;**147**:700–4.
5. Michaud L, Lamblin MD, Mairesse S, Turck D, Gottrand F. Outcome of functional constipation in childhood: a 10-year follow-up study. *Clin Pediatr (Phila)* 2009;**48**:26–31.
6. Abrahamian FP, Lloyd-Still JD. Chronic constipation in childhood: a longitudinal study of 186 patients. *J Pediatr Gastroenterol Nutr* 1984;**3**:460–7.
7. Maffei HVL, Moreira FL, Kissimoto M, Chaves SMF, El Faro S, Aleixo A. Clinical and alimentary history of children attending a pediatric gastroenterology outpatient clinic with functional chronic constipation and its possible complications. *J Pediatr (Rio J)* 1994;**70**:280–6. English abstract available at: http://www.jped.com.br.
8. Aguirre ANC, Vitolo MR, Puccini RF, Morais MB. Constipation in infants: influence of type of feeding and dietary fiber intake. *J Pediatr (Rio J)* 2002;**78**:202–8. English version at: http://www.jped.com.br.
9. Borgo HC, Maffei HVL. Recalled and recorded bowel habits confirm early onset and high frequency of constipation in day–care nursery children. *Arq Gastroenterol (SP)* 2009;**46**:144–50.
10. Mugie SM, Di Lorenzo C, Benninga MA. Constipation in childhood. *Nat Rev Gastroenterol Hepatol* 2011;**8**:502–11.
11. Hofmann AF, Loening–Baucke V, Lavine JE, Hagey LR, Steinbach JH, Packard CA, et al. Altered bile acid metabolism in childhood functional constipation: Inactivation of secretory bile acids by sulfation in a subset of patients. *J Pediatr Gastroenterol Nutr* 2008;**47**:598–606.
12. Weaver LT, Ewing G, Taylor LC. The bowel habit of milk-fed infants. *J Pediatr Gastroenterol Nutr* 1988;**7**:568–71.
13. Roma E, Adamidis D, Nikolara R, Constantipoulos A, Messaritakis J. Diet and chronic constipation in children: the role of fiber. *J Pediatr Gastroenterol Nutr* 1999;**28**:169–74.
14. Daher S, Tahan S, Solé D, Naspitz CK, da Silva Patrício FR, Neto UF, et al. Cow's milk protein intolerance and chronic constipation in children. *Pediatr Allergy Immunol* 2001;**12**:339–42.
15. Borowitz SM, Cox DJ, Tam A, Ritterband LM, Sutphen JL, Penberthy JK. Precipitants of constipation during early childhood. *J Am Board Fam Pract* 2003;**16**:213–28.
16. Kistner M. Dysfunctional elimination behaviors and associated complications in school-age children. *Review J Sch Nurs* 2009;**25**:108–16.
17. Blum NJ, Taubman B, Nemeth N. During toilet training, constipation occurs before stool toileting refusal. *Pediatrics* 2004;**113**:e520–2.
18. Tunc VT, Camurdan AD, Ilhan MN, Sahin F, Beyazova U. Factors associated with defecation patterns in 0- to 24-month-old children. *Eur J Pediatr* 2008;**167**:1357–62.
19. Duman N, Utkutan S, Ozkan H, Ozdoğan S. Are the stool characteristics of preterm infants affected by infant formulas? *Turk J Pediatr* 2000;**42**:138–44.

20. Piemontese P, Giannì ML, Braegger CP, Chirico C, Grüber C, Riedler J, et al. Tolerance and safety evaluation in a large cohort of healthy infants fed an innovative prebiotic formula: a randomized controlled trial. *PLoS One* 2011;**6**:e28010.

21. Souza DS, Tahan S, Morais MB. Constipation and dietary fiber intake in infants: relation with type of feeding, nutritional status and indicators of body iron [in Portuguese]. *Rev Med Minas Gerais* 2012;**22**(suppl. 3):S35.

22. Scalabrin DM, Mitmesser SH, Welling GW, Harris CL, Marunycz JD, Walker DC, et al. New prebiotic blend of polydextrose and galacto–oligosaccharides has a bifidogenic effect in young infants. *J Pediatr Gastroenterol Nutr* 2012;**54**:343–52.

23. Schmelzle H, Wirth S, Skopnik H, Radke M, Knol J, Böckler HM, et al. Randomized double-blind study of the nutritional efficacy and bifidogenicity of a new infant formula containing partially hydrolyzed protein, a high beta-palmitic acid level, and nondigestible oligosaccharides. *J Pediatr Gastroenterol Nutr* 2003;**36**:343–51.

24. Braegger C, Chmielewska A, Decsi T, Kolacek S, Mihatsch W, Moreno L, et al. Supplementation of infant formula with probiotics and/or prebiotics: a systematic review and comment by the ESPGHAN Committee on Nutrition. *J Pediatr Gastroenterol Nutr* 2011;**52**:238–50.

25. Kocaay P, Eğrıtaş O, Dalgiç B. Normal defecation pattern, frequency of constipation and factors related to constipation in Turkish children 0–6 years old. *Turk J Gastroenterol* 2011;**22**:369–75.

26. World Health Organization. The WHO global data bank on infant and young child feeding. Available at: http://www.who.int/nutrition/databases/infantfeeding/en/index.html.

27. Agostoni C, Decsi T, Fewtrell M, Goulet O, Kolacek S, Koletzko B, et al. Complementary feeding: a commentary by the ESPGHAN Committee on Nutrition. *J Pediatr Gastroenterol Nutr* 2008;**46**:99–110.

28. Koletzko B, Dokoupil K, Reitmayr S, Weimert-Harendza B, Keller E. Dietary fat intakes in infants and primary school children in Germany. *Am J Clin Nutr* 2000;**72**:1392–8.

29. Yee J, Smith AM, O'Connor DL, Auestad N, Adamkin D, Connor WF, et al. Introduction of complementary foods in preterm infants varies among countries. *J Am Diet Assoc* 2001;**101**:A76.

30. Fewtrell MS, Lucas A, Morgan JB. Factors associated with weaning in full term and preterm infants. *Arch Dis Child Fetal Neonatal Ed* 2003;**88**:F296–301.

31. Giovannini M, Riva E, Banderali G, Scaglioni S, Veehof SH, Sala M, et al. Feeding practices of infants through the first year of life in Italy. *Acta Paediatr* 2004;**93**:492–7.

32. *Infant Feeding Survey UK*. London: Office for National Statistics 22–11–2012; 2010. Available at: http://www.ic.nhs.uk/statistics-and-data-collections/health-and-lifestyles-related-surveys/infant-feeding-survey/infant-feeding-survey-2010.

33. Nevo N, Rubin L, Tamir A, Levine A, Shaoul RJ. Infant feeding patterns in the first 6 months: an assessment in full-term infants. *J Pediatr Gastroenterol Nutr* 2007;**45**:234–9.

34. Cai X, Wardlaw T, Brown DW. Global trends in exclusive breastfeeding. *Int Breastfeed J* 2012;**7**:12. http://dx.doi.org/10.1186/1746-4358-7-12 Published online.

35. Mattos AP, Brasil ALD, Mello ED, Lopes FA, de Oliveira FLC, Maranhão HS, et al. Manual with dietary guidelines for infants, preschoolers, school children, adolescents and at school [in Portuguese]. In: Paulo São, editor. 2nd ed. Brazil: Department of Nutrition – Brazilian Pediatric Society (SBP); 2008. p. 13–28. Available at: http://www.sbp.com.br/img/manuais/manual_alim_dc_nutrologia.pdf [accessed 22.02.13].

36. Allcutt C, Sweeney M- R. An exploration of knowledge, attitudes and advice given by health professionals to parents in Ireland about the introduction of solid foods. A pilot study. *BMC Public Health* 2010;**10**:201.

37. Forsyth BW, McCarthy PL, Leventhal JM. Problems of early infancy, formula changes, and mothers' beliefs about their infants. *J Pediatr* 1985;**106**:1012–7.

38. Kramer MS, Kakuma R. Optimal duration of exclusive breastfeeding. *Cochrane Database Syst Rev* 2012. http://dx.doi.org/10.1002/14651858.CD003517.pub2 Published online.

39. Zutavern A, Brockow I, Schaaf B, von Berg A, Borte UDM, Kraemer U, et al. Timing of solid food introduction in relation to eczema, asthma, allergic rhinitis, and food and inhalant sensitization at the age of 6 years: results from the prospective birth cohort study LISA. *Pediatrics* 2008;**121**:e44–52.

40. Nwaru BI, Takkinen HM, Niemelä O, Kaila M, Erkkola M, Ahonen S, et al. Timing of infant feeding in relation to childhood asthma and allergic diseases. *J Allergy Clin Immunol* 2013;**131**:78–86.

41. Agostoni C, Riva E, Giovannini M. Dietary fiber in weaning foods of young children. *Pediatrics* 1995;**96**(5 suppl.):1002–5.

42. Koehler S, Sichert-Hellert W, Kersting M. Measuring the effects of nutritional counseling on total infant diet in a randomized controlled intervention trial. *J Pediatr Gastroenterol Nutr* 2007;**45**:106–13.

43. American Academy of Pediatrics Committee on Nutrition. The use and misuse of fruit juice in pediatrics. *Pediatrics* 2001;**107**:1210–3.

44. Nicklas TA, Hayes D. American Dietetic Association. Position of the American Dietetic Association: nutrition guidance for healthy children ages 2 to 11 years. *J Am Diet Assoc* 2008;**108**:1038–44 1046–7.

45. Institute of Medicine. *Food and nutrition board. Dietary Reference Intakes for energy, carbohydrate, fiber, fat, fatty acids, cholesterol, protein, and amino acids*. Washington, DC: National Academy Press; 2002. Available at: http://www.nap.edu.

46. US Department of Agriculture. *The Food Guide Pyramid*. Available at: http://www.cnpp.usda.gov/Publications/MyPyramid/OriginalFoodGuidePyramids/FGP/FGPPamphlet.pdf; 1992 [accessed 22.02.13].

47. Williams CL, Bollella M, Wynder EL. A new recommendation for dietary fiber in childhood. *Pediatrics* 1995;**96**(5 suppl.):985–7.

48. McClung HJ, Boyne LJ, Linsheid T, Heitlinger LA, Murray RD, Fyda J, et al. Is combination therapy for encopresis nutritionally safe? *Pediatrics* 1993;**91**:591–4.

49. Kranz S, Mitchell DC, Siega-Riz AM, Smiciklas-Wright H. Dietary fiber intake by American preschoolers is associated with more nutrient-dense diets. *J Am Diet Assoc* 2005;**105**:221–5.

50. McClung HJ, Boyne L, Heitlinger L. Constipation and dietary fiber intake in children. *Pediatrics* 1995;**96**(5 suppl.):999–1001.

51. Morais MB, Vitolo MR, Aguirre ANC, Fagundes-Neto U. Measurement of low dietary fiber intake as a risk factor for chronic constipation in children. *J Pediatr Gastroenterol Nutr* 1999;**29**:132–5.

52. Gomes RC, Maranhão HS, Pedrosa L de F, Morais MB. Fiber and nutrients intake in constipated children. *Arq Gastroenterol (SP)* 2003;**40**:181–7. English abstract available at: http://www.scielo.br/scielo.php?script=sci.

53. Lee WT, Ip KS, Chan JS, Lui NW, Young BW. Increased prevalence of constipation in pre-school children is attributable to underconsumption of plant foods: A community-based study. *J Paediatr Child Health* 2008;**44**:170–5.

54. Glackin LM, Fraser M, O Neill MB. The adequacy of dietary fibre intake in 5–8 year old children. *Ir Med J* 2008;**101**:118–20.

55. Jennings A, Davies GJ, Costarelli V, Dettmar PW. Dietary fibre, fluids and physical activity in relation to constipation symptoms in pre–adolescent children. *J Child Health Care* 2009;**13**:116–27.

56. Inan M, Aydiner CY, Tokuc B. Factors associated with childhood constipation. *J Paediatr Child Health* 2007;**43**:700–6.

57. Mooren GC, van der Plas RN, Bossuyt PM, Taminiau JA, Büller HA. The relationship between intake of dietary fiber and chronic constipation in children. *Ned Tijdschr Geneesk* 1996;**140**:2036–9.

58. Zaslavsky C, de Barros SG, Gruber AC, Maciel AC, da Silveira TR. Chronic functional constipation in adolescents: clinical findings and motility studies. *J Adolesc Health* 2004;**34**:517–22.

59. de Carvalho EB, Vitolo MR, Gama CM, Lopez FA, Taddei JA, de Morais MB. Fiber intake, constipation, and overweight among adolescents living in São Paulo city. *Nutrition* 2006;**22**:744–9.

60. Maffei HVL, Morais MB. Defining constipation in childhood and adolescence: from Rome, via Boston, to Paris and …? *J Pediatric Gastroenterol Nutr* 2005;**41**:485–6.

61. Hyman PE, Milla PJ, Benninga MA, Davidson GP, Fleisher DF, Taminiau J. Childhood functional gastrointestinal disorders: neonate/toddler. *Gastroenterology* 2006;**130**:1519–26.

62. Rasquin A, Di Lorenzo C, Forbes D, Guiraldes E, Hyams JS, Staiano A, et al. Childhood functional gastrointestinal disorders: child/adolescent. *Gastroenterology* 2006;**130**:1527–37.

63. Hyams J, Colletti R, Faure C, Gabriel-Martinez E, Maffei HV, Morais MB, et al. Functional gastrointestinal disorders: working group report of the first world congress of pediatric gastroenterology, hepatology and nutrition. *J Pediatr Gastroenterol Nutr* 2002;**35**(Suppl. 2):S110–7.

64. Huybrechts I, De Backer G, De Bacquer D, Maes L, De Henauw S. Relative validity and reproducibility of a food–frequency questionnaire for estimating food intakes among Flemish preschoolers. *Int J Environ Res Public Health* 2009;**6**:382–99.

65. Kranz S, Hartman T, Siega-Riz AM, Herring AH. A diet quality index for American preschoolers based on current dietary intake recommendations and an indicator of energy balance. *J Am Diet Assoc* 2006;**106**:1594–604.

66. Jones GP, Briggs DR, Wahlqvist ML, Flentje LM, Shiell BJ. Dietary fiber content of Australian foods 3. Fruits and fruit products. *Food Australia* 1990;**42**:143–5.

67. Pereira AC, Maffei HVL. *Food and dietary fiber intake by children with or without constipation: assessment according to the Food Guide Pyramid and the American Health Foundation. Medimond International Proceedings Pediatric Gastroenterology – Reports from the 2nd World Congress of Pediatric Gastroenterology*. Paris, France: Hepatology and Nutrition; 2004. p. 609–613.

68. McCance RA, Widdowson EM. *The Composition of Foods*. 5th ed. Cambridge, UK: Royal Society of Chemistry-Information Services Ministry of Agriculture; 1991 Fisheries and Food.

69. Association of Official Analytical Chemists. Dietary fiber content of selected food. In: Shils M, Olson JA, Shike M, editors. *Modern Nutrition in Health and Diseases*. 8th ed. Philadelphia, PA: Lea & Febiger; 1994. p. A91–9.

70. Wills RBH. Composition of Australian fresh fruits and vegetables. *Food Technol Aust* 1987;**39**:523–6.

71. Tillotson JL, Bartsch GE, Gorder D, Grandits GA, Stamler J. Food group and nutrient intakes at baseline in the Multiple Risk Factor Intervention Trial. *Am J Clin Nutr* 1997;**65**(1 suppl.):228S–57S.

72. Nakaji S, Sugawara K, Saito D, Yoshioka Y, MacAuley D, Bradley T, et al. Trends in dietary fiber intake in Japan over the last century. *Eur J Nutr* 2002;**41**:222–7.

73. Cummings JH. The effect of dietary fiber on fecal weight and composition. In: Spiller GA, editor. *Handbook of dietary fiber in human nutrition*. Boca Raton, FL: CRC Press; 2001. p. 183–252.

74. Maffei HVL. Chronic functional constipation: which supplementary fiber to choose? *J Pediatr (Rio J)* 2004;**80**:167–8. English version available at: http://www.jped.com.br.

75. Mendez MHM, Derivi SCN, Rodrigues MCR, Fernandes ML. *Food composition table. [in Portuguese]*. Niteroi; Brazil: EDUFF, 1995.

76. Vítolo MR, Aguirre ANC, Fagundes-Neto U, Morais MB. Estimated dietary fiber intake in children according to different food composition reference tables (in Portuguese). *Arch Latinoam Nutr* 1998;**48**:141–5.

77. Guimarães EV, Goulart EM, Penna FJ. Dietary fiber intake, stool frequency and colonic transit time in chronic functional constipation in children. *Braz J Med Biol Res* 2001;**34**:1147–53.

78. Heaton WH. Food, fibre and bowel function. In: Barbara L, Corinaldesi R, Gizzi G, Stanglellini V, editors. *Chronic constipation*. London: Saunders; 1996. p. 79–92.

79. Locke III GR, Pemberton JH, Phillips SF. American Gastroenterological Association (AGA) technical review on constipation. *Gastroenterology* 2000;**119**:1766–78.

80. Nicklas TA, Myers L, Berenson GS. Dietary fiber intake of children: the Bogalusa Heart Study. *Pediatrics* 1995;**96**:988–94.

81. Saldanha LG. Fiber in the diet of US children: results of national surveys. *Pediatrics* 1995;**96**:994–7.

82. Decarli B, Cavadini C, Grin J, Blondel–Lubrano A, Narring F, Michaud PA. Food and nutrient intakes in a group of 11 to 16 year old Swiss teenagers. *Int J Vitam Nutr Res* 2000;**70**:139–47.

83. Royo-Bordonada MA, Gorgojo L, Martín-Moreno JM, Garcés C, Rodríguez-Artalejo F, Benavente M, et al. the Four Provinces Study. Spanish children's diet: compliance with nutrient and food intake guidelines. *Eur J Clin Nutr* 2003;**57**:930–9.

84. Alexy U, Kersting M, Sichert-Hellert W. Evaluation of dietary fibre intake from infancy to adolescence against various references – results of the DONALD Study. *Eur J Clin Nutr* 2006;**60**:909–14.

85. Storey KE, Forbes LE, Fraser SN, Spence JC, Plotnikoff RC, Raine KD, et al. Diet quality, nutrition and physical activity among adolescents: the Web-SPAN (Web-Survey of Physical Activity and Nutrition) project. *Public Health Nutr* 2009;**12**:2009–17.

86. Vadiveloo M, Zhu L, Quatromoni PA. Diet and physical activity patterns of school–aged children. *J Am Diet Assoc* 2009;**109**:145–51.

87. Butte NF, Fox MK, Briefel RR, Siega-Riz AM, Dwyer JT, Deming DM, et al. Nutrient intakes of US infants, toddlers, and preschoolers meet or exceed dietary reference intakes. *J Am Diet Assoc* 2010;**110**:S27–37.

88. O'Neil CE, Nicklas TA, Zanovec M, Cho SS, Kleinman R. Consumption of whole grains is associated with improved diet quality and nutrient intake in children and adolescents: the National Health and Nutrition Examination Survey 1999–2004. *Public Health Nutr* 2011;**14**:347–55.

89. Hampl JS, Betts NM, Benes BA. The "age + 5" rule: comparisons of dietary fiber intake among 4- to 10-year-old children. *J Am Diet Assoc* 1998;**98**:1418–23.

90. US Department of Agriculture. ChooseMyPlate – Daily food plans and worksheets. Available at: http://www.choosemyplate.gov [accessed 22.02.13].

91. Stewart ML, Schroeder NM. Dietary treatments for childhood constipation: efficacy of dietary fiber and whole grains. *Nutr Rev* 2013;**71**:98–109.

92. Cheng G, Libuda L, Karaolis-Danckert N, Alexy U, Bolzenius K, Remer T, et al. Trends in dietary carbohydrate quality during puberty from 1988 to 2007: a cause for concern? *Br J Nutr* 2010;**104**:1375–83.

93. Nurko S, Scott SM. Coexistence of constipation and incontinence in children and adults. *Best Pract Res Clin Gastroenterol* 2011;**25**:29–41.

94. Klauser AG, Voderholzer WA, Heinrich CA, Schindlbeck NE, Müller-Lissner SA. Behavioral modification of colonic function. Can constipation be learned? *Dig Dis Sci* 1990;**35**:1271–5.

95. Voderholzer WA, Schatke W, Mühldorfer BE, Klauser AG, Birkner B, Müller-Lissner SA. Clinical response to dietary fiber treatment of chronic constipation. *Am J Gastroenterol* 1997;**92**:95–8.

96. Walia R, Mahajan L, Steffen R. Recent advances in chronic constipation. *Curr Opin Pediatr* 2009;**21**:661–6.

97. Baker SS, Liptak GS, Colletti RB, Croffie JM, Di Lorenzo C, Ector W, et al. Evaluation and treatment of constipation in infants and children: recommendations of the North American Society for Pediatric Gastroenterology, Hepatology and Nutrition. *J Pediatr Gastroenterol Nutr* 2006;**43**:e1–13.

98. Bautista Casasnovas A, Argüelles Martín F, Peña Quintana L, Polanco Allué I, Sánchez Ruiz F, Varea Calderón V. Guidelines for the treatment of functional constipation. *An Pediatr (Barc)* 2011;**74**:51 e1–7.

99. Olness K, Tobin J. Chronic constipation in children. Can it be managed by diet alone? *Postgrad Med* 1982;**72**:149–54.

100. Anderson AS, Whichelow MJ. Constipation during pregnancy: dietary fiber intake and the effect of fiber supplementation. *Hum Nutr Appl Nutr* 1985;**39**:202–7.

101. Müller-Lissner SA. Effect of wheat bran on weight of stool and gastrointestinal transit time: a meta analysis. *Br Med J* 1988;**296**: 615–7.

102. Badiali D, Corazziari E, Habib FI, Tomei E, Bausano G, Magrini P, et al. Effect of wheat bran in treatment of chronic non organic constipation: a double-blind controlled trial. *Dig Dis Sci* 1995;**40**:349–56.

103. Maffei HVL, Vicentini AP. Prospective evaluation of dietary treatment in childhood constipation: high dietary fiber and wheat bran intake are associated with constipation amelioration. *J Pediatr Gastroenterol Nutr* 2011;**52**:55–9.

104. Suares NC, Ford AC. Systematic review: the effects of fibre in the management of chronic idiopathic constipation. *Aliment Pharmacol Ther* 2011;**33**:895–901.

105. Hongisto S-M, Paajanen L, Saxelin M, Korpela R. A combination of fiber-rich rye bread and yoghurt containing *Lactobacillus GG* improves bowel function in women with self-reported constipation. *Eur J Clin Nutr* 2006;**60**:319–24.

106. Speridião PGL, Tahan S, Fagundes-Neto U, Morais MB. Dietary fiber, energy intake and nutritional status during the treatment of children with chronic constipation. *Braz J Med Biol Res* 2003;**36**:753–9.

107. Loening-Baucke V, Miele E, Staiano A. Fiber (glucomannan) is beneficial in the treatment of childhood constipation. *Pediatrics* 2004;**113**:e259–64.

108. Kokke FT, Scholtens PA, Alles MS, Decates TS, Fiselier TJ, Tolboom JJ, et al. A dietary fiber mixture versus lactulose in the treatment of childhood constipation: A double-blind randomized controlled trial. *J Pediatr Gastroenterol Nutr* 2008;**47**:592–7.

109. Quitadamo P, Coccorullo P, Giannetti E, Romano C, Chiaro A, Campanozzi A, et al. A randomized, prospective, comparison study of a mixture of acacia fiber, psyllium fiber, and fructose vs polyethylene glycol 3350 with electrolytes for the treatment of chronic functional constipation in childhood. *J Pediatr* 2012;**161**:710–5 e1. *Erratum*: 2012; 161: 1180.

110. Ustundag G, Kuloglu Z, Kirbas N, Kansu A. Can partially hydrolyzed guar gum be an alternative to lactulose in treatment of childhood constipation? *Turk J Gastroenterol* 2010;**21**:360–4.

111. González Canga A, Fernández Martínez N, Sahagún AM, García Vieitez JJ, Díez Liébana MJ, Calle Pardo AP, et al. Glucomannan: properties and therapeutic applications (in Spanish). *Nutr Hosp* 2004;**19**:45–50.

112. Kristensen M, Jensen MG. Dietary fibers in the regulation of appetite and food intake. Importance of viscosity. *Appetite* 2011;**56**:65–70.

113. Staiano A, Simeone D, Del Giudice E, Miele E, Tozzi A, Toraldo C. Effect of the dietary fiber glucomannan on chronic constipation in neurologically impaired children. *J Pediatr* 2000;**136**:41–5.

114. Tse PW, Leung SS, Chan T, Sien A, Chan AK. Dietary fiber intake and constipation in children with severe developmental disabilities. *J Paediatr Child Health* 2000;**36**:236–9.

115. Zoppi G, Gobio-Casali L, Deganello A, Astolfi R, Saccomani F, Cecchettin M. Potential complications in the use of wheat bran for constipation in infancy. *J Pediatr Gastroenterol Nutr* 1982;**1**:91–5.

116. Castillejo G, Bulló M, Anguera A, Escribano J, Salas-Salvadó J. A controlled, randomized, double-blind trial to evaluate the effect of a supplement of cocoa husk that is rich in dietary fiber on colonic transit in constipated pediatric patients. *Pediatrics* 2006;**118**:e641–8.

117. Chao HC, Lai MW, Kong MS, Chen SY, Chen CC, Chiu CH. Cutoff volume of dietary fiber to ameliorate constipation in children. *J Pediatr* 2008;**153**:45–9.

118. Pennington JAT, Church HN. *Food values of portions commonly used. Bowes & Church.* 14th ed. Philadelphia, PA: JB Lippincott; 1985.

119. Cullen KW, Baranowski T, Smith SP. Using goal setting as a strategy for dietary behavior change. *J Am Diet Assoc* 2001;**101**:562–6.

120. Houts AC, Mellon MW, Whelan JP. Use of dietary fiber and stimulus control to treat retentive encopresis: a multiple baseline investigation. *J Pediatr Psychol* 1988;**13**:435–45.

121. Sullivan PB, Alder N, Shrestha B, Turton L, Lambert B. Effectiveness of using a behavioural intervention to improve dietary fibre intakes in children with constipation. *J Hum Nutr Diet* 2012;**25**:33–42.

122. Karagiozoglou-Lampoudi T, Daskalou E, Agakidis C, Savvidou A, Apostolou A, Vlahavas G. Personalized diet management can optimize compliance to a high-fiber, high-water diet in children with refractory functional constipation. *J Acad Nutr Diet* 2012;**112**:725–9.

123. Pereira AC, Maffei HVL, Parente TA, Carvalho MA. Weight and height evolution of constipated children receiving wheat bran. *Ciência Investigación Salud (México)* 1998;**3**(special edition):41.

124. Williams CL, Bollella MC, Strobino BA, Boccia L, Campanaro L. Plant stanol ester and bran fiber in childhood: effects on lipids, stool weight and stool frequency in preschool children. *J Am Coll Nutr* 1999;**18**:572–81.

125. Kranz S, Brauchla M, Slavin JL, Miller KB. What do we know about dietary fiber intake in children and health? The effects of fiber intake on constipation, obesity, and diabetes in children. *Adv Nutr* 2012;**3**:47–53.

126. van de Laar RJ, Stehouwer CD, van Bussel BC, te Velde SJ, Prins MH, Twisk JW, et al. Lower lifetime dietary fiber intake is associated with carotid artery stiffness: the Amsterdam Growth and Health Longitudinal Study. *Am J Clin Nutr* 2012;**96**:14–23.

127. Murphy N, Norat T, Ferrari P, Jenab M, Bueno-de-Mesquita B, Skeie G, et al. Dietary fibre intake and risks of cancers of the colon and rectum in the European Prospective Investigation into Cancer and Nutrition (EPIC). *PLoS ONE* 2012:7 e39361.

128. Chuang SC, Norat T, Murphy N, Olsen A, Tjønneland A, Overvad K, et al. Fiber intake and total and cause-specific mortality in the European Prospective Investigation into Cancer and Nutrition cohort. *Am J Clin Nutr* 2012;**96**:164–74.

129. Egger G, Wolfenden K, Pares J, Mowbray G. "Bread: it's a great way to go". Increasing bread consumption decreases laxative sales in an elderly community. *Med J Aust* 1991;**155**:820–1.

130. Clayden GS, Adeyinka T, Kufeji D, Keshtgar AS. Surgical management of severe chronic constipation. *Arch Dis Child* 2010;**95**: 859–60.

F. WHEAT FIBER

Wheat Bran and Cadmium in Human Health

Tatiana Emanuelli[*], *Bruna Gressler Milbradt*[†], *Maria da Graça Kolinski Callegaro*[*], *Paula Rossini Augusti*[**]

[*]Federal University of Santa Maria, Integrated Center for Laboratory Analysis Development (NIDAL), Department of Food Technology and Science, Center of Rural Sciences, Santa Maria, Brazil, [†]Federal University of Santa Maria, Graduate Program in Food Science and Technology, Center of Rural Sciences, Santa Maria, Brazil, [**]Federal University of Rio Grande do Sul, Department of Food Science, Institute of Food Science and Technology, Porto Alegre, Brazil

INTRODUCTION

Cadmium (Cd) is a dangerous environmental contaminant that exerts major toxic effects in the kidneys and in bone; it also affects various other tissues.[1,2] Because of its long half-life in human beings, much effort has been made to reduce human exposure to Cd.[3–5] For the general population, i.e., non-smokers and non-occupationally exposed subjects, diet is the major source of Cd.[1] Although cereals are among the foods that contribute to dietary Cd exposure,[6,7] some cereal constituents have been shown to decrease Cd bioavailability.[8–12]

Wheat bran is one of the most commonly used dietary fiber supplements. It contains approximately 45% total fiber, most of which is insoluble.[13–16] It also contains phytates, which, along with dietary fiber and its associated compounds, mainly the insoluble fiber fraction, have been shown to impair the absorption of essential minerals.[17–20] Thus, despite the higher mineral content of brans, the bioavailability of essential minerals from cereal brans is considered to be low compared to their bioavailability from grain endosperm.[21,22] This low bioavailability has been considered a drawback to the use of wheat bran as a source of essential dietary minerals. However, a number of studies have explored the metal-binding properties of wheat bran as a possible means of reducing the bioavailability of toxic metals in the diet[9,11,23–25] and as a means of removing heavy metals from wastewater.[26–31] In the present chapter, we focus on the interaction between dietary Cd and wheat bran. We first discuss the effects of dietary fiber, phytates, and protein on mineral bioavailability to understand the mechanisms involved in the interactions between bran constituents and dietary minerals. We then review the

sources of Cd exposure as well as the aspects of the toxicokinetics and toxicodynamics of this metal that are relevant to a consideration of dietary exposure to Cd. Later, we review the specific relationship between wheat bran and Cd exposure, including the risk of wheat bran contamination with Cd and the results of *in vitro* and *in vivo* studies of the constituents of wheat that may bind Cd and reduce its gastrointestinal absorption and toxicity.

DIETARY FACTORS AFFECTING MINERAL BIOAVAILABILITY

In the small intestine, the components of food form soluble or insoluble complexes with metals and other trace elements. Some components, such as citric acid and some amino acids, have a positive effect on the bioavailability of minerals, whereas others, such as dietary fiber, its associated compounds, and phytic acid, have negative effects. Interactions between minerals also affect their absorption efficiency. The interactions between inhibitors and enhancers of mineral bioavailability determine the final absorption level of the element in the gut. In this section, we discuss the mechanisms responsible for the effects of dietary fiber, phytates, and protein, which are among the major wheat bran constituents that might affect cadmium absorption.

Dietary Fiber

"Dietary fiber" is a term used to describe a group of substances in plant material that are resistant to digestive enzymes and have various beneficial physiological effects, including laxation and a control of blood

TABLE 19.1 Constituents of Dietary Fiber According to the American Association of Cereal Chemists[32]

Non-Starch Polysaccharides and Resistant Oligosaccharides
Cellulose
Hemicellulose
   Arabinoxylans
   Arabinogalactans
Polyfructoses
   Inulin
   Oligofructans
Galactooligosaccharides
Gums
Mucilages
Pectins
Analogous Carbohydrates
Indigestible Dextrins
   Resistant Maltodextrins (from corn and other sources)
   Resistant Potato Dextrins
Synthesized Carbohydrate Compounds
   Polydextrose
   Methyl cellulose
   Hydroxypropylmethyl Cellulose
Indigestible ("resistant") Starches
Lignin
Substances Associated with the Non-Starch Polysaccharides and Lignin Complex in Plants
Waxes
Phytate
Cutin
Saponins
Suberin
Tannins

Reproduced with permission from the American Association of Cereal Chemists.

cholesterol and glucose levels.[32,33] According to the American Association of Cereal Chemists,[32] "dietary fiber is the edible parts of plants or analogous carbohydrates that are resistant to digestion and absorption in the human small intestine with complete or partial fermentation in the large intestine". As summarized in Table 19.1, the dietary fiber fraction includes polysaccharides, oligosaccharides, lignin, and associated plant compounds.

The composition of dietary fiber of a foodstuff derived from plants varies depending on the plant species and variety, the plant tissue, and the growth stage of the plant, among other factors.[34,35] Dietary fiber constituents can be divided into two fractions based on their chemical, physical, and functional properties. The soluble dietary fiber fraction (SDF) dissolves in water and forms a viscous gel. This fraction includes pectins, gums, inulin-type fructans, and some hemicelluloses. Soluble fiber bypasses digestion in the small intestine and is easily fermented by the microflora of the large intestine. The other fraction, insoluble dietary fiber (IDF), does not form gels due to its water insolubility and undergoes extremely limited fermentation. This fraction includes lignin, cellulose, and some hemicelluloses.[32,33]

The major dietary fiber constituents of wheat grain are hemicelluloses, especially arabinoxylans.[15,36,37] Cellulose, β-glucans, and lignin are also found, but at lower levels.[15,16,38,39] Fiber constituents are mostly located in the outer layers of grains (e.g., aleurone, testa, hyaline, and pericarp); for this reason, they are enriched in the wheat bran,[15] as detailed under Composition of Wheat Bran, below.

Fiber has the capacity to bind various minerals, but this effect depends on the fiber's specific chemical composition. Mineral binding occurs by three mechanisms: chemisorption, physical sorption, and mechanical sorption (Table 19.2). Chemisorption occurs due to the presence of phenolic groups from lignin, phosphate groups from phytic acid, and carboxyl groups from uronic acids. Physical sorption results from Van der Waals forces, which are temperature dependent. Mechanical sorption depends on the degree of porosity of the sorbent and its ability to trap substances within its spatial structure.[40,41] Thus, the metal sorptive properties of fiber are determined by a number of factors: the type of fiber, the degree of graining, the experimental conditions (pH and temperature), the type of ion being absorbed, and others.[22,40–42]

The influence of fiber-rich food products and isolated fiber fractions on mineral absorption has been extensively studied in recent decades, with an emphasis on the essential minerals. The results of these studies vary. Fiber has been reported to have a negative effect,[21,22] to have no effect,[22,43] or even to increase the absorption of minerals,[22,43,44] depending on the experimental conditions and on the fiber source evaluated. The insoluble dietary fiber fraction predominantly decreases mineral absorption.[21,22,45] Conversely, the soluble dietary fiber fraction has a more variable effect; while a few studies have reported that this fiber fraction decreases mineral absorption,[22] most studies have shown that fermentable soluble fiber can increase mineral absorption in animals[46,47] and in humans.[33,48] However, due to the complex composition of food dietary fiber fractions, generalizations should be avoided; it is important to evaluate the effects of each source of dietary fiber.

Table 19.2 summarizes the mechanisms responsible for the effects of various dietary fiber compounds on mineral absorption. Dietary fiber can decrease mineral absorption by several mechanisms; these include the acceleration of intestinal transit, dilution of intestinal content, retention of ions in the pores of the gelatinous structure of some types of fiber, and chemical bonds between fiber and metals.[22,41] Conversely, some digestion-resistant carbohydrates are fermented by microflora in the colon, yielding organic acids such as lactate and short-chain fatty acids, with consequent improvement in mineral absorption by various mechanisms.[46,49–51]

TABLE 19.2 Mechanisms Involved in the Effects of Dietary Fiber or Fiber-Rich Foodstuffs on Mineral Absorption

Effect on Mineral Absorption	Mechanism	Fiber Types
Absorption impairment	Acceleration of intestinal transit, thus reducing the contact time of minerals with their absorption sites	All fiber types
	Dilution of the intestinal content, which delays and possibly reduces absorption	Mainly soluble fibers
	Retention of ions in the pores of the gelatinous structure of some types of fiber (mechanical sorption)	Soluble fibers such as pectins and some hemicelluloses
	Chemical bond between fiber components and metals (chemisorption)	Hemicelluloses and pectins (carboxylic groups) Lignins Phytates (phosphate groups) Oxalates form fiber–metal–oxalate complexes, which are more difficult to disrupt than oxalate– mineral complexes or fiber– mineral complexes Polyphenolic compounds such as tannins
Absorption improvement	Fermentation of digestion-resistant carbohydrates yielding organic acids with consequent: • acidification and increase of mineral solubility • cecum hypertrophy and increase of blood flow • formation of lower-charge metal complexes with short-chain fatty acids	Soluble fibers such as fructans (inulin) and β-glucans Resistant oligosaccharides such as galactooligosaccharides and fructooligosaccharides Resistant starch
	Foodstuffs rich in both fiber and minerals increase the dietary intake of minerals	Seeds in general, especially whole grains and bran

Data compiled from Ruiz-Roso et al.,[21] Torre et al.,[22] Tahiri et al.,[50] and Coudray et al.[51]

Although various mechanisms of action have been proposed for the effects of fiber on mineral absorption, the mechanism of action of arabinoxylans, the major fiber constituents of wheat bran, are still poorly understood. Arabinoxylans can be fermented by human intestinal microbiota *in vitro*, but their fermentation decreases with increased levels of ferrulic acid cross-linking.[52] Soluble corn bran arabinoxylans enhanced the cecal absorption of calcium (Ca) and magnesium (Mg), but only the Mg balance was enhanced by these polysaccharides in rats.[46]

It is also relevant that other components within the fiber matrix, such as phytates, oxalates, and phenolic compounds, can interact strongly with minerals. Because wheat bran contains significant levels of phytates,[16,39] the effect of phytates on mineral bioavailability is discussed in Phytates, below. Furthermore, it is important to emphasize that the effect of dietary fiber on mineral absorption is rarely uniform, i.e., it usually affects a specific mineral or group of minerals.[22,46]

Dietary fiber and its associated compounds are also capable of binding toxic metals and altering their intestinal absorption. Although the mechanisms responsible for the influence of various dietary fiber constituents on heavy metal absorption are still poorly understood, some of the mechanisms proposed for essential minerals also seem to play a role in the absorption of toxic metals. Insoluble fiber usually decreases the accumulation of toxic metals in an organism, whereas soluble fiber

usually increases the retention of toxic metals. Lignin and carboxymethylcellulose reduced Cd retention in the kidneys and liver of rats, but cellulose had no effect.[53] Alginates, pectins, agar, and carrageenans, which are soluble fibers, increased tissue retention of Cd in rats compared to fiber-free diets, whereas cellulose had the opposite effect.[54]

The affinity of soluble and insoluble fiber fractions for toxic metals has been studied *in vitro* and compared among the different fiber constituents. Although most studies show that soluble fiber has a higher binding capacity for heavy metals than insoluble fiber *in vitro*,[12,55] this effect could be abolished *in vivo* because a large portion of these metals can be released by fiber fermentation.[10] Concerning the different fiber constituents, it was shown that neutral polysaccharides such as cellulose and β-glucans exhibit lower heavy metal binding than pectin and hemicellulose.[8,12,56] Along the same line lignin, which is also a neutral compound, binds toxic metal ions, but it has lower binding ability than other fiber constituents.[10,12] In fact, ionizable functional groups such as the carboxyl groups found in pectin have been shown to be important ligands for heavy metals.[10,57]

Phytates

Phytic acid (myoinositol hexaphosphate, IP6) or its salt form, phytate, is the major form of phosphorus storage in many plant tissues. The primary dietary sources of phytates are cereals and legumes, including oil seeds and nuts.[17,58] Phytates are mostly located in the outer membranes of grains, predominantly in the aleurone layer (wheat and barley) or in the embryo (maize).[59,60] For this reason they are enriched in the cereal bran,[58,61] which also has a high content of dietary fiber.

At physiological pH (~6–7), phytate has six negatively charged phosphate groups that strongly bind to metallic cations such as Ca, iron (Fe), Mg, manganese (Mn) and zinc (Zn), rendering them insoluble and thus unavailable for nutritional absorption (Fig. 19.1). Although other food components like fiber and polyphenols may also bind minerals, phytates seem to be the most effective at impairing mineral absorption. *In vitro* studies have demonstrated that the phytates in fiber-rich products are active metal ligands,[62–65] and numerous studies have described the negative effects of phytate on the bioavailability of essential minerals – a subject that has been extensively reviewed in recent decades.[17–20,66]

Zn has been described as the essential mineral most adversely affected by phytate, and the phytate/Zn molar ratio has been proposed as an indicator of Zn bioavailability. Non-heme Fe and Ca absorption are also substantially inhibited by phytate.[20] In addition, phytate can decrease the absorption of other essential minerals, including copper (Cu) and Mn.[17,20,22,58,61,67] Interestingly, a synergistic effect on mineral binding by phytates was observed when two or more types of cations were simultaneously present. For example, Ca-bound phytate shows a higher affinity for Zn and forms co-precipitates, thus reducing its absorption.[20]

Unlike plants and microorganisms, the human small intestine does not synthesize the phytate-degrading enzyme phytase. However, plant and microbial phytase may hydrolyze phytate during food processing (i.e., during germination, soaking, and fermentation), yielding penta-, tetra-, and tri-inositol phosphates, which have a lower binding affinity for minerals.[20,61] In fact, a high degree of phosphorylation of inositol (hexa- and penta-phosphate forms) seems to be necessary to bind minerals.[18,64]

The demonstrated high binding affinity of phytic acid for metal ions raises the question of whether phytates can affect the bioavailability of toxic trace elements such as Cd. An *in vitro* study comparing the ability of phytate to bind Cd and other essential minerals at pH 3–7 showed that binding follows the affinity order Cu > Zn ~ Cd.[8] Due to the co-localization of phytates and fiber in the outer layers of cereal grains, various fiber-rich products also have high phytate content. Persson *et al.*[56] observed that phytate-rich soluble fiber fractions of wheat bran interacted strongly with metal ions, including Cd, and that the incubation of these fractions with phytase reduced Cd binding. Phytate was also identified as an important Cd ligand in soluble dietary fiber fractions isolated from other cereals (e.g., barley, rye, and oats) in the pH range 3.5–7.0.[8]

Based on the *in vitro* studies that demonstrate the binding of minerals to bran phytate, the effect of whole wheat and wheat bran diets on reducing Cd bioavailability in animal studies was assumed to be related to their high phytate content.[9,24] However, the effect of phytates on Cd bioavailability in animals is controversial. Some authors have observed increased Cd retention due to phytate,[68] others have suggested that Cd absorption is reduced by phytates,[69] and still others have found no influence of phytate level on Cd retention.[14] Schlemmer *et al.*[58] reviewed studies of the bioavailability and retention of Cd in animals and concluded that when phytate is an endogenous part of the food matrix it most likely reduces Cd absorption, whereas when the sodium (Na) salt of phytate is provided as a dietary supplement it either has no effect or increases Cd accumulation. Moreover, the concentration of various minerals and the relationship among various minerals and phytate, as well as the type of protein in the diet, play an important role in the effects of phytate on Cd bioavailability and retention.[17,20,58,70]

Protein

Proteins are among the dietary constituents that affect the bioavailability of minerals. Both the amount and type of protein in the diet affect the absorption of essential and toxic minerals.

Increasing the level of dietary protein tends to improve the absorption and bioavailability of Cu by enhancing

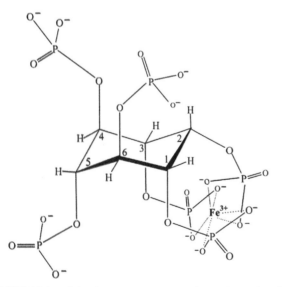

FIGURE 19.1 Molecular structure of monoferric phytate in which iron (Fe^{3+}-ion) is bound to phytic acid such that all six coordination sites are occupied. Under physiological conditions, the negative charges are counterbalanced by protons, sodium ions, or other cations, depending on pH and affinity. *From Schlemmer* et al.[57]; *©2009 WILEY-VCH Verlag GmbH & Co. KGaA, reproduced with permission.*

its solubility (formation of organometallic compounds) and increasing intestinal bulk flow.[71–74] However, when high-protein foods were heated, there was a decrease in Cu absorption that was associated with sugar–amino acid condensation products formed by the Maillard reaction. This reaction reduces the level of free amino acids and available sites for metal–nitrogen bond formation, with a subsequent decrease in the amount of organometallic compounds and, consequently, in the metal bioavailability.[74,75]

Zn absorption is also increased when the total level of dietary protein is increased,[76] but individual proteins may differentially affect Zn absorption. Casein has a modest inhibitory effect on Zn absorption,[76] whereas certain animal protein sources such as beef, eggs, and cheese counteract the inhibitory effect of phytate on Zn absorption from single meals.[77]

The effect of protein consumption on Fe absorption is variable. Non-heme Fe absorption is increased by meat intake but reduced by consumption of plant, milk, and egg proteins.[78] The increased Fe absorption associated with meat intake was explained by the release during protein digestion of peptides that form soluble, low-molecular weight complexes that readily release Fe to mucosal receptors. In contrast, the phosphorylated serine and threonine residues in milk casein bind Fe and other minerals by ionic interactions, and this Fe may be released too slowly in the intestine for efficient absorption.[79,80] The effect of milk protein on Fe absorption can be diminished by enzymatic hydrolysis of casein before its ingestion.[80]

Ca absorption is increased by proteins and phosphopeptides.[81] In particular, phosphopeptides derived from the enzymatic hydrolysis of caseins have been shown to sequester Ca and other cations, protecting them from potentially precipitating anions such as phosphates in the intestine.[82–84] Phosphopeptides therefore help keep Ca in solution until it reaches the distal intestine, thereby facilitating its absorption by passive diffusion.[81]

In addition to affecting the bioavailability of essential minerals, proteins may also directly affect the bioavailability of toxic metals like Cd. This topic is discussed under Cadmium Accumulation and Absorption, below.

CADMIUM

Cd is one of the most important occupational and environmental pollutants, partially due to its long half-life (10–30 years) in the human body.[3–6,85] Although Cd toxicity had been known for many decades,[86] Itai-itai disease revealed the actual dangers of Cd as an environmental pollutant. This endemic bone disease, which is characterized by bone fractures and severe pain, occurred after World War II in Toyama, Japan, due to contamination of the Jinzu River by Cd-containing water from a mine. Itai-itai disease primarily affected elderly Japanese women who had undergone long-term exposure to Cd-contaminated water and rice.[87,88]

During the past 50 years, concerns about Cd toxicity have resulted in many studies of its effects and dangers. The Joint FAO/WHO Expert Committee on Food Additives (JECFA) recently established the provisional tolerable monthly intake of Cd as 25 µg per kg body weight.[89] Furthermore, investigations to elucidate the mode of action of Cd and the mechanisms of its toxicity, to identify biomarkers of its critical effects, and, most importantly, to develop preventive and therapeutic strategies to decrease the body's retention of Cd and, consequently, its toxic effects will continue.[2] Because diet is an important source of Cd for the general population, a great effort has been made to develop strategies to reduce this risk. In this context, some studies have focused on Cd-binding molecules or materials that could be used to reduce the dietary absorption of Cd.[9,90] Numerous studies have also focused on the use of these molecules as biosorbents to reduce the environmental contamination and Cd accumulation in foodstuffs, especially in plant foods.[10,26,28,31,55,91–97]

Cadmium Sources

Important sources of Cd can be grouped into two main categories. Natural sources include the mobilization of naturally occurring Cd in the Earth's crust due to volcanic activity and the weathering of rocks. The second main source of Cd is the anthropogenic mobilization of Cd impurities in raw materials such as phosphate minerals, fossil fuels, and other extracted, treated, and recycled metals, particularly Zn and Cu.[98] Cu and nickel (Ni) smelting and fuel combustion are the most significant anthropogenic sources of Cd. Cd is used in the fabrication of Ni–Cd batteries to protect the steel against corrosion (this application consumes 75% of the overall Cd used in manufacturing), as a pigment, as a plastic stabilizer, and in solders. The International Cadmium Association expects the global production of Ni–Cd batteries to increase, particularly if success is achieved in the production of electric cars.[99]

In areas with industrial facilities that produce Cd emissions (non-ferrous metallurgy plants, coal/oil-fueled power plants, producers of plastics, etc.) and in heavily industrialized cities, Cd levels in the air may reach 0.5 µg/m³. In addition, cigarette smoke also contains Cd (1.2–2.5 µg Cd/g tobacco) because tobacco intensively extracts Cd from soil and accumulates it in leaves. Because the annual global tobacco production reaches about 5.7 million imperial tons, tobacco smoking releases 6.8 to 14.2 tons of Cd to the environment.[99]

Cd is not degraded in the environment and can contaminate water and soil, entering the food chain and increasing the risk of human exposure.[6] For this reason, Cd is present in almost all types of foods. The Cd concentration depends on the type of food, the level of environmental contamination, and the rate of uptake; the latter is influenced by factors such as soil pH, salinity, humus content, crop species and varieties, and the presence of other elements (e.g., Zn).[1,6] The use of fertilizers containing Cd contributes to soil and plant contamination.[2,86] Cereals, especially rice, non-refined wheat products, and vegetables, often contain elevated Cd concentrations, and account for about 80% of Cd intake from foods.[2,6,86]

Cadmium Absorption and Accumulation

As this chapter focuses on the interaction between dietary Cd and wheat bran, only the intestinal absorption of Cd is discussed here.

The absorption of dietary Cd has been reported to range between 0.5% and 37%, depending on animal species and age.[100] However, dietary factors such as minerals, proteins, and dietary fiber and its associated compounds also influence the rate of intestinal absorption and organ retention of Cd.[101]

The rate of Cd absorption from many food sources is reduced if the nutritional status of Zn, Fe, or Ca is high.[101] Conversely, dietary restriction of the essential metals Fe, Zn, and Ca, as well as depletion of Fe or low Zn status, increases the absorption, accumulation, and toxicity of Cd.[4,102–105] Because there is no specific cell entry pathway for Cd, dietary Cd uses the same routes as physiological metals to pass through cell membranes. The essential metal transporters for Fe (divalent metal transporter 1),[106] Zn,[107] and Ca (Ca channel TRPV6),[108] which are located in the duodenum and proximal jejunum, are the sites at which most dietary Cd is absorbed. Thus, the critical determinant of Cd levels in the body is the level and activity of essential metal transporters in the gastrointestinal tract, which are in turn regulated by the body's stores of essential metals and their dietary levels. The body's transport systems for essential metals are upregulated when a nutritional deficiency of Fe, Zn, or Ca exists.[109] In addition, a low dietary level of essential minerals such as Zn, Fe, or Ca reduces the competition of these minerals with Cd for the transporter absorption sites.[109] These mechanisms explain why enhanced Cd absorption occurs in mineral nutritional deficiencies. Thus, the assessment of how Cd toxicity risk depends on the provision of essential minerals must consider these minerals to act as a group and not independently.[4,107]

In addition to the effects of other minerals on intestinal Cd absorption, dietary proteins may also affect Cd absorption and retention. Cd can be found in food in inorganic form (Cd^{2+}, free metal) or in organic form (bound to organic molecules). Proteins are among the organic molecules that bind Cd. In many foods, such as meat, seafood, and vegetables, most Cd is bound to metallothioneins or metallothionein-like proteins such as phytochelatins.[1,6,110,111] Metallothioneins and phytochelatins are inducible low-molecular weight proteins that bind heavy metals due to their uniquely high cysteine content.[112–114] These proteins are widely distributed in animals and plants.[113,114] Various studies in rodents have evaluated differences in the absorption of the inorganic ($CdCl_2$) and organic forms of Cd (Cd bound to metallothionein). Although some studies found no difference in absorption between these two forms of Cd,[115,116] most studies reported lower Cd absorption, accumulation, or toxicity in animals fed metallothionein-bound Cd compared to ionic Cd.[103,117–121] In addition, some studies found a lower accumulation and toxicity of Cd that was physiologically incorporated into animal or plant foods, which is thought to be mainly bound to metallothioneins or metallothionein-like proteins, compared to the ionic form.[122,123] Thus, dietary metallothioneins generally reduce Cd absorption.

In contrast to the dietary metallothioneins, endogenous metallothionein proteins play a minimal role in the gastrointestinal absorption of Cd; however, they have an important role in Cd retention in tissues and dramatically decrease biliary excretion of Cd.[124] Cd binding to endogenous metallothioneins is responsible for Cd accumulation in tissues and for its long biological half-life.[124]

Other studies have focused on the effect of total dietary protein level on Cd absorption. Data from experimental studies in animals and case studies in humans suffering from Itai-itai disease caused by Cd exposure reveal that low protein levels in the diet increase Cd absorption and toxicity.[1,125–127] However, the effect of dietary protein on Cd kinetics is complex. A low-protein diet (11%) administered after Cd exposure and accumulation was shown to enhance the release of Cd from liver and reduce its uptake by the kidneys compared to a control diet containing 24% protein.[128] In fact, high-protein diets may increase Cd body burden.[129,130] Supplementing a non-deficient protein diet (16%) with dried egg protein (2%) increased carcass Cd retention, and led to the preferential accumulation of Cd in the kidneys and liver and a reduction in Cd accumulation in the testes and thigh muscle.[131] Interestingly, the rats fed the high-protein diet also had a higher tissue content of metal-binding metallothioneins and decreased levels of biomarkers of Cd toxicity compared to rats fed the low-protein diet. In fact, endogenous Cd bound to metallothioneins is thought to be non-toxic.[132] Thus, increased synthesis of metallothioneins may prevent Cd binding to other macromolecules and decrease Cd tissue toxicity,[124] even when the overall accumulation of Cd is increased. Accordingly, animals fed a high-protein diet seem to suffer fewer toxic effects than non-supplemented animals or animals fed a low-protein diet,[131,133,134] and this has been assumed to be due to Cd binding to metallothioneins in the body.

Other dietary constituents, including fiber and its associated compounds, may also affect Cd absorption. This is discussed under Wheat Bran and Cadmium Exposure, below.

Cadmium Toxicity

The toxic effects of Cd in animals can occur after either acute or chronic exposure, and affect many organs and tissues, including kidney, liver, lung, testis, brain, bone, and blood.[6] The kidney, which is the main site of Cd storage, has long been considered a primary target of Cd toxicity,[135] and is the critical target organ affected in chronic Cd poisoning.[86,136,137] Cd nephropathy has been described in industrial workers exposed mainly by inhalation, and in the general population exposed through contaminated foods.[137] Urinary levels of Cd are strongly associated with kidney Cd content.[135] Tubule dysfunction may occur if the Cd concentration in the kidney cortex rises above a critical threshold concentration, which is estimated to be $50 \mu g/g$.[3,5]

The long-term inhalation or dietary exposure of humans to Cd can lead to painful and debilitating bone disease in individuals with risk factors such as poor nutrition. The bone effects of Cd that characterize Itai-itai disease were also demonstrated in population studies that found an association between osteoporosis and environmental exposure to low Cd levels.[85] It is generally accepted that Cd-induced kidney damage decreases the reabsorption of Ca in the nephron. The resulting increase in Ca excretion decreases bone mineral density and increases fracture risk, particularly in postmenopausal women and older men.[138] In addition to bone disease characterized by generalized osteomalacia and osteoporosis, Itai-itai disease also produces severe kidney damage.[139]

In addition to its effects on the kidney, Cd also accumulates in the liver,[140] where it induces synthesis of the metal-binding proteins metallothioneins, which are responsible for its long half-life.[3–5] Although Cd binding to metallothioneins is thought to protect against acute toxicity, it also provides an opportunity for toxicity without additional exposure. Subclinical liver inflammation that is characterized by the release of various proinflammatory cytokines, including interleukin 6 and tumor necrosis factor-α, may develop due to the internalization of metallothionein-bound Cd by Kupffer cells.[141] Consistent with the potential effect of Cd on the liver, data from the National Health and Nutrition Examination and Survey from the United States indicate correlations between blood Cd and increased serum alkaline phosphatase (a marker of liver inflammation), increased prevalence of diabetes, and hypercholesterolemia.[142]

A long-term low-level dietary intake of Cd has also been associated with other adverse effects, including decreased lung function, diabetic nephropathy, hypertension, peripheral artery disease, myocardial infarction, periodontal disease, and age-related macular degeneration.[6] Moreover, the International Agency for Research on Cancer (IARC) has classified Cd and its compounds into group 1, meaning that there is sufficient evidence to indicate that they are carcinogenic in humans.[143] Long-term occupational exposure to Cd (e.g., through fumes) contributes to the development of lung cancer, and there is limited evidence that Cd may also cause renal and prostate cancers.[143]

The mechanisms proposed to explain Cd carcinogenicity include expression of aberrant genes, inhibition of DNA repair, inhibition of apoptosis, and induction of reactive oxygen species.[144] Cd changes the homeostasis of essential minerals such as Cu and Zn, and therefore inhibits the activity of antioxidant enzymes such as cytosolic superoxide dismutase.[145,146] It also directly interacts with glutathione, metallothioneins, and DNA.[144] Glutathione is the first line of antioxidant defense in the cell, and its synthesis can be induced by low concentrations of Cd in some cell types.[147] Although an increase in glutathione levels generally protects cells against oxidative stress, the antioxidant systems are overwhelmed and glutathione synthesis decreases at high Cd doses.[144]

WHEAT BRAN AND CADMIUM EXPOSURE

As briefly mentioned above, the risk of human Cd contamination through diet is strongly affected by the dietary content of Cd and its bioavailability. In this section, we review the relationship between wheat bran and Cd exposure, discuss the risk of wheat bran contamination with Cd, and describe *in vitro* and *in vivo* studies of the constituents of wheat that may bind Cd and reduce its gastrointestinal absorption and accumulation.

Composition of Wheat Bran

Wheat bran consists of the multiple layers of the wheat kernel that are external to the wheat grain; altogether, it represents approximately 10–15% of the kernel weight. Figure 19.2 illustrates the different strata of the wheat kernel that constitute the wheat bran: the aleurone layer, the hyaline layer, the testa or seed coat, the inner pericarp, and the outer pericarp.[39] These layers differ in structure and composition.

Table 19.3 shows the major constituents of wheat bran, emphasizing its main fiber components. The concentrations of some constituents may vary widely due to differences in the analytical methods used or in the cultivar

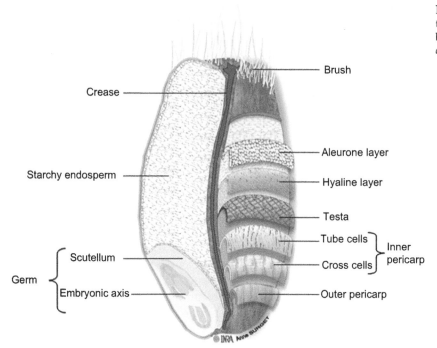

FIGURE 19.2 A histological representation of the wheat grain. See color plate at the back of the book. *From Surget and Barron,*[39] *translated and reproduced with permission from the editor.*

and the growing location of the wheat.[148,149] Nutritionally, wheat bran is a rich source of dietary fiber; it is also a good source of proteins, minerals, vitamins, and antioxidants.[39,150] Wheat bran can contain over 50% fiber, most of which is insoluble dietary fiber (Table 19.3).[13–16] The major fiber components of wheat bran are hemicelluloses, mainly arabinoxylans.[15,36,37] The pericarp and testa are hydrophobic tissues that contain significant amounts of lignin and cellulose.[15,16,39] The aleurone layer is composed of relatively linear arabinoxylans that are highly substituted by ferulic acid.[150,151]

Arabinoxylans possess a linear chain backbone of β-D-xylopyranosyl residues linked through (1→4) glycosidic linkages. α-L-Arabinofuranosyl residues may be attached to some of the β-D-xylopyranosyl residues at O-3, O-4, and/or both O-2,3 positions, resulting in mono-, di- or unsubstituted β-D-xylopyranosyl residues (Fig. 19.3). Ferulic acid or another hydroxycinnamic acid may be esterified to O-5 of α-L-arabinofuranosyl residues linked to O-3 of the xylose residues.[152] These hemicelluloses are often categorized as water-extractable or water-unextractable polysaccharides, the latter being the predominant form in the wheat whole grain and wheat bran.[153]

In addition to arabinoxylans, the aleurone layer also contains β-glucans, which are the main component of the soluble fiber of wheat bran,[38] most of the phytates,[16,39,154] and the essential minerals found in the grain.[36,39]

Cadmium Accumulation in Wheat

The European Community recently established a Cd limit value for wheat grain of 0.2 mg/kg.[155] If wheat and other food products were to reach the maximum allowed Cd levels established by the European Union, 10–25% of the population would be exposed to Cd levels above the provisional tolerable intake.[156] Wheat accumulates more Cd than other commonly grown cereals (the order is rye < barley < oats < wheat).[157] In Sweden, wheat and wheat products contained on average 0.044 mg Cd/kg, and contributed about 43% of the Cd intake.[158] Thus, it is necessary to decrease Cd accumulation in cereals produced for food consumption, particularly in wheat, which is one of the most frequently consumed cereal grains.

In agricultural soils, the primary Cd sources include geological materials, atmospheric deposits, and phosphatic and sewage-sludge fertilizers.[96,97] The rate of Cd accumulation varies among wheat genotypes.[159,160] Because durum wheat genotypes accumulate more Cd in the grain than bread wheat genotypes, Cd accumulation in durum wheat is a growing concern.[161] The genotypic differences in Cd accumulation in wheat strains result from differences in Cd uptake by the plants' roots, and from differences in the plants' internal Cd translocation.[162,163] The transport of Cd may be influenced by various factors such as plant transpiration and the presence of metallothionein-like proteins such as phytochelatins, which act as internal chelators.[110,112,113,164,165] In addition, Cd absorption from the soil is reduced when the pH is increased from 5.0 to 6.0[92–95] and with the use of Zn fertilization.[91,93]

The processing of wheat grain influences its nutritional characteristics as well as the concentration of contaminants in the grain products.[36,166,167] Many studies have shown that Cd is concentrated in the external portion of

TABLE 19.3 Composition of Wheat Bran

Constituent	Amount (g/100 g)	References
Moisture	1.5–2.2	Shenoy and Prakash[13], Callegaro et al.[14]
Protein	13.6–15.9	Shenoy and Prakash[13], Callegaro et al.[14], Bilgicli and Ibanoglu[154]
Fat	4.1–8.1	Shenoy and Prakash[13], Callegaro et al.[14], Bilgicli and Ibanoglu[154]
Carbohydrate	14.7–28.1	Shenoy and Prakash[13], Callegaro et al.[14]
Total ash	4.3–6.1	Shenoy and Prakash[13], Callegaro et al.[14], Bilgicli and Ibanoglu[154]
Total fiber	33.3–52.4	Callegaro et al.[14], Escarnot et al.[15], Stevenson et al.[16], Vitaglione et al.[a]
Insoluble fiber	32.1–48.4	Shenoy and Prakash[13], Callegaro et al.[14], Escarnot et al.[15], Stevenson et al.[16]
Soluble fiber	1.2–4.0	Shenoy and Prakash[13], Callegaro et al.[14], Escarnot et al.[15], Stevenson et al.[16]
DIETARY FIBER CONSTITUENTS AND PHYTATES		
Hemicellulose	22.6–25.0	Escarnot et al.[15], Kasprzak et al.[37]
Arabinoxylan	18.1–25.0	Kasprzak et al.[37], Shewry et al.[153]
Lignin	2.1–7.0	Escarnot et al.[15], Stevenson et al.[16], Suget and Barron[39]
Cellulose	7.5	Escarnot et al.[15]
β-Glucans	2.15–2.51	Li et al.[38]
Phytate	2.18–8.3	Callegaro et al.[14], Stevenson et al.[16], Suget and Barron[39], Bilgicli and Ibanoglu[154]

[a] *Vitaglione P, Napolitano A, Fogliano V. Cereal dietary fibre: a natural functional ingredient to deliver phenolic compounds into the gut. Trends Food Sci Tech 2008; 19: 451–63.*

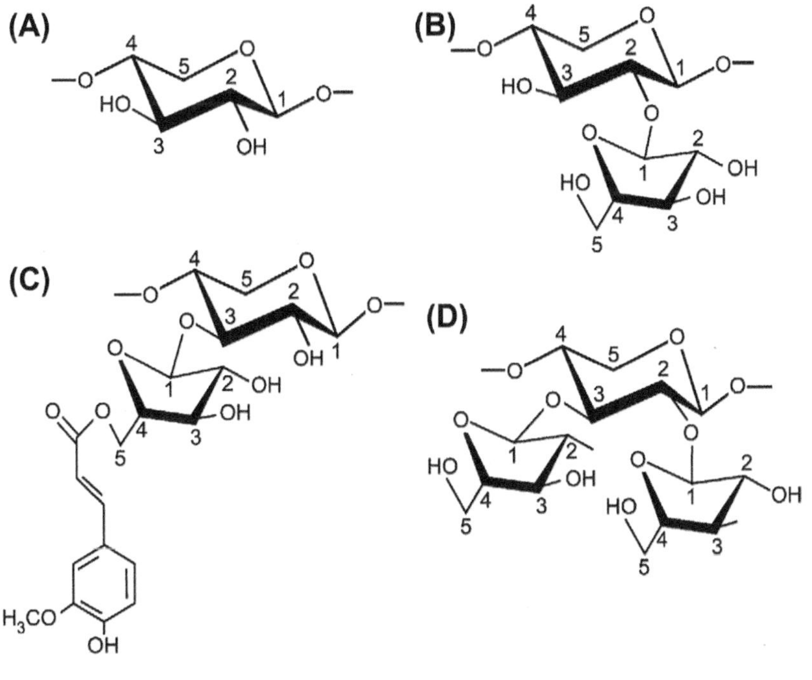

FIGURE 19.3 Structural elements present in arabinoxylans. (A) unsubstituted β-D-xylopyranosyl; (B) β-D-xylopyranosyl monosubstituted at O-2 with α-L-arabinofuranosyl; (C) β-D-xylopyranosyl monosubstituted at O-3 with a ferulic acid residue esterified to O-5 of α-L-arabinofuranosyl, and (D) β-D-xylopyranosyl disubstituted at O-2,3 with α-L-arabinofuranosyl. *From Izydorczyk and Dexter[150], ©2008 Elsevier, with permission.*

the wheat grain, where it is primarily located in the aleurone layer and germ; the lowest concentrations are found in the endosperm.[166–171] The distribution of Cd in different regions of the wheat grain after milling was found to be bran > shorts > flour. Furthermore, Cheli et al.[167] demonstrated that Cd concentration is positively correlated with the fiber content of wheat fractions. However, as will be discussed under *In Vivo* Studies, below, the bioavailability of Cd from wheat bran is reduced compared to its bioavailability from wheat flour (endosperm) and other foods; this may be related to the high fiber and phytate content of bran. Wheat bran has been extensively studied *in vitro* for its capacity to bind toxic minerals, including Cd.

In Vitro Studies

Many *in vitro* studies have demonstrated that wheat bran binds Cd very efficiently; the bran bound up to 85% of the total Cd when this was the only metal ion present in the medium, and over 60% when other heavy metals were also present. The results of these research studies are summarized in Table 19.4. Some of these experiments were performed under temperature and pH conditions similar to those that occur during the physiological absorption of minerals in the human body.[10,55] Because wheat bran has an elevated capacity to bind Cd and other heavy metals, its capacity to act as a biosorbent by removing these ions from wastewater has also been studied. With this purpose in mind, various conditions of temperature, pH, adsorption kinetics, and other factors were tested.[26–31]

The ability of wheat bran to bind Cd was evaluated by our research group (previously unpublished data shown in Fig. 19.4).[172,173] Figure 19.4A illustrates the protocol used, and Figure 19.4B shows the Cd binding to wheat bran that was observed when the metal concentration was increased at pH 6.0 and 37°C. We found that wheat bran binds 40–80% of the added Cd under these conditions, and that Cd binding to wheat bran did not saturate, even when the Cd concentration greatly exceeded the amount usually found in contaminated foods (Fig. 19.4B). There was no difference in the amount of Cd bound to wheat bran that had been subjected to enzymatic digestion with amylase, amyloglucosidase and alkalase, and whole wheat bran (Fig. 19.4C), indicating that the fiber, as well as constituents such as phytate that are linked to fiber, is the main component responsible for Cd binding. Compared to other brans such as rice and oat, wheat bran had an intermediate binding affinity for Cd; rice bran demonstrated a higher affinity for the metal (Fig. 19.4C). However, the observed differences in Cd binding among these brans were small, and they all exhibited high Cd binding capacity.

The binding capacity of Cd for wheat bran was tested under several pH conditions (5, 6, and 7) that fall within the postprandial pH range of the small intestine – the main site of mineral adsorption. The binding of Cd by wheat bran increased from 33% to 85% when the pH was increased from 5 to 7 (Fig. 19.4D). Other studies have found that wheat bran fiber has low affinity for toxic metal cations at gastric pH.[10,55] However, when the pH was neutral, similar to that in the small intestine, the fiber had high maximum binding capacity and high affinity for Cd and was able to bind Cd at very low concentrations.[10,55] This finding suggests that the small intestine is the site where fiber might be able to prevent toxic metal absorption.[55]

The effect of pH on the binding and affinity of wheat bran biomolecules for Cd can be explained by the dissociation of sorption sites such as hydroxyl, carboxyl, sulfhydryl, and phosphate functional groups.[174,175] In acidic medium, the wheat bran surface is highly protonated – a condition that is unfavorable for Cd binding.[28] As the pH increases, the degree of protonation of the bran surface is gradually reduced as functional groups dissociate to anions that show stronger interaction with Cd cations, resulting in increased binding capacity.[28,55]

Ou et al.[10] compared the capacity of water-insoluble and water-soluble dietary fiber isolated from wheat bran to simultaneously bind mercury (Hg), Cd, and lead (Pb) at pH 7.0 at 37°C. The water-insoluble fiber fraction bound these metals at a higher rate than the water-soluble fraction (62% vs 23%). However, the binding capacities of both fractions for toxic metals were reduced by 25% when the essential minerals Ca, Fe, and Zn were added, and they were reduced by 74% when Cu was added. Moreover, because the evaluated fiber fractions had low phytic acid content, this study showed that the dietary fiber fraction is able to bind Cd in a manner that is independent of the presence of phytates. However, phytates from wheat bran also exhibit Cd binding at certain pH values. In this context, a phytate-rich soluble fiber fraction from wheat bran strongly interacted with Cd, and pre-incubation with phytase reduced its Cd-binding ability at pH 3–5 but not at pH 6–7.[56]

Ogata et al.[31] studied the capacity of wheat bran to bind Cd after treatment with pectinase. Although the pectin content of wheat bran has not been quantified, this soluble fiber constituent is known to be present in all plant primary cell walls.[176] Treatment of wheat bran with pectinase reduced the concentration of carboxyl groups. Moreover, microscopic analysis revealed that the cell walls broke down after enzyme treatment, which increased the surface area in the treated bran. These changes were accompanied by a decrease in the amount of Cd bound after pectinase treatment, suggesting that the mechanism of Cd binding by wheat bran partially depends on the concentration of carboxyl groups of pectin present on the wheat surface.[31]

Recently, the *in vitro* binding capacity of whole wheat bran for a mixture of toxic metals (i.e., Pb, Hg, Cd, and arsenic) was compared to that of soy hull and apple peel fibers.[55] The tested fibers had high binding capacities for all four metals, but the apple peel and soy hull fibers were twice as effective as wheat bran at binding Cd. However, *in vivo*, soluble fibers such as those found in apple peel are expected to be extensively fermented by microorganisms in the colon and to release bound metal. In fact, using an *in vitro* colon fermentation model, Ou et al.[10] observed that fermentation partially releases Cd bound to soluble fiber.

Other *in vitro* studies have explored the capacity of wheat bran to bind Cd with a different objective, that of a biosorbent that could be used to remove Cd from

TABLE 19.4 *In Vitro* Studies on the Binding of Cd by Wheat Bran

Adsorbent	Metal	pH	T (°C)	% Adsorption[a]	Effect	References
Wheat, rice, and oat brans	Cd	5.0, 6.0 and 7.0	37	85	Cd adsorption increased significantly as the pH increased from 5 to 7 Cd binding by wheat bran was similar to binding after enzymatic digestion The ratio of affinity of brans for Cd was rice > wheat > oat	Callegaro et al., unpublished data
Water-soluble and water-insoluble dietary fiber from wheat bran	Cd, Hg and Pb	2.0 and 7.0	37	62[b]	Cd adsorption and affinity for wheat bran fiber increased significantly as the pH increased from 2 to 7 Fibers were shown to have similar affinities for different toxic metals Water-insoluble dietary fiber showed higher binding capacity for metals than water-soluble fibers Ca, Fe and Zn moderately reduced the binding of Cd, Hg and Zn; Cu strongly reduced the binding	Ou et al.[10]
Wheat bran, apple peels, and soybean hull fibers	Pb, Hg, Cd and As	2.0 and 7.0	37	45	Binding capacity for every metal tested was influenced by pH and fiber type Soy hull and apple peel fibers bound more Cd than wheat bran	Zhang et al.[55]
Wheat bran and wheat bran treated with pectinase	Cd	7.0	25	55	The amount of Cd adsorbed by wheat bran was greater than the amount adsorbed by pectinase- treated wheat bran	Ogata et al.[31]
Wheat bran	Cd	7.0	30	64	Cd absorption was affected by contact time, wheat bran concentration, pH and temperature	Singh et al.[28]
Wheat bran	Cd	7.0	25	80	Cd adsorption was similar to the adsorption of chromium, Pb, Cu and Hg Maximum adsorption was achieved after 10 minutes Alkali ions do not interfere with the adsorption process	Farajzadeh and Monji[26]

[a] *The ratio of absorption was defined as the percentage of Cd adsorbed by wheat bran relative to the total amount of Cd in contact with the wheat bran at pH 7.*
[b] *Adsorption of Cd by insoluble fiber of wheat bran.*

wastewater, especially industrial effluents.[26–31] Because wheat is a major world food crop, large amounts of straw and bran are produced as waste/by-products during its processing,[177] making their use more cost-effective than that of other products that would need to be grown specifically for this purpose.[178–180] Although both wheat bran and straw could be used as biosorbents, there are more studies of the use of wheat bran for this purpose.[180] In addition to its low cost, wheat bran has other advantages as a potential biosorbent. Equilibrium binding is

achieved within 10 minutes of Cd exposure, making the process very rapid.[26] Wheat bran can remove Cd over a wide range of concentrations ($\mu g/L$ to g/L).[26,31] The process is reversible; thus, the metal can be easily desorbed, permitting recycling of the material.[26,27] In addition, the treatment of wheat bran with NaCl, H_2SO_4, HCl,[26,27] or ultrasound[30] enhances its binding capacity.

Some *in vitro* studies that evaluated the potential of wheat bran as an environmental biosorbent used conditions similar to those found in the gastrointestinal

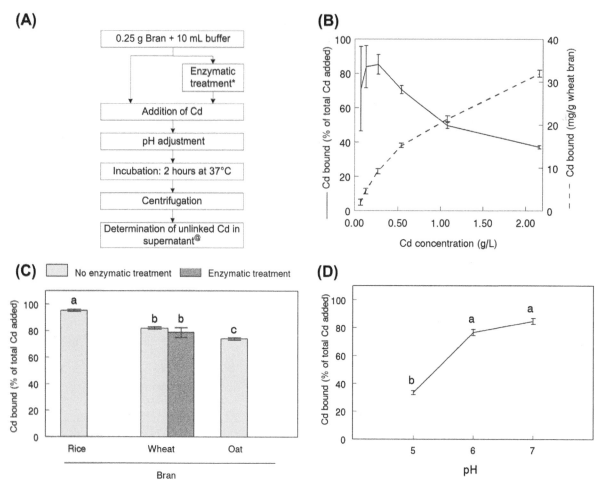

FIGURE 19.4 Cd binding by cereal brans *in vitro* (Callegaro *et al.*, unpublished data; original to this chapter). (A) Simplified protocol for the incubation of brans with Cd. (B) Cd binding to wheat bran at increasing Cd concentration (0.07–2.15 g/L) at pH 6.0. (C) Comparison of the binding capacities of different bran types using 0.135 g Cd/L at pH 6.0. (D) Effect of pH on Cd (0.135 g/L) binding to wheat bran. The results are expressed as the mean values ± standard error of the mean. Mean values followed by different letters are significantly different ($P < 0.01$; one-way ANOVA followed by Duncan's test). *To determine the effect of the enzymatic digestion of starch and proteins on Cd binding, some bran samples were treated with amylase, amyloglucosidase, and alkalase as indicated in method 985.29 of the AOAC[172]. @*The free Cd content of the supernatant was determined using the spectrophotometric method with 4-(2-pyridylazo) resorcinol reagent (PAR).[173] The amount of bound Cd was calculated as the difference between the free Cd and the total amount of Cd added.*

tract.[26,28,31] For this reason, the results of these studies may also be used to understand the physiological interactions between dietary Cd and wheat bran in animals (Table 19.4).

Various studies show that the ratio of Cd adsorption to wheat bran increases rapidly during initial stages but slows during later stages of absorption, continuing until equilibrium is reached.[27–30] Fitting of the wheat bran adsorption data to the Langmuir equilibrium isotherm, the method most commonly used to describe adsorbent systems, indicated the formation of a Cd monolayer on the adsorbent.[28–30,180]

Thus, most studies show that wheat bran has high binding affinity for Cd *in vitro*. The wheat bran dietary fiber fraction clearly contributes to this effect. The insoluble wheat fiber fraction has somewhat higher Cd binding capacity than the soluble fiber fraction.[10] Moreover,

the Cd bound to the soluble fiber fraction can be released *in vivo* during intestinal fermentation. The specific interaction of wheat bran phytates with Cd has not been thoroughly evaluated. Phytates in the soluble fiber fraction of wheat bran were shown to contribute to Cd binding at certain pH values, but the overall contribution of phytate to the Cd-binding capacity of whole wheat bran has not been evaluated.

In Vivo Studies

In addition to the *in vitro* evidence that wheat bran and its constituents bind heavy metals, including Cd, various *in vivo* studies have evaluated whether dietary whole grain wheat, wheat bran, or cereal mixtures containing wheat bran decrease the absorption or toxicity of dietary Cd. These studies are summarized in Table 19.5.

TABLE 19.5 *In Vivo* Studies on the Effect of Dietary Wheat on Cd Absorption, Accumulation, and Toxicity

Dietary Cereal	Dietary Fiber Level (g/kg diet)	Dietary Phytate Level (mmol/kg diet)	Dietary Cd (mg/kg diet)	Animal	Duration (days)	Cereal Effect	References
Whole grain durum wheat (~50% in the single meal diet)	ND	7.5	0.56	Sprague-Dawley rats (75±0.9g body weight)	1	Prior intake of wheat (5% in the diet) for 7 days reduced the absorption of ^{109}Cd from a single meal	House et al.[11]
Whole grain durum wheat (100% in the diet)	ND	ND	0.06–1.6[a]	CD1 mice (22–24g body weight)	11	Reduced the accumulation of Cd in liver and kidney, when compared to the exposure by gavage	Chan and Hale[25]
Whole grain wheat and wheat bran	59 and 82	4.2 and 7.6	~0.035	Sprague-Dawley rats (3 weeks old)	42	Reduction in the accumulation (30–40%) and in the fractional uptake (34–48%) of ^{109}Cd in liver and kidneys compared to the animals fed on a low-fiber wheat-endosperm diet	Wing[24]
Dietary fiber obtained from wheat bran by microbial fermentation was used as a food additive to cookies	80[b]	ND	10[c]	KM mice (25–35g body weight)	4	Increased the rate of fecal Cd excretion (1.27-fold)	Hong et al.[90]
Wheat bran (1.6% in the diet)	16	6.7	0.05	Balb c mice (newly-weaned; 14.9–17.2g body weight)	63	Reduction of 20–30% in the Cd liver accumulation and of 30–35% in the Cd renal accumulation	Lind et al.[9]
Wheat bran (basic diet containing 50% bread crips prepared by replacing half the endosperm wheat flour for wheat bran)	110	8.6	~0.03	Sprague-Dawley rats (66.4±3.7 g body weight)	42	Did not change Cd accumulation after a 6-week exposure compared to an endosperm wheat diet. Reduced the absorption of ^{109}Cd from a single meal compared to an endosperm wheat diet	Moberg et al.[23]
Wheat bran (10% in the diet)	48	12	50	Wistar rats (3 weeks old; 62.4±0.2 g body weight)	30	Prevented Cd-induced decrease of feed intake and body weight gain. Did not reduce Cd absorption or deposition in liver and kidney. Did not prevent Cd damage to hepatic function. Decreased Ca and P absorption and increased Mg absorption in Cd-exposed animals	Callegaro et al.[14]
Cereal bran supplement (10% in the diet, being 3.7% wheat bran)	94	ND	5–25	Wistar rats (3 weeks old; 64±10g body weight)	30	Did not prevent Cd-induced decrease of feed intake and body weight gain. Did not prevent Cd damage on hepatic function or inhibition of renal ALA-D activity. Decreased renal Cd deposition after exposure to 5mg Cd/kg diet, but not after exposure to 25mg Cd/kg diet	Callegaro et al.[182]

a This dose was estimated using the average final body weight (24.9 g) and grain food intake (7.38g/day) and the duration of the experiment (11 days), because authors gave only the total dietary intake of Cd. ND, not determined.
b Expressed as g/kg cookies.
c This value was estimated based on the animal body weight (25–35 g), daily food intake (10% of its body weight food daily), and daily Cd intake, because in this study Cd was administered by gavage at 1mg Cd/kg body weight.

F. WHEAT FIBER

Several *in vivo* studies have shown that consumption of whole grain wheat, and especially wheat bran, reduce the absorption or tissue accumulation of dietary Cd.[9,11,23–25] For similar Cd doses, the Cd accumulation in liver and kidney was greater when the Cd was given by gavage than when it was administered as part of a whole grain wheat diet, regardless of whether Cd was added during preparation of the food or incorporated during plant growth.[25] This study suggests that Cd from contaminated wheat crops is less bioavailable than Cd from water. Moreover, it also suggests that whole grain wheat may decrease the bioavailability of Cd from other food sources. Rats fed a wheat bran diet had lower Cd absorption than rats fed a diet consisting of carrot, lettuce, soybean, spinach, and tomato.[181] In addition, the fractional accumulation of Cd in liver and kidney was 34–48% lower in rats fed whole wheat or wheat bran diets than in rats fed a low-fiber wheat endosperm diet.[24] The protective effect of the whole wheat and wheat bran diets was attributed to their higher fiber or phytate content.[24] The consumption of a cookie enriched with dietary fiber obtained from wheat bran was also shown to increase the rate of fecal Cd excretion.[90] In addition, animals fed wheat bran showed a 20–30% reduction in liver Cd accumulation and a 30–35% reduction in renal Cd accumulation compared to animals fed a control diet or sugar beet- or carrot-containing diets.[9] Compared to the other diets, the wheat bran diet had higher insoluble fiber and phytate contents.[9] Thus, the fraction of Cd in the bran that is available for absorption is 30–40% lower than in the wheat endosperm, which is a low-fiber foodstuff; it is also lower than in diets containing other fiber sources, like sugar beet and carrot, which have a higher soluble fiber content. Cd accumulation was also lower in animals fed a wheat bran diet than in animals fed a flaxseed diet.[14] In this study, both diets had the same amount of total dietary fiber; they differed in that the wheat bran diet contained a greater amount of insoluble dietary fiber and phytates (1.2- and 2-fold, respectively) and less soluble fiber (0.3-fold).[14] Thus, it appears that insoluble dietary fiber fraction and phytates may be responsible for the decrease in the accumulation of dietary Cd triggered by wheat bran. However, in the same study, the effect of a wheat bran diet on Cd accumulation was similar to that of a cellulose diet with the same total and insoluble dietary fiber content but almost no phytates.[14] Thus, the phytate level had no direct relationship to the decrease in Cd accumulation observed in this study. Although most studies have attributed the decrease of Cd absorption and accumulation in animals fed wheat bran diets to the dietary fiber and/or phytates in wheat bran, the effective contributions of each of these factors to the effects of wheat bran on Cd levels have not been evaluated *in vivo*.

The amount of dietary protein has been shown to affect Cd absorption.[125–127,130] However, in most studies, the beneficial effect of whole grain wheat or wheat bran diets on Cd absorption and accumulation was observed by comparison to isoproteic control diets[9,14,182] or to diets with small differences (less than 10%) in protein content.[23,24,183] Thus, it is unlikely that the wheat bran effect is related to its protein content, which is only slightly higher (about 28%) than that of wheat endosperm (food code 4442 vs food code 4501).[184] However, in addition to the total protein content, the quality of the dietary protein could also affect Cd bioavailability because the presence of exogenous Cd-binding proteins like metallothioneins and phytochelatins in the diet reduces Cd absorption.[113,117–121] The possible effects of specific wheat bran proteins on Cd absorption have not been evaluated *in vivo* in animals. *In vitro*, it was observed that treatment of wheat bran with alcalase did not change its binding affinity for Cd (Fig. 19.4C); this would suggest that there is little or no contribution of protein to the Cd binding of wheat bran. However, the efficiency of the protease in hydrolyzing metallothionein-like proteins was not evaluated.

Nutritional deficiencies of Zn, Fe, or Ca have been associated with increased Cd absorption. Thus, the presence of abundant Zn in wheat bran might explain the reduction in Cd absorption that occurs in animals fed wheat bran, especially in the context of mineral-deficient diets. However, the addition of Zn to a wheat endosperm diet to approximately the same levels found in the bran and whole wheat diets had no effect on fractional Cd absorption.[24] Thus, the reduced Cd absorption that occurs with these diets is most likely not due to their higher Zn content but to their higher fiber or phytate content.[24] The relationship of nutritional Fe to wheat bran effects on Cd exposure was also investigated using a different approach. When the effects of wheat bran diets were compared with those of wheat endosperm diets with similar levels of Fe, feeding wheat bran did not reduce the hepatic accumulation of Cd when the diets were low in Fe or marginally Fe-deficient.[183] This finding indicates that when nutritional iron status is less than adequate, the inclusion of wheat bran is not likely to decrease Cd bioavailability. Another concern related to the intake of cereal bran is that it may decrease the absorption of essential minerals. In this context, it was shown that Cd exposure decreased the relative and absolute Ca and phosphorus (P) absorption but that it increased Mg absorption when animals were fed a wheat bran diet, while no such effect was observed in animals maintained on a cellulose diet with similar dietary fiber content. In contrast to cellulose, wheat bran contains excessive amounts of phytate. Each phytate molecule has up to six P atoms and is known to form a complex with Ca, reducing its absorption.[17,185] Therefore, an interaction between phytates and Cd may be responsible for the reduced Ca and P absorption in animals fed wheat bran.[14]

In addition to the various studies that show decreased bioavailability of Cd when wheat bran is consumed at the same meal, it was shown that prior intake of wheat also decreases the absorption and retention of [110]Cd after a single meal compared to animals that had no prior intake.[11] However, the mechanisms responsible for this effect are unknown.

In most studies that reported decreased Cd bioavailability in the presence of dietary whole grain wheat or wheat bran, the Cd level in the diet was less than 0.035 mg/kg; only two studies used dietary Cd levels of 1.6 and 10 mg/kg (Table 19.5). The first concentration range (<0.035 mg/kg) is lower than, while the latter concentration range (1.6 and 10 mg/kg) exceeds, the Cd levels found in food in contaminated areas.[1] In contrast, after animals consumed a diet containing 50 mg Cd/kg, an amount that greatly exceeds the Cd levels found in contaminated food, the amount of Cd deposited in renal tissue was similar whether purified cellulose (control) or wheat bran was used as the fiber source in the diet; flaxseed, however, significantly increased the renal deposition of Cd.[14] In addition, a wheat bran-containing cereal supplement reduced renal Cd accumulation when the metal was added to the diet at 5 mg/kg but not when it was added at 25 mg/kg.[182] Based on these results, it has been proposed that the functional sites on wheat bran that are available to bind Cd are limited, and that they may become saturated when the Cd concentration is increased to 25–50 mg/kg;[14,182] in this case, the amount of metal present exceeds the binding capacity of fibers, and the fiber effect is not detectable. However, in vitro, Cd binding to wheat bran was not observed to saturate (Fig. 19.4B) even at Cd:bran ratios much higher than those used in the in vivo studies (Table 19.5). There are several possible reasons for this difference. First, the amount of water that disperses the dietary Cd and the wheat bran during the digestion process is much lower than that used in the in vitro studies. Moreover, in vivo, essential minerals may also occupy the metal-binding sites of wheat bran and contribute to its saturation. These facts could explain the apparent discrepancy between the in vitro and in vivo studies.

The dietary Cd levels reported in cases of environmental and human contamination are similar to or lower than the Cd levels used in the studies that found beneficial effects of wheat bran on decreasing Cd bioavailability. Thus, consumption of wheat fiber would be expected to decrease Cd absorption at the metal concentrations usually found in non-contaminated and contaminated areas. However, Moberg et al.[23] also used a low dietary Cd level (~0.03 mg/kg) and did not find changes in Cd accumulation in animals fed wheat bran compared with those fed wheat endosperm-containing diets after 6 weeks of exposure. These investigators did find reduced absorption of [109]Cd from a single meal in the animals fed the wheat bran-containing diet compared to those fed the wheat endosperm diet.

Few studies have focused on the possible protective effects of wheat bran against Cd toxicity (Table 19.5). A wheat bran diet prevented the decrease in food intake and body weight gain caused by the addition of 50 mg Cd/kg to the diet.[14] Because the wheat bran diet used in this study was unable to prevent Cd toxicity in liver or reduce Cd bioavailability, the authors proposed that wheat bran protection against Cd-induced body weight loss is related to its ability to prevent the reduction in food intake that is induced by Cd. It was suggested that wheat bran may have masked the metallic flavor of the Cd diet, leading to increased palatability and increased consumption. Another study showed that a wheat bran-containing cereal supplement did not prevent damage to hepatic function or inhibition of renal delta-aminolevulinate dehydratase (ALA-D) activity caused by consumption of a diet containing 25 mg Cd/kg.[182] Although this wheat bran supplement did decrease renal Cd deposition when animals were fed 5 mg Cd/kg, it was not possible to verify whether this decrease resulted in lower toxicity because the biomarkers used to evaluate Cd toxicity were not changed by the Cd diet alone.

Although some wheat varieties have been shown to be Cd-accumulating plants,[186] most studies, summarized in Table 19.5, show that the bioavailability of Cd from wheat bran is reduced compared to its availability from wheat flour (endosperm) and other foods, and that wheat bran is able to reduce the bioavailability of Cd from other food sources. This effect is extremely significant because wheat flour and wheat-based cereals are among the most important food categories contributing to Cd exposure in Europe[7] and the USA.[6] Thus, the consumption of non-contaminated wheat bran may help reduce the bioavailability of dietary Cd. This is particularly important because the half-life of Cd in the organism is elevated (10–30 years in humans),[1,2] and even low-level Cd exposure may pose a risk if it is sustained over a long period. However, more studies are needed to determine whether dietary supplementation with wheat bran helps prevent the toxic effects of Cd. In addition, caution should be exercised in consuming Cd-accumulating wheat varieties cultivated in contaminated areas.

CONCLUSION

Several in vitro studies show that wheat bran has an elevated capacity to bind Cd at physiological conditions of pH and temperature, although this binding capacity may be reduced in the presence of essential minerals and after fermentation. In addition, wheat bran has been suggested as a promising biosorbent agent for removing Cd from wastewater. Further investigations are required to determine the feasibility of large-scale utilization of this method, with special attention to the destination and recycling of the residues generated.

Various studies conducted in rodents have demonstrated that wheat bran reduces Cd bioavailability. Both the insoluble dietary fiber fraction and phytates seem to be responsible for the decrease in the accumulation of dietary Cd triggered by wheat bran. However, the effective contribution of each of these constituents to wheat bran's effects on Cd bioavailability has been incompletely evaluated *in vitro* and has not been evaluated *in vivo*. Because the various constituents of wheat bran exhibit different behaviors when exposed to the pH changes and fermentation processes that occur during gastrointestinal digestion, it is important to study the role of each of these constituents in characterizing the interaction of wheat bran with dietary Cd. The possible contribution of wheat protein to the reduction of Cd bioavailability has not been rigorously evaluated. *In situ* studies could contribute to our understanding of the mechanisms that underlie the reduction of Cd gastrointestinal uptake caused by wheat bran and the role of individual wheat bran constituents in this process. In addition, the possible protective effect of wheat bran against Cd toxicity deserves to be further investigated.

References

1. WHO. *Environmental Health Criteria. 134. Cadmium.* World Health Organization: Geneva, Switzerland; 1992.
2. Järup L, Åkesson A. Current status of cadmium as an environmental health problem. *Toxicol Appl Pharmacol* 2009;**238**:201–8.
3. Satarug S, Nishijo M, Lasker JM, Edwards RJ, Moore MR. Kidney dysfunction and hypertension: Role for cadmium, p450 and heme oxygenases? *Tohoku J Exp Med* 2006;**208**:179–202.
4. Vesey DA. Transport pathways for cadmium in the intestine and kidney proximal tubule: Focus on the interaction with essential metals. *Toxicol Lett* 2010;**198**:13–9.
5. Satarug S. Long-term exposure to cadmium in food and cigarette smoke, liver effects and hepatocellular carcinoma. *Curr Drug Metab* 2012;**13**:257–71.
6. ATSDR. *Agency for Toxic Substances and Disease Registry. Toxicological profile for cadmium.* Atlanta: US Public Health Service; 2012.
7. Sand S, Becker W. Assessment of dietary cadmium exposure in Sweden and population health concern including scenario analysis. *Food Chem Toxicol* 2012;**50**:536–44.
8. Persson H, Nyman M, Önning HLG, Frolich W. Binding of mineral elements by dietary fiber components in cereals – *In vitro* (III). *Food Chem* 1991;**40**:169–83.
9. Lind Y, Engman J, Jorhem L, Glynn AW. Accumulation of cadmium from wheat bran, sugar-beet fibre, carrots and cadmium chloride in the liver and kidneys of mice. *Brit J Nutr* 1998;**80**:205–11.
10. Ou S, Gao K, Li Y. An *in vitro* study of wheat bran binding capacity for Hg, Cd, and Pb. *J Agric Food Chem* 1999;**47**:4714–7.
11. House WA, Hart JJ, Norvell WA, Welch RM. Cadmium absorption and retention by rats fed durum wheat (*Triticum turgidum* L. var. *durum*) grain. *Br J Nutr* 2003;**89**:499–508.
12. Hu GH, Huang SH, Chen H, Wang F. Binding of four heavy metals to hemi-celluloses from rice bran. *Food Res Int* 2010;**43**:203–6.
13. Shenoy AH, Prakash J. Wheat bran (*Tritzcum aestwum*): composition, functionality and incorporation in unleavened bread. *J Food Qual* 2002;**25**:197–211.
14. Callegaro MGK, Milbradt BG, Alves E, Diettrich T, Kemerich DM, Hausen BS. Effect of wheat bran and flaxseed on cadmium effects and retention in rats. *Hum Exp Toxicol* 2010;**30**:981–91.
15. Escarnot E, Agneessens R, Wathelet B, Paquot M. Quantitative and qualitative study of spelt and wheat fibers in varying milling fractions. *Food Chem* 2010;**122**:857–63.
16. Stevenson L, Phillips F, Sullivan K, Walton J. Wheat bran: its composition and benefits to health, a European perspective. *Int J Food Sci Nutr* 2012;**63**:1001–13.
17. Plaami S. Myoinositol phosphates: analysis, content in foods and effects in nutrition. *LWT-Food Sci Tecnol* 1997;**30**:633–47.
18. Urbano G, López-Jurado M, Vidal-Valverde C, Tenorio E, Porres J. The role of phytic acid in legumes: antinutrient or beneficial function? *J Physiol Biochem* 2000;**56**:283–94.
19. Weaver CM, Kannan S. Phytate and mineral bioavailability. In: Reddy NR, Sathe SK, editors. *Food phytates.* Boca Raton: CRC Press; 2002. p. 211–23.
20. Kumar V, Sinha AK, Makkar HPS, Becker K. Dietary roles of phytate and phytase in human nutrition: A review. *Food Chem* 2010;**120**:945–59.
21. Ruiz-Roso B, Péres-Olleros L, García-Cuevas M. Influencia de la fibra dietaria (FD) en la biodisponibilidad de los nutrientes. In: Lajolo FM, Saura-Calixto F, Penna EW, Menezes EW, editors. *Fibra dietética en Iberoamérica: tecnología y salud.* Brazil, Varela: São Paulo; 2001. p. 345–70.
22. Torre M, Rodriguez AR, Saura-Calixto F. Effects of dietary fiber and phytic acid on mineral availability. *Crit Rev Food Sci Nutr* 1991;**30**:1–22.
23. Moberg A, Hallmans G, Sjöström R, Wing KR. The effect of wheat bran on the absorption and accumulation of cadmium in rats. *Br J Nutr* 1987;**58**:383–91.
24. Wing AM. The effects of whole wheat, wheat bran and zinc in the diet on the absorption and accumulation of cadmium in rats. *Br J Nutr* 1993;**69**:199–209.
25. Chan DY, Hale BB. Bioaccumulation of cadmium from durum wheat diets in the livers and kidneys of mice. *Bull Environ Contam Toxicol* 2000;**64**:526–33.
26. Farajzadeh MA, Monji AB. Adsorption characteristics of wheat bran towards heavy metal cations. *Sep Purif Technol* 2004;**38**:197–207.
27. Özer A, Pirinçci HB. The adsorption of Cd(II) ions on sulphuric acid-treated wheat bran. *J Hazard Mater* 2006;**137**:849–55.
28. Singh KK, Singh AK, Hasan SH. Low cost bio-sorbent "wheat bran" for the removal of cadmium from wastewater: Kinetic and equilibrium studies. *Biores Technol* 2006;**97**:994–1001.
29. Nouri L, Ghodbane I, Hamdaoui O, Chiha M. Batch sorption dynamics and equilibrium for the removal of cadmium ions from aqueous phase using wheat bran. *J Hazard Mater* 2007;**149**:115–25.
30. Nouri L, Hamdaoui O. Ultrasonication-assisted sorption of cadmium from aqueous phase by wheat bran. *J Phys Chem* 2007;**111**:8456–63.
31. Ogata F, Tominaga H, Kangawa M, Kawaski N. Adsorption of cadmium ions by wheat bran treated with pectinase. *Chem Pharm Bull* 2011;**59**:1400–2.
32. American Association of Cereal Chemists (AACC). The definition of dietary fiber. *Cereal Food World* 2001;**46**:112–26.
33. Lattimer JM, Haub MD. Effects of dietary fiber and its components on metabolic health. *Nutrients* 2010;**2**:1266–89.
34. Buckeridge MS, Tiné MAS. Composição polissacarídica: estrutura da parede celular e fibra alimentar. In: Lajolo FM, Calixto FS, Penna EW, Menezes EW, editors. *Fibra dietética en Iberoamérica: tecnología y salud.* Varela: São Paulo; 2001. p. 43–60.

35. Dreher ML. Dietary fiber overview. In: Cho SS, Dreher ML, editors. *Handbook of dietary fiber*. New York: Marcel Dekker; 2001. p. 1–16.

36. Hemery Y, Rouau X, Lullien-Pellerin V, Barron C, Abecassis J. Dry process to develop wheat fractions and products with enhanced nutritional quality. *J Food Sci* 2007;**46**:327–47.

37. Kasprzak MM, Lærke HN, Knudsen KEB. Changes in molecular characteristics of cereal carbohydrates after processing and digestion. *Int J Mol Sci* 2012;**13**:16833–52.

38. Li W, Cui SW, Kakuda Y. Extraction, fractionation, structural and physical characterization of wheat β-d-glucans. *Carbohyd Polym* 2006;**63**:408–16.

39. Suget A, Barron C. Histologie du grain de blé. *Industrie des Céréales* 2005;**145**:3–7.

40. Rendleman JA. Metal–polysacharide complexes. Part I. *Food Chem* 1978;**3**:47–79.

41. Borycka B, Stachowiak J. Relations between cadmium and magnesium and aronia fractional dietary fiber. *Food Chem* 2008;**107**:44–8.

42. Rendleman JA. Metal-polysaccharide complexes. Part II. *Food Chem* 1978;**3**:127–58.

43. Callegaro MGK, Diettrich T, Alves E, et al. Supplementation with fiber-rich multimixtures yields a higher dietary concentration and apparent absorption of minerals in rats. *Nutr Res* 2010;**30**:615–25.

44. Cho SS, Clark C, Jenab M. The influence of wheat fiber and bran on mineral nutriture. In: Cho SS, Dreher ML, editors. *Handbook of dietary fiber*. New York, NY: Marcel Dekker; 2001. p. 227–57.

45. Harland BF, Narula G. Dietary fiber and mineral interaction. In: Cho SS, Dreher ML, editors. *Handbook of dietary fiber*. New York, NY: Marcel Dekker; 2001. p. 219–25.

46. Lopez HW, Levrat MA, Guy C, Messager A, Demigné C, Rémésy C. Effects of soluble corn bran arabinoxylans on cecal digestion, lipid metabolism, and mineral balance (Ca, Mg) in rats. *J Nutr Biochem* 1999;**10**:500–9.

47. Weaver CM, Martin BR, Story JA, Hutchinson I, Sanders L. Novel fibers increase bone calcium content and strength beyond efficiency of large intestine fermentation. *J Agric Food Chem* 2010;**58**:8952–7.

48. Bosscher D, Loo JV, Franck A. Inulin and oligofructose as functional ingredients to improve bone mineralization. *Int Dairy J* 2006;**16**:1092–7.

49. Coudray C, Demigné C, Rayssiguier Y. Effects of dietary fibers on magnesium absorption in animals and humans. *J Nutr* 2003;**133**:1–4.

50. Tahiri M, Tressol JC, Arnaud J, et al. Effect of short-chain fructooligosaccharides on intestinal calcium absorption and calcium status in postmenopausal women: a stable-isotope study. *Am J Clin Nutr* 2003;**77**:449–57.

51. Coudray C, Tressol JC, Gueux E, Rayssinguer Y. Effects of inulin-type fructans of different chain length type of branching on intestinal absorption and balance of calcium and magnesium in rats. *Eur J Nutr* 2003;**42**:91–8.

52. Hopkins MJ, Englyst HN, Macfarlane S, Furrie E, Macfarlane GT, McBain A. Degradation of cross-linked and non-cross-linked arabinoxylans by the intestinal microbiota in children. *Appl Environ Microbiol* 2003;**69**:6354–60.

53. Kiyozumi M, Mishima M, Noda S, et al. Studies on poisonous metals. IX. Effects of dietary fibers on absorptions of cadmium in rats. *Chem Pharm Bull* 1982;**30**:4494–9.

54. Rose HE, Quarterman J. Dietary fibers and heavy metal retention in the rat. *Environ Res* 1987;**42**:166–75.

55. Zhang N, Huang C, Ou S. *In vitro* binding capacities of three dietary fibers and their mixture for four toxic elements, cholesterol, and bile acid. *J Hazard Mater* 2011;**186**:236–9.

56. Persson H, Nair BM, Frolich W, Nyman M, Asp NG. Binding of mineral elements by some dietary fiber components – *In vitro* (II). *Food Chem* 1987;**26**:139–48.

57. Nair BM, Asp NG, Nyman M, Persson H. Binding of mineral elements by some dietary fiber components. *Food Chem* 1987;**23**:295–303.

58. Schlemmer U, Frølich W, Prieto RM, Grases F. Phytate in foods and significance for humans: Food sources, intake, processing, bioavailability, protective role and analysis. *Mol Nutr Food Res* 2009;**53**:330–75.

59. Odell BL, Deboland AR, Koirtyohann SR. Distribution of phytate and nutritionally important elements among morphological components of cereal grains. *J Agric Food Chem* 1972;**20**:718–21.

60. Gani A, Wani SM, Masoodi FA, Hameed G. Whole-grain cereal bioactive compounds and their health benefits: A Review. *J Food Process Technol* 2012;**3**:146.

61. Harland BF, Narula G. Food Phytate and its hydrolysis products. *Nutr Res* 1999;**19**:947–61.

62. Nolan KB, Duffin PA, Mcweeny DJ. Effects of phytate on mineral bioavailability – *In vitro* studies on Mg^{2+}, Ca^{2+}, Fe^{3+}, Cu^{2+} and Zn^{2+} also Cd^{2+} solubilities in the presence of phytate. *J Sci Food Agr* 1987;**40**:79–85.

63. Champagne ET, Phillippy BQ. Effects of pH on calcium, zinc, and phytate solubilities and complexes following in vitro digestions of soy protein isolate. *J Food Sci* 1989;**54**:587–92.

64. Sandberg AS, Carlsson NG, Svanberg U. Effects of Inositol tri-, tetra-, penta-, and hexaphosphates on *in vitro* estimation of iron availability. *J Food Sci* 1989;**54**:159–86.

65. Sandberg AS, Svanberg U. Phytate hydrolysis by phytase in cereals: Effects on *in vitro* estimation of iron availability. *J Food Sci* 1991;**56**:1330–3.

66. Gibson RS, Bailey KB, Gibbs M, Ferguson EL. A review of phytate, iron, zinc, and calcium concentrations in plant-based complementary foods used in low-income countries and implications for bioavailability. *Food Nutr Bull* 2010;**31**:134–46.

67. Bohn L, Meyer AS, Rasmussen SK. Phytate: impact on environment and human nutrition. A challenge for molecular breeding. *J Zhejiang Univ Sci B* 2008;**9**:165–91.

68. Rimbach G, Pallauf J, Brandt K, Most E. Effect of phytic acid and microbial phytase on Cd accumulation, Zn status, and apparent absorption of Ca, P, Mg, Fe, Zn, Cu, and Mn in growing rats. *Ann Nutr Metab* 1995;**39**:361–70.

69. Zacharias B, Lantzsch HJ, Drochner W. The influence of dietary microbial phytase and calcium in the accumulation of cadmium in different organs of pigs. *J Trace Elem Med Bio* 1991;**15**:109–14.

70. Yannai S, Sachs KM. Absorption and accumulation of cadmium, lead and mercury from foods by rats. *Food Chem Toxicol* 1993;**31**:351–5.

71. McCall JT, Davis GK. Effect of dietary protein and zinc on the absorption and liver deposition of radioactive and total copper. *J Nutr* 1961;**74**:45–50.

72. Engel RW, Price NO, Miller RF. Copper, manganese, cobalt and molybdenum balance in pre-adolescent girls. *J Nutr* 1967;**92**:197–204.

73. Greger JL, Snedeker SM. Effect of dietary protein and phosphorus levels on the utilization of zinc, copper and manganese by adult males. *J Nutr* 1980;**110**:2243–53.

74. Wapnir RA. Copper absorption and bioavailability. *Am J Clin Nutr* 1998;**67**:1054S–60S.

75. Andrieux C, Sacquet E. Effect of Maillard's reaction products on apparent mineral absorption in different parts of the digestive tract. The role of microflora. *Reprod Nutr Dev* 1984;**25**:379–86.

76. Lönnerdal B. Dietary factors influencing zinc absorption. *J Nutr* 2000;**130**:1378S–83S.

77. Sandström B. Cederblad Å. Zinc absorption from composite meals. II. Influence of the main protein source. *Am J Clin Nutr* 1980;**33**:1778–83.

78. Berner LA, Miller DD. Effects of dietary proteins on iron bioavailability – a review. *Food Chem* 1985;**18**:47–69.

79. West DW. Structure and function of the phosphopyrilated residues of casein. *J Dairy Sci* 1986;**53**:333–52.

80. Amaro López MA, Cámara Martos F. Iron availability: An updated review. *Int J Food Sci Nutr* 2004;**55**:597–606.

81. Guéguen L, Pointillart A. The bioavailability of dietary calcium. *J Am Coll Nutr* 2000;**19**:119S–36S.

82. Mykkänen HM, Wasserman RH. Enhanced absorption of calcium by casein phosphopeptides in rachitic and normal chicks. *J Nutr* 1980;**110**:2141–8.

83. Lee YS, Noguchi T, Naito H. Intestinal absorption of calcium in rats given diets containing casein or aminoacid mixture: The role of casein phosphopeptides. *Br J Nutr* 1983;**49**:67–76.

84. Li Y, Tomé D, Desjeux JF. Indirect effect of casein phosphopeptides on calcium absorption in rat ileum *in vitro*. *Reprod Nutr Dev* 1989;**29**:227–33.

85. Nawrot TS, Staessen JA, Roels HA, et al. Cadmium exposure in the population: from health risks to strategies of prevention. *Biometals* 2010;**23**:769–82.

86. Nordberg NF. Historical perspectives on cadmium toxicology. *Toxicol Appl Pharmacol* 2009;**238**:192–200.

87. Tcuchiya K. Causation of ouch-ouch disease (Itai-itai Byŏ): an introductory review. II. Epidemiology and evaluation. *Keio J Med* 1969;**18**:181–94.

88. Matović V, Buha A, Bulat Z, Đukić-Ćosić D. Cadmium toxicity revisited: focus on oxidative stress induction and interactions with zinc and magnesium. *Arh Hig Rada Toksikol* 2011;**62**: 65–76.

89. WHO. *Summary report of the seventy-third meeting of the Joint FAO/ WHO Expert Committee on Food Additives*. Geneva: World Health Organization; 2010.

90. Hong Y, Zi-jun W, Jian X, Ying-jie D, Fang M. Development of the dietary fiber functional food and studies on its toxicological and physiologic properties. *Food Chem Toxicol* 2012;**50**:3367–74.

91. Oliver DP, Hannam R, Tiller KG, Wilhelm NS, Merry R, Cozens GD. Heavy metals in the environment: the effects of zinc fertilization on cadmium concentration in wheat grain. *J Environ Qual* 1994;**23**:705–11.

92. Oliver DP, Tiller KG, Conyers M, Slattery W, Alston A, Merry R. Effectiveness of liming to minimize uptake of cadmium by wheat and barley grain grown in the field. *Aust J Agr Res* 1996;**47**: 1181–93.

93. Oliver DP, Wilhelm NS, McFarlane JD, Tiller KG, Cozens GD. Effect of soil and foliar applications of zinc on cadmium concentration in wheat grain. *Aust J Exp Agr* 1997;**37**:677–81.

94. Oliver DP, Tiller KG, Alston A, Cozens GD, Merry RH. Effects of soil pH and applied cadmium on cadmium concentration in wheat grain. *Aust J Agr Res* 1998;**36**:571–83.

95. Chaudri A, McGrath S, Gibbs P, et al. Cadmium availability to wheat grain in soils treated with sewage sludge or metal salts. *Chemosphere* 2007;**66**:1415–23.

96. Baize D. Cadmium in soils and cereal grains after sewage-sludge application on French soils. A review. *Agron Sustain Dev* 2009;**29**:175–84.

97. Chaney RL. Food safety issues for mineral and organic fertilizers. In: Sparks D, editor. *Advances in Agronomy*. Waltham: Academic Press; 2012. p. 51–116.

98. UNEP. United Nations Environment Program. *Final review of scientific information on cadmium* 2010.

99. IFCS. *Intergovernmental Forum on Chemical Safety. Global Partnerships for Chemical Safety. The problem of environmental contamination by cadmium, lead and mercury in Russia and Ukraine: a survey*. Available at: http://www.who.int/ifcs/documents/forums/forum6/eco_accord_en.pdf; July 2008 [accessed 25.03.13].

100. Crews HM, Owen LM, Langford N, et al. Use of the stable isotope (106) Cd for studying dietary cadmium absorption in humans. *Toxicol Lett* 2000 112/113: 201–07.

101. Reeves PG, Chaney RL. Bioavailability as an issue in risk assessment and management of food cadmium: A review. *Sci Total Environ* 2008;**398**:13–9.

102. Larsson SE, Piscator M. Effect of cadmium on skeletal tissue in normal and calcium-deficient rats. *Isr J Med Sci* 1971;**7**:495–8.

103. Ohta H, Cherian MG. The influence of nutritional deficiencies on gastrointestinal uptake of cadmium and cadmium-metallothionein in rats. *Toxicology* 1995;**97**:71–80.

104. Tanaka M, Yanagi M, Shirota K, et al. Effect of cadmium in the zinc deficient rat. *Vet Hum Toxicol* 1995;**37**:203–8.

105. WHO. *Cadmium in Drinking-water. Background document for development of WHO Guidelines for Drinking-water Quality*. Geneva, Switzerland: World Health Organization; 2011.

106. Tallkvist J, Bowlus CL, Lonnerdal B. DMT1 gene expression and cadmium absorption in human absorptive enterocytes. *Toxicol Lett* 2001;**122**:171–7.

107. WHO. *Environmental Health Criteria 234. Elemental speciation in human health risk assessment*. Geneva, Switzerland: World Health Organization; 2006. p. 256.

108. Khanal RC, Nemere I. Endocrine regulation of calcium transport in epithelia. *Clin Exp Pharmacol Physiol* 2008;**35**:1277–87.

109. Ryu DY, Lee SJ, Park DW, Choi BS, Klaassen CD, Park JD. Dietary iron regulates intestinal cadmium absorption through iron transporters in rats. *Toxicol Lett* 2004;**152**:19–25.

110. Grill E, Winnacker EL, Zenk M. Phytochelatins: the principal heavy-metal complexing peptides of higher plants. *Science* 1985;**230**:674–6.

111. Günther K, Kastenholz B. Speciation of cadmium in the environment and food. In: Cornelis R, Caruso J, Crews H, Heumann K, editors. *Handbook of Elemental Speciation II. Species in the Environment, Food, Medicine and Occupational Health*. Chichester, UK: John Wiley & Sons; 2005. p. 94–106.

112. Cobbett CS. Phytochelatins and their roles in heavy metal detoxification. *Plant Physiol* 2000;**123**:825–32.

113. Cobbett C, Goldsbrough P. Phytochelatins and metallothioneins: roles in heavy metal detoxification and homeostasis. *Annu Rev Plant Biol* 2002;**53**:159–82.

114. Vašák M, Meloni G. Chemistry and biology of mammalian metallothioneins. *J Biol Inorg Chem* 2011;**16**:1067–78.

115. Sullivan MF, Hardy JT, Miller BM, Buschbom RL, Siewicki TC. Absorption and distribution of cadmium in mice fed diets containing either inorganic or oyster-incorporated cadmium. *Toxicol Appl Pharmacol* 1984;**72**:210–7.

116. Wagner G, Nulty LE, Lefevre M. Cadmium in wheat grain: its nature and fate after ingestion. *J Toxicol Environ Health* 1984;**13**:979–89.

117. Cherian MG. Absorption and tissue distribution of cadmium in mice after chronic feeding with cadmium chloride and cadmium metallothionein. *Bull Environ Contam Toxicol* 1983;**30**:33–6.

118. Groten JP, Sinkeldam EJ, Luten JB, van Bladeren PJ. Cadmium accumulation and metallothionein concentrations after 4-week dietary exposure to cadmium chloride or cadmium-metallothionein in rats. *Toxicol Appl Pharmacol* 1991;**111**:504–13.

119. Ohta H, Cherian MG. Gastrointestinal absorption of cadmium and metallothionein. *Toxicol Appl Pharmacol* 1991;**107**:63–72.

120. Sugawara N, Sugawara C. Gastrointestinal absorption of Cd metallothionein and cadmium chloride in mice. *Arch Toxicol* 1991;**65**:689–92.

121. Groten JP, Koeman JH, Van Nesselrooij JHJ, et al. Comparison of renal toxicity after long-term oral administration of cadmium chloride and cadmium-metallothionein in rats. *Toxicol Sci* 1994;**23**:544–52.

122. Groten JP, Sinkeldam EJ, Luken JB, van Bladeren PJ. Comparison of the toxicity of inorganic and liver incorporated cadmium: A 4-week feeding study in rats. *Food Chem Toxicol* 1990;**28**: 435–41.

123. Lind Y, Wicklund GA, Engman J, Jorhem L. Bioavailability of cadmium from crab hepatopancreas and mushroom in relation to inorganic cadmium: A 9-week feeding study in mice. *Food Chem Toxicol* 1995;**38**:667–73.

124. Klaassen CD, Liu J, Diwan BA. Metallothionein protection of cadmium toxicity. *Toxicol Appl Pharmacol* 2009;**238**:215–20.

125. Suzuki S, Taguchi T, Yokohashi G. Dietary factors influencing upon the retention rate of orally administered $^{105m}CdCl_2$ concentrations in mice with special reference to calcium and protein in the diet. *Ind Health* 1969;**7**:155–9.

126. Friberg L, Piscator M, Nordberg G, Kjellström T. *Cadmium in the environment*. Cleveland: CRC Press; 1974.

127. Friberg L, Kjellström T, Nordberg G, Piscator M. *Cadmium in the Environment. III. A Toxicological and Epidemiological Appraisal*. Washington, DC: Environmental Protection Agency, Office of Research and Development; 1975.

128. Suzuki KT, Tanaka Y, Miyamoto E, et al. Effect of diet on tissue retention of cadmium heavily preaccumulated in rats. *Arch Environ Contam Toxicol* 1984;**13**:609–19.

129. Revis NW. The relationship of dietary protein to metallothionein and cadmium induced renal damage. *Toxicology* 1981;**20**:323–33.

130. Revis NW, Osborne TR. Dietary protein effects on cadmium and metallothionein accumulation in the liver and kidney of rats. *Environ Health Perspect* 1984;**54**:83–91.

131. Grosicki A. Dietary dried egg white protein influences accumulation and distribution of cadmium in rats. *J Toxicol Environ Health A* 2010;**73**:1173–9.

132. Suzuki KT. Metallothionein: analysis in tissues and toxicological significance. *IARC Sci Publ* 1992;**118**:211–7.

133. Itokawa Y, Tomaoko A, Tanaka J. Bone changes in experimental chronic cadmium poisoning. *Environ Health* 1973;**26**:241–4.

134. Mayack LA, Bush PB, Fletcher OJ, Page RK, Fendley TT. Tissue residues of dietary cadmium in wood ducks. *Arch Environ Contam Toxicol* 1981;**10**:637–41.

135. Orlowski C, Piotrowski JK, Subdys JK, Gross A. Urinary cadmium as indicator of renal cadmium in humans: an autopsy study. *Human Exp Toxicol* 1998;**17**:302–6.

136. Järup L, Berglund M, Elinder CG, Nordberg G, Vahter M. Health effects of cadmium exposure - a review of the literature and a risk estimate. *Scand J Work Environ Health* 1998;**24**:1–51.

137. Bernard A. Cadmium and its adverse effects on human health. *Indian J Med Res* 2008;**128**:557–64.

138. Järup L, Alfvén T. Low level cadmium exposure, renal and bone effects-the OSCAR study. *Biometals* 2004;**17**:505–9.

139. Aoshima K, Fan J, Cai Y, Katoh T, Teranishi H, Kasuya M. Assessment of bone metabolism in cadmium-induced renal tubular dysfunction by measurements of biochemical markers. *Toxicol Lett* 2003;**136**:183–92.

140. Satarug S, Baker JR, Reilly PEB, Moore MR, Williams DJ. Cadmium levels in the lung, liver, kidney cortex, and urine samples from Australians without occupational exposure to metals. *Arch Environ Health* 2002;**57**:69–77.

141. Sabolic I, Breljak D, Skarica M, Herak-Kramberger CM. Role of metallothionein in cadmium traffic and toxicity in kidneys and other mammalian organs. *Biometals* 2010;**23**:897–926.

142. Cheung BMY, Ong KL, Wong LYF. Elevated serum alkaline phosphatase and peripheral arterial disease in the United States National Health and Nutrition Examination Survey 1999–2004. *Int J Cardiol* 2009;**135**:156–61.

143. WHO. Exposure to cadmium: A major public health concern. *WHO* 2010.

144. Nzengue Y, Candéias SM, Sauvaigo S, et al. The toxicity redox mechanisms of cadmium alone or together with copper and zinc homeostasis alteration: Its redox biomarkers. *J Trace Elem Med Biol* 2011;**25**:171–80.

145. Martelli A, Rousselet E, Dycke C, Bouron A, Moulis JM. Cadmium toxicity in animal cells by interference with essential metals. *Biochimie* 2006;**88**:1807–14.

146. Liu J, Qu W, Kadiiska MB. Role of oxidative stress in cadmium toxicity and carcinogenesis. *Toxicol Appl Pharmacol* 2009;**238**:209–14.

147. Pathak N, Khandelwal S. Influence of cadmium on murine thymocytes: Potentiation of apoptosis and oxidative stress. *Toxicol Lett* 2006;**165**:121–32.

148. Chao E, Simmons C, Black R. Physiologically functional wheat bran. In: Mazza G, editor. *Functional Foods: Biochemical and Processing Aspects*. Lancaster, UK: Technomic Publication; 1998. p. 39–70.

149. Vitaglione P, Napolitano A, Fogliano V. Cereal dietary fibre: a natural functional ingredient to deliver phenolic compounds into the gut. *Trends Food Sci Tech* 2008;**19**:451–63.

150. Javed MM, Zahoor S, Shaafaat S, et al. Wheat bran as a brown gold: Nutritious value and its biotechnological applications. *Afr J Microbiol Res* 2012;**6**:724–33.

151. Saulnier L, Sado PE, Branlard G, Charmet G, Guillon F. Wheat arabinoxylans: Exploiting variation in amount and composition to develop enhanced varieties. *J Cereal Sci* 2007;**46**:261–81.

152. Izydorczyk MS, Dexter JE. Barley β-glucans and arabinoxylans: Molecular structure, physicochemical properties, and uses in food products – a review. *Food Res Int* 2008;**41**:850–68.

153. Shewry PR, Charmet G, Branlard G, et al. Developing new types of wheat with enhanced health benefits. *Trends Food Sci Tech* 2012;**25**:70–7.

154. Bilgicli N, Ibanoglu S. Effect of wheat germ and wheat bran on the fermentation activity, phytic acid content and colour of tarhana, a wheat flour–yoghurt mixture. *J Food Eng* 2007;**78**:681–6.

155. EC. The Commission of the European Communities. Commission Regulation (EC) No 1881/2006 of 19 December 2006 setting maximum levels for certain contaminants in foodstuffs. *Official J Eur Union* 2006;**L 364**:1–20.

156. Olsson IM, Eriksson J, Oborn I, Skerfving S, Oskarsson A. Cadmium in food production systems: a health risk for sensitive population groups. *Ambio* 2005;**34**:344–51.

157. Jansson G. *Cadmium in Arable Crops. The influence of soil factors and liming. PhD thesis. Department of Soil Sciences*. Uppsala: Swedish University of Agricultural Sciences; 2002. p. 41.

158. Hellstrand S, Landner L. Cadmium Exposure in the Swedish Environment. Part III. Cadmium in fertilizers, soil, crops and foods – the Swedish situation. The Swedish National Chemicals Inspectorate. *Solna* 1998;**1**:98.

159. Oliver DP, Gartrell J, Tiller KG, Correll R, Cozens GD, Youngberg B. Differential responses of Australian wheat cultivars to cadmium concentration in wheat grain. *Aust J Agr Res* 1995;**46**:873–86.

160. Hussan A, Larsson H, Kuktaite R, Johansson E. Concentration of some heavy metals in organically grown primitive, old and modern wheat genotypes: implications for human health. *J Environ Sci Health B* 2012;**47**:751–8.

161. McLaughlin MJ, Parker DR, Clarke JM. Metals and micronutrients: food safety issues. *Field Crops Res* 1998;**60**:143–63.

162. Chaudri AM, Zhao FJ, McGrath SP, Crosland AR. The cadmium content of British wheat grain. *J Environ Qual* 1995;**24**:850–5.

163. Hart JJ, Welch RM, Norvell WA, Sullivan LA, Kochian LV. Characterization of cadmium binding, uptake, and translocation in intact seedlings of bread and durum wheat cultivars. *Plant Physiol* 1998;**116**:1413–20.

164. Jackson PJ, Unkefer CJ, Doolen JA, Watt K, Robinson NJ. Poly (g-glutamylcysteinyl)glycine, its role in cadmium resistance in plant cells. *Proc Natl Acad Sci USA* 1987;**84**:6619–23.

165. Salt DE, Rauser WE. Mg-ATP-dependent transport of phytochelatins across the tonoplast of oat roots. *Plant Physiol* 1995;**107**:1293–301.

166. Sovrani V, Blandino M, Scarpino V, et al. Bioactive compound content, antioxidant activity, deoxynivalenol and heavy metal contamination of pearled wheat fractions. *Food Chem* 2012;**135**:39–46.

167. Cheli F, Campagnoli A, Ventura V, et al. Effects of industrial processing on the distributions of deoxynivalenol, cadmium and lead in durum wheat milling fractions. *LWT-Food Sci Technol* 2010;**43**:1050–7.

168. Mortvedt JJ, Mays DA, Osborn O. Uptake by wheat of cadmium and other heavy metal contaminants in phosphate fertilizers. *J Environ Qual* 1981;**10**:193–7.

169. Pieczonka K, Rosopulo A. Distribution of cadmium, copper and zinc in the caryopsis of wheat *(Triticum aestivum L.)*. *Fresenius Z Anal Chem* 1985;**322**:697–9.

170. Oliver D, Tiller K, Gore P, Moss H. Cadmium in wheat-grain and milling products from some Australian flour mills. *Aust J Agr Res* 1993;**44**:1–11.

171. Radiana TB, Nicolae-Ciprian P, Stela P, Stelica C, Rodica C, Suzana TB. Distribution of some toxic contaminants in the milling products, during the milling process. *Rom Biotech Lett* 2010;**15**:5281–6.

172. *Association of Official Analytical Chemists. Official Methods of Aanalysis of the Association of the Official Analytical Chemists.* 16th ed. Arlington, VA: AOAC; 1995.

173. Fliss H, Ménard M. Oxidant-induced mobilization of zinc from metallothionein. *Arch of Biochem Biophys* 1992;**293**:195–9.

174. Lawther JM, Sun R, Banks B. Extraction, fractionation and characterization of structural polysaccharides from wheat straw. *J Agric Food Chem* 1995;**43**:667–75.

175. Marques PASS, Rosa MF, Pinheiro HM. PH effects on the removal of Cu^{2+}, Cd^{2+} and Pb^{2+} from aqueous solution by waste brewery biomass. *Bioproc Eng* 2000;**23**:135–41.

176. Ridley BL, O'Neill MA, Mohnen D. Pectins: structure, biosynthesis, and oligogalacturonide-related signaling. *Phytochemistry* 2001;**57**:929–67.

177. FAO. Food and Agriculture Organization of the United Nations. Cereal Supply and Demand Brief. Available at: http://www.fao.org/docrep/017/al995e/al995e00.pdf [accessed 01.01.13].

178. Modak JM, Natarajan KA. Biosorption of metals using nonliving biomass – A review. *Miner Metall Proc* 1995;**12**:189–96.

179. Lodiero P, Herrero R, Sastre de Vicente ME. Thermodynamic and kinetic aspects on the biosorption of cadmium by low cost materials: A review. *Environ Chem* 2006;**3**:400–18.

180. Farooq U, Kozinski JA, Khan MA, Athar M. Biosorption of heavy metal ions using wheat based biosorbents – A review of the recent literature. *Bioresource Technol* 2010;**101**:5043–53.

181. Buhler DR. Availability of cadmium from foods and water. In: Calabrese EJ, Tuthill RW, Condie L, editors. *Inorganics in drinking water and cardiovascular disease.* Princeton, NJ: Princeton Scientific Publication; 1985. p. 271–87.

182. Callegaro MGK, Milbradt BG, Diettrich T, et al. Influence of cereal bran supplement on cadmiun effects in growing rats. *Hum Exp Toxicol* 2010;**29**:467–76.

183. Wing AM, Wing K, Tidehag P, Hallmans G, Sjöström R. Cadmium accumulation from diets with and without wheat bran in rats with different iron status. *Nutr Res* 1992;**12**:1205–15.

184. *Canadian Nutrient File.* Available at: http://webprod3.hc-sc.gc.ca/cnf-fce/index-eng.jsp; 2010 [accessed 07.02.13].

185. Harrington ME, Flynn A, Cashman KD. Effects of dietary fibers extracts on calcium absorption in the rat. *Food Chem* 2001;**73**:263–9.

186. Grant CA, Clarke JM, Duguid S, Chaney RL. Selecting and breeding of plant cultivars to minimize cadmium accumulation. *Sci Total Environ* 2008;**390**:301–10.

WHEAT TOXICITY

Wheat Contaminants (Pesticides) and their Dissipation during Processing

Muhammad Atif Randhawa*, *Anwaar Ahmed*†, *Muhammad Sameem Javed**

*National Institute of Food Science & Technology, University of Agriculture, Faisalabad, Pakistan,
†Department of Food Technology, PMAS-Arid Agriculture University, Rawalpindi, Pakistan

INTRODUCTION

Pesticides are recognized as being important for the production of crops. These chemical substances are widely used against plant pests and diseases. The use of pesticides in agriculture has led to an increase in farm productivity by combating a variety of pests that destroy crops, and also improves the quality of the produced food;[1,2] however, post-harvest treatments for protection of raw grain against stored grain pests present potential health risks via both occupational and non-occupational exposure. Different pesticides have been implicated in chronic neurotoxicity, endocrine disruption, immune impacts, genotoxicity, mutagenicity, carcinogenesis, developmental disabilities, and skin and respiratory diseases.[3–8]

Wheat (*Triticum aestivum* L.) is one of the most important staple food grain crops, with a worldwide production of 690 million tons in 2012. Wheat contributes 30% of the world's average crop consumption[9] and is cultivated in most of the countries of the world, but has to compete with insects, weeds, and herbs in the field. The use of insecticides, herbicides, and weedicides plays an important role in the production and storage of wheat, and to date they are irreplaceable. Although insecticides, herbicides, and weedicides have found their way into wide applications and play a significant role in boosting wheat production, the hazards associated with them regarding food safety and human health have increasingly become the focus of world attention. A report regarding pesticide residues in Australian wheat was published on June 27, 2010. This report stated that a total of 770,000 tons of Australian wheat was rejected by the Taiwan government due to the presence of fenitrothion at a concentration of 0.47 ppm, exceeding the maximum residue limit

(MRL) for Taiwan. This is an alarming situation, as if this is the status of a developed nation, then what we should expect from developing countries? Wheat pesticide residues in European countries increased from 0.1% to 0.8% between 2006 and 2009. A total of 1312 samples of wheat were collected throughout the Europe, and of these 0.8% were found to be contaminated with pesticide residues above MRLs, while 31.3% were between MRLs and the level of quantification, and 67.8% samples were well below the level of quantification.[10]

Food safety has been one of the driving forces behind pesticide legislation and regulation. Consumer attitude surveys indicate that 72–82% of Americans consider pesticide residues in food to be a major concern. Nevertheless, in terms of overall food safety the FDA ranks pesticides as its fifth food safety priority and of less concern than microbial contamination of foods, nutritional imbalance, environmental contaminants, and naturally occurring toxins. The need is to balance/harmonize the use of pesticides. The maximum residue limit is fixed for all registered substances – not only whole grain, but also flour, bran, and bread.[11] The control of pesticide residues in grain is generally based on MRLs, which are below the highest residue level expected if the registered dosages of pesticides are applied to crops according to Good Agricultural Practices (GAPs).

Food processing is the post-harvest, value-addition operation of transformation of raw food commodities to a more edible form, and further storage for prolonged periods. According to the Food and Agriculture Organization (FAO), a commodity is said to be processed when it is subjected to physical, chemical, and/or biological transformation processes. Residues of pesticides in food are influenced by the storage, handling, and processing that occurs between harvesting of raw agricultural commodities and consumption of prepared foodstuffs. Regulatory authorities are becoming increasingly interested in the data generated through study of the degradation of pesticides during processing.

MODE OF ENTRY OF PESTICIDE RESIDUES AND THEIR IMPACT ON HEALTH

Excessive use of pesticides particularly in developing nations, their instability and distance transport ultimately ends in extensive environmental issues. Furthermore, traditional, toxic, environmentally persistent, non-patented and inferior quality substances are widely used in developing countries, causing thoughtful health problems having national and international impacts.[12] All pesticides in groundwater and most residues present in surface water enter via the soil.[13,14] There are two main routes by which pesticides enter the soil: spray drift to soil during foliage treatment plus wash-off from treated foliage,[15] and release from granulates applied directly to the soil. Plants take up the pesticides residues from soil, and this route is the most silent means of entry of pesticide residues into food chain. The cycle of pesticide residues and their interaction with biotic and abiotic components of the environment is shown in Figure 20.1.

The indiscriminate use of pesticides leads to higher yields and greater profit, but its negative role is dangerous to humans and all living forms; therefore, instant action and attention is required in order to ensure safety for living organisms. Unfortunately there are a number of barriers to the documentation of systematic and valid data on toxic aspects of pesticide residues in wheat. Residues of pesticides in the food web account for a small but noteworthy portion of acute and chronic human toxicity, and there have been several accidental cases regarding human exposure to pesticides, causing acute poisoning. Toxicological and health effects of some of the most commonly used pesticides are summarized in Table 20.1.[16–24]

Factors Affecting the Mitigation of Pesticide Residues during Storage

Different factors affecting the degradation and breakdown of pesticide residues are summarized below.

Chemical and Environmental Factors

Dissolution, volatilization and co-distillation, temperature, photodegradation, hydrolysis, oxidation, and penetration are the main chemical and environmental factors that are responsible for the degradation of pesticides. All of the above factors, along with the nature of the pesticide, are somewhat correlated with one another. Water activity and kind of stored grains also influence

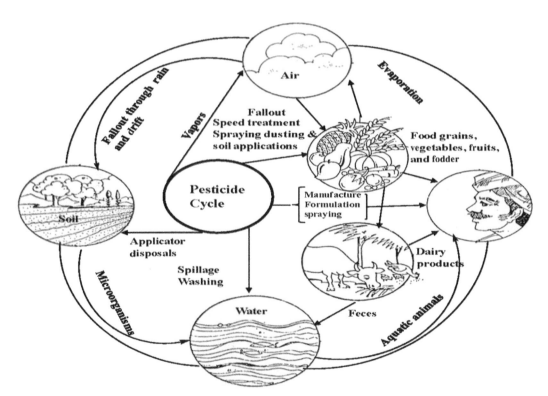

FIGURE 20.1　Pesticide cycle in the environment. (© 2013 Suresh Kumar Kailasa, Hui-Fen Wu and Shang-Da Huang. Originally published in: http://dx.doi.org/10.5772/51929 under CC BY 3.0 license)

TABLE 20.1 Pesticide Exposures Associated with Adverse Effects

Pesticide Class	Active Ingredient	Risks Associated	References
Mixed exposure	Wide variety	Longer time to pregnancy among women whose spouses work in greenhouses Spontaneous abortions in wives and birth defects in children of farmers or pesticide applicators Women with infertility more likely than controls to be exposed to pesticides Risk of childhood leukemia after indoor pesticide exposure during pregnancy Formulations may include organic solvents that exhibit reproductive or developmental toxicity	Ngo et al.[16]
Organophosphates	Chlorpyrifos diazinon, malathion, parathion	Lower birth weight and shorter gestational age among women with residential or agricultural exposure (agents listed left) Neurodevelopmental or childhood behavioral problems (chlorpyrifos diazinon) Altered fetal immune cell function in rats	Kamanyire and Karalliedde[17]
Carbamates	Carbaryl, propoxur	Neurodevelopmental or childhood behavioral problems (carbaryl) Possibly childhood leukemia	Lifshitz et al.[18]
Pyrethroids	Deltamethrin, permethrin	Neurodevelopmental or childhood behavioral problems (deltamethrin) Possibly childhood leukemia	Cantalmessa[19]
Herbicides	Chlorophenoxy herbicides, triazines, glyphosate	Women with infertility more likely to mix and apply herbicides Spontaneous abortions in farm families using certain herbicides Limb and heart defects in children of pesticide applicators or agricultural workers using herbicides Early pregnancy loss and altered fetal immune cell function in rats Possibly human fetal growth restriction from community drinking water (atrazine)	Ashby et al.[20]
Fungicides	Vinclozolin, thiram	Women with infertility more likely to use fungicides supported by some studies in mice and rats Limb defects in children of pesticide applicators using fungicides Pregnant rats exposed during gonadal sex determination had male offspring with decreased sperm concentration that also affected subsequent generations of males (vinclozolin)	Dalvie et al.[21]
Fumigants	Aluminium phosphide, Sulfuryl- fluoride	Significant phosphine-induced inhibition of red blood cell cholinesterase occurs at concentrations of phosphine exceeding 10 µg/ml[22] Sulfuryl fluoride cause neurotoxicology in rats[23]	Potter et al.[22], Hanley et al.[23]
Organochlorines	Dioxin, methoxychlor, DDT, others	Increased rates of endometriosis among women in Seveso Italy (dioxin) supported by studies in mice rats and monkeys Fetal growth restriction in women with diets high in contaminated fish or who have higher blood levels of chlorinated pesticides (DDT and others) Pregnant rats exposed during gonadal sex determination had male offspring with decreased sperm concentration that also affected subsequent generations of males (methoxychlor) Decreased immune cell function at birth and increased middle ear infections after human in utero exposure	Mishra and Sharma[24]

the rate of degradation of insecticide residues during grain storage. The residues also penetrate the grains during storage and accumulate with time.[25,26] Usually, besides the effect of physical and chemical factors such as light, heat, pH, and moisture, the growth dilution factor might have played a significant role in pesticide degradation in plant.[27] However, the factors that influence pesticide persistence in soil are climate, soil properties, and the physical and chemical properties of the pesticide.[28,29]

Processing Factors

Factors affecting rate of pesticide degradation are categorized as washing and wet cleaning; peeling, husking, hulling, and shelling; and cooking.

WASHING AND WET CLEANING

The deduction of pesticide residues via washing of a food commodity may be achieved not only through the dissolution of pesticide residues in tap water but also through rinsing/dipping in chemical baths (i.e., use of detergents, alkalis, acids, hypochlorite, metabisulfite salts, ozonated water, etc.).[26] The process of washing/wet cleaning also results in removal of previously absorbed pesticide residues in the form of dust or soil particles from the outer layer (pericarp) of the commodity.[30–33] However, the removal of pesticide residues is not necessarily correlated with water solubility of the pesticide,[1,32,34,35] and different pesticides may be rinsed from processed units of products by different washing procedures.[32,36–39]

Washing efficiency is associated not only with the water solubility of the pesticide but also with the water activity of the product, thereby reinforcing the view that partition coefficients between the cuticle layer and washing water correlate well with pesticides' water activity.[40] The use of a suitable detergent that solubilizes waxes may dissipate pesticide residues present in the epicuticular wax layer.[32] Washing agents or dipping treatments may also lead to selective removal of pesticide residues with systemic action through similar mechanisms.[39,41,42] Details regarding pesticides in stored cereal grains have been reviewed by some researchers, and a fairly high percentage of the residues can be related to the dust and other fine detritus that is removed when the wheat is cleaned before milling. For instance, deltamethrin levels of 0.52 mg/kg on stored grain were reduced to 0.42 mg/kg after cleaning of grains.[43]

PEELING, HUSKING, HULLING, AND SHELLING

Removal of the outer part of a commodity by peeling, husking, hulling, shelling, or trimming is the most effective food preparation process for eradicating pesticide residues from any product. Most of the fungicides and insecticides which are directly applied to crops, undergo limited diffusion into the cuticle. As a result, residues are restricted to the exterior part and amenable towards removal by hulling, peeling or trimming. Removal of peel

of the food items can thus reduce pesticide residue levels by 70% to 100%.[26,34–36,44–50] Edwards[51] noted that most residues exist in the outer portions of cereal grains, and are amenable to removal by milling operation. For example, with the herbicide glyphosate, which penetrate through translocation, residues are greater in the bran compared to flour. The peeling of potatoes resulted in only 50% reduction of systemic organo-phosphorus pesticides[43] while disyston residues were removed only by 35%.[26] However, the procymidone residues on tomatoes and quinalphos residues on apples were declined by ≥73% each.[34]

COOKING

The processes and conditions employed in food cooking are highly diverse. The details of cooking time, cooking temperature, amount of water loss and type of the system (open or closed pan) are important parameters having quantitative effects on residue levels in the food product. Rates of degradation and volatilization of residues are increased by the heat involved in cooking or pasteurization. For example, in a study on radio-labeled chlorothalonil residues, cooking under open conditions resulted in 85–98% losses by volatilization; however, cooking under closed conditions resulted in hydrolysis, with 50% of the chlorothalonil being recovered unchanged on the crop and hydrolysis products being found in the liquor. For compounds that are of low volatility and relatively stable to hydrolysis, such as dichlorodiphenyltrichloroethane (DDT) and synthetic pyrethroids, reduction of residues through cooking may be low and concentrations may actually increase due to moisture loss.[52]

Organophosphorus (OP) insecticides (3-methyl-4-nitrophenol, fenitrothion oxon, fenitrothion) in raw agriculture products during heating were quite heat stable and hardly any losses occurred on heating for 10–15 min without the addition of water[50,53] and were unsteady to heating in the aqueous medium. After boiling in water 32% decrease in fenitrothion residues and 89.5% decline in triazophos residues occured.[45,54] Nagayama[55] reported that during the cooking process some residual pesticides were translocated into the cooking water from the raw materials, according to their water solubility expression, and the pesticide remained in the processed food according to the water activity expression. Captan was fully declined after cooking of cauliflower in the absence of added water for 15 min and during the preparation of sterilized apple puree (125 °C for 20 min at pH 4), thereby depicting its ability towards thermal degradation. Interestingly, the process of boiling did not reduce chlorpyrifos, diazinon, quinalphos, cypermethrin, λ-cyhalothrin, deltamethrin, fenpropathrin, endosulfan (alpha, beta and endosulfan sulphate), kresoxim methyl, iprodione, and vinclozoline residues on apples.[45] Cooking of cereal in the form of prepared products further reduced residue levels, as described by Joia.[56] However, it is not always clear from the literature whether the amount of residues declined due to cooking, or whether the levels were lower due to dilution because moisture levels in baked products and boiled rice are much higher than in the raw grain/material. Randhawa[36] determined the destiny of the field incurred chlorpyrifos residues and its metabolite 3,5,6-trichloro-2-pyridinol during boiling in six different winter and summer vegetables with water and the decrease of chlorpyrifos ranged from 12% to 48%. The concentration of 3,5,6-trichloro-2-pyridinol was considerably increased during the cooking process, where as chlorpyrifos concentration was substantially decreased with the cooking. This study reveals that all of the degradation products of the pesticide/parent compounds during heating should also be determined in order to evaluate the safety of cooking process. Furthermore, the boiling water that might be used in further cooking/eating must also be analysed for presence of break down products of pesticide residues. Pesticides such as amides, carbamates, thiocarbonyl and having imino groups can be swiftly hydrolyzed particularly in the existence of trace amounts of acid and/or base during the course of boiling or heating.

PESTICIDE RESIDUES IN WHEAT AT HARVEST AND DURING STORAGE

Pesticide residues in crops are serious trade barriers. Unregulated and excessive utilization of pesticides is alarming,[57] due to its uneven distribution and usage on selective crops and the limited reliance on alternative chemicals like biopesticides and botanicals. Twenty-three insect pests have been recorded in the wheat crop, of which termites and, to some extent, Gujhia weevils are recorded as economically important pests.[58,59] Termites damage the crop at all growth stages from planting to harvest, especially in un-irrigated areas with light soils. The Gujhia weevil (*Tanymecus indicus*) causes injury to the plant that resembles termite injury.[60] Different insect pests, diseases, and nematodes of economic significance in wheat are listed in Table 20.2.

By their nature, pesticides are harmful to some forms of life. It is therefore not surprising that, at a certain level of exposure, they may be harmful to humans. The quantity of pollutants in wheat can be extremely high, and may pose a threat to human health.[61] As far as health problems due to pesticide residues in foodstuffs are concerned, several countries have start food contamination monitoring programs and evaluate data regarding pesticide residues according to criteria and guidelines recommended by the Codex Committee on Pesticide Residues, as well as by the European Union. Field-incurred pesticide residues in wheat are summarized in Table 20.3.[10,62–67,68]

Field-incurred pesticide residues in wheat in European countries were determined in 2009, and chlormequat (42.3%) and pirimiphos-methyl (12.02%) residues were found to be higher than all the other pesticides. The pesticides chlormequat, pirimiphos-methyl, mepiquat, chlorpyrifos-methyl, malathion, dithiocarbamates, boscalid, tebuconazole, chlorpyrifos, deltamethrin, carbaryl, spiroxamine, profenofos, chlorpropham, bifenthrin, propamocarb, fenitrothion, phoxim, imazalil, parathion-methyl, bromopropylate, iprodione, pirimicarb, metconazole, cyproconazole, phosmet, thiabendazole, diphenylamine, fludioxonil, phosalone, tolclofos-methyl, metalaxyl, kresoxim-methyl, chlorothalonil, and cypermethrin were all detected in wheat samples. However, chlorpropham, diazinon, difenoconazole, imazalil, and chlorpyrifos residues were found at higher levels and exceeded their respective MRLs.[10] Organochlorine pesticide residues in 36 wheat samples obtained from local farmers and wheat factories in Konya (Turkey) were also determined, and all the examined samples were contaminated by organochlorine pesticide residues of cis-chlordane and methoxychlor. Chlordane isomers, methoxychlor, DDT and its metabolites, aldrin, β-hexachlorocyclohexane (β-HCH), heptachlor, and lindane, were the organochlorine pesticide residues found at the highest levels. In some of these samples, organochlorine pesticide residues were higher than European Community MRLs. The levels of residues of aldrin in one sample, trans-chlordane in one sample,

TABLE 20.2 Insect Pests, Diseases, and Nematodes of Wheat

Insect pests	Diseases	Nematodes
Termite (*Odontotermes obesus*)	Loose smut (*Ustilago tritici*)	Cereal cyst nematode (*Heterodera avenae*)
Aphid (*Macrosiphum avenae*)	Karnal bunt (*Neovossia indica*)	Seed gall nematode (*Anguina tritici*)
Pink stem borer (*Sesamia inferens*)	Leaf blight (*Alternaria triticana, Helminthosporium* spp.)	Root-knot nematode (*Meloidogyne triticoryzae*)
Army worm (*Mythimna separata*)	Leaf rust (*Puccinia recondita*)	
	Stripe rust (*P. striiformis*)	
	Stem rust (*P. graminis*)	
	Powdery mildew (*Erysiphe graminis tritici*)	
	Head blight (*Fusarium* spp.)	

TABLE 20.3   Summary of Pesticide Residues Found in Wheat

Countries	Reference(s)	Product	Sample (no.)	Pesticides Analyzed (no.)	Contaminated Samples (%)	Samples with Residues (%) > MRL Values	Samples with Multiple Residues (%)
USA, 2003	US Food and Drug Administration[62]	USA wheat	69	360	31.9	0	–
		Imported wheat	15	360	6.7	6.7	–
European Union, 2003	CEC[63]	European wheat	1021	185	22	0.5	–
European Union	EFSA[10]	European wheat	1312	38	43	0.8	–
UK, 2005	PRC[64]	UK starchy foods and grains	430	34	58	0	–
		Bran	72	34	90	0	86
		Miscellaneous cereal based foods	72	34	12.5	0	3
		Baby foods cereal based	120	1	1	0	0
	Skrbic[61]	Wheat grain	49	35	–	12.2	–
Kuwait	Sawaya et al.[65]	Cereal products	12	5	58.33	8.3	–
Turkey	Guler et al.[66]	Wheat grain	36	9	36	30	–
Pakistan	Riazuddin et al.[67]	Imported Wheat grain	60	13	22.5	0	–
		Domestic wheat grain	40	13	6.7	0	–
India	Toteja et al.[68]	Wheat grains	1080	5	59.4	1.7	–

oxy-chlordane in eight samples, and methoxychlor in one sample were found to be in excess of European Community MRLs. The level of pesticide residues in wheat grown in Turkey is alarming, as Turkey is a developed nation. Strictly regulated, judicious application of pesticides is required to safeguard humans as well as the environment from their deleterious effects.

The situation regarding pesticide residues in India is no different, as reported by Bakore.[69] A total of 150 wheat samples were collected from Jaipur, Punjab, during the summer, rainy, and winter seasons. All the wheat and water samples were found to be contaminated with various organochlorine pesticide residues of DDT and its metabolites, HCH and its isomers, heptachlor and its epoxide, and aldrin. When wheat flour was analyzed, it was found to contain high levels of residues, warranting the need for corrective action. Furthermore, Jaipur city receives wheat grains from neighboring districts and also from other states such as Punjab, Haryana, and Utter Pradesh; thus the situation is significantly worse because contamination with organochlorine pesticides is clearly widespread throughout India. Similarly, in another multicenter study conducted by the Indian Council of Medical Research, 1712 samples of wheat grain/flour were collected from urban and rural areas in 11 states representing different geographical regions of India. Residues of DDT were detected in about 60% of 1080

samples of wheat grain, and 78% of 632 samples of wheat flour; different HCH isomers were also present in about 45–80% of the samples of wheat grain/flour.[69]

Wheat is usually stored for an extended period, with the potential risk of heavy insect infestation. Storage and transportation of wheat is a critical stage, and must be given full attention; hence spraying or fumigation has become a normal agricultural practice when storing grains. A large number of pesticides are used for the protection of stored grains.[70,71] The grains are treated with degradable pesticides, including organophosphate pesticides, carbamates, synthetic pyrethroids, and insect growth regulators, to prevent insect infestation during storage. There are two principal sources of pesticides in wheat grains: those pesticides sprayed on growing crops,[72,73] and the combination of pesticides added to stored grains.[74] Once pesticides have contaminated the grain, they gain entry into food chain, with consequential health hazards for human beings.[75]

The rice weevil, {Sitophilus oryzae L. (Coleoptera: Curculionidae)} and lesser grain borer, {Rhyzopertha dominica F. (Coleoptera: Bostrychidae)} are the world wide stored grain insect pests which cause more destruction. They are categorized into primary colonies, which indicates that pests of this specie are able to pervading/infesting healthy grains very easily which is impossible for majority of stored grain pests immature stages of these species

TABLE 20.4 Fate of Pesticide Residues (mg/kg) during Wheat Storage

| Pesticides | Storage Interval (Months) | | | | | | | References |
	0	1	2	3	4	6	9	
Chlorpyriphos-methyl	–	–	–	1.11	–	1.01	0.69	Afridi et al., 2001[85]
Pirimiphos-Methyl	–	–	–	2.22	–	1.47	0.61	
Permethrin	–	–	–	1.47	–	1.28	1.04	
Deltamethrin	0.53	0.52	–	0.52	–	0.51	–	Balinova et al.[87]
Deltamethrin	7.35	4.85	3.69	3.09	2.76	–	–	Pal and Shah[78]
Chlorpyrifos	2.84	1.89	1.68	1.92	0.78	–	–	
Fipronil	4.43	2.93	2.73	3.11	2.18	–	–	
α-Endosulfan	2.25	1.35	1.09	1.95	0.90	–	–	
β-Endosulfan	1.25	1.10	0.86	0.77	0.41	–	–	
γ-Endosulfan	3.50	2.45	1.95	2.73	1.31	–	–	
λ-Cyhalothrin	4.24	3.09	2.57	2.61	2.25	–	–	
Malathion	8.89	7.07	6.26	5.60	4.28	–	–	Uygun et al.[89]
Isomalathion	0.31	0.36	0.43	0.42	0.57	–	–	
Fenitrothion	24.5	18.1	17.1	–	–	–	–	
Chlorpyrifos-methyl	1.09	1.08	0.83	0.86	0.76	–	–	Fleurat-Lessard et al.[88]
Permethrin	1.51	1.45	–	1.47	–	–	–	Saka et al.[86]
Piperonyl butoxide	2.41	2.14	–	2.43	–	–	–	
Chlorpyrifos-methyl	2.73	1.60	–	1.48	–	–	–	
Fenitrothion	5.15	3.03	–	2.20	–	–	–	
Malathion	4.15	2.72	–	2.21	–	–	–	
Carbaryl	5.22	4.00	–	3.40	–	–	–	

are not much affected by grain protectants that are applied to the external part of the kernel. However the juvenile of these species are unaffected by the protectants applied on the external side of the grain kernals. The most serious insect pest of the milling industries are the rusty grain beetle, Cryptolestesferrugineus (Stephens) (Coleoptera: Laemophloeidae) and confused flour beetle, Triboliumconfusum (DuVal) (Coleoptera: Tenebrionidae). The species which feed on broken and already infested grains are classified as secondary colonisers.[77]

In most cereal-producing countries, several insecticides are currently registered for application to cereals. Contact insecticide admixture with grain entering stores is widely used to give long-term protection from reinfestation. Active substances with extended persistent insecticidal effects are most commonly used for this purpose. The most commonly used insecticides against insect attack during wheat grain storage are organochlorines, organophosphates, and synthetic pyrethroids.[78] Ability of long time protection of grain protectants is desirable.

In stored wheat, chemicals like pyrethroid, deltamethrin, α-cypermethrin and β-cyfluthrin, provide long-lasting protection for more than 4 month against S. oryzae.[79] Spinosad, a new insecticide cause low mammalian toxicity which based on actinomycete, saccaropolyspora and spinosad metabolites.[80] This pesticides has wide range of target classes and in many parts of the world registered against numerous pests. It proved imperative replacement of conventional grain protectants, as it is already registered in USA for this use.[81] On the exposure to ultra violet radiation, Spinosad breakdown rapidly[82] and its effectiveness varied among different wheat classes.[83] Spinosad dose (rat oral LD50 > 5000 mg/kg of body weight) is measured as harmless because of its low toxicity and very lethal for R. dominica, S. oryzae or C. ferrugineus.[84] The affect of storage on insecticide residues after postharvest application of pesticides show that residues degrade slowly and gradually.[84] (Table 20.4).[78,85–89]

Grain type, water activity, temperature and light govern the rate of insecticide degradation during storage.

Insecticide residues are also found to be penetrating inside the kernals throughout storage and ultimately mount up with passage of time.[25,26] Residues remaining in the grain after treatments can continue to kill insects over a long period of time.[88] It was reported that malathion is less persistant compared to chlorpyrifos-methyl and pirimiphos-methyl.[26] Organophosphate (Malathion and fenitrothion) insecticides are broadly applied as stored grains protectants. During application of insecticide in the form of dust or liquid, substantial quantities of residues persist on surface of wheat while certain amount also penetrate to internal portion. Ultimately, insecticide remains higher in bran compared to wheat flour. In stored wheat and its products the residues of fenitrothion, malathion and isomalathion, have been reported throughout the storage.[89]

Dissipation of pesticide residues during different storage intervals are depicted in Table 20.4.

FATE OF PESTICIDE RESIDUES IN WHEAT MILLING

Whole wheat grains in the form of flour and its milling products have become an essential part of the human diet. Grains are frequently stored for long periods (3–36 months) at ambient temperature in bulk silos, where pesticides may be applied as a post-harvest treatment to reduce losses due to storage pests. Pesticides from a broad range of classes are used widely throughout the world, in various combinations, at different stages of cultivation and during post-harvest storage to protect food commodities against a wide range of pests and to ensure maintenance of quality. The summary of pesticide residues in some milling fractions is presented in Table 20.5.[89–91] Details regarading pesticide residues in milling fractions of wheat are summarized below.

Whole Grain/Whole Wheat Flour

Residues of post-harvest applied pesticides on wheat grains may accumulate and persist during milling and processing. The level of residues depends largely on the type and quantity of the chemical used, the formulation in which it was applied, the temperature and moisture content of the grain during milling, the procedure used in processing of grain during storage, and the length of time elapsing between the application of pesticide and consumption of the food.[92]

Phoxim-methyl residues on wheat were determined by applying at the dose rate of 10 ppm. Very small amounts of residues of phoxim-methyl were found in whole wheat flour as compared to other fractions.[93] Permethrin residues in whole ground grain ranged from 1.378 ± 0.190 to 0.247 ± 0.026 mg/kg in wheat treated at 2 mg a.i. (active ingredient) permethrin/kg, and from 7.40 ± 0.234 to 1.294 ± 0.017 mg/kg in wheat treated at 8 mg a.i. permethrin/kg.[94] The residues in the whole grain were found to be 1.84 ppm after applying deltamethrin which reduced to 1.06 ppm in milled grains.[95] In a separate study, wheat grain was treated with 12 ppm of pirimiphos-methyl and decreased levels of contaminant were shown in processed products as compared to whole grain, whereas whole flour showed about the same level as in grain.[96] Generally, the residue levels of chlorpyrifos-methyl in flour are 1.6- to 5.6-fold lower than in the whole grain.

A study conducted by Fleurat-Lessard and colleagues[91] applied pirimiphos-methyl (PMM) at 10 mg/kg and found that the amounts of PMM measured in whole grain were close to the expected dose – i.e., 10.28 and 9.60 mg/kg for the *Primadur* and *Ardent* cultivars, respectively.

Residues of deltamethrin in the whole grain were 1.84 ppm compared to milled whole grain, which contained 1.06 ppm,[95] and similar results were obtained for phoxim-methyl and pirimiphos-methyl, as described by

TABLE 20.5   Residue Levels of Different Pesticides in Wheat and Milling Fractions (mg/kg)

Pesticide	Whole Grain	Bran	Flour	Semolina	Reference
Malathion	8.89	9.85	0.639	–	Uygun et al.[89]
Isomalathion	0.315	0.133	0.016	–	
Fenitrothion	24.5	34.3	2.35	–	
Malaoxon	0.037	0.027	–	–	
Malathion	61.25	102.50	7.20	–	Uygun et al.[89]
Chlorpyrifos-methyl	18.8	32.9	3.69	–	
Chlorpyrifos-methyl	9.9	5	–	2.7	Balinova et al.[90]
Pirimiphos-methyl	15.6	6.8	–	5.2	
Pirimiphos-methyl	3.49	2.143	0.125	0.417	Fleurat-Lessard et al.[91]

Alnaji and Kadoum.[93] Whole wheat grain was treated with 12 ppm pirimiphos-methyl. Grain processing operations decreased the level of pesticide contamination in processed products, compared to whole grain, as described by Sgarbiero.[97] Ninety five percent reduction in malathion was recorded through milling of wheat to flour from an initial level of 8.89 ppm, as described by Uygun.[89]

Cracked wheat from a local market in Ankara (Turkey) was examined to check residue levels of organochlorine pesticides, including quintozene (PCNB), dichlorodiphenyl trichloroethane (p,p-DDT), dichlorodiphenyl dichloroethylene (p,p-DDE), and dichlorodiphenyl dichloroethane (p,p-DDD). The results of this study revealed that whole wheat enclosed PCNB and lindane residues, although the quantities of residues were found to be within FAO tolerance limits.[98]

Bran

Many pesticide residues are concentrated in the wheat bran and depleted in flour when wheat is milled. As a result higher levels of residues are present in bran compared to wheat, mostly by a factor of about 2–6. Higher residues in bran were observed compared to flour, even for pesticides which pass in through translocation.[26] Residual levels of deltamethrin, permethrin, phenothrin and fenvalerate were noticed to be more persistent on bran. After milling, these residues were highly accumulated in the bran compared to white flour.[99] The bran removal resulted in reduction of malathion significantly due to the presence of chemical residue in the outer surface of the grain.[89]

As already reported, seed coat can retain the pesticides and these residues then concentrate in the bran and germ portions of the grains, which contain significantly higher levels of triglycerides, and resultantly the lipophilicity of the chemical residues in the processed grain can give the idea of their fate during grain milling as well as in the processed food. Residues of the lipophilic pyrethrins tend to remain on the seed coat, although a proportion can migrate through the bran and germ, which contain high levels of triglyceride, to the other milling fractions.[100] Furthermore, Balinova[90] reported that the residues of chlorpyrifos-methyl and pirimiphos-methyl determined in semolina were only slightly lower than the residues in bran, and were, respectively, 2.0- to 3.6-fold and 1.3- to 3.2-fold as high as those on the whole grain.

In the case of recently treated grains, the bran coat contains almost all the PMM residues; the transfer of residues to the semolina and flour fractions can reasonably be attributed to a translocation phenomenon generated by friction and crushing at the beginning of the milling process of the different products that will be separated at a later step of the process. It was also observed by Fleurat-Lessard[91] that most of the PMM residues appeared in bran. The total bran/thirds fractions obtained from milled grain contained 79.5% and 74.5% of the total amount of PMM residue in all the fractions for *Primadur* and *Ardent* varieties, respectively. Higher contamination of semolina by the bran coat fractions observed with the large-kernel cultivar *Ardent* may have been induced by amplified friction during the breaking stage, as described by Skerritt.[101]

White Flour, Semolina, and Related Milling Fractions

In addition to grain handlers and traders, cereal processing companies and regulatory agencies keep a close eye on different fraction of cereals. For processors, analysis of baked or cooked end products and intermediate products such as flours are also important in terms of their safety regarding chemicals.

The distribution of pesticide in different fractions of milled grains was studied by Balinova.[87] Eight fractions of milled grain, including bran, semolina, three types of groats, and three types of flour, were collected and analyzed for pesticide residues. The limits of determination of both pesticides were 0.005 mg/kg, which is good enough for enforcement of the European Commission (EC) Directive that established a MRL of 0.01 mg/kg for any pesticide in cereal-based baby food. He further suggested that milling did not significantly reduce the bulk of the chemicals but resulted in distribution of residues in various processed products. The main part of the insecticides deposited on the grain remained in the outer part of the seed and partly in semolina fractions.

Milling tests were conducted to determine the pesticide residues in white flour derived from wheat. Samples analyzed included flour, bran, shorts, and germs.[102] In most cases, cleaning removed only a small amount of pesticides in all milling fractions. Very little residue was carried over into the flour: 0–0.8 ppm from malathion applied at 2.5–7.5 ppm; 0.8–1.8 ppm from methoxychlor applied at 5–50 ppm; and 1.3–2.6 ppm from lindane applied at 2.5–7.5 ppm.

In the latest studies[78] addressing grain milling and fragmentation of the pesticide residues (malathion, isomalathion, chlorpyrifos-methyl, fenitrothion, pirimiphos-methyl), a substantial portion of the insecticides is found to be dissipated in the semolina fractions. The carryover percentage of malathion, fenitrothion, chlorpyrifos-methyl and pirimiphos methyl from wheat to semolina was 16–28%, 17–22%, 7–8% and 23–28%, respectively.[103] Water activity may adequately explain the varied reductions of pesticides in wheat through milling into white flour; the diminution of fenitrothion and malathion was nearly 95–100%.[89] However, deltamethrin was declined by 57.6%[95] in wheat by converting grain into flour through milling.

In order to determine the behavior of residual dynamics of fenitrothion and melathion (malaoxon and isomalathion) during storage and processing (milling and baking), pesticide free wheat was procured from supervised field trails. Dusting of 2% melathion was done after placing wheat in sealed plastic container. Fenitrothion emulsion (41.6% wettable powder) was applied onto the walls of a pilot-scale container. Results revealed that flour produced by milling of wheat was having lowest residual level compared to other milling fractions. Reduction of malathion residues was about 95% in wheat through milling to flour.[89]

Before using in different form, wheat grains are usually milled into different fractions, therefore mutual effect of milling and storage time is of utmost importance. Deltamethrin applied at 0.5 ppm resulted in residues of between 0.03 and 0.20 ppm in the various types of white flour.[87]

Residues of deltamethrin, fenvalerate, permethrin, and phenothrin were determined during milling and insecticide residues majorly concentrated in the bran and to lesser extent in other fractions.[99] The concentration of pirimiphos-methyl residues in flour is 2.1- to 3.4-fold lower than that of residues on the whole grain.[90] In certain studies, the insecticide residues have been observed to be penetrating inside the grain and ultimately distributed in milling fractions.[25,26]

DISSIPATION OF PESTICIDE RESIDUES IN BAKED WHEAT PRODUCTS

Cereal grains in general, and wheat in particular, provide the raw material for the main food items of all the regional diets in the world. In order to safeguard the wheat against different pests, chemicals are used throughout the world as grain protectants. Consumers are increasingly interested in the fate of pesticide residues during processing of food commodities, requiring realistic estimates of the dietary intake of the pesticides through different processed/refined wheat products (e.g., bread, pasta, cookies, etc). For better protection of the health of consumers, particularly children, there should be particular emphasis on investigating pesticide residues in wheat products, and their dissipation.

Transfer Ratio of Pesticide Residues for Wheat Products

The transfer ratio can be defined as the percentage of pesticide residue in the product divided by the quantity of pesticide residue in the raw material or initial product. Different pesticides exhibit different transfer ratios in different products, depending on differences in the nature and physicochemical properties of pesticides, and also the different unit operations that add value to the produce.

Dissipation of Pesticide Residues in Bread

Bread is a popular leavened baked product which is formulated by two major steps of processing; namely, yeast fermentation of dough, followed by baking at high temperature. Both of these processes contribute to the degradation of residual pesticides. The role of microbes in pesticide degradation is well known. Bakery yeast can degrade most of the pesticides within the organochlorine and pyrethroid groups, as well as organophosphates.[104,105] In baking, when fermented dough is subjected to heat, pesticide residues are dissipated through some physicochemical processes, e.g., co-distillation, evaporation and thermal degradation which vary with the chemical nature of the each insecticide.[106] During this process, the water contained in cells retains pesticide molecules (co-distillation), while heat causes evaporation and degradation.[107] Degradation of pesticides such as hexaconazole, propiaconazole, and deltamethrin depends upon their vapor pressure.[108,109] Contrarily, the binding capability of some pesticides with the medium reduces the activity of microorganisms.[110] Considerable loss of pesticides (47–89%) was observed in the breadmaking process. Pesticide degradation during the process showed negative correlation with the concentration of pesticides in wheat flour. The presence of endosulfan, hexaconazole, and propiaconazole in the matrix also negatively affected the growth of the yeast by 7.5–33.5%, 12.5–44.7%, and 11–40%, respectively. However, other pesticides, such as malathion, chlorpyriphos, and deltamethrin, did not show any significant effect on yeast growth. Such information is critical, and supporting studies are required in order for more realistic estimates to be made regarding the dietary intake of pesticides for humans. Furthermore, it would help in formulating regulatory guidelines regarding the management of residues on such products by fixing or re-evaluating MRLs for quality assurance and control purposes. The level of pesticide degradation is also dependent upon the initial quantity of pesticide residue. Knowledge of this would allow the highest degradation/removal of pesticide residues (75–89%) with the lowest amount of pesticides. However, variation in dissipation of the residues of individual pesticides during the breadmaking process was observed due to differences in physicochemical properties of the pesticides. In this regard, degradation of endosulfan residue was maximal (70%) followed by deltamethrin (63%), malathion (60%), propiaconazole (52%), chlorpyriphos (51%), and hexaconazole (46%) (Table 20.6).[78,103,109,111]

TABLE 20.6 Dissipation of Pesticide Residue (%) in Baked Wheat Products in Comparison to Wheat Grain/Flour*

Product	Pesticide	% Residue Dissipation	References
Bread	Endosulfan	70*	Sharma et al.[109]
	Deltamethrin	63*	
	Malathion	60*	
	Propiaconazole	52*	
	Chlorpyriphos	51*	
	Hexaconazole	46*	
Bread	Chlorpyrifos	25	Pal and Shah[78]
	Fipronil	63	
	Deltamethrin	61	
	Lamda-cyhalothrin	75	
Chapatti	Chlorpyrifos	49	Pal and Shah[78]
	Fipronil	63	
	Deltamethrin	57	
	Lamda-cyhalothrin	71	
Pasta	Malathion	98	Uygun et al.[103]
	Fenitrothion	96	
	Chlorpyrifos methyl	98	
	Pirimiphos methyl	90	
Cookies	Malathion	80	Uygun et al.[111]
	Chlorpyrifos-methyl	76	

Studies without asterisks show the percent dissipation of pesticide residues in baked bread in comparison to the wheat grain used for preparation of bread.
* *Percent dissipation of pesticide residues in baked bread in comparison to flour used for preparing that bread.*

The transfer ratio is also affected by the type of bread – for example, in whole meal bread maximum transfer ratios have been observed in comparison to white bread. On average, in whole meal bread the transfer rate of pesticides residues was more than 50%. A comparative study of white bread and whole meal bread for six applied insecticides (namely permethrin, piperonyl butoxide, chlorpyrifos-methyl, fenithrothion, malathion, and carbaryl) indicated that post-harvest processing of the wheat into whole meal bread had a greater transfer rate of pesticide residues than with white bread (Table 20.7). The transfer ratio of carbofuran was the lowest among all the pesticides studied. These investigations are useful in establishing the maximum residual limits of pesticides as well as helping to determine the authentic/actual levels of pesticide residues in bread.[86] The pesticide residue transfer ratio varies from 1.7–10% for white bread and from 53–101% in whole meal bread.

TABLE 20.7 Transfer Ratio of Pesticide Residues in White and Whole Meal Bread

	Transfer Ratio of Residues (%)	
Pesticide	White Bread	Whole Meal Bread
Permethrin	9.0	93
Piperonyl butoxide	10	101
Chlorpyrifos-methyl	10	98
Fenitrothion	4.4	81
Malathion	5.4	86
Carbaryl	1.7	53

Adapted from Saka et al.[86]

Dissipation of Pesticide Residues in Pasta

Pasta is another important value added food product produced by durum wheat milling into semolina. A considerable amount of pesticides are present in semolina. It is important to investigate the amount of some chemical residues like organophosphates to the consumers through food chain and particularly in the grains.[103] In semolina and spaghetti, pesticides residue levels were investigated during processing of stored wheat at different time periods. After storage of 2 months, residue levels of chlorpyrifos-methyl and malathion in semolina significantly decreased with the same dissipation rate of insecticides as in the stored wheat which can be attributed to the temperature fluctuation. However, the residues level of pirimophos-methyl and fenitrothion reduced slowly, showing that during storage increased temperature did not influenced them. The lowest reduction of pirimophos-methyl residues was reported in semolina. The heating and ventilation process in pasta making increased the volatilization and degradation rate of pesticide residues particularly during time of drying. In the samples of 4 months stored wheat spaghetti, the level of residues, e.g. chlorpyriphos-methyl, malathion and pirimiphos-methyl were not detected and just after 3 months of storage fenitrothion was undetectable. In the spaghetti from 90 and 120 days stored wheat, chlorpyrifos-methyl pesticide was detected with low residue level.[86] The carryover percentages of the pesticides from wheat to semolina and spaghetti are presented in Table 20.8.[111,103] Insecticides of the more lipophilic materials have a tendency to persist on the seed coat.[26] The percent amount of malathion residues were comparatively lower from semolina to spaghetti than that of chemical residues from raw wheat to semolina. Volatilization process, principal phenomena affecting the amount of pesticide residues, can be explained by the higher vapour pressure of malathion. Physicochemical characteristics of malathion affirmed it most affected

TABLE 20.8 Carryover Percentages of the Pesticides from Wheat to Semolina/Flour and Spaghetti/Cookies on Step-Wise Basis

Product	Pesticide	From Wheat to Semolina/Flour (%)	From Semolina/Flour to Spaghetti/Cookies (%)	References
Pasta	Malathion	16	7	Uygun et al.[103]
	Fenitrothion	17	49	
	Chlorpyrifos-methyl	8	21	
	Primiphos-methyl	25	23	
Cookies	Malathion	12	27	Uygun et al.[111]
	Chlorpyrifos-methyl	20	40	

chemical substance during spaghetti making process and considerably during drying at 40°C for 20 hours. For remaining pesticide residues, the residual percent amount was found higher than malathion. Fenitrothion is less persistent than pirimiphos-methyl in wheat. However, the transfer ratio of fenitrothion pesticide residues during spaghetti making from wheat is higher than pirimiphos-methyl. This difference may be due to their methods of application and physic-chemical characteristics. Higher amount of residues were expected when pesticides are directly applied on grains.[112] The carried over residues of chlorpyrifos-methyl from wheat to semolina and spaghetti were less than pirimiphos-methyl residues. Due to physic-chemical characteristics of pirimiphos-methyl, it is less affected during milling and process of spaghetti making. The study of insecticidal behavior revealed that higher amount of pirimiphos-methyl was present in spaghetti due to its low vapour pressure (2 mPa at 20°C).

Dissipation of Pesticide Residues in Cookies

Cookies are one of the best-known snack products. Their consumption is considerable throughout the world, currently running at around 40 packets per person per year,[113] and they are also a significant part of children's diets. Therefore, special emphasis should be placed on the fate of pesticide residues in cookies for better protection of consumers – especially malathion and chlorpyrifos-methyl residues. These pesticides are commonly found in wheat grains and are used as residual insecticides to prevent insect pest attacks on wheat. Therefore, there is a greater chance of their contamination in wheat flour and, ultimately, the cookies. MRLs established by the EC for malathion and chlorpyrifos-methyl in wheat are 8 mg/kg and 3 mg/kg, respectively. Conditions used in the cooking process of cookies, such as high temperature (205°C) and degree of moisture loss, are important for their quantitative effects on residue levels. Chlorpyrifos-methyl is more persistent than malathion and is degraded less, comparatively, during cookie processing due to its physicochemical properties.[111] The carryover

percentage of malathion residues has been found to be about 27% from flour to cookies. Pesticide residues tend to move into the deeper layers of the grain and thereby contaminate the flour.[26] The initial concentration of chlorpyrifos-methyl in wheat has been reported to be significantly lower than that of malathion prior to cookie formulation; this is mainly due to the lipophilic properties of the pesticide, which is retained by the fat in the cookies.

CONCLUSION

The world population is increasing day by day, and wheat is one of the most important cereal crops to satisfy world hunger. In order to achieve greater production of wheat with limited land resources, pesticides play a very important role by preventing wheat from attack by insect pests, weeds, nematodes, etc. Residual pesticides are also applied for safe storage of wheat for later use. The use of pesticides requires great care and control, as they pollute the environment and harm human health. Field-incurred pesticide residues, and residues as a result of post-harvest insecticide treatments on stored grains, generally decline slowly. Data regarding pesticide residues on wheat call for an investigation into the level of pesticide residues in cereal-based foods and for strict regulation by government and industry to ensure public health. The processing of wheat results in reduction of pesticide residues. Mitigation of pesticide residues during processing is affected by the nature of the pesticide, the type of food, and the severity of the processing procedure used; hence, a combination of processing techniques would address the current situation in food safety. Both wheat milling and prerequisites of milling, like wet washing, reduce the pesticide residues in white flour and other milling fractions. However, the situation is much worst with bran. Because bran is a concentrated source of pesticides and much of the pesticides are not able to penetrate deep inside the layers of wheat kernel, the bran is rendered unsafe for human consumption. Conversely, the endosperm is less contaminated by pesticides. Bran should be used with care for human food purposes, as it can contaminate food products with a high load of pesticides, particularly if wheat has been stored and protected by long-acting residual pesticides. Pesticide residues are also dissipated during breadmaking, and manufacture of cookies, pasta, and related products. Pesticides residue in the processed food products are usually much below MRL values.

References

1. Krol WJ, Arsenault TL, Pylypiw HM, Mattina MJI. Reduction of pesticide residues on produce by rinsing. *J Agric Food Chem* 2000;**48**:4666–70.

2. Goto T, Ito Y, Oka H, Saito I, Matsumoto H, Nakazawa H. Simple and rapid determination of N-methylcarbamate pesticides in citrus fruits by electrospray ionization tandem mass spectrometry. *Anal Chim Acta* 2003;**487**:201–9.

3. Maroni M, Fait A. Health effects in man from long-term exposure to pesticides. A review of the 1975–1991 literature. *Toxicology* 1993;**78**:1–3.

4. Dalvie MA, White N, Raine R, Myers JE, Thompson M, London L. Long term respiratory health effects of the herbicide paraquat, among workers in the Western Cape. *Occup Environ Med* 1999;**56**:391–6.

5. Abou-Donia MB. Organophosphorus ester-induced chronic neurotoxicity. *Arch Environ Health* 2003;**58**:484–97.

6. Galloway T, Handy R. Immunotoxicity of organophosphorous pesticides. *Ecotoxicology* 2003;**12**:345–63.

7. Choi SM, Yoo SD, Lee BM. Toxicological characteristics of endocrine disrupting chemicals: developmental toxicity, carcinogenicity, and mutagenicity. *J Toxicol Environ Health B Crit Rev* 2004;**7**:1–24.

8. Solomon G, Ogunseitan OA, Kirsch J. *Pesticides and Human Health: A Resource for Health Care Professionals. Physicians for Social Responsibility.* San Francisco, CA: Los Angeles and Californians for Pesticide Reform; 2000. p. 60.

9. FAO. *FAOSTAT Statistical data*; 2012. Available at: Faostat.fao.org.

10. European Food Safety Authority (EFSA). The 2009 European Union Report on Pesticide Residues in Food. *European food safety authority Journal* 2011;**9**:2430.

11. Fleurat-Lessard F, Wilbert T, Vidal ML. Models linking insecticidal efficacy decline and residues concentration decrease with time, temperature and water activity in chlorpyrifos-methyl treated wheat. In: Credland PF, Armitage DM, Bell CH, Cogan PM, Highley E, editors. Advances in Stored Product Protection. Proceedings of the Eighth International Working Conference on Stored Product Protection, 22-26 July 2002, York, UK. CAB International, Wallingford, UK, pp. 639–645.

12. Ecobichon DJ. Pesticide use in developing countries. *Toxicology* 2001;**160**:27–33.

13. Sondhia S. Leaching behavior of metsulfuron in two texturally different soils. *Environ Monit Assess* 2009;**154**:111–5.

14. Arias-Estevez M, Lopez-Periago E, Mejuto JC, Martınez-Carballo E, Simal-Gandara J, Garcıa-Rıo L. The mobility and degradation of pesticides in soils and the pollution of groundwater resources. *Agriculture, Ecosystems & Environment* 2008;**123**:247–60.

15. Rial-Otero R, Cancho-Grande B, Arias-Estevez M, Lopez-Periago E, Simal-Gandara J. Procedure for the measurement of soil inputs of plant-protection agents washed off through vineyard canopy by rainfalls. *J Agric Food Chem* 2003;**51**:5041–6.

16. Ngo MA, Malley M, Howard I. Maibach. Percutaneous absorption and exposure assessment of pesticides. *J Appl Toxicol* 2010;**30**:91–114.

17. Kamanyire R, Karalliedde L. Organophosphate toxicity and occupational exposure. *Occup Med* 2004;**54**:69–75.

18. Lifshitz M, Shahak E, Sofer S. Carbamate and organophosphate poisoning in young children. *Paediatrics Emerging Care* 1999;**15**:102–3.

19. Cantalamessa F. Acute toxicity of two pyrethroids, permethrin, and cypermethrin in neonatal and adult rats. *Arch Toxicol* 1993;**67**:510–3.

20. Ashby J, Kier L, Wilson A, Green T, Willis GA, Heydens WF, et al. Evaluation of the potential carcinogenicity and genetic toxicity to humans of the herbicide acetochlor. *Hum Exp Toxicol* 1996;**15**:702–35.

21. Dalvie MA, Africa A, London L. Change in the quantity and acute toxicity of pesticides sold in South African crop sectors, 1994-1999. *Environ Int* 2009;**35**:683–7.

22. Potter WT, Rong S, Griffith J, White J, Garry VF. Phosphine-mediated Heinz body formation and hemoglobin oxidation in human erythrocytes. *Toxicol Lett* 1991;**57**:37–45.

23. Hanley Jr TR, Calhoun LL, Kociba RJ, Greene JA. The effects of inhalation exposure to sulfuryl fluoride on fetal development in rats and rabbits. *Fundam Appl Toxicol* 1989;**13**:79–86.

24. Mishra K, Sharma RC. Assessment of organochlorine pesticides in human milk and risk exposure to infants from North-East India. *Sci Total Environ* 2011;**409**:4939–49.

25. Desmarchelier JM. Loss of fenitrothion on grains in storage. *Pesticide Science* 1978;**9**:33–8.

26. Holland PT, Hamilton D, Ohlin B, Skidmore MW. Effects of storage and processing on pesticide residues in plant products. IUPAC Reports on Pesticides (31). *Pure Appl Chem* 1994;**66**:335–56.

27. Tewary DK, Kumar VP, Ravindranath SD, Shanker A. Dissipation behavior of bifenthrin residues in tea and its brew. *Food Contam* 2005;**16**:231–7.

28. Arias-Estevez M. Lo pez-Periago E, Martınez-Carballo E, Simal-Gandara J. Carbofuran absorption kinetics by corn crop soils. *Bull Environ Contam Toxicol* 2006;**77**:267–73.

29. Pateiro-Moure M, Arias-Estevez M, Lopez-Periago E. Martınez-Carballo Elena, Simal-Gandara, Jesus. Occurrence and down slope mobilization of quaternary herbicide residues in vineyard-devoted soils. *Bull Environ Contam Toxicol* 2008;**80**:407–11.

30. Cabras P, Angioni A, Garau VL, Melis M, Pirisi FM, Karim M, et al. Persistence of insecticide residues in olives and olive oil. *J Agric Food Chem* 1997;**45**:2244–7.

31. Guardia RM, Ruiz MA, Molina DA, Canada AMJ. Influence of harvesting mehod and washing on the presence of pesticide residues in olives and olive oil. *J Agric Food Chem* 2006;**54**:8538–44.

32. Angioni A, Schirra M, Garau VL, Melis M, Tuberoso CIG, Cabras P. Residues of azoxystrobin, fenhexamid and pyrimethanil in strawberry following field treatments and the effect of domestic washing. *Food Addit Contam* 2004;**21**:1065–70.

33. Guardia RM, Ruiz MA, Molina DA, Canada AMJ. Multiresidue analysis of three groups of pesticides in washing waters from olive processing by solid-phase extraction-gas chromatograhy with electron capture and thermionic specific detection. *Microchem J* 2007;**85**:257–64.

34. Cengiz MF, Certel M, Karakas B, Goçmen H. Residue contents of captan and procymidone applied on tomatoes grown in greenhouses and their reduction by duration of a re-harvest interval and post-harvest culinary applications. *Food Chem* 2007;**100**:1611–9.

35. Boulaid M, Aguilera A, Camacho F, Soussi M, Valverde A. Effect of household processing and unit-to-unit variability of pyrifenox, pyridaben and tralomethrin residues in tomatoes. *J Agric Food Chem* 2005;**53**:4054–8.

36. Randhawa MA, Anjum FM, Ahmed A, Randhawa MS. Field incurred chlorpyrifos and 3,5,6-trichloro-2-pyridinol residues in fresh and processed vegetables. *Food Chem* 2007;**103**:1016–23.

37. Lentza-Rizos Ch, Kokkinaki K. Residues of cypermethrin in field-treated grapes and raisins produced after various treatments. *Food Addit Contam* 2002;**19**:1162–8.

38. Pugliese P, Molto JC, Damiani P, Marin R, Cossignani L, Manes J. Gas chromatographic evaluation of pesticide residue contents in nectarines after nontoxic washing treatments. *J Chromatogr A* 2004;**1050**:185–91.

39. Cabras P, Angioni A, Garau VL, Melis M, Pirisi FM, Cabitza F. Pesticide residues in raisin processing. *J Agric Food Chem* 1998;**46**:2309–11.

40. Baur P, Buchholz A, Schonherr J. Diffusion in plant cuticles as affected by temperature and size of organic solutes: similarity and diversity among species. *Plant Cell Environ* 1997;**20**:982–94.

41. Randhawa MA, Anjum MN, Butt MS, Yasin M, Imran M. Minimization of imidacloprid residues in cucumber and bell pepper through washing with citric acid and acetic acid solutions and their dietary intake assessment. *International J Food Properties* 2012. doi IJFP-2011-0640.R2.

42. Femenia A, Sanchez ES, Simal S, Rossello C. Effects of drying pretreatments on the cell wall composition of grape tissues. *J Agric Food Chem* 1998;**46**:271–6.

43. Joint Meeting on Pesticide Residues. Refers to the FAO Plant Production and Production Paper series "Pesticide Residues in Food-Evaluations Part 1", published annually by FAO. *Rome* 1992 (Each issue summarizes residue data submitted to the previous JMPR meeting and is organized by pesticide in alphabetical order.).

44. Randhawa MA, Anjum FM, Randhawa MS, Ahmed A, Farooq U, Abrar M, et al. Dissipation of deltamethrin on supervised vegetables and removal of its residue by household processing. *Journal of the Chem Soc Pak* 2008;**30**:227–31.

45. Rasmusssen RR, Poulsen ME, Hansen HCB. Distribution of multiple pesticide residues in apple segments after home processing. *Food Addit Contam* 2003;**20**:1044–63.

46. Burchat CS, Ripley BD, Leishmann PD, Ritcey GM, Kakuda Y, Stephenson GR. The distribution of nine pesticides between the juice and pulp of carrots and tomatoes after home processing. *Food Addit Contam* 1998;**15**:61–71.

47. Clavijo MP, Medina MP, Asensio JS, Bernal JG. Decay study of pesticide residues in apple samples. *J Chromatogr A* 1996;**740**: 146–50.

48. Celik S, Kunc S, Asan T. Degradation of some pesticides in the field and effect of processing. *Analyst* 1995;**120**:1739–43.

49. Rouchaud J, Gustin F, Creemers P, Goffings G, Herrgods M. Fate of the fungicide tolylfluanid in pear cold stored in controlled or non controlled atmosphere. *Bull Environ Contam Toxicol* 1991;**46**:499–506.

50. Fernandez-Cruz ML, Villarroya M, Llanos S, Alonso-Prados JL, Garcia-Baudin JM. Field incurred fenitrothion residues in kakis: comparison of individual fruits, composite samples, peeled and cooked fruits. *J Agric Food Chem* 2004;**52**:860–3.

51. Edwards VT, McMinn AL, Wright AN. In: Hutson D, Roberts T, editors. *Progress in Pesticide Biochemistry*, **vol. 2**. Chichester, UK: Wiley; 1982. p. 71–125.

52. Ahmed A, Randhawa MA, Yusuf MJ, Khalid N. Effect of processing on the pesticide residues in food crops – A Review. *J Agric Res* 2011;**49**:379–90.

53. Fernandez-Cruz ML, Barreda M, Villarroya M, Peruga A, Llanos S, Garcia-Baudin JM. Captan and fenitrothion dissipation in field-treated cauliflowers and effect of household processing. *Pest Manag Sci* 2006;**62**:637–45.

54. Holden AJ, Chen L, Shaw IC. Thermal stability of organophosphorus pesticide triazophos and its relevance in the assessment of risk to the consumer of triazophos residues in food. *J Agric Food Chem* 2001;**49**:103–6.

55. Nagayama T. Behavior of residual organophosphorus pesticides in foodstuffs during leaching or cooking. *J Agric Food Chem* 1996;**44**:2388–93.

56. Joia BS, Webster GRB, Loschiavo SR. Cypermethrin and fenvalerate residues in stored wheat and milled fractions. *J Agric Food Chem* 1985;**33**:618–22.

57. Dhaliwal GS, Arora R. *Principles of insect pest management*. Ludhiana, India: National Agricultural Technology Information Centre; 1996.

58. Bhatia SK. Insect Pests. *Wheat research in India*. ICAR, New Dehli, India: Ramanujam; 1978.

59. Singh VS, Singh RN, Trivedi TP, Sehgal M, Ashok K. Pest management strategies in wheat. *Training mannual No. 6*. New Delhi, India: NCIPM; 1999. p. 40–7.

60. Bindra OS, Singh H. Gujhiaweevil *Tanymecusindicus* Faust (Coleoptera: Curculionidae). *Pesticides* 1970;**4**:16–8.

61. Skrbic B. Organochlorine and organophosphate pesticide residues in wheat varieties from Serbia. *Food Addit Contam* 2007;**24**:695–703.

62. *US Food and Drug Administration (FDA)*. FDA, US: Pesticide Program Residue Monitoring, 2003; 2005.

63. *Commission of the European Communities (CEC)*. Norway, Iceland and Liechtenstein. CEC, Brussels: Monitoring of Pesticide Residues in Products of Plant Origin in the European Union; 2005.

64. *UK. Pesticides Residues Committee (PRC)*. PRC, UK: Annual Review of the Pesticides Residues Committee; 2006.

65. Sawaya WN, Awadhi F, Saeed T, Al-Omair A, Husain A, Ahmad N, et al. Dietary intake of organophosphate pesticides in Kuwait. *Food Chem* 2000;**69**:331–8.

66. Guler GO, Cakmak YS, Dagli Z, Aktumsek A, Ozparlak H. Organochlorine pesticide residues in wheat from Konya region, Turkey. *Food Chem Toxicol* 2010;**48**:1218–21.

67. Riazuddin M, Khan F, Iqbal S, Abbas M. Determination of multiresidue insecticides of organochlorine, organophosphorus, and pyrethroids in wheat. *Bull Envir Contam Toxicol* 2011;**87**:303–6.

68. Toteja GS, Diwakar S, Mukherjee A, Singh P, Saxena BN, Kalra RL, et al. Douressamy. Residues of DDT and HCH in wheat samples collected from different states of India and their dietary exposure: A multicentre study. *Food Addit Contam* 2006;**23**:281–8.

69. Bakore N, John PJ, Bhatnagar P. Organochlorine pesticide residues in wheat and drinking water samples from Jaipur, Rajasthan, India. *Environ Monit Assess* 2004;**98**:381–9.

70. Nayak MK, Daglish GJ. Potential of imidacloprid to control four species of psocids (Psocoptera: Liposcelididae) infesting stored grain. *Pest Manag Sci* 2006;**7**:646–50.

71. Daglish GJ, Wallbank BE, Nayak MK. Synergized bifenthrin plus chlorpyriphos-methyl for control of beetles and psocids (Psocoptera: Liposcelididae) in sorghum in Australia. *J Econ Entomol* 2003;**2**:525–32.

72. Iqbal M, Ali A. Analysis of combining ability for spike characteristics in wheat (*Triticum aestivum* L.). *International J Agric Biol* 2006;**8**:684–7.

73. Jamil A, Ata Z, Khaliq A. Increasing the efficiency of sorghum water extract (sorgaab) by mixing with lower doses of isoproturon to control weeds in wheat. *International J Agric Biol* 2005;**7**:712–8.

74. Wallbank BE. Resisitance to organophosphorus grain protectants in *Oryzaphilus surinamensis* (L.) from off-farm grain storages in New South Wales. *Aus J Entomol* 1996;**35**:193–5.

75. Noble RM, Hamilton DJ, Osborne WJ. Stability of pyrethroids on wheat in storage. *Pesticide Science* 1982;**13**:246–52.

76. Aitken AD. Insect travelers, I: Coleoptera. *Technical Bulletin 31* (H.M.S.O. London). 1975.

77. Arthur FH. Grain protectants: current status and prospects for the future. *J Stored Prod Res* 1996;**32**:293–302.

78. Pal P, Shah PG. Effect of storage and processing on dissipation of five insecticides on wheat. *Pesticide Res J* 2008;**20**:253–8.

79. Athanassiou CG, Papagregoriou AS, Buchelos CT. Insecticidal and residual effect of three pyrethroids against *Sitophilus oryzae* (L.) (Coleoptera: Curculionidae) on stored wheat. *J Stored Prod Res* 2004;**40**:289–97.

80. Mertz EP, Yao RC. *Saccharopolyspora spinosa* sp. *nov* isolated from soil collected in a sugar rum still. *J Sustainable Bacteriol* 1990;**40**:34–9.

81. Subramanyam BH. Performance of spinosad as a stored grain protectant. In: Lorini I, Bacaltchuk B, Beckel H, Deckers E, Sundfeld E, dos Santos JP, Biagi JD, Celaro JC, Faroni LRD, Bortolini LF, Sartori MR, Elias MC, Guedes RNC, da Fonseca RG, Scussel VM, editors. *Proceedings of the 9th International Working Conference for Stored-Product Protection*. Campinas, Brazil: Brazilian Post-Harvest Association, Campinas; 2006. p. 250–7.

82. Saunders DG, Bret BL. Fate of spinosad in the environment. *Down to Earth* 1997;**52**:14–20.

83. Fang L, Subramanyam B, Arthur F. Effectiveness of spinosad against five stored product insects on four classes of wheat. *J Econ Entomol* 2002a;**95**:640–50.

84. Vayias BJ, Athanassiou CG, Milonas DN, Mavrotas C. Persistence and efficacy of spinosad on wheat, maize and barley grains against four major stored product pests. *Crop Protection* 2010;**29**:496–505.

85. Afridi IAK, Parveen Z, Masud SZ. Stability of organophosphate and pyrethroid pesticides on wheat in storage. *J Stored Pro Res* 2001;**37**:199–204.

86. Saka M, Lijima K, Nishida M, Koma Y, Hasegawa N, Sato K, et al. Effects of processing and cooking on the levels of pesticide residues in wheat samples. *Shokuhin Eiseigaku Zasshi* 2008;**49**:150–9.

87. Balinova AM, Mladenova RI, Shtereva DD. Study on the effect of grain storage and processing on deltamethrin residues in post-harvest treated wheat with regard to baby-food safety requirements. *Food Addit Contam* 2007;**24**:896–901.

88. Fleurat-Lessard F, Mary-Laure V, Budzinski H. Modelling Biological Efficacy Decrease and Rate of Degradation of Chlorpyrifos-methyl on Wheat Stored under Controlled Conditions. *J Stored Pro Res* 1998;**34**:341–54.

89. Uygun U, Koksel H, Ali A. Residue levels of malathion and its metabolites and fenitrothion in post-harvest treated wheat during storage, milling and baking. *Food Chem* 2005;**92**:643–7.

90. Balinova A, Mladenova R, Obretenchev DD. Effect of grain storage and processing on chlorpyrifos-methyl and pirimiphos-methyl residues in post-harvest treated wheat with regard to baby food safety requirements. *Food Addit Contam* 2006;**23**:391–7.

91. Fleurat-Lessard F, Chaurand M, Marchega G, Abecassis J. Effects of processing on the distribution of pirimiphos-methyl residues in milling fractions of durum wheat. *J Stored Pro Res* 2007;**43**:384–95.

92. El-Zemaity MS. Degradation Behavior of Malathion and Fenitrothion Residues on Wheat and Barley Under Different Storage Systems in Saudi Arabia. *Bull Environ Contam Toxicol* 1998;**60**:864–71.

93. Alnaji LK, Kadoum AM. Residues on methyl phoxim in wheat and milling fractions. *J Agric Food Chem* 1979;**27**:583–4.

94. Papadopoulou-Mourkidou E, Tomazou T. Persistence and activity of permethrin in stored wheat and its residues in wheat milling fractions. *J Stored Pro Res* 1991;**27**:249–54.

95. Marei AE, Khattab MM, Mansee AH, Youssef MM, Montasser MR. Analysis and dissipation of deltamethrin in stored wheat and milled fractions. *Alexandria J Agric Res* 1995;**16**:275–91.

96. Kaushik G, Santosh S, Naik SN. Food processing a tool to pesticide residue dissipation – A review. *Food Res International* 2009;**42**:26–40.

97. Sgarbiero E, De Baptista GC, Trevizan LRP. Evaluation of degradation and persistence of pirimiphos-methyl residues in wheat grain and derived products. *Revista Brasileira de Toxicologia* 2002;**15**:5–8.

98. Yentur G, Kalay A, Oktem AB. A survey on organochlorine pesticide residues in butter and cracked wheat available in Turkish markets. *Nahrung* 2001;**45**:40–2.

99. Bengston M, Davies RAH, Desmarchelier JM, Henning R, Murray W, Simpson BW. Organophosphorothioates and synergized synthetic pyrethroids as grain protectants on bulk wheat. *Pesticide Science* 1983;**14**:373–84.

100. Anderegg BM, Madisen LG. *Journal of Eco Entomol* 1983;**76**:733–6.

101. Skerritt JH, Simone L, Guihot, Amanda S, Jim D, Peter J. Analysis of Organophosphate, Pyrethroid, and Methoprene Residues in Wheat End Products and Milling Fractions by Immunoassay. *Cereal Chem* 1996;**73**:605–12.

102. Schesser JH, Priddle WE, Farrell EP. Insecticidal Residues in Milling Fractions from Wheat Treated with Methoxychlor, Malathion, and Lindanel. *J Econ Entomol* 1958;**51**:516–8.

103. Uygun U, Senoz B, Koksel H. Dissipation of organophosphorus pesticides in wheat during pasta processing. *Food Chem* 2008;**109**:355–60.

104. Fatichenti F, Farris GA, Deiana P, Cabras P, Meloni M, Pirisi FM. A preliminary investigation into the effect of Saccharomyces cerevisiae on pesticide concentration during fermentation. *Eur J Appl Microbiol Biotechnol* 1983;**1983**(18):323–5.

105. Fatichenti F, Farris GA, Deiana P, Cabras P, Meloni M, Pirisi FM. The effect of *Saccharomyces cerevisiae* on concentration of dicarboximide and acylamide fungicides and pyrethroid insecticides during fermentation. *Microbiol Biotechnol* 1984;**20**: 419–21.

106. Jaggi S, Sood C, Kumar V, Ravindranath SD, Shanker A. Leaching of pesticides in tea brew. *J Agric Food Chem* 2001;**49**:5479–83.

107. Shanker A, Kumar V, Tewary DK. Fate of pesticide residues on tea from leaf to cup. *International J Tea Sci* 2004;**2**:18–26.

108. Kumar V, Ravindranath SD, Shanker A. Fate of hexaconazole residues in tea and its behaviour during brewing process. *Chem Health Saftey* 2004;**11**:21–5.

109. Sharma J, Santosh S, Vipin K, Dhananjay K. Tewary. Dissipation of pesticides during bread-making. *Chem Health Safety* 2005:17–22. http://dx.doi.org/10.1016/j.chs.2004.08.003.

110. Chen ZM, Wan HB. Factors affecting residues of pesticides in tea. *Pesticide Sci* 1986;**23**:109–18.

111. Uygun U, Berrin S, Serpil O, Hamit K. Degradation of organophosphorus pesticides in wheat during cookie processing. *Food Chem* 2009;**117**:261–4.

112. Hassall KA. *The biochemistry and uses of pesticides*. 2nd ed. New York, NY: VCH Publisher; 1990.

113. Anonymous. *Turkish International Food, Beverage, Food Ingredients And Food Processing Exhibition*; 2003. Available at: www.gidasanayii.com.

PART II

RICE AND OTHER WHOLE GRAINS IN HEALTH

SECTION

OVERVIEW OF RICE AND HEALTH

Genetically Modified Rice with Health Benefits as a Means to Reduce Micronutrient Malnutrition: Global Status, Consumer Preferences, and Potential Health Impacts of Rice Biofortification

Hans De Steur*, Joseph Birundu Mogendi*,†, Dieter Blancquaert**, Willy Lambert‡, Dominique Van Der Straeten**, Xavier Gellynck*

*Ghent University, Department of Agricultural Economics, Ghent, Belgium, †Mt Kenya University, Department of Nutrition and Dietetics, Thika, Kenya, **Ghent University, Department of Physiology, Laboratory of Functional Plant Biology, Ghent, Belgium, ‡Ghent University, Department of Bioanalysis, Laboratory of Toxicology, Ghent University, Ghent, Belgium

INTRODUCTION

Within the scope of crop improvement, biofortification of rice is increasingly advocated as a tool to improve human nutrition. By enhancing the micronutrient level of the world's most consumed staple crop, micronutrient malnutrition could be addressed where the need is highest. As rice varieties are mainly characterized by a low vitamin and mineral content, agricultural biotechnology is applied to increase specific micronutrient levels in rice, such as folate and provitamin A (β-carotene). This chapter describes the history of and trends in biofortification and genetically modified (GM) rice, with an emphasis on health benefits in particular. In spite of the potential consumer benefits of this new generation of GM crops, the use of biotechnology in food products remains controversial. As none of these crops are available in the marketplace, they were subject to various *ex-ante* evaluation studies in order to examine consumer demand, potential health benefits, and the cost-effectiveness of their introduction. By reviewing the current state of the art, this study sheds a light on the potential of GM biofortified rice as both a GM food product with health benefits and an alternative policy intervention to tackle micronutrient deficiencies.

As a starting point, the global burden of micronutrient malnutrition and the main micronutrient deficiencies is described. In the following two sections, (GM) biofortification is described within the framework of health interventions to address micronutrient malnutrition, and within the scope of agricultural crop improvement. Next, the global status of the development and commercialization of (GM) biofortified crops and GM rice, as well as GM biofortified rice, is presented. The chapter also contains a section on published research on GM food, GM rice, biofortification, and Golden Rice, and summarizes key research findings regarding consumer preferences for, and the potential cost-effectiveness of, GM biofortified rice. These latter two research topics are crucial to *ex-ante* evaluation of micronutrient interventions and GM foods. Finally, some key challenges and conclusions are formulated (section XI).

WHAT'S AT STAKE? THE GLOBAL BURDEN OF MICRONUTRIENT MALNUTRITION

Micronutrient malnutrition[1] is defined by a chronic lack of micronutrients – i.e., essential vitamins and minerals that are needed in small quantities – and has a large impact on global health while (indirectly) hindering social and economic prosperity through, for example, productivity losses, cognitive impairment, and soaring health care costs.[2,3] Malnutrition is considered one of the principal causes of morbidity and mortality among the poor.[4] There is a clear difference between undernutrition and malnutrition, in that the former is a specific type of the latter. Whereas undernutrition refers to an inadequate intake of specific nutrients, malnutrition covers both under and overnutrition, such as obesity, but also micronutrient deficiency. In the scope of micronutrient malnutrition, "malnutrition" generally refers to undernutrition and, thus, micronutrient deficiencies. In this chapter, therefore, the term "micronutrient malnutrition" is used to define all vitamin and mineral deficiencies.

Most people are not aware of a lack of micronutrients, due to the subclinical character of such deficiencies, and because the underlying causes and health functions of different micronutrients are neglected, poorly addressed, or still undiscovered. Therefore, this form of malnutrition is often referred to as "hidden hunger". Insufficient intake of micronutrients reflects a lack of dietary quality and especially strikes poor people living in rural, less developed areas, because these populations are largely dependent on staple crops (e.g., rice, maize, and wheat), which are known to contain few micronutrients.[2–5] As a consequence, multiple micronutrient deficiency is the rule rather than the exception. Half of malnourished children, for instance, are deficient in several vital micronutrients.[5]

Despite an increasing number of local and global programs to control micronutrient malnutrition, especially the main micronutrient deficiencies (vitamin A, iodine, zinc, and iron),[6] it remains a major public health problem, in particular for children and (pregnant) women. According to global estimates of micronutrient malnutrition, nearly 2 billion people fail to achieve the recommended nutrient intake levels, mainly populations from low-income countries.[2] As a consequence, an annual outlay of US$10.3 billion is still required to fight the global burden of malnutrition successfully, of which at least US$1.5 billion is needed to combat micronutrient deficiencies adequately.[7] The extent of micronutrient malnutrition varies when looking at specific micronutrient deficiencies and different data sources. The number of people with insufficient vitamin A intake, for example, varies between 140,[8] 190,[9] and 254 million.[8,10] Iodine and zinc deficiency figures show that a total of nearly 2 billion people are estimated to be at risk.[3,11,12] Iron deficiency is another widespread type of micronutrient malnutrition, with 1.7 billion people below the recommended intake levels.[3,11] However, the public health significance of a micronutrient deficiency must be evaluated by looking beyond its prevalence – i.e., by estimating its health impacts.

Table 21.1 lists some key figures regarding the devastating health and socioeconomic impacts of global micronutrient malnutrition. Its importance is underpinned by its share in the global burden of disease (GBD). Together, deficiencies of vitamin A, iron, zinc, and iodine accounted for 4% of the GBD in 2004. Regarding regional malnutrition, Southeast Asia is the most problematic region, followed by Africa.[13] However, not all micronutrient deficiencies are included in the current burden analyses of the World Health Organization (WHO), among them folate deficiency. Rough estimations of the global burden of this type of vitamin deficiency (i.e., 4.8 million disability-adjusted life years (DALYs) per year[14]) show that the contribution of micronutrient malnutrition to the GBD is underestimated. According to the Micronutrient Initiative,[15] the total share in the GBD is expected to be around 10%.

Currently, public health programs are primarily targeted towards vitamin A, iodine, zinc, and iron deficiencies,[7,16,17] which are perceived as the four most important types of micronutrient malnutrition. Because children below the age of 5 years are the main sufferers from such deficiencies, it is not surprising that the nutritional targets of the Millennium Development Goals (MDG)[18] and the nutritional challenge of the 2008 Copenhagen Consensus[19] focus on this age group. In the framework of MDG 1 (eradicate extreme poverty and hunger), for instance, the United Nations is striving to halve the prevalence of underweight children (i.e., one of the proxy indicators of poor nutrition) between 1990 and 2015.[20,21] Furthermore, malnutrition needs to be addressed in order to reduce child mortality (MDG 4), maternal health (MDG 5), and, indirectly, other major diseases (MDG 6), and to help achieve the goals on education (MDG 2) and gender equality (MDG 3).[11]

GM BIOFORTIFICATION AS A NOVEL MICRONUTRIENT INTERVENTION

There are currently four main strategies or (potential) policy interventions to address micronutrient malnutrition or particular vitamin or mineral deficiencies: pharmaceutical supplementation, food fortification, dietary diversification, and biofortification (see Table 21.2). Pharmaceutical supplementation refers to micronutrient programs that distribute (multi-) micronutrient supplements for free, or promote the use of supplements. Key supplementation programs are based upon iron, zinc, vitamin A, and/or folic acid supplementation. The latter aims to reduce folate deficiency through increased consumption of folic acid (i.e., the synthetic form of folate). Industrial fortification refers to the addition of micronutrients into staple crops, like rice and wheat; this takes place during flour milling. Dietary diversification

TABLE 21.1 Key Figures Regarding the Estimated Global Impact of Micronutrient Malnutrition, Estimated Burden of Disease in Million DALYs Lost, and as a Percentage of the Global Burden of Disease, per Main Micronutrient Deficiency

| Type of Micronutrient Deficiency | Estimated Burden of Disease[f] | | | |
| | 2000[g] | | 2004 | |
	Millions of DALYs lost	% of GBD	Millions of DALYs lost	% of GBD
Micronutrient malnutrition (MM)	93.2	6.3	60.9	4.0
2 million children may die each year due to MM[a] MM is the world's leading cause of mental impairment[b] MM is responsible for productivity losses of up to 2% of GDP[b]				
Vitamin A deficiency (VAD)	26.6[h]	1.8[h]	22.1[k]	1.5[k]
VAD-related night-blindness and blindness affect 5 million and 350,000 children, respectively[c] VAD is responsible for 0.5 million to 1 million child deaths each year[b,c]				
Iron deficiency (ID)	35.1[d]	2.4[d]	19.7[k]	1.3[k]
ID affects the health and energy of 40% (women)[a] and the mental development of 40–60 % (children)[b,d] in developing countries ID is estimated to result in the annual death of 841,000 persons[g], of which 50,000 are young women dying in pregnancy and child birth[b]				
Zinc deficiency (ZD)	28.0[e]	1.9[e]	15.6[k]	1.0[k]
About 800,000 child deaths per year are related to ZD[e] ZD is associated with approximately 176,000 diarrhea deaths, 406,000 pneumonia deaths, and 207,000 malaria deaths each year[e]				
Iodine deficiency (IOD)	3.5[i]	0.2[i]	3.5[k]	0.2[k]
Each year, IOD leads to an estimated number of 18–20 million mentally impaired babies being born[a,b] IOD is estimated to lower the intellectual capacity of developing countries by 10–15 percentage points[b]				
Folate deficiency (FD)	ND[j]		ND[j]	
FD is estimated to result in approximately 200,000 severe birth defects every year[b] About 1 in 10 adult deaths from heart diseases is attributed to FD[b]				

DALY, disability-adjusted life year; FD, folate deficiency; GBD, global burden of disease; ID, iron deficiency; IOD, iodine deficiency; MM, micronutrient malnutrition; ND, no data available; VAD, vitamin A deficiency; ZD, zinc deficiency.
Note: Figures regarding the global burden of all malnutrition are not presented. According to the FAO report on the state of food insecurity in the world,[3] malnutrition in the developing world leads to a total loss of 220 million (childhood and maternal undernutrition) to 430 million (including nutrition-related risk factors) DALYs.

[a] *Micronutrient Initiative.[15]*
[b] *UNICEF.[5,22]*
[c] *Micronutrient Initiative report.[2]*
[d] *Stoltzfus et al.[23]*
[e] *Caulfield and Black.[24]*
[f] *For more information on the application of DALYs and the DALY approach, see De Steur et al.[25–27]*
[g] *The burden of different micronutrient deficiencies in 2000 is based on the Comparative Risk Factor Assessment (CRA) of the WHO[13] (data are available at the WHO website[28]).*
[h] *Rice et al.[10]*
[i] *WHO World Health Report.[29]*
[j] *Global folate deficiency prevalence is not established, as Kennedy et al.[30] demonstrate, but is expected not to be a marginal phenomenon.[31] Based on the most important outcome of FD (i.e., neural tube defects), calculations by De Steur et al.[14] reveal a global burden of FD of at least 4.8 million DALYs, which is significantly more than the rough 2.3 million estimation of Blencowe et al.[32] However, this is still an underestimation, as other functional outcomes are not included.*
[k] *WHO report on Global Health Risks.[33] The statistics from the report are available at the WHO website.[34]*

A. OVERVIEW OF RICE AND HEALTH

TABLE 21.2   Characteristics of the Key Interventions to Reduce Micronutrient Deficiencies

	Industry-Based Interventions		Natural Micronutrient-Based Interventions	
	Supplementation	Food fortification	Dietary diversification	(GM) Biofortification
Micronutrient dose	RNI dose	Micronutrient enriched staple crops	Micronutrient-rich foods	Micronutrient enriched staple crops
Potential coverage	People taking supplements	Consumers of processed staple crops	Consumers taking part in promotion/education program	Consumers of (GM) staple crops
Target group	(Rural) risk regions	(Urban) populations	Rural risk regions	(Poor) populations
Behavioral changes	Taking pills (correctly)	None	Changing dietary habits	None, unless a product attribute is changed
Funding	Continuous	Continuous	Long term	One-time R&D, continuous labeling and maintenance costs
Funding source	Public	Public or private	Public	Public
Development	Pharmaceutical industry	Food processing industry	Government	Research institutes
Distribution	Health workers/system	Food supply chain (marketing channels)	Health, extension and education system	Seed distribution system

GM, genetically modified; R&D, Research & Development; RNI, recommended nutrient intake.
Source: Own compilation, based on Stein et al.[36]

is considered the most sustainable intervention, and is targeted towards an increased intake of micronutrient-rich foods through nutrition education, promotion of diverse diets, and improved access to locally produced foods rich in vital micronutrients. Although there is the option to address a particular micronutrient intervention through diversifying food habits, such as the promotion of green vegetables and citrus fruits to elevate folate intake levels, the ultimate goal of diversification strategies is usually to improve dietary habits as whole, which encompasses a multi-micronutrient approach.

Biofortification is considered a novel strategy to combat "hidden hunger", by which the nutritional content of staple crops is enhanced. By sharing the advantages of fortification (e.g., wide coverage) and addressing the limitations of supplementation (e.g., short-term strategy, limited coverage, compliance of taking pills), it is intended to be a pro-rural and pro-poor health intervention (see Table 21.2). According to Welch,[35] agricultural approaches are a prerequisite to sustainably control micronutrient malnutrition. Biofortification is considered an agriculture/food-based approach as it uses the regular food chain and goes beyond fortification, because the crops are fortifying themselves,[36,37] This general definition of biofortification does not include agronomic biofortification, where mineral contents are enhanced through the application of fertilizers.[38] Other biofortification strategies focus on the factors that increase the bioavailability of micronutrients rather than enhancing the production of micronutrients.[39] It is also important to note that non-staple crops could also be biofortified. A more exhaustive overview of biofortified staple and

non-staple products, including strawberries (vitamin C), maize and canola (vitamin E), potatoes and mustard (β-carotene), carrots (calcium), and lettuce (iron) is available in Hirschi[40] and in Johns and Eyzaguirre.[37]

Contrary to dietary diversification and supplementation, biofortification uses staple crops as a food vehicle, hence behavioral changes are unlikely to be required. As a consequence, biofortification is self-targeting: as poor malnourished people mainly rely on staple crops, the groups at risk that need to benefit the most from the biofortified crops are addressed.[41] In this way, biofortification can be a complementary policy intervention by fighting micronutrient malnutrition where other interventions fail to do so. First of all, unlike food fortification or pharmaceutical supplementation, biofortification does not rely on an (centralized) industrial food processing sector or accessible public health infrastructures. Although food fortification is often promoted as the primary option to reduce micronutrient malnutrition,[42] the key target group for micronutrient interventions (i.e., poor rural populations) rarely consumes processed foods suitable for fortification.[43] In addition, supplementation programs are often less successful in the long term.[44,45] For example, folic acid supplementation programs in China,[46] Europe,[47–49] and the United States[50] were not sustainable once the program finished, partly due to poor compliance and willingness to take folic acid supplements (correctly).[51] Second, given the technical and practical difficulties, it will be hard to implement fortified rice, such as folic acid fortified rice,[52] successfully in developing malnourished regions. Third, biofortification uses staple crops as its food vehicle and therefore can easily target the micronutrient deficient subgroups without the need to administer pills or promote the consumption of (generally more expensive) micronutrient-rich foods. Furthermore, industrial fortified foods and supplements are often only available in cities and hence cannot reach the poor rural populations. Fourth, possible negative side effects of food fortification, such as the relation between folic acid fortification and masking vitamin B_{12} deficiency, or an increased risk of colorectal cancer, are less likely to occur with biofortification.[53]

Due to the relatively low costs of biofortified crops (a one-time investment in R&D and the ability of farmers to reproduce their own biofortified crop seeds), the cost-effectiveness of biofortified crops is often used as one of the main arguments in favor of this strategy.[36,41,54] Whereas supplementation and fortification have been the two key strategies to control micronutrient malnutrition in the past, biofortification is receiving more and more attention.[2] During the 2008 Copenhagen Consensus, where a panel of economists evaluated the top priorities to counter the world biggest challenges, biofortification was placed fifth.[55]

Notwithstanding the great potential of single biofortified crops, it could be argued that the large prevalence of multiple micronutrient deficiencies and the generally low micronutrient contents of rice and other staple crops requires a combined biofortification strategy. In other words, there is a need to increase the intake of different micronutrients simultaneously through nutritionally complete crops. This is where multi-biofortification enters the public health debate. By enhancing different vitamins and minerals, through conventional or transgenic technologies, multi-biofortification could address micronutrient malnutrition more adequately and efficiently.

In spite of several ongoing initiatives that are attempting to develop multi-biofortified crops, especially those that were or are supported by the Bill & Melinda Gates Foundation under the Grand Challenges in Global Health Initiative, such as rice, sorghum, cassava, and banana,[56,57] evidence of a developed staple crop that stacks different nutrient traits is scarce. Recently, Naqvi et al.[58] published on the development of the first transgenic multi-biofortified crop: maize enriched with vitamin A, vitamin C, and folate. Such gene-stacking applications have already been successfully applied and commercialized in the field of first-generation GM crops, mainly crops that combine herbicide-tolerant and insect-resistant traits.[59] However, these technologies are still in the research pipeline, and little is known about their potential from public health, agricultural and economics perspectives.

Targeting different micronutrient deficiencies simultaneously is a strategy that is also found in other policy interventions, such as pharmaceutical multivitamin supplementation (e.g., iron–folic acid multivitamin pills in India[60] and other Asian countries[61]), multi-micronutrient food fortification (e.g., fortifying grain with folic acid, vitamin B_{12}, and several minerals[62]), and dietary diversification.

Table 21.2 presents an overview of the key characteristics of the different micronutrient interventions. The common objective of these interventions is primary prevention – i.e., tackling micronutrient deficiencies as a risk factor of various diseases. While the two "industry"-based interventions, supplementation and food fortification, aim to reduce micronutrient malnutrition through the enhancement of micronutrient levels in, respectively, supplements (pharmaceutical industry) and staple crops (milling sector), the objective of dietary diversification and biofortification is to increase natural micronutrient levels.

GM BIOFORTIFICATION AS A NOVEL APPROACH TO CROP IMPROVEMENT

Before biofortification, efforts to improve crop content focused mainly on agronomic traits, such as increasing yield potential and productivity, drought resistance, and pest resistance, which primarily benefit the farmer. Table 21.3 gives an overview of the main stages of crop improvement. As these developments in agriculture were based on two different techniques, conventional versus transgenic technology, they marked the Green and Gene Revolutions, respectively.[36,39,63,64] The Green Revolution refers to a broad public sector-led transformation of agricultural sectors in developing countries, mainly between the 1960s and 1980s, which focused on developing high-yielding staple crop varieties (wheat and rice); promoting the utilization of hybridized seeds, pesticides (insecticides), and fertilizers; and providing agricultural extension in order to reduce food shortages and hunger and stimulate overall development.[65] Nobel Peace Prize winner Norman Borlaug is seen as the founding father of this breakthrough in crop development. In the last decennium of the 20th century, a novel privately-led agricultural revolution took place, the Gene (biotech) Revolution, which built upon the previous revolution by implementing GM technology in agriculture to improve productivity and thereby reduce hunger.

The history of biofortification has followed a similar approach, starting with the introduction of conventionally bred nutritionally enriched products in the 2000s (conventional biofortification), and now making progress to commercialize the "gene revolution" in biofortification through private–public partnerships (GM biofortification). What the Green and Gene Revolutions meant for agricultural productivity and hunger (food quantity),

TABLE 21.3   The Main Stages of Crop Improvement

	Crop Improvement			
	Agronomic traits		**Quality traits**	
	Green revolution	**Gene revolution**	**Conventional biofortification**	**GM biofortification**
Breeding technique	Conventional	GM technology	Conventional	GM technology
Timing	1960s–1980s	1990s – ...	2000s – ...	NC – ...
Key beneficiary	Producer (input)		Consumer (output)	
Key objective Long-term objective	Yield improvement Hunger reduction		Health improvement Hidden hunger reduction	
GM crop generation	–	First generation	–	Second generation
Examples	Herbicide tolerance, drought tolerance, pest resistance, and/or virus resistance		Enhanced vitamin and/or mineral contents	

NC, not commercialized; GM, genetic modification.

this biofortification trend hopes to achieve in the field of malnutrition and "hidden hunger" (food quality). In this respect, there has been a shift from producer (input or quantity traits) to consumer (output or quality traits).[66] Although an increased micronutrient content is certainly one of the most advanced improved quality traits in crops, other quality traits can also be addressed, such as the elimination of allergens; improved taste, texture or other sensory characteristics; and prolongation of shelf life. Nevertheless, "GM biofortified crops" and "GM crops with health benefits" are treated as synonyms in this chapter.

Within the scope of crop improvement through GM technology, broadly two product categories can be distinguished: first- versus second-generation GM products. GM biofortified crops belong to the second generation of GM crops, which are primarily designed to benefit the consumer by improving quality traits, among them nutritional properties. The application of GM technology to develop nutrient-dense crops is sometimes referred to as "nutritional genomics".[67] These developments followed the Gene Revolution and its first generation of GM products, which dealt with enhanced agronomic traits, such as insect resistance and herbicide tolerance. In other words, the evolution from first to second generation involves a shift from producer-friendly to consumer-friendly genetic modification.[68] An overview of the consumer and farmer benefits of first- and second-generation GM food products is described in Toenniessen et al.[69] and Lönnerdal,[70] respectively.

Despite these "generation" differences, future GM crops are more likely to combine improved traits from both the first and second generations. In order to make GM biofortified crops attractive to consumers as well as producers, both the health and agronomic benefits have to be addressed. While farmers will be more in favor of

adopting biofortified crops when the yield characteristics are beneficial,[12,71] multi-biofortification will be more likely accepted and consumed by consumers. In this way, stacking refers to the improvement of different output and input traits.

Following this trend, some people argue the need for an "evergreen" revolution, which combines the economic viability of the Green and/or Gene Revolution with a need for ecological sustainability, while improving awareness and knowledge.[72] There is also a third generation of GM crops, where products are developed for industrial or pharmaceutical use. Among the examples are vaccines or biodegradable plastics.[73]

THE GLOBAL STATUS OF (GM) BIOFORTIFICATION AND GM RICE

Biofortification research was accelerated when the international multidisciplinary HarvestPlus (Biofortification Challenge) program was launched in 2004 by the Consultative Group on International Agricultural Research (CGIAR) and the International Food Policy Research Institute (IFPRI).[65,74] It became the key project in development and dissemination of biofortified crops, with an emphasis on iron, zinc, and vitamin A deficiencies in Africa and Asia. Initially, only conventional biofortified crops were explored, until the development in 1999 of Golden Rice as the first biofortified staple crop that was genetically engineered to tackle vitamin A deficiency.[75,76] This was the starting point of the humanitarian HarvestPlus-supported Golden Rice project.[77]

While Africa and Asia fall within the scope of HarvestPlus, AgroSalud coordinates the biofortification efforts in Latin America and the Caribbean (LAC),

TABLE 21.4 A Brief Overview of the Currently Biofortified Products in the World, Developed by Harvestplus or Agrosalud, According to the Improved Micronutrient, Applied Technology, Target Area of First Release, and (Expected) Release Year

Micronutrient	Product	Applied Technology	Target Area[c]	Release Year (# Cultivars Released)	Expected Release Year
Vitamin A (β-carotene)[a]	Cassava	CB	DR Congo and Nigeria		2011–2012
	Maize	CB	Zambia		2012
	Sweet Potato CB		Uganda and Mozambique	2007	
			Brazil, Cuba, Dominican Republic, Haiti and Peru	2009–2010 (8)	
	Rice	TB	Philippines, Bangladesh, India		2012, 2013, 2014[e]
Iron	Pearl Millet	CB	India		2012
	Rice	CB	Bolivia, Cuba and Panama	2009–2010 (8)	
			Brazil, Colombia, Nicaragua and Dominican Republic		2011
	Bean	CB	Bolivia, Brazil, Cuba and Guatemala	2008–2010 (5)	
			Colombia, Costa Rica, El Salvador, Honduras and Nicaragua		2011
Iron, zinc	Wheat	CB	India and Pakistan		2013
	Bean	CB	DR Congo and Rwanda		2011–2012
	Rice	CB	India, Bangladesh		2013
Vitamin B3 (niacin)[b]	Maize	CB	Bolivia, Colombia, El Salvador, Guatemala, Haiti, Honduras, Mexico, Nicaragua and Panama	2008–2010 (21)	ND
Folate	Rice	TB	China[d]		ND[d]

ND, no data.

[a] The human body converts β-carotene or provitamin A into vitamin A.

[b] Niacin or vitamin B_3 is an essential nutrient which is mainly lacking in maize-consuming populations.[82] Niacin is available in different foods, but can also be made in the human body through tryptophan – i.e., an amino acid that is improved by biofortification.

[c] These are the selected countries where the biofortified crops are released, or expected to be tested and released. However, after the first release these crops are intended to also benefit other countries characterized by similar micronutrient deficiencies.

[d] Because these crops are still in a development phase, it is too early to select a target country and a release date. Here, China was selected due to its high folate deficiency prevalence rates, its recent approval of Bt rice, and the potential high impact of the introduction of Folate Biofortified Rice.[14]

[e] Although the transgenic Golden Rice was expected to be released in 2011,[83] field tests and biosafety regulations are still ongoing in the Philippines. The GR trait was also bred into rice varieties in, for example, India, Vietnam, Bangladesh, and Indonesia.

Source: Own compilation, based on Agrosalud[80] for Latin America and the Caribbean, and HarvestPlus[74] for Asia and Africa, except for Golden Rice[77] and Folate Biofortified Rice.[81]

where it aims to increase the iron and zinc content of beans, rice, maize, and sweet potatoes, and develop yellow maize and orange-fleshed sweet potato with higher β-carotene contents.[78,79] Between 2007 and 2010, AgroSalud introduced 42 biofortified cultivars in 13 LAC countries.[80] Depending on each country's policy, the seeds are sold at the full or a subsidized price, or given to farmers free of cost.

The global status of biofortified staple crops, developed and/or released by HarvestPlus or AgroSalud, is shown in Table 21.4.[81–83]

To date, only conventionally bred biofortified staple crops, such as vitamin A enriched sweet potatoes, iron biofortified beans and rice, and maize with a higher vitamin B_3 content, have been released. Future releases will be mainly dominated by conventional breeding techniques, such as vitamin A biofortified cassava and maize, and wheat, rice, and beans with higher zinc and iron levels. However, the progress of Golden Rice or vitamin A biofortified rice shows that transgenic biofortified staple crops are in the pipeline for approval. Other crops, such as banana, barley, cowpeas, groundnuts, lentils, pigeon peas, potatoes, and sorghum, are also expected to become the subject of biofortification.[36] It is important to note that not all R&D efforts in the field of biofortification are presented. In China, for example, a conventional biofortified zinc enriched wheat crop ("Jingdong 8") has been commercialized, but at a very small scale.

Nevertheless, about 16 Chinese crop varieties/lines have been developed, of which 4 have been approved for advanced testing (2011 figures).

The current status and future pipeline of GM biofortified rice – i.e., GM rice with health benefits – are described in Tables 21.5 and 21.6, respectively. When looking at the approval of GM rice events, it is clear that only first-generation GM rice crops, such as herbicide-tolerant and insect-resistant rice, are currently approved for food, feed, and cultivation. There are eight different GM rice events listed. The insect-resistant GM rice in Iran is the only event that has been commercially cultivated in the past, but is currently not authorized.[84] The targeted GM rice traits are insect resistance, herbicide tolerance, and antibiotic resistance. Apart from the Liberty Link rice crops, developed by Bayer Crop Science, all events are approved in only one country (Japan, China and Iran). GM Shanyou 63, as well as LLrice601, LLrice62, and the Iranian event, are approved for food, feed, and cultivation. None of these events is grown or commercialized for food or feed. In other words, GM rice has yet to be commercialized in the world.

Second-generation GM rice crops, and GM biofortified rice in particular, are presently only in the R&D pipeline. According to the study by Stein and Rodriguez,[84] it is expected that by 2015 more or less than 15 GM events will be cultivated, among which are stacked traits. The Chinese traits in particular are expected to be commercialized in the near future, in line with the recent approval of Bt rice.[85] In the field of GM biofortification, only the vitamin A enriched Golden Rice (first and second variants) is currently in an advanced development stage.

Since most of the GM rice products in the R&D pipeline are being developed by Asian providers for direct use at the domestic market, the number of GM rice events that will be approved and commercialized in the future is expected to be low. Today, only LLrice62 has been submitted for approval in the European Union. Despite the positive evaluation of the European Food Safety Authority, this application is currently not moving forward to a decision in the European Commission, leading to a delay in potential authorization (EFSA received the application dossier in August 2004). If this and other GM rice events were to be approved and introduced only into the Asian marketplace, global trade problems would be expected to occur due to the Low Level Presence thresholds for rice imports in the EU.

TABLE 21.5 Approved (Non-Commercialized) GM Rice Events

Event Name	Developer (Institute, Country)	GM Traits	Country	Food[b]	Feed[b]	Cultivation[c]
				Type of Approval (year)		
7Crp#10	National Institute of Agrobiological Sciences (Japan)	Anti-allergy; antibiotic resistance	Japan	2007		2007[d]
7Crp#242-95-7	National Institute of Agrobiological Sciences (Japan)	Anti-allergy; antibiotic resistance	Japan			2007[d]
BTShanyou 63	Huazhong Agricultural University (China)	Insect resistance	China	2009	2009	2009
Huahui-1/TT51-1	Huazhong Agricultural University (China)	Insect resistance	China			2009
LLRICE06[a]	Bayer CropScience (Germany)	Herbicide tolerance	USA	2000	2000	1999
LLRICE601[a]	Bayer CropScience (Germany)	Herbicide tolerance	Colombia	2008		
			USA	2008		2006
LLRICE62[a]	Bayer CropScience (Germany)	Herbicide tolerance	Australia	2008		1999
			Canada	2006	2006	
			Colombia	2008	2011	
			Mexico	2007	2000	
			New Zealand	2008		
			Russia	2007		
			South Africa	2011		
			USA	2000		
Tarom molaii + cry1Ab	Agricultural Biotech Research Institute (Iran)	Insect resistance	Iran	2004	2004	2004

[a] Liberty Link rice.
[b] Direct use or additive.
[c] Domestic or non-domestic use.
[d] Limited cultivation with proper isolation.
Source: ISAAA GM approval database (www.isaaa.org/gmapprovaldatabase/).

GM RICE CROP WITH HEALTH BENEFITS: THE CASE OF RICE BIOFORTIFICATION

In order to tackle micronutrient malnutrition successfully through GM biofortification, care must be taken in selecting the food vehicle for biofortification. In principle, a staple crop such as rice, wheat, corn, or potato should be selected in order to reach the poor rural populations who are most in need of increasing their micronutrient intake levels. There are several reasons that underpin the focus on rice to reduce micronutrient malnutrition. Rice is not only the most consumed and produced product in the world; it is also known to have a low content of micronutrients such as folate and provitamin A. Furthermore, the selection of rice as the food vehicle for biofortification is in line with the technical considerations of fortification (i.e., using an inexpensive, country-wide staple crop) as postulated by the Asian Development Bank.[17,87]

In some cases, it is feasible to increase micronutrient concentrations in rice through conventional breeding techniques, similar to biofortified maize, wheat, beans, and cassava.[41] This is true, for example, for zinc and iron levels in rice.[88] In other cases, however, the application of conventional plant-breeding techniques to enhance the micronutrient content of rice is less successful (e.g., folate) or not possible (e.g., provitamin A). Even though there is a clear potential for conventionally bred folate enriched rice, achieving similar folate improvements to those attained with transgenic techniques will be difficult, because of the low folate levels in natural rice.[89,90] Therefore, folate enriched rice, in this case, is seen as a transgenic biofortified staple crop or second-generation GM crop.

Below, the focus will be mainly on two GM biofortified rice crops, namely Folate Biofortified Rice and provitamin A enriched "Golden Rice". There are three reasons for this choice. First, there are several studies in international peer-reviewed journals that report reconstitution of the folate[79,86,88] and carotenoid biosynthetic pathway.[75,91,92] Second, while rice with a higher folate content, developed by metabolic engineering, is currently the most advanced folate enriched staple crop,[89,93] Golden Rice is the most advanced GM biofortified crop and will most likely be the first to be commercialized.

TABLE 21.6 GM Rice Events in the Pipeline

Event Name (Product Name)	Developer (Institute, Country)	GM Traits	Development Stage
LLRICE62(Liberty Link rice)	Bayer (Germany)	Insect resistance; herbicide tolerance	Commercial pipeline
Bt63 (MH63)	China	Insect resistance	Regulatory pipeline
Xa21	China	Other	Regulatory pipeline
KMD1	China	Insect resistance	Regulatory pipeline
B827	Iran	Insect resistance	Regulatory pipeline
GR1 (Golden Rice 1)	**IRRI (Philippines)**	**Crop composition**	**Advanced development**
Bar68-1	China	Insect resistance; herbicide tolerance	Advanced development
	Bayer (Germany)	Insect resistance; herbicide tolerance	Advanced development
GR2 (Golden Rice 2)	**IRRI (Philippines)**	**Crop composition**	**Advanced development**
Bt	Indonesia	Insect resistance	Advanced development
CP iORF-IV	India	Virus resistance	Advanced development
RTBV-ODs2	India	Virus resistance	Advanced development
	Bayer (Germany)	Insect resistance	Advanced development
chi11 tlp	India	Disease resistance	Advanced development
Bt	Pakistan	Insect resistance	Advanced development
cry1Ac	India	Insect resistance	Advanced development
Glyoxalase I & II	India	Abiotic stress tolerance	Advanced development
Osmotin	India	Abiotic stress tolerance	Advanced development
cry1Ab, cry1C & bar	India	Insect resistance	Advanced development

Note: GM biofortified crops are in bold.
Source: Own compilation, based on Stein and Rodriguez.[86]

(An overview of typical steps in the development process of transgenic biofortified crops – for example, efficacy testing, elite event selection, and trait integration – is available in Dubock.[94] We further refer to several biotechnology studies for a detailed discussion on the technological issues regarding folate biofortification of food plants,[89,95] including rice,[81] wheat,[96] and tomatoes[97].) Third, both GM crops have been subject to various consumer studies on acceptance and willingness to pay, health impact analyses, and cost-effectiveness studies. In addition, the link will be made with multibiofortification. Here, multi-biofortification of rice is understood as rice enriched with folate, β-carotene (provitamin A), zinc, and iron, in line with De Steur and colleagues.[26] Although iron[98,99] and/or zinc[100,101] may also be increased though transgenic approaches, and about 43 genes of 5 protein families are expected to be involved in rice,[102] they are not included in this study due to the lack of socioeconomic studies on these GM biofortified rice crops.

Table 21.7 describes the key characteristics of Folate Biofortified Rice and Golden Rice. Taking into account the biotechnology characteristics, such as the elevated levels of folate and provitamin A in rice, the post-harvest losses (e.g., cooking), and the bioavailability (i.e., the absorption of folate or provitamin A – converted into vitamin A – in the human body), vitamin concentrations after GM biofortification of rice vary between $1.5\,\mu g$ and $3.0\,\mu g$ folate per g rice, and $1.0\,\mu g$ and $6.5\,\mu g$ provitamin A per g rice, depending on the impact scenario. These micronutrient levels are substantially higher than in regular rice varieties. In the case of Folate Biofortified Rice, the total folate intake level after biofortification is 40 times larger than without biofortification. The amount of GM biofortified rice needed in order to recover from folate and vitamin A deficiency depends on the current rice consumption patterns and whether these patterns are still maintained when (partially) switching to GM biofortified rice, and on the current (dietary) vitamin intake. Table 21.7 demonstrates how much GM biofortified rice a consumer needs to consume in order to achieve the daily recommended nutrient intake level (RNI) of the target group. This refers to a theoretical scenario where consumers do not consume any vitamins through their diet. In other words, these figures represent the (GM biofortified) rice consumption threshold to avoid being micronutrient deficient in a situation where only rice could be consumed. In the current situation (i.e., without folate biofortification), about 5 kg of rice should be eaten per day in order to reach the RNI for folate if the consumer depends only on rice. When the same consumer eats Folate Biofortified Rice instead, only 281 g (pessimistic) to 137 g rice (optimistic) is required to achieve adequate folate levels. In the case of Golden Rice, it is not possible to consume vitamin A through a regular rice diet. The

two biofortification scenarios demonstrate that between 500 g and 77 g (children under 5 years) and 800 g and 122 g (pregnant women) of Golden Rice is needed daily to exceed the RNI for vitamin A, and even if the biofortified rice consumption should be below these theoretical thresholds, it should lead to positive health impacts – although full protection from the health outcomes of these micronutrient deficiencies is then impossible. Nevertheless, it could be argued that transgenic lines with a higher micronutrient content could be developed in order to tackle micronutrient deficiencies in regions with medium or low rice consumption. Storozhenko,[81] for example, reported transgenic rice lines with elevated folate levels of up to 17 μg per g rice, as compared to an average of 12 μg folate per g rice.

The aforementioned GM biofortified crops are presented as examples of "single trait" biofortification. However, a multi-biofortification approach might be more likely to occur in the future. Such biofortified crops with enhanced micronutrient concentrations can be developed in two ways. In the so-called "single insertion" approach, the targeted micronutrient traits are stacked as one gene construct. A "back-crossing" approach, where all traits are separately developed and combined through back-crossing,[81,93] is likely to be more costly, due to the high regulatory and financial costs involved in approving all new events as single traits, as well as the time and financial costs required for the testing and approval of each event.[111] Moreover, micronutrient traits are mainly developed by different research institutes, which makes a single-insertion approach the most realistic scenario.

PUBLISHED RESEARCH COVERAGE ON GM FOOD, GM RICE, BIOFORTIFICATION, AND GOLDEN RICE

This section provides a brief overview of the number of publications (2000–2011) in four relevant research domains: GM food, GM rice, biofortification, and Golden Rice. Whereas GM food and (GM or conventional) biofortification are broad food research topics, the topics of GM rice and particularly Golden Rice deal with research applied to a specific staple crop. In this way, this exercise aims to summarize the evolution of international peer-reviewed journal publications in these different but closely related research fields, and particularly in the domain of GM rice crops with health benefits. Golden Rice is selected as it is the GM biofortified crop that has received most attention, at both research and policy levels.

This rudimentary, targeted trend analysis is based on a literature search in the electronic literature database "Web of Knowledge". The database search used the

TABLE 21.7 Characteristics of GM Biofortified Rice, per Product and Impact Scenario

	Indicator	Folate[b] (Folate Biofortified Rice)		Provitamin A[c] (Golden Rice)	
		Pessimistic Scenario	Optimistic Scenario	Pessimistic Scenario	Optimistic Scenario
RICE CHARACTERISTICS					
Initial micronutrient content[a]	µg per g rice	0.08		0	
GM RICE CHARACTERISTICS					
Improved micronutrient content	µg per g rice	12		20	30
Post-harvest losses (e.g., cooking)	%	75	50	80	20
Bioavailability	%	50[d]	50[d]	4:1[e]	2.3:1[e]
Added micronutrient content	µg per g rice	1.4	2.9	1.0	6.5
Total micronutrient content	µg per g rice	1.5	3.0	1.0	6.5
RNI, PER KEY BENEFICIARY					
Women of child-bearing age	µg	400[f]			
Children <5 years	µg			500[g]	
Pregnant women	µg			800[g]	
REQUIRED RICE CONSUMPTION TO ACHIEVE THE RNI					
If current micronutrient intake=0					
Without biofortification	g rice	5000.0		NA[h]	
With biofortification					
Women of child-bearing age	g rice	281.7	137.0		
Children <5 years	g rice			500	76.7
Pregnant women	g rice			800	122.7

NA, not applicable; RNI, recommended nutrient intake

[a] *USDA.[103]*

[b] *Storozhenko et al.[81] and De Steur et al.[27]*

[c] *Zimmerman and Qaim[104], and Stein et al.,[105] updated by Golden Rice Project experts.*

[d] *Bailey.[106]*

[e] *Bioconversion factors refer to the bioavailability of provitamin A and the conversion to vitamin A. Based on Tang et al.,[107] updated by Golden Rice Project experts.*

[f] *WHO.[108] The target group of Folate Biofortified Rice consumption is women of childbearing age, as the health benefits refer to newborns.*

[g] *IOM[109](children) and FAO/WHO[110] (pregnant women).*

[h] *As the initial provitamin A content of rice is non-existent, it is not possible to consume provitamin A through regular rice consumption.*

Source: unless noted otherwise, based on De Steur et al.[26]

following keywords in the topic field: GM food; GM rice; biofortification; and Golden Rice. It is important to notice that the selection of publications is based on studies from various research disciplines, such as biotechnology and genetic engineering (e.g., R&D), agriculture (e.g., impact analyses), politics (e.g., policy level analysis), marketing (e.g., consumer studies), economics (e.g., cost-effectiveness assessment), and so on. Furthermore, some of the selected studies, for example, did not focus on Golden Rice alone but included it as a case study or benchmark exercise, or referred to or built upon this application as a part of the study. Therefore, the extent to which these studies actually explore GM food or another topic (keyword) varies substantially, and hence the total numbers should be interpreted with caution. Nevertheless, as this potential selection bias occurs in each database search,

it is possible to benchmark the importance of these GM related fields in scientific literature. Stated differently, the trends should be evaluated, rather than the absolute figures.

The results in Figure 21.1 show that the number of publications in all four research domains has increased in the last decade. The total research coverage between 2000 and 2011, by numbers, from least to most, is as follows: Golden Rice, 142; GM rice, 362; biofortification, 459; and GM food, 1631. GM food research publications have almost doubled since 2000, while the other topics were still marginal in the beginning of this century. The publications on Golden Rice (i.e., vitamin A enriched GM rice) follow a similar trend to those of GM rice in general; numbers of research topics have increased steadily since 2004. What is more striking is the progression in

A. OVERVIEW OF RICE AND HEALTH

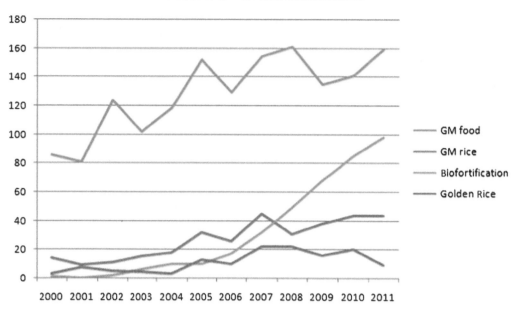

FIGURE 21.1   Number of articles on GM food, GM rice, biofortification and Golden Rice, as derived from the Web of Knowledge literature database (2000–2011). Note: Recent figures (2012) were not included as they were incomplete at the time of the study. See color plate at the back of the book. *Source: own compilation, based on Web of Knowledge (2011).*

biofortification research. While this topic was hardly addressed at the start of the targeted period, with only 3 publications between 2000 and 2002, the number of publications has progressively increased since 2004, rising to about 251 publications in 2009–2011. Together with the figures on biofortification and GM rice, this demonstrates the growing importance of GM crops with health benefits, and GM biofortified rice in particular.

CONSUMER PREFERENCES FOR GM BIOFORTIFIED RICE

As none of the GM biofortified crops is currently approved for cultivation and consumption, it is crucial to determine *ex-ante* the potential demand for such novel crops. Within the large body of literature on biofortification and GM food/rice, there are several studies that aimed to determine consumers' willingness to pay for GM biofortified rice. Given the direct health benefits associated with GM biofortification, due to the enhanced micronutrient content, these studies mainly aimed to assess the extra amount consumers are willing to pay for nutritionally enriched rice. In Table 21.8, seven economic valuation studies on GM biofortified rice crops are presented. While the study of Li *et al.*[112] focuses on GM biofortified rice in general, without making reference to a specific micronutrient trait, the other consumer studies examine either folate or provitamin A enriched Golden Rice. Depending on the applied methodology, Chinese consumers are willing to pay a premium of between 34% (hypothetical method; i.e., contingent valuation)[113] and 72% (nonhypothetical method; i.e., experimental auctions) for

Folate Biofortified Rice.[114] With respect to Golden Rice, willingness-to-pay values vary between 19.5%[115] (India) and 40.0%[116] (Philippines) in Asia. In the United States, premiums for Golden Rice are substantially lower – 16.0 % on average.[117] Besides the GM biofortified rice studies, other studies have obtained economic valuations for conventional biofortified crops. The high consumer preference for vitamin A enriched cassava in North-East Brazil (60–70%),[118] for example, is partly due to the high prevalence of vitamin A deficiency in this region. De Groote *et al.*[119] also elicited valuations for a crop with a higher vitamin content, namely willingness to pay for biofortified corn. Their results showed that consumers in Kenya would be prepared to pay 24% more for corn if it were enriched with provitamin A. Although these findings provide insight into consumer preferences for GM biofortified rice, caution is needed when benchmarking these premiums, due to the study-specific characteristics (e.g., the valuation method, sample selection, targeted product, and selected trait). Nevertheless, when looking at the high premiums, these positive reactions support the high potential demand for GM biofortified crops.

POTENTIAL COST-EFFECTIVENESS OF GM BIOFORTIFIED RICE

As GM biofortified rice is not only an innovative food crop based on agricultural biotechnology but also a potential alternative policy intervention to reduce the burden of micronutrient malnutrition, health-impact and cost-effectiveness analyses are also considered crucial aspects to adequately evaluate its socioeconomic

TABLE 21.8   Willingness to pay for GM Biofortified Rice, Main Characteristics per Study

Study	Trait	Publication Year	Methodology	Country	% Premium (WTP)
Li et al.[112]	Vitamins[a]	2002	DC contingent valuation	Urban China	38.0
De Steur et al.[113]	Folate	2010	OE contingent valuation	Rural China	71.7
De Steur et al.[114]	Folate	2012	Experimental auction	Rural China	33.7
Deodhar et al.[115]	Provitamin A	2008	DC contingent valuation	India	19.5
Depositario et al.[116]	Provitamin A	2009	Experimental auction	Philippines	40.0
Lusk et al.[117]	Provitamin A	2003	DC contingent valuation	United States	16.0

DC, dichotomous choice; ND, no data; OE, open-ended.
Note: In golden rice, provitamin A or β-carotene levels are elevated in order to increase vitamin A consumption.
[a] aluations refer to rice with enhanced vitamin levels in general (without specification of the particular vitamin trait).

TABLE 21.9   Potential Health Impacts and Cost-Effectiveness of GM Biofortified Rice, Main Characteristics per Study

Study	Trait	Country	Health Impact Pessimistic	Optimistic	Cost-Effectiveness Pessimistic	Optimistic
			% Burden Reduction		US$/DALY Saved	
De Steur et al.[26]	Folate	Shanxi Province, Northern China	20	60	120.3	40.1
De Steur et al.[25]		China	20	60	64.2	21.4
De Steur et al.[26]	Provitamin A	China	17	60	18.1	5.0
Stein et al.[105]		India	9	59	23.2	3.7
Zimmerman and Qaim[104]		Philippines	6	32	–	–
De Steur et al.[26]	Multi (GM)[a]	China	11	46	9.6	2.3

DALYs, disability-adjusted life uears; GM, genetically modified; WB, World Bank.
Note: All cost-effectiveness figures are expressed in 2011 dollars, based on the BLS inflation calculator.[123]
[a] Multi-biofortified rice contains higher folate, provitamin A, zinc, and iron levels.

potential.[120] In Table 21.9, five key health-impact studies are described, of which four also assessed the potential health impact. The Chinese regional health impact analysis of De Steur et al.[27] is not included, as the study on multi-biofortification further builds upon their results by including a cost-effectiveness study on folate and three other micronutrient traits in rice (provitamin A, zinc, and iron). For an overview of cost-effectiveness studies on other biofortified crops, see Meenakshi et al.[121]

The potential health benefits of folate, provitamin A, and multi-biofortified rice are measured by their potential contribution to lowering the current burden of micronutrient deficiencies. The results vary between 6% and 20% in the pessimistic scenario, and 32% and 60% in the optimistic scenario. Cost-effectiveness is expressed by the cost (US$) to save a disability-adjusted life year (DALY) that would initially be lost due to the targeted micronutrient deficiency. When looking at the World Bank cost-effectiveness cut-off level for highly cost-effective health interventions[122] (i.e., 258 US$ per DALY saved in 2011),[123] all GM biofortified rice crops fall below this threshold. Due to the combined health impacts of multi-biofortified rice, and the associated cost reductions, the cost-effectiveness of this GM rice crop is substantially lower than that of the so-called single GM biofortified rice crops.

Although these studies differ in their targeted trait and country, and also in data assumptions, Table 21.9 is not intended for comparison of different figures. Instead, evaluation of the introduction of the different GM biofortified rice crops should be interpreted as a whole. Taking together the health-impact and cost-effectiveness figures, GM biofortified rice, regardless of the targeted trait or region, is considered a highly cost-effective intervention to combat micronutrient malnutrition.

KEY CHALLENGES OF THE COMMERCIALIZATION OF GM BIOFORTIFIED RICE

Despite its great potential, GM biofortification has not been the "magic bullet" in the fight against micronutrient deficiencies. According to Hotz and

McClaferty,[124] there are numerous technical, practical, market-oriented, or other concerns that need to be addressed to successfully achieve the goal of biofortifying staple crops. For instance, some target micronutrients need to undergo bioconversion before the body can utilize them, a process that is not 100% effective – for example, provitamin A (β-carotene) needs to be converted to vitamin A. Furthermore, although differences in appearance could be used to position biofortified products in the marketplace,[41] several studies show that acceptance of GM crops will be compromised if they do not resemble the conventional products.[125–127] Rice fortification, for instance, may lead to an intensification of color, which negatively affected its acceptability in Thailand and Bangladesh.[128] With respect to Golden Rice, the visible differences between this GM biofortified rice crop and its regular counterpart could be a constraint to consumer acceptance, because its yellow color may be linked with a longer shelf life and thus lower quality. Similarly, orange provitamin A biofortified maize is less preferred than unfortified white maize.[129,130]

Although scientific evidence is lacking, GM biofortification may also change sensory attributes, which could reduce consumers' willingness to consume such micronutrient enriched crops. The aroma and taste of (conventional) provitamin A enriched maize, for example, was negatively evaluated in Mozambique.[130] Other negative product attribute changes that might be associated with GM biofortification of rice, such as shelf life, and duration and sensory quality of cooking, could also play a role and need to be further investigated.[129]

For a discussion on key issues and challenges in order to advance towards a successful implementation of Folate Biofortified Rice and Golden Rice, we refer to De Steur et al.[120] and the Bertebos Foundation Report,[131] respectively.

CONCLUSIONS

GM biofortified rice as a specific GM crop with health benefits is being increasingly examined as an alternative policy intervention to combat micronutrient malnutrition. At the turn of the century, initial publications on biofortification and Golden Rice as the first GM biofortified crop appeared. From 2004 onwards, the amount of research in the field of GM food, GM rice, and, in particular, biofortification increased dramatically. When looking at consumer studies on GM biofortified rice, the findings show that consumers in target countries are willing to pay for improved micronutrient contents in rice. The high premiums for both Folate Biofortified Rice and Golden Rice indicate that there is a consumer market for GM rice crops with health benefits. The high

cost-effectiveness of single- (folate, provitamin A) and multi- (folate, provitamin A, zinc, and iron) biofortified rice further supports the potential of GM biofortification to tackle a major public health problem such as vitamin A and folate deficiency.

GM biofortification of rice comes at a time when debate is rife regarding the adoption of GM food in many countries in the developing world. Despite its additional health benefits, future research is needed in order to introduce GM biofortified rice, adequately and sustainably, into the marketplace. Even though provitamin A enriched rice is on the verge of being released, it is evident that it will only serve regions where rice is a staple. Moreover, although GM biofortification (of rice) is technically "cost-effective", scientifically underpinned communications and promotion activity are needed to further convince governments and public health agencies of its potential in the developing world.

References

1. Shettya S. Malnutrition and Undernutrition. *Medicine (Baltimore)* 2003;**31**(4):18–22.
2. Micronutrient Initiative. *Investing in the future, a united call to action on vitamin and mineral deficiencies, Global Report 2009*. Ontario, Canada: Micronutrient Initiative; 2009.
3. FAO. *The State of Food Insecurity in the World: monitoring progress towards the World Food Summit and Millennium Development Goals*. Rome, Italy: FAO (Food and Agriculture Organization of the United Nations); 2004.
4. Gwatkin DR, Guillot M. *The burden of disease among the global poor: current situation, future trends, and implications for strategy*. Washington, DC: World Bank; 2000.
5. UNICEF. *Vitamin and Mineral Deficiency: A Global Damage Assessment Report*. New York, NY: UNICEF; 2004.
6. Mason JB, Lotfi M, Dalmiya N, Sethuraman K, Deitchler M, Geibel S, et al. *The Micronutrient Report: Current Progress in the Control of Vitamin A, Iodine, and Iron Deficiencies*. Ottawa, Canada: Micronutrient Initiative/International Development Research Center; 2001.
7. Horton S, Shekar M, McDonald C, Mahal A, Brooks JK. *Scaling Up Nutrition. What Will It Cost?*. Washington DC: World Bank; 2010.
8. West KP. Extent of vitamin A deficiency among preschool children and women of reproductive age. *J Nutr* 2002;**132**:S2857–66.
9. WHO. *Global prevalence of vitamin A deficiency in populations at risk 1995–2005. WHO Global Database on Vitamin A Deficiency*. Geneva, Switzerland: World Health Organization; 2009.
10. Rice AL, West KP, Black RE. Vitamin A deficiency. In: Ezzati M, Lopez AD, Rogers A, Murray CJL, editors. *Comparative Quantification of Health Risks: Global and Regional Burden of Disease Attributable to Selected Major Risk Factors*. Geneva, Switzerland: World Health Organization; 2004.
11. UN. *Fifth report on the world nutrition situation*. Geneva, Switzerland: UN SCN; 2004.
12. Hotz C, Brown KH. Assessment of the Risk of Zinc Deficiency in Populations and Options for its Control. International Zinc Nutrition Consultative Group (IZINCG) Technical Document No. 1. *Food Nutr Bull* 2004;**25**:S91–204.
13. Ezzati M, Lopez AD, Rogers A, Murray CJL. *Comparative quantification of health risks: Global and regional burden of disease attributable to selected major risk factors*. Geneva, Switzerland: World Health Organization; 2004.

14. De Steur H. *Market potential of folate biofortified rice in China. Doctoral thesis.* Ghent University; 2011.

15. *Micronutrient Initiative. About Micronutrient Malnutrition. Fast Facts.* Available at: http://www.micronutrient.org/english/View.asp?x=573; 2011.

16. Fiedler JL, Sanghvi TG, Saunders MK. A review of the micronutrient intervention cost literature: program design and policy lessons. *Int J Health Plann Manage* 2008;23:373–97.

17. Mason JB, Mannar MGV, Mock N. Controlling Micronutrient Deficiencies in Asia. *Asian Development Review* 1999;17(2):66–95.

18. *United Nations. Millennium Development Goals Indicators.* Available at: http://mdgs.un.org/unsd/mdg/Default.aspx; 2011.

19. *Copenhagen Consensus 2008.* Available at: http://www.copenhagenconsensus.com/ 2011.

20. UNICEF. *Progress for Children: A Report Card on Nutrition (No. 4).* New York, NY: UNICEF; 2006.

21. *United Nations. The Millennium Development Goals Report.* New York, NY: United Nations; 2010.

22. UNICEF. *Vitamin and Mineral Deficiency: A Damage Assessment Report for China.* New York, NY: UNICEF; 2004.

23. Stoltzfus RJ, Mullany L, Black RE. Iron deficiency anaemia. In: Ezzati M, Lopez AD, Rogers A, Murray CJL, editors. *Comparative Quantification of Health Risks: Global and Regional Burden of Disease Attributable to Selected Major Risk Factors.* Geneva, Switzerland: World Health Organization; 2004.

24. Caulfield L, Black RE. Zinc deficiency. In: Ezzati M, Lopez AD, Rogers A, Murray CJL, editors. *Comparative Quantification of Health Risks: Global and Regional Burden of Disease Attributable to Selected Major Risk Factors.* Geneva, Switzerland: World Health Organization; 2004.

25. De Steur H, Blancquaert D, Gellynck X, Lambert W, Van Der Straeten D. Ex-ante evaluation of biotechnology innovations: the case of folate biofortified rice in China. *Curr Pharm Biotechnol* 2012;13(15):2751–60.

26. De Steur H, Gellynck X, Blancquaert D, Lambert W, Van Der Straeten D, Qaim M. Potential impact and cost-effectiveness of multi-biofortified rice in China. *New Biotechnology* 2012;29(3):432–42.

27. De Steur H, Gellynck X, Storozhenko S, Liqun G, Lambert W, Van Der Straeten D, et al. The health benefits of folate biofortified rice in China. *Nat Biotechnol* 2010;28(6):554–6.

28. World Health Organization. *Comparative quantification of health risks for the year 2000.* Available at: http://www.who.int/healthinfo/global_burden_disease/risk_factors_2000/en/index.html; 2011.

29. World Health Organization. *World Health Report 2002: reducing risks, promoting healthy life.* Geneva, Switzerland: WHO; 2002.

30. Kennedy G, Natel G, Shetty P. The Scourge of Hidden Hunger: Global Dimensions of Micronutrient Deficiencies. Food *Nutrition and Agriculture* 2003;32:8–16.

31. Mclean E, Benoist B, Allen L. Review of the magnitude of folate and vitamin B12 deficiencies worldwide. *Food Nutr Bull* 2008;29(2):S38–51.

32. Blencowe H, Cousens S, Modell B, Lawn J. Folic acid to reduce neonatal mortality from neural tube disorders. *Int J Epidemiol* 2010;39:110–21.

33. World Health Organization. *Global Health risks. Mortality and burden of disease attributable to selected major risks.* Geneva, Switzerland: WHO; 2009.

34. *World Health Organization Risk factors estimates for 2004.* Available at: http://www.who.int/healthinfo/global_burden_disease/risk_factors/en/index.html; 2011.

35. Welch RM, Graham RD. Breeding for micronutrients in staple food crops from a human nutrition perspective. *Journal of Experimental Botany* 2004;55(396):353–64.

36. Stein AJ. *Micronutrient malnutrition and the impact of modern plant breeding on public health in India: how cost-effective is biofortification?.* Göttingen, Germany: Cuvillier; 2006.

37. Johns T, Eyzaguirre P. Biofortification, biodiversity and diet: A search for complementary applications against poverty and malnutrition. *Food Policy* 2007;32:1–24.

38. Cakmak I. Enrichment of cereal grains with zinc: Agronomic or genetic biofortification? *Plant Soil* 2008;302:1–17.

39. Mayer JE, Pfeiffer WH, Beyer P. Biofortified crops to alleviate micronutrient malnutrition. *Curr Opin Plant Biol* 2008;11:166–70.

40. Hirschi KD. Nutrient biofortification of food crops. *Annu Rev Nutr* 2009;29:401–21.

41. Bouis HE. Plant breeding: a new tool for fighting micronutrient malnutrition. *J Nutr* 2002;132(3):S491–4.

42. Micronutrient Initiative. *Vitamin and Mineral Deficiency. A challenge to the World's Food Companies.* Ontario, Canada: Micronutrient Initiative; 2004.

43. ADB. *Special Evaluation Study for Selected ADB Interventions on Nutrition and Food Fortification.* Manila, Philippines: Asian Development Bank; 2004.

44. Lawrence M, Watkins M, Ershoff D, Petitti D, Chiu V, Postlethwaite D. Design and evaluation of interventions promoting periconceptional multivitamin use. *Am J Prev Med* 2003;25:17–24.

45. Underwood BA, Smitasiri S. Micronutrient Malnutrition: Policies and Programs for Control and their Implications. *Annu Rev Nutr* 1999;19:303.

46. Li Z, Hao L. National Neural Tube Defects Prevention Program in China. *Food Nutr Bull* 2008;29(2):S196–204.

47. Busby A, Armstrong B, Dolk H, Armstrong N, Haeusler M, Berghold A, et al. Preventing neural tube defects in Europe: A missed opportunity. *Reprod Toxicol* 2005;20:393–402.

48. Czernichow S, Noisette N, Blacher J, Galan P, Mennen L, Hercberg S, et al. Case for folic acid and vitamin B12 fortification in Europe. *Semin Vasc Med* 2005;5(2):156–62.

49. Van Der Pal-De Bruin K, De Walle H, De Rover C, Jeeninga W, Cornel M, De Jong-Van Den Berg L. Influence of educational level on determinants of folic acid use. *Paediatr Perinat Epidemiol* 2003;17:256–63.

50. CDC. Use of dietary supplements containing folic acid among women of childbearing age - United States, 2005. *MMWR Morb Mortal Wkly Rep* 2005;54:955–8.

51. Ren A, Zhang L, Li Z, Hao L, Tian Y, Li Z. Awareness and use of folic acid, and blood folate concentrations among pregnant women in northern China – An area with a high prevalence of neural tube defects. *Reprod Toxicol* 2006;22:431–6.

52. Wailes E, Lee T- C. The Status of Rice Fortification in China. In: Alavi S, Bugusu B, Cramer G, Dary O, Lee T-C, Martin L, editors. *Rice Fortification in Developing Countries: A Critical Review of the Technical and Economic Feasibility.* Washington, DC: Academy for Educational Development; 2008. p. 34–45.

53. Smith AD, Kim YI, Refsum H. Is folic acid good for everyone? *Am J Clin Nutr* 2008;87(3):517–33.

54. Meenakshi JV, Johnson N, Manyong V, De Groote H, Yanggen D, Javelosa J, et al. *How cost-effective is biofortification in combating micronutrient malnutrition? An ex-ante assessment. HarvestPlus Working Paper No. 2.* Washington, DC: International Food Policy Research Institute; 2007.

55. Horton S, Alderman H, Rivera J. *Copenhagen Consensus 2008. Malnutrition and hunger. Executive summary.* Copenhagen, Denmark: Copenhagen Business School; 2008.

56. Qaim M, Stein AJ, Meenakshi JV. Economics of biofortification. *Agr Econ* 2007;37(S1):119–33.

57. B&M Gates Foundation. *Global Health Program. Nutrition strategy.* Seattle, WA: Bill & Melinda Gates Foundation; 2009.

58. Naqvi S, Zhu C, Farre G, Ramessar K, Bassie L, Breitenbach J, et al. Transgenic multivitamin corn through biofortification of endosperm with three vitamins representing three distinct metabolic pathways. *Proc Natl Acad Sci USA* 2009;106(19):7762–7.

59. James C. *Global Status of Commercialized Biotech/GM Crops: 2009. ISAAA Brief No. 41.* Ithaca, NY: ISAAA; 2009.

60. Micronutrient Initiative. *India Micronutrient National Investment Plan 2007-2011.* Delhi, India: Micronutrient Initiative; 2006.

61. Sanghvi TG, Harvey PW, Wainwright E. Maternal iron-folic acid supplementation programs: evidence of impact and implementation. *Food Nutr Bull* 2010;**31**(S2):100–7.

62. Alavi S, Bugusu B, Cramer G, Dary O, Lee T-C, Martin L, et al. *Rice Fortification in Developing Countries: A Critical Review of the Technical and Economic Feasibility.* Washington, DC: Academy for Educational Development; 2008.

63. Pingali P, Raney T. *From the Green Revolution to the Gene Revolution: How will the Poor Fare? ESA Working Paper No. 05-09.* Rome, Italy: FAO (Food and Agriculture Organization of the United Nations); 2005.

64. Underwood BA. Overcoming micronutrient deficiencies in developing countries: Is there a role for agriculture? *Food Nutr Bull* 2000;**21**:356–60.

65. Brooks S. *Rice Biofortification: Lessons for Global Science and Development.* London, UK: Earthscan; 2010.

66. GMO EFSA. Safety and nutritional assessment of GM plants and derived food and feed: The role of animal feeding trials. Report of the EFSA GMO Panel Working Group on Animal Feeding Trials. *Food Chem Toxicol* 2008;**46**:S2–70.

67. DellaPenna D. Nutritional genomics: manipulating plant micronutrients to improve human health. *Science* 1999;**285**:375–9.

68. Engel K-H, Frenzel T, Miller A. Current and future benefits from the use of GM technology in food production. *Toxicol Lett* 2002;**127**:329–36.

69. Toenniessen GH, O.Toole JC, DeVries J. Advances in Plant Biotechnology and its Adoption in Developing Countries. *Curr Opin Plant Biol* 2003;**6**:191–8.

70. Lönnerdal B. Genetically Modified Plants for Improved Trace Element Nutrition. *J Nutr* 2003;**133**:S1490–3.

71. Low J, Arimond M, Osman N, Cunguara B, Zano F, Tschirley D. A Food-Based Approach Introducing Orange-Fleshed Sweet Potatoes Increased Vitamin A Intake and Serum Retinol Concentrations in Young Children in Rural Mozambique. *J Nutr* 2007;**137**:1320–7.

72. Seshia S, Scoones I. *Tracing Policy Connections: The Politics of Knowledge in the Green Revolution and Biotechnology Eras in India. IDS Working Paper No. 188.* Brighton: Institute of Development Studies; 2003.

73. Naranjo MA. *Transgenic Plants For The Third Millennium Agriculture Horticulture* 2008;**65**(1):1843–5394.

74. HarvestPlus. *Breeding crops for better nutrition.* Washington, DC: International Food Policy Research Institute (IFPRI); 2009.

75. Beyer P, Al-Babili S, Ye X, Lucca P, Schaub P, Welsch R, et al. Golden Rice: introducing the β-carotene biosynthesis pathway into rice endosperm by genetic engineering. *J Nutr* 2002;**132**:S506–10.

76. Potrykus I. Golden Rice – from idea to reality. In: Foundation Bertebos, editor. *Golden Rice and other Biofortified Food Crops for Developing Countries Challenges and Potential.* Slöige, Sweden: KSLA; 2008. p. 11–6.

77. HUMBO. *The Golden Rice Project.* Available at: http://www.goldenrice.org/index.html; 2011.

78. Agrosalud. *Agrosalud. The development and deployment of biofortified staple crops to reduce nutrient deficiencies and improve food security in Latin America and the Caribbean.* Available at: http://www.agrosalud.org/; 2011.

79. CIAT. *Impact Assessment – Annual Report 2004.* Cali, Colombia: International Center for Tropical Agriculture; 2004.

80. Agrosalud. *Combating Hidden Hunger in Latin America Biofortified Crops with Improved Vitamin A, Essential Minerals and Quality Protein. Final Report to the Canadian International Development Agency.* Cali, Colombia: International Center for Tropical Agriculture (CIAT); 2011.

81. Storozhenko S, De Brouwer V, Volckaert M, Navarrete O, Blancquaert D, Zhang G-F, et al. Folate fortification of rice by metabolic engineering. *Nat Biotechnol* 2007;**25**(11):1277–9.

82. IOM. *Dietary Reference Intakes for Thiamin, Riboflavin, Niacin, Vitamin B6, Folate, Vitamin B12, Pantothenic Acid, Biotin, and Choline.* Washington, DC: National Academy of Sciences; 1998 Institute of Medicine. Food and Nutrition Board.

83. ISAAA. *Philippines Awaits Golden Rice Release in 2011.* Available at: http://www.isaaa.org/kc/cropbiotechupdate/article/default.asp?ID=815; 2007.

84. Stein AJ, Rodríguez-Cerezo E. *The global pipeline of new GM crops. Implications of asynchronous approval for international trade. JRC Scientific and Technical Report EUR 23486 EN.* Luxembourg: Office for Official Publications of the European Communities; 2009.

85. Waltz E. China's GM rice first. *Nat Biotechnol* 2010;**28**(1):8.

86. Stein AJ, Rodríguez-Cerezo E. International trade and the global pipeline of new GM crops. *Nat Biotechnol* 2010;**28**:23–5.

87. Mannar MGV. Food Fortification as a Major Strategy to Address Micronutrient Malnutrition in Asia. In: Wallich C, Hill T, Malaspina A, Mannar MGV, Hunt JM, editors. *The Manila Forum on Food Fortification Policy; 2001.* Manila, Philippines: Asian Development Bank (ADB); 2001. International Life Sciences Institute, and Micronutrient Initiative.

88. Stein AJ, Meenakshi JV, Qaim M, Nestel P, Sachdev HPS, Bhutta ZA. *Health benefits of biofortification: an ex-ante analysis of iron-rich rice and wheat in India.* Providence, RI: Annual meeting of the American Agricultural Economics Association (AAEA); 2005.

89. Bekaert S, Storozhenko S, Mehrshahi P, Bennett M, Lambert W, Gregory J, et al. Folate biofortification in food plants. *Trends Plant Sci* 2008;**13**:28–35.

90. Rébeillé F, Ravanel S, Jabrin S, Douce R, Storozhenko S, Van Der Straeten D. Folates in plants: biosynthesis, distribution, and enhancement. *Physiol Plantarum* 2006;**126**(3):330–42.

91. Paine JA, Shipton CA, Chaggar S, Howells RM, Kennedy MJ, Vernon G, et al. Improving the nutritional value of Golden Rice through increased pro-vitamin A content. *Nat Biotechnol* 2005;**23**(4):482–7.

92. Al-Babili S, Beyer P. Golden Rice – five years on the road – five years to go? *Trends Plant Sci* 2005;**10**:565–73.

93. Blancquaert D, Storozhenko S, Loizeau K, De Steur H, De Brouwer V, Viaene J, et al. Folates and folic acid: from fundamental research towards sustainable health. *Crit Rev Plant Sci* 2010;**29**(1):14–35.

94. Dubock A. Marketing research for optimizing Golden Rice cultivation and consumption. In: Foundation Bertebos, editor. *Golden Rice and other Biofortified Food Crops for Developing Countries Challenges and Potential.* Slöige, Sweden: KSLA; 2008. p. 23–7.

95. DellaPenna D. Biofortification of plant-based food: Enhancing folate levels by metabolic engineering. *Proc Natl Acad Sci USA* 2007;**104**(10):3675–6.

96. McIntosh S, Brushett D, Henry R. GTP cyclohydrolase 1 expression and folate accumulation in the developing wheat seed. *J Cereal Sci* 2008;**48**:503–12.

97. Diaz de la Garza R, Gregory J, Hanson A. Folate biofortification of tomato fruit. *Proc Natl Acad Sci U S A* 2007;**104**:4218–22.

98. Lucca P, Hurrell R, Potrykus I. Genetic engineering approaches to improve the bioavailability and the level of iron in rice grains. *Theoretical and Applied Genetics* 2001;**102**:392–7.

99. Goto F, Yoshihara T, Shigemoto N, Toki S, Takaiwa F. Iron fortification of rice seed by the soybean ferritin gene. *Nat Biotechnol* 1999;**17**(42):282–6.

100. Johnson AAT, Kyriacou B, Callahan DL, Carruthers L, Stangoulis J, Stangoulis J, et al. *Constitutive Overexpression of the OsNAS Gene Family Reveals Single-Gene Strategies for Effective Iron- and Zinc-Biofortification of Rice Endosperm* 2011;**6**(9):1–11.

101. Vasconcelos M, Datta K, Oliva N, Khalekuzzaman M, Torrizo L, Krishnan S, et al. Enhanced iron and zinc accumulation in transgenic rice with the ferritin gene. *Plant Sci* 2003;**164**:371–8.

102. Gross J, Stein R, Fett-Neto A, Palma J. Iron homoestasis related genes in rice. *Genetics and Molecular Biology* 2003;**26**:477–97.

103. USDA. *USDA National Nutrient Database for Standard Reference, release 21.* Available at: Nutrient Data Laboratory home page http://www.ars.usda.gov/ba/bhnrc/ndl; 2008.

104. Zimmermann R, Qaim M. Potential Health Benefits of Golden Rice: a Philippine Case Study. *Food Policy* 2004;**29**:147–68.

105. Stein AJ, Sachdev HPS, Qaim M. Potential impact and cost-effectiveness of Golden Rice. *Nat Biotechnol* 2006;**24**(10):1200–1.

106. Bailey L. Folate and Vitamin B12 Recommended intakes and status in the United States. *Nutr Rev* 2004;**62**(6):14–20.

107. Tang G, Qin J, Dolnikowski GG, Russell RM, Grusak MA. Golden Rice is an effective source of vitamin A. *Am J Clin Nutr* 2009;**89** (1776–1783).

108. WHO. *Standards for Maternal and Neonatal Care. Iron and folate supplementation.* Geneva, Switzerland: World Health Organization; 2006.

109. IOM. *Dietary Reference Intakes for Vitamin A, Vitamin K, Arsenic, Boron, Chromium, Copper, Iodine, Iron, Manganese, Molybdenum, Nickel, Silicon, Vanadium, and Zinc.* Washington, DC: National Academy of Sciences; 2002 Institute of Medicine. Food and Nutrition Board.

110. FAO/WHO. *Vitamin and mineral requirements in human nutrition: report of a joint FAO/WHO expert consultation, Bangkok, Thailand, 21–30 September 1998. 2nd edition.* Geneva, Switzerland: WHO; 2004.

111. Miller HI. The regulation of agricultural biotechnology: science shows a better way. *New Biotechnology* 2010;**27**(5):628–34.

112. Li Q, Curtis K, McCluskey J, Wahl T. Consumer attitudes toward genetically modified foods in Beijing, China. *AgBioForum* 2002;**5**(4):145–52.

113. De Steur H, Gellynck X, Storozhenko S, Liqun G, Lambert W, Van Der Straeten D, et al. Willingness to Accept and Purchase Genetically Modified Rice with High Folate Content in Shanxi Province, China. *Appetite* 2010;**54**:118–25.

114. De Steur H, Gellynck X, Feng S, Rutsaert P, Verbeke W. Determinants of willingness-to-pay for GM rice with health benefits in a high-risk region: Evidence from experimental auctions for folate biofortified rice in China. *Food Qual Prefer* 2012;**25**(2):87–94.

115. Deodhar S, Ganesh S, Chern W. Emerging markets for GM foods: a study of consumer's willingness to pay in India. *Int J Biotechnol* 2008;**10**(6):570–87.

116. Depositario DPT, Nayga RM, Wu X, Laude TP. Effects of Information on Consumers' Willingness to Pay for Golden Rice. *Asian Economic Journal* 2009;**23**(4):457–76.

117. Lusk JL. Effects of Cheap Talk on Consumer Willingness-To-Pay for Golden Rice. *Amer J Agr Econ* 2003;**85**(4):840–56.

118. Gonzalez C, Johnson N, Qaim M. Consumer Acceptance of Second-Generation GM Foods: The Case of Biofortified Cassava in the North-East of Brazil. *J Agr Econ* 2009;**60**(3):604–24.

119. De Groote H, Kimenju S, Morawetz U. Estimating consumer willingness to pay for food quality with experimental auctions: the case of yellow versus fortified maize meal in Kenya. *Agr Econ* 2011;**42**:1–16.

120. De Steur H, Gellynck X, Blancquaert D, Storozhenko S, Liqun G, Lambert W, et al. Market potential of folate biofortified rice in China. In: Preedy VR, Srirajaskanthan R, Patel VB, editors. *Handbook of Food fortification and Health: From Concepts to Public Health Applications (forthcoming).* New York, NY: Springer; 2013.

121. Meenakshi JV, Johnson N, Manyong V, De Groote H, Javelosa J, Yanggen D, et al. How cost-effective is biofortification in combating micronutrient malnutrition? An *ex-ante* assessment. *World Dev* 2010;**38**(1):64–75.

122. *World Bank. World Development Report 1993.* New York, NY: Oxford University Press; 1993.

123. BLS. *Inflation calculator.* Available at: http://data.bls.gov/cgi-bin/cpicalc.pl; 2011.

124. Hotz C, McClafferty B. From harvest to health: Challenges for developing biofortified staple foods and determining their impact on micronutrient status. *Food Nutr Bull* 2007;**28**(2):271–9.

125. Onyango BM, Nayga RM. Consumer Acceptance of Nutritionally Enhanced Genetically Modified Food: Relevance of Gene Transfer Technology. *JARE* 2004;**29**(3):567–82.

126. Siegrist M. Factors influencing public acceptance of innovative food technologies and products. *Trends Food Sci Technol* 2008;**19**:603–8.

127. Tenbült P, De Vries N, Dreezens E, Martijn C. Perceived naturalness and acceptance of genetically modified food. *Appetite* 2005;**45**:47–50.

128. Prom-u-thai C, Rerkasem B, Fukai S, Huang L. Iron fortification and parboiled rice quality: appearance, cooking quality and sensory attributes. *J Sci Food Agric* 2009;**89**:2565–71.

129. De Groote H, Kimenju S. Comparing consumer preferences for color and nutritional quality in maize: Application of a semi-double-bound logistic model on urban consumers in Kenya. *Food Policy* 2008;**33**:362–70.

130. Stevens R, Winter-Nelson A. Consumer acceptance of provitamin A-biofortified maize in Maputo, Mozambique. *Food Policy* 2008;**33**:341–51.

131. Foundation Bertebos. Golden Rice and other Biofortified Food Crops for Developing Countries. Challenges and Potential. Report from the Bertebos Conference in Falkenberg, Sweden, 7–9 September 2008. *Kungl Skogs- och Lantbruksakademiens TIDSKRIFT* 2008(7):1–116.

Rice Bran: A Food Ingredient with Global Public Health Opportunities

Erica C. Borresen*, Elizabeth P. Ryan*,†

*Colorado State University, Department of Environmental and Radiological Health Sciences, Fort Collins, Colorado, USA, †Colorado School of Public Health, Fort Collins, Colorado, USA

INTRODUCTION

Rice is an important staple food crop for human health because it provides the bulk of calories for more than half the world's population. Rice is currently grown in over 100 countries, and more than 1 billion people depend on it for their livelihood.[1] Of the 475 million tonnes of milled rice produced globally, 85% is used for human consumption and the remaining 15% is used for animal feed or is wasted.[2] In developing countries, rice provides roughly 30% of the population's daily diet, and consumption has grown in developed countries to ~27 pounds of rice per person per year.[3] Thus, in order to enhance our understanding of the connections between rice, nutrition, and human health, an overarching recognition of rice is needed in the context of global food security.

Rice is primarily consumed in the polished, white grain form. Unfortunately, the refined white grain has lost many nutritious components with the removal of the bran. The bran portion of the grain contains a rich source of lipids, protein, soluble and insoluble dietary fibers, iron, B vitamins, and a number of small molecules (e.g., phytosterols, phenolic acids, and antioxidants) that can aid in disease prevention, control, and treatment.[4] Figure 22.1 shows paddy rice processing of whole grain rice, and the estimated nutrient contents of the white rice and rice bran parts.

Consumption of the bran portion of whole grain rice is being investigated regarding health attributes relevant to both chronic and infectious diseases. The vast majority of research has focused on chronic disease prevention and control, whereby brown rice and rice bran have been shown to decrease risk of type 2 diabetes,[5,6] regulate lipid metabolism,[7–10] control metabolic syndrome and cardiovascular disease,[11–13] and exhibit anti-cancer activity.[14,15] The effects of rice bran components on the immune response and, more recently, in protection against enteric pathogens such as *Salmonella*,[16] represent areas of research relevant to infectious diseases.[17–19]

Given that many of the world's poorest children and adults eat white rice as their main source of calories, and do not receive the natural health-promoting components found in the bran, they also are at higher risk of malnutrition. Approximately 870 million individuals (or 1 in 8) are considered chronically undernourished in our world today.[20] These individuals can be classified as "food insecure," because they do not have adequate safe and nutritious food because of lack of availability, affordability, accessibility, or some combination of these factors. Although the global population of undernourished people has been steadily declining since the 1990s, there are still more than 2.5 million children under the age of 5 years that die from malnutrition-related complications every year.[20] Achieving food security has become a major global public health priority that relates to the first Millennium Development Goal (MDG) to halve the prevalence of hunger and malnourishment, and the UN Secretary General calling for a "Zero Hunger Challenge" by encouraging all nations to end hunger.[21]

At the same time, obesity has been increasing globally, with rates that have more than doubled since 1980; currently, over half a billion people (or 1 in 10) are obese.[22] The complexity of the obesity epidemic involves individual behaviors, physical inactivity, and dietary choices, as well as socioeconomic influences and psychological conditions apparent in both developed and developing countries. Evidence shows that individuals who have lower birth weights and childhood stunting are at risk for developing co-morbidities associated with

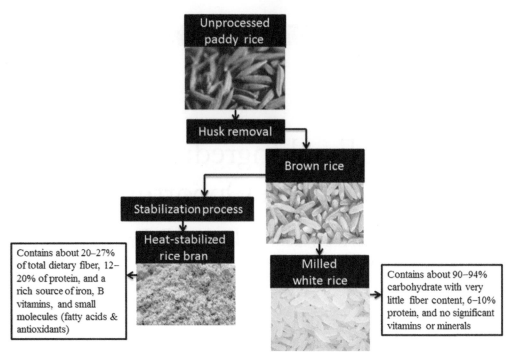

FIGURE 22.1   Whole grain rice processing and a summary of nutrient variations of white rice and rice bran end products.[10,57] See color plate at the back of the book.

abdominal obesity later in life.[23,24] This evolving paradox of malnourished and overweight/obese individuals further stresses the barriers to improve health in our global food system.

Addressing global food security with a multidisciplinary approach and diverse inputs across non-profits, non-governmental organizations (NGOs), academia, private sectors, governments, and even local, small shareholders is challenging. Given that there is an adequate amount of food grown in agriculture to feed the world's population,[25] how do we innovate the rice food system to address issues of hunger, malnutrition, and life-threatening diseases? Specifically, can we develop opportunities for dietary rice bran to simultaneously alleviate the complex problems of malnutrition and obesity-related diseases? The Green Revolution accomplished altering rice genes for improved rice varieties with increased yield to feed the growing population, and now we understand that the increased production of rice does not equate to better nutrition.[26] Tremendous attention has been paid to the development of Golden Rice to combat vitamin A deficiency,[27–29] yet with the rice genome sequenced and the varied cropping systems intact, there still remains a great opportunity to advance dietary rice bran intake as a sustainable solution for human health via improved post-harvest processing (e.g., safe collection and storage of rice bran for human consumption).[30] Furthermore, there continues to be a gap in our knowledge regarding how bran from genetically and geographically diverse rice varieties differs in health attributes.

In this chapter, our objective is to synthesize rice bran's global health opportunities for chronic and infectious disease control and prevention. To this end, we will discuss current challenges, provide an overview of dietary rice bran intake possibilities across the lifespan and address the need for further research on rice health traits and bioactive components from studies using traditional rice varieties.

COMMON TERMINOLOGY FOR DIETARY RICE BRAN AND PUBLIC HEALTH OPPORTUNITIES

There are multiple stakeholders involved in rice food systems that can influence our understanding of nutrition and health benefits. Here, we define a number of commonly used terms throughout the chapter for the purpose of enhancing the clarity of this conceptual framework.

Complementary foods: Foods other than breast milk or infant formula introduced to an infant to provide additional necessary nutrients for proper growth and development.
Chronic diseases: Diseases that progress slowly over time. Examples include obesity, cardiovascular disease, cancer, and type 2 diabetes.[31]
Enteric pathogen: Any bacteria that causes disease in the intestinal tract. Clinical symptoms include greater than or equal to three unformed stools

(diarrhea) in 1 day, and nutrient electrolyte absorption failure by the intestine.[32]

Food security: To attain adequate nutrition so that "… all people, at all times, have physical and economic access to sufficient, safe and nutritious food to meet their dietary needs and food preferences for an active and healthy life".[33]

Food system: All activities, people, and resources utilized from production to consumption, including growing, harvesting, processing, packaging, transporting, marketing, consumption, and disposal.

Green Revolution: An increase in crop yields based on cultivation of high-response varieties of food grains, such as wheat, rice, maize, and millet, and including intensive use of fertilizers, pesticides, irrigation, and machinery.[34]

Gut microbiome: All microbes found in the human gut.[35]

Health: A state of complete physical, mental, and social well-being, and not merely the absence of disease or infirmity.[36]

Infectious diseases: Diseases that are caused by pathogenic microorganisms (e.g., bacteria, viruses, parasites, or fungi) that are spread directly or indirectly between individuals.[37]

Malnutrition: A broad term used to describe people whose food intake does not provide adequate calories and other essential nutrients for growth and health maintenance or when people are not able to fully utilize the food they eat due to illness. This term may also apply to people whose food intake provides more than enough calories, yet from nutrient-depleted sources.[38]

Micronutrients: Nutrients required by humans throughout life in small quantities to orchestrate a range of physiological functions.[39]

Phytochemicals: Chemical compounds found in plant sources that may have biological significance but are not established as essential nutrients.[40]

Public health nutrition: The art and science of promoting population health status via sustainable improvements in the food and nutrition system.[41]

Rice varieties: There are more than 100,000 varieties of rice (*Oryza sativa*), categorized into four major groups: Indica, Japonica, Aromatic, and Glutinous.[42]

Whole grain rice: Rice that contains 100% of the original grain (i.e., germ, endosperm, and bran), and is also known as brown rice.[43]

CURRENT CHALLENGES FOR DIETARY RICE BRAN

After rice is harvested from the field, it goes through a milling process where the hull and bran are removed mechanically, leaving refined white rice (68–70%), rice husk (20%), rice bran (5–10%), and rice germ (2%).[44] Based on current estimates of rice production, there are roughly 66 to 74 million tonnes of bran that can be made available for human consumption.[4] Rice bran contains essential micronutrients and non-essential phytochemicals, and is used as animal feed or becomes agricultural food waste. Consumption of the fully processed white rice grain provides calories that primarily stem from carbohydrates (Fig. 22.1), and white rice consumption as a staple food alone has been shown to lead to malnutrition.[45] Lack of daily intake of essential nutrients can lead to a broad spectrum of risk for infectious and chronic diseases. Individuals suffering from infectious or chronic diseases may experience persistent inflammation and reduced host immune competence, both of which now occur at alarming rates in impoverished and malnourished areas of the world.[46]

Figure 22.2 illustrates a conceptual framework for "rice bran opportunities" in global public health nutrition by means of interrupting the negative cycle between malnutrition and disease (both infectious and chronic). The inner circle displays challenges for achieving adequate nutrition and disease prevention. The rectangles within this circle list causal factors, including nutrient malabsorption, lack of food security, gastrointestinal damage and inflammation, and impaired immune defense.[47,48] The dotted lines outline environmental exposures and damaged gastrointestinal integrity that keep this negative cycle intact. Novel solutions using dietary rice bran include supplementation into culturally acceptable foods and implementation of diverse rice varieties with existing traits of agronomic importance. The outer red squares suggest the utility of rice bran phytochemicals and other bioactive components to improve nutritional status and decrease disease susceptibility (both infectious and chronic). These inputs may in turn reduce obesity, improve growth and cognitive capability, as well as help establish a healthy gut microbiome.

Although the rice bran solution appears conceptually simple, there are challenges to address before rice bran can be sustainably utilized for human consumption. Post-harvest technicalities include the need for heat stabilization (lipase inactivation), ensuring shelf-life and storage conditions in different climates, value-added benefits for rice farmers, cultural taste preferences, and verification of bran nutrient and phytochemical contents across rice varieties. Addressing and overcoming these challenges with innovation represents promising avenues for achieving food security and enhancing human health in global, diverse populations.

Rice Bran Heat Stabilization and Shelf-Life

The main reason why rice bran has been largely limited to animal feed is that it quickly becomes rancid after milling, caused by lipase-mediated oxidation of rice bran

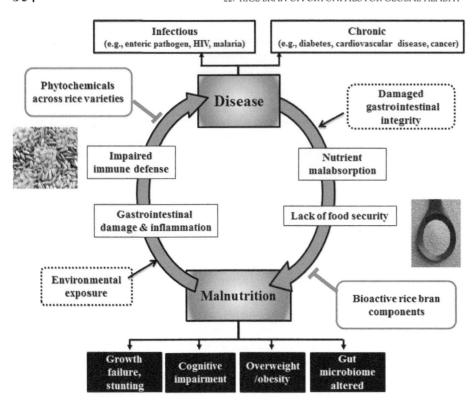

FIGURE 22.2 Conceptual framework for rice bran opportunities in global public health. See color plate at the back of the book. *Adapted from Preidis* et al.[89]

lipids.[49] Milling technology advances have now allowed for stabilized rice bran via cold storage, sun-drying, steaming, and expelling.[50] Countries such as India, Thailand, and the United States have also started to use these stabilization processes to create rice bran oil. Although stabilization is a promising attribute for rice bran products, most of the rice-producing countries do not have this type of technology or current infrastructure. Thus, the immediate challenge is to develop rice bran stabilization methods in areas experiencing food insecurity, malnutrition, and high rates of mortality under the age of 5 years, such as many parts of Sub-Saharan Africa and Asia.

Rice bran has a shorter shelf-life compared to refined white rice due to increases in free fatty lipids during storage.[51] If proper packaging and storage recommendations are followed, white rice can be stored for decades, compared to only about 1 year for the bran fraction. Advancing technology through extrusion cooking (a process of heating the food product under high pressure that results in reduced moisture content and a cooked and dried food product) has allowed for an extended shelf-life of rice bran.[52] Another rice processing technique is parboiling, which deactivates the lipase and allows some minerals and water-soluble vitamins to leak from the bran to the endosperm, which increases the nutrient composition. However, antioxidants are also destroyed in this process, causing the nutrient profile to differ from that of heat-stabilized rice bran.[4] The creation of technology that allows adequate stabilization will result in a longer shelf-life and create an opportunity to develop a market that utilizes rice bran as a common ingredient for human consumption.

Cultural Preferences Regarding Brown Rice or Rice Bran

As traditional diets shift towards convenience around the world, perceptions regarding healthy foods begin to waver and food decisions become based on cost, ease, and preferences. These are important considerations for incorporating rice bran into meals and snacks, and may influence current beliefs or existing knowledge of whole grain, brown rice preferences. For example, individuals in Tanzania are primarily unaware of brown rice; or assume it is part of a diabetic diet.[53] Additionally, participants in a focus group study in southern India commented that eating rice that is not white in color is considered to be inferior.[54]

There is continuing growth in the demand for brown rice by health conscious people in developed countries.[55] Additionally, food scientists and health researchers are aware of the important bioactive compounds in rice bran, yet there continues to be a lack of global consumer awareness regarding the importance of rice bran for chronic disease control and prevention. Limited information has been collected to show the amount of brown rice consumed throughout the world, separately from white rice. Most epidemiological research has to define what exactly a whole grain is, in order to complete analysis on whole grain rice consumption.[5,56] We suggest that collection of data and statistics regarding the dietary intake of brown rice and rice bran (in addition to white rice) is critical for evaluating health properties at a population scale, and for drawing accurate associations between the amounts of brown rice or rice bran intake needed to affect chronic or infectious disease outcomes. As more areas start to face a "double burden of disease", where countries have problems with both infectious and chronic diseases, increased education and lay knowledge regarding the healthy content of brown rice and rice bran may be beneficial for changing nutrition–food behaviors, cultural preferences, and taste perceptions.

Whole Grain Rice Contents of Health Importance

There are some current myths and misconceptions regarding rice bran components that merit clarification and continued investigation. One concern is the level of antinutritional compounds, such as trypsin inhibitors, hemagglutinin (lectin), oryzacystatin, and phytic acid, which can decrease the bioavailability of other nutrients and thus may lead to deficiencies and malnutrition.[57] These compounds are found in rice bran, yet hemagglutinin and oryzacystatin antinutrient activities are inhibited by high heat exposure (such as heat stabilization). Phytic acid, although considered an antinutrient in foods, is a candidate nutraceutical for chemoprevention.[58,59] Continued education from cancer chemoprevention research regarding phytic acid has been helpful, and may be particularly important to areas with minimal access to medicines and healthcare.

Other potential concerns for rice bran that also exist for many other staple food crops include aflatoxin, pesticide residues, and arsenic.[60,61] Recent evaluation of the occurrence and distribution of pesticide residues in brown rice, white rice, and rice bran under controlled field-growing conditions suggests that the lipid content of rice bran may make it more susceptible to uptake of lipophilic pesticides such as difenoconazole and the strobilurins.[62] Greater knowledge of these potential exposures and continued research in this area is necessary not only for raw rice products, but also in combination with water contaminants and cooking conditions. Rice bran arsenic levels appear to be dependent on soil concentrations in specific geographic regions,[63–65] and further research is needed to assess the maximum allowable intake levels from rice, and to accurately differentiate between total, organic, and inorganic forms.

Whole grain consumption across cereal grains has shown promising outcomes for chronic disease prevention, and has been mainly attributed to dietary fiber. In brief, soluble fiber aids in lowering cholesterol, and insoluble fiber helps to decrease gastrointestinal transit time and increase short-chain fatty acid production.[66]

Total dietary fiber makes up about 20% of rice bran, while only 2–3% is soluble fiber.[57] Even though rice bran has generally lower amounts of soluble fiber compared to other brans (such as wheat, corn, or oat brans), it has more compelling cholesterol lowering properties due to its unique lipids.[7–12,67] Mechanisms of action from other bioactive nutrients and compounds (e.g. γ-oryzanol) may also be major driving factors in the disease-fighting activity. Table 22.1 highlights the biological activity associated with some bioactive rice bran components that may also be important for decreasing malnutrition and improving protection against disease. Although these compounds have been reviewed separately for health promotion and disease prevention, our work and that of others suggest that whole food approaches may be more beneficial for health when compared to single-agent dietary supplements.[14,68]

DIETARY RICE BRAN OPPORTUNITIES THROUGHOUT THE LIFESPAN

Addressing the challenges and embracing the opportunities discussed for rice bran in the previous sections is achievable through continued research, public–private partnerships, and global health collaborations. Fortunately, progress has been made through nutrient supplementation programs, breastfeeding promotion, and culturally targeted nutritional education programs. However, focused efforts are still needed for concerns such as iron deficiency and anemia, which continue to be increasingly prevalent in rice-consuming countries.[55] Iron deficiency can be particularly troubling for growing children and for women during pregnancy. Iron and other micronutrients (e.g., potassium, zinc, and magnesium) are detected in the rice grain; however, the amounts vary across varieties.[45] Thus, the untapped resource of rice bran may lead to additional global health achievements for children and adults in rice nutrient enrichment programs, in particular where varieties that contain higher amounts of these essential micronutrients are used.

Rice and health related scientific research that is performed without industry bias is necessary to convey the importance of rice bran for health across the lifespan. Consumers need greater access to knowledge and awareness of rice bran nutritional properties, even though this food rarely reaches our plates. Taste and texture are also important attributes that merit further study for acceptance by consumers, as these features alone have been cited as reasons why brown rice has not been widely accepted.[54] Introduction of rice bran into existing meals is a promising solution that allows individuals to continue eating their preferred foods, while delivering the important bioactive nutrients and phytochemicals. There is an opportunity to enhance health and nutrition

TABLE 22.1   Selected Rice Bran Bioactive Components and Biologic Activity for Human Health

Rice Bran Bioactive Food Components	Examples	Biologic Activity	Reference(s)
Non-saponifiable lipid (i.e., γ-oryzanol)	Combination of ferulic acid, sterol esters, and triterpene alcohols	Antibacterial Antioxidant Reduces cholesterol absorption Cancer chemoprevention	Cicero and Gaddi[8], Ghoneum et al.[18], Rong et al.[90], Seetharamaiah and Chandrasekhara[91]
Vitamin E	α-Tocopherol, γ-tocopherol, tocotrienols	Cancer chemoprevention Antioxidant Antibacterial Reduces cholesterol absorption	Kawakami et al.[92], Minhajuddin et al.[93], Miyazawa et al.[94], Sen et al.[95], Sun et al.[96], Morel et al.[97], Boxer[98], Iqbal et al.[99], Nakashima et al.[100]
Polyphenols	Ferulic acid, α-lipoic acid, caffeic acid, salicylic acid	Antioxidant Antiproliferative effect on cancer Antibacterial Anti-inflammatory	Mori et al.[58], Taniguchi et al.[101], Srinivasan et al.[102]
Phytosterols	β-Sitosterol, campesterol, stigmasterol	Reduces cholesterol absorption Anti-inflammatory Antioxidant Stimulates lymphocyte proliferation Cancer chemoprevention	Basker et al.[103]
Amino acids	Lysine	Growth and development Hypoallergenicity	Khan et al.[70]

across the lifespan with the use of dietary rice bran, and this is explained in greater detail below.

Addition of Rice Bran to Complementary Foods

For the first 6 months of life, it is recommended that infants be exclusively breastfed for proper growth and development.[69] After this period, complementary foods are introduced to an infant's diet; these may include food products based on staples, as well as fruits and vegetables, in liquid to semisolid forms. Acceptable weaning foods may also include higher amounts of protein and fats to continue healthy development into the toddler years, including animal-based sources such as meat, milk, and eggs. However, in areas that lack food security these options may not be available to young members of the family. This can lead to inadequate nutrient uptake and underdevelopment of infants' and toddlers' immune systems, making them more susceptible to diseases such as viral and bacterial associated pneumonia and diarrhea (see Fig. 22.2).[48]

The introduction of rice bran into weaning foods is a tremendous opportunity, because of its exceptional fat and protein content, high digestibility, and hypoallergenic assets.[70] Rice bran lipids can deliver energy needs adjusted based on age. The protein quality of rice bran is more suitable compared to other cereal brans, as it contains a substantial amount of lysine and the amino acid content meets the requirements of growing children.[71] Adding rice bran to complementary foods is a promising approach to improve overall nutritional

quality, and food scientists have been working on creating these rice bran-added products. A recently developed rice bran enriched biscuit included 10% of a rice bran protein concentrate, and was shown to be similarly acceptable when compared to a non-rice bran biscuit.[72] Khan et al. developed a rice bran protein isolate-based formulation that can be used in complementary foods and was tested for acceptability in weaning infants via taste satisfaction.[70] These studies provide compelling evidence for the feasibility of adding rice bran to complementary foods in culturally and socially acceptable ways.

Various strategies, such as micronutrient supplementation, food fortification, and educating mothers about appropriate complementary foods, have proven to be effective in many countries,[20] yet alarming rates of child malnutrition and disease continue. Promising results from a recent Cochrane Review found that those infected with enteric pathogens, have improved outcomes with rice-based medications, such as oral rehydration solutions.[73] Additionally, Intermark Partners Strategic Management, LLC and Sustainable Nutrition International were recently awarded a Patent for Humanity for the development of Nutra-Iso™, a technology that extracts edible protein and other nutrients from rice bran.[74] This product can be used as a nutritional supplement for children and pregnant women. The increasing evidence indicates that practical solutions involving low-cost, energy-rich, and high-nutrition infant products can be developed and implemented in malnourished areas.

Preventing and Treating Malnutrition in Children via a Healthy Gut Microbiome

In addition to delivering a combination of important nutrients, rice bran has also been shown to improve gut health in animal, *in vitro*, and human studies. Henderson *et al.* found that 10% rice bran consumption modulated mucosal immunity by increasing immunoglobin A concentrations and native gut *Lactobacillus* spp. in a mouse model.[19] Martins *et al.* reported improved colon development in malnourished rats with 5% rice bran supplementation.[75] *In vitro* studies have also shown that rice bran can augment phagocytosis and enhance intracellular killing of microbes by human phagocytic cells.[17,18] Additionally, the human gut microbiome has shown to be altered, with immunological benefits, through consumption of whole grains, including brown rice.[76] These studies indicate that rice bran has bioactive properties that modify metabolic properties of the gut microbiome with long-term health improvements that can include, but may not be limited to, improved immune development through proper absorption of nutrients, and protection against enteric infections, especially in high-risk children (Fig. 22.2). The healthcare infrastructure is unstable in many parts of the world and access to medications and medical care may be difficult to obtain; thus, novel, safe and low-cost dietary interventions are crucial to improve global health alongside food security.

Rice Bran for Chronic Disease Prevention and Control

Chronic diseases are increasing in incidence and prevalence in both developed and developing countries. Food quality and eating habits have been implicated in the etiology of these diseases, and whole foods are now being advocated to replace easy-to-distribute, ready-made nutrient-deprived food products that lead to higher caloric intakes. Increased energy intake coupled with sedentary lifestyles contributes to obesity and an increased risk of developing chronic diseases.[77] Numerous *in vitro*, animal, and epidemiological evidences suggest that consuming whole grain rice may be protective against these chronic diseases via unique bioactive nutrients and phytochemicals (e.g., γ-oryzanol and tocotrienols).[55] Vitamin E complex contents in rice bran, which can range from 179–389 mg/kg, are almost three-fourths α- and δ-tocotrienols.[78] Rice bran is also high in fatty acids (oleic, linoleic, and α-linoleic acids) compared with other grains, and includes a vast amount of various compounds such as phytosterols, tocopherols, and γ-oryzanol.[14] These components found in rice bran oil were shown to reduce total cholesterol, low density lipoproteins, and triglycerides, for further protection from cardiovascular disease.[10]

Despite the health advantages and increasing availability of whole grain rice, particularly in developed countries, switching white rice consumers to eating whole grain rice does not seem likely, given cultural connections and taste preferences for white rice. Developing food options with the addition of rice bran allows the populations of rice-consuming countries to continue eating rice in their traditional way but still receive the healthy benefits of eating bran. Our laboratory has completed a placebo-controlled, single-blinded pilot dietary rice bran intervention study in healthy adults with and without a history of colorectal cancer. We developed seven meals and six snacks that include rice bran as a main ingredient. Interim analysis has shown feasibility of consuming 30 g of rice bran daily without complications (data not published). The ability to incorporate rice bran into common meals, such as casseroles, soups, and crackers, indicates an opportunity for the food industry to modify current food products with rice bran, with tremendous potential to result in greater consumer acceptance of these meals and snack foods.[66] Further research on increasing dietary rice bran for health-promoting capabilities will be helpful to endorse these food products.

GLOBAL RICE GENETIC VARIATION

Increased rice yield as a result of the Green Revolution provided substantially more food for a growing global population. These modified rice crops were minimally evaluated for changes in the levels of essential and non-essential nutrients (e.g., certain amino acids, minerals, vitamins, and fatty acids).[79] The grain quantity-over-quality debate (also referred to as the "breeders dilemma") merits continued discussion because rice breeders currently do not include nutritional or health importance as an integrated quantitative trait for crop improvement.[80] With over 100,000 varieties of rice grown throughout the world, substantial opportunities exist to better understand the health importance of and traits associated with bran. Alongside the development and expansion of genetically modified rice to include β-carotene (i.e., Golden Rice), there is still much to learn about traditional rice varieties and how their nutrient profiles, especially regarding the bran component, can address the prevention of malnourishment and disease.

A recent review showed that nutrient make-up of rice varieties differs significantly, and that the varieties with higher nutritional values are used less frequently due to their lower grain yields.[81] The mineral content of 274 rice genotypes has also shown variations,[45] indicating that certain rice varieties should be further evaluated for higher amounts of micronutrients. Rice has been used for medicinal purposes too; for instance, there is a specific variety of rice with red bran that is used to control hypertension and diabetes.[82] Moreover, a medicinal Indian rice variety traditionally used in Ayurveda, called Njavara, has also been scientifically examined.[83–86]

With increasing evidence that rice varieties do not share similar chemical and nutrient compositions,[87] and that the bran component is the most important for delivery of nutrients found in whole grain rice, it is crucial to conduct research on rice varieties for their mechanisms of action to improve a range of health outcomes in people. Studying changes in the human metabolome and gut microbiome will be helpful in this endeavor, as researchers will be able to understand the gut microbial metabolic mechanisms involved and may recommend which rice varieties are optimal for health outcomes in children and adults. Interestingly, different rice cultivars were fed to mice and evaluated for modulation of gut microbiome, allergic reactions, and immune responses.[88] As knowledge continues to increase regarding the connections between rice in the diet, gut microbes, and the human metabolome, there is a strong need to ensure that rice bran is not neglected as a key player, and may serve a major role in food security and global health promotion.

CONCLUSION

This chapter explains how an underutilized food ingredient, namely rice bran, could become the next simple, yet significant, opportunity in global health, nutrition, and food security. Even though challenges are apparent to increase dietary rice bran in the global food market, they merit attention and scientific as well as technological innovation. Additional research and global funding opportunities are necessary to tackle issues of hunger and nutrition-related disease through dietary rice bran interventions. Multidisciplinary, global collaborations are necessary to make sure these solutions are developed in a sustainable, culturally appropriate, and economically sound way. This untapped food source may shed light on how we can feed the world through adequate delivery of nutrients, with an overarching goal of disease prevention and thriving health outcomes.

References

1. *Rice Almanac: source book for the most important economic activity on Earth.* Wallingford, United Kingdom: CABI Publishing; 2002.
2. FAO. *Rice Market Monitor.* 4. Rome: FAO; 2012.
3. *Rice in the global economy: strategic research and policy issues for food security.* Los Banos, Philippines: International Rice Research Institute; 2010.
4. Kahlon TS. Rice Bran: Production, Composition, Functionality and Food Applications, Physiological Benefits. In: Choo SS PS,

editor. *Fiber ingredients: food applications and health benefits.* Boca Raton, FL: Taylor & Francis Group LLC; 2009. p. 305–21.
5. de Munter JS, Hu FB, Spiegelman D, Franz M, van Dam RM. Whole grain, bran, and germ intake and risk of type 2 diabetes: a prospective cohort study and systematic review. *PLoS Med* 2007;**4**(8):e261.
6. Cheng HH, Huang HY, Chen YY, Huang CL, Chang CJ, Chen HL, et al. Ameliorative effects of stabilized rice bran on type 2 diabetes patients. *Ann Nutr Metab* 2010;**56**(1):45–51.
7. Most MM, Tulley R, Morales S, Lefevre M. Rice bran oil, not fiber, lowers cholesterol in humans. *Am J Clin Nutr* 2005;**81**(1):64–8.
8. Cicero AF, Gaddi A. Rice bran oil and gamma-oryzanol in the treatment of hyperlipoproteinaemias and other conditions. *Phytother Res: PTR* 2001;**15**(4):277–89.
9. Gerhardt AL, Gallo NB. Full-fat rice bran and oat bran similarly reduce hypercholesterolemia in humans. *J Nutr* 1998;**128**(5): 865–9.
10. Kahlon TS, Chow FI, Chiu MM, Hudson CA, Sayre RN. Cholesterol-lowering by rice bran and rice bran oil unsaponifiable matter in hamsters. *Cereal Chem* 1996;**73**(1):69–74.
11. Cicero AF, Derosa G. Rice bran and its main components: potential role in the management of coronary risk factors. *Curr Top Nutr Res* 2005;**3**(1):29–46.
12. Jariwalla RJ. Rice-bran products: Phytonutrients with potential applications in preventive and clinical medicine. *Drugs ExpClin Res* 2001;**27**(1):17–26.
13. Kim TH, Kim EK, Lee MS, Lee HK, Hwang WS, Choe SJ, et al. Intake of brown rice lees reduces waist circumference and improves metabolic parameters in type 2 diabetes. *Nutr Res* 2011; **31**(2):131–8.
14. Henderson AJ, Ollila CA, Kumar A, Borresen EC, Raina K, Agarwal R, et al. Chemopreventive Properties of Dietary Rice Bran: Current Status and Future Prospects. *Adv Nutr* 2012;**3**(5): 643–53.
15. Mai HB, Tran VR, Nguyen TT, Le HS, Trinh TD, Le VT, et al. Arabinoxylan Rice Bran (MGN-3) Enhances the Effects of Interventional Therapies for the Treatment of Hepatocellular Carcinoma: A Three-year Randomized Clinical Trial. *Anticancer Res* 2010;**30**(12):5145–51.
16. Kumar A, Henderson AJ, Forster GM, Goodyear AW, Weir TL, Leach JE, et al. Dietary rice bran promotes resistance to Salmonella enterica serovar Typhimurium colonization in mice. *BMC Microbiol* 2012:12.
17. Ghoneum M, Matsuura M. Augmentation of macrophage phagocytosis by modified arabinoxylan rice bran (MGN-3/Biobran). *Int J Immunopath Ph* 2004;**17**(3):283–92.
18. Ghoneum M, Matsuura M, Gollapudi S. Modified arabinoxylan rice bran (MGN-3/Biobran) enhances intracellular killing of microbes by human phagocytic cells *in vitro. Int J Immunopath Ph* 2008;**21**(1):87–95.
19. Henderson AJ, Kumar A, Barnett B, Dow SW, Ryan EP. Consumption of Rice Bran Increases Mucosal Immunoglobulin A Concentrations and Numbers of Intestinal *Lactobacillus* spp. *J Med Food* 2012;**15**(5):469–75.
20. FAO, WFP, IFAD. *The State of Food Insecurity in the World 2012: Economic growth is necessary, but not sufficient to accelerate reduction of hunger and malnutrition.* Rome: FAO; 2012.
21. *United Nations. UN Secretary-General Challenges All Nations To Acheive Zero Hunger.* Rio de Janeiro: United Nations; 2012.
22. Finucane MM, Stevens GA, Cowan MJ, Danaei G, Lin JK, Paciorek CJ, et al. National, regional, and global trends in body-mass index since 1980: systematic analysis of health examination surveys and epidemiological studies with 960 country-years and 9.1 million participants. *Lancet* 2011;**377**(9765):557–67.
23. James PT, Leach R, Kalamara E, Shayeghi M. The worldwide obesity epidemic. *Obesity Res* 2001;**9**:228S–33S.

24. Tanumihardjo SA, Anderson C, Kaufer-Horwitz M, Bode L, Emenaker NJ, Haqq AM, et al. Poverty, obesity, and malnutrition: an international perspective recognizing the paradox. *J Am Diet Assoc* 2007;**107**(11):1966–72.

25. Holt-Gimenez E, Shattuck A, Altieri M, Herren H, Gliessman S. We Already Grow Enough Food for 10 Billion People … and Still Can't End Hunger. *J Sustainable Agric* 2012;**36**(6):595–8.

26. Schneeman BO. Linking agricultural production and human nutrition. *J Sci Food Agric* 2001;**81**(1):3–9.

27. Tang GW, Qin J, Dolnikowski GG, Russell RM, Grusak MA. Golden Rice is an effective source of vitamin A. *Am J Clin Nutr* 2009;**89**(6):1776–83.

28. Stein AJ, Sachdev HPS, Qaim M. Genetic engineering for the poor: Golden Rice and public health in India. *World Development* 2008;**36**(1):144–58.

29. Mayer JE. Delivering Golden Rice to developing countries. *J Aoac Int* 2007;**90**(5):1445–9.

30. International Rice Genome Sequencing P. The map-based sequence of the rice genome. *Nature* 2005;**436**(7052):793–800.

31. WHO. *Chronic Diseases*. Available at: http://www.who.int/topics/chronic_diseases/en/; 2013. (last accessed 22.02.2013).

32. Kolling G, Wu M, Guerrant RL. Enterica pathogens through life stages. *Front Cell Infect Micobiol* 2012;**2**:114.

33. FAO. *Rome Declaration on World Food Security and World Food Summit Plan of Action*. Rome: World Food Summit; 1996.

34. *Glossary of Environment Statistics, Studies in Methods*. New York, NY: United Nations; 1997.

35. Dave M, Higgins PD, Middha S, Rioux KP. The human gut microbiome: current knowledge, challenges, and future directions. *Transl Res* 2012;**160**(4):246–57.

36. Preamble to the Constitution of the World Health Organization as adopted by the International Health Conference. New York, NY; 1946.

37. WHO. *Infectious diseases*. Available at: http://www.who.int/topics/infectious_diseases/en/; 2013. (last accessed 22.02.2013).

38. UNICEF. *Tracking progress on child and maternal nutrition*. New York, NY: A survival and development priority; 2009.

39. UNICEF Canada Committee. Global Child Survival and Health, 2006. UNICEF.

40. FDA. *Guidance for Industry: Evidence-Based Review System for the Scientific Evaluation of Health Claims*. Rockville, MD, FDA; 2009.

41. Hughes R, Somerset S. Definitions and conceptual frameworks for public health and community nutrition: a discussion paper. *Aust J NutrDiet* 1997;**54**:40–5.

42. Hamilton RS. How many rice varieties are there? *Rice Today* 2006:50.

43. Whole Grains Council Definition of whole grains: Oldways Preservation Trust/Whole Grains Council, Boston, MA, 2012.

44. Saunders RM. The properties of rice bran as a foodstuff. *Cereal Foods World* 1990;**35**:632.

45. Jiang SL, Wu JG, Thang NB, Feng Y, Yang XE, Shi CH. Genotypic variation of mineral elements contents in rice (Oryza sativa L.). *Eur Food ResTechnol* 2008;**228**(1):115–22.

46. Boutayeb A. The double burden of communicable and non-communicable diseases in developing countries. *Trans R Soc Trop Med Hyg* 2006;**100**(3):191–9.

47. DeBoer MD, Lima AAM, Oria RB, Scharf RJ, Moore SR, Luna MA, et al. Early childhood growth failure and the developmental origins of adult disease: do enteric infections and malnutrition increase risk for the metabolic syndrome? *Nutr Rev* 2012;**70**(11):642–53.

48. Guerrant RL, Oria RB, Moore SR, Oria MOB, Lima AAM. Malnutrition as an enteric infectious disease with long-term effects on child development. *Nutr Rev* 2008;**66**(9):487–505.

49. Enochian RV, Saunders RM, Schultz WG, Beagle EC, Crowley PR. *Stabilization of rice bran with extrusion cookers, and recovery of edible oil: a preliminary analuysis of operational and financial feasbility*. Washington, DC: USDA/OICD; 1980.

50. Nagendra Prasad MN, Sanjay KR, Shravya Khatokar M, Vismaya MN, Nanjunda Swamy S. Health Benefits of Rice Bran – A Review. *J Nutr Food Sci* 2011;**1**:108.

51. Dhaliwal YS, Sekhon KS, Nagi HPS. Enzymatic-Activities and Rheological Properties of Stored Rice. *Cereal Chem* 1991;**68**(1):18–21.

52. Mujahid A, ul Haq I, Asif M, Gilani AH. Effect of various processing techniques and different levels of antioxidant on stability of rice bran during storage. *J Sci Food Agric* 2005;**85**(5):847–52.

53. Muhihi AJ, Shemaghembe E, Njelekela MA, Gimbi D, Mwambene K, Malik VS, et al. Perceptions, Facilitators, and Barriers to Consumption of Whole Grain Staple Foods among Overweight and Obese Tanzanian Adults: A Focus Group Study. *Int Scholarly Res Netw Public Health* 2012:1–7.

54. Kumar S, Mohanraj R, Sudha V, Wedick NM, Malik V, Hu FB, et al. Perceptions about Varieties of Brown Rice: A Qualitative Study from Southern India. *J Am Diet Assoc* 2011;**111**(10):1517–22.

55. Dipti SS, Bergman C, Indrasari SD, Herath T, Hall R, Lee H, et al. The potential of rice to offer solutions for malnutrition and chronic diseases. *Rice* 2012;**5**:1–18.

56. Sun Q, Spiegelman D, van Dam RM, Holmes MD, Malik VS, Willett WC, et al. White rice, brown rice, and risk of type 2 diabetes in US men and women. *Archintern Med* 2010;**170**(11):961–9.

57. Juliano BO. *Rice Chemistry & Quality*. Philippines: Philippine Rice Research Institute (PhilRice) 2007.

58. Mori H, Kawabata K, Yoshimi N, Tanaka T, Murakami T, Okada T, et al. Chemopreventive effects of ferulic acid on oral and rice germ on large bowel carcinogenesis. *Anticancer Res* 1999;**19**(5A):3775–8.

59. Norazalina S, Norhaizan ME, Hairuszah I, Norashareena MS. Anticarcinogenic efficacy of phytic acid extracted from rice bran on azoxymethane-induced colon carcinogenesis in rats. *Exp Toxicol Pathol* 2010;**62**(3):259–68.

60. Trucksess MW, Abbas HK, Weaver CM, Shier WT. Distribution of aflatoxins in shelling and milling fractions of naturally contaminated rice. *Food Addit Contam A* 2011;**28**(8):1076–82.

61. Bhattacharjee S, Fakhruddin ANM, Chowdhury MAZ, Rahman MA, Alam MK. Monitoring of Selected Pesticides Residue Levels in Water Samples of Paddy Fields and Removal of Cypermethrin and Chlorpyrifos Residues from Water Using Rice Bran. *Bull Environ Contam Toxicol* 2012;**89**(2):348–53.

62. Pareja L, Colazzo M, Perez-Parada A, Besil N, Heinzen H, Bocking B, et al. Occurrence and distribution study of residues from pesticides applied under controlled conditions in the field during rice processing. *J Agric Food Chem* 2012;**60**(18):4440–8.

63. Norton GJ, Islam MR, Deacon CM, Zhao FJ, Stroud JL, McGrath SP, et al. Identification of Low Inorganic and Total Grain Arsenic Rice Cultivars from Bangladesh. *Environ Sci Technol* 2009;**43**(15):6070–5.

64. Ruangwises S, Saipan P, Tengjaroenkul B, Ruangwises N. Total and Inorganic Arsenic in Rice and Rice Bran Purchased in Thailand. *J Food Prot* 2012;**75**(4):771–4.

65. Lombi E, Scheckel KG, Pallon J, Carey AM, Zhu YG, Meharg AA. Speciation and distribution of arsenic and localization of nutrients in rice grains. *New Phytol* 2009;**184**(1):193–201.

66. Alan PA, Ofelia RS, Patricia T, Maribel RSR. Cereal bran and wholegrain as a source of dietary fibre: technological and health aspects. *Int J Food Sci Nutr* 2012;**63**(7):882–92.

67. Bednar GE, Patil AR, Murray SM, Grieshop CM, Merchen NR, Fahey GC. Starch and fiber fractions in selected food and feed ingredients affect their small intestinal digestibility and fermentability and their large bowel fermentability *in vitro* in a canine model. *J Nutr* 2001;**131**(2):276–86.

68. Ryan EP. Bioactive food components and health properties of rice bran. *J Am Vet Med Assoc* 2011;**238**(5):593–600.

A. OVERVIEW OF RICE AND HEALTH

69. WHO. *Global Strategy for Infant and Young Child Feeding.* Geneva, Switzerland: WHO; 2003.

70. Khan SH, Butt MS, Anjum FM, Sameen A. Quality evaluation of rice bran protein isolate-based weaning food for preschoolers. *Int J Food Sci Nutr* 2011;**62**(3):280–8.

71. WHO/FAO/UNU. *Protein and Amino Acid Requirment in Human Nutrition: Report of Joint WHO/FAO/UNU Expert Consultation.* Albany, NY: WHO technical report series; 2007.

72. Yadav RB, Yadav BS, Chaudhary D. Extraction, characterization and utilization of rice bran protein concentrate for biscuit making. *Brit Food J* 2011;**113**(8-9):1173–82.

73. Gregorio GV, Gonzales MLM, Dans LF, Martinez EG. Polymer-based oral rehydration solution for treating acute watery diarrhoea. *Cochrane Database Syst Rev* 2009 (2).

74. U.S. Department of Commerce 2013. *U.S. Department of Commerce Announces Patents for Humanity Winners.* [press release] Retrieved from http://www.uspto.gov/news/pr/2013/13-17.jsp.

75. Martins MSF, Dores EFGC, Aguilar-Nascimento JE, Oyama LM, Latorraca MQ, Gomes-da-Silva MH, et al. Rice bran supplementation during nutritional recovery period of malnourished rats improves colon development. *Nutr Hosp* 2007;**22**(6):648–53.

76. Martinez I, Lattimer J, Hubac K, Case KL, Yang JY, Weber CG, et al. Gut microbiome composition is linked to whole grain-induced immunological improvements. *ISME Journal* 2013;**7**:269–98.

77. Astrup A, Dyerberg J, Selleck M, Stender S. Nutrition transition and its relationship to the development of obesity and related chronic diseases. *Obes Rev* 2008;**9**:48–52.

78. Bergman CJ, Xu Z. Genotype and environment effects on tocopherol, tocotrienol, and gamma-oryzanol contents of Southern US rice. *Cereal Chem* 2003;**80**(4):446–9.

79. Anandan A, Rajiv G, Eswaran R, Prakash M. Genotypic Variation and Relationships between Quality Traits and Trace Elements in Traditional and Improved Rice (Oryza sativa L.) Genotypes. *J Food Sci* 2011;**76**(4) H122–HH30.

80. Sands DC, Morris CE, Dratz EA, Pilgeram A. Elevating optimal human nutrition to a central goal of plant breeding and production of plant-based foods. *Plant Sci Int J Exp Plant Biol* 2009;**177**(5):377–89.

81. Kennedy G, Burlingame B. Analysis of food composition data on rice from a plant genetic resources perspective. *Food Chem* 2003;**80**(4):589–96.

82. Ahuja U, Ahuja SC, Thakrar R, Singh RK. Rice – A Nutraceutical. *Asian Agri-History* 2008;**12**(2):93–108.

83. Mohanlal S, Parvathy R, Shalini V, Helen A, Jayalekshmy A. Isolation, Characterization and Quantification of Tricin and Flavonolignans in the Medicinal Rice Njavara (*Oryza sativa* L.), as Compared to Staple Varieties. *Plant Foods Hum Nutr* 2011;**66**(1):91–6.

84. Shalini V, Bhaskar S, Kumar KS, Mohanlal S, Jayalekshmy A, Helen A. Molecular mechanisms of anti-inflammatory action of the flavonoid, tricin from Njavara rice (*Oryza sativa* L.) in human peripheral blood mononuclear cells: Possible role in the inflammatory signaling. *Int Immunopharmacol* 2012;**14**(1):32–8.

85. Deepa G, Singh V, Naidu KA. Nutrient composition and physicochemical properties of Indian medicinal rice – Njavara. *Food Chem* 2008;**106**(1):165–71.

86. Rao A, Reddy SG, Babu PP, Reddy AR. The antioxidant and antiproliferative activities of methanolic extracts from Njavara rice bran. *Bmc Complement Altern Med* 2010:10.

87. Forster GM, Raina K, Kumar A, Kumar S, Agarwal R, Chen M, et al. Rice varietal differences in bioactive bran components for inhibition of colorectal cancer cell growth. *Food Chem* 2013;**141**(2):1545–52.

88. Sonoyama K, Ogasawara T, Goto H, Yoshida T, Takemura N, Fujiwara R, et al. Comparison of gut microbiota and allergic reactions in BALB/c mice fed different cultivars of rice. *Br J Nutr* 2010;**103**(2):218–26.

89. Preidis GA, Hill C, Guerrant RL, Ramakrishna BS, Tannock GW, Versalovic J. Probiotics, Enteric and Diarrheal Diseases, and Global Health. *Gastroenterology* 2011;**140**(1) 8-+.

90. Rong N, Ausman LM, Nicolosi RJ. Oryzanol decreases cholesterol absorption and aortic fatty streaks in hamsters. *Lipids* 1997;**32**(3):303–9.

91. Seetharamaiah GS, Chandrasekhara N. Studies on hypocholesterolemic activity of rice bran oil. *Atherosclerosis* 1989;**78**(2-3):219–23.

92. Kawakami Y, Tsuzuki T, Nakagawa K, Miyazawa T. Distribution of tocotrienols in rats fed a rice bran tocotrienol concentrate. *Biosci Biotechnol Biochem* 2007;**71**(2):464–71.

93. Minhajuddin M, Beg ZH, Iqbal J. Hypolipidemic and antioxidant properties of tocotrienol rich fraction isolated from rice bran oil in experimentally induced hyperlipidemic rats. *Food Chem Toxicol* 2005;**43**(5):747–53.

94. Miyazawa T, Shibata A, Nakagawa K, Tsuzuki T. Anti-angiogenic function of tocotrienol. *Asia Pac J Clin Nutr* 2008;**17**(Suppl. 1):253–6.

95. Sen CK, Khanna S, Roy S. Tocotrienols in health and disease: the other half of the natural vitamin E family. *Mol Aspects Med* 2007;**28**(5-6):692–728.

96. Sun W, Xu W, Liu H, Liu J, Wang Q, Zhou J, et al. gamma-Tocotrienol induces mitochondria-mediated apoptosis in human gastric adenocarcinoma SGC-7901 cells. *Journal Nutr Biochem* 2009;**20**(4):276–84.

97. Morel S, Didierlaurent A, Bourguignon P, Delhaye S, Baras B, Jacob V, et al. Adjuvant System AS03 containing alpha-tocopherol modulates innate immune response and leads to improved adaptive immunity. *Vaccine* 2011;**29**(13):2461–73.

98. Boxer LA. Regulation of phagocyte function by alpha-tocopherol. *Pro Nutr Soc* 1986;**45**(3):333–44.

99. Iqbal J, Minhajuddin M, Beg ZH. Suppression of 7,12-dimethylbenz[alpha]anthracene-induced carcinogenesis and hypercholesterolaemia in rats by tocotrienol-rich fraction isolated from rice bran oil. *Eur J Cancer Pre* 2003;**12**(6):447–53.

100. Nakashima K, Virgona N, Miyazawa M, Watanabe T, Yano T. The tocotrienol-rich fraction from rice bran enhances cisplatin-induced cytotoxicity in human mesothelioma H28 cells. *Phytother Res* 2010;**24**(9):1317–21.

101. Taniguchi H, Hosoda A, Tsuno T, Maruta Y, Nomura E. Preparation of ferulic acid and its application for the synthesis of cancer chemopreventive agents. *Anticancer Res* 1999;**19**(5A):3757–61.

102. Srinivasan M, Sudheer AR, Menon VP. Ferulic acid: Therapeutic potential through its antioxidant property. *J Clin Biochem Nutr* 2007;**40**(2):92–100.

103. Baskar AA, Ignacimuthu S, Paulraj GM. Al Numair KS. Chemopreventive potential of beta-Sitosterol in experimental colon cancer model – an *in vitro* and *in vivo* study. *BMC Complement Altern Med* 2010;**10**:24.

Rice Bran Oil: Benefits to Health and Applications in Pharmaceutical Formulations

Lucas Almeida Rigo, Adriana Raffin Pohlmann[†], Silvia Stanisçuaski Guterres**, Ruy Carlos Ruver Beck***

*Programa de Pós-Graduação em Ciências Farmacêuticas, Faculdade de Farmácia, Universidade Federal do Rio Grande do Sul, Porto Alegre, Brazil,

[†]Departamento de Química Orgânica, Instituto de Química, Universidade Federal do Rio Grande do Sul, Porto Alegre, Brazil, **Faculdade de Farmácia, Universidade Federal do Rio Grande do Sul, Porto Alegre, Brazil

INTRODUCTION

Rice (*Oryzae Sative* L.) is an important staple food around the world. It represents one of the main foods in the world's dietary energy supply due to its high concentration of starch, and also provides proteins and minerals. Moreover, rice production plays an important role mainly in underdeveloped countries, due to its social and economic relevance.[1] Asia is the world's largest rice producer, accounting for at least 90% of global rice production, which means more than 600 million tonnes (Fig. 23.1). Among Asian countries, China is the greatest producer, followed by India and Indonesia; together these three are responsible for the majority of rice production, producing more than 360 million tonnes/year in total. Outside the Asian region, Brazil is the main rice producer, with yearly production figures in excess of 11 million tonnes/year.[2]

According to the United States Department of Agriculture (USDA), the global growth in domestic consumption of edible vegetable oil increased by approximately 19% between 2008 and 2011, with palm, soybean, and colza oils being the most consumed vegetable oils.[3] Vegetable oils are natural products consisting essentially of lipid compounds, usually obtained from seeds, nuts, or fruits of several types of plants, using different extraction methods. Edible vegetable oils are essential sources of fatty acids, a basic nutrient in the human diet because they perform essential functions for the effective function and maintenance of the body, such as providing the architecture of cell membranes, stimulating hormone production, and supplying energy. Additionally, fatty acids in vegetable oils are composed of lipid fractions with several beneficial effects on health, including antioxidant and anti-inflammatory effects and as vitamins.[4]

Unlike most vegetable oils, rice bran oil (RBO) is not extracted from seeds or nuts such as soybean or groundnut oil, respectively. RBO is obtained from bran, a by-product of the rice grain milling process. Rice bran contains on average 20–25% of RBO, depending on the milling method, geographical origin, and variety of rice,[5] which can influence the quality and nutritional value of rice bran. Because of this low cost and the high nutritional value, rice bran is often used as animal feed.[6]

The protective effect of fruits and vegetables has been attributed to the presence of antioxidants, such as β-carotene, tocopherols and vitamins A and C.[7] Oxidative stress is involved in the triggering of pathological conditions such as cancer and arteriosclerosis, and in cardiovascular risk, as well as in aging processes. Several enzymatic systems in the human body produce reactive oxygen species (ROS), such as the superoxide anion radical and hydrogen peroxide, simply through oxygen consumption.[8] Additionally, exposure to many substances present in the environment, including pollutants, toxic chemical waste, and cigarette smoke (whether inhaled directly or secondhand), contributes to ROS generation. Vegetables, fruits, and their seeds provide a myriad of biological compounds with proven action against several diseases that have been attributed to various antioxidant substances, including tocopherols, vitamin E, β-carotene, and polyphenolic compounds.[9]

Currently, growing interest in the replacement of synthetic antioxidant foods with natural ones has fostered scientific research on new vegetable sources of bioactive compounds. In this context, RBO emerges as a natural

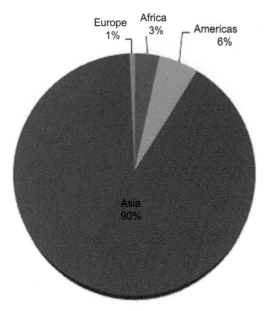

FIGURE 23.1   World-wide rice (paddy) production by region (year 2012).[2]

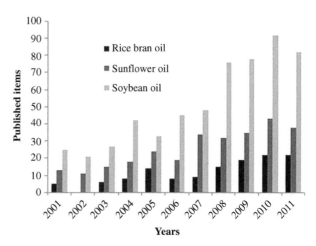

FIGURE 23.2   Published papers on rice bran, sunflower, and soybean oil over the last decade. Searched words: rice bran oil, soybean oil, sunflower oil and health. *ISI Web of Knowledge.*

alternative due to its appreciable content of phytochemical compounds, such as vitamin E and γ-oryzanol, which present antioxidant activities and potential health benefits.[10] Tocotrienols belong to the family of vitamin E compounds, which includes four homologues (α-, β-, δ- and γ-tocopherols and -tocotrienols). Specifically, α-tocopherol is considered the vitamin E homologue of greatest value due to its high level of physiological activity. In addition, tocotrienols have been reported as inhibitors of cholesterol synthesis, lowering serum cholesterol levels in various animal models.[11] γ-Oryzanol, the levels of which in rice bran are 13- to 20-fold (w/w) as high as those of total tocopherols and tocotrienols, decreases animal serum cholesterol levels and has anti-inflammatory activity.[12]

Scientific interest in rice bran oil has emerged recently, compared to major edible vegetable oils, as is revealed by the increasing number of papers published on the subject since the millenium (Fig. 23.2). Although the number may still appear low, the interest of the scientific community in studying RBO for its health benefits is growing due to its chemopreventive agents, which may be used to treat several health disorders. Since the identification of bioactive compounds of RBO, such as those cited above, researchers have concentrated their efforts on the development of new pharmaceutical dosage forms of, or foods containing, rice bran oil or its compounds. The main objectives are to improve treatment strategies and prevent diseases.

Taking all these issues into account, this chapter covers relevant aspects of RBO, including its source and composition, beneficial effects on treating several diseases, and applications in the development of pharmaceutical or cosmetic formulations. The chapter is subdivided into three topics: the first addresses the extraction and composition of RBO, the second the biomedical applications of rice bran oil, and the third the application trends of RBO or its derivates in pharmaceutical, cosmetic, or nutraceutical formulations.

RICE BRAN OIL: EXTRACTION AND COMPOSITION

Rice bran is the main source of rice bran oil, which contains lipids, proteins, tocopherols, and bioactive compounds. Rice bran is obtained from paddy rice in a multistage process, after harvest. The grains are submitted to the milling process, where, first, the kernel is separated from the hull (dehulling).[13] The burnishing step is carried out to remove the brownish layer of the kernel, producing germ and bran. Finally, the whitening process removes residual bran particles and improves the rice grain surface and appearance. Usually the global yield of the milling process, from 100 kg of paddy rice, is about 60 kg of white rice, 10 kg of broken grains, 10 kg of bran and germ, and 20 kg of hulls.[14,15]

RBO is mainly extracted from bran using organic solvents. Hexane has been used as solvent by many researchers and industries due to its good availability, high oil extractability, and the ease of the operation. However, this process has some problems with respect to oil quality, such as higher content of free fatty acids, wax, and other undesirable products. Furthermore, hexane has been identified as an air pollutant. Other methods have been proposed to improve RBO extraction, mainly reducing the use of organic solvents. One such method is an enzymatic process that uses a commercial protease (catalase), giving an extraction yield of 79% and an oil with a quality comparable with that obtained by solvent-based extraction.[16] On the other hand, the aqueous extraction method led to lower free fatty acid content in the oil, compared to that obtained by extraction with hexane.[17] An interesting approach to extracting and refining this oil using supercritical carbon dioxide has been reported to preserve its nutritional phytochemicals and to produce lower quantities of wax, in comparison with organic solvent extraction.[18]

Crude RBO is the first product obtained from the refining process. Crude RBO is dark greenish, and produces a strong smell. Moreover, it has several features, such as acid pH, wastes, and a high concentration of free fatty acids, that make it non-edible. To reach an edible grade, RBO is submitted to either physical or chemical refining. The type of refining process used influences the nutritional composition of RBO.[1] Refining crude rice bran oil involves basically dewaxing, degumming, neutralization of free acids, bleaching to improve color, and steam deodorization. However, large amounts of its phytochemical compounds, especially γ-oryzanol, are lost during this refining process, regardless of the refining method used.[10,19] This loss is attributed to the high lipophilicity of these phytochemical compounds. The refined rice bran oil is light yellow, with a mild background odor and a flavor reminiscent of rice.[20,21]

Vegetable oils are natural products composed essentially of lipids that can be divided into two major classes: saponifiable and non-saponifiable. A saponifiable lipid is one with an ester functional group that can be hydrolyzed under basic conditions and is represented by simple lipids (triglycerides, diglycerides, free fatty acids, and wax). On the other hand, non-saponifiable lipids include the "fat-soluble" vitamins (mainly A and E), and cholesterol. Between 90% and 96% of rice bran oil comprises saponifiable lipids, including oleic (38.4%), linoleic (34.4%), and α-linolenic (2.2%) acids as unsaturated fatty acids, and palmitic (21.5%) and stearic (2.9%) acids as saturated fatty acids.[20] The non-saponifiable fraction of RBO ranges from 2% to 4%, depending on the refining process; this value is higher than that of other vegetable oils, such as sunflower (1.4%), groundnut (0.2%), and safflower (1.3%) oils. This composition underlines the high nutritional value of RBO, and is the fraction that contains the highest number of phytochemical compounds presenting biological activity.[21] The non-saponifiable fraction includes mainly tocopherols, tocotrienols and γ-oryzanol, as well as other compounds that are found at lower concentrations, such as lecithin and carotenoids.[22]

The components of the non-saponifiable fraction (tocotrienols, tocopherols, and phytosterols) have been reported to play a role in the prevention and therapy of dyslipidemia and associated conditions.[23,24] RBO also contains γ-oryzanol, a potent antioxidant. RBO is the only vegetable oil presenting this kind of antioxidant, to which hypocholesterolemic effects have been attributed.

γ-Oryzanol is composed of esters of ferulic acid with phytosterols (sterols and triterpenic alcohols). Among these, cycloartennyl ferulate, 24-methylenecycloartanyl ferulate, campesteryl ferulate, and β-sitostery ferulate are the major constituents of γ-oryzanol.[5]

In plants, phytochemical compounds carry out functions equivalent to those of cholesterol in animals, thus being fundamental compounds for cell membranes and as precursors of sex hormones and vitamins.[25] For this reason, many researchers have devoted their studies to investigating the benefits of RBO for health.

POTENTIAL BIOMEDICAL APPLICATIONS OF RICE BRAN OIL

Studies of RBO and its Components against Free Radicals

At molecular and cellular levels, antioxidants deactivate free radicals, which are natural by-products of many oxidative metabolic processes within cells. Due to their high reactivity, excessive amounts of these products can damage cells walls, cell structures, and genetic material within the cells, which may contribute to triggering several diseases, especially cancer.[26] Unfortunately, cell free-radical production is a continuous process. The human body has some enzymatic mechanisms to minimize free radical production and cell damage, such as superoxide dismutase, catalase, and glutathione peroxidase.[27] On the other hand, natural non-enzymatic antioxidants with known antioxidant activity, including phytochemical compounds such as tocotrienols, tocopherols, and vitamins A and E, can help control free radical production.[28]

Colon carcinogenesis is a multistep process that involves stepwise accumulation of molecular and genetic defects in colonic epithelial cells – i.e., changes in the normal epithelium followed hyperproliferation and, eventually, detectable carcinoma. A recent study using a colon procarcinogen model (1,2-dimethylhydrazine or azoximethane) in rats revealed that the animals fed a rice bran oil diet exhibited significantly reduced colon tumor formation and preneoplastic lesions. In addition, the levels of hepatic enzymes, including glutathione, superoxide dismutase, and catalase, were improved.[29] This effect was linked to the presence of a particular compound in RBO: phytic acid. Phytic acid, with concentrations of between 9.5% and 4.5% by weight in rice bran, is a natural antioxidant, and represents 1–5% of the composition of most cereals, nuts, legumes, and oil seeds. The phytic acid structure presents six phosphate groups, and accounts for 60–90% of the total phosphorus content in seeds. Carcinogenesis involves a metal-mediated reaction, activated mainly by iron. Because the intestine may contain large amounts of potentially reactive iron (particularly in populations that consume diets rich in red meat), phytic acid may act to suppress iron-driven steps in carcinogenesis.[30] Phytic acid was extracted from rice bran and administrated to rats treated with azoximethane. The findings showed that treatment with 0.2% (w/v) phytic acid extract led to the most representative reduction in colon tumor formation. Thus, according to these experimental models, RBO shows potential value in reducing colon cancer.[31]

Physical exercise is generally recognized to have a positive impact on physiological parameters affecting overall health. Even though there are many known health benefits of exercise, there is strong evidence suggesting that strenuous exercise may cause oxidative stress. Exercise can produce an imbalance between free radicals and antioxidants, which leads to a condition of oxidative stress.[32] Rats of the same strain, sex, and weight were subjected to an exercise program (swimming) of 60 min/day, 5 days a week, for 10 weeks to induce oxidative stress. The animals were treated with 125, 250 and 500 mg/kg of emulsions rich in the γ-oryzanol fraction, and antioxidant related genes were determined in rat liver. The results showed that the γ-oryzanol rich fraction has potential antioxidant activity in the regulation of expression of genes associated with oxidative stress, in comparison with untreated groups, regardless of the concentration administered.[33]

Studies on RBO and its Components against Dyslipidemias

Cholesterol is transported in the blood plasma of all mammals by lipoproteins, which have a wide range of molecular sizes. Very low-density lipoprotein (VLDL) is converted to small to low-density lipoprotein (LDL) in the bloodstream. High-density lipoprotein (HDL), the smallest type of lipoprotein, contains the highest proportion of protein to cholesterol. Thus, HDL is able to remove cholesterol from the blood and transport it to the liver for excretion or re-utilization. Hyperlipoproteinemias are lipid disorders associated with increased plasma cholesterol concentrations. LDL cholesterol levels above normal values imply a high risk of cardiovascular disease (CVD) and arteriosclerosis (AT). The risk factors for developing CVD are age, gender, high blood pressure, obesity, tobacco smoking, and, especially, high serum cholesterol levels. These factors affect the circulatory system (arteries, capillaries, and veins), promoting the development of CVDs such as heart failure, cardiomyopathy, and coronary heart disease.[34] Arteriosclerosis is an inflammatory process affecting medium and large-sized blood vessels. If the blood vessels are exposed to high levels of LDL and other substances, such as free radicals, these vessels become more permeable. From this, a series of reactions occurs, which may cause lesions in the

vessel as well as blocking the blood circulation. According to the World Health Organization, more than 17 million people died from cardiovascular disease in 2008. By 2030, this number is estimated to rise to 25 million.[35]

Most therapeutic approaches for the prevention of cardiovascular disease involve a change in lifestyle, regular physical exercise, and improvements in diet such as increasing the intake of foods containing antioxidants. However, drug therapy, including statins, is needed for patients who present with higher levels of cholesterol in the bloodstream.[36]

Regarding the bioactive compounds present in RBO, several studies have demonstrated their ability to improve the lipid status on animal experimental models, reducing the total plasma cholesterol levels. The hypocholesterolemic effect of refined rice bran oil was compared to that of coconut and canola oils. For this purpose, hamsters were used as an animal model and fed for 8 weeks on chow-based diets plus 0.03% of cholesterol and 5% (w/w) of the oils. Both plasma total cholesterol and LDL levels were significantly reduced in the group treated with the diet containing RBO. The same group showed a significant reduction (15–17%) in cholesterol absorption.[37] In another study carried out by the same research group, the effects of different unsaturated vegetable oils on serum lipoprotein levels were evaluated in monkeys.[24] The RBO diet decreased serum total and LDL cholesterols by comparable values (25% and 30%, respectively). These results were not accompanied by the undesired reduction in HDL cholesterol, as occurred with canola and corn oil diets.

The antihyperlipidemic effect of two concentrations (50 mg/kg and 100 mg/kg) of γ-oryzanol administered via the intraperitoneal route was evaluated using hyperlipidemic rats. The groups treated with the phytochemical compound showed a significant decrease in the levels of serum cholesterol, triacylglycerides, LDL, and VLDL, and a significant increase in the level of serum HDL, in comparison with the control group (atorvastatin), regardless of the dose administered. In addition, a significant increase in the level of hepatic antioxidant enzymes showed a high degree of hepatic protection against free radicals.[38]

γ-Oryzanol exerts a hypolipidemic effect even when blended with other vegetable oils. Rats fed a diet containing blends of refined groundnut oil having 3%, 5%, or 10% of γ-oryzanol showed a decrease in total cholesterol in serum (7–16%) and in liver (15%), depending on the γ-oryzanol concentration used, when compared to cholesterol levels of the rats fed on pure groundnut oil. These results demonstrate the feasibility of incorporating this compound as a supplement in other vehicles, if an alternative form of intake is required.[39]

Besides γ-oryzanol, other bioactive components extracted from rice bran have been shown to improve lipid profiles. The effect of a concentrated mixture containing bioactive compounds extracted from rice bran, including γ-oryzanol, phytosterols, tocols, squalene, and octacosanol, on lipid levels was evaluated. Rats were fed a normal diet (without cholesterol), a high cholesterol diet, or a high cholesterol diet with the concentrated mixture. No significant differences in final body weight among groups were observed. However, rats fed a high cholesterol diet showed significant hepatomegaly when compared with rats fed the high cholesterol diet and a mixture containing the bioactive compounds. In contrast, the RBO concentration mixture intake tended to decrease organ weights, especially epididymal fat pads, compared to the group that received the high cholesterol diet. Regarding lipid profiles, the rats fed the diet including the RBO concentration mixture showed an increase in HDL rather than LDL levels, if compared with those levels of rats fed the high cholesterol diet. This result is very important, since HDL reduces the amount of deposited cholesterol in the endothelium, and consequently the risk of arteriosclerosis, by carrying cholesterol from peripheral cells to the liver for excretion in the bile or other pathways. In addition, the RBO mixture diet decreased the atherogenic index, compared with the normal diet. The atherogenic index is one of the most important risk factors for atherosclerotic plaques. Therefore, in the same study the potential antioxidant activity of these compounds in the RBO concentration mixture against oxidative stress was demonstrated.[40]

Humans and animals do not synthesize vitamin E, but primarily acquire tocopherols and tocotrienols from plants, which are the only organisms able to produce vitamin E. Like γ-oryzanol, tocotrienols show high antioxidant and hypolipidemic activities.[41] However, high and prolonged intakes of vitamin E may have pro-oxidant effects.[42] Thus, a minimum dose of tocotrienols was investigated in experimentally challenged hyperlipidemic rats. Animals were treated with different concentrations of a tocotrienol-rich fraction (TRF) extract obtained from RBO, ranging from 0 to 50 mg TRF/kg for 1 week. Treatment with TRF significantly decreased the levels of triglycerides (38–48%) and total cholesterol (around 48%), in comparison with the hyperlipidemic rats, in a dose-dependent manner; however, neither triglycerides nor cholesterol values were altered after treatments using doses higher than 8 mg of TRF/kg per day. Regarding lipoproteins levels, LDL cholesterol decreased by 39%, 60%, and 62% after treatment with 4, 8, and 12 mg TRF/kg, respectively, with a maximum decrease of 74% when 25 mg TRF/kg was administered. In addition, there was no decrease in LDL levels after treatment with 50 mg TRF/kg. According to the authors, the hypocholesterolemic impact of TRF may be associated with the mevalonate-suppressive action of HMG-CoA reductase, which plays a significant role in the metabolic pathway involved in the production of cholesterol. This metabolic route is the same "target" of some drugs available in the market and used to decrease cholesterol levels, such as statins.[12] In addition to lower cholesterol, the same concentration of 8 mg/kg of TRF showed a maximum antioxidant effect. This result is attributed to the ability of TRF to donate electrons to free radicals derived from lipid peroxidation. These results suggest that 8 mg TRF/kg per day is enough to achieve effective hypocholesterolemic and antioxidant activities, under these experimental conditions. Therefore, additional studies extended over longer periods are needed, as well as studies in humans.[43]

Some studies in humans have reported the considerable benefits of RBO and its components against dyslipidemia disorders. A total of 14 healthy subjects were divided into two groups and administered given a lipid diet (one-third of the total dietary fat) for 10 weeks. The fat in the diet was provided in the form of a vegetable oil blend comprised of peanut, olive, corn, canola, and palm oils, or RBO. The RBO diet caused a significant decrease in total and LDL cholesterol levels; however, HDL levels did not change during the evaluation. In addition, levels of apolipoprotein B, a constituent of LDL, were lower in the subjects that received RBO in the fat diet intake.[44]

In another study, 14 subjects aged between 40 and 60 years and with known hyperlipidemia were evaluated to compare the effects of RBO and sunflower oil as cooking oils on their lipid profiles. The subjects were divided in two groups; the first group initially used RBO for 3 months, and the second started the treatment using sunflower oil (period 1). After a washout period of 3 weeks, the groups switched oils for another 3 months (period 2). Both groups showed a consistent reduction in total cholesterol and serum triglycerides in the period when RBO was used in cooking. However, there was no change in the HDL cholesterol values. Since RBO has several advantages and health benefits, the authors suggest that it could be used routinely as a cooking oil.[45]

Both the above studies suggest that these effects in humans may be attributed to the unsaponifiable fraction of RBO, which contains γ-oryzanol. As mentioned above, the refining method can affect the amount of this major compound. In this context, another study was carried out in order to verify whether the concentration of γ-oryzanol makes any difference to cholesterol levels. Thirty hypercholesterolemic men were divided in two groups, which received low (0.05 g/day) or high (0.8 g/day) γ-oryzanol concentrations for 4 weeks. After this period, both groups showed lower total plasma cholesterol, LDL and HDL cholesterol, and triacylglycerol, compared with their basal levels (assessed at the beginning of the study). These results suggest that the γ-oryzanol may improve lipid metabolism, regardless of the concentration used.[23]

The mechanism of action of RBO on lipid metabolism has not been completely elucidated. Its specific content of polyphenols, phytosterols, and other bioactive compounds that belong to the unsaponifiable fraction is supposed to contribute to its antihyperlipidemic action, while other lipids (the saponifiable fraction) do not seem to be fundamental to its activity. As mentioned previously, γ-oryzanol is a natural antioxidant compound composed of four constituents whose ratio varies with the rice cultivation environment and rice species.[19,46] One study has investigated separately the *in vitro* scavenging activity of each form of γ-oryzanol. All constituents have similar scavenging ability, and ferulic acid is the active unit;[47] on the other hand, γ-oryzanol appeared to be a less efficient chain-breaking antioxidant as opposed to tocopherol, which is able to scavenge organic radicals at lower concentrations.[48] In general, all RBOs contain γ-oryzanol and other bioactive compounds mentioned above with antioxidant and hypolipidemic activities. In this sense, the notion that various RBO substances together are accountable for a global effect on lipid balance is the most valid hypothesis regarding the beneficial effects of these bioactive compounds.[49]

Studies on RBO and its Components against Hyperinsulinemias and Other Biomedical Applications

Diabetes mellitus (DM) is a metabolic disorder resulting from a defect in insulin secretion or insulin action, or both, which results in hyperglycemia with disturbances in the metabolism of carbohydrate, fat, and protein. The incidence of DM has increased dramatically in recent years, mainly due to changes in lifestyle, an increase of obesity, and inadequate nutritional dietary intake. The multiple complications in DM include retinopathy, neuropathy, and vascular damage; thus, DM comprises several heterogeneous diseases. DM can be subdivided into two categories, type 1 and type 2, referring to insulin-dependent diabetes mellitus (IDDM) and non-insulin dependent diabetes mellitus (NIDDM), respectively. IDDM is present in patients who have poor or no endogenous insulin secretory ability and require exogenous insulin therapy. In contrast, NIDDM is the most common form of DM, and is characterized by disorders of insulin secretion and insulin resistance. This form arises in individuals over the age of 40 years, is considered to be hereditary, and is often associated with obesity and lack of physical exercise.[50]

Hyperglycemia is also a key factor in the development of renal pathology (nephropathy). Studies have presented evidence that high glucose levels in the bloodstream can lead to the death of renal cells by inducing DNA fragmentation.[51,52] Vitamin E supplementation has been associated with the remission of DM complications.[53] As RBO represents one of the major natural sources of vitamin E, the ability of the tocotrienol-rich fraction (TRF) obtained from RBO extract to improve renal function was evaluated in diabetic rats. After 8 weeks, the group treated with TRF-RBO 200 mg/kg/day showed a significant improvement in glycemic status as well as in renal function in type 1 DM, compared to the untreated group.[54]

The hypoglycemic effect of ferulic acid was evaluated in type 2 diabetic mice. The animals received an oral dose of 0.05 g/kg per day of ferulic acid for 17 days. After this period, blood glucose levels of the treated animals were significantly lower than those of untreated animals. In the same study, the group treated with ferulic acid had significantly lower levels of total plasma cholesterol and LDL, compared with the untreated group.[55]

Human adipose tissue synthesizes and secretes cytokines, a wide range of small structures responsible for intercellular communication. Among cytokines, adiponectin is a protein hormone that modulates a number of metabolic processes, including glucose regulation and fatty acid oxidation. A decrease in plasma adiponectin levels is closely involved in the development of insulin resistance, which may culminate in type 2 DM.[56] High intake of dietary fatty acids, especially from meat, contributes to inducing insulin resistance in adipose cells (adipocyte), which can interfere with the production of adiponectin. The effects of γ-oryzanol regarding reduction in serum cholesterol levels were evaluated in mice by measuring adiponectin serum levels. Hypoadiponectinemia was induced in animals through oral administration of a special diet containing beef tallow, corn oil, or palmitic acid. In addition, two animal groups received beef tallow or corn oil containing 0.025 mmol of γ-oryzanol. After 120 hours, all groups were analyzed. The administration of both γ-oryzanol with corn oil or beef tallow increased adiponectin levels significantly, compared with the group treated only with corn oil. These results are very interesting because stimulation of adiponectin production can be considered a target of a possible drug development, since this cytokine is one of the main factors in obesity and insulin resistance.[57]

A study reported the anti-inflammatory effect of phytochemical compounds from RBO extracts. This effect was evaluated for γ-oryzanol, cycloartenil ferulate, and ferulic acid on severe colitis induced in mice. Both γ-oryzanol and cycloartenyl ferulate significantly inhibited the inflammatory process. Thus, phytosteryl ferulates could be effective as therapeutic or preventive agents for gastrointestinal inflammatory diseases.[58]

Nutrition and the nutritional status of the human body have impacts on immune system function, resistance to infections, and autoimmunity. Immunological cell membranes are provided with fatty acids, which are

TABLE 23.1 Trends of Use of Rice Bran Oil or its Derivates on Pharmaceutical, Cosmetic, and Nutraceutical Formulations

Type of Formulation	Rice Bran Oil/ Bioactive Compound	Use	Main Result	References
Gel-creams containing benzophenone	Rice bran oil at 3% or 5%	Sunscreen	Enhancement of spreadability and no alteration of the sun protection factor	Rigo et al.[60]
Nanoemulsions	Rice bran oil at 10%	Treatment of skin disorders	Improvement of skin moisture in a model of skin psoriasis	Bernardi et al.[70] (2011)
Solid lipid nanoparticles	γ-Oryzanol	Platform for the development of formulations	Particles sizes between 220 and 280 nm, and entrapment efficiency from 15% to 66%	Uracha et al.[73] (2008)
Liposomes	γ-Oryzanol	Natural preservative	In vitro inhibition of free radical generation	Juliano et al.[48]
Gels or creams containing liposomes	Ferulic acid, γ-oryzanol, and phytic acid	Anti-aging in cosmetics	High transdermal accumulation of the compounds in dermis and epidermis	Manosroi et al.[75]
Emulsions containing nanosponges	γ-Oryzanol at 0.06%	Dermal application	Skin retention of γ-oryzanol using a porcine ear skin model	Sapino et al.[77]
Lipid-core nanocapsules	Rice bran oil at 3%	Nanocarrier platform for medicines of cosmetics	Suitability to prepare polymeric nanocapsules to control drug release	Rigo et al.[80]
Hydrogels containing lipid-core nanocapsules	Rice bran oil at 3%	Raw material for sunscreen or skin care formulation	Prevention of edema formation and anti-inflammatory effect in skin damage induced by UVB radiation	Rigo et al.[83]
Chitosan-coated microparticles	γ-Oryzanol at 2.72%	Gastrointestinal drug delivery system	Control of γ-oryzanol either in simulated gastric fluid or in intestinal fluid	Lee et al.[86]
Chitosan-coated microparticles	γ-Oryzanol	Oral administration	Improvement of γ-oryzanol bioavailability after oral administration	Kim et al.[87]

susceptible to free radical damage, and thus a balanced supplementation intake can aid in the maintenance of these cells.[59] Regarding the antioxidant effect of bioactive compounds present in RBO, three different doses of γ-oryzanol (25, 50, and 100 mg/kg) were evaluated regarding immune responses in experimental rats. The results showed that γ-oryzanol may stimulate both cellular and humoral immune responses, regardless of the dose given, making γ-oryzanol a potential immunomodulatory candidate.

TRENDS IN THE USE OF RICE BRAN OIL OR ITS DERIVATES IN PHARMACEUTICAL, COSMETIC, AND NUTRACEUTICAL FORMULATIONS

Many benefits of rice bran oil and its components have been shown in different experimental models, including humans, raising interest in the development of different kinds of products. Several in vitro and in vivo studies have focused on the development of pharmaceutical dosage forms designed for different purposes that cover therapeutic, cosmetic, or nutraceutical applications (Table 23.1).

Gel-creams containing two different concentrations (3% or 5%) of RBO and benzophenone-3 10% (a type of

synthetic sunscreen filter) were prepared. All formulations showed adequate pH for skin application and improved spreadability, compared with formulations without the vegetable oil. The presence of RBO does not alter the sun protection factor, confirming their potential use in preparing cosmetic sunscreen formulations.[60]

Regarding future trends in the development of pharmaceutical dosage forms, which are inclined towards novel drug delivery systems, nanotechnology is playing a key role in the development of therapeutic systems able to control the release of drugs and other active ingredients for cosmetic use.[61,62] The particles used in these systems are less than 1 μm in size and present some advantages in therapeutics, such as the targeting drugs to a specific site of action,[63] increasing drug shelf-life,[64] and improving oral bioavailability of the active ingredients[65] in comparison with conventional approaches. Different types of nanostructured systems have been widely studied in the pharmaceutical field, such as nanoemulsions,[66] liposomes,[67] solid lipid nanoparticles, polymeric nanoparticles, lipid-core nanocapsules,[68] niosomes, and nanosponges.[69] These types of nanostructures are remarkably versatile systems regarding their wide range of application. Figure 23.3 shows the schematic structural representation of different nanostructure systems investigated as drug or cosmetic delivery systems.

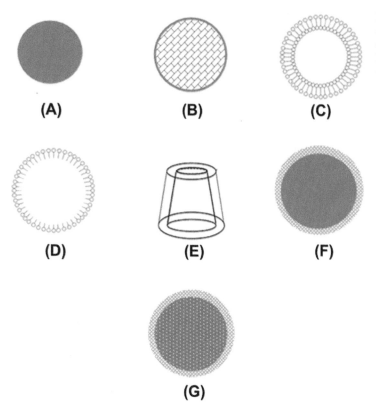

FIGURE 23.3 Schematic structural representation of different nanostructured systems studied as drug or cosmetic delivery systems: (A) nanoemulsion, (B) solid lipid nanoparticles, (C) liposomes, (D) niosomes, (E) cyclodextrins, (F) nanocapsules, (G) lipid-core nanocapsules.

Nanoemulsions (Fig. 23.3A) are composed of small oil globules stabilized by surfactants and dispersed in an aqueous medium. A topical formulation of a nanoemulsion containing RBO 10% was developed to treat skin disorders such as atopic dermatitis and psoriasis. *In vitro* assays showed that this formulation has a low potential; however, when applied to human skin with psoriasis, the formulation improved skin moisture and maintained its normal pH.[70]

Solid lipid nanoparticles (SLNs) consist of solid lipids which are dispersed in an aqueous surfactant solution that becomes solid at room temperature (Fig. 23.3B). This type of nanocarrier has been used for effective controlled release and prolonged stability of lipophilic and hydrophilic drugs. In addition, SLNs are considered safe because they can be prepared from biodegradable materials. Due to its occlusive properties generated by lipid materials, this kind of formulation increases skin hydration.[71] There is a wide range of lipid raw materials used in the preparation of SLNs, such as butter, wax, and phospholipids. Cetyl palmitate is a type of wax of high interest due to its better *in vitro* degradation and lower *in vivo* toxicity as compared with other types of wax.[72] Different concentrations of SLNs prepared from γ-oryzanol and cetyl palmitate were evaluated. The particles were between 220–280 nanometers, and the entrapment efficiency of γ-oryzanol within SLNs varied from 15% to 66% using 9.5% and 8.5% (w/w) of cetyl palmitate. No change in SNL particle size was observed upon storage for 120 days at 25°C. Due to the antioxidant properties of γ-oryzanol, this formulation was considered promising for the development of pharmaceutical, cosmetic, or food products.[73]

Oxidative processes may occur in pharmaceutical dosage forms, particularly in those preparations where high amounts of lipids are used, such as emulsions. Furthermore, preservatives are used in emulsions mostly to prevent the auto-oxidative deterioration of lipid raw material. Similarly to what occurs in the human body, oxidative processes cause destabilization of these preparations, which in turn lose their potential application. Traditionally, synthetic compounds are used for this purpose; however, the safety of some of these compounds is a controversial issue, and thus the investigation of natural antioxidants as an alternative is becoming an important research area in pharmaceutical fields. In this context, the main antioxidant compound of RBO, γ-oryzanol, was evaluated as a preservative in liposomes. Liposomes (Fig. 23.3C) are microscopic vesicles composed of one lipid bilayer or multiple bilayers composed generally of natural phospholipids and cholesterol, dispersed in a liquid medium, which can be designed to deliver drugs or cosmetic substances and may be lipophilic or hydrophilic. However, the lipid composition of the liposomes may destabilize such systems.[67] The antioxidant activity of liposomes prepared from phosphatidylcholine containing γ-oryzanol showed, in an *in vitro* experimental model, that concentrations of 50–100 μM of this compound are able to inhibit free radical generation. As γ-oryzanol is poorly soluble in water, this effect is achieved only when γ-oryzanol is incorporated during liposome preparation; when exogenously added to the formulation, this effect does not exist.[48]

Niosomes (Figure 23.3D) are self-assembly structures similar to liposomes in their architecture. Unlike liposomes, which are prepared with cholesterol, niosomes are made up from a variety of non-ionic surfactants. These kinds of nanocarrier are also biodegradable, biocompatible, and non-toxic, and are able to encapsulate large quantities of material in a relatively small volume of vesicles.[74] Different concentrations of three RBO bioactive compounds (ferulic acid, γ-oryzanol, and phytic acid) entrapped into niosomes prepared with cholesterol and a non-ionic surfactant (polysorbate 61) were incorporated in gel or cream formulations. *In vitro* transdermal permeation properties of these formulations were evaluated, regarding the antioxidant properties of these bioactive compounds. The maximum loadings of compounds in niosomes were 0.5, 1.5, and 1.5% (w/w) of ferulic acid, γ-oryzanol, and phytic acid, respectively. The findings showed that both gel and cream formulations containing RBO bioactive-loaded niosomes can provide high transdermal accumulation of these active substances in the dermis and epidermis, suggesting that these formulations are useful as anti-aging agents in cosmetic formulations.[75]

Cyclodextrins are cyclic oligosaccharides widely used in the pharmaceutical field to improve the solubility of hydrophobic compounds (Figure 23.3E). The most notable feature of cyclodextrins is their ability to form solid inclusion complexes (host–guest complexes) with a very wide range of solid, liquid, and gaseous compounds by molecular complexation. The lipophilic cavity of cyclodextrin provides a microenvironment into which appropriately sized non-polar moieties can enter to form inclusion complexes.[76] In addition, the reaction between cyclodextrin and a suitable cross-linking agent results in cyclodextrin-based nanosponges, which are biocompatible nanoporous nanoparticles. They are spherical solid particles that have been used to increase the solubility of poorly soluble drugs, to protect labile groups and control release. In another study, γ-oryzanol, which is a hydrophobic compound, was associated with nanosponges at 0·06% (w/w). *In vitro* diffusion analyses showed that γ-oryzanol associated with nanosponges exhibited a more controlled release kinetic, in comparison with a solution containing free γ-oryzanol. In addition, this complex also showed *in vitro* antioxidant activity, depending on the γ-oryzanol concentration used. Considering theses results, the complex formed by γ-oryzanol and nanosponges was incorporated in a topical formulation (emulsion). Experiments conducted in porcine ear skin showed that the amount of γ-oryzanol

retained in the skin from an emulsion containing its nano-encapsulated form was higher than the emulsion containing free γ-oryzanol. The nanosponges' inclusion complex with γ-oryzanol suggests that it may have potential topical applications, mainly in the development of sunscreen formulations, regarding their antioxidant properties.[77]

Polymeric nanoparticles have been synthesized using various methods according to their purpose and the type of drugs to be encapsulated. These nanoparticles have been extensively used for the nano-encapsulation of various useful bioactive molecules and drugs in order to develop nanomedicines. Polymeric nanocapsules (Figure 23.3F) are vesicular systems in which a drug is confined in a cavity consisting of an inner liquid oily core surrounded by a polymeric membrane.[78] Regardless of the preparation method, these formulations are obtained as an aqueous suspension. The main type of oil used to compose the oily core of nanocapsules is capric/caprilic triglyceride, because of its ability to solubilize a wide range of active substances.[68] Nowadays, there is a trend to use vegetable oils to prepare polymeric nanocapsules, considering that this kind of oil is rich in phytochemical compounds. As a consequence, such oils could be very interesting for pharmaceutical and cosmetic purposes.

Innovative polymeric nanocapsules, called lipid-core nanocapsules, have been proposed in the past decade. They present a different core compared to the polymeric nanocapsules. Lipid-core nanocapsules (Figure 23.3G) are characterized by a lipid core composed of a mixture of oil and a solid lipid, as sorbitan monostearate, surrounded by a polymeric membrane.[79] Lipid-core nanocapsules prepared with RBO as an oily core (LNC-RBO) have demonstrated potential in the pharmaceutical field. These suspensions prepared using poly(ε-caprolactone) as a polymer and RBO 3% (v/v) present a nanometric mean particle size, low polydispersity, negative zeta potential, and neutral pH values. Rheological analysis showed that these formulations exhibit Newtonian behavior, an appropriate characteristic for the development of parenteral nanomedicines. In addition, an LNC-RBO suspension was able to control drug release. *In vitro* drug release studies showed that LNC-RBO containing clobetasol-propionate 0.05% (w/w) (a corticosteroid used to treat skin disorders) showed a slower release (168 h) compared to an ethanolic solution.[80] This nanometric suspension also presents potential for use in development of sunscreen formulations, considering the potential antioxidant effect of this oil.

Skin exposure to sun radiation (ultraviolet radiation) can generate several complications, such as erythema (sunburn), immunosuppression, or skin cancer. UV exposure is largely responsible for the production of free radicals that damage the antioxidant system of the skin tissue and therefore promote photoaging.[81] Such complications depend on exposure spans, genetic factors, and skin type. Cosmetic formulations have been developed to protect the skin from deleterious effect of UV exposure.[82] The development of sunscreens or skincare products containing bioactive compounds thus raises considerable interest. In an *in vivo* experimental study using mice, LNC-RBO incorporated in a hydrogel formulation prevented edema formation and showed an anti-inflammatory effect in skin damage induced by UVB radiation. These findings suggest that RBO could be used as an interesting raw material in the development of nanomedicines intended for UV protection.[83]

Beyond pharmaceutical technology, the unique properties of RBO make it an attractive ingredient that can provide health benefits in a wide range of food platforms. Thus, the development of products enriched with bioactive compounds obtained from RBO could be of great importance for the treatment of several disorders. To date the application of γ-oryzanol in food systems is limited, since this compound is unstable when heated during food processing and also has poor water solubility.[84]

Entrapment strategies can be used effectively to overcome this drawback, and microencapsulation within a biopolymeric matrix is a promising alternative in the development of food products intended for oral administration. In this sense, the design of oral drug delivery vehicles which effectively carry compounds to the colon site via the oral pathway poses interesting challenges. They need to remain intact when passing through the upper gastrointestinal tract in order to protect the incorporated drugs from chemical and enzymatic degradation. Pectin, one of a number of linear anionic polysaccharides, can form a gel structure by a gelling process involving calcium (Ca) ions. Ca pectinate gel, which is non-toxic, biocompatible, and mechanically strong, has been used as effective oral carrier of many bioactive compounds. Due to its ability to remain intact in the upper gastrointestinal tract, the potential of Ca pectinate as a drug carrier for colon-specific delivery has been associated with several pharmaceutical dosage forms, such as films, gels, creams, and tablets.[85] In this way, Ca pectinate microparticles were developed as a gastrointestinal drug delivery system. However, although they were able to protect the entrapped drug in the stomach, this formulation presented the tendency to a burst of release in intestine, an alkaline medium, because of the macroporous structure formed by gels. To overcome this problem, Ca pectinate microparticles can be reinforced with chitosan, which is another non-toxic and biocompatible polysaccharide that is quite stable under alkaline conditions. Moreover, chitosan presents mucoadhesive properties and is able to stick to the intestinal mucosa. *In vitro* studies carried out using chitosan-coated microparticles containing γ-oryzanol 2.72% revealed that this formulation is effective in suppressing the release of γ-oryzanol in both simulated gastric fluid and intestinal fluid.[86] An *in vivo* study was carried out in rats. In the experiment, 20 mg of γ-oryzanol/kg was administrated orally in rats to evaluate its bioavailability, and the plasma concentration of γ-oryzanol was monitored for 24 hours. The bioavailability of γ-oryzanol from the chitosan-coated microparticle formulation was 47.26 μg/mL per hour compared with the solution containing free γ-oryzanol (17.47 μg/mL per hour), proving that microencapsulation improves the bioavailability of γ-oryzanol. Furthermore, the mucoadhesive properties of chitosan increased the residence time of the formulation in the gastrointestinal tract.[87]

CONCLUSION

This chapter provides an overview of RBO, covering its production and therapeutic applications. Although RBO is less common compared with other vegetable oils (sunflower or soybean oil), this oil is the object of increasing interest due to its versatility in several applications, such as pharmaceutical, cosmetic, or food products. In addition, RBO contains γ-oryzanol, which exists only in this kind of vegetable oil and shows high antioxidant activity. Moreover, RBO contains other phytochemical compounds with anti-inflammatory, anticancer, and hypoglycemic effects. Therefore, development of new platforms of application could increase the number of products containing RBO or its components in the market.

References

1. Kennedy G, Burlingame B, Nguyen N. Nutrient impact assessment of rice in major rice-consuming countries. *International Rice Commission Letters* 2002;**51**:33–42.
2. Food and Agriculture Organization of the United Nations. Available at: http://www.fao.org/index_en.htm. (Last accessed September 2012).
3. United States Department of Agriculture. Available at: http://www.usda.gov/wps/portal/usda/usdahome. (Last accessed September 2012).
4. Siger A, Nogala-Kalucka M, Lampart-Szczapa E. The content and antioxidant activity of phenolic compounds in cold-pressed plant oils. *J Food Lipids* 2008;**15**:137–49.
5. Lerma-García MJ, Herrero-Martínez JM, Simó-Alfonso EF, et al. Composition, industrial processing and applications of rice bran γ-oryzanol. *Food Chem* 2009;**115**:389–404.
6. Nörnberg JL, Stumpf Júnior W, López J, Costa PB. Valor do farelo de arroz integral como fonte de gordura na dieta de vacas Jersey na fase inicial de lactação: digestibilidade aparente de nutrientes. *Rev Bras Zootec* 2004;**33**:2412–21.
7. Kaur C, Kapoor HC. Anti-oxidant activity and total phenolic content of some Asian vegetables. *Int J Food Sci Tech* 2002;**37**:153–61.
8. Bagchi D, Bagchi M, Stohs SJ, Das DK, Ray SD, Kuszynski CA, et al. Free radicals and grape seed proanthocyanidin extract: importance in human health and disease prevention. *Toxicology* 2000;**148**(2-3):187–97.

9. Franco R, Sanchez-Olea R, Reyes-Reyes EM, Panayiotidis MI. Environmental toxicity, oxidative stress and apoptosis: menage a trois. *Mutat Res* 2009;**674**:3–22.

10. Gopala Krishna AG, Hemakumar KH, Khatoon S. Study on the composition of rice bran oil and its higher free fatty acids value. *J Amer Oil Chem Soc* 2006;**83**:117–20.

11. Hasselwander O, Krämer K, Hoppe PP, et al. Effects of feeding various tocotrienol sources on plasma lipids and aortic atherosclerotic lesions in cholesterol-fed rabbits. *Food Res Int* 2002;**35**:245–51.

12. Frank J, Chin W, Schrader C, Eckert GP, Rimbach G. Do tocotrienols have potential as neuroprotective dietary factors? *Ageing Res Rev* 2012;**11**:163–80.

13. Lamberts L, De Bie E, Vandeputte E, Veraverbeke S, Derycke V, De Man W, et al. Effect of milling on colour and nutritional properties of rice. *Food Chem* 2007;**100**:1496–503.

14. Roy P, Ijiri T, Okadome H, Nei D, Orikasa T, Nakamura N, et al. Effect of processing conditions on overall energy consumption and quality of rice (*Oryza sativa* L.). *J Food Eng* 2008;**89**:343–8.

15. Yadav BK, Jindal VK. Changes in head rice yield and whiteness during milling of rough rice (*Oryza sativa* L.). *J Food Eng* 2008;**86**:113–21.

16. Hanmoungjai P, Pyle DL, Niranjan K. Enzymatic process for extracting oil and protein from rice bran. *J Amer Oil Chem Soc* 2001;**78**:817–21.

17. Amarasinghe BMWPK, Kumarasiri MPM, Gangodavilage NC. Effect of method of stabilization on aqueous extraction of rice bran oil. *Food Bioprod Process* 2009;**87**:108–14.

18. Balachandran C, Mayamol PN, Thomas S, Sukumar D, Sundaresan A, Arumughan C. An ecofriendly approach to process rice bran for high quality rice bran oil using supercritical carbon dioxide for nutraceutical applications. *Bioresource Technol* 2008;**99**:2905–12.

19. Krishna AGG, Khatoon S, Shiela PM, Sarmandal CV, Indira TN, Mishra A. Effect of refining of crude rice bran oil on the retention of oryzanol in the refined oil. *J Am Oil Chem Soc* 2001;**78**:127–31.

20. Paucar-Menacho LM, Silva LHd, Santána AdS, Gonçalves LAG. Refino de Óleo de farelo de arroz (*Oryza sativa* L.) em condições brandas para preservação do gamma-orizanol. *Ciênc Tecnol Aliment* 2007;**27**:45–53.

21. Pestana V, Zambiazi R, Mendonça CB, et al. Quality Changes and Tocopherols and γ-Oryzanol Concentrations in Rice Bran Oil During the Refining Process. *J Am Oil Chem Soc* 2008;**85**:1013–9.

22. Chen MH, Bergman CJ. A rapid procedure for analysing rice bran tocopherol, tocotrienol and γ-oryzanol contents. *J Food Comp Anal* 2005;**18**:319–31.

23. Berger A, Rein D, Schafer A, Monnard I, Gremaud G, Lambelet P, et al. Similar cholesterol-lowering properties of rice bran oil, with varied gamma-oryzanol, in mildly hypercholesterolemic men. *Eur J Nutr* 2005;**44**:163–73.

24. Wilson TA, Ausman LM, Lawton CW, Hegsted DM, Nicolosi RJ. Comparative cholesterol lowering properties of vegetable oils: beyond fatty acids. *J Am Coll Nutr* 2000;**19**:601–7.

25. Tham DM, Gardner CD, Haskell WL. Potential Health Benefits of Dietary Phytoestrogens: A Review of the Clinical, Epidemiological, and Mechanistic Evidence. *Am J Clin Nutr* 1998;**83**:2223–35.

26. Valko M, Izakovic M, Mazur M, Rhodes CJ, Telser J. Role of oxygen radicals in DNA damage and cancer incidence. *Mol Cell Biochem* 2004;**266**:37–56.

27. Allen RG, Tresini M. Oxidative stress and gene regulation. *Free Radical Bio Med* 2000;**28**:463–99.

28. Liu RH. Health benefits of fruit and vegetables are from additive and synergistic combinations of phytochemicals. *Am J Clin Nutr* 2003;**78**:517S–20S.

29. Shih C-K, Ho C-J, Li S-C, Yang S-H, Hou W-C, Cheng H-H. Preventive effects of rice bran oil on 1,2-dimethylhydrazine/dextran sodium sulphate-induced colon carcinogenesis in rats. *Food Chem* 2011;**126**:562–7.

30. Graf E, Eaton JW. Antioxidant functions of phytic acid. *Free Radical Bio Med* 1990;**8**:61–9.

31. Norazalina S, Norhaizan ME, Hairuszah I, Norashareena MS. Anticarcinogenic efficacy of phytic acid extracted from rice bran on azoxymethane-induced colon carcinogenesis in rats. *Exp Toxicol Pathol* 2010;**62**:259–68.

32. Urso ML, Clarkson PM. Oxidative stress, exercise, and antioxidant supplementation. *Toxicology* 2003;**189**:41–54.

33. Ismail M, Al-Naqeeb G, Mamat W, Ahmad Z. Gamma-oryzanol rich fraction regulates the expression of antioxidant and oxidative stress related genes in stressed rat's liver. *Nutrition & Metabolism* 2010;**7**:23.

34. Hansson GK. Inflammation, Atherosclerosis, and Coronary Artery Disease. *New Engl J Med* 2005;**352**:1685–95.

35. Celermajer DS, Chow CK, Marijon E, Anstey NM, Woo KS. Cardiovascular Disease in the Developing World Prevalences, Patterns, and the Potential of Early Disease Detection. *J Am Coll Cardiol* 2012;**60**:1207–16.

36. Saklamaz A, Comlekci A, Temiz A, Caliskan S, Ceylan C, Alacacioglu A, et al. The beneficial effects of lipid-lowering drugs beyond lipid-lowering effects: a comparative study with pravastatin, atorvastatin, and fenofibrate in patients with type IIa and type IIb hyperlipidemia. *Metabolism* 2005;**54**:677–81.

37. Ausman LM, Rong N, Nicolosi RJ. Hypocholesterolemic effect of physically refined rice bran oil: studies of cholesterol metabolism and early atherosclerosis in hypercholesterolemic hamsters. *J Nutr Biochem* 2005 Sep;**16**(9):521–9.

38. Ghatak SB, Panchal SJ. Anti-hyperlipidemic activity of oryzanol, isolated from crude rice bran oil, on Triton WR-1339-induced acute hyperlipidemia in rats. *Rev Bras Farmacogn* 2012;**22**:642–8.

39. Chandrashekar P, Kumar PKP, Ramesh HP, Lokesh BR, Krishna AGG. Hypolipidemic effect of oryzanol concentrate and low temperature extracted crude rice bran oil in experimental male wistar rats. *J Food Sci Technol* 2012:1–8.

40. Ha T-Y, Han S, Kim S-R, Kim I-H, Lee H-Y, Kim H-K. Bioactive components in rice bran oil improve lipid profiles in rats fed a high-cholesterol diet. *Nutr Res* 2005;**25**:597–606.

41. Xu Z, Hua N, Godber JS. Antioxidant activity of tocopherols, tocotrienols, and gamma-oryzanol components from rice bran against cholesterol oxidation accelerated by 2,2'-azobis(2-methylpropionamidine) dihydrochloride. *J Agric Food Chem* 2001;**49**:2077–81.

42. Pearson P, Lewis SA, Britton J, Young IS, Fogarty A. The pro-oxidant activity of high-dose vitamin E supplements *in vivo*. *Bio Drugs* 2006;**20**:271–3.

43. Minhajuddin M, Beg ZH, Iqbal J. Hypolipidemic and antioxidant properties of tocotrienol rich fraction isolated from rice bran oil in experimentally induced hyperlipidemic rats. *Food Chem Toxicol* 2005;**43**:747–53.

44. Most MM, Tulley R, Morales S, Lefevre M. Rice bran oil, not fiber, lowers cholesterol in humans. *Am J Clin Nutr* 2005;**81**:64–8.

45. Kuriyan R, Gopinath N, Vaz M, Kurpad AV. Use of rice bran oil in patients with hyperlipidaemia. *Natl Med J India* 2005;**18**:292–6.

46. Bergman CJ, Xu Z. Genotype and Environment Effects on Tocopherol, Tocotrienol, and γ-Oryzanol Contents of Southern US Rice. *Cereal Chem* 2003;**80**:446–9.

47. Akiyama Y, Hori K, Hata K, Kawane M, Kawamura Y, Yoshiki Y, et al. Screening of chemiluminescence constituents of cereals and DPPH radical scavenging activity of gamma-oryzanol. *Luminescence* 2001;**16**:237–41.

48. Juliano C, Cossu M, Alamanni MC, Piu L. Antioxidant activity of gamma-oryzanol: mechanism of action and its effect on oxidative stability of pharmaceutical oils. *Int J Pharm* 2005;**299**:146–54.

49. Cicero AFG, Gaddi A. Rice Bran Oil and γ-Oryzanol in the Treatment of Hyperlipoproteinaemias and Other Conditions. *Phytother Res* 2001;**15**:277–89.

50. Bastak S. Diabetes mellitus and its treatment. *Int J Diabetes Metabolism* 2005;**13**:111–34.

51. Keim AL, Chi MMY, Moley KH. Hyperglycemia-induced apoptotic cell death in the mouse blastocyst is dependent on expression of p53. *Mol Reprod Dev* 2001;**60**:214–24.

52. Allen DA, Harwood S, Varagunam M, Raftery MJ, Yaqoob MM. High glucose-induced oxidative stress causes apoptosis in proximal tubular epithelial cells and is mediated by multiple caspases. *FASEB J* 2003;**17**:908–10.

53. Halim E, Mukhopadhyay AK. Effect of *Ocimum sanctum* (Tulsi) and vitamin E on biochemical parameters and retinopathy in streptozotocin induced diabetic rats. *Indian J Clin Biochem* 2006;**21**:181–8.

54. Siddiqui S, Rashid Khan M, Siddiqui WA. Comparative hypoglycemic and nephroprotective effects of tocotrienol rich fraction (TRF) from palm oil and rice bran oil against hyperglycemia induced nephropathy in type 1 diabetic rats. *Chem Biol Interact* 2010;**188**:651–8.

55. Jung EH, Kim SR, Hwang IK, Ha TY. Hypoglycemic effects of a phenolic acid fraction of rice bran and ferulic acid in C57BL/KsJ-db/db mice. *J Agric Food Chem* 2007;**55**:9800–4.

56. Vettor R, Milan G, Rossato M, Federspil G. Review article: adipocytokines and insulin resistance. *Aliment Pharm Therap* 2005;**22**:3–10.

57. Nagasaka R, Yamsaki T, Uchida A, Ohara K, Ushio H. gamma-Oryzanol recovers mouse hypoadiponectinemia induced by animal fat ingestion. *Phytomedicine* 2011;**18**:669–71.

58. Islam MS, Murata T, Fujisawa M, Nagasaka R, Ushio H, Bari AM, et al. Anti-inflammatory effects of phytosteryl ferulates in colitis induced by dextran sulphate sodium in mice. *Br J Pharmacol* 2008;**154**:812–24.

59. Hodin CM, Visschers RGJ, Rensen SS, Boonen B, Damink SWMO, Lenaerts K, et al. Total Parenteral Nutrition Induces a Shift in the Firmicutes to Bacteroidetes Ratio in Association with Paneth Cell Activation in Rats. *J Nutr* 2012;**142**:2141–7.

60. Rigo L, Rascovetzki R, Beck R. Sunscreen Formulations Containing Rice Bran or Soybean Oil: Rheological Properties, Spreadability and In vitro Sun Protection Factor. *Lat Am J Pharm* 2011;**30**:246–52.

61. Miyazaki K, Islam N. Nanotechnology systems of innovation – An analysis of industry and academia research activities. *Technovation* 2007;**27**:661–75.

62. Alonso MJ. Nanomedicines for overcoming biological barriers. *Biomed Pharmacother* 2004;**58**:168–72.

63. Bernardi A, Zilberstein AC, Jager E, Campos MM, Morrone FB, Calixto JB, et al. Effects of indomethacin-loaded nanocapsules in experimental models of inflammation in rats. *Br J Pharmacol* 2009;**158**:1104–11.

64. Ourique AF, Pohlmann AR, Guterres SS, Beck RC. Tretinoin-loaded nanocapsules: Preparation, physicochemical characterization, and photostability study. *Int J Pharm* 2008;**352**:1–4.

65. He W, Horn SW, Hussain MD. Improved bioavailability of orally administered mifepristone from PLGA nanoparticles. *Int J Pharm* 2007;**334**:173–8.

66. Lu Y, Qi J, Wu W. Absorption, disposition and pharmacokinetics of nanoemulsions. *Curr Drug Metab* 2012;**13**:396–417.

67. Batista CM, Carvalho CMBd, Magalhães NSS. Lipossomas e suas aplicações terapêuticas: estado da arte. *Rev Bras Ciênc Farm* 2007;**43**:167–79.

68. Mora-Huertas CE, Fessi H, Elaissari A. Polymer-based nanocapsules for drug delivery. *Int J Pharm* 2010;**385**:113–42.

69. Kazi KM, Mandal AS, Biswas N, Guha A, Chatterjee S, Behera M, et al. Niosome: A future of targeted drug delivery systems. *J Adv Pharm Technol Res* 2010;**1**:374–80.

70. Bernardi D, Pereira T, Maciel N, Bortoloto J, Viera G, Oliveira G, et al. Formation and stability of oil-in-water nanoemulsions containing rice bran oil: *in vitro* and *in vivo* assessments. *J Nanobiotechnology* 2011;**9**:44.

71. Pardeike J, Hommoss A, Muller RH. Lipid nanoparticles (SLN, NLC) in cosmetic and pharmaceutical dermal products. *Int J Pharm* 2009;**366**:170–84.

72. Lukowski G, Kasbohm J, Pflegel P, Illing A, Wulff H. Crystallographic investigation of cetylpalmitate solid lipid nanoparticles. *Int J Pharm* 2000;**196**:201–5.

73. Uracha R, Surachai L, Siwaporn M, Usawadee S, Nuntavan B, Varaporn J, et al. The effect of cetyl palmitate crystallinity on physical properties of gamma-oryzanol encapsulated in solid lipid nanoparticles. *Nanotechnology* 2008;**19**:095701.

74. Gupta PN, Mishra V, Rawat A, Dubey P, Mahor S, Jain S, et al. Non-invasive vaccine delivery in transfersomes, niosomes and liposomes: a comparative study. *Int J Pharm* 2005;**293**:73–82.

75. Manosroi A, Chutoprapat R, Abe M, Manosroi W, Manosroi J. Transdermal absorption enhancement of rice bran bioactive compounds entrapped in niosomes. *AAPS Pharm Sci Tech* 2012;**13**: 323–35.

76. Del Valle EMM. Cyclodextrins and their uses: a review. *Process Biochemistry* 2004:39.

77. Sapino S, Carlotti ME, Cavalli R, Ugazio E, Berlier G, Gastaldi L, et al. Photochemical and antioxidant properties of gamma-oryzanol in beta-cyclodextrin-based nanosponges. *J Incl Phenom Macrocycl Chem* 2012;**1**:1–8.

78. Kumari A, Yadav SK, Yadav SC. Biodegradable polymeric nanoparticles based drug delivery systems. *Colloid Surface B* 2010;**75**:1–18.

79. Jager E, Venturini CG, Poletto FS, Colome LM, Pohlmann JP, Bernardi A, et al. Sustained release from lipid-core nanocapsules by varying the core viscosity and the particle surface area. *J Biomed Nanotechnol* 2009;**5**:130–40.

80. Rigo L, Coradini K, Ourique AF, Silva C, Guterres S, Pohlmann A, et al. *Study of the type of vegetable oil on the drug release from lipid-core nanocapsules XI.* Brazil: Brazilian MRS Meeting Florianópolis; 2012.

81. Rabe JH, Mamelak AJ, McElgunn PJ, Morison WL, Sauder DN. Photoaging: mechanisms and repair. *J Am Acad Dermatol* 2006; **55**:1–19.

82. Gallagher RP, Lee TK. Adverse effects of ultraviolet radiation: a brief review. *Prog Biophys Mol Biol* 2006;**92**:119–31.

83. Rigo L, Silva C, Ferreira J, Silva CB, Beck RCR. Hydrogels containing rice bran oil-loaded polymeric nanoparticles: protective effect against UVB radiation-induced skin damage in mice. *I° Congresso Brasileiro de Ciências Farmacêuticas* 2012.

84. Parrado J, Miramontes E, Jover M, et al. Preparation of a rice bran enzymatic extract with potential use as functional food. *Food Chem* 2006;**98**:742–8.

85. Liu L, Fishman ML, Kost J, Hicks KB. Pectin-based systems for colon-specific drug delivery via oral route. *Biomaterials* 2003;**24**: 3333–43.

86. Lee J-S, Kim JS, Lee HG. γ-Oryzanol-loaded calcium pectinate microparticles reinforced with chitosan: Optimization and release characteristics. *Colloid Surface B* 2009;**70**:213–7.

87. Kim JS, Lee JS, Chang PS, Lee HG. Optimization, *in vitro* release and bioavailability of gamma-oryzanol-loaded calcium pectinate microparticles reinforced with chitosan. *N Biotechnol* 2010;**27**: 368–73.

Rice Intake, Weight Change and Metabolic Syndrome

Zumin Shi, Anne W. Taylor, Gary A. Wittert

University of Adelaide, Discipline of Medicine, Adelaide, South Australia, Australia

INTRODUCTION

The metabolic syndrome (MetS) is characterized by the clustering of abdominal obesity, raised blood pressure, elevated fasting plasma glucose concentration, and dyslipidemia (high triglycerides, reduced high density lipoprotein [HDL] cholesterol).[1,2] Currently, two definitions of MetS are widely used: the International Diabetes Federation (IDF) definition[1] and the National Cholesterol Education Program Adult Treatment Panel III (NCEP ATP III) definition[3] (Table 24.1). The global burden of MetS is high. In developed countries, it affects more than 20% of the population.[4] In developing countries undergoing rapid nutrition transition, such as China, the prevalence is above 10%. The syndrome is associated with the development of diabetes and cardiovascular disease.[5-10] Different components of the syndrome confer different risks for diabetes or CVD. The risk of diabetes or CVD increases as the number of metabolic abnormalities rises.[11] Obesity and insulin resistance has been proposed as an important mechanism underlying MetS.[2]

Several epidemiological and experimental studies suggest the influence of diet on MetS.[12,13] Consumption of whole grains, fruit, and vegetables are related to a lower risk of MetS.[14] A low-fiber Western dietary pattern is related to an increased risk of MetS.[15] Studies on the association between diet and MetS mainly focus on dietary fat, dietary patterns, fruit, and vegetables. The role of a staple food such as rice, as consumed as part of a traditional lifestyle, or in the context of the adoption of an increasingly Western-type lifestyle, is less studied. A recent large population study from Japan shows that rice consumption is inversely associated with mortality from cardiovascular disease (CVD) in men but not women.[16] The latest evidence-based guideline of the German Nutrition Society thoroughly examines the existing evidence relating to carbohydrate intake and nutrition related diseases, but rice is not specifically addressed.[17]

The aim of this review is to summarize findings from epidemiological studies on the relationship between rice consumption and MetS. We used PubMed to search for existing literature using the key words "rice", "body weight", "overweight", "obesity", "lipids", "dyslipidemia", "glucose", "blood sugar", "insulin resistance", "hypertension", "blood pressure", and "metabolic syndrome". Possible mechanisms linking rice consumption and MetS are also discussed.

HISTORY AND CONSUMPTION OF RICE

Rice is one of the oldest cultivated crops, first mentioned in China in 2800 BC. It is estimated that there are more than 40,000 varieties of cultivated rice; of these, more than 100 grow worldwide.[18] Naturally grown rice has different colors, including white, red, and black. Based on the degree of processing, rice is categorized into two groups: brown rice and white rice. Rice retaining the grain, embryo, and bran is called brown or whole grain rice. White rice is refined rice. The refining process destroys the structure of the grain kernel and removes dietary fiber and other essential micronutrients in grains.

Worldwide, rice provides ~20% of dietary energy.[19] It is the main staple food for more than half of the world's population, mostly in Asian countries. In Western countries, rice consumption is relatively low as compared with Asian countries. For example, the mean daily rice intake in the UK was 92 g in 2010,[18] while it was 280 g in China in 2004.[20] In Japan, rice provides 43% of carbohydrate and 29% of energy intake.[21]

TABLE 24.1 Definition of Metabolic Syndrome

International Diabetes Federation (IDF) criteria (2005)	Central obesity (defined as waist circumference but can be assumed if BMI >30 kg/m²) with ethnicity-specific values*, plus two of the following: 1. Triglycerides 150 mg/dL or greater 2. HDL-cholesterol <40 mg/dL in men and <50 mg/dL in women 3. BP 130/85 mmHg or greater. 4. Fasting glucose 100 mg/dl or greater. *To meet the criteria, waist circumference must be: for Europeans, >94 cm in men and >80 cm in women; and for South Asians, Chinese, and Japanese, >90 cm in men and >80 cm in women. For ethnic South and Central Americans, South Asian data are used; for Sub-Saharan Africans and Eastern Mediterranean and Middle East (Arab) populations, European data are used
National Cholesterol Education Program Adult Treatment Panel III (NCEP:ATPIII) criteria (2001)	Any three or more of the following: 1. Waist circumference >102 cm in men, >88 cm in women 2. Triglycerides 150 mg/dL or greater 3. HDL-cholesterol <40 mg/dL in men and <50 mg/dL in women. 4. BP 130/85 mmHg or greater. 5. Fasting glucose 110 mg/dL* or greater. *In 2003, the American Diabetes Association (ADA) changed the criteria for IFG tolerance from 110 mg/dL to 100 mg/dL.

During the past half century, with the development of food processing technology, highly refined white rice is becoming the dominant form of rice consumed in many Asian countries. For example, in India more than 75% of the refined grain intake is white rice.[22] In China, white rice intake accounts for more than 30% of the daily energy intake.[23]

NUTRITION AND METABOLIC CHARACTERISTICS OF RICE

Rice, especially in the unrefined state, is potentially a very important source of macro- and micronutrients in the human diet, providing carbohydrate, protein, magnesium, zinc, copper, vitamin B6, and dietary fiber.[16] Rice is high in potassium and low in sodium. Moreover, rice is low in fat and free of cholesterol. Table 24.2 shows the nutrient content of rice in China and Australia. A mean of 280 g daily rice consumption in the Chinese diet will provide 20.7 g protein, 216.2 g carbohydrate, 2 g dietary fiber, and 2.2 g fat.

Rice is cooked by boiling or steaming without the addition of butter, margarine, soup, or animal fat in many Asian countries, such as China and Japan. Steamed rice contains twice the amount of water and half the energy compared with steamed bread[24]; 100 g cooked

TABLE 24.2 Nutrient Composition of Rice in China and Australia

Per 100 g	China[a]	Australia[b]	Nutrient Provided by 280 g Rice (Mean Daily Intake in China)
Energy (kJ)	1446	1469	4048
Energy (kcal)	346	351	969
Protein (g)	7.4	6.3	20.7
Carbohydrate (g)	77.2	78.8	216.2
Fat (g)	0.8	0.5	2.2
Cholesterol (mg)	0	0	0
Dietary fiber (g)	0.7	0.7	2.0
Vitamin A (μg)	0	0	0.0
Beta carotene (μg)	0	0	0.0
Beta carotene equivalents (μg)	0	0	0.0
Thiamin (B1) (mg)	0.11	0.08	0.3
Riboflavin (B2) (mg)	0.05	0.02	0.1
Niacin (B3) (mg)	1.9	1.99	5.3
Vitamin C (mg)	0	0	0.0
Vitamin E (mg)	0.46	0.06	1.3
Potassium (mg)	103	49	288.4
Sodium (mg)	3.8	5	10.6
Calcium (mg)	13	7	36.4
Magnesium (mg)	34	34	95.2
Iron (mg)	2.3	0.7	6.4
Manganese (mg)	1.29	1.6	3.6
Zinc (mg)	1.7	1.1	4.8
Copper (mg)	0.3	0.2	0.8
Phosphorus (mg)	110	120	308.0
Selenium (μg)	2.23	8	6.2
Tryptophan (mg)	–	90	

[a] From Chinese Food Composition Table 2004.
[b] From NUTTAB 2010 (http://www.foodstandards.gov.au/consumerinformation/nuttab2010/).

rice contains only 114 kcal energy, while 100 g steamed bread contains 233 kcal energy.[24]

RICE INTAKE AND WEIGHT CHANGE

It is often perceived that starchy foods are associated with weight gain, and a high protein/low carbohydrate diet has become popular for weight loss.[25] The quality of the carbohydrate, however, may be more important than the amount, and cumulative evidence suggests that whole grains are beneficial in terms of body weight regulation.[26]

During the past three decades, the diet in many Asian countries has become Westernized; consumption of plant-based staples has decreased while that of high energy density pre-prepared food has increased. In China between 1989 and 2004, rice intake decreased from 348 g/d to 280 g/d – a 20% decrease over 15 years.[20] During the same period, there was a significant increase in overweight and obesity.[20] However, very few studies have assessed the association between rice intake and body weight status worldwide.

Inverse associations between rice consumption and overweight/obesity have been demonstrated in successive phases of the National Health and Nutrition Examination Survey (NHANES). In NHANES 1999–2004, among those aged 18–50 years, comparing rice eaters (at least 14 g of uncooked white or brown rice per day) with non-rice eaters, the OR was 0.77 (0.65–0.91) for overweight and 0.83 (0.69–1.00) for obesity.[27] This association was independent of ethnicity. In NHANES 2007–2008, it was found that rice consumption was associated with a lower BMI, smaller waist circumference and tricep skinfold thickness, and lower serum insulin concentrations (source: http://www.usarice.com/doclib/198/187/60 77.pdf).

In the Jiangsu Nutrition Study (JIN), we assessed the association between rice intake and weight change by following 1231 Chinese adults aged 20 and older from 2002 to 2007.[28] We found that compared with low rice intake (<200 g/d), weight gain over 5 years was 2 kg less with daily consumption of rice of 400 g/d. Furthermore, in this study the staple food pattern was measured as percentage of rice in staple foods (PRS, PRS=intake of rice/[intake of rice+intake of wheat flour]). Every 10% increase in PRS was associated with 0.28 kg less weight gain. This association holds even if we exclude those consuming predominantly rice or wheat flour as staple foods. When we limit the analysis to those with PRS of between 90% and 10%, the associations between PRS and weight change were not altered. In the study region, rice and wheat flour represented two different staple foods, and therefore the comparison of intake in a geographically small province with a primarily Han population is essentially an ecological study that permits some conclusions to be drawn.

In a 6-week meal replacement trial, 40 overweight/obese Korean women aged between 20 and 35 years were randomly assigned into two low-energy meal replacement groups, consuming either mixed rice (brown and black rice) or white rice. Weight loss occurred in both groups, but it was greater in the mixed rice group compared to the white rice group (−6.75 kg vs −5.37 kg).[29]

ASSOCIATION BETWEEN RICE CONSUMPTION AND INDIVIDUAL COMPONENTS OF METABOLIC SYNDROME

Rice Intake and Central Obesity

The association between rice consumption and central obesity has been assessed in three population studies: one study compared rice eaters with non rice eaters, one study looked at the combination of rice with other food, and one study quantitatively assessed the amount of rice consumption in relation to central obesity.

In NHANES 1999–2004, rice eaters (eating at least 14 g of uncooked white or brown rice per day) had a lower risk of central obesity than non-rice eaters (OR 0.73, 95% CI 0.63–0.86) among those aged 19–50 years after adjusting for age, ethnicity, and energy intake. However, this inverse association was not observed among those aged 51 years and above.[27]

In a large cross-sectional population study in Korean adults (n=21,165), a 103-item food frequency questionnaire was used in the study to calculate energy and nutrient intake, and two questions were asked regarding rice consumption: (1) What kind of cooked rice do you usually eat? (white rice only/rice with other foods/mix of two types); and (2) What kind of foods do you mainly eat cooked rice with? (beans/multigrains). Each participant was categorized into one of four rice eating groups: white rice group, rice with beans, rice with multigrains, and a mixed group.[30] Among men, compared with the white rice group, the mixed group had 18% raised OR of central obesity after adjusting for energy intake, age, physical activity, education, alcohol drinking, and smoking. However, among women, compared with the white rice group, the rice with beans and rice with multigrains groups had a lower risk of central obesity. The association between the amount of rice consumed and central obesity was not assessed, but in both men and women more than 50% of the total energy intake was from cooked rice dishes.[30]

In JIN, among 1231 Chinese adults aged 20 and older, neither a high consumption of rice nor a high PRS were associated with the risk of developing central obesity during a 5-year follow-up after adjusting for potential confounders.[28]

Rice and Hyperglycemia

There are a few cross-sectional and longitudinal studies assessing the association between rice consumption and hyperglycemia or diabetes. Findings from these studies are inconsistent. Results from NHANES 1999–2004 suggest no significant association between rice consumption (comparing rice consumption≥14 g/d and rice consumption <14g/d) and hyperglycemia among those aged 19 years and older after adjusting for age, ethnicity, and energy intake.[27] In a recent 6-year follow-up study in Spain, Soriguer et al. found that those with a frequent rice intake (two or three times per week) had a lower risk of developing diabetes (OR 0.43, 95% CI 0.09–0.95, P=0.04) than those with less frequent rice intake after adjusting for age, sex, obesity, and baseline glucose status.[31] Interestingly, high rice consumption was related to high intake of monounsaturated fatty acids (MUFA), possibly due to the specific rice cooking method of using olive oil. However, adjusting for olive oil intake did not change the association between rice and diabetes. In JIN, rice intake was positively associated with the development of hyperglycemia (blood glucose >5.6mmol/L) after adjusting for socio-demographic and lifestyle factors.[28] ORs for incidence of hyperglycemia across rice intake (≤200, 201–400, ≥401g/d) were 1, 1.96 (1.07–3.60), 2.50 (1.37–4.57) (P for trend 0.005). In the fully adjusted model, each 10% increase of PRS was associated with a 22% increase in the risk of hyperglycemia.

In a recent systematic review based on four prospective cohort studies (including Chinese,[32] Japanese,[33] American,[34] and Australian[34]) with a total of 13,284 incident cases of type 2 diabetes among 352,384 participants, Hu et al.[35] concluded that higher consumption of white rice is associated with a significantly increased risk of type 2 diabetes, especially in Asian countries (China[32] and Japan[33]). The pooled relative risk was 1.55 (95% CI 1.20–2.01) comparing the highest with the lowest category of white rice intake in Asian populations, whereas the corresponding figure was 1.12 (0.94–1.33) in Western populations (P for interaction=0.038). In the total population, for each serving per day increment of white rice intake, the risk of type 2 diabetes increased by 11% (95% CI 8–14%) (P for linear trend <0.001). However, in the four studies included in the review, the reference group of rice intake varied from <5.3g/d to <500g/d – an almost 100-fold difference.[35] Accordingly, aggregated estimates of the effect of rice on diabetes might be misleading even though each study had adjusted for a range of potential confounders. No population studies have assessed the relationship between rice cooking methods and the risk of hyperglycemia, even though it is known that the glycemic index (GI) of rice is affected by how it is cooked.[36]

An ethnic difference in the association between rice consumption and diabetes seems to be supported by the variation in glycemic response to rice between Asian and European populations.

In a study involving 32 Chinese and 31 European healthy volunteers, glycemic response, measured by incremental area under the glucose curve, was over 60% greater for five rice varieties (Jasmine, Basmati, Brown, Doongara, and Parboiled) (P<0.001) amongst Chinese compared with European volunteers.[37] Whether this truly represents genetic variation or reflects some confound associated with the migration process and adoption of a new culture, diet, and lifestyle remains an open question.

Rice and Abnormal HDL

There is convincing evidence showing that a high carbohydrate intake at the expense of total fat and saturated fatty acids reduces the level of total and HDL cholesterol.[17] As a major contributor to carbohydrate intake, rice has been found to be associated with the risk of abnormal HDL.

In JIN, comparing high rice consumption (≥401g/d) with low rice consumption, the OR for developing abnormal HDL was 1.58 (95% CI 1.01–2.48). Every 10% increase of PRS was associated with 7% increased risk of developing abnormal HDL.[28] In NHANES 1999–2004, compared with non-rice eaters, rice eaters had borderline significant increased risk of having abnormal HDL (OR 1.27, 95% CI 0.99–1.63, P=0.059) among those aged 51 years and above.[27] However, among those aged 19–50 years there was no such association. Using cluster analysis, Song and colleagues found that a traditional Korean dietary pattern (high intake of rice and kimchi) was related to a 23% increased risk of low HDL compared with other dietary patterns.[38]

Rice and Triglyceride (TG)

An inverse association between rice intake and TG has been reported in different populations. For example, rice intake was inversely and wheat intake was positively related to the total cholesterol level in the Japanese population.[39] In the aforementioned Korean meal replacement trial, TG levels decreased significantly after 6 weeks among overweight/obese women in the mixed rice meal and white rice groups.[29] In JIN, there was a marginally significant inverse association between rice intake and high TG.[28]

However, an analysis from NHANES 1999–2004 showed no association between rice consumption and elevated TG.[27]

Rice and Blood Pressure

Rice protein has been shown to have an antihypertensive effect in animals,[40] and early in the 1940s a "rice diet" (including rice, sugar, fruit, and fruit juices) was used by Walter Kempner to treat hypertension in patients with chronic glomerulonephritis.[41]

In JIN, there was an inverse association between rice intake, PRS, and hypertension. The group with rice intake

≥401 g/d had 42% less risk of hypertension when compared with the group with rice intake <200 g/d. A consistent association between PRS and hypertension was found with every 10% increase in PRS associated with a 9% decrease in the risk of hypertension. This association cannot be explained by sodium and fat intake, because there was a positive association between rice intake and sodium and sodium intake in the sample. In NHANES 1999–2004, rice eaters had a lower risk of having high blood pressure compared with non-rice eaters (OR 0.66, 95% CI 0.57–0.76) among those aged 19–50 years. However, there was no association between rice consumption and high blood pressure among those aged 51 years and above.[27]

In a clinical trial in Shanghai, among participants with diabetes, a greater reduction in diastolic blood pressure was observed in the brown rice group compared with the white rice group ($P=0.02$).[42]

ASSOCIATION BETWEEN RICE INTAKE AND MetS

Although a number of studies have examined the association between rice intake and individual components of MetS, the association between rice intake and MetS is less studied. There are only three cross-sectional studies, one prospective cohort study, and one randomized clinical trial assessing the relationship between rice intake and MetS (Table 24.3). Among these studies, one Indian study looked at the association between refined grain intake (predominantly rice) and MetS. One Korean study assessed rice eating patterns and MetS.

In a cross-sectional study among 2042 adults aged 20 years and above in urban southern India, refined grain consumption (including white rice, refined wheat flour, and semolina) was positively associated with MetS. Comparing the extreme quartiles of refined grain consumption, the OR for MetS was 7.83 (95% CI 4.72–12.99).[22] Furthermore, high intake of refined grains was associated with insulin resistance.[22] The intake of refined grain was quite high in the study population: the median intake was 218.1 g/d and 448.8 g/d in quartiles 1 and 4, respectively. In total, 46.9% of the total daily energy intake was from refined grains. White rice constituted 75.8% of the refined grain intake with a mean intake of 253.4 g/d, but the study did not specifically assess the association between white rice consumption and MetS.[22]

The Korean diet is high in carbohydrate, mostly rice. Based on data from the Korean Genome and Epidemiology Study (KoGES),[30] Ahn *et al.* assessed the cross-sectional association between rice eating patterns and MetS. Among 26,006 adults with known chronic diseases, four rice eating patterns were indentified: white

rice, rice with beans, rice with multigrains, and a mixed group. Compared with the white group, the other three groups had no significant difference in the OR of MetS in men. The mixed group had an 18% higher OR of central obesity. However, among women, the rice with beans, rice with multigrains, and mixed groups had a lower risk of MetS among postmenopausal but not premenopausal women. The study did not, however, assess whether the total intake of rice was related to MetS.

In NHANES 1999–2004, among those aged 19–50 years, rice eaters (at least 14 g of uncooked white or brown rice per day) had a 21% lower risk of MetS than non-rice eaters ($P<0.05$) after adjusting for age, ethnicity, and sex.[27] No significant association between rice consumption and MetS was found among those aged 51 years and above.

In JIN, we found there was no significant association between rice intake and incident MetS in a 5-year follow-up. Furthermore, the percentage of rice as the staple food was not related to the risk of MetS in our study, despite its positive association with hyperglycemia.

In a randomized trial, 202 middle-aged Chinese adults with diabetes or high risk for diabetes were randomly assigned to a white rice ($n=101$) or brown rice ($n=101$) group and consumed the rice *ad libitum* for 16 weeks. Metabolic risk markers, including BMI, waist circumference, blood pressure, glycated hemoglobin, and serum lipid, glucose, and insulin concentrations, were measured before and after the intervention. The study found that replacing white rice with brown rice had no effect on MetS.[42] Surprisingly, the serum LDL cholesterol concentration decreased more in the white rice group compared to the brown rice group ($P=0.02$) among those with diabetes.[42]

PHYSIOLOGICAL MECHANISMS

Based on the above description, although not consistent, the majority of the epidemiological studies suggest that rice consumption may be beneficial to weight management. Both positive and negative associations between rice and components of MetS were observed. However, the possible mechanisms linking rice and weight and components of MetS are not clear. Based on the effects of single nutrient or physiological characteristics of rice, some hypotheses could be made. In this respect, much attention has been paid to glycemic index, energy density, dietary fiber, and rice protein.

Glycemic Index (GI)

According to the International Table of Glycemic Index (GI) and Glycemic Load (GL) Values, white rice has a relatively higher GI than brown rice, wheat, and

TABLE 24.3 Overview of Studies on Rice Intake and Metabolic Syndrome

Country, Study Name and Reference	Study Population	Dietary Intake Measurement	Rice Intake Level	Exposure Variables	MetS Definition	Main Results	Note
CROSS-SECTIONAL STUDY							
India, Chennai Urban Rural Epidemiology Study 57[2]	2042 urban southern Indian adults aged 20 years and above	FFQ with 222 food items	Mean rice intake 253.4 g/d	Quartiles of refined grain intake	ATP III	Q4 vs Q1 of refined grain intake: OR 7.83 (95% CI 4.72–12.99)	The study focused on refined grain intake; however, 75.8% of refined grain was white rice
Korea, Korean Genome and Epidemiology Study (KeGENS)[30]	26,006 adults aged 20 years and above Exclusion: known chronic diseases	FFQ with 103 food items	No absolute rice intake	Four rice eating patterns: white rice, rice with beans, rice with multigrains, and mixed group	ATP III	Men: no difference between rice eating patterns Women: mixed-group vs white rice group: OR 0.87 (95% CI 0.75–0.99) Rice with beans vs white rice: OR 0.89 (95% CI 0.76–1.04) Rice with multigrains vs white rice: OR 0.93 (95% CI 0.84–1.04)	
USA, NHANES (1999–2004)[27]	25,374 children and adults	24-hour recall		Rice eater (at least 14 g/d white or brown rice) vs non-rice eater	ATP III	Subgroups: 19–50 years, OR 0.79 (0.64–0.97) 51 years and above, OR 1.12 (0.91–1.36)	
COHORT STUDY							
China, Jiangsu Nutrition Study (JIN)[28]	1231 adults aged 20 years and above Follow-up: 5 years	FFQ with 33 food groups	Mean rice intake 321 g/d	Rice intake recoded into three levels: 0–200, 201–400, ≥401 g/d Percentage of rice in staple foods (PRS, PRS=rice intake/(rice intake+wheat flour intake)	IDF	No association between rice intake levels or PRS and incident metabolic syndrome	
RANDOMIZED CLINICAL TRIAL							
China,[42]	202 adults (in two groups), 16 weeks intervention		Participants were provided with 225 g/d cooked rice, either white rice (WR) or brown rice (BR), to eat *ad libitum*	Comparing BR and WR	APT III	Substituting BR for WR did not lead to improvements in metabolic risk factors BP decreased in both groups, with no difference between WR and BR The WR group had a significant decrease in total cholesterol but the BR group did not	

barley.[36] GI values of white rice have a large range (from 40 to 100), and depend on where the rice is grown and how it is cooked. White rice is the main contributor to dietary GL in many Asian populations with rice as staple foods. High GI and GL are found to be related to increased risk of hyperglycemia.[36] A high GI or high GL diet is also related to elevation of plasma TG and lowered HDL levels.[43,44] In Japan, both dietary GI and GL are independently correlated with several metabolic risk factors in subjects whose dietary GI and GL were primarily determined on the basis of the GI of white rice.[21] However in an Indian study it has been found that rice has the least potential to raise postprandial blood glucose and TG compared with other carbohydrates, including commercially prepared whole wheat bread.[45]

Overall diet should be considered when considering the adverse effects of specific individual high GI foods. Because rice-based staple food is often accompanied with high intakes of other plant foods, including vegetables, the detrimental effect of a high glycemic index may be balanced by other beneficial factors in the diet. The interaction between rice, GI, and other components of the diet may be different in relation to the risk of different components of MetS.

Rice Protein

The effects of rice protein on body weight and blood lipids have been studied by a research group in China.[46] The researchers administered two types of rice proteins (RP-A and RP-E, extracted by alkaline and α-amylase, respectively), and casein (control group), to Wistar rats fed a cholesterol-enriched diets for 2 weeks.[46] It was found that compared with casein group, the rice protein groups had significantly reduced hepatic activities of fatty acid synthase (37% reduced in RP-A group, 44% reduced in RP-E group), and increased activities of lipoprotein lipase (55% and 69% increase in RP-A and RP-E groups, respectively) and hepatic lipase (53% and 164% increase in RP-A and RP-E groups, respectively). Furthermore, rats fed with rice protein had 17% less body weight gain than those fed with casein.[46] In another animal study, weanling rats were fed AIN-93G diets made with casein or rice protein isolate (RPI) for 2 weeks. Rats fed with RPI had increased expression of hepatic genes regulated by the peroxisome proliferator-activated receptor (PPAR) and decreased fatty acid synthesis. Rats in the RPI group also had improved glucose and cholesterol homeostasis.[47] Rice protein has been shown to prevent hypertension in an animal study.[40]

As already discussed, in a traditional Asian diet, rice provides a substantial amount of protein. The beneficial effect of rice on blood pressure and body weight may be partly explained by this protein in the daily diet.

Energy Density

As mentioned above, cooked rice is high in water, as a result of which the energy density of a rice staple diet is lower than that of a wheat staple diet; high energy-dense diets are related to obesity[48,49] and MetS.[50] The lower energy density of a rice diet theoretically favors weight control and obesity prevention.

Dietary Fiber, Fat, and Cholesterol

Although the fiber content of refined white rice is lower than that of brown rice, the consumption of large amounts of white rice still results in a relatively high intake of dietary fiber. Rice is the major source of fiber in Asian countries. For example, rice contributes 14% of fiber in the Japanese population.[50] The mean intake of 280 g rice per day in Chinese adults can provide 2 g dietary fiber. It is well-established that fiber has beneficial effects on body weight, blood glucose, blood pressure, blood lipids, and MetS.[51] In addition, rice is low in fat and cholesterol, and has a very low sodium content; together, these favor lower blood pressure and lipid levels.

Lifestyle Factors

Many lifestyle factors may contribute to the observed link between rice and health outcomes. In the USA, data from the Continuing Survey of Food Intakes by Individuals (1994–1996) and NAHNES (2001–2002) suggest that rice eaters have higher consumption of vegetables, dietary fiber, and iron, but a lower percentage of energy from fat, than those who do not consume rice.[52] Rice cultivation is usually a laborious process, and high physical activity levels in these countries may also be linked to the low obesity burden.

CONCLUSION

In conclusion, existing studies suggest both advantages and disadvantages of rice intake. Substitution of rice for flour favors weight control. Overall, there seems no consistent association between rice consumption and the risk of MetS. Very few studies have assessed the association between rice intake, body weight, and MetS. Currently, there is only one prospective study assessing the association between rice consumption and the risk of MetS. More prospective studies in this field are warranted. Further research is needed to elucidate the effects of rice in the context of overall dietary patterns on human health.

References

1. Alberti KG, Zimmet P, Shaw J. Group IDFETFC. The metabolic syndrome–a new worldwide definition. *Lancet* 2005;**366**(9491): 1059–62.

2. Grundy SM, Cleeman JI, Daniels SR, Donato KA, Eckel RH, Franklin BA, et al. Diagnosis and management of the metabolic syndrome: an American Heart Association/National Heart, Lung, and Blood Institute Scientific Statement. *Circulation* 2005;**112**(17):2735–52.

3. Expert Panel on Detection E. Treatment of High Blood Cholesterol in A. Executive Summary of The Third Report of The National Cholesterol Education Program (NCEP) Expert Panel on Detection, Evaluation, And Treatment of High Blood Cholesterol In Adults (Adult Treatment Panel III). *JAMA: J Am Med Assoc* 2001;**285**(19):2486–97.

4. Ford ES. Prevalence of the metabolic syndrome defined by the International Diabetes Federation among adults in the U.S. *Diabetes care* 2005;**28**(11):2745–9.

5. Isomaa B, Almgren P, Tuomi T, Forsen B, Lahti K, Nissen M, et al. Cardiovascular morbidity and mortality associated with the metabolic syndrome. *Diabetes Care* 2001;**24**(4):683–9.

6. Lakka HM, Laaksonen DE, Lakka TA, Niskanen LK, Kumpusalo E, Tuomilehto J, et al. The metabolic syndrome and total and cardiovascular disease mortality in middle-aged men. *JAMA* 2002;**288**(21):2709–16.

7. Wang JJ, Li HB, Kinnunen L, Hu G, Jarvinen TM, Miettinen ME, et al. How well does the metabolic syndrome defined by five definitions predict incident diabetes and incident coronary heart disease in a Chinese population? *Atherosclerosis* 2007;**192**(1):161–8.

8. Ford ES. Risks for all-cause mortality, cardiovascular disease, and diabetes associated with the metabolic syndrome: a summary of the evidence. *Diabetes Care* 2005;**28**(7):1769–78.

9. Lorenzo C, Okoloise M, Williams K, Stern MP, Haffner SM. The metabolic syndrome as predictor of type 2 diabetes: the San Antonio heart study. *Diabetes Care* 2003;**26**(11):3153–9.

10. Hu G, Qiao Q, Tuomilehto J, Balkau B, Borch-Johnsen K, Pyorala K. Prevalence of the metabolic syndrome and its relation to all-cause and cardiovascular mortality in nondiabetic European men and women. *Arch Intern Med* 2004;**164**(10):1066–76.

11. Sattar N, Gaw A, Scherbakova O, Ford I, O'Reilly DS, Haffner SM, et al. Metabolic syndrome with and without C-reactive protein as a predictor of coronary heart disease and diabetes in the West of Scotland Coronary Prevention Study. *Circulation* 2003;**108**(4):414–9.

12. Salas-Salvado J, Fernandez-Ballart J, Ros E, Martinez-Gonzalez MA, Fito M, Estruch R, et al. Effect of a Mediterranean diet supplemented with nuts on metabolic syndrome status: one-year results of the PREDIMED randomized trial. *Arch Intern Med* 2008;**168**(22):2449–58.

13. Esposito K, Marfella R, Ciotola M, Di Palo C, Giugliano F, Giugliano G, et al. Effect of a Mediterranean-Style Diet on Endothelial Dysfunction and Markers of Vascular Inflammation in the Metabolic Syndrome: A Randomized Trial. *JAMA* 2004;**292**(12):1440–6.

14. Sahyoun NR, Jacques PF, Zhang XL, Juan W, McKeown NM. Whole-grain intake is inversely associated with the metabolic syndrome and mortality in older adults. *Am J Clin Nutr* 2006;**83**(1):124–31.

15. Esmaillzadeh A, Kimiagar M, Mehrabi Y, Azadbakht L, Hu FB, Willett WC. Dietary patterns, insulin resistance, and prevalence of the metabolic syndrome in women. *Am J Clin Nutr* 2007;**85**(3):910–8.

16. Eshak ES, Iso H, Date C, Yamagishi K, Kikuchi S, Watanabe Y, et al. Rice intake is associated with reduced risk of mortality from cardiovascular disease in Japanese men but not women. *J Nutr* 2011;**141**(4):595–602.

17. Hauner H, Bechthold A, Boeing H, Bronstrup A, Buyken A, Leschik-Bonnet E, et al. Evidence-based guideline of the German Nutrition Society: carbohydrate intake and prevention of nutrition-related diseases. *Ann Nutr Metab* 2012;**60**(Suppl. 1):1–58.

18. Schenker S. An overview of the role of rice in the UK diet. *Nutr Bull* 2012;**37**(4):309–23.

19. FAO. *Rice is life*; 2004. Available at: http://www.fao.org/rice2004/en/f-sheet/factsheet3.pdf. [accessed 22.01.13].

20. Zhai F, Wang H, Du S, He Y, Wang Z, Ge K, et al. Lifespan nutrition and changing socio-economic conditions in China. *Asia Pac J Clin Nutr* 2007;**16**(Suppl. 1):374–82.

21. Murakami K, Sasaki S, Takahashi Y, Okubo H, Hosoi Y, Horiguchi H, et al. Dietary glycemic index and load in relation to metabolic risk factors in Japanese female farmers with traditional dietary habits. *Am J Clin Nutr* 2006;**83**(5):1161–9.

22. Radhika G, Van Dam RM, Sudha V, Ganesan A, Mohan V. Refined grain consumption and the metabolic syndrome in urban Asian Indians (Chennai Urban Rural Epidemiology Study 57). *Metab Clin Exp* 2009;**58**(5):675–81.

23. Wang L. *Report of China Nationwide Nutrition and Health Survey 2002, Summary Report*. Beijing: People's Medical Publishing House; 2005.

24. Yang Y. *Chinese Food Composition Table 2004*. Beijing: Peking University Medical Press; 2005.

25. Astrup A, Meinert Larsen T, Harper A. Atkins and other low-carbohydrate diets: hoax or an effective tool for weight loss? *Lancet* 2004;**364**(9437):897–9.

26. Karl JP, Saltzman E. The role of whole grains in body weight regulation. *Adv Nutr* 2012;**3**(5):697–707.

27. Fulgoni VLI, Fulgoni SA, Upton JL, Moon M. Diet Quality and Markers for Human Health in Rice Eaters Versus Non-Rice Eaters: An Analysis of the US National Health and Nutrition Examination Survey, 1999-2004. *Nutr Today* 2010;**45**(6):262–72. DOI: 10.1097/NT.0b013e3181fd4f29.

28. Shi Z, Taylor AW, Hu G, Gill T, Wittert GA. Rice intake, weight change and risk of the metabolic syndrome development among Chinese adults: the Jiangsu Nutrition Study (JIN). *Asia Pac J Clin Nutr* 2012;**21**(1):35–43.

29. Kim JY, Kim JH, Lee da H, Kim SH, Lee SS. Meal replacement with mixed rice is more effective than white rice in weight control, while improving antioxidant enzyme activity in obese women. *Nutr Res* 2008;**28**(2):66–71.

30. Ahn Y, Park SJ, Kwack HK, Kim MK, Ko KP, Kim SS. Rice-eating pattern and the risk of metabolic syndrome especially waist circumference in Korean Genome and Epidemiology Study (KoGES). *BMC Public Health* 2013;**13**(1):61.

31. Soriguer F, Colomo N, Olveira G, Garcia-Fuentes E, Esteva I, Ruiz de Adana MS, et al. White rice consumption and risk of type 2 diabetes. *Clin Nutr* 2012.

32. Villegas R, Liu S, Gao YT, Yang G, Li H, Zheng W, et al. Prospective study of dietary carbohydrates, glycemic index, glycemic load, and incidence of type 2 diabetes mellitus in middle-aged Chinese women. *Arch Intern Med* 2007;**167**(21):2310–6.

33. Nanri A, Mizoue T, Noda M, Takahashi Y, Kato M, Inoue M, et al. Rice intake and type 2 diabetes in Japanese men and women: the Japan Public Health Center-based Prospective Study. *Am J Clin Nutr* 2010;**92**(6):1468–77.

34. Sun Q, Spiegelman D, van Dam RM, Holmes MD, Malik VS, Willett WC, et al. White rice, brown rice, and risk of type 2 diabetes in US men and women. *Arch Intern Med* 2010;**170**(11):961–9.

35. Hu EA, Pan A, Malik V, Sun Q. White rice consumption and risk of type 2 diabetes: meta-analysis and systematic review. *BMJ* 2012;**344**:e1454.

36. Foster-Powell K, Holt SH, Brand-Miller JC. International table of glycemic index and glycemic load values: 2002. *Am J Clin Nutr* 2002;**76**(1):5–56.

37. Kataoka M, Venn BJ, Williams SM, Te Morenga LA, Heemels IM, Mann JI. Glycaemic responses to glucose and rice in people of Chinese and European ethnicity. *Diabet Med* 2012.

38. Song Y, Joung H. A traditional Korean dietary pattern and metabolic syndrome abnormalities. *Nutr Metab Cardiovasc Dis* 2012;**22**(5):456–62.

39. Kondo I, Funahashi K, Nakamura M, Ojima T, Yoshita K, Nakamura Y. Association between food group intake and serum total cholesterol in the Japanese population: NIPPON DATA 80/90. *J Epidemiol* 2010;**20**(Suppl. 3):S576–81.

40. Li GH, Qu MR, Wan JZ, You JM. Antihypertensive effect of rice protein hydrolysate with in vitro angiotensin I-converting enzyme inhibitory activity in spontaneously hypertensive rats. *Asia Pac J Clin Nutr* 2007;**16**(Suppl.):275–80.

41. Skyler JS. Walter Kempner: A Biographical Note. *Arch Intern Med* 1974;**133**(5):752–5.

42. Zhang G, Pan A, Zong G, Yu Z, Wu H, Chen X, et al. Substituting white rice with brown rice for 16 weeks does not substantially affect metabolic risk factors in middle-aged Chinese men and women with diabetes or a high risk for diabetes. *J Nutr* 2011;**141**(9):1685–90.

43. Frost G, Leeds AA, Dore CJ, Madeiros S, Brading S, Dornhorst A. Glycaemic index as a determinant of serum HDL-cholesterol concentration. *Lancet* 1999;**353**(9158):1045–8.

44. Liu S, Manson JE, Stampfer MJ, Holmes MD, Hu FB, Hankinson SE, et al. Dietary glycemic load assessed by food-frequency questionnaire in relation to plasma high-density-lipoprotein cholesterol and fasting plasma triacylglycerols in postmenopausal women. *Am J Clin Nutr* 2001;**73**(3):560–6.

45. Ezenwaka CE, Kalloo R. Carbohydrate-induced hypertriglyceridaemia among West Indian diabetic and non-diabetic subjects after ingestion of three local carbohydrate foods. *Indian J Med Res* 2005;**121**(1):23–31.

46. Yang L, Chen JH, Lv J, Wu Q, Xu T, Zhang H, et al. Rice protein improves adiposity, body weight and reduces lipids level in rats through modification of triglyceride metabolism. *Lipids Health Dis* 2012;**11**:24.

47. Ronis MJ, Badeaux J, Chen Y, Badger TM. Rice protein isolate improves lipid and glucose homeostasis in rats fed high fat/high cholesterol diets. *Exp Biol Med* 2010;**235**(9):1102–13.

48. Prentice AM, Jebb SA. Fast foods, energy density and obesity: a possible mechanistic link. *Obes Rev* 2003;**4**(4):187–94.

49. Savage JS, Marini M, Birch LL. Dietary energy density predicts women's weight change over 6 y. *Am J Clin Nutr* 2008;**88**(3):677–84.

50. Eshak ES, Iso H, Date C, Kikuchi S, Watanabe Y, Wada Y, et al. Dietary fiber intake is associated with reduced risk of mortality from cardiovascular disease among Japanese men and women. *J Nutr* 2010;**140**(8):1445–53.

51. Papathanasopoulos A, Camilleri M. Dietary fiber supplements: effects in obesity and metabolic syndrome and relationship to gastrointestinal functions. *Gastroenterology* 2010;**138**(1):65–72 e1–2.

52. Batres-Marquez SP, Jensen HH, Upton J. Rice consumption in the United States: recent evidence from food consumption surveys. *J Am Diet Assoc* 2009;**109**(10):1719–27.

Glycemic Index of Indian Cereal Staple Foods and their Relationship to Diabetes and Metabolic Syndrome

Ruchi Vaidya, Viswanathan Mohan, Mookambika Ramya Bai, Sudha Vasudevan

Madras Diabetes Research Foundation, Dr Mohan's Diabetes Specialties Centre, WHO Collaborating Centre for Non-Communicable Diseases, and International Diabetes Federation (IDF) Centre of Education, Gopalapuram, Chennai, India

INTRODUCTION

India is a land of diversity, not only in culture and geography but also in foods. The two most important cultures that have influenced Indian cuisine and food habits are the Hindu and Muslim religious traditions. Rice has been domesticated in Northern peninsular India since 5000 BC, subsequently spreading to the Indus Valley Civilization (2300–1900 BC) in the Gangetic plain, and later to Southern India (2000–1400 BC). However, wheat and barley were domesticated in both northern and southern regions.[1,2] Cereal staples such as rice and wheat continue to provide the principle source of energy for most of the Indian population.[3]

In earlier days, less refined cereal-based traditional diets were nutrient-dense and high in fiber; however, modern diets have, due to processing and milling technologies, made cereals more refined and energy-dense. A recent national survey in India conducted by the National Sample Survey Organization (NSSO) has reported that there has been a decline in percentage of expenditure on cereal since 1987.[4] Despite the decline, currently cereal staples provide two-thirds of the daily carbohydrates and almost half of the daily calories in Indian diets.[5] Higher intakes of refined cereals probably contribute to India's growing diabetes epidemic. According to a recent national study, currently there are 62.4 million people with diabetes and 77.2 million people with pre-diabetes in India.[6] Diabetes mellitus is mainly characterized by rise in blood glucose level, which can depend on the quality (the glycemic index or GI) and the quantity of ingested carbohydrate. The combination of these two factors is termed the glycemic load (GL), and reflects the total glycemic impact of ingested carbohydrate-rich foods. Indeed, GI has proven to be a more useful nutritional concept than the chemical classifications of carbohydrates, as there is a correlation between physiological effects of carbohydrate-rich foods and diseases like diabetes or cardiovascular disease (CVD). A recent epidemiological study had shown the positive association of high GI and GL foods, like refined grains, with the risk of type 2 diabetes.[7] It is possible that, along with decreased physical activity, diets with higher GI and GL are contributing to India's growing diabetes epidemic.[8] Many Western studies have shown the protective effect of whole grains against chronic diseases such as diabetes and cardiovascular disease.[9]

Additionally, the GI of foods also plays a role in weight management, in sports nutrition, and in the prevalence of childhood obesity. However, the glycemic responses vary for different foods containing the same amount and even type of carbohydrate, depending on processing technologies and food characteristics, such as structure, ripeness (e.g., in fruits), the amylose:amylopectin ratio, the food composition, and cooking methods.[10] Today, there are many food ingredients that can be included in the formulation of foods to lower their GI. Many of these ingredients are natural products of cereals, while others are modified carbohydrates.[11]

The first international GI table was developed by Foster *et al.* in 1995, with values for 565 foods; this was further expanded in 2002.[12,13] In 2008, Atkinson compiled an international table for GI and GL for 2480 individual food items. Although both these tables do provide data on over 100 Indian foods, the GI methodologies used at that time were before the evolution of the standardized GI protocols in 1998.[14,15] Hence, it is important to develop a new database on the GI of Indian foods using the current international GI protocol.

INDIAN CEREAL STAPLE FOODS

History

The agricultural era began about 10,000 BC, when excessive hunting of animal foods led to the decline of meat and emergence of vegetable foods as the staple diet.[16] Food is considered to be a staple when consumed by a community or society daily, and is also that food from which people obtain the major proportion of their daily caloric and nutrient requirements.[1] Biogeographical evidence suggests that peninsular India housed several diverse crop cultivars, including rice, wheat, barley, sorghum, and at least 10 different species of different millets. This clearly reflects the diversity of agricultural and culinary practices in India in ancient times.[17]

Production and Consumption of Cereals and Millets

Cereal and millet production in India is shown in Figure 25.1. Rice production increased 2.5-fold between the 1960s and second decade of this millenium, and India is now the second largest rice producer in the world. Wheat production increased 5.5-fold over the same period (i.e., from 133 to 734 million tonnes).

However, post-Green Revolution, millet consumption has decreased tremendously.[18]

The National Nutrition Monitoring Bureau (NNMB) has recorded the decline in cereal intake from 383 to 344 g/CU per day between 2000 and 2006. Similarly, during the same period the consumption of millet reduced by >50% (from 105 to 52 g/CU per day).[19] In addition, the NSSO noted that the percentage contribution of calories from cereals also decreased between 2005 and 2010 among both rural and urban populations (from 67.5% to 60.4%, and 56.1% to 50.4%, respectively).[20] A recent epidemiological survey among Chennai (a metro city) adults indicated that white rice consumption (median intake of 253 g/d) contributes about 50% of the total calories, similar to other major rice-eating Asian populations (Chinese and Japanese).[7,21,22]

India has the second largest wheat consumption, next to China, and consumption is mostly in the form of homemade chapattis (unleavened flat bread), using custom-milled *atta* (whole wheat flour), and refined wheat flour used for the preparation of various wheat-based bakery products such as bread, biscuits, and processed foods.[23] Though India is the greatest consumer of millet in the world, average millet consumption is lower than that of other cereals.[24]

NUTRITIONAL COMPOSITION OF CEREAL STAPLE FOODS

Nutritional Composition of Cereals and Millets

The macronutrient composition of rice, wheat, and millets is given in Figure 25.2. Rice has good quality protein compared to other cereals,[25] and is rich in

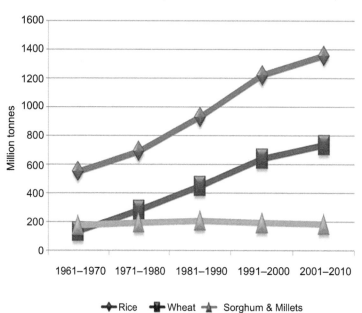

FIGURE 25.1 Production of rice, wheat, sorghum and millets. *Source: Adapted from FAOSTAT 2013.[18]*

branched-chain amino acids such as leucine, isoleucine, and valine. Moreover, rice fat is rich in essential n-6 fatty acids.[26] Rice bran layers consist of non-starchy polysaccharides (cellulose and lignin), fat, and dietary fiber. The aleurone layer and germ contains protein, fat, and good amount of vitamins and minerals.[25] Hence, on polishing there is a decrease in the protein, fat, and dietary fiber content, and a proportionate increase in the available carbohydrate content is more obvious as polishing removes the bran, including the aleurone and germ portions of rice kernel, leaving behind the starchy endosperm.[27]

Wheat is also a good source of trace minerals such as selenium and magnesium – nutrients essential to good health.[28,29] However, when wheat is milled as refined flour, 75% of the dietary fiber is lost (Fig. 25.2B). Millets are far superior to either rice or wheat in terms of nutritive content, and are a rich source of minerals like iron, magnesium, phosphorus, potassium, and dietary fiber.[30] Finger millet (Ragi) has the highest calcium content among all the food grains. The protein content of millet is comparable to that of wheat and maize. The bran layers of millets are good sources of B-complex vitamins.[30]

Traditional hand-pounded rice is known for its nutritional superiority, as less bran is lost during hand pounding and winnowing, compared with polished white rice,

where almost all of the bran is lost. Today, in India, polished white rice and its flour-based preparations are used exclusively. Similarly, wheat in the traditional diet was in the form of coarse flour and grits, but today wheat is used as a refined flour (white flour), refined semolina, and finely pulverized whole wheat flour, all of which could impact carbohydrate quality (GI) and metabolic health.

Glycemic Index and Glycemic Load

The glycemic index (GI), the concept of measuring the glycemic impact of foods primarily from carbohydrates and first developed in 1981 by Jenkins, became popular in the 1990s. However, the GI concept continues to be a controversial subject. GI is a dynamic parameter that reflects the influence of foods in raising blood glucose and the glucose clearance rate.[31] It compares the postprandial glycemic response of 50 g available carbohydrates (measured by capillary blood glucose at intervals of 15 minutes for the first hour, followed by half-hourly for the second hour) of the test food with the standard food (glucose set to a GI scale of 100). The GI is calculated as the incremental area under the curve (IAUC) for the ingested test food over a period of 2 hours expressed as a percentage of the reference standard food area under

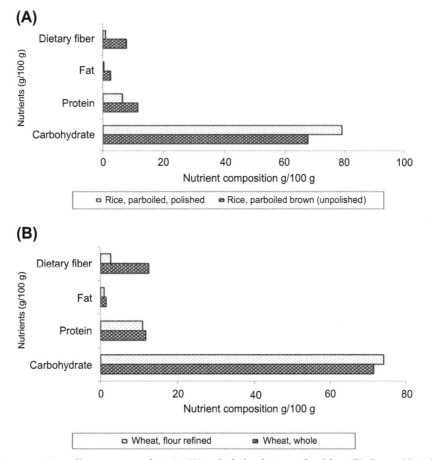

FIGURE 25.2 Proximate composition of brown rice vs white rice (A) and whole wheat vs refined flour (B). *Source: Adapted from Gopalan et al. 2010.[26]*

TABLE 25.1 Description of Indian Foods Planned in Table 25.2

Food Items	Description
HIGH GI MENU ITEMS	
Idly-white rice	It is a white spongy cake made by steaming the fermented batter of rice and black gram dhal in the proportion of 2:1
Chutney onion	Chutneys are ground paste onion and seasoning with mustard seeds is optional
Coffee with milk & sugar	Coffee prepared with 3% fat milk, and sugar and instant coffee powder
Samosa	Dough made from refined wheat flour is folded into triangular shape and stuffed with cooked mixture of potato, peas, carrot, onion and spices and deep fried in oil
White rice	Non parboiled common Indian rice variety *Bapatla* cooked in pressure cooker in the ratio of 1: 2.5
Sambhar	Made out of red gram dhal, tomatoes, onion, vegetables cooked in tamarind pulp along with spices
Potato/dum aloo/shallow fry	Boiled potatoes mixed with turmeric and chilli powder and shallow fried in frying pan ('*kadai*') with oil
Oothapam-white rice	The preparation is similar to dosa but it is cooked as thick pan cake in tava
Kurma vegetable	Vegetables like carrot, peas, potato etc are cooked with spices and coconut paste to thick consistency usually served as accompaniment for rice/chapathi/parotta
LOW GI MENU ITEMS	
Idly brown rice-vegetables	It is a white spongy cake made by steaming the fermented batter of brown rice and black gram dhal in the proportion of 2:1
Onion Sambhar	As mentioned in the high GI menu
Coffee with milk & sugar	As mentioned in the high GI menu
Butter milk	Prepared from whipped curd diluted with water and salt. Asafoetida, curry leaves are optional
White Peas sundal	Dried white peas (bean) soaked for few hours and cooked in pressure cooker and seasoned with Indian spices
Brown rice	Parboiled common Indian brown rice variety *Bapatla* cooked in pressure cooker in the ratio of 1: 2.5
Sambhar	As mentioned in the high GI menu
Dhal-fry	It is made by cooking green gram dhal/red gram dhal/masoor dhal with tomatoes. Ghee is usually used for seasoning with cumin seeds and garnished with coriander leaves and served along with chapathi/ phulka/plain rice
Coffee with milk & sugar	As mentioned in the high GI menu
Masala vadai	It is prepared with coarsely/finely ground paste of split bengal gram and mixed with onion, coriander leaves,ginger and hand pressed into circular shape and then deep fried in oil.
Dosa-brown rice	It is made from fermented batter of parboiled brown rice and split black gram (4:1), and cooked in shallow pan ('*tava*') with oil
Mint chutney	Chutneys are ground paste made greens (mint); seasoning with mustard seeds is optional

Source: Developed from EpiNu database.[50]

the curve for the same duration. Hence, the GI depends on the food characteristics rather than the characteristics of the individual who consumes the food.[32] Capillary blood glucose is recommended because of the ease in obtaining it; also, the capillary rise is higher than the venous rise, and hence the differences between foods are larger and it is easier to detect the significance of GI values.[15] Unfortunately, most of the foods were tested by means of venous samples (Table 25.1).

A study on GI of the same foods tested in India and UK using identical methods showed that the glycemic response to the foods (sweet biscuit, sweet meal biscuit, malted whole wheat cereal, malted wheat cereal, and cereal biscuit) was higher in Asian Indians than in their UK counterparts, despite there being no difference in the GI values of the same foods.[33] Glycemic responses could be ethnic-specific due to the inherent biological variations.[34] In addition to GI, a newer concept, the food insulin index (FII), has also been studied. The basis for the FII is that diets/foods that stimulate less insulin secretion may potentially aid in the prevention and management of diabetes. Foods ranked based

TABLE 25.2 Sample High and Low GI Indian Diet Menu

Meal	High GI Diet				Low GI Diet			
	Menu	Portion Size	GI	GL	Menu	Portion Size	GI	GL
Break Fast	Idly-white rice	50 g	86	12	Idly brown rice-vegetables	50 g	68	4
	Chutney onion	25 g	43	1	Onion Sambar	150 g	24	2
	Coffee with milk & sugar	150 ml	60	8	Coffee with milk & sugar	150 ml	60	8
Mid Morning	Biscuits salt	5 g	85	3	Butter milk	150 ml	36	3
	Coffee with milk & sugar	150 ml	60	8	White Peas sundal	100 g	35	3
Lunch	White rice	250 g	83	54	Brown rice	280 g	59	33
	Sambar	150 ml	24	4	Sambar	150 ml	24	4
	Potato fry	150 g	73	20	Dhal-fry	150 g	24	3
Evening	Coffee with milk & sugar	150 ml	60	8	Coffee with milk & sugar	150 ml	60	8
	Samosa	100 g	83	41	Masala vadai	30 g	10	1
Dinner	Oothapam-white rice	79 g	83	18	Dosa-brown rice	30 g	62	6
	Kurma vegetable	150 g	58	4	Mint chutney	25 g	27	0
Bed Time	Water melon	150 g	76	4	Apple	120 g	36	5
Average			73	184	Average		44	81

Source: Developed from EpiNu database.[50]

on FII could be more precise than carbohydrate counting in adjusting the insulin dosage for type 1 diabetics, since evidence has shown that mixed meals with similar carbohydrate content produce varied insulin response.[35] Sample high and low GI Indian menu plans are shown in Table 25.2.

The glycemic load (GL) estimates the total glycemic impact of the food's carbohydrate on postprandial blood glucose. Thus, GL is calculated as GI% × amount of available carbohydrates provided by the portion of the food eaten.[15] GL foods/meals/diets can be altered either by decreasing the total carbohydrates or by lowering the GI. This indicates the practical challenges each country has in dealing with cultural diets. Perhaps this could be the reason that high GL diets show different physiological effects across countries. For example, we showed that those within the highest quartile of GL had 4-fold increased risk for type 2 diabetes as compared to those within the lowest quartile of GL (OR = 4.25; 2.33–7.7 CI).[7] The variations in GL of Indian diets mainly come from the change in quantity of carbohydrates between those with the lowest and highest quartiles of intake (294 g/d vs 587 g/d, respectively), while GI between these quartiles is less varied (65 vs 71, respectively) due to the unavailability of low GI foods, and hence not reported by this population.[7] It was observed in the US that high-carbohydrate diets were also high in GI, whereas in Scandinavian countries many low GI staples were included in high-carbohydrate diets.[36,37]

Glycemic Index of Indian Foods

Despite increasing evidence of the benefits of low GI foods for many populations, the concept of GI is still not widely accepted. Though the usefulness of the GI is questioned in many developed nations, it appears to be a useful concept in countries such as India, where carbohydrate consumption is high.[5,26] Moreover, low GI foods come with added benefits such as higher fiber and phytonutrient content that are beneficial to overall health. Indeed, there is no scientific evidence to show any deleterious effects of low GI diets. Thus, creating a GI database for Indian foods tested in India will be a valuable resource for dieticians to plan menus and food exchanges effectively, and for food scientists to consider low GI ingredients in food formulation. The recently published international GI table has given values for more than 50 staple cereal-based Indian foods which cannot be considered for application for the various reasons given in Table 25.3.[14,38–49]

GLYCEMIC INDEX AND METABOLIC HEALTH

Blood glucose concentration is tightly regulated by homeostatic regulatory systems in humans. Observational studies indicate that the GI of the diet may have a major influence on glucose homeostasis and metabolic regulations. The major sources of carbohydrate in the

TABLE 25.3   Glycemic Index of Asian Indian Staple Foods as Given in the International GI Table (2008)

Food Items	Authors	GI (Glucose = 100) Normal	Type 2 diabetes	Limitations
RICE AND RICE BASED FOOD ITEMS				
Idiappam, Appam, Puttu, Idli, Pongal, Dosai, Brown Rice boiled, White Rice, Parboiled rice, porridge, Dhokla	Vijayan 1997[38], Urooj 2000[39], Kurup 1992[40], Chaturvedi 1997[41], Kanan W 1998[42], Kavita MS 1997[43], Shobana 2007[44], Pathak P 2000[45]	35–76	31–90	• Half or one hour intravenous samples considered for 2 or 3 hours
Wheat and Wheat Based Food Items				• Portions of test food and reference food provide 75 g of available carbohydrate which was not measured directly as recommended in the new GI protocol.
Wheat Porridge, Chapatti and with different , combinations, Poori , Wheat, Semolina cooked in different forms	Shobana S 2007[44], Chaturvedi 1997[41] Sumathi A 1997[46], Urooj 2000[39], Dilawari JB 1981[47], Kavita MS 1997[43], Mani UV 1992[48]	39–66	46–90	
Other Cereal Based Products				
Upittu , Barley, Chapatti, barley, Maize flour made into chapatti, Varagu, Bajra flour chappati	Urooj 2000[39], Shukla K 1991[49] Mani UV 1993[50]	48–69	37–67	• Handheld Glucometers were used which are not recommended
Millets and Millet Based Products				
Millet/Ragi, Millet/ Ragi flour, Porridge, made from finger millet, and pulses, Jowar, roasted bread, Laddu ; Uppuma kedgeree	Kavita MS 1997 [43], Mani UV 1993[50] Shobana S 2007[44], Pathak P et al 2000[45]	18–77	19–104	

Source: Adapted from Atkinson et al 2008.[14]

diet in India are refined cereals, which have high GI values and have been linked to the widespread occurrence of type 2 diabetes and CVD.[50]

Mechanisms of Action of High GI Foods

Rapid glucose absorption after consuming a high GI meal challenges body homeostasis and disrupts the transition from the postprandial to the post-absorptive phase. Following a high GI meal, during the postprandial phase there is relative hyperglycemia along with increased concentrations of gut hormones such as glucagon-like peptide-1 (GLP-1) and glucose-dependent insulinotropic polypeptide (GIP), which stimulates insulin release from pancreatic beta cells and inhibits glucagon release from pancreatic alpha cells. The resulting high insulin:glucagon ratio aggravates the normal response to eating, including uptake of nutrients by insulin-responsive tissues; stimulation of glycogenesis; lipogenesis; suppression of glycogenolysis; and lipolysis. Beyond 2 hours into the postprandial phase, nutrient absorption in the intestine decreases but the effects of the high insulin:glucagon ratio persist and there is often a drop to the hypoglycemic range. This rapid fall in metabolic fuels results in increased hunger, and increased food intake can lead to obesity.[51–53]

Within 4–6 hours of a high GL meal the decreased concentrations of glucose and free fatty acids trigger certain counter-regulatory hormones, such as glucagon, which restores euglycemia through stimulation of glycogenolysis, gluconeogenesis, and lipolysis, and elevates free fatty acids (FFA) concentrations to higher levels than those observed after a low GI meal. The combined increase in counter-regulatory hormones and FFA resembles the overnight fasting state.[54,55]

Mechanism of Action of Low GI Foods

Ingestion of a low GI meal leads to slow release of glucose and prevents hypoglycemia; elevated hormones and FFA levels do not occur for a 6-hour period due to continued absorption of nutrients from the intestine, paralleled by increasing hepatic glucose output. Low GI foods are associated with increased amounts of carbohydrate escaping digestion in the small intestine (dietary fibers, indigestible oligosaccharides, and resistant starch [RS]) and hence lead to increased colonic fermentation. The short-chain fatty acids (SCFAs) produced during colonic fermentation have local and systematic effects that could contribute to the mechanism for beneficial effects of low GI foods in diabetes, cardiovascular disease, and cancer.[56] Hence, diets containing identical energy and nutrients, but varying in their GI, can elicit markedly different physiological responses.[57]

GI and Chronic Diseases

Non-communicable disorders (NCDs) such as obesity, cardiovascular disease (CVD), diabetes, and its

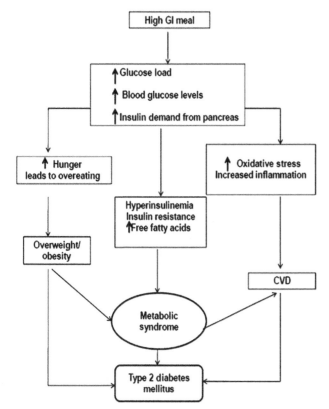

FIGURE 25.3 Physiological effects of high GI foods and link to diabetes. *Source: Adapted from Ludwig DS. The glycemic index: Physiological mechanisms relating to obesity, diabetes and cardiovascular disease. JAMA 2002;287(18):2414–23.*[54]

complications are responsible for over 55% of deaths in India. It is unfortunate that these chronic diseases afflict Indians at a younger productive age, leading to human capital wastage for a growing Indian economy.[58] Evidence has shown that GI has strong relevance to chronic diseases and their associated metabolic regulations (Fig. 25.3).

GI and Diabetes

The links between GI/GL diets and diabetes are related to glucose and insulin responses. High GI diets lead to elevated blood glucose and insulin levels. Hyperinsulinemia further increases β-cell dysfunction and results in insulin resistance, which is a risk factor for type 2 diabetes.[59] On other hand, a low GI diet tends to delay glucose absorption, thereby reducing the peak insulin concentrations and overall insulin demand. Available scientific evidence largely supports that low GI/GL diets, through their effect on postprandial glycemia and glycated proteins, may help in the prevention and treatment of diabetes.[60] A review of randomized control trials, lasting from 4 weeks to 12 months, in diabetic subjects showed that low GI diets compared to high GI diets lowered protein markers of glycemic control measured as HbA1c decreased by 0.5% (95% CI −0.8 to −0.2; $P < 0.001$). This 0.5% reduction is clinically significant, as it corresponds

to a lower dosage of medications for newly diagnosed patients; moreover, the UK Prospective Diabetes Study (UKPDS) suggests that a 1% reduction in mean HbA1c levels corresponds to a 21% reduction in risk for deaths related to diabetes and its complications.[61,62]

Recent GI testing of three popular Indian rice varieties, namely "Sona Masuri," "Ponni" and "Surti Kolam," showed them all to be high GI food choices, because these rice varieties are highly polished (refined grains).[63] A recent epidemiological study among urban adults has shown that higher refined grain consumption is associated with dyslipidemia (low HDL and high TG), metabolic syndrome, and increased risk for type 2 diabetes.[64]

GI and Obesity

A high GI diet results in high insulin and low glucagon levels, inducing glucose storage, inhibiting lipolysis, and consequently reducing glucose availability for metabolic oxidation. This stage could be seen as a fasting state, and triggers glucagon release and hunger signals.[56] Low GI foods, however, tend to maintain glucose and insulin at moderate levels, avoiding the hypoglycemic state. Low GI meals have also shown inverse association with cholecystokinin (CCK) response and satiety.[65] Intervention studies have shown improved fat loss/weight loss with low GI diets compare to high GI diets, the diets having similar nutrient contents.[66] Our study has also shown positive association of GL and refined grains with BMI and waist circumference (WC) among Asian Indians, who have genetic vulnerability to insulin resistance and diabetes.[7,64]

FACTORS INFLUENCING GI OF STAPLE FOODS

The glycemic response of food depends on the rate of gastric emptying, digestion, and absorption of carbohydrates from the small intestine, and in addition on the effects of other food factors in potentiating non-glucose mediated insulin secretion. Various chemical and physical phenomena contribute to differences in carbohydrate digestion and therefore the blood glucose response. A range of food factors have been identified as important determinants of the glycemic response to carbohydrate foods; these are given in Table 25.4.[67]

Particle Size

Particle size affects the digestibility of starch: the larger the particle size, the lower the digestibility of starch. The fibrous coating around cereals and millets serves as a physical barrier delaying the action of enzymes on starch.[67] Further milling, beating, shearing, and refining of foods affects cell and granule integrity. These processes

TABLE 25.4 Factors Contributing to Low and High GI of Foods

Factors/Food Variables	Low GI	High GI
Particle size	Larger particle size, entrapped starch molecules, delays action of digestive enzymes	Small particle size, poor granule integrity, activates action of digestive enzymes
Cell structure/cell wall integrity	Raw foods	Ripe foods
Starch structure	Granular structure, high crystallinity and recrystallinity	Gelatinization
Amylose: Amylopectin ratio	High amylose:amylopectin ratio	Low amylose:amylopectin ratio
Cooking methods	Less exposure to gelatinization	More exposure to gelatinization, grinding, milling
Protein	Increases insulin secretion and lowers GI	–
Fat	Delays gastric emptying and lowers GI	–
Fructose: glucose ratio	High fructose:glucose ratio	Low fructose:glucose ratio
Dietary fibers	Slow gastric emptying and digestion lowers GI	–
Water and carbohydrate in liquid form	–	Higher quantity accelerates gastric emptying and increases GI
Organic acids	Delays gastric emptying and lowers GI	–
Amylase inhibitors	Restricts digestion and lowers GI	–
Chewing	Less chewing	Extended chewing

Source: Adapted from Nord.[55]

decrease particle size and promote absorption of water and breakdown by enzymes.[68] A study comparing four types of wheat – whole grain, cracked grain, coarse and fine whole meal flour – in 10 healthy subjects resulted in glucose responses to whole grain of approximately one-third the response to fine flour. Insulin responses were similar.[69] Studies were carried out to compare breads made of different particle sizes. Consumption of standard white bread and ultrafine ground whole wheat flour breads by middle-aged men and women resulted in lower glycemic indices compared to glucose, but

glycemic indices of whole wheat breads, although lower than white bread, were not different.[70,71]

The only whole grain food with a high GI is rice – specifically, low amylose rice. Rice starch is very easily gelatinized during cooking, and is easily acted upon by digestive enzymes. Along with particle size, the degree of mastication varies significantly between individuals and may be a cause for the considerable interindividual variation observed in the glycemic response (GR) to a single food.[72] A study carried out on factors affecting the GI of barley showed that the GI decreased more significantly in whole grain barley pasta (26 ± 4) than in white pearled barley pasta (35 ± 3); the study also stated that the GI of barley is not predicted by its content of amylose or other starch characteristics.[73]

Processing Conditions

Processing of foods can either increase or decrease the GI of different foods. The nature of starch is influenced by various processing conditions. The gross structure of starch molecules is influenced by grinding, milling, or heat treatment. A study to determine the GI of different varieties of milled and brown rice showed that the Sinandomeng variety, with low dietary fiber, had a GI=75, while its brown rice had a GI=55. Brown rice (IR64) with 23% available carbohydrates and dietary fibers of 2.5g/100g had a low GI=51.[74] Cell wall integrity and cellular structure change with the ripening process, and GI in turn increases with ripening. Green bananas have a high content of RS, and only a negligible amount remains after ripening.[75] The maintenance of high starch crystallinity plays an important role in the low GI of the food. In most ready-to-eat food items the starch crystallinity is greatly reduced during commonly applied food processing conditions, resulting in more or less complete gelatinization. However, pasta is unique in this regard. Pasta has a low GI because of the physical entrapment of ungelatinized starch granules in a sponge-like network of protein (glutein) molecules in pasta dough.[76] A comparative study on the consumption of pasta and bread in 10 type 2 diabetic subjects showed a lower rise in postprandial glucose on consumption of pasta than in bread.[77]

Starch can be indigestible due to its botanical structure (amylose:amylopectin ratio) or become resistant during processing due to retrogradation; this is known as resistant starch (RS). RS formation or digestibility of starch is affected by various processing conditions, and the nature of the starch. When heat and moisture are applied simultaneously (as in normal cooking procedures like boiling, steaming, etc.) to amylopectin-rich starch, it loses its granular definition and gelatinization takes place; this increases the GI of the food. On the other hand, high amylose starch resists gelatinization during most normal food processing methods, like baking and roasting, due to its granular structure; it also contributes to RS formation in the food.[78] Processing conditions like roasting, baking, boiling, and shallow frying have shown high RS formation in commonly consumed cereal and cereal-based products in India, whereas cooking conditions such as steaming and frying showed low RS. When analyzed, the puffed, flaked, and extruded cereal products obtained from the market also showed considerably less retention of RS content.[79]

Dietary Factors

Carbohydrates

Traditionally, carbohydrates have been classified as simple and complex based on the degree of polymerization, and this classification was assumed to reflect their quality. Thus, simple carbohydrates such as simple sugars (mono- and disaccharides) were thought to increase the blood glucose quickly compared to complex carbohydrates such as starchy foods (containing polysaccharides). Further studies on the physiological effects of carbohydrates and fibers, however, showed that not all complex carbohydrates raise blood glucose slowly.[80] Therefore, the quality of carbohydrates is classified based on their glycemic nature. Food composition tables unfortunately do not mention the glycemic nature of carbohydrate foods, such as particle size and nature of the starch.

Available carbohydrates are the carbohydrates that are absorbed in the small intestine and metabolized in the body via pathways which can, at least potentially, yield glucose.[56] Available carbohydrates may influence blood glucose by four major mechanisms: (1) the nature of the monosaccharides absorbed; (2) the quantity carbohydrates absorbed and metabolized; (3) the amount of carbohydrates consumed; and (4) the rate of absorption.

The majority of available carbohydrates are absorbed in the form of glucose (70–85%), while the remainder are a mixture of fructose and galactose. Glucose has a high GI (GI = 100), fructose has a low GI (GI = 23), and sucrose (a combination of glucose and fructose) has a GI = 65.[14] Fructose does not raise blood glucose appreciably because it is converted to glucose in the liver and only a small portion of this glucose is released to circulation.[81] Fructose absorption is also poorly understood, but it is passively absorbed in the intestine through GLUT5 and GLUT 2 transporters.[82] Hence the glycemic indexes of fruit juices are generally lower. Lactose present in milk has a lower GI than sucrose, maybe because the galactose in it elicits a lower glycemic response.[83,84] Polyols or sugar alcohols are naturally present in fruits, but are commercially produced by hydrogenation; those commonly consumed are sorbitol, mannitol, xylitol, lacitol, etc. Polyols elicit a small to moderate rise in plasma glucose in both normals and diabetics compared to glucose.[85]

Certain carbohydrates are not digested or absorbed in the human intestine, and are termed "unavailable carbohydrates." Carbohydrates can be unavailable because humans lack the enzymes necessary to hydrolyze them into their component monosaccharides – for example, fructooligosaccharides, non-starch polysaccharides (NSP), and resistant starch (RS). Monosaccharides, such as sorbitol and xylose, may be unavailable because they are incompletely transported into the intestinal cells and bloodstream. The term RS is defined as the fraction of dietary starch that escapes digestion in the small intestine,[86] and is of five types, namely RS1 (physically confined and mainly found in whole and fractionally milled grains, seed, and legumes); RS2 (resistant ungelatinized granules with type B crystallinity that is gradually hydrolyzed by α-amylase; food sources include raw potatoes, green bananas, and a few legumes and high amylase corn); RS3 (retrograded starch found in potatoes that are cooked and cooled, bread, cornflakes, and food products that have undergone repeated moist heat treatment); RS4 (starches that are chemically modified as a result of cross-linking chemical agents and are present in breads, cakes etc.); and RS5 (an amylase lipid complexed starch as a result of extended retrogradation, with reduced enzyme susceptibilities to pancreatic α-amylase and amyloglucosidase found in fried foods).[87,88]

The glycemic response is also affected by the rate of carbohydrate absorption, which can be reduced by the addition of viscous fibers, correlation between rates of digestion of starches *in vitro*, use of digestive enzyme inhibitors, the euglycemic hyperinsulinemic clamp, and oral carbohydrate loading.

Protein

Protein is an insulinotrophic substance that stimulates or affects the production of insulin when consumed along with a diet rich in carbohydrate.[89] This synergism was reported in type 2 DM adults where 50 g glucose with 50 g protein was found to increase the insulin secretion and reduce the plasma glucose level.[90] However, this effect varies with different types of amino acids and protein. Branched-chain amino acids that are found in animal protein (e.g., whey protein hydrolyzate) show an increased insulinemic response and glucose uptake. In diabetic adults, this type of response prevents lipolysis and excessive release of FFA, thereby reducing the risk for CVD.[91] Similarly, diets rich in leucine, tyrosine (non-essential amino acid), and phenylalanine (essential amino acid) increase the insulin responses when ingested along with carbohydrates.[89] In a randomized control study, protein in the form of soya protein concentrate was shown to increase the effect of maintaining glucose homeostasis three-fold compared with fat consumed in the form of corn oil, and this effect of protein was associated with high waist circumference and high dietary fiber intake.[92] It is known from evidence that food proteins also affect glucose metabolism due to their varied nutrient composition.[93–97] Milk contains 80% casein, which is insulinogenic, and 20% whey, which acts as an insulin secretagogue, although the factors that are responsible for this effect (such as rapid release of amino acids, release of bioactive peptide, and glucose-dependent insulinotropic polypeptide [GIP] secretion) are yet to be studied.[98] However, in the urban component of the Chennai Urban Rural Epidemiological Study (CURES) it was observed that intake of dairy products was inversely associated with the risk of type 2 diabetes among Asian Indians.[7] This finding needs further research to identify the mechanisms and factors related to milk composition.

Apart from the quality and quantity of protein, the rate of digestion also impacts the glycemic response. Proteins that are slowly absorbed do not show a rise in plasma amino acids, and thus do not stimulate the production of insulin. In 1990, Nuttall and Gannon proposed a study of this effect by supplementing the normal subjects with 50 g of egg white protein and cottage cheese protein, where the former reduced the insulin response and the latter increased the insulin response. On the other hand, the conversion of protein to urea was found to be lowered by 50% in subjects who consumed egg white protein compared to the cottage cheese protein.[99] On the contrary, protein also increases the plasma glucose concentration by stimulating glucagon secretion. A reduced percentage of energy from protein (12% to 0%) reduces the insulin requirement by 25% in type 1 DM, reduces hepatic glucose output and fasting insulin by 20%, and increases glucagon secretion by 24% in normal subjects.[100] However, the insulinogenic effect of protein also depends on individual insulin sensitivity.[101]

Fat

The postprandial glycemic response is determined mainly by the rate of gastric emptying.[102–105] Nutrients such as fat interact with the receptors in the small intestine to slow down gastric emptying, possibly due to their high calorie content and reduced absorption rate.[106] Gut incretin hormones such as glucagon-like peptide (GLP-1) and glucose-dependent insulinotropic polypeptide (GIP), which accounts for 50% rise in plasma insulin level, can, after an oral glucose load,[107] be attenuated by fat.[108] In a randomized cross-over study, fat in the form of olive oil ingested before a carbohydrate meal (potato meal) delayed gastric emptying and attenuated the postprandial glucose level, and insulin and GIP secretion. However, this effect of fat also depends on the lipolysis of triglycerides to fatty acids.[109] The effect of fatty acids such as SFA, MUFA, and PUFA on the insulinemic response has also been studied.[110,111] Diets high in linoleic acid (LA) (n-6 PUFA) and low in (n-3 PUFA) could increase the risk of metabolic syndrome in Asian Indians;[112] moreover, according to American Diabetes Association (ADA), the percentage of energy

derived from oleic acid or EPA and DHA that is usually recommended for individuals with type 2 diabetes only leads to a modest reduction in the postprandial insulin response, compared to diets rich in palmitic acid or linoleic acid.[113] Similarly, the impact of different fat sources on the glycemic response has been studied, and results showed that safflower or olive oil decreased, and butter increased, the plasma glucose level, whereas triacylglycerol concentration increased with safflower oil;[114,115] this is consistent with the study result of Mekki et al. on the effect of postprandial lipemia after supplementation of a mixed meal containing 40 g fat as butter, olive oil, or sunflower oil.[116] This may possibly be due to the difference in the binding of specific fatty acids to FABP2 (fatty acid binding protein), which is then formed into chylomicrons in the endoplasmic reticulum. Fatty acids in butter (contains 25% fat as short- and medium-chain fatty acids) bind to FABP2 to a lesser extent than olive oil (75% oleic acid) or safflower oil (75% linoleic acid) because of its varied fat content and the type of fatty acids present in it. As a result, butter is more absorbed into the portal vein rather than transported for chylomicron synthesis, and this further increases the hepatic glucose output and thereby results in a high plasma glucose level.[117] Diets rich in MUFA help in stimulating GLP secretion by enhancing L cell sensitivity,[118] and these incretin hormones (including GIP) are being used as a new therapeutic approach in the treatment of type 2 diabetes.[119]

Fiber

Fiber comprises the edible parts of cereals, fruits, and vegetables that are resistant to digestion and absorption in the human small intestine.[120,121] Interest in the association of dietary fiber and risk for chronic diseases arose as early as 1970s, when Burkitt and Trowell hypothesized that lack of fiber in the diet was associated with increased incidence of obesity, type 2 diabetes, coronary heart disease, and some cancers among the Western population. Recent epidemiological studies have also confirmed this hypothesis and shown a protective role of dietary fiber in reducing the risk of chronic diseases.[122–125] Dietary fiber is a complex mixture of polysaccharides that has been shown to exert several physiological effects in the human gastrointestinal tract and hence may have an influence on disease risk. However, the effect of dietary fiber in foods on the glycemic response is undecided. Dietary fiber delays gastric emptying and decreases the absorption of nutrients, resulting in lower postprandial glucose and insulin response. Recent research has shown that the soluble versus insoluble fraction of fiber in foods may give a clear insight regarding the efficacy of dietary fiber on GI.[126]

The carbohydrate metabolism of grains is influenced by several factors, such as differences in structure and composition (particle size), amount and type of fiber, viscosity, presence of antinutrition factors, and cooking method and temperature.[127] The fiber content of rice has shown no positive correlation with its GI.[80] However, the

GI of brown rice is lower compared to that of its counterpart, polished white rice. This may be attributed to the differences in physiochemical properties, longer cooking time, and lesser gelatinization of brown rice, and the presence of other antinutritional factors such as phytates and polyphenols in brown rice which slow starch digestion and delay glucose absorption.[128,129]

Potential Ingredients to Lower GI

Today, many functional ingredients are available for exploitation in food formulation to lower the GI of processed foods. These functional ingredients come from grains, fruits and vegetables (β-glucans, non-digestible oligosaccharides and RS), and modified carbohydrates.[11]

Recent research has focused on the effect of viscous soluble fiber on the carbohydrate metabolism and blood glucose response. Two recent studies have demonstrated that a novel functional viscous fiber, PGX®, added to commonly consumed starchy foods, one of which was rice, resulted in a dose-dependant reduction in the GI (PGX added to rice = 19% for a 2.5-g dose and 30% for a 5-g dose).[130,131] Recent studies from our center have also shown that when fenupower (a soluble dietary fiber rich in galactomannan extracted from fenugreek seeds) was incorporated into commonly consumed breakfast meal choices of Indians (idly- and whole wheat-flour pulkha), the GI dropped by 30% for idly- and 8.4% for whole wheat-flour pulkha compared to their controls tested without fenupower. Similarly, in another study the GI of whole wheat flour roti and atta mix roti was tested and it was found that although both had low GI values, the GI of the atta mix was considerably lower than that of the whole wheat flour mix. In this study, the galactomannan from bengal gram, psyllium, and fenugreek seeds present in atta mix may change the physical availability of carbohydrate to hydrolytic enzymes, thus converting the carbohydrates to a slow release form, resulting in lowering of the plasma glucose level.[132] In another study, the effect of 4 g and 8 g β-glucan added to Indian flat breads (chapatti) showed 43% and 47% reduction in GI values compared to control chapattis made from whole wheat flour.[10]

Thus, the effect of inherent fiber on the GI is still not well established. However, incorporation of viscous fiber products has shown their potential to reduce the GI. Further well-designed studies with respect to different components of fiber and its mechanisms are still needed, considering its effects in the prevention of diabetes and metabolic syndrome.

CONCLUSIONS

Cereal staples have served as major calorie contributors to Indian diets since ancient times. The recent shift to refined grains with a high GI could be one of the reasons for the increasing prevalence of diabetes and metabolic syndrome in India. It is unlikely that the total carbohydrate content of Indian diets could be altered, due to traditional dietary habits. It is thus reasonable to encourage the introduction of low GI foods and to promote high-fiber foods to reduce the GL of Indian meals. Moreover, low GI foods come with added benefits, such as a higher fiber and phytonutrient content, that are beneficial to overall health. Several mechanistic, prospective, and randomized clinical trials globally have proved that a low GI has beneficial effects on glycemic and insulinemic responses, but there are limited studies with Indian diets.

There is thus an urgent need to create a database of the GI of Indian foods using standardized methodology. This will enable those engaged in public health and clinical practice in health advocacy and counseling. Use of newer functional ingredients could help lower the GI, and hence better formulations of such foods need to be developed. Low GI foods could possibly help to tackle the epidemic of type 2 diabetes and metabolic syndrome in India, but randomized clinical trials are needed on this subject.

Acknowledgements

The authors thank R. Gayathri, Manobala, Dr S. Shobana, Dr Sandhya, and Sahithya, Nutrition and Dietetics Research Department, Madras Diabetes Research Foundation for their support in the preparation of the manuscript.

References

1. *Dimensions of need – An atlas of food and agriculture.* Italy: Food and Agriculture organization of the United Nations Rome; 1995. Available at: http://www.fao.org/docrep/U8480E/U8480E00.htm [accessed 09.02.13].
2. *Achaya, Konganda Thammu. The Illustrated Foods of India: AZ.* New Delhi, India: Oxford University Press; 2009 2–4.
3. Ramachandran P. *FAO The double burden of malnutrition: Case studies from six developing countries.* Rome: Food and agriculture organization of the United Nations (FAO); 2006.
4. NSSO. *National Sample Survey Organization Household Expenditure Survey. 66th Round – A Critique;* 2011. Available at: http://re-emergingworld.com/blog/wp-content/uploads/2011/08/20-07-2011-NSSO-Household-Consumer-Expenditure.Survey_Blog-Writeup-V1-1.pdf [accessed 07.03.13].
5. Radhika G, Sathya RM, Ganesan A, Saroja R, Vijayalakshmi P, Sudha V, et al. Dietary profile of urban adult population in South India in the context of chronic disease epidemiology (CURES–68). *Public Health Nutr* 2010;**14**(4):591–8.
6. Anjana RM, Pradeepa R, Deepa M, Sudha V, Unnikrishnan R, Bhansali A, et al. Prevalence of diabetes and prediabetes (impaired fasting glucose and/or impaired glucose tolerance) in urban and rural India: Phase I results of the Indian Council of Medical Research–INdia DIABetes (ICMR–INDIAB) study. *Diabetol* 2011;**54**(12):3022–7.
7. Mohan V, Radhika G, Sathya RM, Tamil SR, Ganesan A, Sudha V. Dietary carbohydrates, glycaemic load, food groups and newly detected type 2 diabetes among urban Asian Indian population in Chennai, India (Chennai Urban Rural Epidemiology Study 59). *Br J Nutr* 2009;**102**(10):1498–506.

8. Mohan V, Radhika G, Vijayalakshmi P, Sudha V. Can the diabetes/cardiovascular disease epidemic in India be explained, at least in part, by excess refined grain (rice) intake. *Ind J Med Res* 2010;**131**:369–72.

9. Mellen PB, Walsh TF, Herrington DM. Whole grain intake and cardiovascular disease: a meta-analysis. *Nutr, Metab Cardiovas Dis* 2008;**18**(4):283–90.

10. Henry CJK, Thondre PS. *The glycaemic index: concept, recent developments and its impact on diabetes and obesity*. London, UK: Smith-Gordon Pub; 2011 Chapter 15, pp. 154–75.

11. Henry CJK. *Novel food ingredients for weight control*. Cambridge, England: Woodhead Publishing Ltd; 2007.

12. Foster-Powell K, Miller J. International tables of glycemic index. *Am J Clin Nutr* 1995;**62**(Suppl.):871S–90S.

13. Foster-Powell K, Holt SH, Brand-Miller JC. International table of glycemic index and glycemic load values. *Am J Clin Nutr* 2002;**76**(1):5–56.

14. Atkinson FS, Foster-Powell K, Brand-Miller JC. International tables of glycemic index and glycemic load values. *Diab Care* 2008;**31**(12):2281–3.

15. FAO. *WHO report on Carbohydrates in human nutrition. Paper 66*. Rome: Report of a Joint FAO/WHO Expert Consultation; 1997.

16. Eaton SB, Konner M. Paleolithic nutrition: A consideration of its nature and current implications. *New Engl J Med* 1985;**312**(5):283–9.

17. Fuller Dorian Q. Ceramics, seeds and culinary change in prehistoric India. *Antiquity* 2005;**79**(306):761–77.

18. FAO. Food and agricultural organization of the United Nations. Available at: http://faostat.fao/site/399/default.aspx [accessed 20.02.13].

19. NNMB. National nutrition monitoring bureau. Diet and Nutritional status of population and prevalence of hypertension among adults in rural areas. National Institute of Nutrition. *Indian Council Med Res* 2006.

20. NNMB. *National Sample Survey Organisation. Nutritional intake in India. 61st Round. Report No. 513(61/1.0/6). July 2004–June 2005*. Ministry of Statistics & Programme Implementation Government of India; 2007.

21. Villegas R, Liu S, Gao YT, Yang G, Li H, Zheng W, et al. Prospective study of dietary carbohydrates, glycemic index, glycemic load, and incidence of type 2 diabetes mellitus in middle-aged Chinese women. *Arch Intern Med* 2007;**167**:2310–6.

22. Nanri A, Mizoue T, Noda M, Takahashi Y, Kato M, Inoue M, et al. Rice intake and type 2 diabetes in Japanese men and women: the Japan Public Health Center– based Prospective Study. *Am J Clin Nutr* 2010;**92**(6):1468–77.

23. National Multi-Commodity Exchange of India Ltd. Report on Wheat. 4th Floor H.K. House, B/h Jivabhai Chambers, Ashram Road, Ahmedabad, Gujarat, India. Available at: www.nmce.com/files/study/wheat.pdf [accessed 12.03.13].

24. Millets–Future of Food and Farming. Millet Network of India, Deccan Development Society, FIAN, India. Available at: www.swaraj.org/shikshantar/millets. pdf [accessed 12.03.13].

25. Juliano BO. *Rice in human nutrition*. Rome, Italy: Food and Agriculture Organization; 1993.

26. Gopalan C, Rama Sastri BV, Balasubramaniam SC. *Nutritive value of Indian Foods*. Hyderabad, India: National Institute of Nutrition, Indian Council of Medical Research; 2010.

27. Singh N, Singh H, Kaur K, Bakshi MS. Relationship between the degree of milling, ash distribution pattern and conductivity in brown rice. *Food Chem* 2000;**69**:147–51.

28. Adams ML, Lombi E, Zhao FJ, McGrath SP. Evidence of low selenium concentrations in UK bread-making wheat grain. *J Sci Food and Agr* 2002;**82**:1160–5.

29. Topping D. Cereal complex carbohydrates and their contribution to human health. *J Cereal Sci* 2007;**46**:220–9.

30. Food and Agriculture Organization of the United Nations. *Sorghum and millets Hum Nutr FAO* 1995.

31. Chiu CJ, Liu S, Willett WC, et al. Informing food choices and health outcomes by use of the dietary glycemic index. *Nutr Rev* 2011;**69**(4):231–42.

32. Jenkins DJ, Wolever TM, Taylor R, Barker H, Fielden H, Baldwin JM, et al. Glycemic index of foods: a physiological basis for carbohydrate exchange. *Amr J Clin Nutr* 1981;**34**(3):362–6.

33. Henry CJK, Lightowler HJ, Newens K, Sudha V, Radhika G, Sathya RM, et al. Glycaemic index of common foods tested in the UK and India. *Br J Nutr* 2008;**99**(4):840–5.

34. Sharp PS, Mohan V, Levy JC, Mather HM, Kohner EM. Insulin resistance in patients of Asian Indian and European origin with non-insulin dependent diabetes. *Horm Metab Res* 1987;**19**(2):84–5.

35. Bao J, de Jong V, Atkinson F, Petocz P, Brand-Miller JC. Food insulin index: physiologic basis for predicting insulin demand evoked by composite meals. *Am J Clin Nutr* 2009;**90**(4):986–92.

36. Chan HMS, Brand-Miller J, Holt SHA, Wilson D, Rozman M, Petocz P. The glycaemic index values of Vietnamese foods. *Eur J Clin Nutr* 2001;**55**:1076–83.

37. Ball SD, Keller KR, Moyer-Mileur LJ, Ding Y, Donaldson D, Jackson WD. Prolongation of satiety after low versus moderately high glycaemic index meals in obese adolescents. *Paediatrics* 2003;**111**:488–94.

38. Vijayan L, Sumathi S. Glycaemic response to selected Kerala breakfast items in people with diabetes. *Asia Pacific J Clin Nutr* 1997;**6**(2):80–3.

39. Urooj A, Puttaraj S. Glycaemic responses to cereal-based Indian food preparations in patients with non-insulin-dependent diabetes mellitus and normal subjects. *Br J Nutr* 2000;**83**:483–8.

40. Kurup PG, Krishnamurthy S. Glycemic Index of Selected Foodstuffs commonly used in South India. *Int J Vit Nutr Res* 1992;**62**:266–8.

41. Chaturvedi A, Sarojini G, Nirmala G, Nirmalamma N, Satyanarayana D. Glycemic index of grain amaranth, wheat and rice in NIDDM subjects. *J Plant Foods Hum Nutr* 1997;**50**:171–8.

42. Kanan W, Biljani RL, Sachdeva U, Mahapatra SC, Shah P, Karmarkar MG. Glycaemic and insulinaemic responses to natural foods, frozen foods and their laboratory equivalents. *Ind J Physiol Pharmacol* 1998;**42**(1):81–9.

43. Kavita MS, Prema L. Glycaemic response to selected cereal-based South Indian meals in non-insulin dependent diabetics. *J Nutr Environ Med* 1997;**7**:287–94.

44. Shobana S, Usha Kumari SR, Malleshi NG, Ali SZ. Glycemic response of rice, wheat and finger millet based diabetic food formulations in normoglycemic subjects. *Int J Food Sci Nutr* 2007;**58**:363–72.

45. Pathak Feldman N, Norenberg C, Voet H, Manor E, Berner Y, Madar Z. Enrichment of an Israeli ethnic food with fibres and their effects on the glycaemic and insulinaemic responses in subjects with non-insulin-dependent diabetes mellitus. *Br J Nutr* 1995;**74**:681–8.

46. Sumathi A, Vishwanathan S, Malleshi NG, Rao SV. Glycemic response to malted, popped and roller dried wheat-legume based foods in normal subjects. *Int J Food Sci and Nutr* 1997;**48**(2):103–7.

47. Dilawari JB, Kamath PS, Batta RP, Mukewar S, Raghavan S. Reduction of postprandial plasma glucose by Bengal gram dhal (Cicer arietinum) and Rajmah (*Phaseolus vulgaris*). *Am J Clin Nutr* 1981;**34**:2450–3.

48. Mani UV, Pradhan SN, Mehta NC, Thakur DM, Iyer U, Mani I. Glycaeimc index of conventional carbohydrate meals. *B Jr Nutr* 1992;**68**:445–50.

49. Shukla K, Narain JP, Puri P, Gupta A, Bijlani RL, Mahapatra SC, et al. Glycaemic response to maize, bajra and barley. *Ind J Physiol Pharmacol* 1991;**35**:249–54.

50. Aston LM. Glycemic index and metabolic disease risk. *Proc Nutr Soc* 2006;**965**:125–34.

51. Ludwig DS, Majzoub JA, Al-Zahrani A, Dallal GE, Blanco I, Roberts SB. High glycemic index foods, overeating, and obesity. *Pediatrics* 1999;**103**(3):E26.

52. Jenkins DJ, Wolever TM, Vuksan V, Brighenti F, Cunnane SC, Rao AV, et al. Nibbling versus gorging: metabolic advantages of increased meal frequency. *N Engl J Med* 1989;**321**(14):929–34.

53. Jenkins DJ, Wolever TM, Ocana AM, Vuksan V, Cunnane SC, Jenkins M, et al. Metabolic effects of reducing rate of glucose ingestion by single bolus versus continuous sipping. *Diabetes* 1990;**39**(7):775–81.

54. Ludwig DS. The glycemic index: Physiological mechanisms relating to obesity, diabetes and cardiovascular disease. *JAMA* 2002;**287**(18):2414–23.

55. Wolever TM, Bentum-Williams A, Jenkins DJ. Physiological modulation of plasma free fatty acid concentrations by diet. Metabolic implications in non diabetic subjects. *Diab Care* 1995;**18**(7):962–70.

56. Wolever TMS. *The glycemic index: A physiological classification of dietary carbohydrates*. UK: CAB Internationls; 2006:160–164.

57. Ritz P, Krempf M, Cloarec D, Champ M, Charbonnel B. Comparative continuous-indirect-calorimetry study of two carbohydrates with different glycemic indices. *Am J Clin Nutr* 1991;**54**(5):855–9.

58. World Health Organization (WHO). *Global Status Report on Noncommunicable Diseases 2010 – Description of the Global Burden of NCDs, Their Risk Factors and Determinants*. Geneva, Switzerland: WHO; 2011. Available at: http://whqlibdoc.who.int/publications/2011/9789240686458_eng.pdf [accessed 10.01.13].

59. Virkamaki A, Ueki K, Kahn C. Protein–protein interaction in insulin signaling and molecular mechanisms of insulin resistance. *Rev J Clin Invest* 1999;**103**:931–43.

60. Esfahani A, Wong JM, Mirrahimi A, Srichaikul K, Jenkins DJ, Kendall CW. The glycemic index: physiological significance. *J Am Col Nutr* 2009;**28**(Suppl. 1):439–45.

61. United Kingdom Prospective Diabetes Study (UKPDS). Relative efficacy of randomly allocated diet, sulphonylurea, insulin, or metformin in patients with newly diagnosed non-insulin dependent diabetes followed for three years. *BMJ* 1995;**310**:83–8.

62. Sievenpiper JL, Kendall CW, Esfahani A, et al. Effect of non-oilseed pulses on glycaemic control: a systematic review and meta-analysis of randomised controlled experimental trials in people with and without diabetes. *Diabetol* 2009;**52**:1479–95.

63. Shobana S, Kokila A, Lakshmipriya N, Subhashini S, Ramya Bai M, Mohan V, et al. Glycaemic index of three Indian rice varieties. *Int J Food Sci Nutr* 2012;**63**(2):178–83.

64. Holt S, Brand J, Soveny C, Hansky J. Relationship of satiety to postprandial glycaemic, insulin and cholecystokinin responses. *Appetite* 1992;**18**(2):129–41.

65. Bouche C, Rizkalla SW, Luo J, Vidal H, Veronese A, Pacher N, et al. Five week low glycemic index diet decreased total fat mass and improves plasma lipid profile in moderately overweight nondiabetic men. *Diab Care* 2002;**25**:822–8.

66. Radhika G, Dam Van, Rob M, Sudha V, Ganesan A, Mohan V. Refined grain consumption and the metabolic syndrome in urban Asian Indians (Chennai Urban Rural Epidemiology Study 57). *Metab* 2009;**58**(5):675–81.

67. Nord T. *Glycemic index from research to nutrition recommendations*. Denmark: Nordic Council of Ministers; 2005:21–22.

68. Miller B, Wolever TMS, Colaguiri S, Powell KF. *The glycemic index – the glucose revolution*. NewYork, NY: Marlowe and Company; 2001:37–39.

69. Behall KM, Scholfield DJ, Hallfrisch J. The effect of particle size of whole grain flour on plasma glucose, insulin, and TSH in human subjects. *J Am Col Nutr* 2000;**18**:591–7.

70. Holt SH, Miller JB. Particle size, satiety and the glycaemic response. *Eur J Clin Nutr* 1994;**48**:496–502.

71. Holm J, Björck I. Bioavailability of starch in various wheat-based bread products: evaluation of metabolic responses in healthy subjects and rate and extent of *in vitro* starch digestion. *Am J Clin Nutr* 1992;**55**:420–9.

72. Ranawana V, Monro JA, Mishra S, Henry CJK. Degree of particle size breakdown during mastication may be a possible cause of interindividual glycaemic variability. *Nutr Res* 2010;**30**(4):246–54.

73. Aldughpassi A, Abdel-Aal ESM, Wolever TM. Barley Cultivar, Kernel Composition, and Processing Affect the Glycemic Index. *J Nutr* 2012;**142**(9):1666–71.

74. Trinidad TP, Mallillin AC, Encabo RR, Sagum RS, Felix AD, Juliano BO. The effect of apparent amylose content and dietary fibre on the glycemic response of different varieties of cooked milled and brown rice. *Int J Food Sci Nutr* 2013;**64**(1):89–93.

75. Brouns F, Björck I, Frayn KN, Gibbs AL, Lang V, Wolever TMS. Glycaemic index methodology. *Nutr Res Rev* 2005;**18**(1):145.

76. Granfeldt Y, Björck I. Glycemic response to starch in pasta: a study of mechanisms of limited enzyme availability. *J Cereal Sci* 1991;**14**(1):47–61.

77. Järvi AE, Karlström BE, Granfeldt YE, Björck IM, Vessby BO, Asp NG. The influence of food structure on postprandial metabolism in patients with non-insulin-dependent diabetes mellitus. *Am J Clin Nut* 1995;**61**(4):837–42.

78. Brown MA, Storlien LH, Brown IL, Higgins JA. Cooking attenuates the ability of high-amylose meals to reduce plasma insulin concentrations in rats. *Bri J Nutr* 2003;**90**(04):823–7.

79. Vaidya RH, Sheth MK. Processing and storage of Indian cereal and cereal products alters its resistant starch content. *J Food Sci Technol* 2011;**48**(5):622–7.

80. Jenkins DJ, Wolever TM, Taylor RH, Barker H, Fielden H, Baldwin JM, et al. Glycemic index of foods: a physiological basis for carbohydrate exchange. *Am J Clin Nutr* 1981;**34**(3):362–6.

81. Nuttall FQ, Khan MA, Gannon MC. Peripheral glucose appearance rate following fructose ingestion in normal subjects. *Metab Clin Exp* 2000;**49**(12):1565–71.

82. Corpe CP, Burant CF, Hoekstra JH. Intestinal fructose absorption: clinical and molecular aspects. *J Ped Gastroenterol Nutr* 1999;**28**(4):364–74.

83. Přibylová J, Kozlová J. Glucose and galactose infusions in newborns of diabetic and healthy mothers. *Neonatol* 1979;**36**(3–4):193–7.

84. Gannon MC, Khan MA, Nuttall FQ. Glucose appearance rate after the ingestion of galactose. *Met Clin Exp* 2001;**50**(1):93–8.

85. Macdonald I, Keyser A, Pacy D. Some effects, in man, of varying the load of glucose, sucrose, fructose, or sorbitol on various metabolites in blood. *Am J Clin Nutr* 1978;**31**:1305–11.

86. Englyst HN, Wiggins HS, Cummings JH. Determination of the non-starch polysaccharides in plant foods by gas-liquid chromatography of constituent sugars as alditol acetates. *Analyst* 1982;**107**:307–18.

87. Sajilata MG, Singhal RS, Kulkarni PR. Resistant starch – a review. *Comprehensive rev Food Science and Food safety* 2006;**5**(1):1–17.

88. Eerlingen RC, Jacobs H, Delcour J. Enzyme-resistant starch. 5. Effect of retrogradation of waxy maize starch on enzyme susceptibility. *Cereal Chem* 1994;**71**(4):351–5.

89. van Loon LJ, Saris WH, Verhagen H, Wagenmakers AJ. Plasma insulin responses after ingestion of different amino acid or protein mixtures with carbohydrate. *Am J Clin Nutr* 2000;**72**(1):96–105.

90. Nuttall FQ, Mooradian AD, Gannon MC, Billington C, Krezowski P. Effect of protein ingestion on the glucose and insulin response to a standardized oral glucose load. *Diab Care* 1984;**7**(5):465–70.

91. Blaak EE. Prevention and treatment of obesity and related complications: a role for protein? *Int J Obes* 2006;**30**:S24–7.

92. Moghaddam E, Vogt JA, Wolever TM. The effects of fat and protein on glycemic responses in nondiabetic humans vary with waist circumference, fasting plasma insulin, and dietary fiber intake. *J Nutr* 2006;**136**(10):2506–11.

93. Holt SH, Miller JC, Petocz P. An insulin index of foods: the insulin demand generated by 1000-kJ portions of common foods. *Am J Clin Nutr* 1997;**66**(5):1264–76.

94. Nuttall FQ, Gannon MC. Plasma glucose and insulin response to macronutrients in nondiabetic and NIDDM subjects. *Diab Care* 1991;**14**(9):824–38.

95. Lang V, Bellisle F, Alamowitch C, Craplet C, Bornet FR, Slama G, et al. Varying the protein source in mixed meal modifies glucose, insulin and glucagon kinetics in healthy men, has weak effects on subjective satiety and fails to affect food intake. *Eur J Clin Nutr* 1999;**53**(12):959.

96. Floyd Jr JC, Fajans SS, Conn JW, Knopf RF, Rull J. Insulin secretion in response to protein ingestion. *J Clin Invest* 1966;**45**(9):1479.

97. Nuttall FQ, Gannon MC, Wald JL, Ahmed M. Plasma glucose and insulin profiles in normal subjects ingesting diets of varying carbohydrate, fat, and protein content. *J Am Coll Nutr* 1985;**4**(4):437–50.

98. Nilsson M, Stenberg M, Frid AH, Holst JJ, Björck IM. Glycemia and insulinemia in healthy subjects after lactose-equivalent meals of milk and other food proteins: the role of plasma amino acids and incretins. *Am J Clin Nutr* 2004;**80**(5):1246–53.

99. Nuttall FQ, Gannon MC. Metabolic response to egg white and cottage cheese protein in normal subjects. *Metab* 1990;**39**(7):749–55.

100. Larivière F, Chiasson JL, Schiffrin A, Taveroff A, Hoffer LJ. Effects of dietary protein restriction on glucose and insulin metabolism in normal and diabetic humans. *Metab* 1994;**43**(4):462–7.

101. Brand-Miller JC, Colagiuri S, Gan ST. Insulin sensitivity predicts glycemia after a protein load. *Metab* 2000;**49**(1):1–5.

102. Rayner CK, Samsom M, Jones KL, Horowitz M. Relationships of upper gastrointestinal motor and sensory function with glycemic control. *Diab Care* 2001;**24**(2):371–81.

103. Horowitz M, Edelbroek MA, Wishart JM, Straathof JW. Relationship between oral glucose tolerance and gastric emptying in normal healthy subjects. *Diabetol* 1993;**36**(9):857–62.

104. Schwartz JG, Guan D, Green GM, Phillips WT. Treatment with an oral proteinase inhibitor slows gastric emptying and acutely reduces glucose and insulin levels after a liquid meal in type II diabetic patients. *Diab Care* 1994;**17**(4):255–62.

105. Jones KL, Horowitz M, Carney BI, Wishart JM, Guha S, Green L. Gastric emptying in early noninsulin-dependent diabetes mellitus. *J Nuclear Med: official publication, Society of Nuclear Med* 1996;**37**(10):1643.

106. Lin HC, Zhao XT, Wang LIJIE. Fat absorption is not complete by midgut but is dependent on load of fat. *Am J Physiol-Gastrointestinal Liver Physiol* 1996;**271**(1):G62–7.

107. Nauck MA, Baller B, Meier JJ. Gastric inhibitory polypeptide and glucagon-like peptide-1 in the pathogenesis of type 2 diabetes. *Diab* 2004;**53**(suppl. 3):S190–SS96.

108. Feinle C, O'Donovan D, Doran S, Andrews JM, Wishart J, Chapman I, et al. Effects of fat digestion on appetite, APD motility, and gut hormones in response to duodenal fat infusion in humans. *Am J Physiol-Gastrointestinal Liver Physiol* 2003; **284**(5):G798–807.

109. Gentilcore D, Chaikomin R, Jones KL, Russo A, Feinle-Bisset C, Wishart JM, et al. Effects of fat on gastric emptying of and the glycemic, insulin, and incretin responses to a carbohydrate meal in type 2 diabetes. *J Clin Endocrinol Metab* 2006;**91**(6):2062–7.

110. Shah M, Adams-Huet B, Brinkley L, Grundy SM, Garg A. Lipid, glycemic, and insulin responses to meals rich in saturated, cis-monounsaturated, and polyunsaturated (n-3 and n-6) fatty acids in subjects with type 2 diabetes. *Diab Care* 2007;**30**(12):2993–8.

111. MacIntosh CG, Holt SH, Brand-Miller JC. The degree of fat saturation does not alter glycemic, insulinemic or satiety responses to a starchy staple in healthy men. *J Nutr* 2003;**133**(8):2577–80.

112. Lakshmipriya N, Gayathri R, Praseena K, Vijayalakshmi P, Geetha G, Sudha V, et al. Type of vegetable oils used in cooking and risk of metabolic syndrome among Asian Indians. *Int J Food Sci Nut* 2013;**64**(2):131–9.

113. Shah M, Adams-Huet B, Brinkley L, Grundy SM, Garg A. Lipid, glycemic, and insulin responses to meals rich in saturated, cis-monounsaturated, and polyunsaturated (n-3 and n-6) fatty acids in subjects with type 2 diabetes. *Diab Care* 2007;**30**(12):2993–8.

114. Dworatzek PD, Hegele RA, Wolever TM. Postprandial lipemia in subjects with the threonine 54 variant of the fatty acid-binding protein 2 gene is dependent on the type of fat ingested. *Am J Clin Nutr* 2004;**79**(6):1110–7.

115. Gatti E, Noe D, Pazzucconi F, Gianfranceschi G, Porrini M, Testolin G, et al. Differential effect of unsaturated oils and butter on blood glucose and insulin response to carbohydrate in normal volunteers. *Eur J Clin Nutr* 1992;**46**(3):161.

116. Mekki N, Charbonnier M, Borel P, Leonardi J, Juhel C, Portugal H, et al. Butter differs from olive oil and sunflower oil in its effects on postprandial lipemia and triacylglycerol-rich lipoproteins after single mixed meals in healthy young men. *J Nutr* 2002;**132**(12):3642–9.

117. Dworatzek PD, Hegele RA, Wolever TM. Postprandial lipemia in subjects with the threonine 54 variant of the fatty acid-binding protein 2 gene is dependent on the type of fat ingested. *Am J Clin Nutr* 2004;**79**(6):1110–7.

118. Rocca AS, LaGreca J, Kalitsky J, Brubaker PL. Monounsaturated fatty acid diets improve glycemic tolerance through increased secretion of glucagon-like peptide-1. *Endocrinol* 2001; **142**(3):1148–55.

119. Baggio LL, Drucker DJ. Biology of incretins: GLP-1 and GIP. *Gastroenterol* 2007;**132**(6):2131–57.

120. Slavin JL, Savarino V, Paredes-Diaz A, Fotopoulos G. A review of the role of soluble fiber in health with specific reference to wheat dextrin. *J Int Med Res* 2009;**37**(1):1–17.

121. Burkitt DP, Trowell HC. *Refined carbohydrate foods and disease. Some implications of dietary fibre. UK.* London: Academic Press Inc; 1975.

122. Pereira MA, O'Reilly E, Augustsson K, Fraser GE, Goldbourt U, Heitmann BL, et al. Dietary fiber and risk of coronary heart disease: a pooled analysis of cohort studies. *Arch Inter Med* 2004;**164**(4):370.

123. Stevens J, Ahn K, Houston D, Steffan L, Couper D. Dietary Fiber Intake and Glycemic Index and Incidence of Diabetes in African-American and White Adults The ARIC Study. *Diab Care* 2002;**25**(10):1715–21.

124. Hodge AM, English DR, O'Dea K, Giles GG. Glycemic index and dietary fiber and the risk of type 2 diabetes. *Diab Care* 2004;**27**(11):2701–6.

125. Spiller GA, editor. *CRC Handbook of dietary fiber in human nutrition.* CRC; 2001.

126. Jenkins DJ, Wolever TM, Leeds AR, Gassull MA, Haisman P, Dilawari J, et al. Dietary fibres, fibre analogues, and glucose tolerance: Importance of viscosity. *Br Med J* 1978;**1**:1392–4.

127. Henry CJK. *Novel food ingredients for weight control.* Cambridge, UK: Woodhead Publishing Ltd; 2007.

128. Panlasigui LN, Thompson LU, Juliano BO, Perez CM, Yiu SH, Greenberg GR. Rice varieties with similar amylose content differ in starch digestibility and glycemic response in humans. *Am J Clin Nutr* 1991;**54**(5):871–7.

129. Yoon JH, Thompson LU, Jenkins DJ. The effect of phytic acid on in vitro rate of starch digestibility and blood glucose response. *Am J Clin Nutr* 1983;**38**(6):835–42.

130. Jenkins AL, Kacinik V, Lyon M, Wolever TM, Vuksan V. Effect of adding the novel fiber, PGX®, to commonly consumed foods on glycemic response, glycemic index and GRIP: a simple and effective strategy for reducing post prandial blood glucose levels – a randomized, controlled trial. *Nutr J* 2010;**9**:58.

131. Brand-Miller JC, Atkinson FS, Gahler RJ, Kacinik V, Lyon MR, Wood S. Effects of PGX, a novel functional fibre, on acute and delayed postprandial glycaemia. *Eur J Clin Nutr* 2010;**64**(12):1488–93.

132. Radhika G, Sumathi C, Ganesan A, Sudha V, Henry CJK, Mohan V. Glycaemic index of Indian flatbreads (rotis) prepared using whole wheat flour and "atta mix"-added whole wheat flour. *Br J Nutr* 2010;**103**(11):1642–7.

Rice and Type 2 Diabetes

Akiko Nanri, Tetsuya Mizoue

Department of Epidemiology and Prevention, Center for Clinical Sciences, National Center for Global Health and Medicine, Tokyo, Japan

INTRODUCTION

In Japan, the respective prevalence of probable and possible diabetes increased respectively from 6.9 to 8.9 and from 6.8 to 13.2 million cases between 1997 and 2007.[1] Probable diabetes cases are characterized either by high levels of glycated hemoglobin (≥6.1%) or by receiving medication for type 2 diabetes. Possible diabetes cases are characterized by glycated hemoglobin levels ranging from 5.6% to 6.1%.[1] Within populations of Japanese men and women aged over 50 years, the prevalence of probable and possible diabetes has been reported to be as high as 30–40%.[1] Although the prevalence of obesity (an important risk factor for type 2 diabetes) is lower in Japanese than in Western populations,[2] the prevalence of type 2 diabetes is not dramatically lower.[3] This might be attributed to not only genetic differences, but also dietary differences between Asian and Caucasian populations. Japanese traditionally consume white rice, and the percentage of energy from carbohydrate is higher whereas the percentage of energy from fat is lower in comparison with Western populations.[1,4] Compared with brown rice, white rice contains less dietary fiber and fewer of the vitamins and minerals [5] that are potentially protective against type 2 diabetes. In addition, white rice has a high glycemic index (GI),[6] which is a measure of the effect of food intake on blood glucose concentrations,[7–9] and has been shown to predict type 2 diabetes risk.[7–9] Among not only Asian populations which consume rice as a staple food, but also Western populations which consume a lesser amount of rice, white rice has been reported to be associated with increased risk of type 2 diabetes.

RICE INTAKE IN JAPAN

According to the National Health and Nutrition Survey conducted in Japan in 2011,[10] the daily intake of rice and processed rice for adult Japanese men and women is 395.6 g

and 267.7 g, respectively. Rice and processed rice contributes 46.4% of the total carbohydrate intake. Although rice consumption and percent of carbohydrate from rice and processed rice in Japan has decreased over the past several decades (Fig. 26.1), nearly 30% of total energy intake for Japanese people is still derived from rice. Moreover, in a study among 1354 Japanese female farmers aged 20–78 years by Murakami *et al.*,[11] white rice was the major contributor to dietary GI and GL (58.5%), followed by confectioneries (10.6%), fruit (6.7%), sugars (5.5%), bread (4.3%), noodles (3.4%), other rice (3.2%), and potatoes (2.6%).

RICE INTAKE AND TYPE 2 DIABETES RISK IN THE JAPAN PUBLIC HEALTH CENTER-BASED PROSPECTIVE (JPHC) STUDY

To date, six prospective studies have reported the association between rice intake and type 2 diabetes. Of these, three studies have been conducted among Western populations (Australia, US, and Spain),[12–14] two among Chinese,[15,16] and one among Japanese (Table 26.1). In the US study, in spite of lower consumption of rice, rice intake was associated with increased risk of type 2 diabetes.[14] Because the Japanese population consumes more rice, a higher risk of type 2 diabetes associated with rice intake is predicted. In our previous study, we prospectively investigated the association of rice intake with the risk of developing type 2 diabetes using data from the large-scale population based cohort study in Japan.[17]

The JPHC Study

The JPHC Study was launched in 1990 for cohort I and in 1993 for cohort II.[18] The participants of cohort I included residents aged 40 to 59 years, in five Japanese public health center areas (Iwate, Akita, Nagano, Okinawa, and Tokyo); the participants of cohort II included residents aged 40 to 69 years in six Japanese public health center areas (Ibaraki, Niigata, Kochi, Nagasaki, Okinawa, and Osaka). A questionnaire survey was conducted at baseline (in 1990 for cohort I and in 1993 for cohort II), 5-year follow-up (in 1995 for cohort I and in 1998 for cohort II), and 10-year follow-up (in 2000 for cohort I and in 2003 for cohort II). Information on medical

histories and health-related lifestyle, smoking, drinking, and dietary habits was obtained at each survey.

Study Participants

From the study population at baseline ($n = 140,420$), we excluded those who resided in two public health center areas because of the differences in recruitment criteria. Of the remaining 116,672 eligible participants, 95,373 (81.7%) responded to the questionnaire survey at baseline. Of these, 80,128 (84.0%) also responded to the 5-year follow-up survey, which is the baseline of the present analysis. Of these, 71,075 (88.7%) responded to the 10-year follow-up survey. We excluded participants who reported a history of type 2 diabetes ($n = 5183$) or severe disease ($n = 6284$), including cancer, cerebrovascular disease, myocardial infarction, chronic liver disease, and renal disease, at baseline or 5-year follow-up surveys. An additional 556 subjects with missing information for rice intake and 537 subjects who reported extreme total energy intake were excluded, leaving a total of 59,288 participants (25,666 men and 33,622 women) ultimately enrolled in this analysis.

Dietary Assessment

At baseline, 5-year follow-up, and 10-year follow-up surveys, participants completed a self-administered questionnaire on lifestyle and health. In this analysis, we used data from the 5-year follow-up survey as baseline

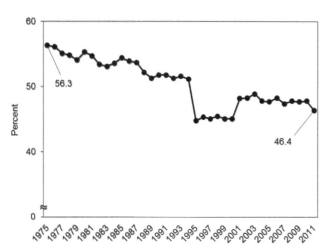

FIGURE 26.1 Trend in percentage of carbohydrate from rice and processed rice in Japan.

TABLE 26.1 Previous Prospective Studies that Examined the Association between Rice Intake and Type 2 Diabetes

First Author	Year	Country	No of Subjects	Age of Subjects (y)	Follow-up Period (y)	Rice Intake Category to Compare	RR or OR of Type 2 Diabetes (95% CI)
Hodge et al.[12]	2004	Australia	31,641 men and women	40–69	4	The highest quartile (≥2.5 times/week) vs. the lowest quartile (<1 times/week)	OR 0.93 (0.68–1.27); P for trend = 0.90
Villegas et al.[15]	2007	China (Shanghai)	64,227 women	40–70	4	≥750 g/day vs. <500 g/day	RR 1.78 (1.48–2.15)
Sun et al.[14]	2010	US	39,765 men 157,463 women	32–87 26–65	14–22	≥5 serving/week vs. <1 serving/month	HPFS RR: 1.02 (0.77–1.34); P for trend = 0.08 NHS I RR: 1.11 (0.87–1.43); P for trend = 0.02 NHS II RR: 1.40 (1.09–1.80); P for trend = 0.01 All RR: 1.17 (1.02–1.36); P for trend < 0.001
Nanri et al.[17]	2010	Japan	25,666 men and 33,622 women	45–75	5	The highest quartile (700 g/day in men; 560 g in women) vs. the lowest quartile (280g/day in men; 165 g in women)	Men: OR 1.19 (0.85–1.68); P for trend = 0.32 Women: OR 1.65 (1.06–2.57); P for trend = 0.005
Yu et al.[16]	2011	China (Hong Kong)	690 men and women	25–74	9–14	1 SD increase	OR 0.87 (0.67–1.13)
Soriguer et al.[13]	2013	Spain	605 men and women	18–65	6	2–3 times/week vs ≤1 time/week	OR 0.43 (0.19–0.95)

Abbreviations: CI, confidence interval; HPFS, Health Professionals Follow-Up Study; NHS, Nurses' Health Study; OR, odds ratio; RR, relative risk; SD, standard deviation.

data because the questionnaire used for the 5-year fol-low-up survey inquired more comprehensively about food intakes than that used for the baseline survey. At the 5-year follow-up survey, a food frequency question-naire (FFQ) was used to assess the average intake of 147 food and beverage items over the previous year.[19] For rice, participants were asked to provide their usual rice-bowl size from three options (small, medium, and large) and the number of bowls consumed daily from nine options (<1 bowl, 1 bowl, 2 bowls, 3 bowls, 4 bowls, 5 bowls, 6 bowls, 7–9 bowls, or ≥10 bowls). We calculated the daily intake of rice by multiplying daily consumption frequency by the typical rice-bowl size. The valid-ity of the FFQ was subsampled by using either 14- or 28-day dietary records. Spearman's correlation coef-ficients between rice intake derived from the FFQ and those derived from dietary records were 0.67 in men and 0.55 in women. With regard to the reproducibility of estimations between the two FFQs administered 1 year apart, the respective Spearman's correlation coefficients for rice intake were 0.79 in men and 0.69 in women.

Ascertainment of Type 2 Diabetes

Type 2 diabetes newly diagnosed during the 5-year period after the 5-year follow-up survey was determined by a self-administered questionnaire at the 10-year fol-low-up survey. At the 10-year follow-up survey, study participants were asked if they had ever been diagnosed with diabetes and, if so, when the initial diagnosis had been made. Because the 5-year follow-up survey was

used as the starting point of observation for the inci-dence of type 2 diabetes, only those participants who were diagnosed after 1995 for cohort I and 1998 for cohort II were regarded as incident cases during follow-up. In a validation study that we conducted, 94% of self-reported diabetes cases were confirmed as such by medical records.[20]

Results and Discussion

During the 5-year period, 1103 participants were newly diagnosed with diabetes (625 men and 478 women). Among women, rice intake was significantly and positively associated with incidence of type 2 dia-betes with adjustment for covariates other than BMI (*P* for trend = 0.003); the multivariable-adjusted odds ratio for the highest versus lowest quartile category was 1.69 (95% confidence interval: 1.08–2.63). Even after additional adjustments for BMI, the significant positive association was observed (*P* for trend = 0.05); the corresponding value was 1.65 (95% CI: 1.06–2.57) (Fig. 26.2). Among men, the odds ratios of type 2 dia-betes for the higher quartile categories of rice intake were higher compared with the lowest quartile cat-egory, though the association was not statistically sig-nificant (*P* for trend = 0.32). Participants with a higher intake of rice tended to have a lower BMI compared to those with a lower intake of rice; the mean BMI for the lowest through the highest quartile categories of rice intake were 23.8 kg/m², 23.5 kg/m², 23.5 kg/m², and 23.4 kg/m² in men (*P* for trend < 0.01) and 23.6 kg/m²,

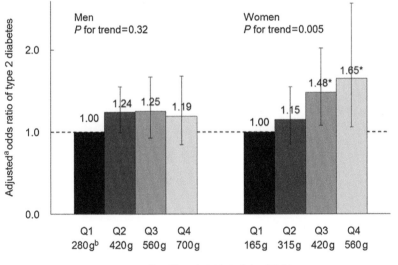

FIGURE 26.2 Multivariable-adjusted odds ratios of type 2 diabetes according to quartile categories of rice intake in the JPHC Study.[17]

[a]Adjusted for age, study area, body mass index, smoking status, alcohol consumption, family

history of diabetes, total physical activity, history of hypertension, occupation, total energy

intake, coffee consumption, and intakes of calcium, magnesium, dietary fiber, fruit,

vegetables, fish, bread, and noodles.

[b]Median of the category.

23.5 kg/m^2, 23.5 kg/m^2, and 23.4 kg/m^2 in women (P for trend = 0.02). This suggested that rice or a rice-based diet, probably because of its low fat content, may aid in obesity prevention better than a diet with low rice consumption, at least from an ecologic standpoint. Nevertheless, we noted an increased risk of type 2 diabetes in persons who consumed greater amounts of rice, which suggested that a high intake of rice may increase type 2 diabetes independent of BMI. High rice intake may increase the risk of type 2 diabetes through mechanisms other than obesity-related ones.

In an analysis stratified by physically strenuous activity at work or during leisure-time (Fig. 26.3), a marginally significant trend association between rice intake and type 2 diabetes was observed among men not engaged in strenuous physical activity (P for trend = 0.08), whereas such a trend association was not observed among men who were engaged in strenuous physical activity (P for trend = 0.85; P for interaction = 0.23). Likewise, a marginally significant, positive trend association between rice intake and type 2 diabetes was observed among women not engaged in any strenuous physical activity (P for trend = 0.08), but not among those engaged in such activity (P for trend = 0.30; P for interaction = 0.27). This finding underscored the importance of physical activity in assessment of the diet–diabetes risk relationship. More specifically, low physical activity may be a prerequisite condition for

rice consumption to influence type 2 diabetes risk. If a large proportion of glucose is taken up and metabolized in muscle, high levels of physical activity may counterbalance elevated rice intake.

We further repeated the analysis by age, BMI, smoking status (men only), and menopausal status (women only). The positive association between rice intake and type 2 diabetes was observed among both women aged <60 and ≥60 years; the multivariable-adjusted odds ratios (95% CI) of type 2 diabetes for the highest versus the lowest quartile category of rice intake were 1.64 (0.90–2.98) among women aged <60 (P for trend = 0.02) and 1.51 (0.75–3.02) among women aged ≥60 years (P for trend = 0.18). In stratified analysis by BMI, the positive association between rice intake and type 2 diabetes became strong among non-obese women (BMI <25 kg/m^2); the multivariable-adjusted odds ratios (95% CI) of type 2 diabetes across the quartile categories of rice intake were 1.00 (reference), 1.46 (0.88–2.40), 2.59 (1.55–4.32), and 2.78 (1.38–5.59) (P for trend <0.001). In contrast, among obese women (BMI ≥25 kg/m^2), such association was not observed. Among men, there was no association between rice intake and type 2 diabetes among non-smokers, whereas risk of type 2 diabetes tended to increase with rice intake among smokers. The adjusted odds ratios (95% CI) of type 2 diabetes for the lowest through the highest quartile categories were 1.00 (reference), 1.59 (1.12–2.25), 1.70 (1.11–2.59),

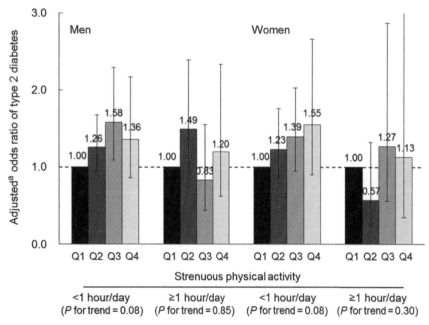

FIGURE 26.3 Multivariable-adjusted odds ratios of type 2 diabetes according to quartile categories of rice intake by strenuous physical activity in the JPHC Study.[17]

^{a}Adjusted for age, study area, body mass index, smoking status, alcohol consumption, family history of diabetes, history of hypertension, occupation, total energy intake, coffee consumption, and intakes of calcium, magnesium, dietary fiber, fruit, vegetables, fish, bread, and noodles.

and 1.55 (0.94–2.57) among smokers (P for trend = 0.11). In stratified analysis by menopausal status, rice intake was significantly associated with increased risk of type 2 diabetes among both premenopausal and postmenopausal women (P for trend = 0.02 in both). The increased risk of type 2 diabetes associated with rice intake was higher among premenopausal women than among postmenopausal women. The adjusted odds ratios (95% CI) of type 2 diabetes for the highest versus the lowest quartile of rice intake were 2.62 (0.93–7.41) among premenopausal women and 1.55 (0.92–2.62) among postmenopausal women.

In women but not men, the association was strengthened after excluding subjects who sometimes or always added minor cereals to rice; fully-adjusted odds ratios (95% CI) of type 2 diabetes for the lowest to highest quartile categories of rice intake were 1.00 (reference), 1.29 (0.85–1.97), 1.67 (1.08–2.58), and 1.81 (1.03–3.18), respectively (P for trend = 0.01). Because minor cereals are rich in magnesium and fiber and are potentially important food factors in the regulation of glucose absorption and metabolism,[21] the addition of these to rice is expected to help reduce type 2 diabetes risk.

In this large-scale prospective study, rice intake was associated with increased risk of developing type 2 diabetes in Japanese women. Although the association between rice intake and type 2 diabetes was not clear among men, rice intake was suggestively associated with increased risk of type 2 diabetes in physically inactive men.

RICE INTAKE AND TYPE 2 DIABETES: RESULT OF META-ANALYSIS

A meta-analysis was conducted using data from six prospective cohort studies of the association between rice intake and type 2 diabetes risk.[22] Two of the six cohort studies were conducted in Asia (including the Japanese study mentioned above) while the others were conducted in the US and Australia. Among a total of 352,384 participants, 13,284 cases of type 2 diabetes were identified during the 4–22 years of follow-up. The summary relative risk for the highest versus lowest category of rice intake was 1.27 (95% CI: 1.04–1.54), though significant heterogeneity was observed among studies. In stratified analysis by ethnicity, the association was stronger for Asian populations than for Western populations; the summary relative risks (95% CI) were 1.55 (1.20–2.01) for the former and 1.12 (0.94–1.33) for the latter. Moreover, a dose–response association between white rice intake and type 2 diabetes was observed; the relative risk for each serving per day increment of

white rice consumption was 1.11 (95% CI: 1.08–1.14; P for linear trend < 0.001). This meta-analysis suggests that higher white rice intake is associated with an increased risk of type 2 diabetes, especially among Asian populations. The authors ascribed the relatively weaker association for Western populations to much lower white rice intake, and thus a minor contribution of white rice to dietary glycemic load.

Since publication of the above meta-analysis, two prospective studies have reported the association between rice intake and type 2 diabetes.[13,16] In the Hong Kong Dietary Survey among 690 men and women aged 25–74 years,[16] 74 cases of type 2 diabetes were identified during the 9–14 years of follow-up. The mean (SD) of rice intake was 827.8 (867.3) g/week. The odds ratio of developing type 2 diabetes for 1 SD increase of rice intake (g/week) was 0.87 (95% CI: 0.67–1.13) after adjustment for sex, age, BMI, waist-to-hip ratio, current smoking status, alcohol intake, exercise/sports, and family history of diabetes. In another study among 605 Spanish adults (aged 18–65 years),[13] 54 cases of type 2 diabetes were diagnosed 6 years later. The odds ratio of a new diagnosis diabetes for category of rice intake two to three times per week was 0.43 (95% CI: 0.19–0.95) compared with category of rice intake once or less a week after adjustment for age, sex, obesity, and presence of impaired fasting glucose and/or impaired glucose tolerance at baseline. The two studies might have some limitations. First, the number of study subjects was small. Second, some important factors associated with type 2 diabetes were not adjusted for. For example, the latter study did not adjust for physical activity, smoking status, alcohol consumption, family history of diabetes, and total energy intake.[13]

Brown rice or whole grains have a lower GI than white rice.[6] Only one study examined the association for white rice and brown rice separately.[14] In that study, white rice was associated with increased risk of type 2 diabetes (P for trend < 0.001) (Fig. 26.4); the multivariable-adjusted odds ratio of type 2 diabetes for ≥ 5 servings/week was 1.17 (95% CI: 1.02–1.36) compared to < 1 serving/month. In contrast, brown rice intake was associated with decreased risk of type 2 diabetes (P for trend = 0.005); the multivariable-adjusted odds ratio for ≥ 2 servings/week was 0.89 (95% CI: 0.81–0.97) compared to < 1 serving/month. Moreover, when 50 g of white rice intake was replaced with the same amount of brown rice, the relative risk of type 2 diabetes decreased by 16%. The beneficial effect of brown rice might be explained by the fact that brown rice has lower GI and is rich in insoluble fiber, magnesium, other minerals, and vitamins than white rice. Insoluble fiber and magnesium have shown to be associated with decreased risk of type 2 diabetes.[21]

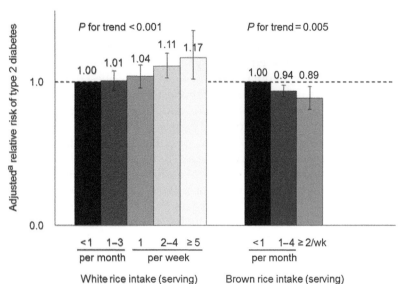

[a]Adjusted for age, ethnicity, body mass index, smoking status, alcohol intake, multivitamin use, physical activity, family history of diabetes, total energy intake, and intake of red meat, fruits and vegetables, whole grains, and coffee.

GLYCEMIC INDEX AND GLYCEMIC LOAD AND TYPE 2 DIABETES

The glycemic index, developed by Jenkins *et al.*,[8] is a measure of the effect of food intake on blood glucose concentrations. It is determined by comparison of the increase of postprandial blood glucose between each carbohydrate-containing food and a standard food (glucose or white bread per 50 g available carbohydrate). Glycemic load (GL) is the GI multiplied by the amount of carbohydrate. The GI of white rice varies by the species and cooking method, and ranges from 37–104 as a standard food of glucose.[6] A diet with a high GI increases blood glucose concentration and insulin demand, and could then contribute to higher risk of type 2 diabetes.[9] In addition, high intake of high GI carbohydrate is suggested to increase insulin resistance, at least in the short term.[9]

In 2011, the result of a meta-analysis was reported on the association between dietary GI or GL and type 2 diabetes risk.[7] Of 13 prospective studies included in that analysis, eight were conducted in the US, two in Europe, two in Australia, and one in China. Of 12 studies examining the association with GI, six observed a significant positive association. As regards GL, four studies out of 12 reported an increased risk of type 2 diabetes associated with higher GL. The summary relative risk of type 2 diabetes for the highest versus lowest category of GI was 1.16 (95% CI: 1.06–1.26; heterogeneity $I^2 = 50.8\%$; $P = 0.02$). The corresponding value for GL was 1.20 (95% CI: 1.11–1.30; heterogeneity $I^2 = 34.8\%$; $P = 0.10$). When

the analysis was limited to studies which adjusted for total fiber or cereal fiber, the significant positive association with GI or GL remained; the summary relative risks (95% CI) of type 2 diabetes for the highest versus lowest category of GI and GL were 1.14 (1.03–1.26) and 1.16 (1.05–1.29), respectively. The authors concluded that reducing the intake of high GI foods, particularly refined carbohydrates, may bring potential benefits in diabetes prevention among the general population.

After the publication of this meta-analysis, a Japanese study reported a prospective association between GI or GL and type 2 diabetes.[23] In that study, of 1995 male employees aged 35–55 years, 133 cases of diabetes were identified during 6 years of follow-up. Dietary GI was significantly associated with an increased risk of type 2 diabetes; the multivariable-adjusted hazard ratios (95% CI) of type 2 diabetes across quintile category of GI were 1.00 (reference), 1.71 (0.94–3.10), 1.66 (0.89–3.10), 1.86 (1.01–3.44), and 1.96 (1.04–3.67) after adjustment for age, BMI, family history of diabetes, smoking, alcohol intake, habitual exercise, and presence of hypertension and hyperlipidemia, total energy intake, and dietary total fiber intake. Dietary GL was not associated with type 2 diabetes risk. In stratified analyses by BMI (<22.0 kg/ m^2, 22.0–<25.0 kg/m^2, or ≥25.0 kg/m^2), insulin resistance (tertile of homeostasis model assessment-insulin resistance [HOMA-IR]), or insulin secretion (pancreatic β-cell function; tertile of HOMA-β) at baseline, high GI was significantly associated with increased risk of type 2 diabetes among men with BMI <22 kg/m^2 or the lowest tertile of HOMA-IR or HOMA-β. The multivariable-adjusted hazard ratios (95% CI) of type 2 diabetes across tertile of GI were 1.00 (reference), 4.09 (1.13–14.9), and 5.78 (1.63–20.5) among men with BMI < 22.0 kg/m^2 (P for trend = 0.005). The corresponding values were 1.00 (reference), 2.07 (0.61– 6.95), and 3.67 (1.21–11.2) among men in the lowest category of HOMA-IR (P for trend = 0.015), and 1.00 (reference), 1.64 (0.86–3.13), and 1.86 (1.01–3.44) among men in the lowest category of HOMA-β (P for trend = 0.049). In contrast, among men with BMI 22–< 25.0 kg/m^2 and ≥ 25.0 kg/m^2 or the middle and highest tertile of HOMA-IR or HOMA-β, such association was not observed.

CARBOHYDRATE INTAKE AND TYPE 2 DIABETES

Previously, 11 prospective studies have examined the association between carbohydrate intake and type 2 diabetes (Table 26.2). Of these, six studies were conducted in the US, three in Europe, one in Australia, and one in China. There was no study among Japanese. Most of these studies observed no association between carbohydrate intake and type 2 diabetes,[12,24–29] whereas some reported a positive[15,30,31] or inverse association.[32] In some studies, however, the results changed between models with and without adjustment for BMI, waist circumference, and dietary factors.[12,24,28,29,31] For example, in a study presenting no association in a fully adjusted model,[12] carbohydrate intake was significantly associated with decreased risk of type 2 diabetes before adjustment for BMI and waist circumference. This finding suggests that carbohydrate intake may increase type 2 diabetes risk via obesity. In another study,[31] carbohydrate intake was not associated with type 2 diabetes with adjustment for non-dietary factors. After additional adjustment for dietary factors such as total fiber, protein, saturated fat, polyunsaturated fat, and total energy intake, however, carbohydrate intake was significantly associated with increased risk of type 2 diabetes. The association between carbohydrate intake and type 2 diabetes risk might be confounded by other dietary factors.

These studies, except for the Chinese study, were conducted among Western populations, which have a much lower percentage of energy from carbohydrate than among Asian populations. The energy from carbohydrate intake was 60% of total energy intake in Japanese adults,[10] whereas it was around 40% of total energy intake among the Western populations.[24,28,29,32] Furthermore, as mentioned above, not only quantity but also quality of carbohydrate (GI and GL) may play a role in development of type 2 diabetes or glucose intolerance. The sources of carbohydrate were different between Asian and Western populations. In Japan, rice and processed rice account for 46.4% of the total carbohydrate intake. In contrast, among US adults, the major sources of carbohydrate were soft drinks and soda (13.9%), yeast breads and rolls (10.0%), cakes, cookies, quick bread pastry, and pie (8.3%), and candy, sugars and sugary foods (7.6%), while rice and cooked grains contribute 3.1% of the total carbohydrate intake. Given these differences in the amount and sources of carbohydrate between Asian and Western populations, the association among Asian populations may differ from that among Western populations. However, only one Asian study in China observed an increased risk of type 2 diabetes associated with carbohydrate intake,[15] and further studies to examine whether carbohydrate is associated with type 2 diabetes risk is required among Asian populations.

TABLE 26.2 Previous Prospective Studies that Examined the Association between Carbohydrate Intake and Type 2 Diabetes

First Author	Year	Country	No of Subjects	Age of Subjects (y)	Follow-up Period (y)	Type 2 Diabetes Risk Associated with Carbohydrate Intake
Salmeron et al.[26]	1997	US	42,759 men	40–75	6	No association
Salmeron et al.[27]	1997	US	65,173 women	40–65	6	No association
Meyer et al.[25]	2000	US	35,988 women	55–69	6	No association
Hodge et al.[12]	2004	Australia	36,787 men and women	40–69	4	No association
Schulze et al.[28]	2004	US	91,249 women	24–44	8	No association
Villegas et al.[15]	2007	China	64,227 women	40–70	4.6	Increased risk
Halton et al.[30]	2008	US	85,059 women	30–55	20	Increased risk
Schulze et al.[29]	2008	Germany	9702 men and 15,365 women	35–65	7–11	No association (in both sexes)
Sluijs et al.[31]	2010	The Netherlands	37,846 men and women	21–70	10	Increased risk
Simila et al.[32]	2012	Finland	25,943 non-smoker men	50–69	12	Decreased risk
Ericson et al.[24]	2012	US	10,550 men and 16,590 women	45–74	12	No association (in both sexes)

LOW-CARBOHYDRATE DIET SCORE AND TYPE 2 DIABETES

As mentioned previously, the association between carbohydrate intake and type 2 diabetes risk remains controversial. Nevertheless, low-carbohydrate diets are popular for weight loss. Recently, three studies have reported the association between low-carbohydrate diet score developed by Halton et al.[33] and type 2 diabetes risk.[30,34,35] As regards calculation of low-carbohydrate diet score,[33,34] first the percentages of energy from carbohydrate, protein, and fat were divided into 11 categories with equal sample sizes. Second, the carbohydrate categories were scored from 10 (lowest intake) to 0 (highest intake), whereas protein and fat categories were scored from 0 (lowest intake) to 10 (highest intake). Finally, ranks were added to create a total score with a maximum value of 30, which represented the highest intake of total protein and total fat and the lowest intake of carbohydrate.

In the Nurses' Health Study,[30] the low-carbohydrate diet score was significantly associated with increased risk of type 2 diabetes after adjustment for age, smoking status, postmenopausal hormone use, physical activity, alcohol intake, and family history of type 2 diabetes (P for trend <0.0001). However, the significant association disappeared after additional adjustment for BMI (P for trend=0.26). In that study, low-carbohydrate diet score was associated with higher BMI, and it is suggested that higher BMI is mediator of the association between low-carbohydrate diet and type 2 diabetes. Moreover, when separate scores were created for animal protein and fat and vegetable protein and fat, a low-carbohydrate and high-animal protein and fat score was not associated with increased risk of type 2 diabetes (P for trend=1.0), whereas a low-carbohydrate and high-vegetable protein and fat score was significantly associated with decreased risk (P for trend=0.001). In the Health Professionals Follow-Up Study,[34] although a low-carbohydrate diet score was significantly associated with increased risk of type 2 diabetes after adjustment for covariates including BMI (P for trend <0.01), the association was largely attenuated after adjustment for BMI. In addition, a low-carbohydrate and high-animal protein and fat score was significantly positively associated with type 2 diabetes risk. These findings suggest that replacing carbohydrate with protein and fat from animal food might be associated with increased risk of type 2 diabetes, but replacing carbohydrate with protein and fat from vegetable might be associated with decreased risk. However, a Chinese study did not support these findings in Western populations; a low-carbohydrate diet score was significantly associated with increased risk of type 2 diabetes, and a low-carbohydrate and high-plant protein and fat score was also associated with increased risk of type 2 diabetes risk.[35] Because few studies examined the association of low-carbohydrate diet score with type 2 diabetes risk, further investigation is required.

CONCLUSION

White rice intake may be associated with increased risk of developing type 2 diabetes, especially among Asian populations who consume a high amount of rice. Although rice is rich in carbohydrates, the association between carbohydrate intake and type 2 diabetes is controversial. There are very few studies which examined the association between rice or carbohydrate intake and type 2 diabetes among Asian populations including Japanese. In addition, it is possible that the association between rice or carbohydrate intake and type 2 diabetes risk among Asian populations might differ from that in Western populations due to the differences in the amount of rice intake and the amount or sources of carbohydrate intake between them. Therefore, further investigation in Asian populations is needed to confirm whether or not rice and carbohydrate intake contributes to the risk of developing type 2 diabetes. Moreover, for Japanese or other populations who consume rice as a major staple food, dietary modification strategies should be explored to prevent type 2 diabetes.

References

1. Kenko Eiyo Joho Kenkyukai. *The National Health and Nutrition Survey in Japan, 2007*. Tokyo, Japan: Daiichi-shuppan; 2010.
2. Huxley R, Omari A, Caterson ID. Obesity and diabetes. In: Ekoe JM, Rewers M, Williams R, Zimmet P, editors. *The epidemiology of diabetes mellitus*. 2nd ed. Oxford, UK: Wiley-Blackwell; 2008.
3. International Diabetes Federation. *IDF Diabetes Atlas* 4th ed. Available at: http://atlas.idf-bxl.org/map; 2009. [accessed 14.01.10].
4. Wright JD, Wang CY. Trends in intake of energy and macronutrients in adults from 1999–2000 through 2007–2008. *NCHS Data Brief* 2010;49:1–8.
5. Science and Technology Agency. *Standard Tables of Food Composition in Japan. 5th revised and enlarged ed*. Tokyo, Japan: Printing Bureau of the Ministry of Finance; 2005.
6. Foster-Powell K, Holt SH, Brand-Miller JC. International table of glycemic index and glycemic load values. *Am J Clin Nutr* 2002;76:5–56.
7. Dong JY, Zhang L, Zhang YH, Qin LQ. Dietary glycaemic index and glycaemic load in relation to the risk of type 2 diabetes: a meta-analysis of prospective cohort studies. *Br J Nutr* 2011;106:1649–54.
8. Jenkins DJ, Wolever TM, Taylor RH, Barker H, Fielden H, Baldwin JM, et al. Glycemic index of foods: a physiological basis for carbohydrate exchange. *Am J Clin Nutr* 1981;34:362–6.
9. Willett W, Manson J, Liu S. Glycemic index, glycemic load, and risk of type 2 diabetes. *Am J Clin Nutr* 2002;76:274S–80S.
10. Ministry of Health. Labour and Walfare, Japan. *The National Health and Nutrition Survey in Japan* 2011. Available at http://www.mhlw.go.jp/bunya/kenkou/eiyou/dl/h23-houkoku.pdf [accessed 27.03.13].
11. Murakami K, Sasaki S, Takahashi Y, Okubo H, Hosoi Y, Horiguchi H, et al. Dietary glycemic index and load in relation to metabolic risk factors in Japanese female farmers with traditional dietary habits. *Am J Clin Nutr* 2006;83:1161–9.

12. Hodge AM, English DR, O'Dea K, Giles GG. Glycemic index and dietary fiber and the risk of type 2 diabetes. *Diabetes Care* 2004;**27**:2701–6.

13. Soriguer F, Colomo N, Olveira G, Garcia-Fuentes E, Esteva I, Ruiz de Adana MS, et al. White rice consumption and risk of type 2 diabetes. *Clin Nutr* 2013;**32**:481–4.

14. Sun Q, Spiegelman D, van Dam RM, Holmes MD, Malik VS, Willett WC, et al. White rice, brown rice, and risk of type 2 diabetes in US men and women. *Arch Intern Med* 2010;**170**:961–9.

15. Villegas R, Liu S, Gao YT, Yang G, Li H, Zheng W, et al. Prospective study of dietary carbohydrates, glycemic index, glycemic load, and incidence of type 2 diabetes mellitus in middle-aged Chinese women. *Arch Intern Med* 2007;**167**:2310–6.

16. Yu R, Woo J, Chan R, Sham A, Ho S, Tso A, et al. Relationship between dietary intake and the development of type 2 diabetes in a Chinese population: the Hong Kong Dietary Survey. *Public Health Nutr* 2011;**14**:1133–41.

17. Nanri A, Mizoue T, Noda M, Takahashi Y, Kato M, Inoue M, et al. Rice intake and type 2 diabetes in Japanese men and women: the Japan Public Health Center-based Prospective Study. *Am J Clin Nutr* 2010;**92**:1468–77.

18. Tsugane S, Sobue T. Baseline survey of JPHC study – design and participation rate. Japan Public Health Center-based Prospective Study on Cancer and Cardiovascular Diseases. *J Epidemiol* 2001;**11**(Suppl. 6):S24–9.

19. Sasaki S, Kobayashi M, Ishihara J, Tsugane S. Self-administered food frequency questionnaire used in the 5-year follow-up survey of the JPHC Study: questionnaire structure, computation algorithms, and area-based mean intake. *J Epidemiol* 2003;**13**(Suppl. 1):S13–22.

20. Kato M, Noda M, Inoue M, Kadowaki T, Tsugane S. Psychological factors, coffee and risk of diabetes mellitus among middle-aged Japanese: a population-based prospective study in the JPHC study cohort. *Endocr J* 2009;**56**:459–68.

21. Schulze MB, Schulz M, Heidemann C, Schienkewitz A, Hoffmann K, Boeing H. Fiber and magnesium intake and incidence of type 2 diabetes: a prospective study and meta-analysis. *Arch Intern Med* 2007;**167**:956–65.

22. Hu EA, Pan A, Malik V, Sun Q. White rice consumption and risk of type 2 diabetes: meta-analysis and systematic review. *BMJ* 2012:**344** e1454.

23. Sakurai M, Nakamura K, Miura K, Takamura T, Yoshita K, Morikawa Y, et al. Dietary glycemic index and risk of type 2 diabetes mellitus in middle-aged Japanese men. *Metabolism* 2012;**61**:47–55.

24. Ericson U, Sonestedt E, Gullberg B, Hellstrand S, Hindy G, Wirfalt E, et al. High intakes of protein and processed meat associate with increased incidence of type 2 diabetes. *Br J Nutr* 2013;**109**:1143–53.

25. Meyer KA, Kushi LH, Jacobs Jr DR, Slavin J, Sellers TA, Folsom AR. Carbohydrates, dietary fiber, and incident type 2 diabetes in older women. *Am J Clin Nutr* 2000;**71**:921–30.

26. Salmeron J, Ascherio A, Rimm EB, Colditz GA, Spiegelman D, Jenkins DJ, et al. Dietary fiber, glycemic load, and risk of NIDDM in men. *Diabetes Care* 1997;**20**:545–50.

27. Salmeron J, Manson JE, Stampfer MJ, Colditz GA, Wing AL, Willett WC. Dietary fiber, glycemic load, and risk of non-insulin-dependent diabetes mellitus in women. *JAMA* 1997;**277**:472–7.

28. Schulze MB, Liu S, Rimm EB, Manson JE, Willett WC, Hu FB. Glycemic index, glycemic load, and dietary fiber intake and incidence of type 2 diabetes in younger and middle-aged women. *Am J Clin Nutr* 2004;**80**:348–56.

29. Schulze MB, Schulz M, Heidemann C, Schienkewitz A, Hoffmann K, Boeing H. Carbohydrate intake and incidence of type 2 diabetes in the European Prospective Investigation into Cancer and Nutrition (EPIC) – Potsdam Study. *Br J Nutr* 2008;**99**:1107–16.

30. Halton TL, Liu S, Manson JE, Hu FB. Low-carbohydrate-diet score and risk of type 2 diabetes in women. *Am J Clin Nutr* 2008;**87**:339–46.

31. Sluijs I, van der Schouw YT, van der AD, Spijkerman AM, Hu FB, Grobbee DE, et al. Carbohydrate quantity and quality and risk of type 2 diabetes in the European Prospective Investigation into Cancer and Nutrition-Netherlands (EPIC-NL) study. *Am J Clin Nutr* 2010;**92**:905–11.

32. Simila ME, Kontto JP, Valsta LM, Mannisto S, Albanes D, Virtamo J. Carbohydrate substitution for fat or protein and risk of type 2 diabetes in male smokers. *Eur J Clin Nutr* 2012;**66**:716–21.

33. Halton TL, Willett WC, Liu S, Manson JE, Albert CM, Rexrode K, et al. Low-carbohydrate-diet score and the risk of coronary heart disease in women. *N Engl J Med* 2006;**355**:1991–2002.

34. de Koning L, Fung TT, Liao X, Chiuve SE, Rimm EB, Willett WC, et al. Low-carbohydrate diet scores and risk of type 2 diabetes in men. *Am J Clin Nutr* 2011;**93**:844–50.

35. He YN, Feskens E, Li YP, Zhang J, Fu P, Ma GS, et al. Association between high fat-low carbohydrate diet score and newly diagnosed type 2 diabetes in Chinese population. *Biomed Environ Sci* 2012;**25**:373–82.

Rice and the Glycemic Index

*Un Jae Chang**, *Yang Hee Hong*[†], *Eun Young Jung****, *Hyung Joo Suh*[†]

*Dongduk Women's University, Department of Food and Nutrition, Seoul, South Korea, [†]Korea University, Department of Food and Nutrition Seoul, South Korea, **Jeonju University, Department of Home Economic Education, Jeollabuk-do, South Korea

INTRODUCTION

Carbohydrates should provide most of the total caloric intake, indicating their role as an essential macronutrient in human health. However, the calories provided by a specific glycemic carbohydrate component cannot be accurately assessed based on its quantity alone due to variations in the rate and extent of its digestion and absorption.[1] Therefore, the concept of the glycemic index (GI), a scale that ranks carbohydrate-rich foods by how much they raise blood glucose levels, was proposed by Jenkins et al.[2] to represent the physiological effect of carbohydrates in foods.

The GI is defined as the incremental area under the blood glucose curve (IAUC) of a 50-g carbohydrate portion of a test food expressed as a percentage of the response to 50 g carbohydrate of a standard food taken by the same subject, on a different day. The GI means how much each gram of available carbohydrate in a food raises blood glucose levels following consumption of the food, relative to consumption of pure glucose.[2] It can be used to describe scientifically the effects of carbohydrate-rich food on postprandial glucose in the blood. Although the GI of a food is determined by *in vivo* tests in which both food and human factors are involved, the digestion property of the carbohydrate component in the food is the ultimate determinant of the food's GI value.[3] Since the appearance of the GI concept, there have been extensive clinical and nutritional investigations on carbohydrates.[4] In general, low GI foods have been shown to have beneficial effects on glucose control, hyperinsulinemia, insulin resistance, blood lipids, and satiety, and hence could be helpful in preventing and managing obesity and diabetes.[5]

Starch is one of the most important glycemic carbohydrate components in foods, as it is supplied by traditional staple food materials and the many ingredients made from them that are incorporated into foods. The glycemic response to starchy foods has been the subject of much interest. The rates of digestion and absorption of glucose in the small intestine determine the GI of starchy foods.[6,7] For nutritional purposes, starch can be classified into rapidly digestible starch (RDS), slowly digestible starch (SDS), and resistant starch (RS) according to *in vitro* digestion.[8] The rate of starch digestion is directly related to glycemic responses, and the GI of food products is positively correlated with the amount of RDS.[9] SDS and RS will lead to slower glucose release and a lower glycemic response. RS in particular, being the indigestible starch portion in the stomach and digested in the small intestine, can help in body weight management, and in the prevention of heart disease, cancer, diabetes, and cardiovascular disease, as well as providing functional control of the GI.[10]

Rice (*Oryza sativa*) is of particular interest when assessing variability in starch digestibility. Rice contains about 76–78% starch, and is one of the primary dietary sources of carbohydrate worldwide.[11] Rice has delivered a wide range of results in the GI studies; the glycemic indexes of rice varieties have ranged from as low as 48 for the Australian Doongara white rice variety to 109 for Thailand Jasmine polished white long grain rice.[12–14] This wide variability in the GI of rice makes it impossible to state categorically that rice is either a low GI food or a high GI food. In some of these studies rice was classified as a low GI food, whereas others assigned it to the high GI category. This variation has been attributed to a multitude of factors, including amylose content, dietary fiber content, physical size and form, post-harvest treatments (parboiling and milling), and cooking (gelatinization).[13,15,16] The awareness of the general public regarding health foods

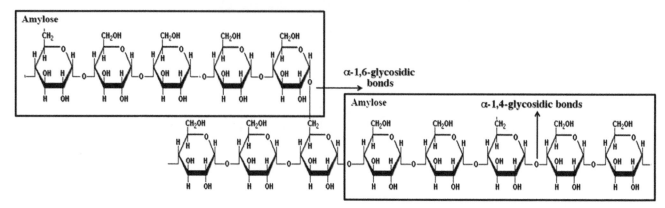

FIGURE 27.1   Structures of amylose and amylopectin.

has been on the rise recently, and people are looking for the right variety of rice and more efficient methods of cooking it.

GI and the Amylose Content of Rice

Rice contains two types of starch; amylose and amylopectin (Fig. 27.1). High amylose starch is reported to be more resistant than amylopectin to starch digestion because of its compact linear structure.[17,18] Amylose is a long, straight starch molecule that does not gelatinize during microwave cooking, and hence rice with a greater amylose content tends to be fluffy, with separate grains, after cooking. Moreover, amylose hardens and forms crystals during cooking and melts when the rice is reheated.[19] Rice varieties with a high amylose content are reported to raise blood glucose less than rice with a higher amylopectin content; rice that is high in amylose has a lower GI.[14] This is because amylose is harder to break down than simple sugars such as glucose, etc., and ensures a sustained release of sugar into the blood without spiking immediately after a meal. Studies have demonstrated that the structure of amylose affects the digestibility rate (Table 27.1).[20,21] Long-chain amylose is associated with slowly digestible starch. It is thought that much of the variation in the GI of rice is due to differences in the proportion of starch present as amylose – i.e., the amylose:amylopectin ratio.

The amylose content of rice varies between 0% and 40%. Most rices contain 20% amylase, but varieties that contain a higher proportion of amylose have been shown to have a slower rate of digestion and produce lower glycemic responses.[22] Miller *et al.*[23] determined the GI for three commercial varieties of rice (two varieties with a normal amylose content of 20%, and the other with 28% amylase) and a waxy rice (0–2% amylose). They observed that the rice with a higher amylose content (Doongara, 28% amylose) gave a significantly lower GI than did the normal amylase rice varieties (Calrose and Pelde, 20% amylose). The waxy rice with 0–2% amylose had a GI

TABLE 27.1   Amylose Content and Starch Digestibility Values (% of Total Starch) of Various Rices[20,21]

Rice	Amylose	TS	RDS	SDS	RS	Reference
Doongara	31.1	82.1	12.7	56.5	12.9	Sagum and Arcot[21]
Inga	20.2	83.6	21.7	52.7	9.2	
Japonica	11.5	83.2	60.1	14.6	8.6	
RU0201142	16.5	79.7	61.7	10.9	7.0	Benmoussa *et al.*[20]
CCDR	15.8	75.3	48.5	19.1	8.5	

TS, total starch; RDS, rapidly digestible starch; SDS, slowly digestible starch; RS, resistant starch. Values are mean ± standard deviation.

similar to that of those containing normal amounts of amylose. The relationship between amylose content and the GI of rice may be exponential rather than linear.[14] Rice varieties high in amylose have been shown to have lower starch digestion rates and glycemic responses than do rice varieties low in amylose[19,23,24] (Table 27.2).

Processing may alter amylose properties in the rice and affect the GI. Rashmi and Urooj[25] reported an inverse correlation between the amylose content and the starch digestion index of rice. They observed a qualitative alteration in amylose when rice was cooked by pressure-cooking, boiling, steaming, and straining, suggesting a processing effect on amylose. Amylose values in cooked rice are lower than the values for raw rice. This may be due to the redistribution of starch fractions that is known to occur during processing, including cooking.[22,26]

GI AND THE DIETARY FIBER CONTENT OF RICE

The correlation between the dietary fiber and the glycemic index was reported[14] (Fig. 27.2). It was suggested that the dietary fiber as well as the amylose in rice has a significant role on the GI. Amylose has a linear structure

TABLE 27.2 Correlation between Amylose Content and Glycemic Index of Rice[24]

Amylose Content	Glycemic Index
High	Low glycemic index, and the rice grains will show high volume expansion (not necessarily elongation) and a high degree of flakiness. The rice grains cook dry, are less tender, and become hard upon cooling.
Low	High glycemic index, and the rice grains will cook moist and sticky.

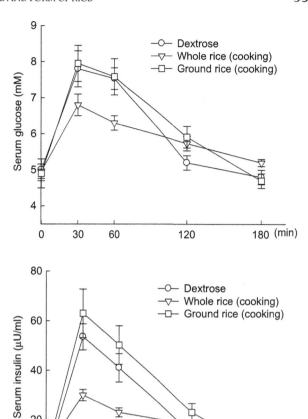

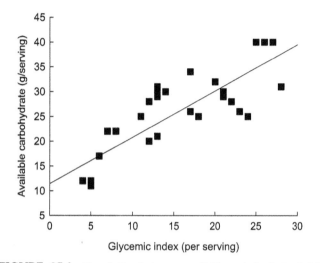

FIGURE 27.2 Correlation between available carbohydrate (total carbohydrate minus the dietary fiber) and the glycemic index.[14]

FIGURE 27.3 Serum glucose and insulin concentrations after ingestion of whole rice and ground rice.[34] Values are means ± standard deviation.

and readily undergoes staling after cooking. The resultant resistant starch is then metabolized similarly to the dietary fiber in the large intestine or colon. In conclusion, the presence of amylose and dietary fiber in rice affects glucose response and the GI. The combined effect of amylose and dietary fiber contributes significantly to the low glycemic response and the GI in rice.[14,27]

High dietary fiber was shown to produce lower blood glucose responses than low dietary fiber.[28,29] Perhaps the most important feature of the dietary fiber hypothesis is that it focused attention on events occurring in the gastrointestinal tract and provided a rationale for the relationship between the rate of starch digestion and the glycemic response.[17] The low glycemic response to high dietary fiber was thought to be due to a reduced rate of gastric emptying and a reduced rate of small intestinal absorption.[30,31] In an *in vitro* digestion system designed by Jenkins *et al.*,[32] it was shown that the rate of release of starch digestion products from a dialysis bag containing a sample of the food and digestive enzymes was related to the glycemic response. Soluble fiber in particular provides a better predictive capability of the glycemic response than does total dietary fiber content or insoluble fiber content.[33]

GI AND THE PARTICLE SIZE AND FORM OF RICE

The particle size and form of rice are other factors that may affect the GI, resulting in a change in the rate of digestion and the subsequent blood glucose profile of rice[17,34] (Fig. 27.3). O'Dea *et al.*[35] noted that ground rice resulted in a significantly higher glycemic response than that seen with whole rice. They suggested that a higher surface area–starch ratio resulted in an increased rate of starch hydrolysis *in vivo*. *In vitro* digestion of ground and unground rice showed that ground rice was digested more quickly than unground rice. After incubation with pancreatic amylase for 30 minutes, unground rice was 30.8% hydrolyzed while ground rice was 71.8% hydrolyzed.[6] Booher *et al.*[36] also reported that conditions which increase the digestibility of rice include modifications that produce obvious hydration of the granules, and disruption of the organized granule structure.

GI AND POST-HARVEST TREATMENT OF RICE: PARBOILING AND MILLING

The GI of pretreated rice may vary depending on the degree of processing. Parboiling, the steam-pressure treatment, is an optional processing step prior to milling. Parboiling includes soaking of the rice until it reaches saturation, heat treatment until the starch is gelatinized, then slow drying before the husk is removed. Various modernized processes have been developed in which the processing time is reduced by using warmer soaking temperatures and applying pressure during the heat treatment. Parboiling leads to profound changes in the rice kernels, including alterations in the starch fraction, which may affect the rate of digestion and absorption as well as the overall digestibility. Moreover, it appears that the type and degree of these alterations depend on the severity of the method applied.[37,38] Parboiling is generally believed to lower the GI of rice. Wolever and Jenkuns[39] were the first to bring attention to the subject. They investigated two commercially obtained rice samples and found a lower GI in the parboiled rice sample compared to the non-parboiled sample. Later studies compared parboiled and non-parboiled rice of the same variety. The finding was confirmed by that of Larsen et al.,[40] where a severely pressure-parboiled rice showed a significant reduction in the GI as compared with its non-parboiled counterpart. Casiraghi et al.[41] also observed that parboiling lowered the GI of rice. Milling is the process that creates the difference between brown and white rice. Limited studies regarding the effects of brown rice (unmilled or partly milled rice) compared with white rice (milled rice) on GI have shown contradictory results; some indicated that brown rice had a lower rate of starch digestion and glycemic response, while others reported no difference.[2,6,23] Brand-Miller et al.[23] (Table 27.3) reported the same GI for both white and brown Calrose rice, and the same GI for both white and brown Doongara rice, while the GI of Pelde brown rice was lower at 76 and higher for white rice at 93. In these studies, rice samples were not controlled; that is,

commercially available white rice was taken at random and not milled from the same batch of brown rice. Hence the variety and physicochemical properties of the rice samples may have differed. Cooking conditions for both white rice and brown rice were also widely different, with no given basis for such conditions. Recently, Panlasigui and Thompson[42] determined the rate of starch digestion and blood glucose response to white and brown rice prepared from the same batch and variety of rough rice and cooked, based on their physicochemical properties. They observed that in healthy volunteers the GI was 12.1% lower in brown rice than white rice, while in diabetics the GI was 35.6% lower in brown rice. The effect was partly due to the higher amounts of phytic acid, polyphenols, dietary fiber, and oil in brown rice compared to white rice, and the difference in some physicochemical properties of the rice samples, such as minimum cooking time and degree of gelatinization. White rice has shorter minimum cooking time and higher volume expansion than brown rice, indicating that white rice is more easily hydrated and gelatinized compared with brown rice. This was confirmed by the lower amylograph viscosity peak and consistency of brown rice compared with white rice. Evidently, the bran that envelops the rice kernels can act as a barrier against entry of water and impede the swelling of the starch granules during heat treatment. It is likely that the dietary fiber-rich bran fraction continues to serve as a barrier to digestive enzyme action.[42] Phytic acid and polyphenols, which are more concentrated in the bran layer, may also have contributed to the slow starch digestion rate and lower blood glucose response. Previous studies have shown a negative relationship between phytic acid intake and blood glucose response.[43,44] The removal of phytic acid from navy beans has been shown to increase the starch digestion rate and blood glucose response, while the addition of phytic acid to the dephytinized navy bean or white bread[43,44] has been shown to decrease it. Phytic acid is thought to reduce the starch digestion rate by binding the amylase enzyme (which needs calcium for its activity) either with proteins closely associated with the starch, or with the starch through phosphate links.[39,45] Polyphenol intake has also been shown to relate negatively to glycemic response[46] and may act in a similar manner to the phytic acid by binding with proteins closely associated with the starch or with the luminal and brush border enzymes.[39] Phytosterols, gammaoryzanols, tocopherols, and tocotrienols, which are high in rice bran and oil, have also been suggested to have hypoglycemic and hypoinsulinemic effects.[47] A greater significant effect was observed *in vivo* than *in vitro*, indicating the involvement of physiological mechanisms for the reduced blood glucose response other than just reduced starch digestibility. That the above components, rich in the bran, may influence glycemic response was

TABLE 27.3 Glycemic Indexes of Brown Rice and White Rice[23]

	Rice	Glycemic Index
Calrose	Brown	87 ± 8
	White	83 ± 13
Pelde	Brown	76 ± 6
	White	93 ± 11
Doongara	Brown	66 ± 7
	White	64 ± 9

Values are means ± standard error of the mean.

also evident when reduced GI was observed when rice bran was fed to healthy[23] or diabetic volunteers.[47]

GI AND THE COOKING OF RICE: GELATINIZATION

Rice is processed for consumption in a variety of ways, such as boiling, pressure-cooking, and steaming.[48] Cooking of rice usually results in gelatinization of the granules.[49–51] Disruption of the structure of native starch by gelatinization (i.e., swelling of the granules in the presence of heat and water) increases its susceptibility to enzymatic degradation *in vitro* and its availability for digestion and absorption in the small intestine.[49,50] A more prominent rise in blood glucose has thus been reported with consumption of cooked as opposed to raw starch. Consequently, the glucose response was found to be significantly higher after ingestion of cooked starch but not raw starch from wheat,[52] corn,[49] or potato,[53] as well as rice.[54,55] The rice with a relatively low degree of gelatinization resulted in low metabolic responses with the GI[56] (Table 27.4). The cooking of rice seems to be affected sufficiently to render the starch easily available for digestion and absorption in the small intestine, thus resulting in high glucose responses. Sajilata *et al.*[57] reported that boiling, pressure-cooking, and steaming increase the resistant starches that resist digestion by α-amylase in the small intestine. Lee and Oh[58] reported a significant reduction in the GI of resistant starch-containing meals when compared with a white wheat bread diet. The level of resistant starches present in carbohydrate foods depends on several factors, such as processing (treatment temperature, time of heat exposure, rate of cooling) and storage conditions (temperature).[57] Numerous processing conditions and storage in a cool environment may result in up to 30% starch retrogradation – that is, crystallization of the amorphous system created by gelatinization.[59] Ranawana *et al.*[16] suggested that the gelatinized starch has not undergone sufficient retrogradation, resulting in a higher availability of digestible starch for gastrointestinal enzymes.

Rice varieties, even those with similar amylose content, were shown to vary widely in their gelling properties when heat treated.[60–62] Panlasigui *et al.*[54] determined the rate of starch digestion and the blood glucose responses to three varieties of long grain, non-waxy (non-glutinous) rice (IR62, IR36, and IR42), all with comparable high amylose contents, and whether the differences were related to their physicochemical properties. They observed that the starch digestion rate and glycemic responses were highest in IR42, followed by IR36 and then IR62. The differences were not due to unabsorbed carbohydrate but were related to their physicochemical properties, such as gelatinization temperature, minimum cooking time, amylograph consistency, and volume expansion upon cooking.[16,54,63] They concluded that amylose content alone was not a good predictor of the starch digestion rate or glycemic response. Rice varieties with similar high amylose contents can differ in physicochemical (gelatinization) properties, and these in turn can influence starch digestibility and the blood glucose response.

These results indicate that amylose content alone may not be a good predictor of the digestion rate and the GI of rice; the physicochemical properties of rice may also exert an influence. There are many other factors that influence the GI of rice, including amylose content, dietary fiber content, physical size and form, post-harvest treatments (parboiling and milling), and cooking (gelatinization). Because rice is a staple food in many parts of the world, it is important to study the factors that may help predict its GI. The GI of rice cannot be predicted easily; *in vivo* studies conducted on humans are the only way to accurately determine the GI of rice. We suggest that the identification and classification of the commonly consumed rice varieties into low GI, medium GI, or high GI foods will enable selection rice with a low GI, thereby minimizing and/or preventing the development of chronic diseases, notably diabetes.

TABLE 27.4 Glycemic Indexes of Cooked Rice (CR), Uncooked Rice Powder (UP), and Uncooked Freeze-Dried Rice Powder (UFP)[56]

	CR	UP	UFP
Carbohydrate (g)	50	50	50
Degree of gelatinization (%)	76.9 ± 1.8	3.5 ± 1.4	5.4 ± 2.2
Glycemic index (%)	72.4 ± 9.5	49.7 ± 7.7	59.8 ± 9.2
Insulin index (%)	94.8 ± 5.1	74.4 ± 8.2	68.0 ± 9.7

Values are mean ± standard deviation.

References

1. Englyst KN, Vinoy S, Englyst HN, Lang V. Glycaemic index of cereal products explained by their content of rapidly and slowly available glucose. *Br J Nutr* 2003;**89**(3):329–40.

2. Jenkins D, Wolever T, Taylor RH, et al. Glycemic index of foods: a physiological basis for carbohydrate exchange. *Am J Clin Nutr* 1981;**34**(3):362–6.

3. Wolever TMS, Yang M, Zeng XY, et al. Food glycemic index, as given in glycemic index tables, is a significant determinant of glycemic responses elicited by composite breakfast meals. *Am J Clin Nutr* 2006;**83**(6):1306–12.

4. Wolever T. Carbohydrate and the regulation of blood glucose and metabolism. *Nutr Rev* 2003;**61**:S40–8.

5. Augustin L, Franceschi S, Jenkins D, et al. Article 31: Glycemic index in chronic disease: a review. *Eur J Clin Nutr* 2002;**56**:1049–71.

6. O'Dea K, Snow P, Nestel P. Rate of starch hydrolysis *in vitro* as a predictor of metabolic responses to complex carbohydrate *in vivo*. *Am J Clin Nutr* 1981;**34**(10):1991–3.

7. Englyst HN, Veenstra J, Hudson GJ. Measurement of rapidly available glucose (RAG) in plant foods: a potential *in vitro* predictor of the glycaemic response. *Br J Nutr* 1996;**75**(3):327–38.

8. Englyst HN, Hudson GJ. The classification and measurement of dietary carbohydrates. *Food Chem* 1996;**57**(1):15–21.

9. Englyst KN, Englyst HN, Hudson GJ, et al. Rapidly available glucose in foods: an *in vitro* measurement that reflects the glycemic response. *Am J Clin Nutr* 1999;**69**(3):448–54.

10. Nugent A. Health properties of resistant starch. *Nutr Bull* 2005;**30**(1):27–54.

11. Frei M, Siddhuraju P, Becker K. Studies on the *in vitro* starch digestibility and the glycemic index of six different indigenous rice cultivars from the Philippines. *Food Chem* 2003;**83**(3):395–402.

12. Brand JC, Nicholson PL, Thorburn AW. Food processing and the glycemic index. *Am J Clin Nutr* 1985;**42**(6):1192–6.

13. Jenkins DJA, Wolever T, Jenkins AL. Starchy foods and glycemic index. *Diabetes care* 1988;**11**(2):149–59.

14. Foster-Powell K, Holt SHA, Brand-Miller JC. International table of glycemic index and glycemic load values: 2002. *Am J Clin Nutr* 2002;**76**(1):5–56.

15. Ludwig DS. The glycemic index. *JAMA* 2002;**287**(18):2414–23.

16. Ranawana D, Henry C, Lightowler H, Wang D. Glycaemic index of some commercially available rice and rice products in Great Britain. *Int J Food Sci Nutr* 2009;**60**(s4):99–110.

17. Thorne MJ, Thompson L, Jenkins D. Factors affecting starch digestibility and the glycemic response with special reference to legumes. *Am J Clin Nutr* 1983;**38**(3):481–8.

18. Hoover R, Manuel H. Effect of heat–moisture treatment on the structure and physicochemical properties of legume starches. *Food Res Int* 1996;**29**(8):731–50.

19. Chiu CJ, Liu S, Willett WC, Wolever T. Informing food choices and health outcomes by use of the dietary glycemic index. *Nutr Rev* 2011;**69**(4):231–42.

20. Benmoussa M, Moldenhauer KAK, Hamaker BR. Rice amylopectin fine structure variability affects starch digestion properties. *J Agric Food Chem* 2007;**55**(4):1475–9.

21. Sagum R, Arcot J. Effect of domestic processing methods on the starch, non-starch polysaccharides and *in vitro* starch and protein digestibility of three varieties of rice with varying levels of amylose. *Food Chem* 2000;**70**(1):107–11.

22. Juliano BO, Goddard MS. Cause of varietal difference in insulin and glucose responses to ingested rice. *Plant Foods Hum Nutr (Formerly Qualitas Plantarum)* 1986;**36**(1):35–41.

23. Miller JB, Pang E, Bramall L. Rice: a high or low glycemic index food? *Am J Clin Nutr* 1992;**56**(6):1034–6.

24. Jain A, Rao SM, Sethi S, et al. Effect of cooking on amylose content of rice. *Eur J Exp Biol* 2012;**2**(2):385–8.

25. Rashmi S, Urooj A. Effect of processing on nutritionally important starch fractions in rice varieties. *Int J Food Sci Nutr* 2003;**54**(1):27–36.

26. Goddard MS, Young G, Marcus R. The effect of amylose content on insulin and glucose responses to ingested rice. *Am J Clin Nutr* 1984;**39**(3):388–92.

27. Björck I, Liljeberg H, Östman E. Low glycaemic-index foods. *Br J Nutr* 2000;**83**(S1):S149–55.

28. Jenkins D, Leeds AR, Gassull MA, Cochet B, Alberti GM. Decrease in postprandial insulin and glucose concentrations by guar and pectin. *Ann Intern Med* 1977;**86**(1):20.

29. Potter JG, Coffman KP, Reid RL, et al. Effect of test meals of varying dietary fiber content on plasma insulin and glucose response. *Am J Clin Nutr* 1981;**34**(3):328–34.

30. Leeds A, Ebied F, Ralphs D, et al. Pectin in the dumping syndrome: reduction of symptoms and plasma volume changes. *Lancet* 1981;**317**(8229):1075–8.

31. Elsenhans B, Süfke U, Blume R, Caspary W, et al. The influence of carbohydrate gelling agents on rat intestinal transport of monosaccharides and neutral amino acids *in vitro*. *Clin sci* 1980;**59**(5):373.

32. Jenkins DJA, Ghafarai H, Wolever TMS, et al. Relationship between rate of digestion of foods and post-prandial glycaemia. *Diabetologia* 1982;**22**(6):450–5.

33. Wolever TMS, Jenkins DJA. Effect of dietary fiber and foods on carbohydrate metabolism. *CRC Handb Dietary Fiber Hum Nutr* 1993;**1993**:111–52.

34. Im SS, Kim MH, Sung CJ, Lee JH. The effect of cooking form of rice and barley on the postprandial serum glucose and insulin responses in normal subject. *J Korean Soc Food Nutr* 1991;**20**(4):293–9.

35. O'Dea K, Nestel P, Antonoff L. Physical factors influencing postprandial glucose and insulin responses to starch. *Am J Clin Nutr* 1980;**33**(4):760–5.

36. Booher LE, Behan I, McMeans E, Boyd H. Biologic Utilizations of Unmodified and Modified Food Starches Ten Figures. *J Nutr* 1951;**45**(1):75–99.

37. Biliaderis CG, Tonogai JR, Perez CM, Juliano BO. Thermophysical properties of milled rice starch as influenced by variety and parboiling method. *Cereal chem* 1993:**70**.

38. Ong M, Blanshard J. Texture determinants of cooked, parboiled rice. II: Physicochemical properties and leaching behaviour of rice. *J Cereal Sci* 1995;**21**(3):261–9.

39. Wolever TM, Jenkins D. The use of the glycemic index in predicting the blood glucose response to mixed meals. *Am J Clin Nutr* 1986;**43**(1):167–72.

40. Larsen H, Rasmussen O, Rasmussen PH, et al. Glycaemic index of parboiled rice depends on the severity of processing: study in type 2 diabetic subjects. *Eur J Clin Nutr* 2000;**54**(5):380–5.

41. Casiraghi MC, Brighenti F, Pellegrini N, et al. Effect of Processing on Rice Starch Digestibility Evaluated by *in vivo* and *in vitro* methods. *J Cereal Sci* 1993;**17**(2):147–56.

42. Panlasigui LN, Thompson LU. Blood glucose lowering effects of brown rice in normal and diabetic subjects. *Int J Food Sci Nutr* 2006;**57**(3–4):151–8.

43. Yoon JH, Thompson LU, Jenkins D. The effect of phytic acid on *in vitro* rate of starch digestibility and blood glucose response. *Am J Clin Nutr* 1983;**38**(6):835–42.

44. Thompson LU, Button CL, Jenkins D. Phytic acid and calcium affect the *in vitro* rate of navy bean starch digestion and blood glucose response in humans. *Am J Clin Nutr* 1987;**46**(3):467–73.

45. Thompson L. Antinutrients and blood glucose. *Food Technol* 1988;**42**(4):123–32.

46. Thompson L, Yoon J, Jenkins D, et al. Relationship between polyphenol intake and blood glucose response of normal and diabetic individuals. *Am J Clin Nutr* 1984;**39**(5):745–51.

47. Qureshi AA, Sami SA, Khan FA. Effects of stabilized rice bran, its soluble and fiber fractions on blood glucose levels and serum lipid parameters in humans with diabetes mellitus Types I and II. *J Nutr Biochem* 2002;**13**(3):175–87.

48. Juliano BO, Hicks PA. Rice functional properties and rice food products. *Food Rev Int* 1996;**12**(1):71–103.

49. Collings P, Williams C, MacDonald I. Effects of cooking on serum glucose and insulin responses to starch. *BMJ (Clinical research edn)* 1981;**282**(6269):1032–1032.

50. Annison G, Topping DL. Nutritional role of resistant starch: chemical structure vs physiological function. *Annu Rev Nutr* 1994;**14**(1):297–320.

51. Sakuma M, Yamanaka-Okumura H, Naniwa Y, et al. Dose-dependent effects of barley cooked with white rice on postprandial glucose and desacyl ghrelin levels. *J Clin Biochem Nutr* 2009;**44**(2):151.

52. Marangoni F, Poli A. The glycemic index of bread and biscuits is markedly reduced by the addition of a proprietary fiber mixture to the ingredients. *Nutrition, Metab Cardiovasc Dis* 2008;**18**(9):602–5.

53. Vaaler S, Hanssen KF, Aagenæs Ø. The effect of cooking upon the blood glucose response to ingested carrots and potatoes. *Diabetes care* 1984;**7**(3):221–3.

54. Panlasigui LN, Thompson LUl, Juliano BO, et al. Rice varieties with similar amylose content differ in starch digestibility and glycemic response in humans. *Am J Clin Nutr* 1991;**54**(5):871–7.

55. Wallace AJ, Monro JA, Brown RC, Frampton CM. A glucose reference curve is the optimum method to determine the glycemic glucose equivalent values of foods in humans. *Nutr Res* 2008;**28**(11):753–9.

56. Jung EY, Suh HJ, Hong WS, et al. Uncooked rice of relatively low gelatinization degree resulted in lower metabolic glucose and insulin responses compared with cooked rice in female college students. *Nutr Res* 2009;**29**(7):457–61.

57. Sajilata M, Singhal RS, Kulkarni PR. Resistant starch–a review. *Compr Rev food sci food saf* 2006;**5**(1):1–17.

58. Lee YH, Oh SH. Effect of resistant starch on human glycemic response. *Korean J Community Nutr* 2004;**9**(4):528–35.

59. Faraj A, Vasanthan T, Hoover R. The effect of extrusion cooking on resistant starch formation in waxy and regular barley flours. *Food Res Int* 2004;**37**(5):517–25.

60. Juliano BO, Perez CM. Major factors affecting cooked milled rice hardness and cooking time. *J texture Stud* 2007;**14**(3):235–43.

61. Bhattacharya M, Zee S, Corke H. Physicochemical properties related to quality of rice noodles. *Cereal Chem* 1999;**76**(6):861–7.

62. Perez CM, Juliano BO. Indicators of eating quality for non-waxy rices. *Food Chem* 1979;**4**(3):185–95.

63. Brouns F, Bjorck I, Frayn K, et al. Glycaemic index methodology. *Nutr Res Rev* 2005;**18**(1):145.

Arsenic in Rice: Sources and Human Health Risk

Mohammad Azizur Rahman[*], *Mohammad Mahmudur Rahman*[†], *Ravi Naidu*[†]

[*]University of Technology, Centre for Environmental Sustainability, Faculty of Science, Sydney, New South Wales, Australia, [†]University of South Australia, Center for Environmental Risk Assessment and Remediation (CERAR), Mawson Lakes, South Australia, Australia; and Cooperative Research Centre for Contamination Assessment and Remediation of the Environment (CRC-CARE), Salisbury South, South Australia, Australia

INTRODUCTION

Arsenic is ubiquitous in the environment,[1] and is released to it through natural phenomena and anthropogenic inputs. Arsenic is also redistributed in the environment by rain, underground water, and human activities. Although arsenic in the environment comes mainly from minerals and geogenic sources, human activities such as mining, burning of fossil fuels, and indiscriminate use of arsenical pesticides during the early to mid-1900s resulted in extensive soil contamination.[2] A large number of sites around the globe have been reported to be contaminated by arsenic from natural and anthropogenic sources.[3,4] Widespread human exposure to arsenic from drinking water and foods, and associated incidences of human health hazards (non-carcinogenic effects, including dermal symptoms, respiratory problems, neurologic complications, obstetric effects, etc., and carcinogenic effects on different organs, affecting the skin, lung, bladder, liver etc.) have been a growing concern during the past three decades globally.[4,5] Arsenic in groundwater has been reported in many parts of the world, including North America, Europe, Australia, and several Latin American countries.[5–8] However, groundwater contamination with elevated levels of arsenic and associated health problems has reached critical levels in recent years in several South (S) and Southeast (SE) Asian countries.[9]

Arsenic-contaminated groundwater is used not only for drinking purposes but also for the irrigation of crops in these countries, particularly for the staple food, paddy rice (*Oryza sativa* L.), in Bangladesh and other S and SE Asian countries.[10,11] Groundwater has been used extensively, particularly during the dry season, to irrigate rice in Bangladesh.[11] Background levels of arsenic in paddy soils range from 4 to 8 mg/kg,[12,13] and can reach up to 83 mg/kg in areas where the paddy field has been irrigated with elevated levels of arsenic-contaminated groundwater.[13] Other countries in S and SE Asia affected with arsenic in groundwater include several states of India, Nepal, Myanmar, Pakistan, Vietnam, Lao People's Democratic Republic, Cambodia, Taiwan, and several provinces of China,[6,9,14–16] and, more recently, the lowlands of Sumatra in Indonesia.[17] Surface-water contamination of arsenic in Thailand is mainly due to industrial activities.[4] In Bangladesh and the West Bengal state of India, arsenic in groundwater has been recognized as the widest environmental and human health disaster, with an estimate of more than 100 million people at risk from arsenic poisoning,[4,18] while about 700,000 people have already been affected by arsenic-related diseases in S and SE Asia.[19]

Because of high levels of arsenic in paddy soils, from contaminated underground irrigation water,[11,13] rice contains relatively higher amounts of arsenic[20–22] compared to other agricultural crops.[23,24] The concentration of arsenic and its chemical forms in rice varies considerably depending on rice variety[25] and geographical variation.[20,26] Inorganic arsenic (iAs) species dominate over organo-arsenic (orgAs) species in both uncooked rice and cooked rice,[27] and the dietary intake of arsenic in the human body depends on the type of rice consumed and on the cooking process used.[28–32] A large population in Asian arsenic-endemic areas lives on a subsistence diet of rice. As well as daily water consumption of 4–6 L,[33] the average daily rice consumption by an adult of this region, particularly in Bangladesh and West Bengal (India), is between 400 and 650 g.[34] Therefore, second to water, rice constitutes the largest dietary source of arsenic for humans.[35] When the high concentration of iAs,[36] cooking method, and high consumption rate are taken into account, rice is considered to be a major threat to human health in arsenic-endemic S and SE Asia.

Arsenic poisoning is greatest in Bangladesh, followed by West Bengal, India. However, numerous cases have now been reported from many countries, including Chile, Cambodia, Laos, Burma, Pakistan, Nepal, Vietnam, Taiwan, Iran, Argentina, Finland, the United States, several provinces in China, and several other Indian states. Arsenic exposure to humans is not restricted to the arsenic-contaminated countries. Hundreds of thousands of people worldwide are also facing slow poisoning and risk of death from arsenic in their daily diets. The possibility of human exposure to arsenic is increasing with the expansion of the global food trade. Arsenic in foods from arsenic-endemic areas will pose a potential health risk for the people of those countries where arsenic contamination of drinking water is not reported. Thus, arsenic in foods and its subsequent impacts on human health is not a regional issue but an important global issue. In this chapter, the sources of arsenic in rice and the health risk of arsenic from a rice diet are discussed.

ARSENIC IN RICE GRAIN

The significant number of articles published on arsenic concentrations in rice grain in recent years implies that the dietary intake of arsenic form rice has received the attention of the wider scientific community.[13,27,30,36–42] The high arsenic content in rice is a significant concern for arsenic-affected countries, as well as for countries that import rice from arsenic-affected countries. Arsenic concentrations in rice grain from diverse origins is presented in Table 28.1.[11,13,20,21,23,27,39,43–54]

Bangladesh is one of the highly arsenic-contaminated countries.[55] Rice grain collected from the arsenic-contaminated western part of Bangladesh had arsenic levels of 0.03–1.84 µg/g dry weight (dry wt).[11] In another study, arsenic concentrations in rice collected from the fields of the southern part of Bangladesh were found to be between 0.04 and 0.92 µg/g dry wt.[13] However, arsenic concentrations in rice collected from markets across the country were found to be 0.18–0.31 µg/g dry wt.[13] It is interesting that arsenic concentrations in rice vary with the sampling site and rice growing season, both of which are related to the arsenic concentration in irrigation water. Other studies also showed high levels of arsenic in Bangladeshi rice. For example, Islam et al.[56] reported 0.05–2.05 µg/g dry wt of arsenic in rice grain collected from southern Bangladesh, while Rahman

et al.[30] reported 0.57–0.69 µg/g dry wt of arsenic in rice collected from a highly arsenic-contaminated area of the country. All these studies have revealed high arsenic levels in Bangladeshi rice grain.

Rice from the Indian state of West Bengal also contains high levels of arsenic. Williams et al.[27] reported 0.05 µg/g dry wt of arsenic (0.03–0.08 µg/g dry wt) in white basmati rice collected from Indian supermarkets. Meharg et al.[20] found 0.07 µg/g dry wt of arsenic (0.07–0.31 µg/g dry wt, $n = 133$) in Indian white rice. Other studies also reported high levels of arsenic in rice grain from West Bengal (0.11–0.44 µg/g dry wt[53] and 0.03–0.48 µg/g dry wt).[52] The Nadia district in West Bengal is one of the highly arsenic-contaminated areas in India, and arsenic concentrations in rice grain (either collected directly from farmers or purchased from local markets) ranged between 0.02 and 0.17 µg/g dry wt with a mean of 0.13 µg/g dry wt ($n = 50$).[39]

A number of studies have shown high levels of arsenic in Taiwanese rice. Rice collected directly from Taiwanese farms was reported to have an arsenic concentration of 0.76 µg/g dry wt.[49] A market basket survey, conducted by Lin et al.,[50] reported <0.10–0.63 µg/g dry wt of arsenic in Taiwanese rice, which is a comparable level to that reported by Williams et al.[27] The concentration of arsenic in Vietnamese rice was found to be 0.03–0.47 µg/g dry wt.[27,51] Thai rice has also been reported to contain high levels of arsenic (0.11 ± 0.01 µg/g dry wt).[27] A recent market basket survey reported that arsenic concentrations in Thai rice ranged between 0.01 and 0.39 µg/g dry wt, with a mean of 0.14 µg/g dry wt ($n = 54$).[20] Comparing this with the previous reports of Williams et al.[27], the higher arsenic concentrations in Thai rice found in a recent study by Meharg et al.[20] suggest that arsenic levels in Thai rice have increased in recent years. A considerable amount of arsenic has also been found in rice from the USA. A market basket survey conducted by Schoof et al.[23] reported that total arsenic concentrations in rice from the USA ("American rice") were 0.20–0.46 µg/g dry wt, while Heitkemper et al.[45] found levels of 0.11–0.34 µg/g dry wt. A recent study reported 0.03–0.66 µg/g dry wt of arsenic in American rice,[20] which is much higher than that reported by Williams et al.[27] The studies reveal that arsenic-contaminated rice is a significant source of dietary arsenic for the people of arsenic-affected areas, as well as for people of those countries that import rice from contaminated regions.

ARSENIC SPECIATION IN RICE GRAIN

Inorganic arsenic (iAs) species are more toxic than orgAs species.[57,58] Pentavalent methylarsenic species (DMAA^V and MMAA^V) are considered to be non-toxic.[59] Therefore, arsenic speciation in rice is considered to be

TABLE 28.1 Total (tAs), Inorganic (iAs), and Organic (orgAs) Arsenic Concentrations (μg/g dry wt.) in Rice Grain from Different Countries.

Origin	tAs		iAs		orgAs		% of iAs		Reference
	Mean	Range	Mean	Range	Mean	Range	Mean	Range	
Australia	0.03	0.02–0.04	–	–	–	–	–	–	Williams et al.[13]
	1.25	–	0.18	–	1.07	–	86	–	Juhasz et al.[43]
Bangladesh	0.13	0.02–0.33	0.08	0.01–0.21	–	–	61	–	Meharg et al.[20]
	0.50	0.03–1.84	–	–	–	–	–	–	Meharg and Rahman[11]
	0.34	0.15–0.59	–	–	–	–	–	–	Williams et al.[27]
	0.39	0.26–0.58	0.39	0.26–0.58	0.005	0.001–0.010	100	–	Williams et al.[27]
	0.23	0.18–0.31	0.16	0.11–0.22	–	–	65	60–71	Williams et al.[13]
	0.24	0.21–0.27	0.20	0.17–0.22	–	–	82	81–83	Williams et al.[13]
	0.13	0.03–0.30	0.08	0.01–0.21	0.02	<LOD–0.05	60	44–86	Ohno et al.[44]
	0.69	0.41–0.98	0.31	0.23–0.39	0.23	0.05–0.43	44	45–59	Sun et al.[21]
Canada	0.11	–	0.08	–	0.01	–	76	–	Heitkemper et al.[45]
	0.02	–	<LOD	–	0.01	–	71	–	Ohno et al.[44]
China	0.14	0.02–0.46	0.16	0.07–0.38	–	–	87	–	Williams et al.[27]
	0.12	0.07–0.19	–	–	–	–	–	–	Williams et al.[13]
	0.82	0.46–1.18	0.50	0.25–0.76	0.10	0.07–0.12	60	55–64	Sun et al.[21]
	0.49	0.31–0.70	–	–	–	–	–	–	Xie and Huang[46]
	0.93	–	–	–	–	–	–	–	Liu et al.[47]
Egypt	0.05	0.01–0.58	–	–	–	–	–	–	Williams et al.[27]
Europe	0.15	0.13–0.20	0.08	0.06–0.10	0.04	0.04–0.06	52	44–62	Ohno et al.[44]
France	0.28	0.09–0.56	–	–	–	–	–	–	Williams et al.[27]
India	0.07	0.07–0.31	0.03	0.02–0.07	–	–	43	–	Williams et al.[27]
	0.05	0.03–0.08	0.04	0.02–0.05	up to 0.01	<LOD–0.01	56	36–67	Ohno et al.[44]
Italy	0.15	0.07–0.33	0.11	0.07–0.16	–	–	73	–	Williams et al.[27]
	0.21	0.19–0.22	0.12	0.10–0.14	0.07	0.05–0.09	57	53–65	Ohno et al.[44]
Japan	0.19	0.07–0.42	–	–	–	–	–	–	Williams et al.[27]
Philippines	0.07	0.00–0.25	–	–	–	–	–	–	Williams et al.[13]
Spain	0.20	0.05–0.82	–	–	–	–	–	–	Williams et al.[27]

(Continued)

TABLE 28.1 Total (tAs), Inorganic (iAs), and Organic (orgAs) Arsenic Concentrations (µg/g dry wt.) in Rice Grain from Different Countries—cont'd

Origin	tAs Mean	tAs Range	iAs Mean	iAs Range	orgAs Mean	orgAs Range	% of iAs Mean	% of iAs Range	Reference
	0.34	0.29–0.41	0.14	0.10–0.20	–	–	41	34–48	Laparra et al.[48]
	0.17	–	0.08	–	0.05	–	48	–	Ohno et al.[44]
Thailand	0.14	0.01–0.39	–	–	–	–	–	–	Williams et al.[27]
	0.10	0.06–0.14	–	–	–	–	–	–	Williams et al.[13]
Taiwan	0.11	–	0.08	–	0.03	–	74	–	Ohno et al.[44]
	0.76	–	0.51	–	0.11	–	67	–	Schoof et al.[49]
	0.05	<0.10–0.14	–	–	–	–	–	–	Lin et al.[50]
	0.10	<0.10–0.63	–	–	–	–	–	–	Lin et al.[50]
	0.19	0.06–0.17	0.12	–	0.04	–	61	–	Schoof et al.[49]
	0.20	0.19–0.22	0.11	–	0.05	–	58	–	Schoof et al.[49]
USA	0.25	0.03–0.66	0.10	0.05–0.15	–	–	40	–	Williams et al.[27]
	0.30	0.2–0.46	–	–	–	–	–	–	Schoof et al.[23]
	0.28	0.21–0.34	0.10	0.02–0.11	0.18	0.17–0.24	35	9–32	Heitkemper et al.[45]
	0.26	0.11–0.40	0.08	0.02–0.14	0.14	0.04–0.26	35	10–41	Ohno et al.[44]
Vietnam	0.21	0.03–0.47	–	–	–	–	–	–	Phuong et al.[51]
West Bengal (India)	0.14	0.02–0.40	–	–	–	–	–	–	Pal et al.[52]
	0.25	0.14–0.48	–	–	–	–	–	–	Pal et al.[52]
	0.08	0.03–0.16	–	–	–	–	–	–	Pal et al.[52]
	0.13	0.02–0.17	–	–	–	–	–	–	Mondal and Polya[39]
	0.21	0.11–0.44	–	–	–	–	–	–	Roychowdhury et al.[53]
	0.33	0.18–0.43	–	–	–	–	–	–	Roychowdhury et al.[53]

LOD, Level of detection.
Adapted from Rahman and Hasegawa[54], with permission from Elsevier.

important for its possible impacts on human health. Arsenic concentration in rice grain is higher than in other cereal grains (by up to 10-fold[42]) because rice plants are generally grown in flooded conditions where arsenic mobility and bioavailability is high.[60] On average, around 50% of the total arsenic in rice grain is iAs (varying from 10% to 90%), while the remaining fraction is DMAA, with trace amounts of MMAA is some samples.[60] Asian rice mainly contains toxic iAs, while American and Australian rice contains non-toxic methylarsenicals.[27,43,61] Therefore, the high arsenic concentration in Asian rice makes it a threat to human health compared to rice from other arsenic-contaminated areas.[54] The concentration of arsenic speciation in rice grain from different origins is also presented in Table 28.1.

Although As^{III} predominates over As^V in rice in most cases,[27,62] arsenic speciation in rice showed significant inconsistency with origin, types, and varieties.[20,27] With the exception of rice from the USA, iAs is the main species in rice grain from other geographical areas around the world.[13,20,21,23,25,27,60,63,64] The ratios of iAs species in American, European, Bangladeshi, and Indian rice were reported to be about 42 ($n=12$), 64 ($n=7$), 80 ($n=11$), and 81% ($n=15$), respectively, of the recoverable arsenic.[27] A number of studies reported that approximately 44–86% of the total arsenic in Bangladeshi rice is inorganic,[13,20,21,27] while a field study conducted by Ohno et al.[44] reported up to 100% iAs in Bangladeshi rice. Up to 67% of the total arsenic has been reported to be inorganic in Taiwanese rice,[49] while Thai rice contained about 91% iAs.[27] The ratio of iAs in Chinese rice was found to be about 60–87%,[20,21] while the concentrations of iAs species in European and Italian rice were about 44–62% and 57–73%, respectively.[20,27] Spanish rice also contained a higher percentage of iAs (about 34–48%),[27,48] but this was less than in French and Italian rice. The fractions of iAs in Australian and American rice were about 14% and 40%, respectively – the lowest levels compared to rice from other countries (Table 28.1).

Methylarsenic species are the only orgAs species that have been found in rice. Australian and American rice mostly contained less/non-toxic methylarsenic species,[27,43] whereas European and Asian rice contained highly toxic iAs species.[62,65] A market basket survey conducted by Williams and colleagues[27] showed that methylarsenic (almost entirely as DMAA^V) is the major species (between 36–65%, with a mean of 54%) in American rice. Another study by Heitkemper and colleagues[45] reported a much higher percentage (70–80%, with a mean of 64%) of methylarsenic (mainly DMAA^V) in North American rice. Australian rice also contains mainly orgAs species (86%).[43] Levels of methylarsenic species were found to be 12–43% in Bangladeshi rice,[21,27] 9–50% in Canadian rice,[27,45] 10–15% in Chinese rice,[21] 30% in European rice,[27] 12% in Indian rice,[27] 26–40% in Italian rice,[27] 29%

in Spanish rice,[27] 27% in Thai rice,[27] and 14–25% in Taiwanese rice.[49] The variations in orgAs concentration in rice are related to the sources of arsenic contamination and the uptake efficiency of arsenic species by rice varieties.

ARSENIC IN COOKED RICE

Arsenic concentration and speciation in cooked rice depends on the cooking method,[66] which differs from country to country and even region to region of a country. People of the South Asian countries usually cook rice with excess water, whereas Southeast Asians do not use excess water when cooking rice. A number of studies showed that the cooking methods influence the retention of total as well as arsenic species in cooked rice.[30,31,37,52,67,68] For example, elevated levels of total arsenic were found in cooked rice in arsenic-contaminated areas of Bangladesh.[69] The additional arsenic in cooked rice is supposed to come from arsenic-contaminated cooking water, resulting either from chelation by rice grains or due to evaporation during the cooking process.[70] However, it was found that if the cooking water contained a low level of arsenic, the total arsenic concentration in cooked rice was less in cooked rice than in rice grain.[37,52] A study by Sengupta et al.[67] showed that cooking rice with a high volume of low-arsenic water and discarding the gruel after cooking (the traditional cooking method in India) removed up to 57% of the total arsenic in cooked rice. This removal of arsenic occurred irrespective of the concentration of arsenic in the rice grain; this may be because the water-soluble arsenic in rice, which was released into the cooking water during cooking process, was discarded with the gruel after cooking. However, the arsenic concentration in cooked rice increases significantly when the arsenic concentration in the cooking water is high.[30,67] This is because arsenic is absorbed by rice (through osmosis) from cooking water during the cooking process.

A large number of people in South Asian countries use parboiled rice (i.e., rice that has been boiled and dried before dehusking/milling), while the people of East and Southeast Asian countries and Japan use only non-parboiled rice for cooking. In some countries, people cook rice with excess water and discard the gruel after cooking. This cooking procedure is popular in South Asian countries. On the other hand, cooking rice with limited water (hence no gruel remains after cooking) is a popular method worldwide. The preparation of rice for cooking, and the cooking methods, have a substantial influence on arsenic retention in cooked rice.[30,31,67] The arsenic concentration in non-parboiled rice cooked with limited water was found to be 0.75 ± 0.04 to $1.09\pm0.06\,\mu g/g$ dry wt, which was about 13–37% higher than that in rice grain and 27–60% higher than that in rice cooked with excess water.[30] Cooking rice with excess water results in a decrease in the concentrations of total and iAs in cooked rice when the gruel is discarded, while arsenic concentration increases significantly when rice is cooked with limited water and the gruel is not discarded after cooking. For example, Raab and colleagues[68] found that cooking rice with excess water reduced total and iAs in cooked rice by 35% and 45%, respectively, while cooking with limited water did not remove arsenic substantially.

ARSENIC SPECIATION IN COOKED RICE

Arsenic speciation in cooked rice depends mainly on its speciation in the rice grain and in cooking water. In a study by Laparra et al.,[48] the effect of arsenic in cooking water on total and iAs retention in cooked rice was investigated. Total arsenic concentrations in raw basmati and white rice collected from Spanish supermarkets were 0.05 ± 0.001 and $0.13 \pm 0.008 \mu g/g$ dry wt, respectively. No substantial modifications or changes in total and iAs concentrations in cooked rice were found when the rice was cooked with uncontaminated water. When the rice was cooked with water containing $0.6 \mu g/L$ of As^V, total arsenic concentrations in cooked basmati and round white rice were increased to 2.36 ± 0.08 and $2.29 \pm 0.05 \mu g/g$ dry wt, of which iAs were 96 and 81%, respectively. Total and iAs concentrations were 1.96 ± 0.01 and 1.66 ± 0.002 $\mu g/g$ dry wt, respectively, when the rice was cooked with water containing $0.4 \mu g/L$ As^V, and thire concentrations were 4.21 ± 0.09 and $3.73 \pm 0.04 \mu g/g$ dry wt, respectively, when the rice was cooked with water containing $1.0 \mu g/L$ As^V. The results indicate that arsenic speciation is not changed substantially during the cooking process, and the total arsenic concentration in cooked rice is proportional to its concentration in cooking water. The retention of total and iAs in cooked rice also varies for rice type.

SOURCES OF ARSENIC IN RICE

Rice, the main cereal crop in many countries, including arsenic-endemic Bangladesh, West Bengal (India), Thailand, and Vietnam, needs a substantial amount of water for cultivation. In many S and SE Asian countries, underground water is the main source for rice cultivation during the dry season. Recently, it has become apparent that arsenic-contaminated underground irrigation water is adding a significant amount of arsenic to paddy soils and to rice, which poses a serious threat to sustainable rice cultivation in this region.[11,55,61–74] Due to the decreased rainfall, even in the monsoon season, the dependency on groundwater for rice cultivation is considered likely to increase in this region in the coming years in order to increase crop production to meet the demands of the increasing population. This practice may increase additional arsenic deposition in paddy soil. Thus, inorganic arsenic-rich underground irrigation water is the main source of arsenic in rice in Asian arsenic-endemic countries. On the other hand, arsenical pesticides are the main source of arsenic for American rice. In addition, microbial methylation of inorganic arsenic to orgAs in the rice field (in water and rhizosphere soil) would also contribute to the orgAs content in rice.

HUMAN HEALTH RISK OF ARSENIC FROM RICE DIET

Although there are many possible pathways of human exposure to arsenic,[39] epidemiological data published over the past few years have revealed that contaminated drinking groundwater is the major source of dietary arsenic in many countries, especially in S and SE Asia, followed by rice.[23,44,50,75–78] It was estimated that, in a typical Bangladeshi diet, the daily consumption of rice with a total arsenic level of $0.08 \mu g/g$ dry wt would be equivalent to a drinking water arsenic level of $10 \mu g/L$.[13] A number of arsenic speciation studies showed that 42–91% of the total arsenic in S and SE Asian rice consists of toxic inorganic species,[20,23,27,45,49,60,79] while the major species in American rice is DMAA.[27] Other studies also showed that iAs in rice products such as breakfast cereals, rice crackers, rice milk, baby rice, and other rice condiments is also high (75–90%).[64,80,81] Total[30,37,48,52,67,70] and iAs[48,82] concentrations in cooked rice were found to be increased due to cooking with arsenic-rich water.[48,68]

The bioaccessibility and bioavailability of arsenic in rice are two important factors that have substantial influence on arsenic toxicity in humans. The bioaccessibility and bioavailability mainly depend on the arsenic speciation in rice, and the toxic iAs species is readily assimilated into bloodstream.[11] Therefore, the health risk of iAs is greater than that of orgAs species. Laparra et al.[48] investigated the bioavailability and bioaccessibility of iAs in cooked rice to assess the potential toxicological risk of this species to human. Total and iAs concentrations in the bioaccessible fraction of cooked rice were $1.06–3.39 \mu g/g$ dry wt (>90% of the total arsenic in cooked rice) and $0.80–3.10 \mu g/g$ dry wt, respectively, indicating that a significant fraction of iAs can be available for intestinal absorption. To estimate the bioavailability (retention, transport, and uptake) of iAs to humans, bioaccessible fractions of arsenic in cooked rice were added to Caco-2 cells.[48] Results showed that arsenic retention, transport, and uptake by Caco-2 cells from cooked rice were 0.60–6.40, 3.30–11.40, and 3.90–17.80%, respectively. Considering the lowest (3.90%) and the

TABLE 28.2 Total (tAs) and Inorganic (iAs) Arsenic Concentrations (µg/g dry wt) in Rice Grain, and the Contribution of iAs to the WHO's Recommended Maximum Tolerable Daily Intake (MTDI) of iAs for Humans (2.1 µg/d per kg body wt.)[13]*

Origin of rice	tAs	iAs	iAs (%)	Contribution of iAs to MTDI (%)	Reference(s)
Bangladesh	0.21–0.31	0.14–0.22	71–83	48–79	Williams et al.[13]
Canada	0.11	0.08	76	26	Heitkemper et al.[45]
China	0.22	0.07	32	25	Williams et al.[13]
Europe	0.15	0.08	52	29	Williams et al.[27]
India	0.07	0.03	43	11	Meharg et al.[20]
Italy	0.15–0.21	0.11–0.12	57–73	39–43	Meharg et al.[20], e
Spain	1.21–2.36	1.49–2.28	81–98	82–99	Laparra et al.[48]
Thailand	0.11	0.08	74	29	Williams et al.[27]
Taiwan	0.19–0.76	0.11–0.51	58–67	39–182	Schoof et al.[49]
USA	0.25–0.28	0.08–0.10	35–40	29–36	Heitkemper et al.[45], Meharg et al.[20], Williams et al.[27]

* The WHO recommended MTDI value of iAs has been withdrawn recently. The MTDI is based on iAs concentration (%) in rice grain, a body weight of 60 kg, a consumption rate of 0.5 kg rice grain per day, and bioavailability of iAs in cooked rice (90%).[48]

highest (17.80%) total arsenic uptake values in the study, it was estimated that daily consumption of 5.7 kg or 1.2 kg cooked rice containing 4.21 ± 0.09 or 2.29 ± 0.05 µg/g dry wt, respectively, would be required to reach the WHO recommended maximum tolerable daily intake (MTDI) of iAs (2.1 µg/d per kg body weight[13]). However, the WHO recommended MTDI value of iAs has been withdrawn recently. An adult male consumes about 1.5 kg cooked rice (0.5 kg rice grain) a day in arsenic-endemic South Asian countries, indicating that the people of this region may reach the MTDI of arsenic just from their rice diet. The contribution of iAs to MTDI, in rice from a range of countries, is listed in Table 28.2.[13,20,27,45,47,48] Another study by Williams et al.[13] showed that the contribution of iAs in rice to the MTDI of arsenic for a Bangladeshi adult (assuming the body weight is 60 kg) would be 55–79%, depending on iAs concentration in rice and rice type. The MTDI may exceed the 100% level when the concentration of iAs in rice is high.[21,44,49]

In another study, Juhasz et al.[43] investigated the bioavailability of arsenic in rice and its significance for human health risk. In that study, the absolute bioavailability of arsenic species (As^V, As^{III}, MMAA, and DMAA) was determined using a swine animal model. The absolute bioavailability of iAs was highest (103.9% and 92.5% for As^{III} and As^V, respectively) followed by DMAA (33.3%) and MMAA (16.7%).[43] The contribution of rice consumption to MTDI was also estimated in cooked rice of different varieties from diverse origins. Results showed that the consumption of Quest rice of Australian origin may contribute 438% of the arsenic MTDI based on tAs concentration. However, the arsenic MTDI value would be about 185% for Quest if the MTDI calculation were based on arsenic speciation and bioavailability data, which is comparable to white rice of Taiwan origin (190%; Table 82.3[43]) even though the tAs concentration in Quest rice is two-fold greater than that in white rice. Thus, calculation of MTDI values considering the tAs concentration in rice grain significantly overvalues arsenic intake for varieties that mainly contain orgAs species (e.g., Quest rice contains 86% orgAs).[43] On the other hand, if only iAs concentration in rice is considered in the MTDI, the calculation would not reflect the real amount of arsenic intake from high iAs-containing rice varieties (e.g., Asian rice). Therefore, the MTDI should be calculated based on arsenic concentration, speciation, and the bioavailability of arsenic species.

MITIGATION OF ARSENIC EXPOSURE FROM RICE

It has been confirmed by a number of research groups that rice represents a major route of arsenic exposure in populations that depend on a rice diet,[38,39,41] and consumption of rice containing a high level of arsenic, particularly the highly toxic and bioavailable iAs species, poses a potential health risk to human.[54,83] Therefore, how to mitigate or reduce arsenic exposure from rice is an important concern in the scientific community. A range of methods, from agronomic measures and plant breeding to genetic modification, may be employed to mitigate arsenic exposure from rice. Some of the important and effective methods of arsenic exposure mitigation

TABLE 28.3   Assessment of the Contribution of Rice Consumption to Maximum Tolerable Daily Intake (MTDI Based on the Bioavailability of Arsenic Species) *

Rice Variety	Origin	tAs	iAs	orgAs	Contribution of MTDI (%) Based on:		
					tAs	iAs	As Bioavailability
Parija	Bangladesh	0.21	0.12	0.05	74	43	49
Miniket	Bangladesh	0.22	0.19	0.04	77	66	70
BRRIdhan29	Bangladesh	0.30	0.21	0.03	105	75	78
White	Taiwan	0.76	0.51	0.11	266	178	190
Long White	USA	0.40	0.08	0.26	140	28	58
Long Brown	USA	0.34	0.14	0.15	119	49	66
Basmati White	India	0.05	0.03	0.01	18	12	13
Basmati Brown	India	0.07	0.04	0.004	25	15	16
Medium Risotto	Italy	0.22	0.14	0.08	77	50	60
Arborio	Italy	0.21	0.14	0.07	74	49	56
Paella	Spain	0.17	0.08	0.05	60	29	35
Long Jasmine	Thailand	0.11	0.08	0.03	39	28	31
Long Wild	Canada	0.11	0.08	0.009	39	29	30
Quest	Australia	1.25	0.18	1.08	438	61	185

* The contribution to MTDI (%) was calculated based on the concentration (μg/g dry wt) of arsenic species in rice grain, a body weight of 60 kg, a consumption rate of 0.42 kg dry rice grain per day, and bioavailability factors of 0.33 and 1.0 for organic arsenic (orgAs) and inorganic arsenic (iAs), respectively, in cooked rice.[43]

involve agronomic measures, breeding rice varieties, and cooking methods.

Agronomic Measures

The main sources of arsenic in rice grain are arsenic-rich paddy soils and irrigation water. Arsenic chemistry in paddy soils is extremely complex because of frequent redox cycles in the soil, and arsenic uptake in rice from soil is influenced by a range of factors, including bioavailability, rhizosphere processes, and metabolism in rice plants.[84] Therefore, agronomic measures such as water management[55,85,86] and fertilization practices[86–88] would be effective methods to reduce arsenic uptake in rice grain.

Rice is usually grown in anaerobic (flooded) conditions in which arsenic exists mainly as dissolve As^{III} form and is readily taken up by the rice plant. Therefore, rice grown under flooded conditions was found to accumulate much more arsenic than that grown under aerobic conditions.[89] As^{V} was found to be the main arsenic species in the aerobic soil, and arsenic accumulation in rice grain was observed to be 10- to 15-fold higher in flooded than in aerobically grown rice.[89] Maintaining aerobic conditions during either the vegetative or the reproductive stage of rice growth decreases arsenic accumulation in rice grain significantly compared with rice grown under flooded conditions.[86]

Iron is believed to be an important factor in regulating arsenic bioavailability and uptake in rice.[90–92] Rice plants carry oxygen from the air down their stems, and discharge it in the rhizosphere through the roots.[71] This creates an oxidized zone around the roots in which iron is oxidized and precipitated to form a coating.[92] As^{V} has a high binding affinity with precipitated iron hydroxides, which act as an arsenic filter to reduce arsenic uptake in rice.[90] However, sulfur was found to enhance the formation of iron plaque in the rhizosphere and reduce arsenic accumulation in rice.[87] In another study, phosphate fertilizer was found to decrease iron plaque formation on rice roots and increase arsenic uptake in rice plant.[88] The addition of nitrate also decreases iron plaque formation on the rice root surface; however, the addition of nitrate reduced arsenic uptake by rice plant. These results suggest that nitrate may inhibit Fe(III) reduction and/or stimulate nitrate-dependent Fe(II) oxidation, leading to arsenic co-precipitation with, or adsorption to, Fe(III) minerals in the soil.[84] Two silicon transporter proteins, Lsi1 and Lsi2, which are highly expressed in rice roots, can transport As^{III}. Lsi2 in particular plays an important role in the root-to-shoot transport of As^{III} and arsenic accumulation in rice grains.[93] Therefore, silicon is another important nutrient that controls arsenic uptake in rice grains. Silicon fertilization decreases the total arsenic concentration in straw and grain by 78% and 16%, respectively, even though the addition of silicon increases arsenic concentration in the soil solution. Silicon decreases the iAs concentration in grain by 59% while increasing the concentration of DMAA by 33%.[86]

Breeding Rice Varieties

Significant genetic variations in the arsenic concentration of rice grain have been reported,[94] and breeding rice varieties with low arsenic uptake would be an effective way to reduce arsenic exposure risk from rice. It has been reported that rice cultivars with red bran had significantly more grain arsenic than cultivars with brown bran,[94] indicating that rice cultivars with red bran were associated with higher arsenic concentrations. A number of Bangladeshi local rice cultivars with low grain arsenic content were also identified.[94] It has been suggested that some tropical japonica cultivars with low grain arsenic levels would have the potential to be used in breeding programs to develop rice varieties with low arsenic uptake, and genetic studies aiming to identify genes which decrease grain arsenic. Genetic variation in As^{III} tolerance has been reported in rice.[95] Breeding of arsenic-tolerant rice varieties would be a useful method, for highly contaminated environments, that may reduce the risk of arsenic exposure.

Cooking Methods

The risk of arsenic exposure from rice grain can be reduced by cooking rice following the best method to reduce the arsenic burden in cooked rice. A number of studies have shown that the arsenic concentration in cooked rice is influenced by cooking methods.[22,30–32,67,68] Rice is usually cooked with a substantial amount of water in South Asian regions. Approximately 10–35% higher arsenic levels were found in cooked rice compared to that in raw rice in arsenic-endemic areas of Bangladesh.[69] The additional arsenic is considered to come from arsenic-contaminated cooking water, and the increase in total arsenic concentration in cooked rice was a result of either chelation by rice grains or evaporation during the cooking process.[70] On the other hand, parboiling (boiling and drying raw rice before dehusking/milling) of raw rice decreases the arsenic concentration in rice grain. In addition, cooking rice with excess water and disposing of the gruel (concentrated cooking water) after cooking also reduces arsenic concentration in cooked rice.[30] Another study which showed that cooking rice with a high volume (excess) of water (water:rice = 6:1) reduced tAs and iAs content in cooked rice by 35% and 45%, respectively.[68] Irrespective of the concentration of arsenic concentration in the raw rice and cooking water, cooking rice with low-arsenic water following the traditional cooking method in India (washing rice three or four times, cooking with a rice:water ratio of 1:6, and discarding the excess water [gruel] after cooking) has been reported to remove up to 57% of tAs from cooked rice[65]. The removal of tAs may be due to the release of water-soluble arsenic fractions from rice into the gruel, which is then discarded.

References

1. Tamaki S, Frankenberger WTJ. Environmental chemistry of arsenic. *Rev Environ Contam Toxicol* 1992;**124**:79–110.
2. Smith E, Naidu R, Alston AM. Arsenic in the soil environment: A review. *Adv Agron* 1998;**64**:149–95.
3. Mandal BK, Suzuki KT. Arsenic round the world: A review. *Talanta* 2002;**58**(1):201–35.
4. Rahman MM, Naidu R, Bhattacharya P. Arsenic contamination in groundwater in the Southeast Asia region. *Environ Geochem Health* 2009;**31**:9–21.
5. Chatterjee D, Halder D, Majumder S, Biswas A, Nath B, Bhattacharya P, et al. Assessment of arsenic exposure from groundwater and rice in Bengal Delta Region, West Bengal, India. *Water Res* 2010;**44**(19):5803–12.
6. Nordstrom DK. Worldwide occurrences of arsenic in ground water. *Science* 2002;**296**(5576):2143–5.
7. Smith E, Smith J, Smith L, Biswas T, Correll R, Naidu R. Arsenic in Australian environment: An overview. *J Environ Sci Health A* 2003;**38**(1):223–39.
8. Smith JVS, Jankowski J, Sammut J. Natural occurrences of inorganic arsenic in the Australian coastal groundwater environment. In: Naidu R, Smith E, Owens G, Bhattacharya P, Nadebaum P, editors. *Managing Arsenic in the Environment: From Soil to Human Health*. Melbourne, Australia: CSIRO; 2006. p. 129–53.
9. Mukherjee A, Sengupta MK, Hossain MA, Ahamed S, Das B, Nayak B, et al. Arsenic contamination in groundwater: A global perspective with emphasis on the Asian scenario. *J Health Popul Nutr* 2006;**24**(2):142–63.
10. Ninno Cd, Dorosh PA. Averting a food crisis: Private imports and public targeted distribution in Bangladesh after the 1998 flood. *Agric Eco* 2001;**25**(2-3):337–46.
11. Meharg AA, Rahman M. Arsenic contamination of Bangladesh paddy field soils: Implications for rice contribution to arsenic consumption. *Environ Sci Technol* 2003;**37**(2):229–34.
12. Alam MB, Sattar MA. Assessment of arsenic contamination in soils and waters in some areas of Bangladesh. *Water Sci Technol* 2000:185–92.
13. Williams PN, Islam MR, Adomako EE, Raab A, Hossain SA, Zhu YG, et al. Increase in rice grain arsenic for regions of Bangladesh irrigating paddies with elevated arsenic in groundwaters. *Environ Sci Technol* 2006;**40**(16):4903–8.
14. Dahal BM, Fuerhacker M, Mentler A, Karki KB, Shrestha RR, Blum WEH. Arsenic contamination of soils and agricultural plants through irrigation water in Nepal. *Environ Pollut* 2008;**155**(1):157–63.
15. Winkel LHE, Trang PTK, Lan VM, Stengel C, Amini M, Ha NT, et al. Arsenic pollution of groundwater in Vietnam exacerbated by deep aquifer exploitation for more than a century. *Proc Natl Acad Sci* 2011;**108**(4):1246–51.
16. Pokhrel D, Bhandari BS, Viraraghavan T. Arsenic contamination of groundwater in the Terai region of Nepal: An overview of health concerns and treatment options. *Environ Int* 2009;**35**(1):157–61.
17. Winkel L, Berg M, Stengel C, Rosenberg T. Hydrogeological survey assessing arsenic and other groundwater contaminants in the lowlands of Sumatra, Indonesia. *Appl Geochem* 2008;**23**(11):3019–28.
18. Sun G, Li X, Pi J, Sun Y, Li B, Jin Y, et al. Current research problems of chronic arsenicosis in China. *J Health Popul Nutr* 2006;**24**(2):176–81.

19. Kemper K, Minnatullah K. *Towards a More Effective Operational Response Arsenic Contamination of Groundwater in South and East Asian Countries.* Water and Sanitation Program: World Bank; 2005.

20. Meharg AA, Williams PN, Adomako E, Lawgali YY, Deacon C, Villada A, et al. Geographical variation in total and inorganic arsenic content of polished (white) rice. *Environ Sci Technol* 2009;**43**(5):1612–7.

21. Sun GX, Williams PN, Carey AM, Zhu YG, Deacon C, Raab A, et al. Inorganic arsenic in rice bran and its products are an order of magnitude higher than in bulk grain. *Environ Sci Technol* 2008;**42**(19):7542–6.

22. Torres-Escribano S, Leal M, Velez D, Montoro R. Total and inorganic arsenic concentrations in rice sold in Spain, effect of cooking, and risk assessments. *Environ Sci Technol* 2008;**42**(10):3867–72.

23. Schoof RA, Yost LJ, Eickhoff J, Crecelius EA, Cragin DW, Meacher DM, et al. A market basket survey of inorganic arsenic in food. *Food Chem Toxicol* 1999;**37**(8):839–46.

24. Das HK, Mitra AK, Sengupta PK, Hossain A, Islam F, Rabbani GH. Arsenic concentrations in rice, vegetables, a fish in Bangladesh: A preliminary study. *Environ Int* 2004;**30**(3):383–7.

25. Booth B. Arsenic speciation varies with type of rice. *Environ Sci Technol* 2008;**42**(10):3484–5.

26. Booth B. Arsenic in US rice varies by region. *Environ Sci Technol* 2007;**41**(7):2075–6.

27. Williams PN, Price AH, Raab A, Hossain SA, Feldmann J, Meharg AA. Variation in arsenic speciation and concentration in paddy rice related to dietary exposure. *Environ Sci Technol* 2005;**39**(15):5531–40.

28. Musaiger AO, D'Souza R. The effects of different methods of cooking on proximate, mineral and heavy metal composition of fish and shrimps consumed in the Arabian Gulf. *Arch Latinoam Nutr* 2008;**58**(1):103–9.

29. Ohno K, Matsuo Y, Kimura T, Yanase T, Rahman MH, Magara Y, et al. Effect of rice-cooking water to the daily arsenic intake in Bangladesh: Results of field surveys and rice-cooking experiments. *Water Sci Technol* 2009;**59**(2):195–201.

30. Rahman MA, Hasegawa H, Rahman MA, Rahman MM, Miah MAM. Influence of cooking method on arsenic retention in cooked rice related to dietary exposure. *Sci Total Environ* 2006;**370**(1):51–60.

31. Signes A, Mitra K, Burlo F, Carbonell-Barrachina AA. Effect of cooking method and rice type on arsenic concentration in cooked rice and the estimation of arsenic dietary intake in a rural village in West Bengal, India. *Food Addit Contam: Part A* 2008;**25**(11):1345–52.

32. Signes A, Mitra K, Burlo F, Carbonell-Barrachina AA. Contribution of water and cooked rice to an estimation of the dietary intake of inorganic arsenic in a rural village of West Bengal, India. *Food Addit Contam: Part A* 2008;**25**(1):41–50.

33. Farmer J, Johnson L. Assessment of occupational exposure to inorganic arsenic based on urinary concentrations and speciation of arsenic. *Br J Ind Med* 1990;**47**(5):342.

34. Duxbury JM, Mayer AB, Lauren JG, Hassan N. Food chain aspects of arsenic contamination in Bangladesh: Effects on quality and productivity of rice. *J Environ Sci Health A* 2003;**38**(1):61–9.

35. Chen S, Yeh S, Yang M, Lin T. Trace element concentration and arsenic speciation in the well water of a Taiwan area with endemic Blackfoot disease. *Biol Trace Elem Res* 1995;**48**(3):263–74.

36. Meharg AA. Arsenic in rice – understanding a new disaster for South-East Asia. *Trends Plant Sci* 2004;**9**(9):415–7.

37. Bae M, Watanabe C, Inaoka T, Sekiyama M, Sudo N, Bokul MH, et al. Arsenic in cooked rice in Bangladesh. *Lancet* 2002;**360**(9348):1839–40.

38. Mondal D, Banerjee M, Kundu M, Banerjee N, Bhattacharya U, Giri AK, et al. Comparison of drinking water, raw rice and cooking of rice as arsenic exposure routes in three contrasting areas of West Bengal, India. *Environ Geochem Health* 2010;**32**(6):463–77.

39. Mondal D, Polya DA. Rice is a major exposure route for arsenic in Chakdaha block, Nadia district, West Bengal, India: A probabilistic risk assessment. *Appl Geochem* 2008;**23**(11):2987–98.

40. Rahman MA, Hasegawa H, Rahman MM, Miah MA. Accumulation of arsenic in tissues of rice plant (*Oryza sativa* L.) and its distribution in fractions of rice grain. *Chemosphere* 2007;**69**(6):942–8.

41. Rahman MA, Hasegawa H, Rahman MM, Miah MAM, Tasmin A. Arsenic accumulation in rice (*Oryza sativa* L.): Human exposure through food chain. *Ecotoxicol Environ Saf* 2008;**69**(2):317–24.

42. Williams PN, Villada A, Deacon C, Raab A, Figuerola J, Green AJ, et al. Greatly enhanced arsenic shoot assimilation in rice leads to elevated grain levels compared to wheat and barley. *Environ Sci Technol* 2007;**41**(19):6854–9.

43. Juhasz AL, Smith E, Weber J, Rees M, Rofe A, Kuchel T, et al. *In vivo* assessment of arsenic bioavailability in rice and its significance for human health risk assessment. *Environ Health Persp* 2006;**114**(12):1826–31.

44. Ohno K, Yanase T, Matsuo Y, Kimura T, Hamidur Rahman M, Magara Y, et al. Arsenic intake via water and food by a population living in an arsenic-affected area of Bangladesh. *Sci Total Environ* 2007;**381**(1–3):68–76.

45. Heitkemper DT, Vela NP, Stewart KR, Westphal CS. Determination of total and speciated arsenic in rice by ion chromatography and inductively coupled plasma mass spectrometry. *J Anal Atomic Spectrom* 2001;**16**(4):299–306.

46. Xie ZM, Huang CY. Control of arsenic toxicity in rice plants grown on an arsenic-polluted paddy soil. *Commun Soil Sci Plant Anal* 1998;**29**(15):2471–7.

47. Liu H, Probst A, Liao B. Metal contamination of soils and crops affected by the Chenzhou lead/zinc mine spill (Hunan, China). *Sci Total Environ* 2005;**339**(1–3):153–66.

48. Laparra JM, Velez D, Barbera R, Farre R, Montoro R. Bioavailability of inorganic arsenic in cooked rice: Practical aspects for human health risk assessments. *J Agric Food Chem* 2005;**53**(22):8829–33.

49. Schoof RA, Yost LJ, Crecelius E, Irgolic K, Goessler W, Guo HR, et al. Dietary arsenic intake in Taiwanese districts with elevated arsenic in drinking water. *Hum Ecol Risk Ass* 1998;**4**(1):117–35.

50. Lin HT, Wong SS, Li GC. Heavy metal content of rice and Shellfish in Taiwan. *J Food Drug Anal* 2004;**12**(2):167–74.

51. Phuong TD, Chuong PV, Khiem DT, Kokot S. Elemental content of Vietnamese rice. Part 1. Sampling, analysis and comparison with previous studies. *Analyst* 1999;**124**(4):553–60.

52. Pal A, Chowdhury UK, Mondal D, Das B, Nayak B, Ghosh A, et al. Arsenic burden from cooked rice in the populations of arsenic affected and nonaffected areas and Kolkata city in West-Bengal, India. *Environ Sci Technol* 2009;**43**(9):3349–55.

53. Roychowdhury T, Uchino T, Tokunaga H, Ando M. Survey of arsenic in food composites from an arsenic-affected area of West Bengal, India. *Food Chem Toxicol* 2002;**40**(11):1611–21.

54. Rahman MA, Hasegawa H. High levels of inorganic arsenic in rice in areas where arsenic-contaminated water is used for irrigation and cooking. *Sci Total Environ* 2011;**409**(22):4645–55.

55. Khan MA, Islam MR, Panaullah GM, Duxbury JM, Jahiruddin M, Loeppert RH. Accumulation of arsenic in soil and rice under wetland condition in Bangladesh. *Plant Soil* 2010;**333**(1–2):263–74.

56. Islam M, Jahiruddin M, Islam S. Assessment of arsenic in the water-soil-plant systems in Gangetic floodplains of Bangladesh. *Asian J Plant Sci* 2004;**3**(4):489–93.

57. Ng JC. Environmental contamination of arsenic and its toxicological impact on humans. *Environ Chem* 2005;**2**(3):146–60.

58. Meharg AA, Hartley Whitaker J. Arsenic uptake and metabolism in arsenic resistant and nonresistant plant species. *New Phytol* 2002;**154**(1):29–43.

59. Jain CK, Ali I. Arsenic: Occurrence, toxicity and speciation techniques. *Water Res* 2000;**34**(17):4304–12.

60. Zhu YG, Williams PN, Meharg AA. Exposure to inorganic arsenic from rice: A global health issue? *Environ Pollut* 2008;**154**(2):169–71.

61. Zavala YJ, Gerads R, Gürleyük H, Duxbury JM. Arsenic in rice: II. Arsenic speciation in USA grain and implications for human health. *Environ Sci Technol* 2008;**42**(10):3861–6.

62. Zavala YJ, Gerads R, Gurleyuk H, Duxbury JM. Arsenic in Rice: II. Arsenic speciation in USA grain and implications for human health. *Environ Sci Technol* 2008;**42**(10):3861–6.

63. Potera C. US rice serves up arsenic. *Environ Health Persp* 2007;**115**(6) A296-A.

64. Sun GX, Williams PN, Zhu YG, Deacon C, Carey AM, Raab A, et al. Survey of arsenic and its speciation in rice products such as breakfast cereals, rice crackers and Japanese rice condiments. *Environ Int* 2009;**35**(3):473–5.

65. Zavala YJ, Duxbury JM. Arsenic in rice: I. Estimating normal levels of total arsenic in rice grain. *Environ Sci Technol* 2008;**42**(10):3856–60.

66. Rahman MA, Hasegawa H, Rahman MM, Miah MA. Influence of cooking method on arsenic retention in cooked rice related to dietary exposure. *Sci Total Environ* 2006;**370**(1):51–60.

67. Sengupta MK, Hossain MA, Mukherjee A, Ahamed S, Das B, Nayak B, et al. Arsenic burden of cooked rice: Traditional and modern methods. *Food Chem Toxicol* 2006;**44**(11):1823–9.

68. Raab A, Baskaran C, Feldmann J, Meharg AA. Cooking rice in a high water to rice ratio reduces inorganic arsenic content. *J Environ Monit* 2009;**11**(1):41–4.

69. Misbahuddin M. Consumption of arsenic through cooked rice. *Lancet* 2003;**361**(9355):435–6.

70. Rahman MA, Ismail MMR, Hasegawa H. Cooking: Effects on dietary exposure to arsenic from rice and vegetables. In: Nriagu JO, editor. *Encyclopedia of Environmental Health*. Burlington, VT: Elsevier; 2011. p. 828–33.

71. Brammer H, Ravenscroft P. Arsenic in groundwater: A threat to sustainable agriculture in South and South-east Asia. *Environ Int* 2009;**35**(3):647–54.

72. Khan MA, Stroud JL, Zhu YG, McGrath SP, Zhao FJ. Arsenic bioavailability to rice is elevated in Bangladeshi paddy soils. *Environ Sci Technol* 2010;**44**(22):8515–21.

73. Dittmar J, Voegelin A, Maurer F, Roberts LC, Hug SJ, Saha GC, et al. Arsenic in soil and irrigation water affects arsenic uptake by rice: Complementary insights from field and pot studies. *Environ Sci Technol* 2010;**44**(23):8842–8.

74. Khan MA, Islam MR, Panaullah GM, Duxbury JM, Jahiruddin M, Loeppert RH. Fate of irrigation-water arsenic in rice soils of Bangladesh. *Plant and Soil* 2009;**322**(1-2):263–77.

75. Bhattacharya P, Samal AC, Majumdar J, Santra SC. Arsenic contamination in rice, wheat, pulses, and vegetables: A study in an arsenic affected area of West Bengal India. *Water Air Soil Poll* 2010;**213**(1-4):3–13.

76. Roychowdhury T, Tokunaga H, Ando M. Survey of arsenic and other heavy metals in food composites and drinking water and estimation of dietary intake by the villagers from an arsenic-affected area of West Bengal, India. *Sci Total Environ* 2003;**308**(1-3):15–35.

77. Signes-Pastor AJ, Deacon C, Jenkins RO, Haris PI, Carbonell-Barrachina AA, Meharg AA. Arsenic speciation in Japanese rice drinks and condiments. *J Environ Monit* 2009;**11**(11):1930–4.

78. Signes-Pastor AJ, Mitra K, Sarkhel S, Hobbes M, Burló F, de Groot WT, et al. Arsenic speciation in food and estimation of the dietary intake of inorganic arsenic in a rural village of West Bengal, India. *J Agric Food Chem* 2008;**56**(20):9469–74.

79. Meharg AA, Lombi E, Williams PN, Scheckel KG, Feldmann J, Raab A, et al. Speciation and localization of arsenic in white and brown rice grains. *Environ Sci Technol* 2008;**42**(4):1051–7.

80. Meharg AA, Deacon C, Campbell RCJ, Carey AM, Williams PN, Feldmann J, et al. Inorganic arsenic levels in rice milk exceed EU and US drinking water standards. *J Environ Monit* 2008;**10**(4):428–31.

81. Meharg AA, Sun G, Williams PN, Adomako E, Deacon C, Zhu YG, et al. Inorganic arsenic levels in baby rice are of concern. *Environ Pollut* 2008;**152**(3):746–9.

82. Smith NM, Lee R, Heitkemper DT, DeNicola Cafferky K, Haque A, Henderson AK. Inorganic arsenic in cooked rice and vegetables from Bangladeshi households. *Sci Total Environ* 2006;**370**(2–3):294–301.

83. Rahman MM, Owens G, Naidu R. Arsenic levels in rice grain and assessment of daily dietary intake of arsenic from rice in arsenic-contaminated regions of Bangladesh - implications to groundwater irrigation. *Environ Geochem Health* 2009;**31**:179–87.

84. Chen X-P, Zhu Y-G, Hong M-N, Kappler A, Xu Y- X. Effects of different forms of nitrogen fertilizers on arsenic uptake by rice plants. *Environ Toxicol Chem* 2008;**27**(4):881–7.

85. Arao T, Kawasaki A, Baba K, Mori S, Matsumoto S. Effects of water management on cadmium and arsenic accumulation and dimethylarsinic acid concentrations in Japanese rice. *Environ Sci Technol* 2009;**43**(24):9361–7.

86. Li RY, Stroud JL, Ma JF, McGrath SP, Zhao FJ. Mitigation of arsenic accumulation in rice with water management and silicon fertilization. *Environ Sci Technol* 2009;**43**(10):3778–83.

87. Hu Z-Y, Zhu Y-G, Li M, Zhang L-G, Cao Z-H, Smith FA. Sulfur (S)-induced enhancement of iron plaque formation in the rhizosphere reduces arsenic accumulation in rice (*Oryza sativa* L.) seedlings. *Environ Pollut* 2007;**147**(2):387–93.

88. Hu Y, Li JH, Zhu YG, Huang YZ, Hu HQ, Christie P. Sequestration of As by iron plaque on the roots of three rice (*Oryza sativa* L.) cultivars in a low-P soil with or without P fertilizer. *Environ Geochem Health* 2005;**27**(2):169–76.

89. Xu XY, McGrath SP, Meharg AA, Zhao FJ. Growing rice aerobically markedly decreases arsenic accumulation. *Environ Sci Technol* 2008;**42**(15):5574–9.

90. Liu WJ, Zhu YG, Smith FA, Smith SE. Do phosphorus nutrition and iron plaque alter arsenate (As) uptake by rice seedlings in hydroponic culture? *New Phytol* 2004;**162**(2):481–8.

91. Chen Z, Zhu YG, Liu WJ, Meharg AA. Direct evidence showing the effect of root surface iron plaque on arsenite and arsenate uptake into rice (*Oryza sativa*) roots. *New Phytologist* 2005;**165**(1):91–7.

92. Liu WJ, Zhu YG, Hu Y, Williams PN, Gault AG, Meharg AA, et al. Arsenic sequestration in iron plaque, its accumulation and speciation in mature rice plants (*Oryza sativa* L.). *Environ Sci Technol* 2006;**40**(18):5730–6.

93. Ma JF, Yamaji N, Mitani N, Xu XY, Su YH, McGrath SP, et al. Transporters of arsenite in rice and their role in arsenic accumulation in rice grain. *Pro Natl Acad Sci* 2008;**105**(29):9931.

94. Norton GJ, Islam MR, Deacon CM, Zhao FJ, Stroud JL, McGrath SP, et al. Identification of low inorganic and total grain arsenic rice cultivars from Bangladesh. *Environ Sci Technol* 2009;**43**(15):6070–5.

95. Norton GJ, Lou-Hing DE, Meharg AA, Price AH. Rice-arsenate interactions in hydroponics: Whole genome transcriptional analysis. *J Exp Bot* 2008;**59**(8):2267–76.

Arsenic in Rice-Based Infant Foods

Sandra Munera-Picazo*, Amanda Ramírez-Gandolfo*, Claudia Cascio[†],
Concha Castaño-Iglesias**, Antonio J. Signes-Pastor*, [†], Francisco Burló*,
Parvez I. Haris[†], Ángel A. Carbonell-Barrachina*

*Universidad Miguel Hernández, Departamento Tecnología Agroalimentaria, Grupo Calidad y Seguridad Alimentaria,
Alicante, Spain, [†]De Montfort University, Faculty of Health and Life Sciences, Leicester, UK, **Universidad Miguel
Hernández, Departamento de Farmacología, Pediatría y Química Orgánica, Alicante, Spain

INTRODUCTION

Arsenic (As) occurs naturally in the environment in a broad variety of compounds, of which inorganic arsenic (iAs) is the most toxic form. Inorganic arsenic has been classified by the International Agency for Research on Cancer[1] in Group 1, as carcinogenic to humans. This was based on the induction of primary skin cancer, as well as the induction of lung and urinary bladder cancer. The Joint FAO/WHO Expert Committee on Food Additives (JECFA) established a Provisional Tolerable Weekly Intake (PTWI) for iAs of 0.015 mg/kg of bodyweight/week in 1988. However, the European Food Safety Agency (EFSA) has recently concluded that this PTWI is no longer appropriate as iAs produces cancer of the lung and urinary bladder in addition to skin cancer, and a range of adverse health effects have been reported at exposures lower than those reviewed by the JECFA.[2]

The main exposure route to iAs in the EU is dietary,[2] particularly for young infants, with toxicological concerns exacerbated by the high food consumption per body mass that typifies infants. It is only in the last few years that As speciation in foods has become more robust. The urgent need for speciation data is evident, especially in those foods that can represent emerging risks, such as rice-based infant foods.

The national iAs exposures from food and water across 19 European countries have been estimated to range from 0.1 to 0.6 μg/kg body weight (bw) per day for average consumers.[2] The minimum and maximum dietary exposure varied by a factor of 2–3 across the 19 European countries, based on different dietary habits rather than different occurrence data. The food subclasses of cereal grains and cereal-based products, followed by food for special dietary uses; bottled water, coffee and beer; rice grains and rice-based products; fish; and vegetables were identified as the main contributors to iAs exposure in the general European population. The idea that early-life exposure to iAs via baby rice may increase the risk for adverse health effects was first reported by Meharg and colleagues.[3] They demonstrated that the median consumption (0.2 mg/kg per day) of iAs intake from rice products for babies was higher than the maximum exposures in the region. The need for legislation on As in baby food in order to prevent excessive As exposure in infants consuming rice-based products has been already highlighted.[4]

Arsenicals were widely used in agriculture as pesticides or plant defoliants for many years. Currently, the use of both inorganic and organic arsenicals is legally forbidden or reduced to the minimum. However, a legacy of contaminated orchard soils has been left behind due to the extensive use of inorganic forms in the past; this is of great importance because residues from the application of these compounds can produce phytotoxic effects long after application has ceased. It is also important to highlight that the most popular fertilizers (nitrogen, phosphorus, potassium) will incorporate trace amounts of As into agricultural soils as contaminants, due to the high chemical similarity between phosphorus and As.

High As accumulation in rice occurs due to paddy cultivation (i.e., anaerobic conditions), where soil As is highly available for plant uptake.[5] Signes-Pastor et al.[6] analyzed tAs in agricultural products from West Bengal (North 24 Parganas district): vegetables, cereals, and spices (Table 29.1). The vegetables group presented a

TABLE 29.1 Arsenic Speciation (µg/kg dry wt) in Vegetables, Cereals, and Spices from Kasimpur (West Bengal), Analyzed by HPLC-HG-AFS[6]

Sample	Inorganic As	Organic As	Total As
VEGETABLES (DRY WT)			
Carrot	90	22	1120
Kidney beans	42	nd	42
Radish	94	60	154
Tomato	54	nd	54
Onion	56	nd	56
Betel nut	26	nd	26
Cauliflower	60	nd	60
Brinjal	48	nd	48
Potatoes	47	34	81
CEREALS (DRY WT)			
Paddy rice	243	242	488
Atab rice	121	147	268
Boiled rice	380	91	471
Puffed rice	40	80	120
SPICES (DRY WT)			
Coriander seeds	41	35	76
Turmeric powder	24	47	71
Cumin seeds	76	nd	76
Mustard	48	nd	48
Ginger mango	148	60	208
Fenugreek seeds	5	23	28

nd, not detected.

mean of 75 µg/kg, with radish having the highest tAs concentration at 167 µg/kg. The mean tAs concentration for the cereal group was the highest, 339 µg/kg, with paddy rice and boiled rice showing the highest concentrations at 496 µg/kg and 469 µg/kg, respectively. Finally, the mean tAs concentration for the spice group was 90 µg/kg. A similar trend to that described for tAs was also observed for iAs, with the highest content corresponding to rice samples.

Within plants, the highest As residues are found in roots, with intermediate contents being found in green vegetables, and edible seeds and fruits containing the lowest As levels.[5] Thus, As content seems to be restricted during upward transport within the plant system. Consequently, As content in cereals, including rice, is expected to be low. However, Williams *et al.*[7] demonstrated that this statement is not true for rice. These authors reported

that in rice the median shoot/soil transfer factors were nearly 50-fold higher than those in wheat and barley, but median grain/shoot transfer factors for wheat and barley were 4-fold higher than those of rice. Under similar farming conditions, the tAs content reached mean values of 188, 60, and 50 µg/kg in rice, barley, and wheat, respectively.[7] Additionally, several authors have clearly demonstrated that methylated orgAs are rapidly moved from the roots into shoot tissues in different plants, including turnip,[8] tomato,[9] and beans.[10] The differences in these transfer factors among rice, wheat, and barley are probably due to differences in As speciation and dynamics in anaerobic rice soils, compared to aerobic soils for barley and wheat. In summary, transfer of As from soil to grain is an order of magnitude greater in rice than in wheat and barley, despite lower rates of shoot-to-grain transfer in rice.[7]

European rice has high tAs and iAs contents,[11] and recent studies have reported high tAs and iAs in rice products from the European Union (EU) or marketed in the EU. Sun *et al.*[12] conducted a survey of As and its speciation in rice products such as breakfast cereals, rice crackers, and Japanese rice condiments, and reported tAs contents ranging from 14 to 280 µg/kg, with most of the As being present as iAs (75–90%). Signes-Pastor *et al.*[13] studied As speciation in Japanese rice drinks and condiments sold in the UK. These authors concluded that (1) rice-based products displayed higher iAs contents than did those from barley and millet; (2) most of the tAs in the rice products was iAs (63–83%), and (3) high consumers of Japanese products could be at serious risk. High consumers of rice in Europe, such as certain ethnic groups, are estimated to have a daily dietary exposure to iAs of about 1 µg/kg bw.[2] Ethnic differences in As exposure within Europe and the USA have been reported in the literature.[14] Whilst studies on exposure to iAs from foods, and especially water consumption, are widely available, very little work has been done to investigate exposure to As from rice consumption. In one of the few studies conducted in this area, Pearson *et al.*[15] reported increased urinary excretion of iAs after consumption of rice, reflecting increased exposure. High iAs exposure from consumption of rice-based food is therefore of concern.

In contrast to adults, our understanding of As metabolism and kinetics in infants is much more limited although some important studies have been conducted with infants exposed to iAs through drinking water in South America and Asia.[16] Concha *et al.*[17] were among the first to raise concerns that children may be more vulnerable to exposure to iAs. Later, Fängström *et al.*[18] demonstrated that the urinary metabolite pattern of children (18 months of age) in Bangladesh is indicative of decreased As methylation efficiency during weaning.

The next section describes how, and in what quantities, rice As previously absorbed, transported, and accumulated in the rice grains will reach the bodies of infants worldwide.

ARSENIC CONTENTS IN RICE-BASED INFANT PRODUCTS

Most children are weaned using, initially, pure rice porridge, a precooked, dried and milled product.[11,19] As the child develops, this porridge is used for the basis of meals by mixing it with puréed fruit or vegetables – either homemade mixtures with baby rice, or pre-prepared commercial products. Rice biscuits are used during teething. Many common food items eaten by infants are also rice-based, such as cereals and biscuits.[12] This dependence on rice is exacerbated for those with food intolerances. Rice milk is often used as an animal milk substitute for those with milk intolerance,[19] while rice-based products are the staple for those with gluten intolerances.[20]

The wide use of rice after months 5–6 could explain, at least in part, why the arsenic content in 1-year-old weaned babies' hair was found to be 10-fold greater than in 1-month-old infants.[3,21]

Because of high food consumption rates per body mass, children are at higher risk of exposure of dietary contaminants, including As.[2,3,19] The UK Food Standards Agency (UK FSA) has already issued advice that children under 4.5 years do not take rice milk,[22] as typical consumption patterns would lead to iAs intakes exceeding WHO Permissible Maximum Tolerable Daily Intakes (PMTDI). However, this tolerable intake has been found to be no longer appropriate in the recent As assessment of As in food by the EFSA,[2] based on updated toxicological data.[2] EU baby rice itself has elevated As levels and may lead to high dietary exposure.[3] Similarly, rice-based products pose a risk to young children due to high iAs content.[3,12,19] Research indicates that young children are more sensitive receptors to iAs than adults;[18] consequently, ensuring that infants' exposure to iAs is minimized is an imperative. The EFSA As review[2] concluded that (1) iAs levels in EU diets are at a level consistent with the possibility of risk to consumers, (2) rice is one of the most important sources of iAs, and (3) young children have the highest exposures with respect to the general population.

Food propensity questionnaire studies regarding infant diet have revealed that by the age of 3 months 18% of infants were being fed cereals, rising to 40% at 4 months of age.[23] This study also revealed that 71–86% of infants aged between 5 and 10.5 months are fed baby cereals. A significant proportion of the baby cereal is represented by rice-based products. Due to the fast growth and development within the first year of life, and the consequent need for energy supply, the average food intake by infants is much greater (relative to their body weight) compared to that of adults and older children.

The problem of exposure to iAs from rice-based products is likely to increase as the demand for rice-based baby foods continues to grow and change. For example, in 2008 the number of baby food product launches containing rice ingredients almost doubled as food manufacturers continued to respond to consumers' demand for natural, organic, and hypoallergenic products.[23] In 2007, more than 30 baby food products containing rice ingredients launched worldwide were tracked. Since the shift in focus to "all things natural" there has been a significant jump, and the number of products launches more than doubled in 2008. This trend has continued. For instance, during the first quarter of 2009, and in Eastern Europe alone, there was a considerable increase in interest in baby foods containing rice ingredients; new product launches jumped from 7% of the year's total in 2007 to 37% in 2008.

The EFSA[2] pointed out that studies quantifying tAs and especially iAs are needed to allow European authorities to legislate regarding proper maximum contents of iAs in food, including rice-based products. Up to now several countries, such as China, have legislated regarding these thresholds; however, a solid scientific base to set up these limits remains to be established.

As a brief introduction, Figure 29.1 shows the mean contents of both tAs and iAs in the main groups of infant foods according to studies by the main research groups dealing with As occurrence in infant foods (University of Aberdeen, UK; Karolinska Institutet, Sweden; De Montfort University, UK; and Universidad Miguel Hernández, Spain). In general, the highest contents of iAs were found in baby rice, followed by cereals, rice milk, and special foods (e.g., milk for lactose intolerance). In contrast, breast milk and infant formula showed the lowest contents of tAs.

Breast Milk and Formula

Breast milk is recommended as the sole source of infant nutrition for the first 6 months of life because it has the ideal nutritional properties to fulfil babies' requirements. However, less than 35% of the world's infants are exclusively breastfed at this age.[24] Substitutes for breast milk include other milks, sweetened liquids, and solid foods in the developing world,[25] while infant formula is the most common substitute in the USA and in Europe for infants younger than 4 months.[26] Feeding patterns differ between formula- and breast-fed infants, with higher milk intakes in formula-fed infants from the sixth week of life.[27]

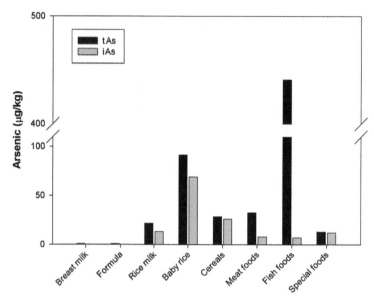

FIGURE 29.1   Total arsenic (tAs) content in the main groups of rice-based infant foods.

Ljung *et al.*[28] mentioned that Sweden has one of the highest rates of breastfeeding in Europe, with 12% exclusively breast fed at 6 months; however, breastfeeding has declined in recent years and the use of substitutes is increasing.[29,30]

Infant formula and foods may contain toxic elements as a result of their natural presence in raw materials, of contamination, or of food processing. Ljung *et al.*[28] evaluated the concentrations of essential and toxic elements, including tAs, in infant formula and infant foods. They proved that extensively hydrolyzed milks have significantly higher As concentration, up to 1.18 μg/L (extensively hydrolyzed whey), than does breast milk, 0.6 μg/L. The tAs ranged from 0.17 μg/L in regular milk up to 1.58 μg/L in soy protein, with mean and median values of 0.73 and 0.60 μg/L, respectively.[28] No data are available on iAs for these products, breast milk, or infant formula; however, if it is considered that approximately 60% of tAs in infant foods is present as inorganic species,[31] the mean and median values for iAs can be estimated at 0.44 and 0.36 μg/L.

Rice Milk

Rice milk is an alternative to cow's milk and, similar to soy milk, it is marketed for vegans and vegetarians, those following macrobiotic diets, lactose intolerance sufferers, and sufferers from cancer-related illness who wish to avoid the hormones present in animal milk.[32,33] The milk can be prepared enzymatically (for commercial products) – for instance, by liquefaction of the whole grain with α-amylase in an aqueous medium to form a liquid slurry, and then with glucosidase in a saccharification step – or mechanically (for homemade products) by extracting ground rice with hot water.[19] Commercial formulations tend to be fortified with minerals and vitamins to account for deficiencies compared to animal milks, although the low protein

and fat content of rice milk products makes them unsuitable alternatives for infants and toddlers, unless the fat and protein is supplemented in other forms.[32,34]

Meharg and colleagues[19] evaluated the tAs contents and As speciation in rice milk sold on the market in the UK, and concluded that iAs levels in rice milk exceed EU and US drinking water standards. The tAs contents in rice milks ranged from 10.2 to 33.2 μg/L, with mean and median values of 21.6 and 22.2 μg/L, respectively; the iAs contents ranged from 7.1 to 20.0 μg/L, with mean and median values of 13.2 and 13.4 μg/L, respectively. Oat and soya milks were considered as control samples, and their tAs concentrations were 3.5 and 3.0 μg/L, respectively, indicating the high impact of rice on the As content in foods.

Weaning Foods Based on Rice

Although the WHO[24] recommends that infants should be breast fed until they are 6 months old, a high percentage of babies start taking solid foods from month 4.[35] This early consumption is mainly induced by the information included in labeling of the infant foods, which recommends that, in general, gluten-free infant rice be introduced into the infant's diet at month 4.[20,36] Later, at month 6, the infant body is ready to enjoy more complex foods, such as cereals containing gluten (wheat, oat, etc.). Finally, puréed infant foods containing meat (mainly chicken) and fish (mainly hake) are introduced at 6 and 8 months of age, respectively.[20,36] However, infants with celiac disease have little option than to consume rice or maize flour instead of the more popular wheat flour.[31]

Baby Rice and Baby Cereals

Due to the high dependence of infants on rice foods during their first year, several studies.[20,28,31] have quantified both tAs and iAs contents in baby rice (gluten-free items) and baby cereals containing gluten. At month 6 the infant stomach is able to digest gluten, and gluten-containing cereals are introduced, replacing in part the intake of rice. Ljung et al.[28] studied Swedish infant foods, reporting values of tAs ranging from 1 to 33 μg/kg in semolina and wholegrain rice. Swedish spelt flour and oats showed low levels of tAs, while relatively high levels (17–18 μg/kg) were found in samples of rice plus banana. Simultaneously, Burló et al.[20] showed significant differences among Spanish baby rice (gluten-free) and baby cereals with gluten (mixture of several cereals, wheat, barley, oat, rye, sorghum and millet). The total As content in rice-based products ranged from 43 to 80 μg/kg, with a mean value of 57 μg/kg; on the other hand, tAs ranged from 9 to 39 μg/kg, with a mean of 24 μg/kg in infant cereals. More recently, Carbonell-Barrachina et al.[31] studied a higher number of samples from Spain and performed As speciation; similar patterns to those reported by Burló et al.[20] for tAs were found for iAs, and mean values for gluten-free infant rice and infant cereals with gluten were 69 and 26 μg/kg, respectively (tAs values were 126 and 33 μg/kg). A clear correlation was proven by Burló et al.[20] between the percentage of rice in Spanish baby rice and tAs content; the higher the rice content in the formulation of baby rice, the higher was the tAs content (Fig. 29.2).

In summary, both tAs and iAs contents are significantly higher in baby rice compared to baby cereals, and this is certainly due to the greater participation of rice in the formulation of baby rice products (almost 100% compared to ~10%).

Apart from the rice percentage, other important factors in determining the occurrence of As in infant foods are the rice cultivar,[37,38] the geographical origin,[11] and rice processing.[39] In this respect, Meharg et al.[11] studied the tAs in polished (white) rice from 10 countries (Bangladesh, China, Egypt, France, India, Italy, Japan, Spain, Thailand, and the USA) covering 4 continents, and found significant differences among samples, with Egypt and India having the lowest tAs contents and France the highest. It is possible that this geographical variation in the As content of rice is also reflected in significant differences in As content in infant foods from different geographical origins. This was the main hypothesis behind the study of Carbonell-Barrachina et al.,[31] who quantified both tAs and iAs in infant rice from four countries (China, the USA, the UK, and Spain). These authors found statistically significant differences among the tAs contents and the speciation as affected by the country of origin. US and UK products showed the highest mean values of tAs (~240–250 μg/kg), while Spain and China had the lowest contents of both tAs (181 and 135 μg/kg, respectively) and, more importantly, iAs (85 and 114 μg/kg, respectively). The US and Spanish samples had the

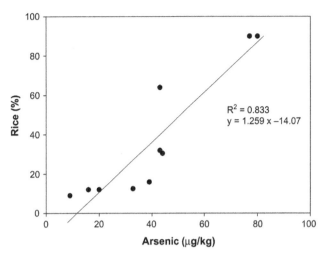

FIGURE 29.2 Relationship between total arsenic (tAs) content and rice percentage in samples of Spanish infant rice and cereals.

highest contents of DMA (~45%), perhaps related to previous use of organic pesticides in agriculture, while the As from the Chinese and UK samples seems to have come from inorganic sources, mainly from irrigation water.

Meat and Fish Puréed Baby Foods

At approximately 6 months of age, an additional source of proteins is included in the baby's diet: meat. Normally the first type of meat introduced is chicken, although it is possible to find, on the market, beef foods recommended for 6-month-old infants. Meat is always prepared mixed with vegetables, rice, legumes, and potatoes. Later, at approximately 8 months of age, white fish is introduced into the diet and again combined with vegetables, rice, and potatoes. Recent studies by Burló et al.[20] and Carbonell-Barrachina et al.[31] have quantified the amount of both tAs and iAs in Spanish puréed meat and fish infant foods, and results clearly proved that tAs was drastically higher in fish products (content higher than 2000 μg/kg was found in a sole product) than in any other infant food. However, when As speciation was performed[31] it was demonstrated that cationic species, mainly arsenobetaine, accounted for about 95% of the tAs present, leaving the content of iAs below 10 μg/kg. It is generally considered that arsenobetaine, mainly derived from seafood and fish,[40–42] is relatively non-toxic compound that is excreted by humans without transformation.[43,44] Total As in meat products was low, ranging from 9 to 55 μg/kg, with less than 10 μg/kg being present as iAs. The main source for this iAs was probably rice, the percentage of which in puréed infant foods is reduced to a content ranging from 5% to 10%.

Daily Intake of Inorganic Arsenic

Millions of people worldwide consume rice, which is generally naturally elevated in As compared to other cereal staples, and anthropogenic pollution further elevates grain As content. However, little is known about the bioaccessibility and bioavailability of As in cooked rice and processed rice products. The toxicology of As is independent of source once it crosses the gut membrane. Laparra et al.[45] studied the bioaccessibility of As(III) and As(V) in cooked rice and, after simulating gastrointestinal digestion, the bioaccessibility of iAs ranged between 63% and 93%. Juhasz et al. [46] assessed the bioavailability of As in rice using the *in vivo* swine assay. They reported that DMA was poorly absorbed, resulting in low bioavailability values (only 33% of the tAs from rice was bioavailable). On the other hand, iAs was efficiently absorbed, resulting in high bioavailability (89% of rice-bound As was bioavailable). From these results, it seems that bioaccessibility and bioavailability of As in cooked rice is high, and it is highly dependent on As speciation.[47] However, there are major differences among As species, and the effects of more complex matrices, such as those of rice-based infant foods, on both the bioaccessibility and bioavailability need elucidation.

Infants

According to the WHO,[24] after 6 months of age it becomes difficult to meet infants' nutrient needs just from human milk. Consequently, it is recommended that at 6 months of age complementary food is introduced. However, despite these guidelines, weaning occurs at an early age in most countries[48] – for example, Santamaria-Orleans et al.[49] reported that Spanish infants started with weaning foods at 4.4 months of life instead of 6 months. Briefel et al.[50] reported that, in the period from 4–6 months, US infants are introduced to infant cereals and puréed infant foods, mostly based on fruits and vegetables.

In this review, the daily As intake will be discussed, according to the infant nutrition (main types of foods being consumed), in the period from 1 to 12 months of age. The daily food intake for an infant in this period will be calculated according to the recommendations made by the companies that manufacture infant foods – for instance:

4 *months*: five feeds of breast milk (140 mL/feed),[27] 35 g of gluten-free infant rice, and 50 g fruit-rice

6 *months*: three feeds of breast milk (240 mL/feed), 98 g of infant rice, and 100 g of meat-based infant food

8 *months*: two feeds of breast milk (240 mL/feed), 98 g of gluten-free infant rice or infant cereals with gluten, 200 g of meat-based infant food, and 200 g of fish-based infant food

12 *months*: two feeds of breast milk (240 mL/feed), 98 g of infant rice or infant cereals, 250 g of meat-based infant food, and 250 g of fish-based infant food.

It must be pointed out that it was assumed that infants were taking only breast milk (ideal scenario) until the fourth month of age, the water used to reconstitute infant rice/cereals was As-free (which is the normal situation in most of the European Union countries), and body weights considered were on the 50th percentile.[51]

Figure 29.3 summarizes the daily intake of tAs for infants aged from 1 to 12 months, and it can easily be observed that the daily intake significantly increased at month 8 of age – without any doubt related to the consumption of fish-based puréed foods. However, as mentioned previously, about 95% of the tAs present in fish foods is in the form of arsenobetaine, a non-toxic compound that is easily eliminated by the human organism. Therefore, the need for speciation data in this type of foods is of the utmost importance in order to refine the risk assessment studies. If the data presented in Figure 29.3 were considered for risk assessment, it would lead to considerable overestimation of the health risk related to dietary As exposure. In fact, the only study in the literature to date that presents As speciation data for a complete range of infant foods is that by Carbonell-Barrachina et al.[31] for Spanish products. The maximum daily intake of iAs was estimated in the period from 8 to 12 months of age, with 0.41 and 0.26 μg/kg bw per day for infants consuming products without or with gluten, respectively. Until 6 months of age the daily intake was 0.30 μg/kg bw per day, increasing significantly thereafter.

However, the CONTAM Panel of the EFSA[2] modeled the dose–response data from key epidemiologic studies and selected a benchmark response of 1% extra risk. The lowest $BMDL_{01}$ values were for lung cancer, and this EFSA Panel concluded that the overall range of $BMDL_{01}$ values of 0.3–8.0 μg/kg bw per day should be used instead of a single reference point in the risk characterization of iAs. The estimated dietary exposures to iAs of

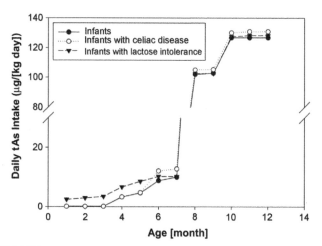

FIGURE 29.3 Daily intake of total arsenic (tAs) for infants aged up to 1 year and belonging to normal (with no food intolerances) and special groups (with celiac disease or with lactose intolerance).

Spanish children[31] were close to or higher than those of adults, but this does not necessarily indicate that children are at greater risk, because the exposure estimates were within the range of $BMDL_{01}$ values. Moreover, the negative effects of As are due to long-term exposure,[2] although infants seem to be very susceptible to the toxic effects of iAs.[52]

Special Communities

As previously mentioned, infant diets tend to differ according to the digestive assimilation of nutrients. Babies or infants with gastrointestinal alterations or dysfunctions, such as lactose intolerance or celiac disease, will significantly increase the daily intake of rice-based foods. Consequently, it is important to evaluate whether changes in the diets of these special groups (e.g., substitution of wheat by rice) will result in significant changes in the daily intake of tAs and/or iAs.

LACTOSE INTOLERANCE

Lactose intolerance is the inability to digest and metabolize lactose caused by a lack of lactase, the enzyme required to break down lactose in the digestive system. The symptoms of lactose intolerance include abdominal pain, bloating, flatulence, diarrhea, and acid reflux.[53] This disorder is normally detected after the third year of age, because babies produce a huge amount of lactase at birth.[54] An alternative to breast milk and animal milk (e.g., cow's milk) are soybean or rice milks.[19,55] An increase in the intake of rice products can imply an increase in the intake of As. Data compiled in Figure 29.3 show that, following the replacement of breast milk and/or formula by rice milk, there is a significant increase in the daily iAs intake up to month 6 of age.

CELIAC DISEASE

Celiac disease is a digestive illness that damages the small intestine and interferes with the absorption of nutrients from food.[56] The only treatment for celiac disease is a gluten-free diet, which involves excluding foods that contain wheat, rye, and barley. Despite these restrictions, people with celiac disease can eat a well-balanced diet with a variety of foods, including rice, maize, potato, soy, amaranth, quinoa, buckwheat, or bean flour instead of wheat flour.[56] Celiac disease may start at any age, including both childhood and adolescence, and is also relatively common in adulthood.[57]

Rice-based foods are ideal for feeding infants with celiac disease, and these particular infants will not make the change from gluten-free products (consumed mainly during the period 4–6 months of age) to cereals containing gluten. The daily tAs intake of infants from this group is higher than in other infants of the same age after 6 months (Fig. 29.3). A similar situation, as described by Carbonell-Barrachina et al.,[31] occurs when the daily

intake of iAs is considered. These authors reported mean iAs intakes of 0.05, 0.16, 0.25, and 0.26 μg/kg bw per day for infants with no food-related illnesses at 4, 6, 8, and 12 months of age, respectively. However, if the infants suffered from celiac disease and could consume only gluten-free products, mainly rice, their daily intakes were significantly increased to 0.26, 0.27, 0.41, and 0.40 μg/kg bw per day for the same ages. In summary, infants with celiac disease, who are "forced" to consume gluten-free products, with high percentages of rice, are at serious risk due to the most elevated intakes of iAs. This situation is even worse when it is considered that this high dependence of infants with celiac disease on rice-based foods will be lifelong, and the exposure to high levels of iAs from foods will become a chronic condition.

ASIAN COMMUNITIES – FOR EXAMPLE, BANGLADESHIS

In 2009, the European Food Safety Authority estimated that certain ethnic groups with heavy rice consumption living in Europe have a 7.8-fold higher iAs daily intake than the average European consumer.[2] Asian communities are well known to consume high quantities of rice. Bangladeshis consume 445 g per person per day (dry weight) in their country of origin; once they move to the Europe this consumption decrease to 251 g per day of rice (dry wt).[58] Nevertheless, the Bangladeshi population still represents the largest rice consumer group in the UK, with an average of 30-fold more rice consumed than in white Caucasians.[58] It has previously been reported that Bangladeshis in the UK may be in danger of being exposed to higher levels of As through their diet.[59] Meharg[58] highlighted the need for a survey on rice consumption habits of this ethnic group. It is documented that UK Bangladeshis suffer disproportionately from diabetes and cardiovascular disease compared to other groups,[60] and that Bangladeshi men have a standardized mortality ratio for stroke of 249, according to the 2001 census. In light of these studies, Cascio et al.[14] carried out a biomonitoring study on 49 volunteers regarding the effect of rice consumption on urinary arsenicals in a general population group of UK Bangladeshis and UK Caucasians. Results (Fig. 29.4) have shown that even if total urinary As did not significantly differ in the two groups, the sum of the medians of DMA (dimethylarsinic acid), MMA (monomethylarsonic acid), and iAs for the Bangladeshi group was found to be over three-fold higher than for the Caucasian group. Urinary DMA was significantly higher ($p < 0.001$) in UK Bangladeshis than in the white Caucasians as well as iAs ($p < 0.001$). In contrast, cationic compounds were significantly lower in the Bangladeshis than in the Caucasians. Significant positive correlations were found for both iAs and DMA, and the daily consumption of rice. The higher DMA and iAs levels in the

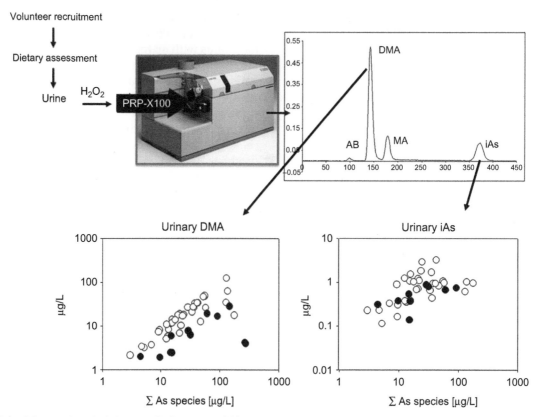

FIGURE 29.4   Scheme of methodology applied to screen differences in urinary arsenicals among UK Caucasian and UK Bangladeshi volunteers.[14] Volunteers were asked to complete a questionnaire to assess their rice intake. HPLC-ICP-MS was performed to screen main arsenicals in urine. Urinary dimethylarsonic acid (DMA), and inorganic arsenic (iAs) were significantly higher in UK Bangladeshis (indicated by white dots) than in UK Caucasians (black dots).

Bangladeshis were considered by the authors[14] to be the consequence of higher rice consumption in this community. Rice in fact accumulates both iAs and orgAs. Once ingested, iAs can be metabolized (through MMA) to DMA by humans. Furthermore, DMA is largely present in American long grain rice, and may be excreted unchanged in urine. A previous study by Pearson et al.[15] demonstrated that, for a single volunteer, consumption of rice resulted in increased urinary excretion of DMA. The study by Cascio et al.[14] showed that a higher dietary intake of DMA from rice can alter the DMA/MMA ratio in urine, and highlights the fact that the DMA/MMA ratio as an indication of methylation capacity in populations consuming large quantities of rice should be applied with caution.

ARSENIC TOXICITY AND METABOLISM IN THE HUMAN BODY

The carcinogenic and toxic properties of As in humans and in the environment strongly depend on chemical species, with inorganic forms generally more toxic than organic ones (orgAs), and trivalent forms more toxic than pentavalent ones.

The general population can be exposed to iAs through food and water consumption. Once As is ingested, the extent of absorption in the gastrointestinal tract depends on its chemical species (and essentially water solubility) and the complexity of the food matrix: about 95% of arsenite and arsenate present in drinking water is rapidly absorbed after ingestion in humans.[61] Unfortunately, there is a lack of human data on the bioavailability of organic arsenicals. Once absorbed, the iAs enters the bloodstream and is distributed between the plasma and erythrocytes, binding to globin chains of the hemoglobin molecule.[2] From the bloodstream As can reach several target organs, including the liver, kidney, spleen, and lung. Several weeks later, As is transported to high sulfur-containing proteins in tissues such as hair, nails, and skin.[2,62,63] *Post mortem* analysis on humans with long-term As exposure showed the highest As concentrations in the skin and lungs (0.01–1 mg/kg dry wt), as well as the hair and nails.[64,65] In subjects exposed to high concentrations of As in drinking water (0.2–2 mg/L), the As content in the liver was found to be 3.75- to 37.5-fold higher than in unexposed people.[66] In the case of fatal arsenic trioxide (As_2O_3) poisoning, the kidney and liver showed the highest concentrations of tAs, with values 63- and 350-fold higher, respectively, than those in the blood. In all organs, As(III) was the predominant species, and MMA(V) occurred at higher concentrations than DMA(V). MMA and DMA were more prevalent in lipid-rich organs (49% and 45% of tAs in cerebellum and in brain, respectively) compared with other organs (20% of tAs). As(V) was found in small quantities in the liver, kidney, and blood (2% of tAs).[67]

In the human body, iAs undergoes enzyme-mediated biotransformation resulting in sequential methylation. In humans, As biomethylation occurs mainly in the liver,[68] and the enzyme arsenic(+III) methyltransferase (As3MT) has been isolated from cytosol in hepatocytes. On the contrary, fibroblasts and urothelial cells do not express As3MT, so As is mainly accumulated as iAs in these cells. The cyto- and genotoxicity of As in hepatocytes is confirmed by its accumulation in nuclei and mitochondria.[69] Other methylation sites are the kidney, testis, and lung.

Different hypotheses have been postulated about As metabolism in humans, but despite the large number of studies carried out there is still no universally approved mechanism for the metabolic pathways of As *in vivo*.

Once As(V) enters the cells via the active phosphate transport mechanisms,[70] it is reduced to As(III) thanks to the activity of glutathione reductase[71] or by purine nucleoside phosphorylase.[72,73] According to Cullen's model[40] (Fig. 29.5), As(III) is then methylated to methylarsonate (MMA[V]) with an oxidative methylation reaction catalyzed by arsenic(+III) methyltransferase coded by the gene As3MT[74] that corresponds to Cyt19 in the Human Proteome Organization's classification. As3MT exploits S-adenosyl-L-transferase (SAM) as a methyl donor. This

methylation reaction is considered to be a detoxification step. Methylarsonate [MMA(V)]. is converted to methylarsonite [MMA(III)] by glutathione S-transferase (GST O).This step is considered an activation step, with the trivalent methylated species of As being more reactive and toxic than the pentavalent precursors. A further oxidative methylation step is performed by As3MT with the production of dimethylarsinousus acid [DMA(V)]. In light of this model, some authors report the primary methylation index (PMI) as the ratio MMA(V)/[As(III)+As(V)] in urine and a secondary methylation index (SMI) as the ratio DMA(V)/MMA(V) in urine.[75] The first methylation step is considered to be the limiting methylation step in humans. Some studies correlate urinary As methylation profile to the activity of the enzyme arsenic(+III) methyltransferase, and levels of expression and SNPs of As3MT.[76] More recently criticism has been directed at this pathway based on the experimental evidence that arsenic(+III) methyltransferase produces more DMA(V) using As(III) as a substrate than from MMA(III). Hayakawa[77] has proposed an alternative pathway (see dotted lines in Fig. 29.5) in which arsine triglutathione (ATG) can be generated non-enzymatically from arsine As(III) and glutathione. ATG then becomes a substrate for the enzyme As(+III) methyltransferase that uses SAM to generate arsenic diglutathione (ADG). ADG will either first give MMA(III) and finally MMA(V), or become a substrate for a second methylation reaction catalyzed by the As3MT leading to the production of arsenic monoglutathione (AMG). To support this evidence that arsenic triglutathione and methylarsenic diglutathione have been found in bile of rats,[78] Hayakawa's model is

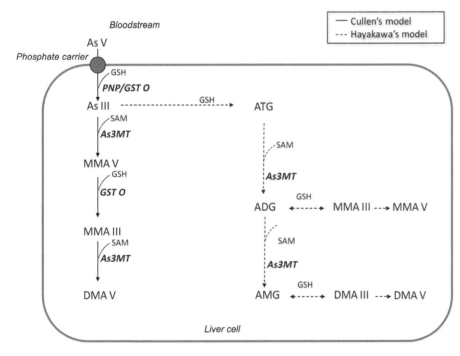

FIGURE 29.5 Arsenic methylation in human hepatocytes according to Cullen's model (continuous arrows)[40] and Hayakawa's model (dotted arrows).[77] ATG, arsenic triglutathione; ADG, arsenic diglutathione; AMG, arsenic monoglutathione; As(III), arsenite; As(V), arsenate; MMA(V), monomethylarsonate; MMA(III), monomethylarsonite; DMA(III), dimethylarsinite; DAM(V), dimethylarsinate; PNP, purine nucleoside phosphorylase; GST O, glutathione-s-transferase; As3MT, arsenic(III) methyltransferase; GSH, glutathione.

compatible with the idea that methylation is a detoxification mechanism because the final products are just pentavalent methylated species.

The main metabolites excreted in human urine are organic species, DMA(V) and MMA(V), with a typical proportion 60–80% DMA, 10–20% MMA, and 10–20% iAs[79] in individuals who do not eat food of marine origin, such as fish, shellfish, and algae. Marine organisms are generally rich in organic arsenicals, including arsenobetaine (AB) and arsenosugars, the latter mostly found in marine algae and in mussels and oysters.[80] Fish consumption increases urinary excretion of AB and DMA in the few days after consumption. In addition, arsenosugars that can be present in fish are metabolized to urinary thio-arsenicals, including oxo-dimethylarsenoethanol (oxo-DMAE), trimethylarsine oxide, oxo-dimethylarsenoacetate (oxo-DMAA), and thio-dimethlyarsenoacetate (thio-DMAA).[81] Moreover, arsenic fatty acids have been found in urine after ingestion of cod liver, which contains arsenolipids.[82] DMA(III) and MMA(III) are highly reactive and unstable compounds that can be found in urine by means of sophisticated analytical approaches.[83] For instance, DMA(III) in urine is converted to DMA(V) in 17 hours even at −20°C. Cationic compounds in urine, such us arsenocholine (AC), trimethylarsine oxide (TMAO), and the tetramethylarsonium ion (TETRA), are present at very low levels.[83]

It has also been reported that arsenobetaine, which is considered to be non-toxic and excreted unchanged through urine, may be stored in the human body, raising potential health concerns.[84]

SOLUTIONS TO REDUCE ARSENIC CONTENT DURING RICE PROCESSING

Rice Processing, Types and Co-Products

Rice is the staple food for nearly two-thirds of the world's population.[85] It has been reported that as much as 75% of the daily calorie intake of the people in some Asian countries is derived from rice.[85,86] Rice varieties are divided in two types: (1) Japonica, a broad, thick, short, round grain which tends to be sticky and soft-cooking, and (2) Indica, an elongated, thin, slightly flattened grain that remains separate and is firmer-cooking.[87]

Rice processing is a combination of several operations to convert paddy into well-milled silky-white rice, which has superior cooking quality attributes.[85,88]

Rice properties are known to be dependent on the variety of rice, methods of cultivation, and processing and cooking conditions. Proteins, fats, vitamins, and minerals are concentrated in the germ and outer layer of the starchy endosperm,[85,89,90] and these parts of the rice grain are removed by milling operations. Usually, between 5% and 10% by weight of brown rice is removed (outer layers) during milling.

Rice can be classified, according to its different processing, into paddy, wholegrain brown, and milled white rice. During rice processing, different by- or co-products are produced including hull and bran (Fig. 29.6). Moreover, white rice (the final product) can also reach its final commercial stage in different forms: large broken rice, small broken rice, and rice flour. The following provides basic details regarding these rice types and co-products.

Paddy: Heads of rice form as tiny clusters of flowers in the base of the rice plant. The fertilized flower closes to become a protective hull, which the rice plant fills with liquid starch and protein. Later, the liquid consolidates to form a starchy inner grain attached to a seed embryo, all encased in nutrient-, enzyme-, and oil-rich layers. This complete grain, encased in its hull, is called paddy.[87]

Rice hull: This hard, protective shell of the grain is high in silica and is inedible for humans. Removal of the hull is the first stage of rice milling. Whole ungrounded rice hulls are used for animal bedding, stock-feeds, fruit juice extraction, and horticultural purposes. Ground and processed hulls are used in stock-feeds, potting mixes, pet litter, and industrial ashes.[87]

Wholegrain brown rice is the complete form of the rice grain, and is either sold as natural brown rice or, value-added, as quicker cooking rice.[87]

FIGURE 29.6 **Processing of rice from paddy (1) to wholegrain or brown (2) and to white polished (3).** a, hull; b, bran; c, polish; d, aleurone layer; e, starchy endosperm; f, embryo.

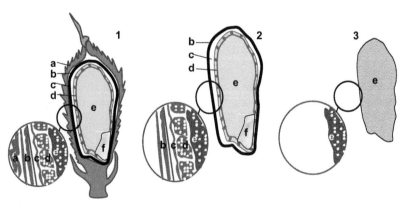

Rice bran is a byproduct of polishing the whole grain rice, comprising the pericarp, aleurone layer, embryo, and some endosperm.[91] It is used as a traditional ingredient in Japanese cooking such as rice bran pickling. It can be added to products such as rice crackers to increase the fiber content. Stabilized rice bran extract, known as rice bran soluble, is sold as a natural superfood and premier health food product, as it is high in antioxidants, vitamins, mineral nutrients, and soluble fiber.[92–94] A number of companies producing this product also supply food aid programs where malnourished children are given a daily ration of the product.[92–94] The supplement has already been used in Malawi, Guatemala, and El Salvador, with plans to expand further into Latin America, India, and the Caribbean.[92–94]

With the volatile, nutritious bran layers and germ removed, the starchy center of the grain has a longer storage life and quicker cooking period; this is called *milled white rice*. This is the most common form of rice for human consumption around the world. During rice milling some grains break and the large broken pieces are separated from small broken ones. *Large broken rice* grains are used in the manufacture of breakfast cereals, confectionery, pet foods, and formulated rice-based livestock feeds.[87] On the other hand, *small broken rice* is used extensively as an ingredient in snack foods, small goods, and formulated rice-based livestock feeds. Finally, small broken rice grains are ground to produce a fine powder called *rice flour*. This is used extensively for baby food manufacture, for baking applications, and as a bulking agent and flavor carrier in many manufactured food products.[87]

Effects of Rice Processing on Arsenic Content

Signes *et al.*[39] were probably the first researchers to investigate the As content in the hull of rice. They compared the main two dehusking processes used in rural villages of West Bengal (India) – the wet process (soaking of rice, boiling, and mechanical hulling) and the dry process (mechanical process) – and made recommendations about when to use one or the other, mainly according to the availability of As-free water for rice processing. Their conclusions were that hulling of paddy rice, containing 373 µg tAs/kg, significantly decreased the As content in the rice grain to 311 µg tAs/kg, and that it is not recommended that the rice husk or hull be used for feeding animals because the As content was highly elevated, at close to 950 µg tAs/kg.

Sun *et al*[92] proved that the pattern of tAs concentration in rice grain fractions was endosperm < whole grain < bran, with mean values being 560, 760, and

3300 µg/kg in rice samples from China and Bangladesh. This pattern in the As concentration leads to whole grain (brown) rice having higher As levels than polished (white) samples. Rice bran, both commercially purchased and specifically milled at a laboratory, had levels of iAs reaching 1000 µg/kg.

Later, Lombi *et al.*[94] reported striking differences in As distribution and speciation among husk, bran, and endosperm. The high As content in the bran is probably the most important result, because rice bran is widely used as food additive and as a premier health food product.[95] Total As concentrations significantly increased from the endosperm (540 µg/kg) to the bran (6240 µg/kg) and husk (12,420 µg/kg). A high concentration of As was also observed in the embryo in comparison with inner parts of the endosperm. The large majority of the As extracted was present as inorganic species; however, speciation was affected by localization within the rice grain. In the bran and endosperm, the major As species identified by XANES were DMA and As(III)-thiol complexes, while DMA appeared to be the main organic species in all rice parts.

Sun and colleagues[92] also analyzed five rice bran soluble products from the USA and Japan, and values for iAs ranged between 610 and 1900 µg/kg. It is necessary to highlight that although pure rice bran is used as a health food supplement, perhaps of more concern is rice bran soluble, which is marketed as a superfood and as a supplement to malnourished children in international aid programs without having undergone adequate toxicological research.

In summary, the pattern for the As content in different rice types is paddy rice > brown rice > white rice, and this pattern is due to the fact that As content follows the pattern hull >> bran > endosperm (Fig.29.7).

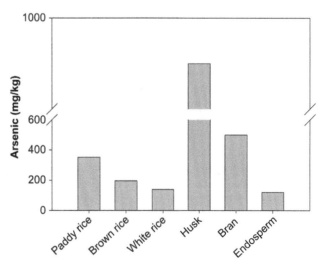

FIGURE 29.7 Total arsenic (tAs) content in different types of rice and rice parts.

Organic Foods and New Fashion Rice Products

In general, the majority of consumers worldwide prefer well milled rice (WMR) with little or no bran remaining on the endosperm. It has also been reported that consumer preferences vary from country to country and region to region. For instance, Japanese like sticky rice,[85,96] but Americans prefer semi-milled long grain or even brown rice (BR), whereas people in the India subcontinent prefer well milled parboiled rice.[85]

Nowadays, growing health consciousness has led consumers to start preferring rice milled to a lower degree (partially milled rice, PMR) or even brown rice in some countries. In addition, various value-added rice products, such as germinated brown rice (GBR) or rice bread (RB) have also been developed.[85] This is the general fashion among consumers worldwide, and some parents may want to transfer this fashion to their babies' diet and might therefore be considering feeding them with brown organic rice. In the absence of adequate research in this area, the wisdom of such a trend is questionable and health policymakers need to act to provide sound advice to parents of young babies and adults suffering from celiac disease.

Germinated brown rice (GBR) is produced by soaking rice kernels in warm water (30–40°C) until they just begin to bud. The potential health benefits and superior quality of GBR have attracted public attention, and GBR has become a popular healthy food. As a result of this popularity, modern rice cookers have also been developed to facilitate the production of GBR at the household level.[85] GBR contains more fiber, the essential amino acid, lysine, and γ-aminobutyric acid (GABA) than conventional BR. GBR contains more nutrients compared to milled rice – for instance, 10-fold more GABA; about 4-fold more dietary fiber, vitamin E, niacin and lysine; and about 3-fold more B$_1$, B$_2$, and magnesium.[85,97] All these nutrients may have positive effects in human health, and, according to some studies, they will help in preventing major diseases such as cancer, heart disease, etc.[85,97–99] However, no investigation is yet available quantifying the contents of tAs and iAs in this type of food and their impact on human health.

Rice bran soluble products are specifically marketed to food aid programs as nutritional supplements for undernourished children, who have low body weights. Children appear to be especially prone to disease resulting from As exposure,[100,101] and poor nutrition is thought to increase the severity of arsenical disease.[100,102]

It is of the highest priority that, before including any product in a child's diet, a wide range of analyses is conducted to prove their safety and quality. It is obvious that special attention must be paid when considering any rice-based food, due to the elevated As content of rice compared to other cereals.

CONCLUSIONS

The most important conclusion of the Scientific Opinion on Arsenic in Food of the EFSA[2] was that dietary exposure to iAs should be reduced. It has also been proved that both tAs and iAs contents are highly elevated in rice-based infant/baby foods. There are three main strategies to solve this situation: (1) questioning whether rice is suitable for infant foods and, if the answer is no, removing rice from infant food formulations; (2) reducing the intake of rice through diversification of the diet, such as including other cereals that do not contain high levels of As; and/or (3) trying to reduce the As content in rice intended for infant foods. Until the latter option comes into effect, some governments have chosen the former two options.[20] For instance, in the UK, children younger than 4.5 years are advised against consuming rice milk because of concern regarding high As exposure. Similarly, in Denmark children below 10 kg are also advised against consuming rice milk. However, these two options are not possible for certain groups of our society: *infants with celiac disease*, who have few other options than consuming rice flour; and *rice farmers*, because these options seriously jeopardize their markets. Therefore, research needs to be carried out to identify approaches that significantly reduce the high As contents in rice. Current research is focused on: (1) screening of As levels in existing rice to identify varieties that have low As levels, (2) breeding rice to obtain rice cultivars with restricted As uptake and upward transport to the edible grain, and (3) modifying current anaerobic growing practices in rice fields, moving towards more aerobic conditions, which will reduce As availability to rice plants but perhaps also their yields.[5] However, and considering the fact that safety of infants and babies needs to be addressed immediately, the only way of ensuring low As content in rice-based baby foods is to use exclusively white polished rice in the manufacture of these products. Therefore, the final conclusion of this review is that only white polished rice with proven low levels of iAs should be used in the manufacturing of infant/baby foods until "almost" As-free rice is available through other options.

References

1. IARC. IARC monographs on arsenic in drinking water. Available at: http://monographs.iarc.fr/ENG/Monographs/vol84/mono84-6.pdf.
2. EFSA Panel on Contaminants in the Food Chain (CONTAM), Scientific opinion on arsenic in food. *EFSA J* 2009;**7**:1351.
3. Meharg AA, Sun G, Williams PN, Adamako E, Deacon C, Zhu YG, et al. Inorganic arsenic levels in baby rice are of concern. *Environ Pollut* 2008;**152**:746–9.
4. Masotti A, Da Sacco L, Bottazzo G. Risk assessment of inorganic arsenic pollution on human health. *Environ Pollut* 2009;**157**:1771–2.

5. Carbonell-Barrachina AA, Signes-Pastor AJ, Vázquez-Araújo L, Burló F, Sengupta B. Presence of arsenic in agricultural products from arsenic-endemic areas and strategies to reduce arsenic intake in rural villages. *Mol Nutr Food Res* 2009;**53**:531–41.

6. Signes-Pastor AJ, Mitra K, Sarkhel S, Hobbes M, Burló F, de Groot WT, et al. Arsenic speciation in food and estimation of the dietary intake of inorganic arsenic in a rural village of West Bengal, India. *J Agric Food Chem* 2008;**56**:9469–74.

7. Williams PN, Villada A, Deacon C, Raab A, Figuerola J, Green AJ, et al. Greatly enhanced arsenic shoot assimilation in rice leads to elevated grain levels compared to wheat and barley. *Environ Sci Technol* 2007;**41**:6854–9.

8. Carbonell-Barrachina AA, Burló F, Valero D, López E, Martinez-Romero D, Martinez-Sanchez F. Arsenic toxicity and accumulation in turnip as affected by arsenic chemicals speciation. *J Agri Food Chem* 1999;**47**:2288–94.

9. Burló F, Guijarro I, Carbonell-Barrachina AA, Valero D, Martinez-Sánchez F. Arsenic species: Effects on and accumulation by tomato plants. *J Agric Food Chem* 1999;**47**:1247–53.

10. Lario Y, Burló F, Aracil P, Martínez-Romero D, Castillo S, Valero D, et al. Methylarsonic and dimethylarsinic acids toxicity and total arsenic accumulation in edible bush beans, *Phaseolus vulgaris. Food Addit Contam* 2002;**19**:417–26.

11. Meharg AA, Williams PN, Adamako E, Lawgali YY, Deacon C, Villada A, et al. Geographical variation in total and inorganic arsenic content of polished (white) rice. *Environ Sci Technol* 2009;**43**:1612–7.

12. Sun GX, Williams PN, Zhu YG, Deacon C, Carey AM, Raab A, et al. Survey of arsenic and its speciation in rice products such as breakfast cereals, rice crackers and Japanese rice condiments. *Environ Int* 2009;**35**:473–5.

13. Signes-Pastor AJ, Deacon C, Jenkins RO, Haris PI, Carbonell-Barrachina AA, Meharg AA. Arsenic speciation in Japanese rice drinks and condiments. *J Environ Monit* 2009;**11**:1930–4.

14. Cascio C, Raab A, Jenkins RO, Feldmann J, Meharg AA, Haris PI. The impact of a rice based diet on urinary arsenic. *J Environ Monit* 2011;**13**:257–65.

15. Pearson GF, Greenway GM, Brima EI, Haris PI. Rapid arsenic speciation using ion pair LC-ICPMS with a monolithic silica column reveals increased urinary DMA excretion after ingestion of rice. *J Anal Atom Spectrom* 2007;**22**:361.

16. Vahter M. Effects of arsenic on maternal and fetal health. *Ann Rev Nutr* 2009;**29**:381–99.

17. Concha G, Vogler G, Lezcano D, Nermell B, Vahter M. Exposure to inorganic arsenic metabolites during early human development. *Toxicol Sci* 1998;**44**:185–90.

18. Fängström B, Hamadani J, Nermell B, Grander M, Palm B, Vahter M. Impaired arsenic metabolism in children during weaning. *Toxicol Appl Pharmacol* 2009;**239**:208–14.

19. Meharg AA, Deacon C, Campbell RCJ, Carey AM, Williams PN, Feldmann J, et al. Inorganic arsenic levels in rice milk exceed EU and US drinking water standards. *J Environ Monitor* 2008;**10**:428–31.

20. Burló F, Ramírez-Gandolfo A, Signes-Pastor AJ, Haris PI, Carbonell-Barrachina AA. Arsenic contents in Spanish infant rice, pureed infant foods, and rice. *J Food Sci* 2012;**71**:T15–9.

21. Gibson RS, Cage L. Changes in hair arsenic levels in breast and bottle fed infants during the 1st year of infancy. *Sci Total Environ* 1982;**26**:33–40.

22. UK FSA (Food Standard Agency). Arsenic in rice: research published. Available online at: http://www.food.gov.uk/news/newsarchive/2009/may/arsenicinriceresearch [accessed 30.11.11].

23. Beneo-Remy. Available online at: http://www.beneo-remy.com [accessed 19.09.13].

24. WHO (World Health Organization). *Infant and Young Child Feeding. Model Chapter for Textbooks for Medical Students and Allied Health Professionals*. Geneva, Switzerland: WHO; 2009.

25. Marriott BM, Campbell L, Hirsch E, Wilson D. Preliminary data from demographic and health surveys on infant feeding in 20 developing countries. *J Nutr* 2007;**137**:518S–23S.

26. Freeman V, Van't Hof M, Haschke F. Patterns of milk and food intake in infants from birth to age 36 months: the Euro-growth study. *J Pediatr Gastroenterol Nutr* 2000;**31**(Suppl. 1):S76–85.

27. Sievers E, Oldigs HD, Santer R, Schaub J. Feeding patterns in breast-fed and formula-fed infants. *Ann Nutr Metab* 2002;**46**:243–8.

28. Ljung K, Palm B, Grandèr M, Vahter M. High concentrations of essential and toxic elements in infant formula and infant foods – A matter of concern. *Food Chem* 2011;**127**:943–51.

29. Socialstyrelsen. *Breast-Feeding and Smoking Habits among Parents of Infants Born in 2007*. Stockholm, Sweden: Official Statistics of Sweden; 2009.

30. Socialstyrelsen. *Breast-Feeding and Smoking Habits among Parents of Infants Born in 2008*. Stockholm, Sweden: Official Statistics of Sweden; 2010.

31. Carbonell-Barrachina AA, Xiangchun W, Ramírez-Gandolfo A, Norton GJ, Burló F, Deacon C, et al. Inorganic arsenic contents in rice-based infant foods from Spain, UK, China and USA. *Environ Pollut* 2012;**163**:77–83.

32. Cavalho NE, Kenney RD, Carrington PH, Hall DE. Severe nutritional deficiencies in toddlers resulting from health food milk alternatives. *Pediatrics* 2001;**107**:1–7.

33. Cockell KA, Bonacci G, Belonje B. Manganese content of soy or rice beverages is high in comparison to infant formulas. *J Am Coll Nutr* 2004;**23**:124–30.

34. Hill DJ, Roy N, Heine RG, Hosking CS, Francis DE, Brown J, et al. Effect of a low-allergen maternal diet on colic among breastfed infants: a randomized, controlled trial. *Pediatrics* 2005;**116**:709–15.

35. Mennella JA, Ziegler P, Briefel R, Novak T. Feeding infants and toddlers study: The types of foods fed to Hispanic infants and toddlers. *Am Diet Assoc* 2006;**106** S96-S-106.

36. Fenwick E. *Guía Completa de la Madre y el Bebé*. Barcelona, Spain: Ediciones Medici, S.A; 2005.

37. Norton GJ, Islam MR, Deacon CM, Zhao FJ, Stroud JL, McGrath SP, et al. Identification of low inorganic and total grain arsenic rice cultivars from Bangladesh. *Environ Sci Technol* 2009;**43**:6070–5.

38. Norton GJ, Duan G, Dasgupta T, Islam MR, Lei M, Zhu Y, et al. Environmental and genetic control of arsenic accumulation and speciation in rice grain: comparing a range of common cultivars grown in contaminated sites across Bangladesh, China and India. *Environ Sci Technol* 2009;**43**:8381–6.

39. Signes A, Mitra K, Burlo F, Carbonell-Barrachina AA. Effect of two different rice dehusking procedures on total arsenic concentration in rice. *Eur Food Res Technol* 2008;**226**:561–7.

40. Cullen WR, Reimer KJ. Arsenic speciation in the environment. *Chem Rev* 1989;**89**:713–64.

41. Edmonds JS, Francesconi KA. Arsenic in seafoods: Human health aspects and regulations. *Mar Pollut Bull* 1993;**26**:665–74.

42. Sharma VK, Sohn M. 2009. Aquatic arsenic: Toxicity, speciation, transformations, and remediation. *Environ Int* 2009;**35**:743–59.

43. Navas-Acien A, Francesconi KA, Silbergeld EK, Guallar E. Seafood intake and urine concentrations of total arsenic, dimethylarsinate and arsenobetaine in the US population. *Environ Res* 2011;**111**:110–8.

44. Sabbioni E, Fischbach M, Pozzi G, Pietra G, Gallorini M, Piette JL. Cellular retention, toxicity and carcinogenic potential of seafood arsenic I. Lack of cytotoxicity and transforming activity of arsenobetaine in the BALB/3T3 cell line. *Carcinogenesis* 1991;**12**:1287–91.

45. Laparra JL, Vélez D, Barberá R, Farré R, Montoro R. Bioavailability of inorganic arsenic in cooked rice: Practical aspects for human risk assessments. *J Agric Food Chem* 2005;**53**:8829–33.

46. Juhasz AL, Smith E, Weber J, Rees M, Rofe A, Kuchel T, et al. *In vivo* assessment of arsenic bioavailability in rice and its impact on human health risk assessment. *Environ Health Persp* 2006;**114**:1826–31.

47. Ackerman AH, Creed PA, Parks AN, Fricke MW, Schwegel CA, Creed JT, et al. Comparison of a chemical and enzymatic extraction of arsenic from rice and an assessment of the arsenic absorption from contaminated water by cooked rice. *Environ Sci Technol* 2005;**39**:5241–6.

48. Synnott K, Bogue J, Edwards CA, Scott JA, Higgins S, Norin E, et al. 2007. Parental perceptions of feeding practices in five European countries: an exploratory study, Eur. *J Clin Nutr* 2007; **61**:946–556.

49. Santamaria-Orleans A, Miranda-León MT, Rivero-Urgell M, Campoy-Folgoso C. Infant formula feeding pattern and weaning introduction in Spanish infants. *Early Nutrition and its Later Consequences: New Opportunities, Perinatal Nutrition Programmes Adults Health*. New York, NY: E-Publishing Inc; 2005. p. 199–200.

50. Briefel RR, Reidy K, Karwe V, Devaney B. Feeding infants and toddlers study: improvements needed in meeting infant feeding recommendations. *J Am Diet Ass* 2004;**104**:S31–7.

51. WHO (World Health Organization). Child growth standards. Available online at: http://www.who.int/childgrowth/standards/curvas_por_indicadores/en/index.html [accessed 30.11.11].

52. Rahman A, Vahter M, Smith AH, Nermell B, Yunus M, El Arifeen S, et al. 2009. Arsenic exposure during pregnancy and size at birth: A prospective cohort study in Bangladesh,. *Am J Epidemiol* 2009;**169**:304–12.

53. Cynthia N, Gil IL, Pereira-Scromeda MC, Torres EE. Intolerancia a la lactosa en pediatría, Rev. Post. Catedr. *Med* 2010;**198**:16–20.

54. David CD. Lactose intolerance. Available online at: http://www.nlm.nih.gov/medlineplus/ency/article/000276.htm [accessed 30.11.11].

55. WHO (World Health Organization). *The Treatment of Diarrhea. A Manual for Physicians and other Senior Health Workers, fourth edn*. Geneva, Switzerland: WHO; 2005.

56. NIDDK (National Institute of Diabetes and Digestive and Kidney 491 Diseases). Celiac disease. Available online at: http://digestive.niddk.nih.gov/ddiseases/pubs/celiac/celiac.pdf [accessed 30.11.11].

57. Rodrigo L. Celiac disease. *World J Gastroenterol* 2006;**12**:6585–93.

58. Meharg AA. Levels of arsenic in rice – literature review, Food Standard Agency – literature review. *FSA* 2007.

59. Al Rmalli SW, Haris PI, Harrington CF, Ayub M. A survey of arsenic in foodstuffs on sale in the United Kingdom and imported from Bangladesh. *Sci Total Environ* 2005;**337**:23–30.

60. NHS, Health Survey for England 2004: health of minorities-full report. Available online at: http://www.ic.nhs.uk/pubs/hse04ethnic [accessed 30.11.11].

61. ATSDR. Toxicological profile for arsenic. *U. S. Department of Health and Human Services*. Atlanta, GA: Public Health Service; 2007.

62. Hughes MF, Kenyon EM, Edwards BC, Mitchell CT, Del Razo LM, Thomas DJ. Accumulation and metabolism of arsenic in mice after repeated oral administration of arsenate. *Toxicol App Pharmacol* 2003;**191**:202–10.

63. Vahter M. Metabolism of arsenic. In: Fowler B, editor. *Biological and environmental effects of arsenic*. Oxford, UK: Elsevier Science; 1983. p. 171–97.

64. Liebscher K, Smith H. Essential and Nonessential Trace Elements. A Method of Determining Whether an Element is Essential or Nonessential in Human Tissue. *Health Criteria 18 – Arsenic* 1968.

65. Cross JD, Dale IM, Smith H. A suicide by ingestion of a mixture of copper, chromium and arsenic compounds. *Forensic Sci Int* 1979;**13**:25–9.

66. Guha Mazumder DN, Haque R, Ghosh N, De BK, Santra A, Chakraborty D, et al. Arsenic levels in drinking water and the prevalence of skin lesions in West Bengal, India. *Int J Epidemiol* 1998;**27**:871–7.

67. Benramdane L, Accominotti M, Fanton L, Malicier D, Vallon J-J. Arsenic speciation in human organs following fatal arsenic trioxide poisoning - A case report. *Clin Chem* 1999;**45**:301–6.

68. Dopp E, Hartmann LM, von Recklinghausen U, Florea AM, Rabieh S, Zimmermann U, et al. Forced uptake of trivalent and pentavalent methylated and inorganic arsenic and its cyto-/genotoxicity in fibroblasts and hepatoma cells. *Toxicol Sci* 2005;**87**:46–56.

69. Dopp E, Von Recklinghausen U, Hartmann LM, Stueckradt I, Pollok I, Rabieh S, et al. Subcellular distribution of inorganic and methylated arsenic compounds in human urothelial cells and human hepatocytes. *Drug Metab Dispos* 2008;**36**:971–9.

70. Rossman TG. Mechanism of arsenic carcinogenesis: an integrated approach. *Mutat Res-Fund Mol Mech Muta* 2003;**533**:37–65.

71. Aposhian HV, Zakharyan RA, Avram MD, Sampayo-Reyes A, Wollenberg ML. A review of the enzymology of arsenic metabolism and a new potential role of hydrogen peroxide in the detoxification of the trivalent arsenic species. *Toxicol Appl Pharmacol* 2004;**198**:327–35.

72. Gregus Z, Németi B. Purine nucleoside phosphorylase as a cytosolic arsenate reductase. *Toxicol Sci* 2002;**70**:13–9.

73. Radabaugh TR, Sampayo-Reyes A, Zakharyan RA, Aposhian HV. Arsenate reductase II. Purine nucleoside phosphorylase in the presence of dihydrolipoic acid is a route for reduction of arsenate to arsenite in mammalian systems. *Chem Res Toxicol* 2002;**15**:692–8.

74. Aposhian HV. Enzymatic methylation of arsenic species and other new approaches to arsenic toxicity, Ann. Rev. Pharmacol. *Toxicol* 1997;**37**:397–419.

75. Engström KS, Broberg K, Concha G, Nermell B, Warholm M, Vahter M. Genetic polymorphisms influencing arsenic metabolism: Evidence from Argentina, Environ. *Health Perspect* 2007;**115**:599–605.

76. Engström K, Vahter M, Mlakar SJ, Concha G, Nermell B, Raqib R, et al. Polymorphisms in Arsenic(+III Oxidation State) Methyltransferase (AS3MT) Predict Gene Expression of AS3MT as Well as Arsenic Metabolism, Environ. *Health Perspect* 2011;**119**:182–8.

77. Hayakawa T, Kobayashi Y, Cui X, Hirano S. A new metabolic pathway of arsenite: arsenic–glutathione complexes are substrates for human arsenic methyltransferase Cyt19. *Arch Toxicol* 2005;**79**:183–91.

78. Kala SV, Neely MW, Kala G, Prater CI, Atwood DW, Rice JS, et al. The MRP2/cMOAT transporter and arsenic-glutathione complex formation are required for biliary excretion of arsenic. *J Biol Chem* 2000;**275**:33404–8.

79. Buchet JP, Lauwerys R, Roels H. Comparison of the urinary excretion of arsenic metabolites after a single oral dose of sodium arsenite, monomethylarsonate, or dimethylarsinate in man, Int. Arch. Occup. Environ. *Health* 1981;**48**:71–9.

80. Sanchez-Rodas D, Geiszinger A, Gómez-Ariza JL, Francesconi KA. Determination of an arsenosugar in oyster extracts by liquid chromatography-electrospray mass spectrometry and liquid chromatography-ultraviolet photo-oxidation-hydride generation atomic fluorescence spectrometry. *Analyst* 2002;**127**:60–5.

81. Raml R, Goessler W, Traar P, Ochi T, Francesconi KA. Novel Thioarsenic Metabolites in Human Urine after Ingestion of an Arsenosugar, 2',3'-Dihydroxypropyl 5-Deoxy-5-dimethylarsinoyl-B-d-riboside. *Chem Res Toxicol* 2005;**18**:1444.

82. Schmeisser E, Rumpler A, Kollroser M, Rechberger G, Goessler W, Francesconi KA. Arsenic fatty acids are human urinary metabolites of arsenolipids present in cod liver. *Angew Chem Int Ed* 2006;**45**:150.

83. Francesconi KA, Kuehnelt D. Determination of arsenic species: A critical review of methods and applications, 2000-2003. *Analyst* 2004;**129**:373–95.

84. Newcombe C, Raab A, Williams PN, Deacon C, Haris PI, Meharg AA, et al. Accumulation or production of arsenobetaine in humans? *J Environ Monit* 2010;**12**:832.

85. Roy P, Orikasa T, Okadome H, Nakamura N, Shiina T. Processing conditions, rice properties, health and environment. *Int J Environ Res Public Health* 2011;**8**:1957–76.

86. FAO (Food and Agricultural Organization). Rice in the world. Available online at: http://www.fao.org/wairdocs/tac/x5801e/x5801e08.htm [accessed 30.11.11].

87. SunRice. SunRice rice grain poster. Available online at: http://www.sunrice.com.au/uploads//documents/education/SunRice GrainPoster.pdf [accessed 30.11.11].

88. Roberts LR. Composition and taste evaluation of rice milled to different degrees. *J Food Sci* 1979;**44**:127–9.

89. Juliano BO, Bechtel DB. The rice grain and its gross composition. In: Juliano BO, editor. *Rice Chemistry and Technology, 2nd Ed., 57 American Association of Cereal Chemists, Inc.* St Paul, MN: USA; 1985. p. 17–57.

90. Itani T, Tamaki M, Arai E, Horino T. Distribution of amylase, nitrogen, and minerals in rice kernels with various characters. *J Agric Food Chem* 2002;**50**:5326–32.

91. Meharg AA, Williams PN, Schekel K, Lombi E, Feldmann J, Raab A, et al. Speciation of arsenic differs between white and brown rice grain. *Environ Sci Technol* 2008;**42**:1051–7.

92. Sun GX, Williams PN, Carey AM, Zhu YG, Deacon C, Raab A, et al. Inorganic arsenic in rice bran and its products are an order of magnitude higher than in bulk grain. *Environ Sci Technol* 2008;**42**:7542–6.

93. NutraCea Inc. Food ingredients. Available online at: http://www.nutracea.com/FoodIngredients [accessed 30.11.11].

94. Lombi E, Scheckel KG, Pallon J, Carey AM, Zhu YG, Meharg AA. Speciation and distribution of arsenic and localization of nutrients in rice grains. *New Phytol* 2009;**184**:193–201.

95. Sun GX, Williams PN, Carey AM, Zhu YG, Deacon C, Raab A, et al. Speciation and distribution of arsenic and localization of nutrients in rice grains. *New Phytol* 2008;**184**:193–201.

96. Deshpande SS, Bhattacharya KR. The texture of cooked rice. *J Text Stud* 1982;**13**:31–42.

97. Kayahara H, Tsukahara K. Flavor, health and nutritional quality of pre-germinated brown rice, in: Proceeding of the International Chemical Congress of Pacific Basin Societies. *Hawaii, USA* 2000.

98. Ito Y, Mizukuchi A, Kise M, Aoto H, Yamamoto S, Yoshihara R, et al. Postprandial blood glucose and insulin responses to pre-germinated brown rice in healthy subjects. *J Med Invest* 2005;**52**:159–64.

99. Miura D, Ito Y, Mizukuchi A, Kise M, Aoto H, Yagasaki K. Hypocholesterolemic action of pre-germinated brown rice in hepatoma-bearing rats. *Life Sci* 2006;**79**:259–64.

100. Vahter ME. Interactions between arsenic-induced toxicity and nutrition in early life. *J Nutr* 2007;**137**:204–11.

101. Vahter M. Health effects of early life exposure to arsenic. *Basic Clin Pharm Toxicol* 2008;**102**:204–11.

102. Li L, Ekstrom EC, Goessler W, Lonnerdal B, Nermell B, Yunus M, et al. Nutritional status has marginal influence on the metabolism of inorganic arsenic in pregnant Bangladeshi women. *Environ Health Perspect* 2008;**116**:315–21.

Inorganic Arsenic in Rice and Rice Bran: Health Implications

Suthep Ruangwises*, *Piyawat Saipan*†, *Nongluck Ruangwises***

*Chulalongkorn University, Department of Veterinary Public Health, Bangkok, Thailand, †Khon Kaen University, Department of Veterinary Public Health, Khon Kaen, Thailand, **Mahidol University, Department of Pharmaceutical Chemistry, Bangkok, Thailand

INTRODUCTION

Rice is a staple food for people in many countries, especially in Asia, Africa, and South America. *Oryza sativa* is the most widely grown rice in Asia, while *O. glaberrima* is the major rice in Africa. At present, *O. glaberrima* is grown only in some regions of African countries, as it is being replaced by *O. sativa*.[1] The world's annual paddy rice production between 2008 and 2011 was fairly stable, at 686.1, 686.9, 683.4, and 702.2 million tons, respectively.[2-5] Daily rice consumption varied considerably – from more than 600 g/day in Myanmar and Laos to less than 50 g/day in some countries in Europe.[6]

Arsenic is a semi-metallic element occurring naturally in the Earth's crust in more than 200 mineral compounds. Arsenic compounds have been widely used in many industries, and as components in pesticides for agricultural use. Both natural processes and human actions cause arsenic contamination in the air, water, soil, and food. In the environment, arsenic compounds do not break down into elemental arsenic but can change form, particularly from inorganic to organic arsenic, due to natural metabolism of the biota.[7] Inorganic and organic arsenic compounds found in foods are summarized in Table 30.1. It should be noted that MMA and DMA in foods generally refer to monomethylarsonic acid and dimethylarsinic acid, respectively. The inorganic arsenic species (As^{III} and As^{V}) are the most toxic forms of arsenic, and are carcinogenic in humans. It has been shown that plants, including rice, can accumulate arsenic at different concentrations in various edible parts.[8-12] Since rice is consumed in large quantities in several countries, there have been increasing health concerns regarding exposure to inorganic arsenic through rice consumption.

INORGANIC ARSENIC TOXICITY

Acute Toxicity of Inorganic Arsenic

Ingestion of large quantities of inorganic arsenic (70–180 mg) can be fatal to humans.[13] Several physiological systems are affected in inorganic arsenic intoxication. Acute manifestations include irritation of the gastrointestinal tract, anorexia, hepatomegaly, fever, and disturbances of cardiovascular and nervous system functions. Cardiac failure has been reported in fatal cases.[13] The acute oral LD$_{50}$ of arsenic trioxide (As$_2$O$_3$) in mice and in rats was 26–39 and 15–293 mg As/kg body weight (bw), respectively.[14-16] The acute oral LD$_{50}$ of calcium arsenate and of lead arsenate in rats was 53 and 231 mg As/kg bw, respectively.[17]

Chronic Toxicity and Carcinogenicity of Inorganic Arsenic

Chronic oral exposure to inorganic arsenic affects almost all organ systems in the body, including cardiovascular, gastrointestinal, hematological, immune, nervous, reproductive, and respiratory systems. Recent reports by the World Health Organization and the US Department of Health and Human Services have indicated that increased risks of skin cancers and cancers of internal organs are related to chronic exposure to high inorganic arsenic levels in drinking water.[7,18]

The World Health Organization International Agency for Research on Cancer (IARC) has evaluated the carcinogenicity of inorganic arsenic compounds several times. The IARC first evaluated inorganic arsenic in 1973, finding that there was an association

TABLE 30.1   Inorganic and Organic Arsenic Present in Foods

Arsenic Compound	Abbreviation
INORGANIC ARSENIC	
Arsenate	As^V
Arsenite	As^{III}
ORGANIC ARSENIC	
Arsenobetaine	AB
Arsenocholine	AC
Dimethylarsinic acid (dimethylarsinite, cacodylic acid)	DMA^V
Dimethylarsinous acid	DMA^{III}
Dimethylarsionylethanol	DMAE
Dimethylarsionylribosides	Oxo-arsenosugars
Dimethyldithioarsinic acid	$DMDTA^V$
Dimethylmonothioarsinic acid	$DMMTA^V$
Methylarsonic acid (monomethylarsonic acid, methylarsonate)	MMA^V
Tetramethylarsonium ion	TMA^+
Trimethylarsine oxide	TMAO
Trimethylarsoniopropionate	TMAP

between skin cancer incidence and exposure to inorganic arsenic in drugs, in contaminated drinking water, or in the occupational environment. The IARC also concluded that the risk of lung cancer was significantly increased in smelter workers who worked in an occupational environment with high concentrations of arsenic trioxide. At that time, the mechanism of actions of inorganic arsenic was not extensively described. In 1980, the IARC, based on further studies, concluded that there was sufficient evidence that inorganic arsenic compounds are skin carcinogens; consequently inorganic arsenic, but not organic arsenic, was classified in Group 1 as carcinogenic to humans. It should be noted that evidence for the carcinogenicity of inorganic arsenic in experimental animals was inadequate. The IARC has further evaluated the carcinogenicity of inorganic arsenic in other organs. In 2004, the IARC again concluded that there was sufficient evidence to indicate that inorganic arsenic was carcinogenic in humans, although there was limited evidence for carcinogenicity in experimental animals. In 2009, the IARC confirmed that inorganic arsenic in drinking water causes cancers of the lung, skin, and urinary bladder in humans; however, the evidence for cancers of the kidney, liver, and prostate was limited.[19,20]

Metabolism of Inorganic Arsenic

Metabolism of inorganic arsenic in humans involves reduction from As^V to As^{III} and oxidative methylation from inorganic arsenic to MMA and DMA, respectively.[21–23] It has been shown that most of the MMA and DMA is excreted in the urine without further metabolism.

$$H_3As^VO_4 \rightarrow H_3As^{III}O_4 \rightarrow CH_3As^VO(OH)_2$$
$$\rightarrow CH_3As^{III}O(OH)_2 \rightarrow (CH_3)_2As^VOOH$$
$$\rightarrow (CH_3)_2As^{III}OOH$$

RISK ASSESSMENT FOR INORGANIC ARSENIC

Risk assessment consists of four steps: hazard identification, dose–response assessment, exposure assessment, and risk characterization. For the dose–response assessment, two major approaches are generally used to evaluate threshold and non-threshold endpoints. In the United States, threshold approaches have been used for non-cancer endpoints, and non-threshold approaches have been used for cancer endpoints. The United States Environmental Protection Agency (US EPA) has applied the reference dose (RfD) for threshold approaches, and the carcinogenic slope factor (CSF) for non-threshold approaches. For threshold approaches, the process involves identification of the "no observed adverse effect level" (NOAEL) of a chemical. The NOAEL refers to the highest dose of a chemical that produces no statistically significant increase in the frequency of adverse effects in humans or experimental animals. The obtained NOAEL is in turn used for estimation of a reference dose (RfD). For non-threshold approaches, the US EPA has used a linearized multistage (LMS) model for calculation of a cancer slope factor.[24]

US EPA Oral Reference Dose (RfD$_o$)

The US EPA estimated the oral reference dose (RfD$_o$) for inorganic arsenic based on the studies of Tseng and colleagues[25,26] The studies were conducted on 40,421 Taiwanese (19,269 males and 21,152 females), residing in an endemic area on the southwest coast of Taiwan, who were exposed to arsenic in artesian well water. The studies showed that the incidence of blackfoot disease, hyperpigmentation, and keratosis increased with age and the dose of inorganic arsenic. Blackfoot disease was used as the endpoint for estimation of the RfD$_o$. The prevalences of blackfoot disease in both males and females for the three age groups (20–39 years, 40–59 years, and more than 60 years) were 4.6, 10.5, and 20.3 per 1000, respectively. Tseng *et al.* showed increased incidences of hyperpigmentation and keratosis with age.[26] The overall prevalences of hyperpigmentation and keratosis in the exposed groups were 184 and 71 per 1000, respectively. The text states that incidence increases with dose, but data for the individual doses are not shown. These data show that skin lesions are the most sensitive endpoint.

The control (NOAEL) group consisted of 2,552 individuals. The amount of inorganic arsenic consumed by the NOAEL group was calculated from drinking water and food. Concentrations of inorganic arsenic in well water ranged between 0.001 and 0.017 mg/L, with an arithmetic mean of 0.009 mg/L. Due to limited available data on inorganic arsenic concentrations in food, only sweet potatoes and rice were used to estimate the amount of ingested arsenic. The average amount of dietary inorganic arsenic ingested by the NOAEL group was 0.002 mg/day. Daily water consumption of 4.5 L/day and an average body weight of 55 kg were used for calculation of NOAEL of inorganic arsenic. NOAEL of inorganic arsenic was calculated using the equation:

$$NOAEL = ([C_W \times IR_W] + IF)/BW$$

where C_W = arithmetic mean of inorganic arsenic in well water (0.009 mg/L), IR_W = intake rate of water (4.5 L/day), IF = dietary intake of inorganic arsenic (0.002 mg/day), and BW = the average body weight of Taiwanese (55 kg). NOAEL is ([0.009 mg/L × 4.5 L/day] + 0.002 mg/day)/50 kg = 0.000814 mg/kg per day.

For calculation of RfD_O, the US EPA has applied an uncertainty factor (UF) of 3 to account for the lack of data precluding reproductive toxicity as a critical effect, and to account for some uncertainty as to whether the NOAEL of the critical study accounts for all sensitive individuals. However, the US EPA has not applied a modifying factor (MF) in the calculation. The RfD_O for inorganic arsenic is 0.000814 mg/kg per day/3 = 2.71×10^{-4} mg/kg per day. This value was rounded up to 3×10^{-4} mg/kg per day.

US EPA Oral Carcinogenic Slope Factor

The US EPA Risk Assessment Forum has completed a reassessment of the carcinogenicity risk associated with ingestion of inorganic arsenic, using the studies of Tseng and colleagues.[25,26] A multistage model with time was used to estimate dose-specific and age-specific skin cancer prevalence rates associated with ingestion of inorganic arsenic; both linear and quadratic model fitting of the data were performed. The oral carcinogenic slope factor of skin cancer for a 70-kg person consuming 2 L/day of drinking water was estimated to be 1.5 mg/kg bw per day. The maximum likelihood estimate (MLE) of skin cancer risk ranged from 1×10^{-3} to 2×10^{-3} for an arsenic intake of 1 μg/kg per day, and the cancer unit risk for drinking water was 5×10^{-5} μg/L.

JECFA Benchmark Dose

At the meeting of the 72nd Joint FAO/WHO Expert Committee on Food Additives (JECFA), the committee re-evaluated and reviewed the "provisional tolerable weekly intake" (PTWI) of 15 μg/kg bw per day for inorganic arsenic. Two studies by Chen et al.[27,28] were selected for dose–response modeling for inorganic arsenic, since they were prospective studies with an average 11.5-year follow-up time. The JECFA used the US EPA benchmark software (BMDS version 2.1.1) with nine dichotomous models to fit the data. The nine dichotomous models were: gamma, logistic, log-logistic, log probit, multistage, multistage (cancer), probit, Weibull, and quantal-linear. The JECFA has calculated the benchmark dose ($BMD_{0.5}$), and the lower limit of a one-sided 95% confidence interval on the benchmark dose ($BMDL_{0.5}$), with 0.5% increased incidence for inorganic arsenic. The lowest $BMDL_{05}$ of 3.0 μg/kg bw per day for lung cancer was generated by the quantal-linear model. Therefore, the committee determined that the previous PTWI of 15 μg/kg bw per day (provisional tolerable daily intake, PTDI = 15/7 = 2.1 μg/kg bw per day) was in the range of the $BMDL_{05}$, and withdrew the PTWI.[20]

It should be noted that the $BMDL_{0.5}$ of 3.0 μg/kg bw per day is not actually safety standard for inorganic arsenic. An approach using the margin of safety (MOE) should be applied to evaluate the risk of inorganic arsenic from dietary exposure. The MOE is defined as the ratio of $BMDL_{0.5}$ to the dietary intake of inorganic arsenic.[29,30]

ACCUMULATION OF ARSENIC IN RICE

It has been reported that rice grains can accumulate arsenic from the soil. Rice accumulates arsenic in approximately 13- and 20-fold greater amounts compared with wheat and barley, respectively. Williams et al. reported that the average transfer factors (TF) of arsenic from soil to grain for rice, wheat, and barley were 0.04, 0.003, and 0.002, respectively.[31] The transfer factor is defined as the ratio of arsenic concentration in the grain to its concentration in soil. Besides inorganic arsenic, the major organic arsenic species found in rice are MMA and DMA. The percentages of inorganic with respect to total arsenic vary considerably, ranging from 11% to 96%.[32,33] Recently, Meharg et al. utilized synchrotron-based X-ray fluorescence (S-XRF) to investigate the location of arsenic in polished (white) and unpolished (brown) rice grains.[34] Laser ablation inductively coupled plasma mass spectrometry was used to confirm the location of arsenic. The study showed that most arsenic is localized on the surface, consisting of the pericarp and aleurone layer, of brown rice. The polishing process removes all of the pericarp and most of the aleurone layer, thus producing rice bran containing higher levels of total and inorganic arsenic than found in the endosperm (white rice).

INORGANIC ARSENIC IN RICE

Concentrations of Inorganic Arsenic in Rice

Concentrations of total and inorganic arsenic in rice are highly variable, depending on the types of rice and arsenic concentrations in soil and irrigating water. Some of the total and inorganic arsenic concentrations

in rice from various countries, presumably grown in uncontaminated soil, from published reports are presented in Table 30.2. Guzmán Mar *et al.* reported concentrations of total and inorganic arsenic in rice purchased from local markets in Pennsylvania, USA; the samples were basmati rice from India, jasmine rice from Thailand, and white rice grown in the USA. Basmati rice samples had concentrations of total and inorganic arsenic of 204 and 142 ng/g, respectively, while the values found in the jasmine rice samples were 137 and 111 ng/g. Total and inorganic arsenic levels of 225 and 169 ng/g, respectively, were found in the white rice samples grown in Texas.[35]

TABLE 30.2 Total Arsenic, Inorganic Arsenic, and Percentages of Inorganic Arsenic with Respect to Total Arsenic in Rice from Various Countries

Country	Sample	Origin of Rice	n	Total Arsenic (ng/g)	Inorganic Arsenic (ng/g)	% Inorganic Arsenic[a]	Reference
USA	Basmati	India	1	204 ± 5[b]	142[c]	69.6[d]	Guzmán et al.[35]
					(105 ± 4, 37 ± 3)		
	Jasmine	Thailand	1	137 ± 3[b]	111[b]	81.0[d]	
					(86 ± 4, 25 ± 1)		
	White	USA	1	225 ± 6[b]	169	75.1[d]	
					(161 ± 5, 8 ± 4)		
Spain	White basmati	India	2	62.5	28.5	46.0	Torres-Escribano et al.[36]
	White	Spain	11	211	94.6	50.3	
	Brown	Spain	10	207	161	78.6	
	White	Thailand	3	148	89	59.7	
Scotland	White basmati	India	9	45.6	26.7	54.9	Williams et al.[37]
	Brown basmati	India	1	70	40	61	
	White	Taiwan	3	383	247	62.0	
	Jasmine	Thailand	1	110	80	74.0	
	White	USA	8	276	76.3	27.3	
	Brown	USA	4	225	105	37.3	
Thailand	Polished – White	Thailand	30	125 ± 30.3	68.3 ± 17.6	54.9 ± 7.94	Ruangwises et al.[38]
	Polished – Jasmine	Thailand	30	124 ± 21.4	68.4 ± 15.6	55.2 ± 8.26	
	Polished – Sticky	Thailand	30	136 ± 43.9	75.9 ± 24.8	56.4 ± 9.18	
	Brown – White	Thailand	30	194 ± 38.9	124 ± 34.4	63.6 ± 8.77	
	Brown – Jasmine	Thailand	30	186 ± 40.6	120 ± 31.6	64.2 ± 8.07	
	Brown – Sticky	Thailand	30	198 ± 57.4	131 ± 35.6	66.9 ± 9.08	
USA	White	USA	15	265	102	42.3	Zavala et al.[10]
	Brown	USA	9	331	137	47.8	

[a] *% Inorganic arsenic = (mean concentration of inorganic arsenic × 100)/mean concentration of total arsenic.*
[b] *Values are the means of three determinations ± 95% CL.*
[c] *Values are the summation of As(III) and As(V) reported in the literature, which are shown in parentheses.*
[d] *% Inorganic arsenic was calculated from inorganic arsenic and total arsenic concentrations reported in the literature.*

Torres-Escribano *et al.* determined concentrations of total and inorganic arsenic in rice purchased from local markets in Spain. Rice samples consisted of 2 samples of white basmati rice from India, 3 samples of Thai white rice, and 10 samples of white rice grown in Spain. Total and inorganic arsenic levels in Indian rice were 62.5 and 28.5 ng/g, respectively, while the levels in Thai white rice were 148 and 89 ng/g, respectively. White rice grown in Spain contained total and inorganic arsenic levels of 211 and 94.6 ng/g, respectively.[36]

Williams *et al.* reported concentrations of total and inorganic arsenic in 21 rice samples from India, Thailand, Taiwan, and the USA, which were purchased from supermarkets in the city of Aberdeen, Scotland. White basmati rice from India ($n = 9$) had total and inorganic arsenic levels of 45.6 and 26.7 ng/g, respectively, while the levels in Thailand jasmine rice ($n = 1$) were 110 and 80 ng/g, respectively. White rice from Taiwan ($n = 3$) and the USA ($n = 8$), respectively, contained total and inorganic arsenic levels of 383 and 247 ng/g, and 276 and 76.3 ng/g.[37]

Ruangwises *et al.* determined concentrations of total and inorganic arsenic in polished and brown rice of three different types – white, jasmine, and sticky – collected from the 10 provinces in Thailand with the highest rice production. Brown rice of all three rice types contained significantly higher levels of both total and inorganic arsenic than polished rice of the same rice types. Total arsenic levels found in polished rice (white, jasmine, and sticky) were 125, 124, and 136 ng/g, respectively, while the concentrations of inorganic arsenic were 68.3, 68.4, and 75.9 ng/g, respectively. For brown rice samples, total arsenic concentrations in white, jasmine, and sticky rice were 194, 186, and 198 ng/g, respectively, whereas inorganic arsenic concentrations were 124, 120, and 131 ng/g, respectively.[38]

Zavala *et al.* reported the levels of total and inorganic arsenic in 24 rice samples grown in three states in the USA. Total arsenic concentrations found in white ($n = 15$) and brown rice were 265 and 331 ng/g, respectively, while inorganic arsenic levels in both rice types were 102 and 137 ng/g, respectively.[10] Zavala *et al.* also reported that As[III] and DMA were the major arsenic species detected in all 24 rice samples. Concentrations of DMA increased linearly with increasing levels of total As, but As[III] concentrations were fairly constant, at approximately 0.1 mg/kg. Together with other published data, rice could be categorized into DMA and inorganic arsenic types. Rice from the USA was predominantly the DMA type.

Concentrations of Inorganic Arsenic in Rice Bran

In general, rice bran contains concentrations of total and inorganic arsenic higher than those found in the corresponding polished rice. Sun *et al.* reported

concentrations of total and inorganic arsenic in polished rice and rice bran freshly produced from whole grain rice samples from China and Bangladesh.[39] Average concentrations of total and inorganic arsenic in rice bran from China ($n = 2$) and from Bangladesh ($n = 4$) were 4445 and 2515 ng/g, and 2733 and 1538 ng/g, respectively. Mean concentrations of total and inorganic arsenic in polished rice from China and from Bangladesh were 510 and 250 ng/g, and 578 and 190 ng/g, respectively. The arsenic bran/rice ratio may be described as the quotient of the concentration of (total or inorganic) arsenic in rice bran to the concentration in polished rice. The total and inorganic arsenic bran/rice ratios for Chinese rice were 4445/510 = 8.72 and 2515/250 = 10.1, respectively, while the values for Bangladeshi rice were 2733/578 = 4.73 and 1538/190 = 8.09, respectively.

Ruangwises *et al.* reported that the concentrations of total and inorganic arsenic in rice bran from white, jasmine, and sticky rice were 894, 832, and 963 ng/g, respectively, while inorganic arsenic levels were 633, 599, and 673 ng/g, respectively.[38] The arsenic bran/rice ratio for white rice was 894/125 = 7.15. The ratios for jasmine and sticky rice were 832/124 = 6.71 and 963/136 = 7.08, respectively. The inorganic arsenic ratios for the three rice types were 9.27, 8.75, and 8.87, respectively. Data from two independent studies showed that, regardless of concentrations of total and inorganic arsenic in rice bran and polished rice, the bran/rice ratios for total and inorganic arsenic are approximately 7 and 9, respectively. Total and inorganic arsenic levels in rice bran and polished rice are shown in Table 30.3.

Sun *et al.* also determined concentrations of total arsenic in nine rice bran products, ranging from 710 to 1980 ng/g, and inorganic arsenic, ranging between 480 and 1880 ng/g.[39] Rice bran is sold as a nutritional supplement for humans and is also used as an ingredient in other foods, including rice cakes, muffins, and breakfast cereals.

It should be noted that the US FDA has analyzed total arsenic in rice for more than 20 years. At present, the US FDA is determining total and inorganic arsenic in rice and rice products, including infant rice cereal, breakfast cereal, rice cakes, and rice beverages. The first analytical results of 192 samples of rice and rice products have been posted on its website. The US FDA will post additional data on more than 1000 rice types and rice products as the results become available.

The Effects of Cooking Methods on the Contents of Inorganic Arsenic in Cooked Rice

It has been demonstrated that the methods of rice cooking (traditional and modern methods) with uncontaminated water can affect arsenic concentrations in cooked rice. In the traditional cooking method, rice

TABLE 30.3   Total Arsenic, Inorganic Arsenic, and Arsenic Bran/Rice Ratios in Rice Bran from Various Countries

Country	Rice Type	Origin of Rice	N	Total Arsenic (ng/g)[a]	Total Arsenic Bran/Rice Ratio	Inorganic Arsenic (ng/g)[a]	Inorganic Arsenic Bran/Rice Ratio	% Inorganic Arsenic	Reference
Scotland	White	China	2	4,445 (510)	8.72	2,515 (250)	10.1	57	Sun et al.[39]
	White	Bangladesh	4	2,733 (578)	4.73	1,538 (190)	8.09	57.8	
Thailand	White	Thailand	15	894 (125)	7.15	633 (68.3)	9.27	70.5	Ruangwises et al.[38]
	Jasmine	Thailand	15	832 (124)	6.71	599 (68.4)	8.75	72.2	
	Sticky	Thailand	14	963 (136)	7.08	673 (75.9)	8.87	69.9	

[a] *Values in parentheses are concentrations of total or inorganic arsenic in polished rice.*

is boiled with a large amount of water in a metal container (pot). After the rice is well cooked, excess water is drained from the container. The traditional rice cooking method can reduce inorganic arsenic content by approximately 30%.[40] In the modern cooking method, a small volume of water is added to rice in an electric rice cooker or, alternatively, simply boiled in an open pan. The volume of water added to the container should be just enough for cooking the rice, with very little excess water for drainage. This rice cooking method retains all of the inorganic arsenic in cooked rice.[41,42]

Bioavailability of Inorganic Arsenic in Rice

An interesting arsenic research study in recent years concerned the bioavailability of arsenic in food products. Bioavailability is defined as the amount of a chemical that actually enters the systemic circulation, compared to the amount that enters the body. The bioavailability for the oral route could be divided into two phases: bioaccessibility and absorption. Bioaccessibility refers to the maximum soluble amount of a chemical in the gastrointestinal medium available for absorption into the bloodstream.[43] Bioaccessiblity results from the enzymatic digestion of food within the gastrointestinal tract to release soluble chemicals. This process of digestion by gastrointestinal enzymes also releases arsenic from food. Recently, Laparra *et al.* studied the bioaccessibility of total and inorganic arsenic in cooked rice using simulated gastrointestinal digestion.[43] The *in vitro* digestion system consisted of two steps: gastric and intestinal. The first step consisted of digestion with a gastric enzyme, pepsin, while the second step involved digestion with pancreatin and bile extract. The bioaccessibility of arsenic in cooked rice was approximately 100% for both total and inorganic arsenic.[43]

Absorption refers to the process whereby a chemical moves from the gastrointestinal tract into the circulatory system. In general, investigation of the absorption process requires studies using experimental animals. An alternative *in vitro* absorption system using human colon

carcinoma Caco-2 cells has been extensively utilized to study absorption of chemicals, including arsenic. A study using a Caco-2 cell system showed that only 3.9–17.8% of the total soluble arsenic added into the experimental system was taken up by Caco-2 cells.[43] The study results suggested that not all of the digested inorganic arsenic in the gastrointestinal tract is entirely absorbed into the bloodstream and elicits toxicity.

HEALTH IMPLICATIONS

An extensive review of published reports has shown that no epidemiological studies have indicated the health effects associated with the ingestion of inorganic arsenic through consumption of rice. In the process of evaluating the risk of inorganic arsenic, bioavailability should be included in the assessment. Several studies have suggested that drinking water containing high levels of inorganic arsenic plays a major role in health risk among people residing in contaminated areas. It has been reported that approximately 25 million people in Bangladesh live in polluted areas and consume water containing arsenic at levels above 50 ppb (five times the WHO standard of 10 ppb).[44,45]

Meharg and Zhao also suggested that "Even if epidemiological studies were to be initiated, it would take decades to understand how elevated arsenic in rice affects lifetime health outcomes."[6] Zavala *et al.* concluded that "At present, it is impossible to fully assess the health risk of arsenic in rice."[10]

References

1. Linares OF. African rice (*Oryza glaberrima*): history and future potential. *Proc Nat Acad Sci* 2002;**99**:16360–5.
2. FAO Rice Market Monitor. Trade and Market Division. *Food Agric Organ United Nations* 2010;**vol. XIII**(1).
3. FAO Rice Market Monitor. Trade and Market Division. *Food Agric Organ United Nations* 2011;**vol. XIV**(1).
4. FAO Rice Market Monitor. Trade and Market Division. *Food Agric Organ United Nations* 2012;**vol. XV**(1).

5. FAO Rice Market Monitor. Trade and Market Division. *Food Agric Organ United Nations* 2013;**vol. XVI**(1).

6. Meharg AA, Zhao FJ. Risk from arsenic in rice grain. In: Meharg AA, Zhao FJ, editors. *Arsenic & rice*. New York, NY: Springer; 2012. p. 31–50.

7. World Health Organization. *Environmental Health Criteria 224. Arsenic and arsenic compounds*. 2nd ed. Geneva, Switzerland: World Health Organization; 2001.

8. Baroni F, Boscagli A, Di Lella LA, Protano G, Riccobono F. Arsenic in soil and vegetation of contaminated areas in southern Tuscany (Italy). *J Geochem Explor* 2004;**81**:1–14.

9. Helgesen H, Larsen EH. Bioavailability and speciation of arsenic in carrots grown in contaminated oil. *Analyst* 1998;**123**:791–6.

10. Zavala YJ, Gerads R, Gorleyok H, Duxbury JM. Arsenic in rice: II. Arsenic speciation in USA grain and implications for human health. *Environ Sci Technol* 2008;**42**:3861–6.

11. Zhao R, Zhao M, Wang H, Taneike Y, Zhang X. Arsenic speciation in moso bamboo shoot – a terrestrial plant that contains organo-arsenic species. *Sci Total Environ* 2006;**371**:293–303.

12. Carbonell-Barrachina AA, Burló F, Burgos-Hernández A, López E, Mataix J. The influence of arsenite concentration on arsenic accumulation in tomato and bean plants. *Sci Hort* 1997;**71**:167–76.

13. Liu J, Goyer RA, Waalkes MP. Toxic effects of metals. In: Klaassen CD, editor. *Casarett & Doull's toxicology: the basic science of poisons*. 7th ed. New York, NY: McGraw-Hill; 2008. p. 931–79.

14. Harrison JWE, Packman EW, Abbott DD. Acute oral toxicity and chemical and physical properties of arsenic trioxides. *AMA Arch Ind Health* 1958;**17**:118–23.

15. Kaise T, Watanabe S, Itoh K. The acute toxicity of arsenobetaine. *Chemosphere* 1985;**14**:1327–32.

16. Done AK, Peart AJ. Acute toxicities of arsenical herbicides. *Clin Toxicol* 1971;**4**:343–55.

17. Gaines TB. The acute toxicity of pesticides to rats. *Toxicol Appl Pharmacol* 1960;**2**:88–99.

18. Agency for Toxic Substances and Disease Registry. *Toxicological profile for arsenic*. Atlanta GA, U.S: Department of Health and Human Services; 2007.

19. Straif K, Benbrahim-Talla L, Baan R, Grosse Y, Secretan B, El Ghissassi F, et al. A review of human carcinogens—Part C: metals, arsenic, dusts, and fibres. *Lancet Oncol* 2009;**10**:453–4.

20. Joint FAO/WHO Expert Committee on Food Additives (JECFA). *Safety evaluation of certain contaminants in food. WHO Food Additives Series 63*. Geneva, Switzerland: World Health Organization; 2011.

21. Gebel TW. Arsenic methylation is a process of detoxification through accelerated excretion. *Int J Hyg Environ Health* 2002;**205**:505–8.

22. Buchet JP, Lauwerys R, Roels H. Comparison of the urinary excretion of arsenic metabolites after a single oral dose of sodium arsenite, monomethylarsenate, or dimethylarsenate in man. *Int Arch Occup Environ Health* 1980;**48**:71–9.

23. Marafante E, Vahter M. The effect of methyltransferase inhibition on the metabolism of [^{74}As] arsenite in mice and rabbits. *Chem Biol Interact* 1984;**50**:4–57.

24. Faustman EM, Omenn GS. Risk assessment. In: Klaassen CD, editor. *Casarett & Doull's toxicology: the basic science of poisons*. 7th ed. New York, NY: McGraw-Hill; 2008. p. 107–28.

25. Tseng WP. Effects and dose–response relationships of skin cancer and blackfoot disease with arsenic. *Environ Health Perspect* 1977;**19**:109–19.

26. Tseng WP, Chu HM, How SW, Fong JM, Lin CS, Yeh S. Prevalence of skin cancer in an endemic area of chronic arsenicism in Taiwan. *J Natl Cancer Inst* 1968;**40**:453–63.

27. Chen CL, Chiou HY, Hsu LI, Hsueh YM, Wu MM, Wang YH, et al. Arsenic in drinking water and risk of urinary tract cancer: a follow-up study from northeastern Taiwan. *Cancer Epidemiol Biomarkers Prev* 2010;**14**:2984–90.

28. Chen CL, Chiou HY, Hsu LI, Hsueh YM, Wu MM, Chen CJ. Ingested arsenic, characteristics of well water consumption and risk of different histological types of lung cancer in northeastern Taiwan. *Environ Res* 2010;**110**:455–62.

29. European Union Member States Working Group. Discussion paper on guidance for risk management options on how to deal with the results from new risk assessment methodologies. 5th Session of the Codex Committee on Contaminants in Food. The Hague, The Netherlands, 21-25 March 2011. Available at: ftp://ftp.fao.org/codex/cccf5/cf05_11e.pdf [accessed 10.01.13].

30. Wong WW, Chung SW, Chan BT, Ho YY, Xiao Y. Dietary exposure to inorganic arsenic of the Hong Kong population: results of the first Hong Kong total diet study. *Food Chem Toxicol* 2013;**51**:379–85.

31. Williams PN, Villada A, Deacon C, Raab A, Figuerola J, Green AJ, et al. Greatly enhanced arsenic shoot assimilation in rice leads to elevated grain levels compared to wheat and barley. *Environ Sci Technol* 2007;**41**:6854–9.

32. Heitkemper DT, Vela NP, Stewart KR, Westphal CS. Determination of total and speciated arsenic in rice by ion chromatography and inductively coupled plasma mass spectrometry. *J Anal At Spectrom* 2011;**16**:299–306.

33. Zhu YG, Sun GX, Lei M, Teng M, Liu YX, Chen NC, et al. High percentage inorganic arsenic content of mining impacted and non-impacted Chinese rice. *Environ Sci Technol* 2008;**42**:5008–13.

34. Meharg AA, Lombi E, Williams PN, Scheckel KG, Feldmann J, Raab A, et al. Speciation and localization of arsenic in white and brown rice grains. *Environ Sci Technol* 2008;**42**:1051–7.

35. Guzmán Mar JL, Reyes LH, Rahman GMM, Kingston HM. Simultaneous extraction of arsenic and selenium species from rice products by microwave-assisted enzymatic extraction and analysis by ion chromatography–inductively coupled plasma-mass spectrometry. *J Agric Food Chem* 2009;**57**:3005–13.

36. Torres-Escribano S, Leal M, Vélez D, Montoro R. Total and inorganic arsenic concentrations in rice sold in Spain, effect of cooking, and risk assessments. *Environ Sci Technol* 2008;**42**:3867–72.

37. Williams PN, Price AH, Raab A, Hossain SA, Feldmann J, Meharg AA. Variation in arsenic speciation and concentration in paddy rice related to dietary exposure. *Environ Sci Technol* 2005;**39**:5531–40.

38. Ruangwises S, Saipan P, Tengjaroenkul B, Ruangwises N. Total and inorganic arsenic in rice and rice bran purchased in Thailand. *J Food Prot* 2012;**75**:771–4.

39. Sun GX, Williams PN, Carey AM, Zhu YG, Deacon C, Raab A, et al. Inorganic arsenic in rice bran and its products are an order of magnitude higher than in bulk grain. *Environ Sci Technol* 2008;**42**:7542–6.

40. Raab A, Baskaran C, Feldmann J, Meharg AA. Cooking rice in a high water to rice ratio reduces inorganic arsenic content. *J Environ Monit* 2008;**11**:41–4.

41. Rahman MA, Hasegawa H, Rahman MA, Rahman MM, Miah MAM. Influence of cooking method on arsenic retention in cooked rice related to dietary exposure. *Sci Total Environ* 2006;**370**:51–60.

42. Sengupta MK, Hossain MA, Mukherjee A, Ahamed S, Das B, Nayak B, et al. Arsenic burden of cooked rice: traditional and modern methods. *Food Chem Toxicol* 2006;**44**:1823–9.

43. Laparra JM, Vélez D, Barberá R, Farré R, Montoro R. Bioavailability of inorganic arsenic in cooked rice: practical aspects for human health risk assessments. *J Agric Food Chem* 2005;**53**:8829–33.

44. International Agency for Research on Cancer. *Some drinking-water disinfectants and contaminants, including arsenic. IARC Monographs on the Evaluation of Carcinogenic Risks to Humans* vol. 84. Lyon, France: IARC; 2004. pp. 269–477.

45. Anawar HM, Akai J, Mostofa KMG, Safiullah, Tareq SM. Arsenic poisoning in groundwater: health risk and geochemical sources in Bangladesh. *Environ Int* 2002;**27**:597–604.

Apoptosis and Arabinoxylan Rice Bran

Mamdooh Helal Ghoneum

Charles Drew University of Medicine and Science, Department of Otolaryngology, Los Angeles, California, USA

THE MANUFACTURE OF MGN-3/ BIOBRAN®

The main chemical structure of MGN-3/BioBran® is an arabinoxylan, containing a xylose main chain and an arabinose polymer side chain (Fig. 31.1).[1] MGN-3/ BioBran is manufactured and provided by Daiwa Pharmaceutical Co, Ltd, Tokyo, Japan.

Rice bran is the portion of rice that remains after removal of the husk and edible endosperm. The cell walls of the rice seed endosperm consist of polysaccharides such as cellulose, water-soluble hemicelluloses, and pectin. Rice bran hemicellulose contains a large number of different polysaccharides, including pentoses such as arabinoxylan and xyloglycan. The bioreactivity of these polysaccharide molecules is enhanced by treating the hemicellulose extract with multiple carbohydrate-hydrolyzing enzymes obtained from the shiitake mushroom. The product produced via this process is called MGN-3/BioBran.

The method of manufacturing MGN-3/BioBran consists of three steps: (1) extraction of polysaccharides from defatted rice bran hemicellulose; (2) manufacture of multiple shiitake-derived carbohydrate-hydrolyzing enzymes used to treat the extracted polysaccharides; and (3) partial hydrolysis reaction of rice bran hemicellulose polysaccharides by the carbohydrate-hydrolyzing enzymes obtained from shiitake mushrooms. Finally, a powder is obtained after the compound is treated with high heat and pressure. A synopsis of the manufacturing process is presented in Figure 31.2.

SYNERGY OF MGN-3/BIOBRAN WITH INTERLEUKIN-2 FOR THE ACTIVATION OF HUMAN NK CELLS

MGN-3/BioBran has been proven to be a potent biological response modifier (BRM), as indicated by its ability to activate human dendritic cells (DC) and to increase T- and B-cell mitogen response.[1–3] In addition, we have presented evidence for the role of MGN-3/BioBran as a potent activator of natural killer (NK) cells. Oral administration of MGN-3/BioBran stimulated NK cell activity at 1–2 weeks post-treatment in healthy subjects and in cancer patients.[4–6] It is interesting to note that the NK cell immunomodulatory effect of MGN-3/BioBran was evaluated for 4 years in patients with breast cancer, and results revealed NK cell activity was maintained at a high level for the entirety of the treatment period.[5,7] This suggests that MGN-3/BioBran does not have hyporesponsiveness, which is known to be a serious problem associated with many BRMs.[8–11] In addition, MGN-3/ BioBran enhancement of NK cell activity is associated with an increase in NK cell granular content and an increase of activated NK cell surface markers CD69, CD25, and CD54.[12,13] Each of these receptors is indicative of an activated lymphocyte; CD69 is the earliest receptor to be expressed, CD54 (ICAM-1) is an adhesion molecule highly expressed in activated cells, and CD25 is the receptor for interleukin-2 (IL-2), an immune stimulatory cytokine.

Due to the high NK cell augmentary effect of MGN-3/ BioBran alone and its lack of hyporesponsiveness, it was thought that combining MGN-3/BioBran with IL-2, known to be an NK cell activator, might have a synergistic effect on the activation of human NK cells. IL-2 is a 15-kD protein secreted by antigen-activated T cells.[14] NK cells form a unique lymphocyte subset in that they constitutively express IL-2 receptors (IL-2R) and therefore are always IL-2 reactive.[15–19] IL-2 is frequently used as a treatment for metastatic cancer, such as renal cell carcinoma, and also for the treatment of viral infection.[20–26] However, IL-2 administered intravenously in high doses produces undesirable side effects, including a systemic delayed-type hypersensitivity (DTH) response with delayed onset of the signs and symptoms of severe infection, including fever, rigors, malaise, myalgia, nausea/ vomiting, and hypotension.[27] In order to examine the

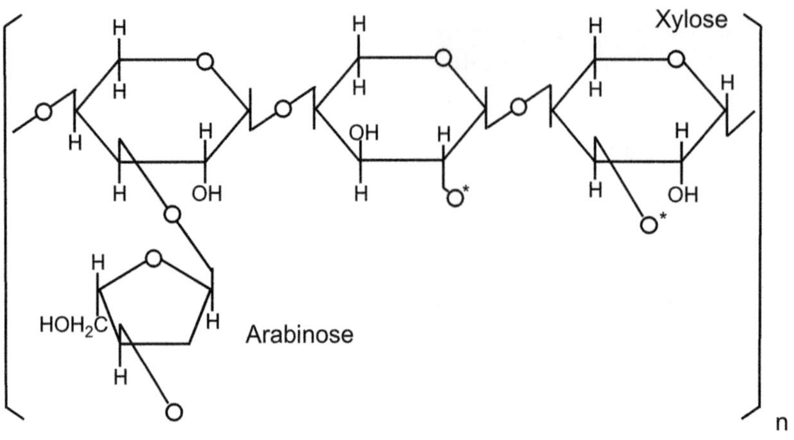

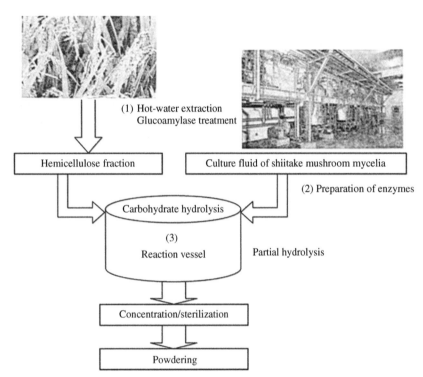

FIGURE 31.1 Chemical structure of MGN-3/Bio-Bran®. MGN-3/BioBran consists of a xylose main chain with an arabinose side chain.

FIGURE 31.2 The three main steps in manufacturing of MGN-3/BioBran. Using hot water and glucoamylase, the hemicellulose fraction is isolated for further processing. Shiitake mushroom carbohydrate-hydrolyzing enzymes are extracted from a culture of mycelia. The hemicellulose fraction and shiitake mushroom extract are hydrolyzed together to form the product MGN-3/BioBran.

synergistic effect of MGN-3/BioBran and IL-2, human NK cells were cultured with MGN-3/BioBran in the presence and absence of IL-2, and cytotoxicity of NK cells against K562 target cancer cells was examined by chromium release assay.[13] Figure 31.3 summarizes the results of the NK cell augmentary effect by MGN-3/Bio-Bran and IL-2. NK cells treated with both agents killed over 80% of K562 cells – higher than either treatment alone. The enhancement of NK cell activity was associated with a several-fold increase in tumor necrosis factor (TNF-α) and interferon-γ (IFN-γ) secretions. TNF-α production may inhibit tumorigenesis, and IFN-γ is an important cytokine for the induction and modulation of immune responses.[28,29] These results show that MGN-3/BioBran in conjunction with IL-2 maximizes NK cell

activation and the production of IFN-γ and TNF-α, suggesting their possible therapeutic effects against cancer and viral infection.

SYNERGY OF MGN-3/BIOBRAN WITH OTHER THERAPEUTIC MODALITIES FOR THE INDUCTION OF CANCER CELL APOPTOSIS

MGN-3/BioBran has a direct effect on tumor cell growth and has been shown to be a safe, non-toxic agent. *In vitro* studies showed that MGN-3/BioBran arrests the growth of cutaneous squamous cell carcinoma (SCC13) cells, in conjunction with increasing intracellular levels

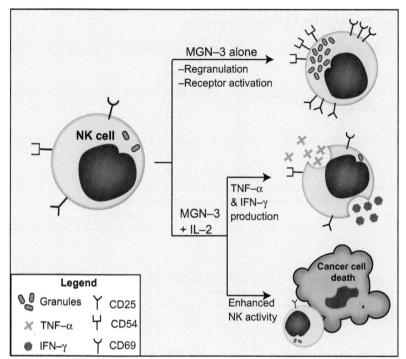

FIGURE 31.3 **Natural killer augmentory effects by MGN-3/BioBran alone and its synergy with IL-2.** Treatment with MGN-3/BioBran alone resulted in regranulation and receptor activation of NK cells. In addition, treatment of NK cells with MGN-3/BioBran and IL-2 increased TNF-α and IFN-γ secretions and enhanced NK cell activity. See color plate at the back of the book.

of IL-10 and IL-12, and also induces apoptosis of human breast cancer MCF-7 cells.[30–32] In additional studies with animals bearing tumors, treatment with MGN-3/Bio-Bran resulted in a significant reduction of tumor volume, which was associated with extensive apoptosis of the tumor tissue.[33] Many anticancer drugs also function by inducing apoptosis; however, these drugs are toxic.[34–40] It is therefore of particular interest to examine the synergy of MGN-3/BioBran with chemotherapy for the induction of cancer cell apoptosis to minimize the side effects associated with these drugs. We have also evaluated the synergistic effect of MGN-3/BioBran used in conjunction with other anticancer agents, such as curcumin, caffeine, and baker's yeast.

Chemotherapeutics

Multidrug resistance (MDR) in cancer cells is a major obstacle for the chemotherapeutic cure of cancer. MDR cells exhibit decreased drug accumulation inside cancer cells, and hence are less susceptible to chemotherapy.[41,42] As a result, the doses must be increased, leading to severe toxicities such as congestive heart failure, myelosuppression, mucositis, diarrhea, alopecia, myalgias, neutropenia and thrombocytopenia, neurotoxicity, immunosuppression, and mutagenic and carcinogenic effects.[43–51] Many attempts have already been made to develop agents that can inhibit or reverse multidrug resistance, such as cyclosporin A, PSC833 and verapamil, difloxacin and probencid, cepharanthin, and drug-coated polymer nanospheres and nanoparticles.[52–58] However,

many of these agents possess side effects. Therefore, it is of particular interest to explore alternative therapeutic approaches that reduce the toxicity of chemotherapy.

MGN-3/BioBran has been shown to be a chemosensitizing agent that possesses great potential for adjuvant therapy in the treatment of cancer. We have demonstrated that MGN-3/BioBran sensitizes human leukemic HUT 78 cells to the anti-CD95 antibody-induced apoptosis. MGN-3/BioBran treatment caused a 200% increase in cancer cell apoptosis with increased activation of caspases 8, 9, and 3.[59] Further experiments examined the sensitizing ability of MGN-3/BioBran toward chemotherapeutic drugs such as daunorubicin and adriamycin.[31,32] Breast cancer MCF-7 cells were cultured with different concentrations of daunorubicin or adriamycin (1×10^{-9} to 1×10^{-6} M) in the presence or absence of different concentrations of MGN-3/BioBran for 3 days. Cancer cell survival was determined by MTT assay. Cells cultured with MGN-3/BioBran and low concentrations of daunorubicin or adriamycin showed an equivalent percentage of apoptosis compared to cells treated with high concentrations of these chemotherapeutic drugs alone. Enhancement of cancer cell apoptosis by MGN-3/BioBran was associated with increased accumulation of chemotherapeutics within cancer cells. Results suggest that MGN-3/BioBran enhances cancer cell apoptosis and thereby reduces the toxicity associated with chemotherapy.

Other studies have shown that MGN-3/BioBran is beneficial for increasing the quality of life (QOL) for animals and cancer patients undergoing chemotherapeutic

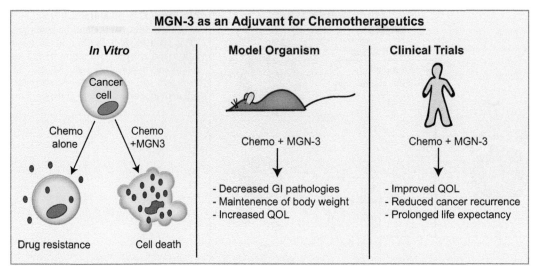

FIGURE 31.4　MGN-3/BioBran acts as an adjuvant for chemotherapeutic drugs in three different models; *in vitro*, and in animal and cancer patients. For *in vitro* studies, treatment with MGN-3/BioBran increased the accumulation of chemotherapy drugs (red ovals) in cancer cells, which ultimately induced apoptosis. In animal studies, MGN-3/BioBran improved QOL and maintained body weight, and in cancer patients it reduced cancer recurrence and prolonged life expectancy. See color plate at the back of the book.

treatment. Results depicted in Figure 31.4 show that MGN-3/BioBran acts as an adjuvant for chemotherapeutic drugs in three different models; *in vitro*, and in animal and cancer patients. One study, using rats, investigated the gross pathologies and weight loss associated with treatment with the chemotherapeutic drugs cisplatin and doxorubicin. Rats that received co-treatment with MGN-3/BioBran plus chemotherapy demonstrated maintenance of body weight, less signs of gross gastrointestinal pathologies, and reduced incidence of diarrhea.[60] In another study, MGN-3/BioBran was beneficial in inhibiting cisplatin-induced weight loss in mice.[61] The beneficial role of MGN-3/BioBran was further confirmed in clinical trials which showed that MGN-3/BioBran treatment enhanced NK cell activity, reduced cancer recurrence, improved QOL, and prolonged life expectancy following surgery and chemotherapy in patients with metastatic cancer and hepatocellular carcinoma.[6,62] These data demonstrate that in addition to its chemosensitizing effects, MGN-3/BioBran also aids in recovery and improves QOL in animals and patients undergoing conventional therapies.

Curcumin

Curcumin, commonly known as turmeric, has been used in Eastern medicine for quite some time. However, it's only in the past 20 years or so that the medicinal properties of curcumin have been investigated in the laboratory and clinics. Several studies have shown that curcumin exhibits antioxidant, anti-inflammatory activity, as well as being a regulator of cell growth. These properties indicate that curcumin could be a strong candidate for the treatment of disease.[63]

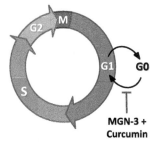

FIGURE 31.5　MGN-3/BioBran and curcumin treatment may cause an arrest in cell cycle progression. Evidence suggests that this combination of therapies arrests the cell cycle in G0–G1 transition, thus inhibiting cancer cell proliferation and growth. See color plate at the back of the book.

These properties, in conjunction with the ability of MGN-3/BioBran to exert an apoptotic effect on cancer cells, have led us to investigate the potential synergistic effects of these two products for the treatment of multiple myeloma.

Multiple myeloma (MM) is a B-cell malignancy which, despite many treatment options, remains incurable. We have shown that a combined treatment of MGN-3/BioBran and curcumin increased the apoptotic rate of the MM cell line U266 (57%) in comparison to either product alone (25% for MGN-3/BioBran and 24% for curcumin), using the MTT assay.[64] The mechanism underlying this effect seems to be related to control of the cell cycle. Cells treated with both products were arrested before G0–G1 transition (Fig. 31.5). In addition, the anti-apoptotic factor Bcl-2 was decreased and the pro-apoptotic factor Bax was upregulated. The change in the Bax:Bcl-2 ratio indicates that the arrested cells were also initiating programmed cell death. This study shows that combination treatment with curcumin and MGN-3/BioBran increases apoptosis in MM cells and may provide an alternative treatment option for MM patients.

Caffeine

Caffeine is a crystalline xanthine alkaloid that acts as a stimulant in the brain. Caffeine is found in many plants and natural products around the globe. The two most common sources of caffeine for human consumption are coffee and tea. While primarily used for increased energy, several studies have shown that an increase in caffeine also provides a reduced risk of many types of cancers, including colon, skin, and endometrial cancers.[65–67] Further studies have shown that combination treatment with caffeine and the chemotherapeutic drug cisplatin increased apoptosis in breast cancer MCF-7 cells compared to treatment with cisplatin alone.[68] In addition, chemopreventative effects of coffee extract and a rice germ product on the development of colorectal cancer were reported.[69]

We investigated the synergistic effect of MGN-3/BioBran and caffeine for the induction of apoptosis in MCF-7 cells. MCF-7 cells were treated with MGN-3/BioBran (100 µg/ml) and caffeine at concentrations of 1.25 mM and 5 mM, and cell survival was determined using an MTT assay. Treatment with a combination of MGN-3/BioBran and caffeine induced apoptosis in cancer cells more than either treatment alone.[32] These results suggest that combination treatments of caffeine and MGN-3/BioBran have the potential to be effective adjuvant treatments to current chemotherapies.

Baker's yeast, S. cerevisiae

Saccharomyces cerevisiae, better known as brewer's or baker's yeast, is a unicellular eukaryotic organism that has been commonly used for several centuries in baking and brewing of wine or beer, due to its ability to ferment sugar into CO_2 gas and ethanol. This yeast strain has also been used in scientific research for decades to better understand eukaryotic cell functions.[70] We have recently introduced the non-pathogenic baker's yeast as a novel approach for cancer therapy. In *in vitro* studies, various tumor cells showed the ability to phagocytize yeast, after which the tumor cells underwent apoptosis (Fig. 31.6). These cancer cells included those of the breast, tongue, colon, and skin.[71–75] *S. cerevisiae* induces apoptosis in human breast cancer cells by mechanisms that involve altering intracellular Ca^{2+} and the ratio of Bax:Bcl-2.[74] In animals bearing tumors, intratumoral injections of heat-killed yeast resulted in increased levels of apoptotic cancer cells and a significant decrease in tumor volume.[76,77]

Exploration of the synergistic apoptotic effect of yeast and MGN-3/BioBran revealed increased levels of cancer cell apoptosis. Human breast cancer cells (BCCs) such

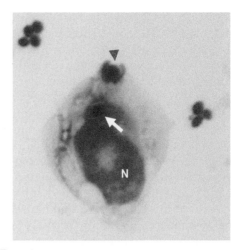

FIGURE 31.6 **Breast cancer cells phagocytize baker's yeast.** This image shows a Giemsa-stained cytospin preparation of MCF-7 cells at two different stages of yeast phagocytosis. One yeast is in the process of phagocytosis (red arrowhead), while the other has already been phagocytosed into the cancer cell (white arrow). Notice that the nucleus (N) is condensing and the nucleus to cytoplasm ratio is increasing. See color plate at the back of the book.

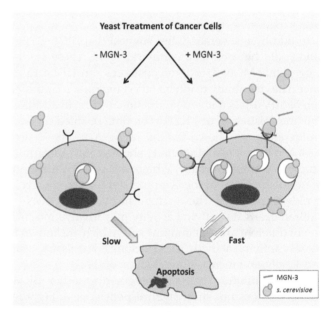

FIGURE 31.7 The co-culture of cancer cells with yeast in the presence of MGN-3/BioBran. MGN-3/BioBran enhances binding of yeast, leading to an increase in phagocytosis of yeast and subsequent increase in cancer cell apoptosis. See color plate at the back of the book.

as MCF-7 and HCC70 were cultured *in vitro* with heat-killed yeast at a ratio of 1:10 in the presence or absence of MGN-3/BioBran. The percent of apoptotic cells was assessed by MTT assay. Results depicted in Figure 31.7 showed that BCCs treated with MGN-3/BioBran exhibited increased percentages of attachment and uptake of yeast by MCF-7 cells. MGN-3/BioBran also increased apoptosis of BCCs.[78–81] The MGN-3/BioBran effect was dose-dependent, and was associated with increased activation of caspases 8 and 9 in MCF-7 cells and caspases 9 and 3 in HCC70 cells.[78] These data demonstrate that MGN-3/BioBran accelerates yeast-induced apoptosis of BCCs, which may represent a novel therapeutic strategy for the treatment of breast cancer.

CONCLUSION

Over the past 20 years, MGN-3/BioBran has been the focus of research to explore its biotherapeutic activities on cancer and viral infection and the mechanisms underlying its effects. In this chapter, we summarized several studies that demonstrate the ability of MGN-3/BioBran to sensitize cancer cells to chemotherapy, thus leading to their demise, and suggest the use of MGN-3/BioBran as an adjuvant for the treatment of cancer. Further studies have shown that MGN-3/BioBran exerts an antioxidant activity, as indicated by modulation of lipid peroxidation, augmenting the antioxidant defense system and protecting against oxidative stress. Thus, it appears that daily supplementation with MGN-3 may have therapeutic potential in apoptotic disorders associated with excess oxidative stress, such as cancer.

In addition, several studies suggest that MGN-3/BioBran could be used as an antiviral agent. These studies suggest that MGN-3/BioBran possesses anti-HIV activity, since it has the ability to inhibit HIV-1 replication by inhibition of HIV-1 p24 antigen production *in vitro*. In addition, oral administration of MGN-3/BioBran resulted in T-cell proliferation, as shown by the mitogen response with PHA and Con A.[1] Another study showed that oral administration of arabinoxylan rice bran was effective in shortening the duration of the symptoms of the common cold in elderly people.[82] The mechanism by which MGN-3/BioBran exerts its antiviral activity may involve modulation of different arms of immune cells which are known to possess antiviral activity. These include NK cells, DC cells, and T cells, and increased production of IFN-γ.

MGN-3/BioBran has advantages over other BRMs because it does not show hyporesponsiveness. Hyporesponsiveness is known to be a serious problem associated with many BRMs. The results of our studies show that NK cell activity is maintained at a high level throughout the continuation of treatment with MGN-3/BioBran over 4 years.[5,7] In addition, MGN-3 has been shown to be a safe and non-toxic agent, as manifested by the following: the LD_{50} of MGN-3 is greater than 36 g/kg; the Ames test for mutagenicity was negative; and the subchronic toxicity study in rats, antigenicity study, and genotoxic testing all demonstrated that MGN-3 is non-toxic. Furthermore, MGN-3 was safe when examined in humans by means of blood chemistry analysis, which included liver enzymes (SGOT and SGPT), and in clinical trials on cancer patients.

We conclude that MGN-3/BioBran is a safe agent that could be used as an effective adjuvant to the conventional therapeutic regimens used for the treatment of cancer and viral infection. More clinical trials are needed to validate and improve cancer treatment options by utilizing MGN-3 and its unique anticancer properties.

References

1. Ghoneum M. *Anti-HIV activity in vitro of MGN-3, an activated arabinoxylane from rice bran* 1998;**243**:25–29.
2. Cholujova D, Jakubikova J, Sedlak J. BioBran-augmented maturation of human monocyte-derived dendritic cells. *Neoplasma* 2009;**56**:89–95.
3. Ghoneum M, Agrawal S. Activation of human monocyte-derived dendritic cells *in vitro* by the biological response modifier arabinoxylan rice bran (MGN-3/BioBran). *Int J Immunopathol Immunopharmacol* 2001;**24**:941–8.
4. Ghoneum M. Enhancement of human natural killer cell activity by modified arabinoxylane from rice bran (MGN-3). *Int J Immunother* 1998;**14**:89–99.
5. Ghoneum M, Brown J. NK immunorestoration of cancer patients by MGN-3, a modified arabinoxylan rice bran (study of 32 patients followed for up to 4 years). In: Klatz R, Goldman R, editors. *Anti-aging Medical Therapeutics*. Marina del Rey, CA: Health Quest Publications; 1999. p. 217–26. vol. III.
6. Takahara K, Sano K. The life prolongation and QOL improvement effect of rice bran arabinoxylan derivative (MGN-3. Bio-Bran) for progressive cancer. *Clin Pharmacol Therapy* 2004;**14**:267–71.
7. Ghoneum M. *Immunostimulation and Cancer Prevention*. Las Vegas, NV: 7th International Congress on Antiaging and Biomedical Technologies; Dec 11–13, 1999.
8. Brahmi Z. Nature of natural killer cell hyporesponsiveness in the Chediak-Higashi syndrome. *Hum Immunol* 1983;**6**:45–52.
9. Talmadge JE, Herberman RB, Chirigos MA, et al. Hyporesponsiveness to augmentation of murine natural killer cell activity in different anatomical compartments by multiple injections of various immunomodulators including recombinant interferons and interleukin 2. *J Immunol* 1985;**135**:2483–91.
10. Saito T, Welker RD, Fukui H, et al. Development of hyporesponsiveness to augmentation of natural killer cell activity after multiple doses of maleic anhydride divinyl ether: association with decreased numbers of large granular lymphocytes. *Cell Immunol* 1985;**90**:577–89.
11. Saito T, Ruffman R, Welker RD, et al. Development of hyporesponsiveness of natural killer cells to augmentation of activity after multiple treatments with biological response modifiers. *Cancer Immunol Immunother* 1985;**19**:130–5.
12. Ghoneum M, Abedi S. Enhancement of natural killer cell activity of aged mice by modified arabinoxylan rice bran (MGN-3/BioBran). *J Pharm Pharmacol* 2004;**56**:1581–8.
13. Ghoneum M, Jewett A. Production of tumor necrosis factor-alpha and interferon-gamma from human peripheral blood lymphocytes by MGN-3, a modified arabinoxylan from rice bran, and its synergy with interleukin-2 *in vitro*. *Cancer Detect Prev* 2000;**24**:314–24.
14. Smith KA. Interleukin 2: Inception, impact, and implications. *Science* 1988;**240**:1169–76.
15. Phillips JH, Takeshita T, Sugamura K, Lanier LL. Activation of natural killer cells via the p75 interleukin 2 receptor. *J Exp Med* 1989;**170**:291–6.
16. Caligiuri MA, Zmuidzinas A, Manley TJ, et al. Functional consequences of IL-2 receptor expression on resting human lymphocytes: Identification of a novel NK cell subset with high affinity receptors. *J Exp Med* 1990;**171**:1509–26.

17. Siegel JP, Sharon M, Smith PL, Leonard WJ. The IL-2 receptor beta chain (p70): Role in mediating signals for LAK, NK, and proliferative activities. *Science* 1987;**238**:75–8.

18. Tsudo M, Goldman CK, Bongovanni KF, et al. The p75 peptide is the receptor for interleukin 2 expressed on large granular lymphocytes and is responsible for the interleukin 2 activation of these cells. *Proc Natl Acad Sci* 1987;**84**:5394–8.

19. Kehrl JH, Dukovich M, Whalen G, et al. Novel interleukin 2 (IL-2) receptor appears to mediate IL-2-induced activation of natural killer cells. *J Clin Invest* 1988;**81**:200–5.

20. Rosenberg SA, Lotze MT, Muul LM, et al. A progress report on the treatment of 157 patients with advanced cancer using lymphokine-activated killer cells and interleukin-2 or high-dose interleukin-2 alone. *N Engl J Med* 1987;**316**:889–97.

21. West WH, Tauer KW, Yannelli JR, et al. Constant-infusion recombinant interleukin-2 in adoptive immunotherapy of advanced cancer. *N Engl J Med* 1987;**316**:898–905.

22. Parkinson DR, Fisher RI, Rayner AA, et al. Therapy of renal cell carcinoma with interleukin-2 and lymphokine-activated killer cells: Phase II experience with a hybrid bolus and continuous infusion interleukin-2 regimen. *J Clin Oncol* 1990;**8**:1630–6.

23. Weiss GR, Margolin KA, Aronson FR, et al. A randomized phase II trial of continuous infusion interleukin-2 or bolus injection interleukin-2 plus lymphokine-activated killer cells for advanced renal cell carcinoma. *J Clin Oncol* 1992;**10**:275–81.

24. Khatri VP, Baiocchi RA, Bernstein ZP, Caligiuri MA. Immunotherapy with low-dose interleukin-2: rationale for prevention of immune-deficiency-associated cancer. *Cancer J Sci Am* 1997;**3**(Suppl. 1):S129–36.

25. Clark AGB, Holodniy M, Schwartz DH, et al. Decrease in HIV provirus in peripheral blood mononuclear cells during zidovudine and human rIL-2 administration. *J AIDS* 1992;**5**:52–9.

26. Pahwa S, Morales M. Interleukin-2 therapy in HIV infection. *AIDS Patient Care STDS* 1998;**12**:187–97.

27. Lotze ME, Matory YL, Ettinghausen SE, et al. *In vivo* administration of purified human interleukin 2. 11. Half life, immunologic effects, and expansion of peripheral lymphoid cells *in vivo* with recombinant IL-2. *J Immunol* 1985;**135**:2865–75.

28. Williams GM. Antitumor necrosis factor-alpha therapy and potential cancer inhibition. *Eur J Cancer Prev* 2008;**17**:169–77.

29. Gattoni A, Parlato A, Vangieri B, et al. Interferon-gamma: biologic functions and HCV terapy (type I/II) (2 of 2 parts). *Clin Ter* 2006;**157**:457–68.

30. Ghoneum M, Tachiki Uyemura K, et al. *Natural biological response modifier (MGN-3) shown to be effective against tumor cell growth.* Las Vegas, NV: Eighth Congress Anti-aging and Biomedical Technologies; 2000 14–17 December.

31. Gollapudi S, Ghoneum M. MGN-3/BioBran, modified arabinoxylan from rice bran, sensitizes human breast cancer cells to chemotherapeutic agent, daunorubicin. *Cancer Detect Prev* 2008;**32**:1–6.

32. Ghoneum M, Gollapudi S. *Modified arabinoxylan rice bran (MGN-3/BioBran) potentiates apoptosis in cancer cells induced by multiple anti-cancer agents in vitro.* Nice, France: International Symposium on Predictive Oncology & Intervention Strategies; February 7–10, 2004 Cancer Detect Prev.

33. Badr El-Din NK, Noaman E, Ghoneum M. In vivo tumor inhibitory effects of nutritional rice bran supplement MGN-3/BioBran on Ehrlich carcinoma-bearing mice. *Nutr Cancer* 2008;**60**:235–44.

34. Eastman A. Activation of programmed cell death by anticancer agents: cisplatin as a system model. *Cancer Cells* 1990;**2**:275–80.

35. Friesen C, Herr I, Krammer PH, et al. Involvement of the CD95 (APO-1/FAS) receptor/ligand system in drug-induced apoptosis in leukemia cells. *Nat Med* 1996;**2**:574–7.

36. Marchetti P, Mortier L, Beauvillain V, et al. Are mitochondria targets of anticancer drugs responsible for apoptosis? *Ann Biol Clin (Paris)* 2002;**60**:391–403.

37. Sorenson CM, Barry MA, Eastman A. Analysis of events associated with cell cycle arrest at G2 phase and cell death induced by cisplatin. *J Natl Cancer Inst* 1990;**82**:749–55.

38. Andersson A, Fagerberg J, Lewensohn R, et al. Pharmacokinetics of cisplatin and its monohydrated complex in humans. *J Pharm Sci* 1996;**85**:824–7.

39. Hickman JA. Apoptosis induced by anticancer drugs. *Cancer Metastasis Rev* 1992;**11**:121–39.

40. Sanderson BJ, Ferguson LR, Denny WA. Mutagenic and carcinogenic properties of platinum-based anticancer drugs. *Mutat Res* 1996;**355**:59–70.

41. Persidis A. Cancer Multidrug Resistance. *Nat Biotech* 1999;**17**:94–5.

42. Perez EA. Impact, mechanisms, and novel chemotherapy strategies for overcoming resistance to anthracyclines and taxanes in metastatic breast cancer. *Breast Canc Res and Treat* 2009;**114**: 195–201.

43. Singal PK, Iliskovic N. Doxorubicin-induced cardiomyopathy. *N Engl J Med* 1999;**339**:900–5.

44. Lorigan P, Lee SM, Betticher D, et al. Chemotherapy with vincristine/ifosfamide/carboplatin/etoposide in small cell lung cancer. *Semin Oncol* 1995;**22**:32–41.

45. Francis PA, Kris MG, Rigas JR, et al. Paclitaxel (Taxol) and docetaxel (Taxotere): active chemotherapeutic agents in lung cancer. *Lung Cancer* 1995;**12**:S163–72.

46. Fossella FV, Lee JS, Berille J, Hong WK. Summary of phase II data of docetaxel (Taxotere), an active agent in the first- and second-line treatment of advanced non-small cell lung cancer. *Semin Oncol* 1995;**22**:22–9.

47. Strauss GM, Lynch TJ, Elias AD, et al. A phase I study of fosfamide/carboplatin/etoposide/paclitaxel in advanced lung cancer. *Semin Oncol* 1995;**22**:70–4.

48. Grisold W, Cavaletti G, Windebank AJ. Peripheral neuropathies from chemotherapeutics and targeted agents: diagnosis, treatment, and prevention. *Neuro Oncol* 2012(Suppl. 4) iv45–54.

49. Lucchetta M, Lonardi S, Bergamo F, et al. Incidence of atypical acute nerve hyperexcitability symptoms in oxaliplatin-treated patients with colorectal cancer. *Cancer Chemother Pharmacol* 2012;**70**:899–902.

50. Mills KH, Greally JF, Temperley IJ, et al. Haematological and immune suppressive effects of total body irradiation in the rat. *Ir J Med Sci* 1980;**149**:201–8.

51. Sanderson BJ, Ferguson LR, Denny WA. Mutagenic and carcinogenic properties of platinum-based anticancer drugs. *Mutat Res* 1996;**355**:59–70.

52. Santin AD, Hermonat PL, Ravaggi A, et al. Effects of concurrent cisplatinum administration during radiotherapy vs. radiotherapy alone on the immune function of patients with cancer of the uterine cervix. *Int J Radiat Oncol Biol Phys* 2000;**48**:997–1006.

53. Barrand MA, Rhodes T, Center MS, Twentyman PR. Chemosensitisation and drug accumulation effects of cyclosporin A, PSC833 and verapamil in human MDR large cell lung cancer cells expressing a 190 K membrane protein distinct from P-glycoprotein. *Eur J Cancer* 1993;**29A**:408–15.

54. Gollapudi S, Thadepalli F, Kim CH, et al. Difloxacin reverses multidrug resistance in HL60/AR cells that overexpress multi drug resistance related protein (MRP) gene. *Oncol Res* 1995;**7**: 73–85.

55. Gollapudi S, Kim CH, Tran B, et al. Probencid reverses multidrug resistance in multidrug resistance associated protein-associated protein overexpressing HL/AR and H69/AR cells but not in P-glycoprotein overexpressing HL60/Tax and P388/ADR cells. Cancer Chemother. *Pharmacol* 1997;**40**:150–8.

56. Nishikawa K, Asaumi J, Kawasaki S, et al. Influence of cepharanthin on the intracellular accumulation of adriamycin in normal liver cells and spleen cells of mice *in vitro* and *in vivo*. *Anticancer Res* 1997;**17**:3617–21.

57. Astier A, Doat B, Ferrer MJ. Enhancement of adriamycin antitumor activity by its binding with an intracellular sustained-release form, polymethacrylate nanospheres, in U-937 cells. *Cancer Res* 1835-1841;**1988**;48.

58. Lambert G, Fattal E, Pinto-Alphandary H, et al. Polyisobutylcyanoacrylate nanocapsules containing an aqueous core as a novel colloidal carrier for the delivery of oligonucleotides. *Pharm Res* 2000;**17**:707–14.

59. Zhang R, Wang X, Wu C, et al. Synergistic enhancement effect of magnetic nanoparticles on anticancer drug accumulation in cancer cells. *Nanotechnol* 2006;**17**:3622–6.

60. Ghoneum M, Gollapudi S. MGN-3 sensitizes human T cell leukemia cells to death receptor (CD95)-induced apoptosis. *Cancer Letter* 2003;**201**:41–9.

61. Jacoby HI, Wnorowski G, Sakata K, et al. The effect of MGN-3 on cisplatin and doxorubicin induced toxicity in the rat. *J Nutraceuticals Funct Med Foods* 2001;**3**:3–11.

62. Endo Y, Kambayashi H. Modified rice bran beneficial of weight loss of mice as a major and acute adverse effect of Cisplatin. *Pharmacol and Toxicol* 2003;**92**:300–3.

63. Bang MH, Van Riep T, Thinh NT, et al. Arabinoxylan rice bran (MGN-3) enhances the effects of interventional therapies for the treatment of hepatocellular carcinoma: a three-year randomized clinical trial. *Anticancer Res* 2010;**30**:5145–51.

64. Joe B, Vijaykumar M, Lokesh BR. Biological properties of curcumin-cellular and molecular mechanisms of action. *Crit Rev Food Sci Nutr* 2004;**44**:97–111.

65. Ghoneum M, Gollapudi S. Synergistic apoptotic effect of arabinoxylan rice bran (MGN-3/BioBran) and curcumin (turmeric) on human multiple myeloma cell line U266 *in vitro*. *Neoplasma* 2011;**58**:118–23.

66. Sinha R, Cross AJ, Daniel CR, et al. Caffeinated and decaffeinated coffee and tea intakes and risk of colorectal cancer in a large prospective study. *Am J Clin Nutr* 2012;**96**:374–81.

67. Song F, Qureshi A, Han J. Increased caffeine intake is associated with reduced risk of basal cell carcinoma of the skin. *Cancer Res* 2012;**72**:3282–9.

68. Gunter MJ, Schaub JA, Xue X, et al. A prospective investigation of coffee drinking and endometrial cancer incidence. *Int J Cancer* 2012;**131**:E530–6.

69. Niknafs B. Induction of apoptosis and non-apoptosis in human breast cancer cell line (MCF-7) by cisplatin and caffeine. *Iran Biomed J* 2011;**15**:130–3.

70. Mori H, Kawabata K, Matsunaga K, et al. Chemopreventive effects of coffee bean and rice constituents on colorectal carcinogenesis. *Biofactors* 2000;**12**:101–5.

71. Kataoka T, Powers S, Cameron S, et al. Functional homology of mammalian and yeast RAS genes. *Cell* 1985;**40**:19–26.

72. Ghoneum M, Gollapudi S. Induction of apoptosis in human breast cancer cells by Saccharomyces cerevisiae, the baker's yeast, *in vitro*. *Anticancer Res* 2003;**24**:1455–63.

73. Ghoneum M, Gollapudi S, Hamilton J, et al. Human squamous cell carcinoma of the tongue and colon undergoes apoptosis upon phagocytosis of *Saccharomyces cerevisiae*, the baker's yeast, *in vitro*. *Anticancer Res* 2005;**25**:981–9.

74. Ghoneum M, Gollapudi S. Apoptosis of breast cancer MCF-7 cells *in vitro* is induced specifically by yeast and not by fungal mycelia. *Anticancer Res* 2013-2022;**2006**:26.

75. Ghoneum M, Matsuura M, Braga M, et al. *S. cerevisiae* induces apoptosis in human metastatic breast cancer cells by altering intracellular Ca2+ and the ratio of Bax and Bcl-2. *Int J Oncology* 2008;**33**:533–9.

76. Ghoneum M. *Baker's yeast, S. cerevisiae, exerts anti-metastatic effects on skin cancer in lungs of mice*. San Diego, CA: The American Association of Cancer Research (AACR), special Conference on Cell Death Mechanisms and Cancer Therapy; February 1–4, 2010.

77. Ghoneum M, Wang L, Agrawal S, et al. Yeast therapy for the treatment of breast cancer: A nude mice model study. *In Vivo* 2007;**21**:251–8.

78. Ghoneum M, Badr El-Din N, Noaman E, et al. *Saccharomyces cerevisiae*, the Baker's yeast, suppresses the growth of Ehrlich carcinoma-bearing mice. *Cancer Immunol Immunother* 2008;**57**:581–92.

79. Ghoneum M, Gollapudi S. Synergistic role of arabinoxylan rice bran (MGN-3/BioBran) in *S. cerevisiae*-induced apoptosis of monolayer breast cancer MCF-7 Cells. *Anticancer Res* 2005;**25**:4187–96.

80. Ghoneum M, Gollapudi S. Modified arabinoxylan rice bran (MGN-3/BioBran) enhances yeast-induced apoptosis in human breast cancer cells *in vitro*. *Anticancer Res* 2005;**25**:859–70.

81. Ghoneum M, Brown J, Gollapudi S. Yeast therapy for the treatment of cancer and its enhancement by MGN-3/BioBran, an arabinoxylan rice bran. Cellular Signaling and Apoptosis Research. In: Demasi AR, editor. New York, NY: Nova Science Publishers, Inc; 2007. p. 185–200.

82. Tazawa K, Ichihashi K, Fujii T, et al. The orally administration of the Hydrolysis Rice Bran prevents a common cold syndrome for the elderly people based on immunomodulatory function. *J Trad Med* 2003;**20**:132–41.

γ-Oryzanol: An Attractive Bioactive Component from Rice Bran

Christelle Lemus, Apostolis Angelis, Maria Halabalaki, Alexios Leandros Skaltsounis

University of Athens, Division of Pharmacognosy and Natural Products Chemistry, Department of Pharmacy, Athens, Greece

INTRODUCTION

Oryza sativa L. seeds of the Poaceae family, commonly known as Asian rice or simply rice, could be considered as one of the most important grains since it is consumed by the half of the world population. According to a United States Department of Agriculture (USDA) report,[1] 453.4 million tonnes of rice was consumed worldwide in 2010/2011.

In Asia in particular rice comprises a basic component of the daily diet,[2] and it occupies one of the top positions of commodities with the highest worldwide production according to FAOSTAT (the Statistics Division of the Food and Agriculture Organization of the United Nations).[2] As expected, Asia is by far the main producer and China the most representative country, producing 200 million tonnes of rice and paddy in 2010 (Fig. 32.1).

The oil deriving from rice, namely rice bran oil (RBO), is one of the most commonly used cooking oils in Asia, and the major by-product of the rice milling industry. RBO represents a rich source of high added-value phytochemicals of nutritional, pharmaceutical, and cosmetic interest, such as tocopherols and tocotrienols (tocols or vitamin E), lecithin, carotenoids, and γ-oryzanol, and has therefore attracted considerable interest in recent years.[3,4] γ-Oryzanol is of particular significance because it is abundant in RBO compared to other vegetable oils.[5]

γ-Oryzanol was first isolated in 1954 by Kaneko and Tsuchiya[6] from the unsaponifiable fraction of rice bran as a crystalline substance; it was considered to be a single compound and was named oryzanol in reference to the botanical species of rice, *Oryza sativa*. Three years later,

Shimizu *et al.*,[7] using a different extraction method, discovered that γ-oryzanol was not a single entity and suggested that it was composed of three ferulic acid esters of triterpene alcohols, which were designated oryzanol A, B, and C. Subsequently the same scientific team identified oryzanol A as cycloartenyl ferulate,[8] and in 1958 oryzanol C was identified as 24-methylene cycloartanyl ferulate.[9] Finally, oryzanol B was found to be a mixture of oryzanol A and C. Since then, various studies have been carried out investigating the composition of γ-oryzanol, allowing the identification of more than 20 ferulic acid esters of triterpene alcohols and sterols by different methods.[10]

Given that RBO is an important by-product in the rice industry, much attention has been paid to optimization of its production and further treatment processes. In the standard industrial procedure of RBO production a refining process takes place through a deacidification treatment with alkali, giving rise to soapstock. This residue is quite valuable, since the highest percentage of γ-oryzanol contained in the crude oil is lost in the soapstock (83%–95%, according to Krishna *et al.*[11]). Therefore soapstoack is the richest source of γ-oryzanol and probably the most important by-product of rice processing.

γ-Oryzanol generally exhibits a wide spectrum of health-beneficial effects, including anticarginogenic, anti-inflammatory, antihyperlipidemic, antidiabetic, and neuroprotective, which are mainly attributed to its antioxidant capacity.[4] This pleiotropic biological profile of γ-oryzanol, together with its high availability in industrial by-products, has contributed significantly to the observed increasing interest from academia and industry, especially in recent years.

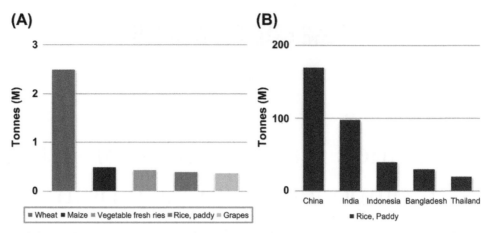

FIGURE 32.1 (A) Whole world production: proportion of rice amongst other grains (average 1961–2010). (B) Production of top five producers of rice (average 1961–2010). *Food and Agriculture Organization of the United Nations* (http://faostat3.fao.org/home/index.html#VISUALIZE). Please see color plate at the back of the book.

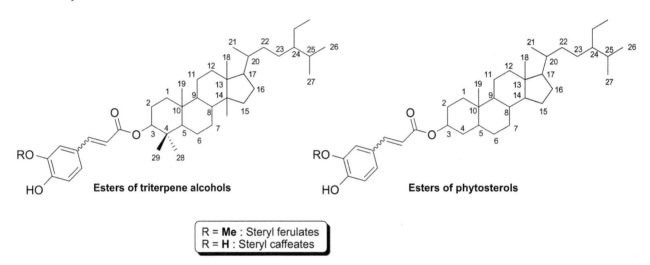

FIGURE 32.2 General structures and numeration of γ-oryzanol compounds.

CLASSIFICATION AND BIOSYNTHESIS OF γ-ORYZANOL

Chemically, γ-oryzanol is a mixture of structurally related components, and specifically esters of ferulic acid with phytosterols and triterpene alcohols, also referred as steryl ferulates. Steryl ferulates have been identified in rye, corn, triticale, barley, and wheat, but their richest source is rice, and specifically RBO.[12] The most abundant steryl ferulates in RBO, comprising almost 95% of γ-oryzanol, are campesterol, β-sitosterol, cycloartenol, and 24-methylenecycloartenol esters (Fig. 32.2). Although the constituents of γ-oryzanol were identified as steryl esters of ferulic acid, Fang's work has recently revealed the presence of caffeate esters of cycloartenol and campesterol as well.[13]

Numerous others steryl ferulates have been reported to be present in γ-oryzanol in low concentrations, detected and identified via several spectroscopic methods, and most of these are presented in Table 32.1.

With regard to the structural composition, it seems clear that steryl ferulates biogenetically originated from the esterification of ferulic acid with sterols and/or triterpene alcohols. The steryl ferulates principally differ at the triterpenoid moiety, which represents the bulkier part of the molecule, while both sterols and triterpene alcohols consist of a four-ring cyclopentanophenanthrene skeleton with a hydroxyl group at position 3. Their biosynthesis initiates with acetyl-CoA and implicates the enzymatic controlled formation of isopentenyl diphosphate (IPP) via mevalonic acid. IPP is then involved in the production of prenyl diphosphate homologues (DMAPP, GPP) by a succession of elongation reactions. Condensation of three molecules of IPP from geranyl diphosphate (GPP) produces squalene, which is epoxided to oxidosqualene, a common precursor of sterols and triterpene alcohol[14] (Fig. 32.3). Several labeled experiments led to the determination of pathways involved in triterpene biogenesis via lanosterol or cycloartenol.[15]

TABLE 32.1 Basic γ-Oryzanol Components Identified Using MS and NMR Techniques

	R_1	R_2	Name	Formula	M (g/mol)	Ref(s)
	F		24-Methylenecycloartanyl ferulate	$C_{41}H_{60}O_4$	616.45	Fang et al.[13], Akihisa et al.[22], Xu and Godber[75], Berger et al.[187]
	F		Cycloartenyl ferulate	$C_{40}H_{58}O_4$	602.43	Fang et al.[13], Akihisa et al.[22], Xu and Godber[75], Berger et al.[187]
	C		Cycloartenyl caffeate	$C_{39}H_{56}O_4$	588.42	Fang et al.[13]
	F		Cycloartanyl ferulate	$C_{40}H_{60}O_4$	604.45	Fang et al.[13]
	F		Cyclobranyl ferulate	$C_{41}H_{60}O_4$	616.45	Berger et al.[187]
	F		(24)-cycloart-25-ene-3β, 24-diol-3β-*trans* ferulate	$C_{39}H_{56}O_5$	604.41	Angelis et al.[17]
	F		Cycloart-23-Z-ene-3β, 25-diol-3β-*trans* ferulate	$C_{39}H_{56}O_5$	604.41	Angelis et al.[17]
	F		Cycloeucalenyl ferulate	$C_{40}H_{58}O_4$	602.43	Fang et al.[13], Akihisa et al.[22]
	F		Campesteryl ferulate	$C_{38}H_{56}O_4$	576.42	Fang et al.[13], Xu and Godber[75], Berger et al.[187]
	C		Campesteryl caffeate	$C_{37}H_{54}O_4$	562.40	Fang et al.[13]
	F		Sitosteryl ferulate	$C_{39}H_{58}O_4$	590.43	Fang et al.[13], Akihisa et al.[22], Xu and Godber[75], Berger et al.[187]
	F		Stigmasteryl ferulate	$C_{39}H_{56}O_4$	588.42	Fang et al.[13], Akihisa et al.[22], Xu and Godber[75], Berger et al.[187]
	F		Δ^7-Stigmastenyl ferulate	$C_{39}H_{56}O_4$	588.42	Xu and Godber[75]
	F		Δ^7-Sitostenyl ferulate	$C_{39}H_{58}O_4$	590.43	Fang et al.[13], Xu and Godber[75]
	F		Δ^7-Campestenyl ferulate	$C_{39}H_{56}O_4$	576.42	Fang et al.[13], Xu and Godber[75]
	F		Gramisteryl ferulate	$C_{39}H_{56}O_4$	588.42	Akihisa et al.[22]
	F		Citrostadienyl ferulate	$C_{40}H_{58}O_4$	602.43	Akihisa et al.[22]

(Continued)

TABLE 32.1　Basic γ-Oryzanol Components Identified Using MS and NMR Techniques—cont'd

	R₁	R₂	Name	Formula	M (g/mol)	Ref(s)
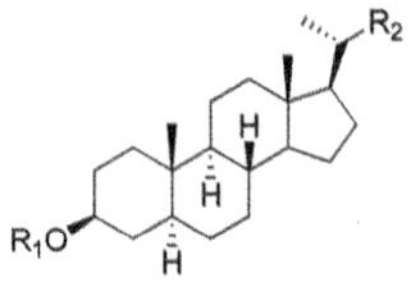	F	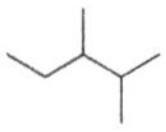	Campestanyl ferulate	$C_{38}H_{58}O_4$	578.43	Fang et al.[13], Xu and Godber[75]
	F	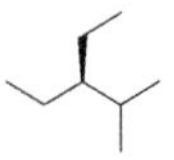	Sitostanyl ferulate	$C_{39}H_{60}O_4$	592.45	Fang et al.[13], Akihisa et al.[22], Xu and Godber[75]

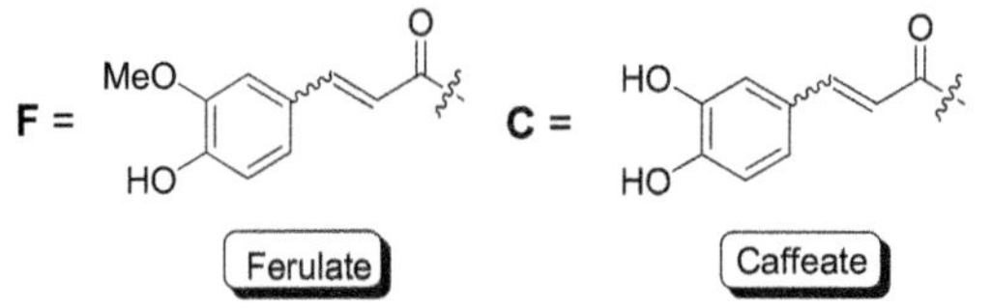

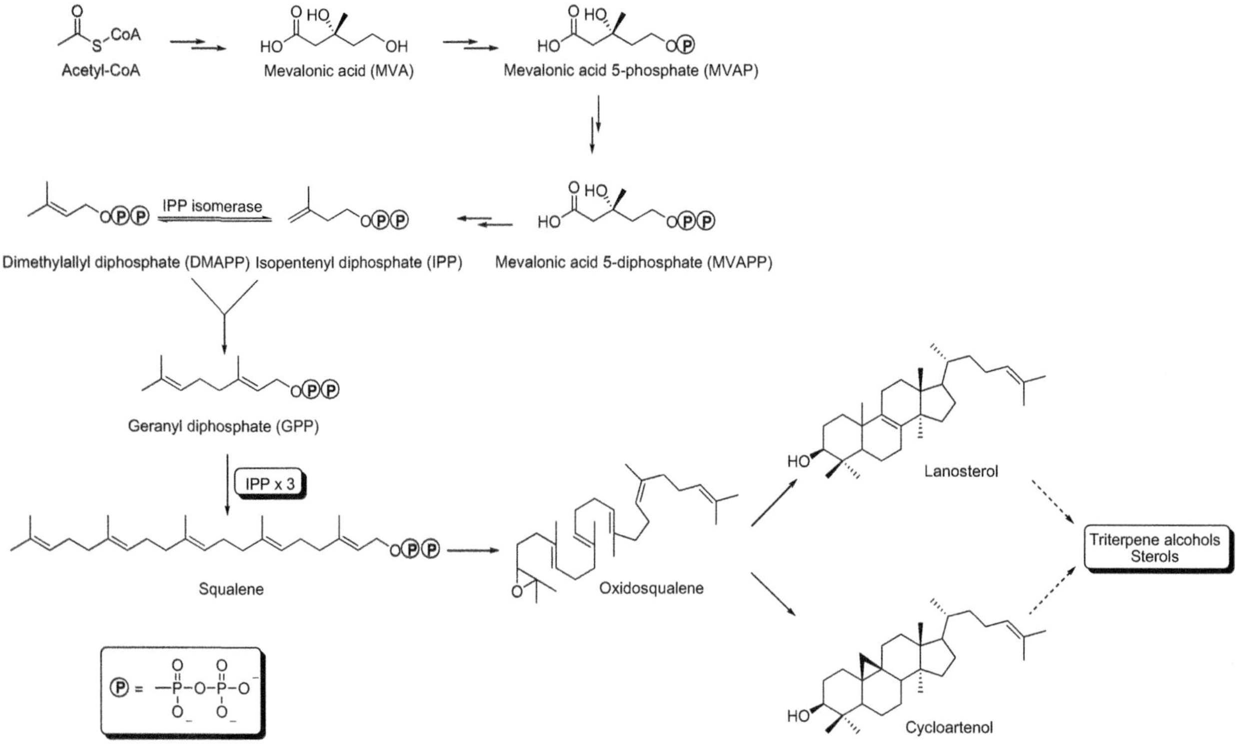

F = Ferulate　　C = Caffeate

FIGURE 32.3　Biogenetic synthesis of sterols.

Structurally, the number of methyl groups attached on C-4 allows differentiation of the sterol ferulates from the triterpene alcohol ferulates, the former having no methyl or just one methyl (4-methylsterol) group on C-4, and the latter containing two methyl groups at the tetracyclic ring system. In the case of triterpene alcohol ferulate esters, a cyclopropane in position C-9/C-10 is also usually present.[16] The composition of the side chain of sterols and triterpene alcohols of γ-oryzanol varies with the different derivatives (Table 32.1). Recently, a new group of γ-oryzanol, designated as polar γ-oryzanol

has been suggested by Angelis et al. and generally it concerns hydroxylated derivatives characterized by alkyl groups attached to C-24. Specifically, three hydroxylated triterpene alcohol ferulates ([24R] and [24S]-cycloart-25-ene-3β,24-diol-3β-trans ferulate, and cycloart-23Z-ene-3β,25-diol-3β-trans ferulate) have been isolated and identified.[17] The presence of such hydroxylated ferulates was also mentioned previously by Fang et al.[13]

The γ-oryzanol ferulates are characterized by the trans configuration of the ferulic acid part. Ferulic acid (FA) is a derivative of cinnamic acid

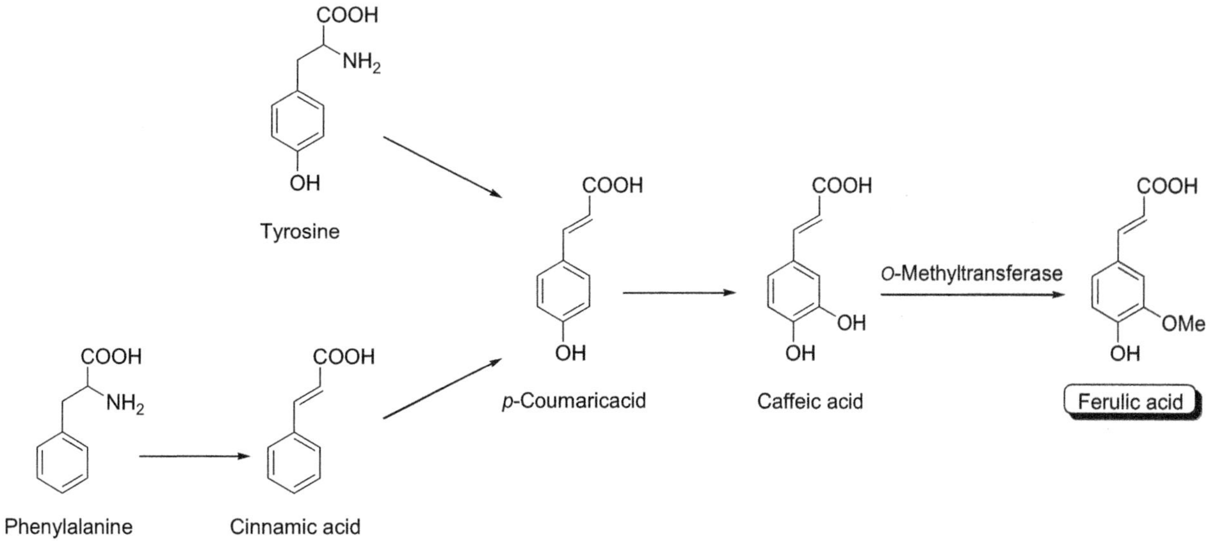

FIGURE 32.4 Biogenetic formation of ferulic acid.

(4-hydroxy-3-methoxycinnamic acid), and is one of the most abundant phenolic acids in plants. FA is rarely found in its free form, but is generally linked to sugars, polysaccharides, or proteins.[18] This moiety is also responsible for the characteristic ultraviolet absorption observed in RBO. Biogenetically, this phenolic unit comes from the methoxylation of the *m*-hydroxyl group of caffeic acid, catalyzed by the enzyme *O*-methyltransferase.[19] This suggests that the enzyme involved in the biosynthesis of steryl ferulates could accept caffeic acid as a substrate and thus explain the presence of caffeate esters in γ-oryzanol (Fig. 32.4). As with many natural phenols, FA possesses antioxidant activity,[20] and has been found to exhibit beneficial effects against cancer, diabetes, and Alzheimer disease.[21] Although the steryl ferulates are generally characterized by a *trans* configuration of the ferulic acid, several authors have also shown the presence of *cis* derivatives.[13,17,22] However, Fang *et al.* suggest the possibility that these *cis* derivatives might be artifacts due to a *cis–trans* isomerization which may occur during the production of rice bran because of the long wavelength UV radiation.[13]

As mentioned previously, γ-oryzanol compounds are formed through esterification between ferulic (or caffeic) acid and a triterpene (sterol or triterpene alcohol). In order to investigate this hypothesis, Sato[23] performed synthesis of the γ-oryzanol steryl ferulates (^{14}C labeled), starting with the formulation of guaiacol with ^{14}C-labeled formaldehyde to give vanillin-[14]C. Condensation of this latter with malonic acid followed by acetylation gave 4′-acetylferulic acid-^{14}C, which was treated with 2SOCl2 forming 4′-acetylferulic acid chloride-[14]C. The nucleophilic reaction between the triterpenyl alcohols (obtained by saponification of γ-oryzanol) and the chloride-^{14}C produced γ-oryzanol-^{14}C with

a yield of 97% after crystallization. Akihisa[22] has also proposed a synthesis of eight steryl ferulates contained in γ-oryzanol. Thus, 4-propionyl ferulate, obtained by condensation of *trans*-ferulic acid and propionic anhydride in an alkaline medium, was added to stigmasterol, yielding a 4-propionyl ferulate of stigmasterol. Finally, basic hydrolysis of the propionyl ester moiety gave *trans*-stigmasteryl ferulate. Using the same synthetic pathway, *trans*-gramisteryl ferulate and *trans*-citrostadienyl ferulate were prepared from the corresponding free sterols. It should be mentioned that the author has also prepared the corresponding *cis* derivatives, by irradiation at 365 nm, under N2 with a 100-W mercury vapor discharge lamp, of the *trans*-ferulates. In this manner, *cis*-stigmasteryl ferulate, *cis*-gramisteryl ferulate, *cis*-citrostadienyl ferulate, *cis*-cycloeucalenyl ferulate, and *cis*-24-methylenecycloartanyl ferulate were synthesized. It is important to note that recently a patent has been filed concerning the preparation of steryl ferulates.[24] The synthesis involves the acetylation of ferulic acid followed by esterification with a phytosterol in the presence of N,N′-dicyclohexylcarbodiimide (DCC) and 4-dimethylaminopyridine (DMAP). Finally, deprotection of the acetate gave the desired phytosteryl ferulate.

EXTRACTION AND ISOLATION OF γ-ORYZANOL

Rice bran comprises the outer layers of the brown rice kernel (pericarp, tegmen, aleurone, and sub-aleurone) and is obtained as a by-product of the rice milling process. Rice bran constitutes approximately 8–10% of paddy rice, which leads in huge production of this added-value material globally.[25] The high nutritious value of rice bran is due to its high contents of protein (14–16%), dietary fiber (8–12%), phytic acid (8.7%), and oil (16–23%). The extraction of rice bran leads to RBO, which contains an important amount of biologically active nutraceuticals such as γ-oryzanol, vitamin E (tocopherols and tocotrienols), and phytosterols.[26,27] Apart from neutral lipids (88–90%), crude RBO contains a rich unsaponifiable fraction (4–5%), free fatty acids (2–4%), and small amounts of gum and waxes. The unsaponifiable fraction contains mainly γ-oryzanol and tocols, while other bioactive compounds, such as carotenoids, squalene, lecithin, tricin, and long-chain alcohols, are also present in lower concentrations.[4,28–30]

The use of RBO as food product depends on the quality of the bran, the extraction method used, and the refining process. Rice bran contains several types of lipases which are activated during the milling process, leading to hydrolysis of lipids into free fatty acids (FFA). This deterioration gives the products a rancid smell and bitter taste, making them unsuitable for consumption.[31] Although direct extraction of freshly milled rice bran leads to good quality RBO, the commonly used procedure includes initial stabilization of the bran prior to oil extraction. The stabilization of rice bran aims to avoid the process of hydrolytic rancidity by destruction or inhibition of lipases. A variety of methods, such as sun-drying, cold storage, steaming, and ohmic heating, as well as chemical treatments, has been used for this purpose. It should be noted that the chosen method has a significant effect on the lipase's activity, the extraction yield, and the levels of bioactive compounds.[32,33] The stored stabilized bran retains standard FFA levels for about 2 months, while food-grade n-hexane is the solvent of choice for commercial extraction of RBO.[34–36] The major advantage of this solvent is its high stability and capacity for dissolving oil, and it is considered by FDA as safe for extraction of edible oils from oil seeds or oil-bearing materials.[37] n-Hexane is mixed directly with the stabilized rice bran in maceration or percolation type extractors, and the miscella, after removal of the solvent by vacuum evaporation or distillation, yields crude RBO. Although n-hexane is an effective solvent for extraction of oil from rice bran, it poses some disadvantages, such as toxicity at high concentrations and flammability, and is also environmentally hazardous. For these reasons, the bran oil industry has shown an increased interest in alternative solvents as well as in solvent-free processes such as ohmic heating and supercritical fluid extraction.

The crude RBO obtained from solvent extraction of rice bran is unsuitable for edible use due to its high levels of FFA, waxes, gums, and pigments. The removal of these components by chemical or physical refining leads to food-grade RBO. Chemical refining produces good quality RBO regarding color and cloud point, and thus is generally preferred over physical refining. However, chemical refining causes significant losses of bioactive components, which are removed into the soapstock, in contrast to physical refining, which leads to RBO rich in phytochemicals. Regarding γ-oryzanol content, physical refining removes only 1.1–5.9% of γ-oryzanol while chemical refining almost completely removes the γ-oryzanol content (93–95%) from crude RBO.[11,38] The beneficial properties of γ-oryzanol and tocopherols in human health means that high commercial value has been added to rice products. Thus, the factors that influence these phytochemicals' extraction rates are of great importance and have been extensively studied. More than 50 research articles have been reported worldwide investigating the main factors and their impact on the levels of constituents of rice. Both genetic and environmental factors seem to affect significantly the γ-oryzanol content in rice and rice bran. Particular attention should be given to the milling, extraction, and refining processes due to the direct impact of those procedures on γ-oryzanol levels.[4,10] Generally, the γ-oryzanol content in rice ranges significantly in different genotypes and growing environments. Bergman and Xu reported a study on seven rice cultivars of the Southern US over 2 years, and demonstrated that γ-oryzanol's content ranged from 2510 to 6864 mg/kg, while the growing environment had a greater effect than the genotype.[3] Another study, performed by Miller et al., on 30 brown rice cultivars of European origin grown at different areas and in different seasons showed approximately the same γ-oryzanol content (26–63 mg/100 g) and indicated that environmental conditions were the main factor for this range. Moreover, it was found that the degree of maturity of rice grains has no significant influence on γ-oryzanol levels.[39]

On the other hand, Heinemann et al. analyzed 32 genotypes of brown rice belonging to the indica and japonica subspecies, cultivated in Brazil, and found that the mean content of γ-oryzanol across all samples was significantly higher in japonica (246.3 mg/kg) compared to indica (190.1 mg/kg) rice subspecies.[40] Japonica varieties were found to be richer in γ-oryzanol compared to indica varieties, as demonstrated in a few more studies conducted in commercial rice varieties growing in Taiwan and Pakistan. Beyond the above result the authors found that: (1) no obvious difference in γ-oryzanol content was noted between black- and red-colored rice varieties; (2) γ-oryzanol was affected significant by crop year; and (3) basmati rice cultivars are a good source of γ-oryzanol.[41–43]

The impact of growing temperature on phytochemical levels was the subject of research reported by Britz and coworkers. In this study, the seeds from six different rice lines grown in replicate greenhouses were analyzed. The results showed that the γ-oryzanol levels increased by 35–57% at an elevated temperature in five of six lines, but the levels of tocols were not affected. Moreover, the study demonstrated that the increased temperature was the main factor altering the γ-oryzanol content.[44] On the contrary, the application of organic and inorganic fertilizers and pesticides to the rice crop had no particular impact on the content of γ-oryzanol and vitamin E.[45]

Another critical factor that significantly modifies the levels of several rice bioactive components is germination. The investigation of its influence and studies related to the development of functional foods have been the subject of several published research articles. For instance, Lee et al. found that during germination of rough rice of four Korean varieties the γ-oryzanol content increased 0.8- to 1.5-fold,[46] while Kim et al. reported that the γ-oryzanol contents in rough rice and brown rice were increased 1.13- and 1.20-fold, respectively, after germination.[47] The effect of germination time on the levels of biochemical compositions and antioxidant activity has been also explored. For instance, Moongngarm and Khomphiphatkul showed that 2- to 3-day germination of rough rice was the optimum time for the increase in γ-oryzanol content and determined antioxidant activity,[48] while Kiing et al. demonstrated that some Sarawak cultivars are characterized by the highest concentration of γ-oryzanol after 16 hours of germination.[49]

The change in γ-oryzanol, relative to other nutritional components of paddy rice and brown rice during the germination process, was also investigated by Oh and coworkers. The results showed significant concentration differences throughout germination, whilst brown rice exhibited a higher γ-oryzanol content than paddy rice.[50] Moreover, Sungsopha et al. investigated the influence of germination and enzymatic treatment on the levels of the bioactive contents and antioxidant activity of rice bran. Among other findings, they discovered that both germination of rough rice and enzymatic treatment improved the levels of γ-oryzanol two-fold, compared to untreated rice bran.[51]

The milling process itself also seems to have a significant impact on the levels of rice bioactive compounds. Since the outer layers of the rice kernel contain almost the total amount of γ-oryzanol in rice, the degree of milling leads to products with different levels of these compounds. Thus, the influence of the milling process on the levels of γ-oryzanol has been reported in a few studies. Overall, findings demonstrate that the concentrations of γ-oryzanol in rice, as well as the levels of other compounds, are significantly decreased as the degree of milling is increased.[30,52] For instance, Tuncel and Yilmaz showed that the γ-oryzanol content obtained from different steps of milling procedure ranged from 12.19 to 3296.5 mg/kg, while the whitening and polishing processes led to the loss of approximately 94% of the γ-oryzanol compared to brown rice.[53]

Critical factors for γ-oryzanol content, and rice bioactives in general, are the extraction and refining methods. These affect both the yield of the produced oil and the levels of the biological active compounds significantly. The most commonly used method for extraction of RBO is solvent extraction, while soxhlet and supercritical fluid extraction (SFE) are, so far, used mainly in laboratory-scale production. Although n-hexane is the solvent of choice, especially in large-scale extraction of RBO, numerous attempts have been made to find alternative solvents that are able to increase the overall yield of RBO and its phytochemical content. As for other factors, the influence of the solvent and the extraction method on the levels of γ-oryzanol has been extensively investigated. For example, Xu and Godber compared the ability of supercritical CO_2 and organic solvents to extract lipids and γ-oryzanol from rice bran. They assayed several organic solvents and found that the mixture of 50% n-hexane and 50% isopropanol (vol/vol), at a temperature of 60°C for 45–60 minutes, produced the highest yield (1.68 mg/g of rice bran) of γ-oryzanol. On the other hand, the use of SFE under a temperature of 50°C and pressure of 68,901 kPa (680 atm) for 25 minutes led to 5.39 mg γ-oryzanol/g of rice bran – an amount approximately four times greater than the highest yield achieved using solvent extraction. Moreover, it was possible to obtain an extract with a high concentration of γ-oryzanol (50–80%) after 15–20 minutes of extraction under optimized conditions.[54]

Along these lines, Imsanguan and coworkers reported a comparative study in which the effects of operating mode, temperature, pressure, and solvent on α-tocopherol and γ-oryzanol extraction yield from rice bran were investigated. They also compared the efficiency of SFE-CO_2, solvent, and soxhlet extraction in respect to the recovery of these compounds. The authors found that the best conditions for SFE-CO_2 extraction of γ-oryzanol were 65°C and 48 MPa, in continuous operating mode, while, regarding solvent extraction, ethanol at 55–60°C was found to be the most suitable choice. Furthermore, they concluded that SFE-CO_2 was the most effective method for extracting both α-tocopherol and γ-oryzanol from rice bran.[55]

In another study, Lai et al. found that both methanol and ethyl acetate extracts of japonica rice bran exhibited a higher γ-oryzanol content (1.6–1.8 g/kg bran) compared to the n-hexane extract.[56] Using three different solvents, Chen and Chiu tried to characterize the major phytochemicals and antioxidant properties of taro-scented rice bran and found that ethyl acetate can extract γ-oryzanol more efficiently (1.55 ± 0.20 g/kg rice bran) while the use of methanol leads to higher yields (15.42 ± 1.41 g/kg bran).[57] Moreover, Rodrigues and Oliveira demonstrated that ethanol is an efficient solvent for extraction of γ-oryzanol and the influence of temperature is important when a low level of water is added to ethanol.[58] In a second work on the same subject, Oliveira et al. showed that it is possible to obtain 1527–4164 mg of γ-oryzanol/kg of fresh rice bran when ethanol is used as an extraction solvent and when particular attention is given to solvent hydration, temperature, solvent-to-rice bran mass ratio, and stirrer speed.[59]

Chemical and physical refining of RBO affects the concentration of γ-oryzanol in the final product differently. A complete work on this influence has been carried out by Gopala Krishna and coworkers.[11] Specifically, the effects of chemical and physical refining as well as the different processing steps of chemical refining on the content of γ-oryzanol were investigated. Initially, the authors compared physical and chemical refining methods regarding the concentration of γ-oryzanol in refined oil, and found that the oil derived by the physical refining process retained the original amount of γ-oryzanol (1.60% and 1.74%), while the chemically refined oil showed a considerably lower amount (0.19%). Subsequently, they studied the effect of the chemical refining steps and found that the alkali treatment removed 93.0–94.6% of the total amount from crude oil, while the degumming and dewaxing steps removed only 1.1% and 5.9% of the total amount, respectively. On the other hand, bleaching and deodorization of RBO did not affect the content of γ-oryzanol. Finally, the quantitative analysis of by-products of the chemical refining process showed that the soapstock and acid oil contained high levels of γ-oryzanol (6.3–6.9% and 3.3–7.4% respectively), indicating that they are a good source of these compounds.[11] In another study, Pestana-Bauer et al. evaluated the contents of γ-oryzanol and tocols in all the residues produced during RBO refining. Results showed that the precipitated soap had the highest γ-oryzanol concentration (14.2 mg/g, representing 95.3% of the total γ-oryzanol in crude RBO) while distillation of the residue after fatty acid recovery from soap was the best source of γ-oryzanol (43.1 mg/g, representing 11.5% of the total γ-oryzanol in crude RBO).[60] Similarly, Scavariello and Barrera-Arellano explored the influence of temperature and the molar ratio of sulfuric acid/soaps on γ-oryzanol content during the acidulation process of soapstock. They found that temperature does not significantly influence the concentration of γ-oryzanol in the acid oil, whereas the different ratios of sulfuric acid/soaps gave concentrations of γ-oryzanol varying between 3.13% and 3.74%.[61]

Optimization of the refining process in order to produce food-grade RBO rich in phytochemicals has been the subject of several studies as well. Dunford and King used SFE-CO$_2$ fractionation as an alternative process to reduce the free fatty acid (FFA) content and minimize phytosterol loss in RBO. They stated that RBO fractions with <1% FFA and 1.8% γ-oryzanol could be obtained

when particular attention was given to pressure and temperature conditions.[62] Van Hoed et al. reported an optimized physical refining method to produce RBO with an acceptable color and high γ-oryzanol content. The developed process consisted of an acid degumming, prebleaching, dewaxing, physical removal of free fatty acids using packed column technology, a modified washing step, conventional bleaching, and deodorization. The refined RBO produced had a color similar to that obtained from chemical refining, and γ-oryzanol recovery of 39%.[63] Along these lines, Sereewatthanawut and coworkers reported two-step nanofiltration processing of crude RBO to produce refined oil enriched in γ-oryzanol. The final product was acceptable for consumption (FFA <0.20 wt%) while the γ-oryzanol level was increased from 0.95% (in commercial oil) to 4.1 wt%.[64]

Due to its commercial importance, many attempts have been made to isolate and purify γ-oryzanol, mainly from rice industry by-products. There is particular interest in its recovery from RBO soapstock, as is clearly demonstrated by the approximately 40 patents that have been filed worldwide for this purpose. Published reports cited in the literature use a wide range of methods and techniques, including simple extraction, crystallization, and silica-based chromatography, as well as more advanced procedures such as countercurrent chromatography (CCC). An overview of the different methods used for the isolation and purification of γ-oryzanol, as well as the advantages and limitations of each process, is presented below.[65]

Solvent Extraction Processes

Tsuchiya and colleagues reported a process based on liquid–liquid extraction for the isolation of 60% pure γ-oryzanol from a high starting amount of RBO (100 kg). This process requires five individual steps, including two saponification reactions, hydrolysis with HCl, and two liquid–liquid extractions with ether and aqueous alkali. The low yield of γ-oryzanol and the number of steps are the main disadvantages of this process.[66] Likewise, Masao and Yoshizane reported a patent in which a two-step leaching process for isolation of γ-oryzanol from RBO is used. Initially, the soapstock is leached with methanol or ethanol and carbon dioxide is transmitted. As a result, removal of the major impurities and the soap is accomplished, leaving γ-oryzanol in the purified medium. A second leaching step is then required, and methanol or ethanol washing are used to remove weak alkali salts from the dry residue. This process led to efficient removal of impurities from the soapstock and recovery of 85% pure γ-oryzanol.[67] Takeshi reported a patented process for obtaining γ-oryzanol from soapstock which includes two main parts and a total of eight successive steps. In the first part, FFAs were esterified to methyl esters (FAMEs) and continuously removed from the soapstock by distillation, while in the second part of the procedure the residue that remained after distillation of FAMEs was leached consecutively with n-hexane, methanol, and methanolic alkali. The drawback of this process is the high number of steps involved.[68] Finally, Indira et al. have reported a simple, rapid and easy to scale process for the recovery of γ-oryzanol from the saponified and dehydrated soapstock. In this process γ-oryzanol was directly extracted from the raw material by leaching, using solvents such as ethyl acetate, acetone, or mixtures thereof. It was noted that the operating conditions, such as temperature and pH, should be controlled in order to minimize the degradation of γ-oryzanol during processing. The main disadvantages are the varying purity (33–43% w/w) and the low recovery rate (57–80% w/w) of the obtained γ-oryzanol.[69]

Crystallization Methods

Koji and Tokuo reported a two-step procedure to purify γ-oryzanol. Initially, a mixture of alcohols (methanol, propanol, or butanol) and hydrocarbons (n-hexane, cyclohexane), or toluene was used in a multistage crystallization procedure, while in a second step the obtained material was submitted to a recrystallization step using the same solvent mixture. However, the original raw material, the final purity, and the yield of γ-oryzanol were not recorded.[70] Similarly, Mingzhi and Yanyan reported a patent in which a four-step crystallization procedure for extraction of high purity γ-oryzanol (98%) from RBO is described. The second alkali-refining soapstock was used as a starting material, and a multiphase fractional crystallization procedure was carried out.[71] Along the same lines, Narayan et al. described a crystallization process for the recovery of 65% pure γ-oryzanol from a γ-oryzanol enriched fraction. The initial material was obtained by leaching of pretreated and dehydrated soapstock, and treated with mixtures of acetone and methanol in different proportions. With cooling of the eluent at room temperature mucilaginous impurities were precipitated, while further cooling to 5–10°C overnight led to γ-oryzanol crystallization.[72] Another example is the work of Zullaikah et al.; these authors achieved isolation of γ-oryzanol from RBO by a two-step crystallization process. The first crystallization step resulted in the removal of mainly triacylglycerol (TG) and steryl esters, while γ-oryzanol remained in the liquid phase along with FFA, monoacylglycerol, squalene, tocols, and phytosterols. At the second crystallization step, the liquid phase (γ-oryzanol-rich product) was kept at room temperature (20.5 ± 1.5°C) for 24h, and after addition of n-hexane as an antisolvent was further kept at 5 ± 1°C for another 48h and crystal γ-oryzanol was precipitated. This crystallization process resulted to 93–95% pure γ-oryzanol,

but with a total recovery rate of only 59%.[73] Likewise, starting with RBO soapstock, Kaewboonnum and coworkers have recently reported a method for the recovery of γ-oryzanol using a two-step crystallization procedure. The initial material was obtained from soapstock after saponification, dehydration, and extraction of residue by ethyl acetate. At the first crystallization step, a mixture of ethyl acetate/methanol was used at 30°C for 1h, while the second crystallization step was carried out at 5°C for 24h. At the end of the procedure the yield and purity of γ-oryzanol were 55.17 ± 0.59 wt% and 74.60 ± 4.12 wt%, respectively. The drawbacks of this process were the low purity and recovery of the target compounds.[5]

Silica-Based Chromatographic Methods

Several methods have been also reported for the isolation of γ-oryzanol using silica-based chromatographic methods. For instance, Tsuchiya and Okubo reported an attempt to extract γ-oryzanol from rice bran acid oil. The process included, first esterification of FFAs to methyl esters followed by distillation of the esters, and, secondly, treatment of the residue by column chromatography using a mixture of alcohol and ether as eluent. The main drawback of this process was the low yield (1.75%), while the purity of the γ-oryzanol was not mentioned.[74] Likewise, Xu and Godber have used preparative normal-phase HPLC to isolate γ-oryzanol of high purity from crude RBO and, subsequently, reverse-phase HPLC to separate individual components.[75] Lai et al. reported an efficient chromatographic method to obtain 90–98% pure γ-oryzanol from RBO using a preparative normal-phase column chromatography. As the stationary phase a silica gel packed with small particles (12 μm) was used, while the mobile phase (n-hexane and ethyl acetate) was used in a three-step gradient elution program starting from 85:15 v/v, continuing with 50:50 v/v, and completed with pure ethyl acetate. As stated by the authors, it is an easy to scale-up method in order to achieve high recovery (about 90%) of γ-oryzanol. However, the major disadvantage of this procedure was the solubility limit of RBO (about 30–35 wt/vol%), which allowed a maximum production of 10mg per injection.[76] Moreover, Stöggl et al. reported a comparative study for the utilization of C18 and C39 silica stationary phases in the detection and separation of tocopherols, carotenoids, and γ-oryzanol in a single run. According to the results, it was demonstrated that higher resolution between all target compounds was obtained using the C30 stationary phase.[77]

Countercurrent Chromatography (CCC)

Recently, Angelis and coworkers described an advanced method for the isolation of high purity γ-oryzanol from crude RBO using CCC. This process includes one-step fractionation and isolation of high purity (97%) γ-oryzanol from RBO using a non-aqueous biphasic solvent system (heptane–acetonitrile–butanol 1.8:1.4:0.7, v/v/v). Additionally, a fraction containing hydroxylated triterpene alcohol ferulates or polar γ-oryzanol was obtained. Scale-up from the analytical to preparative chromatographic column was also successfully achieved, revealing the advantage of CCC for large-scale operations compared to other isolation techniques.[17] To our knowledge, this is the only study so far concerning the use of CCC for the isolation of γ-oryzanol.

Combined Approaches

Apart from the abovementioned methods, there are several studies that incorporate different chromatographic methods for the isolation of highly pure γ-oryzanol. For instance, Yasuo et al. described a four-step procedure to recover γ-oryzanol from RBO. First, the FFAs were esterified and FAMEs were removed from RBO by molecular distillation. The remaining unsaponified fraction was subjected to liquid–liquid extraction using a mixture of n-hexane and tetrahydrofurane. The tetrahydrofurane phase, in which the unsaponified fraction was partitioned, was concentrated and an amount of water was added. The γ-oryzanol was precipitated and recovered in the aqueous phase. Finally, crystallization with n-hexane resulted in highly pure γ-oryzanol (98.3%). However this process has the disadvantage of low recovery of γ-oryzanol.[78] Similarly, Masao and Yoshizane used RBO as the raw material for the extraction of γ-oryzanol via a procedure containing two leaching steps and two liquid–liquid extraction steps. For the leaching, solvents such as trichloroethylene, benzene, n-hexane, or a mixture of benzene and n-hexane and gas CO_2 were used, resulting in the elimination of impurities (mainly soap) from the soapstock. Regarding the liquid–liquid extraction phase, the residual mixture obtained after a second leaching step took place using the same solvent mixture. This process led to the recovery of γ-oryzanol with purity of up to 90% (w/w). The use of chlorinated or aromatic solvents could be considered the major negative aspect of this method.[67]

Seetharamiah and Prabhakar reported a process that includes liquid–liquid extraction, column chromatography, and crystallization techniques for the isolation of γ-oryzanol from RBO. In the leaching step a mixture of diethyl ether and methanol was used, and the ether-rich phase was extracted repeatedly with aqueous alkali. The alkaline γ-oryzanol extracts were neutralized with acetic acid, and γ-oryzanol was extracted with diethyl ether. Subsequently, the γ-oryzanol rich fraction was subjected to column chromatography on alumina as stationary phase, and n-hexane, petroleum ether/methanol (9:1 vol/vol) and diethyl ether/methanol (20:1 vol/vol) were used for elution. As a result, a recovery rate of 75.7% (w/w) γ-oryzanol with a purity of 51.4% (w/w) was achieved. Finally, this fraction was subjected to a two-step crystallization process in order to improve the purity of γ-oryzanol. The weakness of this method is the number of repeated liquid–liquid extraction steps and the column chromatography, which hinders its use for large-scale purposes.[79]

Saska and Rossiter described a two-step procedure for the isolation of γ-oryzanol from degummed and dewaxed RBO. Primarily, the use of a simulated moving bed chromatography separator resulted in enhancement of γ-oryzanol, from 1.2–1.6% to 12–15%. Subsequently, crystallization of the crude product with heptanes led to 90–95% pure γ-oryzanol, with a recovery rate of 85–90%. The drawbacks of this method are the high investment cost and complexity related to the use of simulated moving bed chromatography separators.[80] Similarly, Das et al described a two-step method for the isolation of γ-oryzanol from RBO. At the first step, the initial material was subjected to vacuum distillation for FFA elimination. Afterwards, aqueous alkaline hydrolysis of the residue was carried out and anionic micellar aggregates containing solubilized γ-oryzanol were formed. The addition of calcium ions to this aqueous micellar aggregate induced instant coprecipitation of the calcium salts of the fatty acids and the aggregate-associated γ-oryzanol. The dried precipitate was then extracted with ethyl acetate and evaporated. At a second step, γ-oryzanol rich residue was purified by silica gel column chromatography.[81]

An interesting approach was presented by Rao et al., who compared four techniques in a six-step procedure in order to isolate γ-oryzanol from RBO. The process included saponification of the neutral oil present in the soapstock, leaching of residue, crystallization, and column chromatography and recrystallization of the γ-oryzanol fraction. The overall outcome was the attainment of 90% (w/w) pure γ-oryzanol, with a recovery rate of 56–70% (w/w). The limitation of this process is the number of steps required, as well as the use of column chromatography, which makes the scaling-up very complex.[82] Moreover, Kasim et al. described the isolation of γ-oryzanol from residue obtained during the production of biodiesel from RBO using a series of steps in a three-phase procedure. Initially, the residue obtained during the production of biodiesel from RBO was subjected to a degumming and dewaxing procedure, acid-catalyzed esterification, and vacuum distillation. The derived residue was then extracted, leading to an increase in γ-oryzanol content from 16% to 47%, with a recovery rate of 97%. Finally, silica gel column chromatography was used for the purification of γ-oryzanol to 83.79%, with a recovery rate of 81.75%, while the overall recovery was estimated to be approximately 69.82%.[83]

An innovative and easy method for the rapid separation of γ-oryzanol in non-aqueous systems was recently proposed by Kaewchada *et al.* The process includes synthesis of molecularly imprinted polymers (MIPs) with selectivity for γ-oryzanol. Polymeric materials were synthesized via a thermal polymerization method, using γ-oryzanol as a template, anacardic acid (AnAc) as a functional monomer, toluene as a porogen, benzoyl peroxide (BPO) as the initiator, and divinylbenzene as the cross-linker. Different parameters that affect the absorption capacity of MIPs have been described. However, further investigations are required in order for this method to find wider application in the separation of γ-oryzanol.[84]

γ-ORYZANOL ANALYSIS AND CHARACTERIZATION – IDENTIFICATION OF DIFFERENT COMPONENTS

The particular chemical nature of γ-oryzanol, consisting of numerous components together with their high quantitative alternations and close structures, complicates considerably its characterization and identification. Moreover, the lipophilicity of γ-oryzanol, which could be considered as a relative polar entity in a highly lipophilic environment such as RBO, allows the utilization of several techniques but at the same time complicates the selection of suitable analytical methods. The presence of several substrates, such as crude oil and RBO fractions, etc., as well as the complicated isolation procedure required for the delivery of high purity γ-oryzanol further hinders its analysis; this is of major importance due to the increasing interest in γ-oryzanol and its multiple applications. Therefore, since its initial identification[6] several analytical methods have been proposed for the determination of different γ-oryzanol constituents and for their quantitation in different materials. It is also noticeable that new components are constantly being suggested.[13,17,85,86] The first published reports regarding γ-oryzanol were focused mainly on the separation and characterization of γ-oryzanol components, incorporating several chromatographic methods such as thin layer chromatography (TLC), liquid chromatography (LC), gas chromatography (GC), GC-mass spectrometry (MS), and high performance liquid chromatography (HPLC) – mainly reversed phase (RP).[8,9,87] Regarding identification, much information was first derived from research studies carried out on steryl and triterpene alcohol ferulates isolated from other sources. CG and GC-MS were used as methods of choice for the identification thereof, usually after derivatization.[88,89] Later on, most studies were related to the detection of γ-oryzanol in multiple rice-related

materials and in particular in RBO, and its separation from other components such as lipids, tocopherols, and tocotrienols, while a number of methods were suggested for γ-oryzanol quantitation.

One of the first complete methods for the separation, identification, and quantitation of γ-oryzanol was proposed by Rogers *et al.* in 1993. Specifically, a reversed phase (RP) high-performance liquid chromatography (HPLC) device connected to a photodiode array detector (PDA) was utilized. The mobile phase consisted of acetonitrile/methanol/isopropanol/water (45:45:5:5 by volume) and was linearly modified to acetonitrile/methanol/isopropanol/water (50:45:5 by volume) for 4 minutes, after the first 6 minutes, and was kept constant for 15 minutes before a return to the initial conditions. The selected wavelength for monitoring γ-oryzanol was 325 nm. Moreover, chemical ionization (CI) MS was incorporated for the elucidation of the structure of γ-oryzanol components. Cycloartenyl ferulate, 24-methylene cycloartanyl ferulate, campesteryl ferulate, β-sitosteryl ferulate, and cycloartanyl ferulate were first proposed as the major constituents.[90] Additionally, the developed methods were applied to several fully processed edible RBOs from different manufacturers. After approximately a year, and due to the lipophilic nature of RBO, a new method was suggested for the same purposes using normal phase (NP)-HPLC.[91] Five commercial silica-based columns were assayed and several chromatographic parameters, such as mobile phase, temperature, and flow rate, were optimized. For the same reason, a method using HPLC connected to evaporative light-scattering detector (ELSD) has been proposed.[92] In parallel, some reports regarding the qualitative and quantitative characterization of γ-oryzanol in biological fluids appeared more than three decades ago, following the first evidence regarding its biological properties, and were related to its metabolism and absorption in animals[93,94] as well as the determination of ferulic acid, a main metabolite of γ-oryzanol.[95,96] Of high importance is the work of Norton, who investigated the separation, isolation, and identification of steryl and triterpene alcohol ferulates, cinnamates, and coumarates in corn bran and rice bran, published in 1994 and 1995. An optimized RP-HPLC-PDA method was proposed for their separation and quantification, and a GC-MS method was developed, after derivatization, for the identification of γ-oryzanol components.[97,98] A very significant contribution was that of Xu and Godber, mainly to the separation of high purity γ-oryzanol from RBO and the identification of additional minor constituents. Using a combination of NP and RP-HPLC, the isolation of several compounds of satisfactory purity was achieved, while GC-MS using the electron impact (EI) ionization method was utilized for the identification thereof. More than 10 different steryl ferulates were suggested: Δ7-stigmastenyl ferulate, stigmasteryl ferulate, cycloartenyl ferulate, 24-methylenecycloartanyl ferulate, Δ^7-campestenyl ferulate, campesteryl ferulate, Δ^7-sitostenyl ferulate, sitosteryl ferulate, compestanyl ferulate, and sitostanyl ferulate. Three (cycloartenyl ferulate, 24-methylenecycloartanyl ferulate, and campesteryl ferulate) were found to be the major components of γ-oryzanol, verifying previous reports. Moreover, useful structural information was derived for the identification of steryl ferulates after TMS (trimethylsilylane) derivatization based on their fragmentation patter, via GC-EI-MS analysis.[75] It is noteworthy that the work of Xu and Godber was integrated to a significant degree by Akihisa *et al.* in 2000.[22] Six novel steryl ferulates, two *trans-* and four *cis-*ferulates, together with five known *trans-*ferulates and one known *cis-*ferulate, respectively, were isolated using preparative TLC, NP-HPLC, and RP-HPLC. The preparation of synthetic derivatives and the corresponding free forms have assisted considerably in the identification procedure and the evaluation of their anti-inflammation properties, and resulted in valuable NMR data. It is important to note that this work unambiguously confirmed the presence of *cis-*derivatives in RBO, which could comprise artifacts of the refining procedure.[99,100]

Generally, using ^{1}H NMR analysis, the identification of steryl ferulates among other chemical classes can be performed easily if the purity level is satisfactory. Based on the structural characteristics of the core skeleton, the signals could be divided in two groups: one corresponding to the aromatic part of the molecule (ferulate), and the other corresponding to the triterpenoid part (sterol and/or tritepene alcohol).[101] The protons of the two parts of the molecule are resonated in different chemical shift areas. In particular, the aromatic ones are resonated in low fields (approximately 6.5–7.5 ppm) and the aliphatic ones in high fields (~0.5–2.5 ppm). The signals of the double bonds of the aliphatic part, which are resonated in the area between (~4.5–5.5 ppm), are very characteristic and could be utilized as indicative in the identification process. Also, rather characteristic are the signals of the double bond of the ferulate moiety.[102] The signals of these two protons of the double bond are resonated in low fields, separately, as two double peaks. In particular, the proton closer to the aromatic ring appears very deshielded (~7.6 ppm) while the other one is resonated in higher fields (@6.3 ppm), in respect to the deuterated solvent used. However, most indicative is the coupling constant value (J) of these peaks, which could be used for the identification of *trans-* and *cis-*ferulates since they are at approximately 15–16 Hz and 12–13 Hz, respectively. Finally, quite indicative are the signals of the methyl groups, which could be used for the determination of subgroups and further structural details.[22,89,103]

Furthermore ^{13}C NMR data could be rather useful for the structure elucidation of steryl ferulates. Based on the degree of substitution (mainly methyl groups), the number of rings (4- or 5-rings derivatives) and the length of the side chain (usually C_5 or C_6), the total number of carbon signals detected are 40, in average (37 to 41 for the identified RBO steryl ferulates so far). Similarly to the ^{1}H NMR spectra, the signals could be split in two main groups. The first set of signals (approx. 30) is resonated in high fields (10 to 60 ppm, approx.) corresponding to the triterpenoid part of the basic structure while the rest, approximately 10 signals are appeared rather deshielted (100 to 170 ppm, approx.) and correspond to the ferulic moiety. Specifically, characteristic are the signals of the carbonyl group (~ 165–170 ppm), the oxygenated methane carbon (~ 80 ppm) as well as the methyl group of the ferulate resonated at around 55 ppm. Nevertheless, for detailed structure information, 2D NMR analysis is required.[102–104]

The available structural information was enriched by the contribution of Fang *et al.*, who gave new insight in MS-based identification of steryl ferulates. The use of an Ion Trap (IT) analyzer equipped with an electrospray ionization probe (ESI), hyphenated to a HPLC enabled the determination of several MS/MS fragments and revealed fragmentation partners of steryl ferulates.[13] Both ionization modes, negative and positive, were used with the last being more effective. Most of the data regarding useful fragments of steryl ferulates were in accordance with previous studies using conventional GC-EI-MS platforms. However, the major advantage of this approach is that no treatment of the sample e.g. RBO (saponification) and/or derivatization (sililation, acetylation) is required prior analysis. Furthermore, hydroxylated derivatives of steryl ferulates were suggested for the first time and were further analyzed afterwards from the same group.[13,105] The same year, an interesting approach was proposed from Miller *et al.* for the rapid analysis and comparative studies of γ-oryzanol, in different rice varieties using coupled liquid-gas chromatography (LC-GC).[106] Pre-separated fractions using HPLC, of γ-oryzanol were transferred on line to GC analysis while the identity of the detected compounds was also confirmed by off-line GC-MS.

The following years, several analytical methodologies focusing mostly to the simultaneous characterization of different chemical classes of secondary metabolites occurring in RBO were suggested. Different analytical parameters, alternative platforms and/or materials were incorporated for this reason.[28,107,108] For instance, Stoggl *et al.* reported an approach for the concurrent analysis of β-carotene, tocopherols, and γ-oryzanol, using RP-HPLC-PDA, in a single run of 20 min, using methanol/tert-butyl methyl ether (75:25 v/v) as a mobile phase. A study comparing HPLC C18 and C30 columns, was also carried out and the last found more efficacious. Additionally, an IT analyzer equipped with an atmospheric pressure chemical ionization (APCI) probe was used for the verification of steryl ferulates identity while both direct infusion and LC-MS methodologies were employed.[77] Another example is the RP-HPLC-PDA method proposed by Huang and Ng, in 2011 aiming to the simultaneous determination of tocopherols, tocotrienols and γ-oryzanol in rice; however, focusing mainly on the first two classes.[109] The last 3 years limited additional methods have been proposed giving new alternatives at γ-oryzanol analysis and characterization. Zaima *et al.*, in 2010 presented a matrix-assisted laser desorption/ionization (MALDI)-imaging mass spectrometry (IMS) method for analyzing rice grains and the distribution of different metabolites. According to this study, γ-oryzanol is localized in the bran (germ and seed coat) together with phoshatidylcholine and phytic acid while α-tocopherol is mainly present in the germ, especially in the scutellum.[110]

Furthermore, in 2011 a new LC-MS method was suggested by Angelis *et al.*, employing a high resolution (HR) MS analyzer and, specifically, the relatively newly invented Orbitrap analyzer (Orbital trap), equipped with an APCI probe, in both modes. To our knowledge, this was the first time that a HRMS platform was utilized for the analysis of steryl ferulates, verifying previous findings but also revealing new structural data for the identification of γ-oryzanol. Additionally, a new class of γ-oryzanol, the so-called polar γ-oryzanol, was determined, eluting similarly to γ-oryzanol as a set of compounds and presenting higher hydrophilicity. According to the authors, the utilization of APCI methods in both modes assisted the detection of possible impurities and, specifically, the presence of glycerol esters, which are highly abundant in RBO and usually co-eluted with γ-oryzanol components.[17]

In general, considering the elucidation of the structure of steryl ferulates using MS, most of the information available has been derived by GC-MS methodologies using traditional derivatization techniques such as acetylation or silylation of γ-oryzanol or its basic components after isolation. Interpretation of the spectra usually follows primarily the identification of diagnostic peaks of the ferulic moiety (with or without the derivatization unit, e.g., Ac, TMS) and afterwards identification of the triterpenoid part based on the corresponding fragmentation pattern.[88] In particular, under EI conditions, characteristic ions at m/z 177 and 193 (underivatized forms) are observed as indicative for the ferulic moiety, which could also be used for the differentiation of steryl and stanyl ferulates. Also, in most cases the fragment ions which correspond to the triterpenoid part of the molecule are present after cleavage of the ferulic acid. Similar observations have been made by Das *et al.*, using the LSIMS method, in positive mode, while they also noticed the presence of pseudomolecular ions corresponding

to adducts with sodium.[81] Moreover, the detection of $[M-C_{10}H_{10}O_4+H]^+$ ions and their utilization as being indicative for the identification of steryl ferulates was also confirmed from Stoggle *et al.*, using LC-APCI-MS methods without prior derivatization.[77]

On the other hand, when using atmospheric pressure ionization (API) methods such as ESI or APCI, the fragmentation is less extensive compared to hard ionization techniques such as EI or chemical ionization (CI), and specifically in the negative mode pure spectra are delivered most of the time. More detailed information could be derived by the use of LC-MS-MS methods in both modes. In the negative mode, the ions are characteristic; these are formed after the elimination of one and/or two methyl groups from the ferulic and the triterpenoid part, respectively, while the [feruloyl]⁻ fragment ion is also evident. In contrast, no fragment ions corresponding to the triterpenoid part of the molecules were detected, implying that the negative mode is less pronounced for the identification of steryl ferulates. In the positive mode, basic ions are the intact alcohol moiety (triterpene alcohols or sterols), which are derived from the cleavage of feruloyl and alcohol moieties. Also indicative are the ions yielded by the loss of different numbers of methyl and methylene groups.

These data, as well as other MS information regarding more in-depth characterizations of steryl ferulates, have been discussed by Fang *et al.*[13] In particular, the author reported that *cis*-isomers have longer retention times than the corresponding *trans*-isomers using C18 RP-HPLC (e.g., campesterol *cis*-ferulate vs campesterol *trans*-ferulate). Also highlighted was the presence of hydroxylated steryl ferulates based on the highly intense $[M+H-194-H_2O]^+$ ions. Moreover, they reported for the first time the presence of caffeate esters of STAFs in RBO based on the presence of fragment ions at m/z 179 in negative CID spectra and $[M+H-180]^+$ ions for intact alcohol moieties (triterpene alcohols or sterols) in positive mass spectra together with the absence of $[M-H-Me]^-$ ions.

Along the same lines, the utilization of HR-MS platforms for the identification of steryl ferulates could be considered of high importance. Accurate mass measurements, high resolution spectra, and additional spectrometric features provide high confidence in the identification procedure.[111] Until now, there is only one publication, by Angelis *et al.*, that reports the characterization of steryl ferulates in RBO using the LC-HR-MS platform, equipped with an APCI probe, in both modes. Utilization of the extraction ion method (XIC chromatograms) has revealed the presence of both *cis*- and *trans*-isomers and therefore facilitated significantly the characterization of γ-oryzanol. Moreover, the use of a suggested elemental composition (EC) for every ion of interest measured accurately ($\Delta m \leq 2-3$ ppm) together with ring double bond equivalent (RDBeq) values has led to identification of steryl ferulates with high confidence.[17] Furthermore, additional possible derivatives were suggested by the authors, while the ion [M+H–H₂O]⁺, present in full scan spectra, was proposed as indicative for the identification of polar γ-oryzanol.

Apart from the traditional and most commonly utilized analytical methods, a few others have been incorporated for the analysis, quantification, and characterization of γ-oryzanol for various purposes. For instance, Deepam and coworkers reported the development of a high-performance thin layer chromatography (HPTLC) method for the constituents of RBO[112], while Kumar et al. proposed a thin-layer chromatographic (TLC) method for the detection of RBO in other vegetable oils monitoring γ-oryzanol components.[113] Furthermore, alternative, non-chromatography-based techniques have also been proposed for the determination of γ-oryzanol in RBO. For instance, spectrophotometric methods such as fixed wavelength, and second-derivative and multicomponent analysis, have been reported for the quantitation of γ-oryzanol.[114]

After reviewing the previous and current trends in the analysis and characterization of γ-oryzanol, it will be useful to cite and briefly discuss the most common applications where these methods are utilized. Thus, the methodologies mentioned have been used in the evaluation of the extraction and isolation procedure of γ-oryzanol or its components from different materials, such as RBO and soapstock, since the efficient and fast procumbent thereof remains an important challenge, mainly for industry.[5,56,59,101,115–117] Known or slightly modified methods have also been incorporated for quality assessment of the RBO production procedure and the corresponding derived materials, as well as for the appraisal of oils from different sources and for adulteration issues.[118,119] In particular, different parameters, mainly regarding the refining process, related to the content of γ-oryzanol still comprise an important research topic.[11,60,63,120-126] Numerous studies dealing with the stability of γ-oryzanol, mainly during storage or cooking,[127–129] have been performed, for the identification of optimal or alternative sources[130] and the isolation of γ-oryzanol, as well as comparative studies between different rice varieties,[39,40,42,43,131–136] commercial rice varieties,[41,137] and conventional and organic rice[102] mutant species.[138–140] An interesting research topic would include localization of γ-oryzanol in the different parts of rough rice seed,[47,141] its content in paddy and brown rice,[50,142] and its quantitative differentiation during maturation and development.[44,46,49,52,143–145] Finally, the existing methods have also been incorporated to detect and or quantify γ-oryzanol in biological samples in order to further investigate its biological properties and role; for instance, the work by Lubinus et al. is related to the fate of steryl ferulates upon consumption by healthy humans.[146] However, such studies are rather limited and further investigation is required.

PHARMACOLOGICAL ACTIVITIES AND APPLICATIONS OF γ-ORYZANOL

Since the discovery of γ-oryzanol in the 1950s, numerous studies have been performed exploring the pharmacological potentials of γ-oryzanol.[4,26,147] Widely used in Asia as a therapeutical agent to treat clinical disorders involved with the menopause,[148] stimulation of the sebaceous glands,[149] or ulcers,[150] γ-oryzanol has attracted much interest throughout the world. According to Cicero and Gaddi,[151] early studies on the biological profile of γ-oryzanol started with the work by Nakamura[152] in the 1960s regarding the influence of γ-oryzanol on hepatic cholesterol biosynthesis. Since then, according to the PubMed database, more than 180 research articles have been published, presenting a wide spectrum of biological activities. In addition, several reports investigating the biological properties of γ-oryzanol rich extracts and commercial or purified γ-oryzanol, using various in vitro or in vivo models, have also been presented.

The larger proportion of these biological studies concerns the antioxidant activity of this γ-oryzanol, due to the presence of the phenol moiety in its composition. By definition, reactive oxygen species (ROS) are free radicals which, when they are overproduced in the organism, may cause oxidative stress by oxidation of biological macromolecules such as proteins, nucleic acids, and cell membranes. This oxidative damage is the origin of many chronic diseases, and cell aging. Thus, over recent decades the research into new antioxidants has been considerably increased.

In this context, due to the presence of the ferulic/caffeic acid part, which enables donation of electrons and destroys the action of free radicals, γ-oryzanol has been widely studied for its antioxidant properties.[153–155] For example, Kim's work shows that γ-oryzanol inhibits pyrogallol autoxidation and is more effective than the well-known synthetic antioxidants (BHA, BHT, and TBHQ) against hydroperoxide formation.[156] Moreover, Hiramitsu et al. have suggested that γ-oryzanol inhibits lipid peroxidation induced from porcine retinal homogenates using ferric ion or UV light,[157] and thus could be employed in retinotoxic evaluation of ophthalmic drugs. On the other hand, Xu and Godber were more interested in the antioxidant properties of the individual three major compounds of γ-oryzanol (cycloartenyl ferulate, 24-methylenecycloartanyl, and campesteryl ferulate), using a linoleic acid-based peroxidation model. Their results indicated that these components are able to significantly reduce the production of hydroperoxides.[158]

The antioxidant activities of γ-oryzanol against cholesterol oxidation have also been investigated.[159] Cholesterol oxidation products (COPs) lead to the formation of several toxic atherogenic, mutagenic, and carcinogenic compounds,[160] which cause cell membrane damage and are responsible for many pulmonary and cardiovascular diseases.[161,162] It has been shown that γ-oryzanol is capable of reducing the production of COP considerably, with higher activity than that of vitamin E.[163] It is noteworthy that a significant correlation between oxidative stress and various diseases, such as malignancies, diabetes, atherosclerosis, chronic inflammation, human immunodeficiency virus (HIV) infection, ischemia reperfusion injury, and sleep apnea has been highlighted.[164] Overall, given this background, much interest has focused on investigation of the therapeutic properties of γ-oryzanol against several health complications and diseases, using numerous models and assays.

Anti-Ulcer Effect

In the 1970s–1980s, the anti-ulcerogenic properties of γ-oryzanol were extensively investigated in Japan, using rat models. Nevertheless, further studies are needed to identify its inhibitory effect and establish its real clinical efficacy.[165–168]

Anti-Inflammatory Effect

Recently, many researchers have investigated the capacity of γ-oryzanol to treat inflammation. γ-Oryzanol has been found to inhibit the increase in swelling of the hind paw in adjuvant-induced arthritis in rats in a dose-dependent manner (1–100 mg/kg),[169] and to possess a strong anti-inflammatory effect on sodium dextran sulfate-induced colitis[170] and ethanol-induced liver damage[171] in mice, via inhibition of NF-κB activity.

Anti-Allergic Effect

Oka and colleagues have demonstrated, for the first time, a possible anti-allergenic effect of γ-oryzanol using a fraction extracted from domestic Japanese rice, according to the Bligh and Dyer method. Using the passive cutaneous anaphylaxis (PCA) reaction model on rats, the authors observed a significant anti-allergic effect determined by the inhibition of mast cell degranulation.[172] Moreover, using the same methodology they also assayed the effect of major components of the fraction, such as cycloartenyl ferulate (28.2%), 24-methylene cycloartanyl ferulate (22.4%), β-sitosteryl ferulate (12.3%), and cyclobranyl ferulate (<10%), and similar inhibition of mast cell degranulation with a greater potential for cyclobranyl ferulate was assisted. Finally, they investigated the possible mechanism of action proposing that γ-oryzanol is able to capture immunoglobulin E (IgE), preventing its cross-linking to the high-affinity IgE receptor (FcεRI), involved in the allergic disorder.

Antidiabetic Effect

Several experiments have been conducted in order to analyze the potential of γ-oryzanol as a therapeutic agent against diabetes mellitus. In different trials, mainly carried out on diabetic rats, γ-oryzanol was found to possess an antidiabetic effect, improving insulin sensitivity and reducing the blood glucose level.[173–175]

Anticancer Properties

γ-Oryzanol and its components have been evaluated for their anticancer properties. Yasukawa et al. reported an inhibitory effect of the four major components of oryzanol (cycloartenyl ferulate, 24-methylene cycloartanyl ferulate, campesteryl ferulate and sitosteryl ferulate) on tumor promotion in two-staged carcinogenesis in mouse skin.[176] Furthermore, the recent work by Kim has shown that γ-oryzanol significantly reduced the tumor mass in mice inoculated with CT-26 colon cancer. Oral administration of 1% γ-oryzanol resulted in a dose-dependent reduction of the tumor growth by 44% without affecting the weight of other organs.[177] In addition, some studies have been performed in order to explore safety regarding the carcinogenic properties of γ-oryzanol, using F344 rat and B6C3F$_1$ mouse lung carcinogenesis models.[178,179] A tumor progression effect was observed with γ-oryzanol, but it was weak and occurred only with high doses.[180,181]

Antihyperlipidemic Effect

Owing to the structural analogy of γ-oryzanol compounds with cholesterol, another important research area concerns its ability to lower cholesterol levels. The first scientific study on this topic was carried out in humans in 1970. Specifically, Suzuki and Oshima[182] observed a decrease of total cholesterol (TC), within 7 days, in the plasma of 50 healthy young women who consumed 60 g of a combination of 70% RBO and 30% safflower oil. Later, in 1982, Ishihara et al.[148,183] focused particularly on γ-oryzanol, showing that after four to eight treatments of 300 mg of this component per day in hyperlipoproteinemic subjects, there was a decrease in total cholesterol (TC), low density lipoprotein cholesterol (LDL-C), and triglyceride (TG) plasma levels, together with an increase in high density lipoprotein cholesterol (HDL-C) concentration, with no side effects. Similar results have been published since in humans,[184–189] rats,[190–193] rabbits,[194] and hamsters.[195–197] This information is well reviewed by Cicero and Gaddi,[151] with particular attention to the treatment of hyperlipoproteinemias, indicating that γ-oryzanol could be utilized as a therapeutic agent for hyperlipidemia and atherosclerosis.[198,199]

Effect on Menopausal Disorders

In Japan, two studies have investigated the effect of γ-oryzanol on menopausal disorders. In the first, in the 1960s, 100 mg of γ-oryzanol was administered to 13 women who had undergone hysterectomy ("surgical menopause") three times a day for 38 days. According to the findings, 67% of the women reported a significant reduction in menopausal symptoms such as hot flushes.[200] In 1982, in another study, 40 women with climacteric disturbances were administered 300 mg of γ-oryzanol, daily for 4–8 weeks. In 90% of the cases a general improvement concerning reduction of menopausal disorders was observed.[148] Since then, studies have been conducted investigating the effect on γ-oryzanol on menopausal disorders compared with other approaches such as acupuncture.[201-204] Even if acupuncture presents a better outcome, Tian indicated that a combined use of acupuncture and Chinese medicine is more effective for treating the menopausal syndrome.[205]

APPLICATIONS

As discussed previously, γ-oryzanol exhibits a wide range of biological activities as a natural antioxidant product. Thereby, it has found numerous applications as a sunscreen and as an anti-aging agent in the cosmetics industry, as well as being a natural additive to improve food stability and a pharmaceutical raw material. For example, due to its antioxidant properties, γ-oryzanol is widely employed and patented as a sunscreen agent in cosmetic formulations. A non-chemical sunscreen composition including γ-oryzanol together with proanthocyanidins, ferulic acid, titanium oxide, and *Scutellaria* extract has been patented.[206] Recently, γ-oryzanol has also been incorporated in an aqueous cosmetic composition intended for the photoprotection of skin and hair against UV radiation.[207] Furthermore, Manosroi has investigated the anti-aging effect of creams and gels containing rice bran bioactive compounds including γ-oryzanol on human skin.[208] Promising results regarding the amelioration of thickness, roughness, and elasticity of the skin have indicated the potential of γ-oryzanol for protection against skin aging. Apart from its application as a skin protecting agent, γ-oryzanol has also been introduced as antioxidant in preparations for eyebrows and eyelashes, in skin cream, shampoo, and lip balm, and in nail color products and products for the surrounding skin.[12,209]

Additionally, due to γ-oryzanol's ability to significantly reduce production of toxic cholesterol oxidation products (COPs) it has been used as a food additive. During the cooking process or storage of foods, formation of COPs occurs with the action of air, light, or heat. In this context, it has been reported that the addition of γ-oryzanol delayed the formation of COP in refrigerated cooked beef[210] and improved the oxidative stability of vegetable oils at frying temperatures.[154,211] Additionally, Khuwijtjaru's works have revealed a possible degradation of γ-oryzanol in stripped rice bran oil during thermal

oxidation.[212] Accordingly, the effect of γ-oryzanol microencapsulation, aiming to achieve stability against heat-induced lipid oxidation, has been studied.[213,214] In exploring the antilipoperoxidation efficacy of γ-oryzanol when incorporated into nanosponges, it was found that γ-oryzanol retains a significant antilipoperoxidative activity even when it is encapsulated. Consequently, encapsulation could be used to protect γ-oryzanol from photochemical degradation and thus the loss of its antioxidant effect.[10] This high resistance to heat resulted in the approval and classification of γ-oryzanol in Japan as an "oxidation inhibitor" in the Food Additive List, and therefore several food stabilization techniques using γ-oryzanol have been patented.

Another activity that is attributed to γ-oryzanol concerns its metabolic effect on the body. Throughout the world γ-oryzanol is commonly used by athletes and bodybuilders as a sports supplement, with many papers and websites reporting muscle bulk growth in athletes by the increase in testosterone production and stimulation of human growth hormone release. However, as pointed out by several authors,[215] there is no solid valid scientific evidence for these effects, and the performance claims that are advertised are only supported by the conviction from athletes that γ-oryzanol is an excellent ergogen. Faced with this lack of data, two studies have focused on the possible ergogenic effects of γ-oryzanol, but neither has supported this assertion. According to Wheeler,[216] γ-oryzanol is poorly absorbed and its intravenous or subcutaneous injection in rats was found to reduce hormone synthesis and release, while an increase in the release of catecholamines, dopamines and norepinephrine in the brain was also observed, leading to the conclusion that this metabolic milieu may actually reduce testosterone production. Fry studied the improvement in muscular power or strength of weight-trained males who consumed 500 mg/day of γ-oryzanol, after 9 weeks of an endurance exercise program.[217] No significant differences between the supplemented and the control placebo groups were observed for measures of circulating concentrations of hormones, minerals, binding protein, or blood lipids, suggesting that more research is needed regarding this possible anabolic effect.

CONCLUSION

Unquestionably, γ-oryzanol is a natural entity of high scientific interest and industrial value. The significant health-beneficial effects of γ-oryzanol, as well as its pleotropic nature, have resulted in numerous applications in nutrition, medicine, and cosmetics. Nowadays, two main research topics related to γ-oryzanol concentrate the interest of the scientists. The first concerns characterization of γ-oryzanol's components, and biological evaluation of the activity of both γ-oryzanol and its components while the second focuses mainly on the efficient extraction, isolation, and exploitation of its commercial potentials. Several new techniques and methodologies have contributed considerably to both research axes in the recent years. Sophisticated analytical concepts have been incorporated for the detection and elucidation of γ-oryzanol's constituents and their isolation, as well as its fast, simple, and reproducible production. However, more effort should be invested in the unambiguous and complete characterization of γ-oryzanol, while purity issues still remain relatively unresolved. Furthermore, attention should be concentrated on the assessment of γ-oryzanol's pharmacological properties and exploration of its biological role.

References

1. United States Department of Agriculture. Grain. *World Markets and Trade*. Available at: http://www.fas.usda.gov/grain/circu lar/2010/05-10/grainfull05-10.pdf 2010.

2. *Food and Agriculture Organization of the United Nations (FAOSTAT)*. Available at: http://faostat.fao.org/ 2007.

3. Bergman CJ, Xu Z. Genotype and environment effects on tocopherol, tocotrienol, and γ-oryzanol contents of Southern US rice. *Cereal Chem* 2003;**80**(4):446–9.

4. Patel M, Naik SN. γ-oryzanol from rice bran oil – a review. *J Sci Ind Res* 2004;**63**:569–78.

5. Kaewboonnum P, Vechpanich J, Santiwattana P, Shotipruk A. γ-Oryzanol recovery from rice bran oil soapstock. *Sep Sci Technol* 2010;**45**(9):1186–95.

6. Kaneko R, Tsuchiya T. New compound from rice bran oil. *J Soc Chem Ind Japan* 1954;**57**:526–9.

7. Shimizu M, Ohta G, Kitahara S, Tsunoo G, Sasahara S. Studies on the constituents of rice bran oil. I. Isolation of phenolic substances. *Pharm Bull* 1957;**5**:36–9.

8. Ohta G, Shimizu M. Studies on the constituents of rice bran oil. II. Structure of oryzanol A. *Pharm Bull* 1957;**5**:40–3.

9. Shimizu M, Ohta G. A New Triterpenoid Alcohol, 24-methylene cycloartanol as its Ferulate from Rice Bran Oil. *Pharm Bull* 1958;**6**:325–6.

10. Lerma-Garcia MJ, Herrero-Martinez JM, Simo-Alfonso EF, Mendonca CRB, Ramis-Ramos G. Composition, industrial processing and applications of rice bran γ-oryzanol. *Food Chem* 2009;**115**(2):389–404.

11. Gopala Krishna AG, Khatoon S, Shiela PM, Sarmandal CV, Indira TN, Mishra A. Effect of refining of crude rice bran oil on the retention of oryzanol in the refined oil. *J Am Oil Chem Soc* 2001;**78**(2):127–31.

12. Mandak E, Nyström L. Steryl ferulates, bioactive compounds in cereal grains. *Lipid Technol* 2012;**24**(4):80–2.

13. Fang N, Yu S, Badger TM. Characterization of Triterpene Alcohol and Sterol Ferulates in Rice Bran Using LC-MS/MS. *J Agric Food Chem* 2003;**51**(11):3260–7.

14. Croteau R, Kutchan TM, Lewis NG. Natural products (Secondary metabolites). In: Buchanan B, Gruissem W, Jones R, editors. *Biochemistry & Molecular Biology of Plants*. Hoboken, NJ: John Wiley & Sons; 2002. p. 1250–318.

15. Wu TK, Griffin JH. Conversion of a plant oxidosqualene-cycloartenol synthase to an oxidosqualene-lanosterol cyclase by random mutagenesis. *Biochemistry* 2002;**41**(26):8238–44.

16. Harrabi S. Sterols. *Handbook of Analysis of Active Compounds in Functional Foods*. Boca Raton, FL: CRC press; p. 787–804.

17. Angelis A, Urbain A, Halabalaki M, Aligiannis N, Skaltsounis AL. One-step isolation of γ-oryzanol from rice bran oil by nonaqueous hydrostatic countercurrent chromatography. *J Sep Sci* 2011;**34**(18):2528–37.

18. Rosazza JPN, Huang Z, Dostal L, Volm T, Rousseau B. Review: Biocatalytic transformations of ferulic acid: An abundant aromatic natural product. *J Ind Microbiol Biotechnol* 1995;**15**(6):457–71.

19. Negishi O, Sugiura K, Negishi Y. Biosynthesis of vanillin via ferulic acid in Vanilla planifolia. *J Agric Food Chem* 2009;**57**(21):9956–61.

20. Graf E. Antioxidant potential of ferulic acid. *Free Radical Biol Med* 1992;**13**(4):435–48.

21. Srinivasan M, Sudheer AR, Menon VP. Ferulic acid: Therapeutic potential through its antioxidant property. *J Clin Biochem Nutr* 2007;**40**(2):92–100.

22. Akihisa T, Yasukawa K, Yamaura M, et al. Triterpene alcohol and sterol ferulates from rice bran and their anti-inflammatory effects. *J Agric Food Chem* 2000;**48**(6):2313–9.

23. Sato A, Awata N. Synthesis of γ-oryzanol (triterpenyl esters of ferulic acid)-[14]C. *Radioisotopes* 1981;**30**(3):156–8.

24. Devi BLAP, Kanjilal S, Ramakrishna S, Madhusudhana K, Diwan PV, Prasad RBN. A process for the preparation of phytosteryl ferulate (WO/2010/097810A2). India; 2010.

25. Ju YH, Vali SR. Rice bran oil as a potential resource for biodiesel: A review. *J Sci Ind Res* 2005;**64**(11):866–82.

26. Nagendra Prasad MN, Sanjay KR, Shravya Khatokar M, Vismaya MN, Nanjunda Swamy S. Health benefits of rice bran – A review. *J Nutr Food Sci* 2011;**1**(3):1–7.

27. Taniguchi H, Hashimoto H, Hosoda A, Kometani T, Tsuno T, Adachi S. Functionality of compounds contained in rice bran and their improvement. *Nippon Shokuhin Kagaku Kogaku Kaishi* 2012;**59**(7):301–18.

28. Chen MH, Bergman CJ. A rapid procedure for analysing rice bran tocopherol, tocotrienol and γ-oryzanol contents. *J Food Compos Anal* 2005;**18**(2–3):139–51.

29. Renuka Devi R, Arumughan C. Antiradical efficacy of phytochemical extracts from defatted rice bran. *Food Chem Toxicol* 2007;**45**(10) 2014-21.

30. Ha TY, Ko SN, Lee SM, et al. Changes in nutraceutical lipid components of rice at different degrees of milling. *Eur J Lipid Sci Tech* 2006;**108**(3):175–81.

31. Yoon SH, Kim SK. Oxidative stability of high-fatty acid rice bran oil at different stages of refining. *J Am Oil Chem Society* 1994;**71**(2):227–9.

32. Thanonkaew A, Wongyai S, McClements DJ, Decker EA. Effect of stabilization of rice bran by domestic heating on mechanical extraction yield, quality, and antioxidant properties of cold-pressed rice bran oil (*Oryza saltiva* L.). *Food Sci Technol-LEB* 2012;**48**(2):231–6.

33. Loypimai P, Moonggarm A, Chottanom P. Effects of ohmic heating on lipase activity, bioactive compounds and antioxidant activity of rice bran. *Aus J Basic Appl Sci* 2009;**3**(4):3642–52.

34. Johnson LA, Lusas EW. Comparison of alternative solvents for oils extraction. *J Am Oil Chem Soc* 1983;**60**(2):229–42.

35. Talwalker RT, Garg NK, Krishnamurti CR. Rice bran – a source material for pharmaceuticals. *J Food Sci Technol* 1965;**2**:117–9.

36. *American Association of Cereal Chemists. Approved methods of the American Association of Cereal Chemists*. 9th ed. St Paul, MN: American Association of Cereal Chemists; 1995.

37. Wakelyn PJ, Wan PJ. Edible oil extraction solvents: FDA regulatory considerations. *Inform* 2004;**15**(1):22–3.

38. Van Hoed V, Depaemelaere G, Ayala JV, Santiwattana P, Verhe R, De Greyt W. Influence of chemical refining on the major and minor components of rice bran oil. *J Am Oil Chem Soc* 2006;**83**(4):315–21.

39. Miller A, Engel KH. Content of γ-oryzanol and composition of steryl ferulates in brown rice (*Oryza sativa* L.) of European origin. *J Agric Food Chem* 2006;**54**(21):8127–33.

40. Heinemann RJB, Xu Z, Godber JS, Lanfer-Marquez UM. Tocopherols, tocotrienols, and γ-oryzanol contents in Japonica and Indica subspecies of rice (*Oryza sativa* L.) cultivated in Brazil. *Cereal Chem* 2008;**85**(2):243–7.

41. Huang SH, Ng LT. Quantification of tocopherols, tocotrienols, and γ-oryzanol contents and their distribution in some commercial rice varieties in Taiwan. *J Agric Food Chem* 2011;**59**(20):11150–9.

42. Lu TJ, Chen HN, Wang HJ. Chemical constituents, dietary fiber, and γ-oryzanol in six commercial varieties of brown rice from Taiwan. *Cereal Chem* 2011;**88**(5):463–6.

43. Anwar F, Zubair M, Ashraf M, Uddin MK. Characterization of high-value bioactives in some selected varieties of Pakistani rice (*Oryza sativa* L.). *Int J Mol Sci* 2012;**13**(4):4608–22.

44. Britz SJ, Prasad PV, Moreau RA, Allen Jr LH, Kremer DF, Boote KJ. Influence of growth temperature on the amounts of tocopherols, tocotrienols, and γ-oryzanol in brown rice. *J Agric Food Chem* 2007;**55**(18):7559–65.

45. Tuano APP, Xu Z, Castillo MB, et al. Content of tocols, γ-oryzanol and total phenolics and grain quality of brown rice and milled rice applied with pesticides and organic and inorganic nitrogen fertilizer. *Philippine Agric Scientist* 2011;**94**(2):211–6.

46. Lee YR, Kim JY, Woo KS, et al. Changes in the chemical and functional components of Korean rough rice before and after germination. *Food Sci Biotechnol* 2007;**16**(6):1006–10.

47. Kim HY, Hwang IG, Kim TM, et al. Chemical and functional components in different parts of rough rice (*Oryza sativa* L.) before and after germination. *Food Chem* 2012;**134**(1):288–93.

48. Moongngarm A, Khomphiphatkul E. Germination time dependence of bioactive compounds and antioxidant activity in germinated rough rice (*Oryza sativa* L.). *Am J Appl Sci* 2011;**8**(1):15–25.

49. Kiing SC, Yiu PH, Rajan A, Wong SC. Effect of germination on γ-oryzanol content of selected sarawak rice cultivars. *Am J Appl Sci* 2009;**6**(9):1658–61.

50. Oh SK, Hwang PS, Kim KJ, Kim YK, Lee JH. Changes in nutritional components throughout germination in paddy rice and brown rice. *J Food Sci Nutr* 2010;**15**(2):113–9.

51. Sungsopha J, Moongngarm A, Kanesakoo R. Application of germination and enzymatic treatment to improve the concentration of bioactive compounds and antioxidant activity of rice bran. *Aus J Basic Appl Sci* 2009;**3**(4):3653–62.

52. Chen MH, Bergman CJ. Influence of kernel maturity, milling degree, and milling quality on rice bran phytochemical concentrations. *Cereal Chem* 2005;**82**(1):4–8.

53. Tuncel NB, Yilmaz N. γ-oryzanol content, phenolic acid profiles and antioxidant activity of rice milling fractions. *Eur Food Res Technol* 2011;**233**(4):577–85.

54. Xu Z, Godber JS. Comparison of supercritical fluid and solvent extraction methods in extracting γ-oryzanol from rice bran. *J Am Oil Chem Soc* 2000;**77**(5):547–51.

55. Imsanguan P, Roaysubtawee A, Borirak R, Pongamphai S, Douglas S, Douglas PL. Extraction of α-tocopherol and γ-oryzanol from rice bran. *Food Sci Technol-LEB* 2008;**41**(8):1417–24.

56. Lai P, Li KY, Lu S, Chen HH. Phytochemicals and antioxidant properties of solvent extracts from Japonica rice bran. *Food Chem* 2009;**117**(3):538–44.

57. Chen HH, Chiu TH. Phytochemicals characterization of solvent extracts from taro-scented japonica rice bran. *J Food Sci* 2011;**76**(4) C656–C62.

58. Rodrigues CEC, Oliveira R. Response surface methodology applied to the analysis of rice bran oil extraction process with ethanol. *Int J Food Sci Technol* 2010;**45**(4):813–20.

59. Oliveira R, Oliveira V, Aracava KK, Rodrigues CEDC. Effects of the extraction conditions on the yield and composition of rice bran oil extracted with ethanol – A response surface approach. *Food Bioprod Process* 2012;**90**(1):22–31.

60. Pestana-Bauer VR, Zambiazi RC, Mendonça CRB, Beneito-Cambra M, Ramis-Ramos G. γ-Oryzanol and tocopherol contents in residues of rice bran oil refining. *Food Chem* 2012;**134**(3):1479–83.

61. Scavariello EMS, Barrera-Arellano D. Optimisation of the acidulation process of soapstock from the neutralisation of rice bran oil. *Grasas y Aceites* 2004;**55**(2):155–9.

62. Dunford NT, King JW. Phytosterol enrichment of rice bran oil by a supercritical carbon dioxide fractionation technique. *J Food Sci* 2000;**65**(8):1395–9.

63. Van Hoed V, Ayala JV, Czarnowska M, De Greyt W, Verhe R. Optimization of physical refining to produce rice bran oil with light color and high oryzanol content. *J Am Oil Chem Soc* 2010;**87**(10):1227–34.

64. Sereewatthanawut I, Baptista IIR, Boam AT, Hodgson A, Livingston AG. Nanofiltration process for the nutritional enrichment and refining of rice bran oil. *J Food Engineering* 102(1): 16–24.

65. Narayan AV, Barhate RS, Raghavarao KSMS. Extraction and purification of oryzanol from rice bran oil and rice bran oil soapstock. *J Am Oil Chem Soc* 2006;**83**(8):663–70.

66. Tsuchiya T, Kaneko R, Tanaka A, inventors. *Separation of γ-oryzanol from rice bran oil or rice embryo oil (JP4895).* Japan; 1957.

67. Masao N, Yoshizane S, inventors. *γ-oryzanol from alkaline cake of rice oil (JP6812730).* Japan; 1968.

68. Takeshi Y, inventor. *γ-oryzanol (DE130102).* Germany; 1969.

69. Indira TN, Narayan AV, Barhate RS, et al., inventors. *Process for the production of oryzanol enriched fraction from rice bran oil soapstock (US6896911).* USA; 2005.

70. Koji T, Tokuo F., inventors. *Concentration and purification of constituent component of γ-oryzanol (JP63104948).* Japan; 1986.

71. Mingzhi L, Yanyan L., inventors. *Study of γ-oryzanol extracted from the second soapstock of rice bran oil (CH330029).* China; 1997.

72. Narayan AV, Barhate RS, Indira TN, et al., inventors. *A simple process for the crystallization of γ-oryzanol from γ-oryzanol enriched fraction (WO/2004/055040).* Brazil; 2004.

73. Zullaikah S, Melwita E, Ju YH. Isolation of oryzanol from crude rice bran oil. *Bioresour Technol* 2009;**100**(1):299–302.

74. Tsuchiya T, Okubo O., inventors. *γ-oryzanol (JP13649).* Japan; 1961.

75. Xu Z, Godber JS. Purification and identification of components of γ-oryzanol in rice bran oil. *J Agric Food Chem* 1999;**47**(7):2724–8.

76. Lai SM, Hsieh HL, Chang CW. Preparative separation of γ-oryzanol from rice bran oil by silica gel column chromatography. *J Liquid Chromatogr Relat Technol* 2005;**28**(1):145–60.

77. Stoggl W, Huck C, Wongyai S, Scherz H, Bonn G. Simultaneous determination of carotenoids, tocopherols, and γ-Oryzanol in crude rice bran oil by liquid chromatography coupled to diode array and mass spectrometric detection employing silica C30 stationary phases. *J Sep Sci* 2005;**28**(14):1712–8.

78. Yasuo W, Tsukasa A, Tomisei I., inventors. *γ-oryzanol (JP6812731).* Japan; 1968.

79. Seetharamaiah GS, Prabhakar JV. γ-oryzanol Content of Indian Rice Bran Oil and Its Extraction from Soapstock. *J Food Sci Technol* 1986;**23**:270–3.

80. Saska M, Rossiter CJ. Recovery of γ-oryzanol from rice bran oil with silica-based continuous chromatography. *J Am Oil Chem Soc* 1998;**75**(10):1421–7.

81. Das PK, Chaudhuri A, Kaimal TNB, Bhalerao UT. Isolation of γ-oryzanol through calcium ion induced precipitation of anionic micellar aggregates. *J Agric Food Chem* 1998;**46**(8):3073–80.

82. Rao KVSA, Rao BVSK, Kaimal TNB., inventors. *Process for the isolation of γ-oryzanols from rice bran oil soapstock (US6410762).* USA; 2002.

83. Kasim NS, Chen H, Ju YH. Recovery of γ-oryzanol from biodiesel residue. *J Chinese Inst Chem Eng* 2007;**38**(3-4):229–34.

84. Kaewchada A, Borvornpongsakul C, Jaree A. Synthesis of molecularly imprinted polymers from AnAc for the separation of γ-oryzanol. *Korean J Chem Eng* 2012;**29**(9):1279–84.

85. De Deckere EAM, Korver O. Minor constituents of rice bran oil as functional foods. *Nutr Rev* 1996;**54**(11 II) S120–S1S6.

86. Scavariello EM, Arellano DB. γ-oryzanol: an important component in rice brain oil. *Arch Latinoam Nutr* 1998;**48**(1):7–12.

87. Endo T, Ueno K, Inaba Y. Studies on the ferulates contained in rice bran oil. I. Analysis of the ferulates by means of GLC and TLC. *J Jpn Oil Chem Soc* 1968;**17**:344–8.

88. Evershed RP, Spooner N, Prescott MC, John Goad L. Isolation and characterisation of intact steryl ferulates from seeds. *J Chromatogr A* 1988;**440**(C):23–35.

89. Seitz LM. Stanol and sterol esters of ferulic and *p*-coumaric acids in wheat, corn, rye, and triticale. *J Agric Food Chem* 1989;**37**(3):662–7.

90. Rogers EJ, Rice SM, Nicolosi RJ, Carpenter DR, McClelland CA, Romanczyk Jr LJ. Identification and quantitation of γ-oryzanol components and simultaneous assessment of tocols in rice bran oil. *J Am Oil Chem Soc* 1993;**70**(3):301–7.

91. Diack M, Saska M. Separation of vitamin E and γ-oryzanols from rice bran by normal-phase chromatography. *J Am Oil Chem Soc* 1994;**71**(11):1211–7.

92. Moreau RA, Powell MJ, Hicks KB. Extraction and quantitative analysis of oil from commercial corn fiber. *J Agric Food Chem* 1996;**44**(8):2149–54.

93. Fujiwara S, Sakurai S, Noumi K, Sugimoto I, Awata N. Metabolism of γ-oryzanol in rabbit. *Yakugaku Zasshi* 1980;**100**(10):1011–8.

94. Fujiwara S, Sakurai S, Sugimoto I, Awata N. Absorption and metabolism of γ-oryzanol in rats. *Chem Pharm Bull* 1983;**31**(2):645–52.

95. Fujiwara S, Noumi K, Sugimoto I, Awata N. Mass fragmentographic determination of ferulic acid in plasma after oral administration of γ-oryzanol. *Chem Pharm Bull* 1982;**30**(3):973–9.

96. Fujiwara S, Honda S. Determination of cinnamic acid and its Analogues by electrophoresis in a fused silica capillary tube. *Anal Chem* 1986;**58**(8):1811–4.

97. Norton RA. Isolation and identification of steryl cinnamic acid derivatives from corn bran. *Cereal Chem* 1994;**71**:111–7.

98. Norton RA. Quantitation of steryl ferulate and *p*-coumarate esters from corn and rice bran. *Lipids* 1995;**30**:269–74.

99. Hartley RD, Jones EC. Effect of ultraviolet light onsubstituted cinnamic acids and the estimation of their *cis* and *trans* isomers by gas chromatography. *J Chromatogr* 1975;**107**:213–8.

100. Van Boven M, Daenens P, Tytgat J, Cokelaere M. Determination of simmondsin and simmondsin ferulates in jojoba meal and feed by High-Performance Liquid Chromatography. *J Agric Food Chem* 1996;**44**(8):2239–43.

101. Kumar RR, Tiku PK, Prakash V. Preferential extractability of γ-oryzanol from dried soapstock using different solvents. *J Sci Food Agric* 2009;**89**(2):195–200.

102. Cho JY, Lee HJ, Kim GA, et al. Quantitative analyses of individual γ-Oryzanol (steryl ferulates) in conventional and organic brown rice (*Oryza sativa* L.). *J Cereal Sci* 2012;**55**(3):337–43.

103. Thompson MJ, Dutky SR, Patterson GW, Gooden EL. NMR spectra of C-24 isomeric sterols. *Phytochem* 1972;**11**(5):1781–90.

104. Manik CD, Shashi BM. *Rev Triterpernoids* 1983;**22**(5):1071–95.

105. Luo H-F, Li Q, Yu S, Badger TM, Fang N. Hydroxylated triterpene alcohol ferulates from rice bran. *J Nat Prod* 2005;**68**:94–7.

106. Miller A, Frenzel T, Schmarr HG, Engel KH. Coupled liquid chromatography-gas chromatography for the rapid analysis of γ-oryzanol in rice lipids. *J Chromatogr A* 2003;**985**(1-2):403–10.

107. Monsoor MA, Proctor A. Tocopherol, tocotrienol, and oryzanol content of rice bran aqueous extracts. *J Am Oil Chem Soc* 2005;**82**(6):463–4.

108. Yoshie A, Kanda A, Nakamura T, Igusa H, Hara S. Comparison of γ-oryzanol contents in crude rice bran oils from different sources by various determination methods. *J Oleo Sci* 2009;**58**(10):511–8.

109. Huang SH, Ng LT. An improved high-performance liquid chromatographic method for simultaneous determination of tocopherols, tocotrienols and γ-oryzanol in rice. *J Chromatogr A* 2011;**1218**(29):4709–13.

110. Zaima N, Goto-Inoue N, Hayasaka T, Setou M. Application of imaging mass spectrometry for the analysis of *Oryza sativa* rice. *Rapid Commun Mass Spectrom* 2010;**24**(18):2723–9.

111. Tchoumtchoua J, Njamen D, Mbany J, Skaltsounis A, Halabalaki M. Structure-oriented UHPLC-LTQ Orbitrap-based approach as a dereplication strategy for the identification of isoflavonoids from *Amphimas pterocarpoides* crude extract. *J Mass Spectrom* 2013 (in press).

112. Afinisha Deepam LS, Soban Kumar DR, Sundaresan A, Arumughan C. A new method for simultaneous estimation of unsaponifiable constituents of rice bran oil using HPTLC. *J Sep Sci* 2007;**30**(16):2786–93.

113. Kumar A, Sharma V, Lal D. Thin layer chromatographic method for the detection of rice bran oil in other vegetable oils. *J Food Sci Tech* 2009;**46**(1):85–6.

114. Bucci R, Magri AD, Magri AL, Marini F. Comparison of three spectrophotometric methods for the determination of γ-oryzanol in rice bran oil. *Anal Bioanal Chem* 2003;**375**(8):1254–9.

115. Kaewboonnum W, Wachararuji K, Shotipruk A. Value added products from byproducts of rice bran oil processing. *Chiang Mai J Sci* 2008;**35**(1):116–22.

116. Lilitchan S, Tangprawat C, Aryusuk K, Krisnangkura S, Chokmoh S, Krisnangkura K. Partial extraction method for the rapid analysis of total lipids and γ-oryzanol contents in rice bran. *Food Chem* 2008;**106**(2):752–9.

117. Abidi SL, Rennick KA. Determination of nonvolatile components in polar fractions of rice bran oils. *J Am Oil Chem Soc* 2003;**80**(11):1057–62.

118. Ravikumar Patil HS, Haraprasad N, Makari HK, Gurumurthy H, Chetan DM, Anil Kumar HS. Polyphenol composition of nutraceutical concentrate obtained from edible vegetable oil seeds. *Electron J Environ Agric Food Chem* 2008;**7**(8):3181–98.

119. Mishra R, Sharma HK, Sengar G. Quantification of rice bran oil in oil blends. *Grasas y Aceites* 2012;**63**(1):53–60.

120. Mayamol PN, Samuel T, Balachandran C, Sundaresan A, Arumughan C. Zero-trans shortening using palm stearin and rice bran oil. *J Am Oil Chem Soc* 2004;**81**(4):407–13.

121. Rajan RGR, Krishna AGG. Refining of high free fatty acid rice bran oil and its quality characteristics. *J Food Lipids* 2009;**16**(4):589–604.

122. Pestana VR, Zambiazi RC, Mendonça CRB, Bruscatto MH, Ramis-Ramosc G. The influence of industrial processing on the physicochemical characteristics and lipid and antioxidant contents of rice bran. *Grasas y Aceites* 2009;**60**(2):184–93.

123. Pestana VR, Zambiazi RC, Mendonça CRB, Bruscatto MH, Lerma-Garcia MJ, Ramis-Ramos G. Quality changes and tocopherols and γ-oryzanol concentrations in rice bran oil during the refining process. *J Am Oil Chem Soc* 2008;**85**(11):1013–9.

124. Schramm R, Abadie A, Hua N, Xu Z, Lima M. Fractionation of the rice bran layer and quantification of vitamin E, oryzanol, protein, and rice bran saccharide. *J Biol Eng* 2007;**1**:9.

125. Yu F, Kim SH, Kim NS, Lee JH, Bae DH, Lee KT. Composition of solvent-fractionated rice bran oil. *J Food Lipids* 2006;**13**(3):286–97.

126. Renuka Devi R, Arumughan C. Phytochemical characterization of defatted rice bran and optimization of a process for their extraction and enrichment. *Bioresource Technol* 2007;**98**(16):3037–43.

127. Pascual CdSCI, Massaretto IL, Kawassaki F, Barros RMC, Noldin JA, Marquez UML. Effects of parboiling, storage and cooking on the levels of tocopherols, tocotrienols and γ-oryzanol in brown rice (*Oryza sativa* L.). *Food Res Int* 2011.

128. Gertz C, Klostermann S, Kochhar SP. Testing and comparing oxidative stability of vegetable oils and fats at frying temperature. *Eur J Lipid Sci Tech* 2000;**102**(8-9):543–51.

129. Krishna AGG, Khatoon S, Babylatha R. Frying performance of processed rice bran oils. *J Food Lipids* 2005;**12**(1):1–11.

130. Nagasaka R, Shinoda A, Ushio H, Ohshima T. γ-Oryzanol in laminarian seaweeds. *Nippon Suisan Gakkaishi [Japanese Edition]* 2008;**74**(1):61–5.

131. Deepa G, Singh V, Naidu KA. Characterization of antioxidant compounds and antioxidant activity of Indian rice varieties. *J Herbs Spices Med Plants* 2012;**18**(1):18–33.

132. Biswas S, Sircar D, Mitra A. de B. Phenolic constituents and antioxidant properties of some varieties of Indian rice. *Nutr Food Sci* 2011;**41**(2):123–35.

133. Boonsit P, Pongpiachan P, Julsrigival S, Karladee D. Gamma oryzanol content in glutinous purple rice landrace varieties. *Chiang Mai Univ J Natu Sci* 2010;**9**(1):151–8.

134. Przybylski R, Klensporf-Pawlik D, Anwar F, Rudzinska M. Lipid components of North American wild rice (*Zizania palustris*). *J Am Oil Chem Soc* 2009;**86**(6):553–9.

135. Anwar F, Anwer T, Mahmood Z. Methodical characterization of rice (*Oryza sativa*) bran oil from Pakistan. *Grasas y Aceites* 2005;**56**(2):125–34.

136. Khatoon S, Gopalakrishna AG. Fat-soluble nutraceuticals and fatty acid composition of selected indian rice varieties. *J Am Oil Chem Soc* 2004;**81**(10):939–43.

137. Gopala Krishna AG, Hemakumar KH, Khatoon S. Study on the composition of rice bran oil and its higher free fatty acids value. *J Am Oil Chem Soc* 2006;**83**(2):117–20.

138. Seo WD, Kim JY, Park DS, et al. Comparative analysis of physicochemicals and antioxidative properties of new giant embryo mutant, YR23517Acp79, in rice (*Oryza sativa* L.). *J Korean Soc Appl Biolog Chem* 2011;**54**(5):700–9.

139. Jeng TL, Ho PT, Shih YJ, Lai CC, Wu MT, Sung JM. Comparisons of protein, lipid, phenolics, γ-oryzanol, vitamin E, and mineral contents in bran layer of sodium azide-induced red rice mutants. *J Sci Food Agric* 2011;**91**(8):1459–65.

140. Azrina A, Maznah I, Azizah AH. Extraction and determination of oryzanol in rice bran of mixed herbarium UKMB; AZ 6807: MR 185, AZ 6808: MR 211, AZ6809: MR 29. *ASEAN Food J* 2008;**15**(1):89–96.

141. Yu S, Nehus ZT, Badger TM, Fang N. Quantification of vitamin E and γ-oryzanol components in rice germ and bran. *J Agric Food Chem* 2007;**55**(18):7308–13.

142. Moongngarm A, Saetung N. Comparison of chemical compositions and bioactive compounds of germinated rough rice and brown rice. *Food Chem* 2010;**122**(3):782–8.

143. Shallan MA, El-Beltagi HS, Mona AM, Amera TM. Chemical evaluation of pre-germinated brown rice and whole grain rice bread. *Electron J Environ Agric Food Chem* 2010;**9**(5):958–71.

144. Lin PY, Lai HM. Bioactive compounds in rice during grain development. *Food Chem* 2011;**127**(1):86–93.

145. Banchuen J, Thammarutwasik P, Ooraikul B, Wuttijumnong P, Sivongpaisal P. Increasing the bio-active compounds contents by optimizing the germination conditions of southern Thai brown rice. *Songklanakarin J Sci Technol* 2010;**32**(3):219–30.

146. Lubinus T, Barnsteiner A, Skurk T, Hauner H, Engel KH. Fate of dietary phytosteryl-/-stanyl esters: analysis of individual intact esters in human feces. *Eur J Nutr* 2012:1–17.

147. Sugano M, Koba K, Tsuji E. Health benefits of rice bran oil. *Anticancer Res* 1999;**19**(5 A):3651–7.

148. Ishihara M, Ito Y, Nakakita T, et al. Clinical effect of γ-oryzanol on climacteric disturbance on serum lipid peroxides. *Nihon Sanka Fujinka Gakkai Zasshi* 1982;**34**(2):243–51.

149. Ueda H, Hayakawa R, Hoshino S, Kobayashi M. The effect of topically applied γ-Oryzanol on sebaceous glands. *J Dermatol* 1976;**3**(1):19–24.

150. Itaya K, Kiyonaga J. Studies on γ-oryzanol: effects of γ-oryzanol on stress ulcer. *Folia Pharmacol Jap* 1976;**72**(4):475–81.

151. Cicero AF, Gaddi A. Rice bran oil and γ-oryzanol in the treatment of hyperlipoproteinaemias and other conditions. *Phytother Res* 2001;**15**(4):277–89.

152. Nakamura H. Effect of gamma-oryzanol on hepatic cholesterol biosynthesis and faecal excretion of cholesterol metabolites. *Radioisotopes* 1966;**15**:371–4.

153. Vorarat S, Managit C, Iamthanakul L, Soparat W, Kamkaen N. Examination of antioxidant activity and development of rice bran oil and γ-oryzanol microemulsion. *J Health Res* 2010;**24**(2):67–72.

154. Wang T, Hicks K, Moreau R. Antioxidant activity of phytosterols, oryzanol, and other phytosterol conjugates. *J Am Oil Chem Soc* 2002;**79**(12):1201–6.

155. Juliano C, Cossu M, Alamanni MC, Piu L. Antioxidant activity of γ-oryzanol: mechanism of action and its effect on oxidative stability of pharmaceutical oils. *Int J Pharm* 2005;**299**(1-2):146–54.

156. Kim JS. Antioxidant activity of γ-oryzanol and synthetic phenolic compounds in an oil/water (O/W) emulsion system. *J Food Sci Nutr* 2007;**12**(3):173–6.

157. Hiramitsu T, Armstrong D. Preventive effect of antioxidants on lipid peroxidation in the retina. *Ophthalmic Res* 1991;**23**(4):196–203.

158. Xu Z, Godber JS. Antioxidant activities of major components of γ-oryzanol from rice bran using a linoleic acid model. *J Am Oil Chem Soc* 2001;**78**(6):645–9.

159. Kim J-S, Godber JS, King JM, Prinyawiwatkul W. Inhibition of cholesterol autoxidation by the nonsaponifiable fraction in rice bran in an aqueous model system. *J Am Oil Chem Soc* 2001;**78**(7):685–9.

160. Woods JA, O'Brien NM. Investigation of the potential genotoxicity of cholesterol oxidation products in two mammalian fibroblast cell lines. *Nutr Cancer* 1998;**31**(3):192–8.

161. Ansari GAS, Walker RD, Smart VB, Smith LL. Further investigations of mutagenic cholesterol preparations. *Food Chem Toxicol* 1982;**20**(1):35–41.

162. Kumar N, Singhal OP. Cholesterol oxides and atherosclerosis: A review. *J Sci Food Agr* 1991;**55**(4):497–510.

163. Xu Z, Hua N, Godber JS. Antioxidant activity of tocopherols, tocotrienols, and γ-oryzanol components from rice bran against cholesterol oxidation accelerated by 2,2′-azobis(2-methylpropionamidine) dihydrochloride. *J Agric Food Chem* 2001;**49**(4):2077–81.

164. Dröge W. Free Radicals in the Physiological Control of Cell Function. *Physiol Rev* 2002;**82**(1):47–95.

165. Ichimaru Y, Moriyama M, Ichimaru M, Gomita Y. Effects of γ-oryzanol on gastric lesions and small intestinal propulsive activity in mice. *Nihon Yakurigaku Zasshi* 1984;**84**(6):537–42.

166. Itaya K, Isikawa M. Effect of γ-oryzanol on experimental gastric ulcer and duodenal ulcer in rat. *Pharmacometrics* 1978;**16**(3):493–501.

167. Itaya K, Kitonaga J, Ishikawa M. Studies of γ-oryzanol. (2). The antiulcerogenic action. *Nihon Yakurigaku Zasshi* 1976;**72**(8):1001–11.

168. Itaya K, Kiyonaga J. Studies of γ-oryzanol. (1). Effects on stress-induced ulcer. *Nihon Yakurigaku Zasshi* 1976;**72**(4):475–81.

169. Sumio T, Kazuhiko H. Anti-inflammatory effects of γ-oryzanol. *Natu Med* 2003;**57**(3):95–9.

170. Islam MS, Murata T, Fujisawa M, et al. Anti-inflammatory effects of phytosteryl ferulates in colitis induced by dextran sulphate sodium in mice. *Br J Pharmacol* 2008;**154**(4):812–24.

171. Chotimarkorn C, Ushio H. The effect of *trans*-ferulic acid and γ-oryzanol on ethanol-induced liver injury in C57BL mouse. *Phytomedicine* 2008;**15**(11):951–8.

172. Oka T, Fujimoto M, Nagasaka R, Ushio H, Hori M, Ozaki H. Cycloartenyl ferulate, a component of rice bran oil-derived γ-oryzanol, attenuates mast cell degranulation. *Phytomedicine* 2010;**17**(2):152–6.

173. Ghatak S, Panchal S. Anti-diabetic activity of oryzanol and its relationship with the antioxidant property. *Int J Diabetes Dev Ctries* 2012;**32**(4):185–92.

174. Cheng HH, Ma CY, Chou TW, Chen YY, Lai MH. γ-oryzanol ameliorates insulin resistance and hyperlipidemia in rats with streptozotocin/nicotinamide-induced type 2 diabetes. *Int J Vitam Nutr Res* 2010;**80**(1):45–53.

175. Ghatak SB, Panchal SS. Protective effect of oryzanol isolated from crude rice bran oil in experimental model of diabetic neuropathy. *Rev Bras Farmacogn* 2012;**22**:1092–103.

176. Yasukawa K, Akihisa T, Kimura Y, Tamura T, Takido M. Inhibitory effect of cycloartenol ferulate, a component of rice bran, on tumor promotion in two-stage carcinogenesis in mouse skin. *Biol Pharm Bull* 1998;**21**(10):1072–6.

177. Kim SP, Kang MY, Nam SH, Friedman M. Dietary rice bran component γ-oryzanol inhibits tumor growth in tumor-bearing mice. *Mol Nutr Food Res* 2012;**56**(6):935–44.

178. Tamagawa M, Otaki Y, Takahashi T, Otaka T, Kimura S, Miwa T. Carcinogenicity study of γ-oryzanol in B6C3F1 mice. *Food Chem Toxicol* 1992;**30**(1):49–56.

179. Tamagawa M, Shimizu Y, Takahashi T, et al. Carcinogenicity study of γ-oryzanol in F344 rats. *Food Chem Toxicol* 1992;**30**(1):41–8.

180. Hirose M, Ozaki K, Takaba K, Fukushima S, Shirai T, Ito N. Modifying effects of the naturally occurring antioxidants gamma-oryzanol, phytic acid, tannic acid and n-tritriacontane-16, 18-dione in a rat wide-spectrum organ carcinogenesis model. *Carcinogenesis* 1991;**12**(10):1917–21.

181. Hirose M, Fukushima S, Imaida K, Ito N, Shirai T. Modifying effects of phytic acid and γ-oryzanol on the promotion stage of rat carcinogenesis. *Anticancer Res* 1999;**19**(5A):3665–70.

182. Suzuki S, Oshima S. Influence of blending of edible fats and oils on human serum cholesterol level. 1. Blending of rice bran oil and safflower oil. *Jpn J Nutr* 1970;**28**:3–6.

183. Ishihara M. Effect of γ-oryzanol on serum lipid peroxide level and clinical symptoms of patients with climacteric disturbances. *Asia Oceania J Obstet Gynaecol* 1984;**10**(3):317–23.

184. Yoshino G, Kazumi T, Amano M, et al. Effects of γ-oryzanol and probucol on hyperlipidemia. *Curr Ther Res Clin Exp* 1989;**45**(6):975–82.

185. Yoshino G, Kazumi T, Amano M, et al. Effects of γ-oryzanol on hyperlipidemic subjects. *Curr Ther Res Clin Exp* 1989;**45**(4):543–52.

186. Sasaki J, Takada Y, Handa K, et al. Effects of γ-oryzanol on serum lipids and apolipoproteins in dyslipidemic schizophrenics receiving major tranquilizers. *Clin Ther* 1990;**12**(3):263–8.

187. Berger A, Rein D, Schafer A, et al. Similar cholesterol-lowering properties of rice bran oil, with varied γ-oryzanol, in mildly hypercholesterolemic men. *Eur J Nutr* 2005;**44**(3):163–73.

188. Lichtenstein AH, Ausman LM, Carrasco W, et al. Rice bran oil consumption and plasma lipid levels in moderately hypercholesterolemic humans. *Arterioscler Thromb* 1994;**14**(4):549–56.

189. Moriyama N, Shinozaki T, Kanayama K, Yatomi S. Development of the processing rice which added new functionality. *Nippon Nogeikagaku Kaishi* 2002;**76**(7):614–21.

190. Ghatak SB, Panchal SJ. Anti-hyperlipidemic activity of oryzanol isolated from crude rice bran oil on triton WR-1339-induced acute hyperlipidemia in rats. *Brazilian J Pharmacognosy* 2012;**22**(3):642–8.

191. Nakayama S, Kurishima H, Kobayashi K, Tsuji T. Effects of γ-oryzanol and its related compounds on triton induced hyperlipidemia in rats. *J Showa Med Association* 1986;**46**(3):359–64.

192. Nakayama S, Manabe A, Suzuki J, Sakamoto K, Inagaki T. Comparative effects of two forms of γ-oryzanol in different sterol compositions on hyperlipidemia induced by cholesterol diet in rats. *Jpn J Pharmacol* 1987;**44**(2):135–43.

193. Sakamoto K, Tabata T, Shirasaki K, Inagaki T, Nakayama S. Effects of γ-oryzanol and cycloartenol ferulic acid ester on cholesterol diet induced hyperlipidemia in rats. *Jpn J Pharmacol* 1987;**45**(4):559–65.

194. Hiramatsu K, Tani T, Kimura Y, Izumi S, Nakane PK. Effect of γ-oryzanol on atheroma formation in hypercholesterolemic rabbits. *Tokai J Exp Clin Med* 1990;**15**(4):299–305.

195. Negm CS, Silliman K. the effects of rice bran oil and oryzanol on plasma levels of total cholesterol and HDLcholesterol in male golden hamsters. *J Am Diet Association* 1995(9 Suppl.):95.

196. Rong N, Ausman LM, Nicolosi RJ. Oryzanol decreases cholesterol absorption and aortic fatty streaks in hamsters. *Lipids* 1997;**32**(3):303–9.

197. Wilson TA, Nicolosi RJ, Woolfrey B, Kritchevsky D. Rice bran oil and oryzanol reduce plasma lipid and lipoprotein cholesterol concentrations and aortic cholesterol ester accumulation to a greater extent than ferulic acid in hypercholesterolemic hamsters. *J Nutr Biochem* 2007;**18**(2):105–12.

198. Inoue Y, Horinuki R, Kimura Y. Suppression of experimental atherosclerosis in rats by γ-oryzanol. *J Jpn Atherosclerosis Soc* 1989;**17**(3):499–507.

199. Zhang Q, Yang X, Li Y. Effects of γ-oryzanol on experimental coronary atherosclerosis in rats. *Chinese J Cardiol* 1986;**14**(5) 287–90+319.

200. Murase Y, Lishima H. Clinical studies of oral administration of γ-oryzanol on climacteric complaints and its syndrome. *Obstet Gynecol Prac* 1963;**12**:147–9.

201. Borud E, Grimsgaard S, White A. Menopausal problems and acupuncture. *Autonomic Neuroscience: Basic and Clinical* 2010;**157**(1-2):57–62.

202. Cho SH, Whang WW. Acupuncture for vasomotor menopausal symptoms: A systematic review. *Menopause* 2009; **16**(5):1065–73.

203. Ma XP, Wu FD, Shan QH. Clinical observation on treating menopause syndrome with acupuncture therapy. *J Acupunct Tuina Sci* 2009;**7**(1):51–4.

204. Zhang H. Influence of acupuncture on the clinical manifestation and beta-endorphin level in female patients with menopausal symptoms. *Chinese J Clin Rehabil* 2006;**10**(31):1–3.

205. Tian H, Zhang C. The combined use of acupuncture and Chinese medicines for treatment of menopausal syndrome - A clinical report of 63 cases. *J Tradit Chinese Med* 2008;**28**(1):3–4.

206. Manirazman A, inventor. *Non-chemical sunscreen composition (US005817299A)*. USA; 1996.

207. Grare C, Marion C, Philippon C. inventors; *Aqueous cosmetic composition containing composite material particles and γ-oryzanol (WO2012110303A2)*. France; 2012.

208. Manosroi A, Chutoprapat R, Abe M, Manosroi W, Manosroi J. Anti-aging efficacy of topical formulations containing niosomes entrapped with rice bran bioactive compounds. *Pharm Biol* 2012;**50**(2):208–24.

209. Riedel JH, Petsitis X. inventors; Eur Patent 945120, assignee. *Mascara and eyebrow pencils containing γ-oryzanol and calcium salt.* Germany; 1999.

210. Kim JS, Suh MH, Yang CB, Lee HG. Effect of γ-oryzanol on the flavor and oxidative stability of refrigerated cooked beef. *J Food Sci* 2003;**68**(8):2423–9.

211. Kochhar SP. Stabilisation of frying oils with natural antioxidative components. *Eur J Lipid Sci Tech* 2000;**102**(8-9):552–9.

212. Khuwijitjaru P, Yuenyong T, Pongsawatmanit R, Adachi S. Degradation kinetics of γ-oryzanol in antioxidant-stripped rice bran oil during thermal oxidation. *J Oleo Sci* 2009;**58**(10):491–7.

213. Suh MH, Yoo SH, Lee HG. Antioxidative activity and structural stability of microencapsulated gamma-oryzanol in heat-treated lards. *Food Chem* 2007;**100**(3):1065–70.

214. Sapino S, Carlotti ME, Cavalli R, et al. Photochemical and antioxidant properties of γ-oryzanol in beta-cyclodextrin-based nanosponges. *J Incl Phenom Macro* 2012:1–8.

215. Grunewald KK, Bailey RS. Commercially Marketed Supplements for Bodybuilding Athletes. *Sports Medicine* 1993;**15**(2):90–103.

216. Wheeler KB, Garleb KA. γ-Oryzanol-plant sterol supplementation: metabolic, endocrine, and physiologic effects. *Int J Sport Nutr* 1991;**1**(2).

217. Fry AC, Bonner E, Lewis DL, Johnson RL, Stone MH, Kraemer WJ. The effects of γ-oryzanol supplementation during resistance exercise training. *Int J Sport Nutr* 1997;**7**(4):318–29.

Evaluation of Physical and Nutritional Properties of Extruded Products Based on Brown Rice and Wild Legume Mixtures

Elena Pastor-Cavada*, Silvina R. Drago†, Rolando J. González†

*Instituto de la Grasa (CSIC), Sevilla, Spain, †Universidad Nacional del Litoral, Instituto de Tecnología de Alimentos, Santa Fe, Argentina

INTRODUCTION

Rice

Rice ranks second in world crop production after maize, and provides more than 20% of the total energy consumed by the world population.[1] Although rice is consumed mainly as polished grain, consumption of brown or whole grain rice is highly recommended. Mature rice grain is harvested as a covered grain (rough rice or paddy), in which the caryopsis is enclosed in a tough siliceous hull (husk). The caryopsis itself is a single-seeded fruit, wherein the pericarp is fused to the seed (composed of seed coat, nucellus, endosperm, and embryo).[2] Dehulling separates the hull (husk) from the brown rice, which still retains the bran layers that give it a tan color, chewy texture, and nut-like flavor. Retaining the nutrient-dense bran layer makes brown rice a 100% whole grain food, rich in minerals and vitamins, especially the B-complex group.

Different cultivars of waxy and non-waxy rice are usually classified according to their grain dimensions, amylose content, and amylograph consistency, the gelatinization properties of the extracted starches, and the texture (from both Instrom hardness and sensory measurements) of cooked rice.[2] The different types of rice are used according to their physicochemical and functional characteristics. For example, in baking products those with an amylose content below 20% are recommended due to low retrogradation effects,[3] particularly for cakes and puddings, and waxy rices are preferred.[4] Moreover, it is well known that low retrogradation is an advantageous property for starchy cooked products that have

to be kept at a low temperature. On the other hand, for expanded-type products, such as cereal snacks, high amylose rice is preferred.[5]

In the present work, a commercial sample of low amylose long wide-grain rice was used. This selection of rice was based on previous laboratory experience. As will be explained later, it has been observed that whole rice grains are processed in a single-screw extruder, such the Brabender 20 DN design (the one used in this study), and at the extrusion conditions normally used for expanded products it was found that the best extrusion performance and the most homogeneous cooking degree were achieved with low amylose rice.

Legumes

Among legumes, the family *Fabaceae* is one of the most important from the economical point of view, since plants of high protein value, such as peas, beans, and lentils, belong to it. Legumes are considered nutritious foods for their content of carbohydrates, lipids, fiber, minerals, vitamins, and good quality proteins.[6–8] Protein content varies between 20% and 40%.[9] These proteins are rich in lysine, but have some deficit in tryptophan and methionine.[10,11] At present the study of legumes is a matter of significant interest, with the inclusion of wild taxons being important so as not only to extend our knowledge about them but also to contribute to the broadening of the genetic reserve. With regard to this, the ONU declared 2010 as the year of "Biological Diversity," citing several reasons concerning the need to conserve biodiversity and promote both the revalorization of marginally grown legume species and the study of wild species.

The high level of good protein content and mineral composition of legumes makes them an excellent ingredient to be included in food feeding programs, particularly to complement cereal-containing menus.[12] The addition of legumes to cereals is a known practice to improve protein value and increase fiber content without increasing lipid content.[13,14] Moreover, it has been observed that the addition of legumes can improve product texture.[15,16]

Regarding the nutritional improvement of foods, not only content and protein quality and the bioavailability of nutrients but also the organoleptic quality of the product should be considered. It is known that the presence of active lipoxigenase impairs the sensory properties of legume flour, particularly for those people not accustomed to legumes in their daily diet. Lipoxygenase inactivation before legume grain grinding has been proved to be a necessary step for improvement of the sensory characteristics of legume-based products.[17] This methodology was verified in a previous work in our laboratory, where expanded products were obtained without impairment of their sensory characteristics. Sosa Moguel and colleagues[18] studied the influence of lipoxygenase inactivation and extrusion cooking on the physical and nutritional properties of corn/cowpea blends, and concluded that extrusion and lipoxygenase inactivation are promising options for developing corn/cowpea extruded snack products with good physical properties and nutritional quality.

Extrusion

Modern consumers are willing to buy healthy, novel, and convenient foods. They also like as wide a variety of foods as possible so that they can chose freely according to their own wishes. The wide variety of cereal food products present in the market nowadays is directly related to the above concept, and extrusion technology has allowed cereal processors to produce such a variety as a response to consumer demand.

Food extrusion has been practiced for over 60 years. It was initially used in the manufacture of macaroni and ready-to-eat cereal products. In these operations, relatively little heating or cooking was accomplished within the extruder. Extruders are used to mix and pressurize high-moisture food dough and force it through a shaping die at temperatures below the boiling point of water, where little or no puffing occurs. It is an efficient processing technique to produce new products from starchy and proteinous raw materials. It is a thermomechanical process which converts a non-cohesive material (flour) into a cooked homogeneous textured one, in a very short residence time (HTST process).[19–21]

Screw cooking extruders were developed in the 1940s for the purpose of making puffed snacks from cereal flours or grits. Now, food extrusion includes a variety of extruder designs, which allow the manufacture of a large number of products of different shapes, colors, and appearances. In fact, cooking extrusion of starchy materials has become a very commonly used technique to obtain a wide range of products, such as snacks, breakfast cereals, etc.[22] An extrusion process is also used to produce textured vegetables and special foods for feeding programs.[23–25] The future of this technology appears to lie in its ability to produce novel foods.[22,26]

The advantages of the extrusion process and the physicochemical changes which take place have been discussed by several authors.[26–33] During the extrusion process, structural changes occur in the material fed into the extruder (flour or grits): starch granules lose their crystalline structure (gelatinization); proteins are denatured; and biologically active components, such as protease inhibitor and lipoxigenase, are inactivated.[34–37] The microbial population is almost eliminated, and protein–lipid complexes are formed.[38] All of these changes affect flavor and texture.[39–41]

An important concept in extrusion cooking is the "cooking degree" reached by the starchy material during the process. The quality of extrusion cooked products is very much dependent on the cooking degree of the starch fraction. Other factors are the physical properties and size distribution of the particles. The meaning of the term "cooking degree" (CD) is directly related to the proportion of starch structure (either crystalline or granular) that has been lost during the cooking process. The transport of particles inside the extruder is characterized by its residence time distribution (RTD), which presents some dispersion and contributes to the heterogeneity of the degree of granular structure destruction. Even though the temperature level is high enough to accomplish starch gelatinization at a particular moisture level, it is possible to find, in the extrudate, native starch granules together with gelatinized granules, fragments of them, and dispersed amylose and amylopectin in several degrees of aggregation. The former correspond to those particles that, having the shortest residence time, could not be cooked because their residence time was not long enough for the cooking process to be accomplished. The proportion of each type of starch structure will affect hydration properties.[42] Thus, an extrusion cooking process converts starch granules in different "structural states" (native, gelatinized, fragments of granules, and macromolecular aggregates), which have to be taken into account when the effects of factors such as temperature (T) and moisture (M) are being analyzed. These two factors act in opposing directions on the friction exerted inside the extruder, and consequently the effect of T and M on cooking degree will depend on the relative magnitude of the effect of each factor. For extrusion conditions corresponding to low CD, native and gelatinized granules predominate, while fragments of granules and macromolecule dispersions predominate for conditions corresponding to high CD.

Maize is the most common raw material used to produce extrusion expanded snacks, but in recent years rice has become important because of its neutral flavor, white color, high digestibility, and hypoallergenic characteristics.[43–45] On the other hand, it is known that cereal proteins are deficient in lysine but have a good content of methionine, and because young people, particularly children, are the main consumers of these kind of products, efforts have been made to improve their nutritional value.[15,46–49]

A variety of legumes have been used in extruded cereal products, including, for example, *Cicer* arietinum,[37,50–52] *Glycine* max,[53,54] *Lupinus albus*,[54–56] *Phaseolus* lunatus,[57] and, mainly, *Phaseolus vulgaris*.[50,58–66] In the case of the *Fabae* family, only *L. sativus* and *V. faba* have been studied in extruded products.[50,55,56,60,67–69] Therefore, this work will be about obtaining and studying extrudates from some wild species of the *Lathyrus* and *Vicia* genera because extrusion not only produces nutritional food combining cereals and legumes but is also a good way to remove antinutritional components from legumes.[60,70–74] Lipoxygenase inactivation before legume grain grinding has been proved to be a necessary step for improvement of the sensory characteristics of legume-based extruded products.[17]

Even though the use of extrusion has been recognized as appropriate technology for the production of precooked cereal-based products, some restrictions have to be mentioned, particularly for the case of the single-screw extruder: (1) the particle size of the material fed to the extruder has to be controlled, so as to avoid a broad particle size distribution; (2) a maximum limit exists for oil and moisture content, depending on the extruder design. In our case, long wide-grain low amylose brown rice and the wild legumes selected were converted into grits, and then mixtures of rice/legume at a ratio of 85:15 were prepared for extrusion experiments. This ratio was considered appropriate for a good quality product, according to previous work, since an improvement in protein value is obtained without impairing the sensory attributes of the expanded product.

EXTRUDED PRODUCTS

Among wild taxons of the genera *Lathyrus* and *Vicia* studied, those corresponding to *L. annuus, L. clymenum, V. lutea* subsp. *lutea* var. *hirta*, and *V. sativa* subsp. *sativa*, were selected to be used in the production of brown rice-based expanded products which, besides their nutritional improvement, would be suitable for those suffering from celiac disease.

Each legume sample was treated to inactivate lipoxygenase, by immersing the beans in boiling water for 2 minutes and then immediately cooling them with tap water. Treated beans were dried in an oven at 50°C until they reached 9–10% moisture, and then ground with a rolling mill (Vario Miag, Germany), care being taken not to produce too many fine particles (below <250 μm). The particle size of the final grits was 420–250 μ, with less than 1% of the particles being below 250 μm.

In addition, a commercial sample of low amylose long wide-grain brown rice, having 13% moisture content, was milled according to a milling diagram developed in our laboratory;[75] this produced grits with a particle size of 1190–420 μm, which is considered adequate for the extrusion process.

The extrusion process was carried out with a Brabender 20 DN single-screw extruder, using a 4:1 compression ratio screw, a 3/20-mm (diameter/length) die, and a screw speed of 150 rpm. Each rice/legume grits mixture (85:15) sample was conditioned to 14% moisture 1 hour before each run. The feeding rate of the extruder was at full capacity. While the extruder feeding section was kept cool by circulating water through the jacketed device, the metering and die sections were both maintained at 175°C by using the heat control device of the extruder. These extrusion conditions were also previously tested so as to obtain a good expansion level.

Extruded Products: Physical Characterization

Extruded samples were obtained as soon as the stationary condition was reached, torque and mass output being measured simultaneously. Torque (exerted on the extruder axle as the material is being transported through the extruder) and mass output are extrusion responses which depend not only on the processing extrusion conditions but also on the material being extruded. These responses are used to determine the specific mechanical energy consumption (SMEC)[26,76] using the following formula: $SMEC\ (J/g) = k \times T \times N/Qa$, where k is 61.6×10^{-3}; T is torque in Brabender units (BU); N is screw rpm, and Qa (g/min) is the mass output, referred to as the feeding moisture level. The value of k takes into account unit conversion and constants. Table 33.1 shows that SMEC decreases as legume is added to rice, the effect corresponding to R+LC showing the highest values. Pérez-Navarrete and colleagues[57] and Ruíz-Ruíz and colleagues[77] observed a similar tendency when *Phaseolus lunatus* or *Phaseolus vulgaris* was added to maize grits. This effect could be attributed to the lower mechanical hardness of legume particles in comparison to rice particles, which in turn would reduce friction inside the extruder, and consequently a lower amount of mechanical energy would be consumed.[78] A reduction in SMEC would indicate a reduction of cooking degree (CD) in the starch fraction and, presumably, a lower degree of starch granule destruction.[26]

TABLE 33.1 Physical Characteristics Corresponding to Rice/Legume Extruded Samples[†]

Sample	SMEC (J/g)	Expansion	Density (g/cm³)	Hard-ness	Solubility (%)
Rice	689.7[d]	3.46 ± 0.09[b]	0.143 ± 0.01[a]	7	39.3 ± 0.22[ab]
R+LA	611.4[b]	3.20 ± 0.06[a]	0.147 ± 0.01[c]	8	40.6 ± 0.41[b]
R+LC	577.5[a]	3.22 ± 0.04[a]	0.146 ± 0.00[bc]	8	42.5 ± 0.10[c]
R+VH	626.9[bc]	3.26 ± 0.14[a]	0.145 ± 0.01[b]	8	40.4 ± 0.60[b]
R+VS	656.1[c]	3.36 ± 0.06[ab]	0.142 ± 0.00[a]	8	38.7 ± 0.24[a]

R, rice; LA, *L. annuus*; LC, *L. clymenum*; VH, *V. lutea* var. *hirta*; VS, *V. sativa* subsp. *sativa*.

[†] *Average ± SD; different letters indicate significant differences (P < 0.05) within the same column.*

Physical characterization of expanded products has to be performed in order to estimate consumer acceptability.[29,79–81] Some of these characteristics are expansion rate, density, and texture (determined on extrudates) and water solubility (determined on extrudate flour). All are related to the cooking degree reached by the starch fraction.[78,82] Before physical characterization, samples were air-dried in an oven at 50°C until a moisture content of about 8% was reached, this moisture level being considered adequate for physical evaluations. The dried samples were divided into several portions and each portion kept in a hermetically sealed plastic bag until its evaluation.

Expansion

Expansion is one of the most important physical characteristics for expanded snack-like products. It is determined as the ratio between extrudate diameter (D) and die diameter (d): E = D/d. The average of 10 measurements is normally used.[26] The expansion process occurs very rapidly, and is the consequence of "water flashing" from the viscoelastic mass coming out of the extruder die. This process has been discussed by several authors.[78,83–86] During extrusion, pressure inside the extruder is high enough to keep water (moisture) as a liquid. As soon the mass comes out of the extruder die (atmospheric pressure), water is converted into vapor ("flash off") and escapes from the mass, leaving air bubbles in the extrudates; simultaneously, the mass is cooled down and consequently solidifies. The light, porous structure formed is characteristic of expanded products. Wall porous thickness, size, and distribution are affected by several factors, the main ones being the cooking degree (CD) reached by the starch during extrusion, moisture content, and extrudate temperature. All of them affect viscoelasticity and, consequently, the degree of expansion.[78,86] Expansion (E) is not a good indicator of CD because, initially, as CD increases E also increases, but E reaches a maximum value at a certain value of CD, after which E decreases as CD increases further. This effect is attributed to the fact that as CD increases, the porous walls become thinner as a result of a decrease in extrudate viscoelasticity, which in turn leads to a reduction in E.

It is observed (Table 33.1) that the addition of legume to rice reduces expansion, the effect being significant except with *V. sativa* subsp. *sativa*. This reduction effect produced by the addition of legume to cereal was also found by Pérez-Navarrete *et al.*,[57] Anton *et al.*,[65] Patil *et al.*,[87] and Shirani and Ganesharanee[88] working with the legumes *Phaseolus vulgaris*, *Lens culinaris*, *Phaseolus lunatus*, and *Cicer arietinum*, respectively. Although no significant effect was observed among the different legumes used, the same explanation given for SMEC could also be applied to expansion. Another explanation was offered by Martínez-Serna *et al.*[89] and Onwulata *et al.*[90] They suggested that as protein legumes have high hydrophily, they could negatively affect extruding mass elasticity by reducing the available water for starch gelatinization, and so reducing expansion. Nevertheless, expansion values shown by the extruded rice/legumes are in the range of those of commercial snack products.

Density

Extrudate density (D) is obtained by calculating the weight db/volume ratio (g/cm³), corresponding to an extrudate section of about 15 cm long. The average of 10 determinations is normally used. Density is inversely related to the cooking degree of the starch component.[78,91] This effect is attributed to the fact that as CD increases, the porous walls became thinner as a result of a decrease in extrudate viscoelasticity, and as a result a lighter product is obtained. Taking into account the SMEC results and the comments just made, the observed increase in extrudate density as a consequence of legume addition (Table 33.1) was as expected. Such effect was significant in all cases, except for the R+VS sample. A similar tendency was found by other authors – for example, the addition of *Lens culinaris*, *Phaseolus lunatus*, or *Phaseolus vulgaris* to maize produced an increase in extrudate density.[57,65,77,87] Similar results were obtained by Suknark *et al.*[92] and Yagci and Gögüs,[93] working with peanut and hazelnut. Onwulata *et al.*[47,48] and Veronica *et al.*[16] have suggested that any addition of protein and/or fiber to starchy materials would increase density. As in the case of expansion, D values shown by these extruded rice/legumes are in the range of those of commercial snack products.

Texture

Product texture was evaluated by a trained panel (three judges), according to Fritz and colleagues.[17] The score given to each sample was obtained by consensus among the judges. A hardness scale from 1 to 9 (soft to hard) was used, the extremes of which were established using extruded samples. Table 33.1 shows that addition of legumes produced a hardening effect on the extrudate texture, which is in agreement with the result obtained corresponding to expansion and density, and confirming a decrease of cooking degree, in comparison with extruded rice alone. This hardening effect has been also observed by Ruíz-Ruíz et al.,[77] working with maize–*Phaseolus vulgaris* blends; they showed that hardness reflects alveolar wall resistance and the number of alveoli per unit of extrudate thickness, and that these characteristics vary greatly depending on material composition and degree of protein denaturalization.

Water Solubility

Water solubility (S) determination is based on water-dispersible solids and is expressed as the percentage of solids dispersed from a given flour sample. The procedure is well known:[26] 100 g of extruded sample is first ground with a laboratory hammer mill (Retsch GmbH & Co. KG, Haan, Germany) with a 2-mm sieve, and then with a Cyclotec (FOSS, Hillerød, Denmark) mill through a 1-mm sieve. Next, 2.5 g of flour is dispersed in 50 ml water, shaken for 30 minutes and centrifuged at $2000g$; soluble solids are obtained after evaporation in an oven at 105°C.

It has been suggested that water solubility (S) of extruded starchy materials is a good indicator of CD. Several works have shown that S is directly related to SMEC and inversely related to density.[26,78,94,95] In

our case, the addition of legume usually produced an increase in S (Table 33.1), the effect significant being only for R + LC samples. This apparent contradiction in the results of SMEC and D could be explained by considering that the legume itself can supply soluble solids (protein and sugar) to the water phase, contributing to the total solid dispersed from the extruded sample. Although the differences in S values among the extruded samples are small, a correspondence among S, SMEC, and D is observed. For example, rice and R + VS samples, which showed the lowest values of S, also showed the highest SMEC and lowest D, indicating that a reduction in soluble solid coming from the legume is produced as CD increases.

Chemical and Nutritional Characterization of Extruded Samples

Chemical Composition

Table 33.2 shows the differences between the composition of rice flour and rice after extrusion.

In previous experiments, it was observed that extrusion of brown rice under the same extrusion conditions corresponding to those values shown in Table 33.2 caused a decrease in total fiber content. The effect of extrusion on fiber content has been discussed by several researchers. Kasprzack and Rzedzicki,[46] Ruíz-Ruíz et al.,[77] and Frias et al.[96] pointed out that extrusion produces a decrease in total fiber, explaining that during extrusion some components of fiber, such as pectic polymers and cellulose, would undergo degradation reactions, and their fragments, having low molecular weight, may not be determined as fiber with the methodology used. On the other hand, Vasanthan et al.[97] and Pérez-Navarrete et al.[57] found that an increase in fiber occurred after extrusion.

Table 33.3 shows the proximate analysis corresponding to rice and rice/legume extruded samples. There are differences between rice and the rice/legume mixture. Moisture content was around 8%, with some small differences among samples. On the other hand, ash, soluble

TABLE 33.2 Proximate Analysis (% in db) Corresponding to Rice Flour and Rice fter Extrusion[†]

Component	Brown Rice	Extruded Brown Rice
Ash	0.73 ± 0.01^a	1.19 ± 0.01^b
Fat	2.38 ± 0.02^b	0.53 ± 0.15^a
Fiber	4.8 ± 0.01^b	3.81 ± 0.15^a
Protein (N × 6.25)	6.0 ± 0.1^a	7.38 ± 0.1^b

[†] *Average ± SD; different letters indicate significant differences (P < 0.05) within the same column.*

TABLE 33.3 Proximate Analysis (% in db) Corresponding to Rice and Rice/Legume Extruded Samples[†]

	Rice	Rice + LA	Rice + LC	Rice + VH	Rice + VS
Moisture	8.2 ± 0.0^b	8.1 ± 0.1^b	7.9 ± 0.1^a	8.2 ± 0.1^b	8.1 ± 0.0^b
Ash	1.19 ± 0.01^a	1.42 ± 0.02^b	1.44 ± 0.01^c	1.46 ± 0.02^c	1.41 ± 0.15^b
Fat	0.53 ± 0.15^a	0.54 ± 0.14^a	0.81 ± 0.0^{ab}	0.53 ± 0.14^a	1.07 ± 0.0^b
Fiber	3.81 ± 0.1^a	7.51 ± 0.16^c	7.96 ± 0.2^c	7.3 ± 0.02^b	8.16 ± 0.15^c
Solube sugars	0.23 ± 0.0^a	0.32 ± 0.0^b	0.31 ± 0.0^b	0.33 ± 0.0^{bc}	0.35 ± 0.0^c
Protein (N × 6.25)	7.38 ± 0.1^a	10.5 ± 0.5^b	10.1 ± 0.1^b	11.32 ± 0.3^b	10.89 ± 0.3^b

LA, *L. annuus*; LC, *L. clymenum*; VH, *V. lutea* var. *hirta*; VS, *V. sativa* subsp. *sativa*. All expressed in db, except moisture.

[†] *Average ± SD; different letters indicate significant differences (P < 0.05) within the same column.*

sugars, and protein and fiber content increased with the addition of legume, as expected, since legumes are richer in these components in comparison with rice. Even though some significant changes among samples were observed, the values corresponding to each component were in the range expected according to the composition of rice and rice/legume average mixture (85:15) before extrusion. It is important to point out that extruded rice/legume mixtures showed an increase of almost 50% in protein and about twice the fiber content in comparison with extruded rice, confirming that a significant nutritional improvement could be obtained in rice extruded products by only 15% rice replacement.

Amino Acid Content

Table 33.4 shows the difference between amino acid content (g/100) of brown rice before and after extrusion (average±SD) and the FAO[98] reference for essential amino acids (proposed for preschool children). It is observed that some essential amino acids (phenylalanine, histidine, isoleucine, leucine, lysine, and valine) decreased significantly after extrusion, while other essential amino acids remained unchanged.

Even though these results indicate that extrusion processes affect the amino acid pattern of brown rice, under the conditions used in this experiment, FAO[98] requirements (proposed for preschool children) are satisfied for all essential amino acids except for lysine and, to some extent, histidine.

When the protein quality of a mixture of cereals and legumes is analyzed, special attention has to be given to the content of the sulfur amino acids (methionine and cysteine), lysine, and tryptophan with respect to the FAO[98] reference proposed for preschool children, since legume proteins would be deficient in sulfur amino acids and tryptophan, and cereal proteins deficient in lysine.[10,11] As is well known, a more balanced protein is obtained when cereal and legumes are mixed.[13–15,49]

Table 33.5 shows how much the amino acid pattern of extruded rice is affected by a 15% replacement with each of the wild legumes used. Two of the genus Lathyrus (L. annuus and L. clymenum) and two of the genus Vicia (V. lutea subsp. lutea var. hirta and V. sativa subsp. sativa) showed no significant differences except in methionine, tryptophan, cysteine, and lysine. Methionine and cysteine content decreased in all cases. However, the level reached for total sulfur amino acids does not differ too much from FAO[98] requirements. The same comment applies to tryptophan. In the case of lysine, its content increased by about 30% but the level reached was still not enough to satisfy FAO[98] requirements, indicating that a higher replacement level should be used; however, this could impair the sensory properties of the final expanded products and, furthermore, may result in a deficiency in sulfur amino acids. Regarding the content of the other essential amino acids, it can be said that the FAO[98] requirement is satisfied.

In the case of non-essential amino acids, only arginine showed significant differences between Rice + VH and the other samples. The only exception was Rice + VS, where there were no significant differences. These non-homogeneous effects on the amino acid patterns of extruded rice mixtures, resulting from the addition of wild legumes and also observed with essential amino acids, are difficult to explain. Singh et al.[99] have suggested that each amino acid would respond in a different manner according to the extrusion conditions and for each particular sample. These comments tend to explain why the amino acid patterns of extruded mixtures do not follow exactly the arithmetical rules that would be used to calculate the amino acid content of mixtures using amino acid values of the corresponding raw materials.

TABLE 33.4 Amino Acid Composition (g/100 g) of Brown Rice Before and After Extrusion and FAO Reference for Essential Amino Acids (Proposed for Preschool Children)[†]

		Rice	Extruded Rice	FAO
Essential amino acids	Cys	1.6±0.3	2.0±0.1	
	Phe*	5.4±0.0[b]	5.0±0.0[a]	
	His**	2.2±0.0[b]	1.7±0.1[a]	1.9
	Ile*	3.5±0.1[b]	2.8±0.0[a]	2.8
	Leu*	9.2±0.1[b]	8.9±0.0[a]	6.6
	Lys*	3.8±0.0[b]	3.3±0.4[a]	5.8
	Met	1.8±0.3	1.6±0.0	2.5 (Met+Cys)
	Tyr*	2.2±0.5[a]	3.2±0.1[b]	6.3 (Phe+Tyr)
	Thr	4.2±0.0	3.9±0.1	3.4
	Trp	1.2±0.0	1.5±0.1	1.1
	Val*	5.5±0.1[b]	4.5±0.2[a]	3.5
Non-essential amino acids	Ala	6.3±0.1	6.3±0.1	
	Arg	8.3±0.1	8.2±0.1	
	Asp	9.9±0.3	10.7±0.2	
	Gly*	5.8±0.1[b]	5.2±0.0[a]	
	Glu	21.2±0.2	20.8±0.0	
	Pro	3.8±0.7	4.8±0.4	
	Ser	5.6±0.1	5.7±0.3	

Cys, cysteine; Phe, phenilanine; His, histidine; Ile, isoleucine; Leu, leucine; Lys, lysine; Met, methionine; Tyr, tyrosine; Thr, threonine; Trp, thryptophane; Val, valine; Ala, alanine; Arg, arginine; Asp, aspartic acid; Gly, glycine; Glu, glutamic acid; Pro, proline; Ser, serine.

[†] Average ± SD; different letters indicate significant differences within the same column.
* P < 0.05, **P < 0.01.

TABLE 33.5 Amino Acid Composition (g/100 g) of Extruded Samples and FAO Reference for Essential Amino Acids (Proposed for Preschool Children)[†]

	Amino Acid	Rice	Rice + *LA*	Rice + *LC*	Rice + *VH*	Rice + *VS*	FAO
Essential amino acids	Cys*	2.0 ± 0.1^b	1.3 ± 0.4^a	1.3 ± 0.1^a	1.5 ± 0.1^a	1.2 ± 0.3^a	
	Phe	5.0 ± 0.1	4.9 ± 0.4	4.6 ± 0.1	4.9 ± 0.0	4.8 ± 0.2	
	His	1.7 ± 0.1	2.2 ± 0.3	1.8 ± 0.0	2.0 ± 0.1	2.0 ± 0.0	1.9
	Ile	2.8 ± 0.0	3.7 ± 1.1	2.9 ± 0.0	3.0 ± 0.1	2.9 ± 0.0	2.8
	Leu	8.9 ± 0.0	8.4 ± 0.5	8.9 ± 0.1	8.3 ± 0.2	8.5 ± 0.1	6.6
	Lys**	3.3 ± 0.3^a	4.4 ± 0.1^b	4.7 ± 0.1^b	4.6 ± 0.1^b	4.6 ± 0.8^b	5.8
	Met*	1.6 ± 0.0^b	1.1 ± 0.2^a	1.0 ± 0.0^a	1.1 ± 0.0^a	0.9 ± 0.2^a	2.5 (Met + Cys)
	Tyr	3.2 ± 0.1	2.9 ± 0.1	3.0 ± 0.1	2.9 ± 0.1	2.9 ± 0.1	6.3 (Phe + Ter)
	Thr	3.9 ± 0.1	4.4 ± 0.3	4.0 ± 0.0	4.3 ± 0.1	4.3 ± 0.1	3.4
	Trp**	1.5 ± 0.1^b	1.0 ± 0.0^a	1.1 ± 0.0^{ab}	1.0 ± 0.1^a	1.0 ± 0.1^a	1.1
	Val	4.5 ± 0.2	4.4 ± 0.4	4.1 ± 0.0	4.6 ± 0.1	4.3 ± 0.3	3.5
Non-essential amino acids	Ala	6.3 ± 0.1	6.6 ± 1.1	5.7 ± 0.1	5.4 ± 0.1	5.6 ± 0.1	
	Arg*	8.2 ± 0.1^a	8.5 ± 0.3^a	8.4 ± 0.1^a	9.4 ± 0.3^b	8.6 ± 0.2^{ab}	
	Asp	10.7 ± 0.2	11.0 ± 0.4	11.6 ± 0.2	11.1 ± 0.6	11.6 ± 0.4	
	Gly	5.2 ± 0.0	5.2 ± 0.0	5.1 ± 0.0	5.0 ± 0.1	5.2 ± 0.2	
	Glu	20.8 ± 0.0	20.4 ± 1.7	21.0 ± 0.2	20.3 ± 0.1	21.6 ± 0.2	
	Pro	4.8 ± 0.4	3.8 ± 0.2	4.8 ± 1.3	4.6 ± 1.4	4.2 ± 0.5	
	Ser	5.7 ± 0.3	5.8 ± 0.1	6.0 ± 0.0	6.0 ± 0.2	5.8 ± 0.2	

Cys, cysteine; Phe, phenilanine; His, histidine; Ile, isoleucine; Leu, leucine; Lys, lysine; Met, methionine; Tyr, tyrosine; Thr, threonine; Trp, thryptophane; Val, valine; Ala, alanine; Arg, arginine; Asp, aspartic acid; Gly, glycine; Glu, glutamic acid; Pro, proline; Ser, serine.

[†] *Average ± SD; different letters indicate significant differences within the same column.*

* $P < 0.05$, **$P < 0.01$.

In Vitro Protein Digestibility

According to the FAO,[98] protein digestibility (PD) is considered one of the most important properties of protein quality. In general, the cooking process positively affects protein digestibility; Table 33.6 shows values of *in vitro* protein digestibility (PDiV) corresponding to extruded samples (brown rice and its wild legume mixtures). It is observed that the addition of legumes did not significantly affect the PDiV of extruded brown rice. However, extrusion cooking produced an increase in the PDiV of brown rice, since its value before extrusion was 80%. This positive effect was attributed to the heat and shear treatments involved during extrusion, which would cause protein denaturation and, consequently, an improvement in protease accessibility.[99–102]

These results are in agreement with those of other workers.[57–59] For example, the PDiV in "snacks" obtained from *V. faba, Phaseolus vulgaris*, or maize–*Phaseolus lunatus* mixture varied between 81% and 84.8%. However, Van der Poel *et al.*[103] and Alonso *et al.*[59] reported

TABLE 33.6 *In Vitro* Protein Digestibility (PdiV) Corresponding to Extruded Samples (Brown Rice and Wild Legume Mixtures)[†]

Extruded Samples	PDiV (%)
Rice*	84.1 ± 0.5
Rice + *L. annuus*	82.5 ± 1.7
Rice + *L. clymenum*	82.8 ± 0.2
Rice + *V. lutea* var. *hirta*	82.6 ± 2.1
Rice + *V. sativa* subsp. *sativa*	85.3 ± 0.9

[†] *Average ± SD.*

* *Protein digestibility of brown rice before extrusion was 80%.*

values for *V. faba* of 94.8% and 87.4%, respectively. These differences can be attributed to differences in the methodology and raw material used, and also to different extrusion conditions. Nevertheless, the PDiV values obtained for the extruded whole rice–wild legume mixture are high enough for a good protein quality.

Total Phenolic Compound Contents

Table 33.7 shows the phenolic compound contents corresponding to extruded samples. Addition of legume did not produce significant changes to extruded rice, although the extrusion process significantly reduced phenolic content, since the original content of brown rice was 1.07 mg/g and those of legumes were even much higher. Pastor-Cavada et al.[104,105] reported values for *L. annuus* (4.6 mg/g), *L. clymenum* (6.2 mg/g), *V. lutea* subsp. *lutea* var. *hirta* (2.1 mg/g), and *V. sativa* subsp. *sativa* (21.3 mg/g). This negative effect of extrusion was also observed by others,[65,106–108] indicating that phenolic compounds undergo degradation reactions under the extrusion conditions used in this study.

Potential Availability of Minerals

Table 33.8 shows the results of iron and zinc content (mg/kg), their potential availability (%), and their potential supply (PS, %) for a 30-g portion corresponding to extruded samples.

The RDI (recommended daily intake) of a nutrient is always above its actual requirement, since the nutritional recommendation is calculated using factors related to environmental factors, and the individual variability and bioavailability of such nutrients in the diet.[109] The expression of the potential supply of a nutrient takes into account the availability and thus the contribution from a particular food.

Iron content increased significantly ($P < 0.01$) with the addition of legumes, since legumes are considered to be iron-rich materials. Several researchers have also observed this positive effect of the addition of legumes to cereals.[110–112] DFe% also increased with the addition of legumes, although no significant differences ($P < 0.05$) were observed for the Rice + LA and Rice + VS samples. Drago et al.[63] also observed an improvement in iron dialyzability when dehulled *P. vulgaris* was added to whole corn flour in a 50:50 ratio (11.6% vs 10.5%).

It is estimated that 1.8 mg of iron per day is necessary to meet the needs of 80–90% of adult women, and adolescents of both sexes.[113] This value was used to estimate the potential supply of Fe (PS_{Fe}). Regarding these values, extruded rice–legume mixtures would provide from 2.6–5.7% of the requirements per 30-g serving.

Zinc content, similarly to iron, increased significantly ($P < 0.01$) with the addition of legumes, as was expected, since the Zn content of legumes is higher than that of cereals. Several researchers have also observed this positive effect of the addition of legumes to cereals.

It is also observed that DZn% values corresponding to extruded mixtures were higher than that of extruded rice, although no significant differences ($P < 0.01$) were found for Rice + VC and Rice + VH samples. Regarding the potential supply of Zn (PS_{Zn}), the values were higher in extruded mixtures than in extruded rice. In the case of this mineral, the daily requirements for adults are 2.2 mg/day.[114] A 30-g portion of extruded mixture would supply about 3.6% of those recommendations.

It is interesting to point out that the DFe% and DZn% values obtained for extruded samples (whole rice and its mixtures with wild legumes) are not low, despite the presence of phytates, which are known as mineral absorption inhibitors.[115–117] Drago et al.[63] have demonstrated the positive effect of extrusion cooking on mineral dialyzability, explaining that during extrusion a

TABLE 33.7 Total Phenolic Compound Contents (mg/g) Corresponding to Extruded Samples[†]

Extruded Samples	Polyphenols Content (mg/g)
Rice	0.36 ± 0.02
Rice + *L. annuus*	0.28 ± 0.02
Rice + *L. clymenum*	0.47 ± 0.10
Rice + *V. lutea* var. *hirta*	0.39 ± 0.03
Rice + *V. sativa* subsp. *sativa*	0.42 ± 0.03

[†] *Average ± SD.*

TABLE 33.8 Mineral Content (mg/kg), Potential Mineral Availability (%) and % Potential Mineral Supply (in 30 g portion) Corresponding to Extruded Samples[†]

Extruded Samples	Fe (mg/kg)	DFe (%)	PS Fe (%)*	Zn (mg/kg)	DZn (%)	PS_{Zn} (%)**
Rice	14.8 ± 1.4^a	7.4 ± 0.0^a	1.7	17.6 ± 0.8^a	10.0 ± 1.3^a	2.1
Rice + LA	22.5 ± 1.2^c	9.3 ± 0.0^{ab}	3.26	19.4 ± 0.3^{ab}	14.6 ± 0.4^c	3.6
Rice + LC	17.2 ± 0.5^b	10.0 ± 0.5^b	2.6	20.1 ± 0.6^b	13.8 ± 0.1^{bc}	3.5
Rice + VH	21.0 ± 0.8^c	16.3 ± 2.8^c	5.7	23.9 ± 1.7^c	12.4 ± 0.5^{ab}	3.7
Rice + VS	24.6 ± 1.2^c	9.4 ± 2.6^{ab}	3.5	24.1 ± 1.1^c	12.3 ± 0.2^{ab}	3.7

Potential availability of Zn and Fe, DZn% and DFe%; potential supply of Zn and Fe, PS_{Zn} and PS_{Fe}. LA, L. annuus; LC, L. clymenum; VH, V. lutea subsp. lutea var. hirta; VS, V. sativa subsp. sativa.

* P < 0.05, **P < 0.01.

[†] *Average ± SD; different letters indicate significant differences within the same column.*

partial degradation of phytates occurs and polyphenols would also lose their chelating properties.[118]

CONCLUSIONS

Extruded products based on whole rice with the addition of wild legumes offer four main advantages: they are whole grain food grade, they have a better nutritional quality than traditional extruded cereal products, they are made with grains with such a small amount of gluten that they can almost be considered "gluten-free" cereals, and, finally, the fact that they are made with wild legumes makes them innovative products.

References

1. Smith BD. *The Emergence of Agriculture*. New York, NY: W H Freeman & Co; 1998.
2. Juliano BO. *The rice grain and its gross composition. Rice: Chemistry and Technology*. St Paul, MN: AACC; 1985. p. 17–57.
3. Bean MM, Nishita KD. Rice flours for baking. In: Juliano BO, editor. *Rice Chemistry and Technology*. St Paul, MN: AACC; 1985. p. 539–56.
4. Juliano BO, Sakurai J. Miscellaneous rice products. In: Juliano BO, editor. *Rice Chemistry and Technology*. St Paul, MN: AACC; 1985. p. 569–18.
5. González RJ, Torres RL, De Greef DM. Comportamiento a la cocción de variedades de arroz y maíz utilizando el amilógrafo y dos diseños de extrusores. *Inform Tecnol* 1998;9:35–43.
6. Deshpande SS, Campbell CG. Genotype variation in BOAA, condensed tannins, phenolics and enzyme inhibitors of grass pea (*Lathryus sativus*). *Can J Plant Sci* 1992;72:1037–47.
7. Boateng J, Verghese M, Walker L, Ogutu S. Effect of processing on antioxidant contents in selected dry beans (*Phaseolus* spp. L.). *LWT-Food Sci Technol* 2008;41:1541–7.
8. Tosh SM, Yada S. Dietary fibers in pulse seeds and fractions: characterization, functional attributes and applications. *Food Res Int* 2010;43:450–60.
9. Gepts P, Beavis WD, Brummer EC, Shoemaker RC, Stalker HT, Weeden NF, et al. Legumes as a model plant family. Genomic for food and feed report of the Cross-Legume Advances through Genomics Conference. *Plant Physiol* 2005;137:1228–35.
10. Farzana W, Khalil IA. Protein quality of tropical food legumes. *J Sci Technol* 1999;23:13–9.
11. Wang TL, Domoney C, Hedley CL, Casey R, Grusak MA. Can we improve the nutritional quality of legume seeds? *Plant Physiol* 2003;131:886–91.
12. Drago SR, González RJ, Chel-Guerrero L, Valencia ME. Evaluación de la Disponibilidad de Minerales en Harinas de Frijol y en Mezclas de Maíz/Frijol Extrudidas. *Rev Inform Tecnol* 2007;18(1):41–6.
13. Cheftel JC, Cuq JL, Lorient D. *Proteínas alimentarias*. Acribia S.A: Zaragoza; 1989.
14. Berrios JJ. Extrusion cooking of legumes: Dry bean flours. *Enc Agr Food Biol Engn* 2006;1:1–8.
15. Liu Y, Hsieh F, Heymann H, Huff HE. Effect of process conditions on the physical and sensory properties of extruded oat-corn puff. *J Food Sci* 2000;65:1253–9.
16. Veronica AO, Olusola OO, Adebowale EA. Qualities of extruded puffed snacks from maize/soybean mixture. *J Food Proc Engn* 2006;29:149–61.
17. Fritz M, González RJ, Carrara C, De Greef DM, Torres RL, Chel L. Selección de las condiciones de extrusión, para una mezcla maíz-frijol: aspectos sensoriales y operativos. *Braz J Food Technol* 2006: 3–7 Edición Especial III JIPCA.
18. Sosa-Moguel O, Ruíz-Ruíz J, Martínez-Ayala A, González R, Drago S, Betancur-Ancona D, et al. Effect of extrusion conditions and lipoxygenase inactivation treatment on the physical and nutritional properties of corn/cowpea (*Vigna unguiculata*) blends. *Int J Food Sci Nutr* 2009;60(S7):341–54.
19. Linko P, Colonna P, Mercier C. High temperature, short time extrusion-cooking. *Adv Cereal Sci Technol* 1981;4 145–35.
20. Wiedman W, Strobel E. Processing and economic advantages of extrusion cooking in comparison with conventional processing in the food industry. In: O'Connor C, editor. *Extrusion technology for the food industry*. New York, NY: Elsevier Applied Science; 1987. p. 132–69.
21. Anton AA, Luciano FB. Instrumental textural evaluation of extruded snack foods: A review. *Ciencia Tecnol Alime* 2007;54:245–51.
22. Bouzaza D, Arhaliass A, Bouvier JM. Die design and dough expansion in low moisture extrusion cooking procesess. *J Food Engn* 1996;29(2):139–52.
23. Fornal L, Majewska K, Wicklund T. The quality of oat extrudates. *Acta Acad Agric Tech Olst Technol Aliment* 1998;30:119–26.
24. Huber G. Snack foods from cooking extruders. In: Lucas RW, Rooney LW, editors. *Snacks Food Processing*. Boca Raton, FL: CRC Press; 2001.
25. Pansawat N, Jangchud K, Jangchud A, Wuttijumnong P, Saalia FK, Eitenmiller RR, et al. Effects of extrusion condition on secondary extrusion variables and physical properties of fish, rice-based snacks. *LWT-Food Sci Technol* 2008;41:632–41.
26. González RJ, Torres RL, De Greef DM. Extrusión-Cocción de Cereales. *Bol Soc Bras Cienc Tecnol Alime* 2002;36(2): 104–15.
27. Harper JM. *Extrusion of food*. Boca Raton, FL: CRC Press; 1981.
28. Fast RB. Manufacturing technology of ready to eat cereals. In: Fast RB, Caldwell EF, editors. *Breakfast cereals and how they are made*. St Paul, MN: AACC; 1991. p. 15–42.
29. Tahnoven R, Hietanen A, Sankelo T, Kortaniemi VM, Laakso P, Kallio H. Snack foods. *Lebensm Unter Forsch* 1998;206:360–3.
30. Colonna P, Buleon A, Mercier C. Physically modified starches. In: Galliard T, editor. *Starch: Properties and Potential*. London, UK: J. Wiley & Sons; 1987. p. 79–114.
31. Biliaderis C. The structure and modification of starch with food constituent. *Can J Physiol Pharm* 1991;69:60–78.
32. Kokini JL, Chang CN, Lai LS. The rol of rheological properties on extrudate expansion. In: Kokini JL, Ho CT, Karwe MV, editors. *Food Extrusion Science and Technology*. New York, NY: Marcel Dekker; 1992. p. 631–51.
33. Rhee KS, Kim ES, Kim BK, Jung BM, Rhee KC. Extrusion of minced catfish with corn and defatted soy flours for snack foods. *J Food Process Pres* 2004;28:288–90.
34. Rackis JJ, Wolf WJ, Backer EC. Protease inhibitors in plants food: Content and inactivation. In: Friedman M, editor. *Nutritional and toxicological significance of enzymes inhibitors in food*. New York, NY: Plenum; 1986. 299–47.
35. Edwards RH, Becker R, Mossman AP, Gray GM, Whiteland LC. Twin extrusion cooking of small white beans (Phaseolus vulgaris). *LWT-Food Sci Technol* 1994;27(5):472–81.
36. Steel CJ, Sgarbieri VC, Jackis MH. Use of extrusion technology to overcome undersirable properties of hard-to-cook dry beans (*Phaseolus vulgaris* L.). *J Agr Food Chem* 1995;43:2487–92.
37. Ummadi P, Chenoweth WL, Uebersax MA. The influence of extrusion processing on iron dialyzability, phytates and tannins in legumes. *J Food Process Pres* 1995;19:119–31.

38. Torres RL. *Estudio de las Características Fisicoquímicas de diferentes Genotipos (Cultivares) de Maíz y el Comportamiento durante la Extrusión Termoplástica*. Master Thesis on Food Science and Technology. Chemical Engineering Faculty. Santa Fe, Argentina: Universidad Nacional del Litoral; 2005.

39. Ramírez JL, Wanderlei C. Efecto de los parámetros de extrusión, características de pasta y textura de pellets (snacks de tercera generación) producidos a partir de trigo y maíz. *Alimentaria* 1998;9:93–7.

40. González RJ, De Greef DM, Torres RL, Robuti J, Borrás F. Effects of endosperm hardness and extrusion temperature on properties of products obtained with grits from two commercial maize cultivars. *LWT-Food Sci Technol* 2003;37:193–8.

41. Fernandes dos Santos M, Sin-Huei W, Ascheri JL, Ramírez C. Puffed extruded corn-grits and soybean mixtures for snack use. *Pesqui Agropecu Bras* 2002;37(10):1495–501.

42. Haller D, González RJ, Drago S, Torres RL, De Greef DM. *Harina de maíz para tortillas: Efectos de la dureza del endospermo y de las variables de extrusión, revista de la Facultad de Ingeniería Química (Vol. 52, in press)*. Mexico: Chel Guerrero, UADY, Yucatan; 2012.

43. Bryant RJ, Kadan RS, Champagne TE, Vinyard BT, Boykin D. Functional and digestive characteristics of extruded rice flour. *Cereal Chem* 2001;78:131–7.

44. Kadan RS, Bryant RJ, Pepperman AB. Functional properties of extruded rice flours. *Cereal Chem* 2003;68:1669–72.

45. Saccheti G, Pinnavaia GG, Guidolin E, Dalla Rosa M. Effects of extrusion temperature and feed composition on the functional, physical and sensory properties of chestnut and rice flour-based snack-like products. *Food Res Int* 2004;37:527–34.

46. Kasprzack M, Rzedzicki Z. Application of everlasting pea goléemela in extrusion-cooking technology. *Int Agrophys* 2008;22:339–47.

47. Onwulata CL, Konstance RP, Smith PW, Holsinger VH. Co-extrusion of dietary fiber and milk proteins in expanded corn products. *LWT-Food Sci Technol* 2001;34:424–9.

48. Onwulata CL, Smith PW, Konstance RP, Hosinger VH. Incorporation of whey products in extruded corn, potato or rice snacks. *Food Res Int* 2001;34:679–87.

49. Rampersad R, Badrie N, Comissiong E. Physico-chemical and sensory characteristics of flavoured snacks from extruded cassava/pigeonpea flour. *J Food Sci* 2003;68:363–7.

50. Abd El-Hady EA, Habiba RA. Effect of soaking and extrusion conditions on antinutrients and protein digestibility of legume seeds. *LWT-Food Sci Technol* 2003;36:285–93.

51. Lazou AE, Michailidis PA, Thymi S, Krokida MK, Bisharat GI. Structural properties of corn-legume based extrudates as a function of processing conditions and raw material characteristics. *Int J Food Prop* 2007;10:721–38.

52. Brenes A, Viveros A, Centeno C, Arija I, Marzo F. Nutritional value of raw and extruded chickpeas (*Cicer arietinum* L.) for growing chickens. *Span J Agric Res* 2008;6(4):537–45.

53. Baskaran V, Bhattacharaya S. Nutritional status of the protein of corn-soy based extruded products evaluated by rat bioassay. *Plant Food Hum Nutr* 2004;59:101–4.

54. Solanas EM, Castrillo C, Jover M, de Vega A. Effect of extrusion on *in situ* ruminal protein degradability and *in vitro* digestibility of undergraded protein from different feedstuffs. *J Sci Food Agr* 2008;88:2589–97.

55. Masoero F, Pulimeno AM, Rossi F. Effect of extrusion, espansion and toasting on the nutritional value of peas, faba beans and lupins. *Ital J Anim Sci* 2005;4:177–89.

56. Díaz D, Morlacchini M, Masoero F, Moschini M, Fusconi G, Piva G. Pea seeds (*Pisum sativum*), faba beans (*Vicia faba* var *minor*) and lupin seeds (*Lupinus albus* var *multitalia*) as protein sources in broiler diets: effect of extrusion on growth performance. *Ital J Anim Sci* 2006;5:43–53.

57. Pérez-Navarrete C, González R, Chel-Guerrero L, Betancur-Ancona D. Effect of extrusion on nutritional quality of maize and lima bean flour blends. *J Sci Food Agr* 2006;86:2477–84.

58. Balandrán-Quintana RR, Barbosa-Cánovas GV, Zazueta-Morales JJ, Anzaldúa-Morales A, Quintero-Ramos A. Functional and nutritional properties of extruded whole pinto bean meal (*Phaseolus vulgaris* L.). *J Food Sci* 1998;63(1):113–6.

59. Alonso R, Grant G, Dewey P, Marzo F. Nutritional assesment *in vitro* and *in vitro* of raw and extruded peas (*Pisum sativum* L.). *J Agr Food Chem* 2000;68:2286–90.

60. Alonso R, Aguirre AF. Effects of extrusion and traditional processing methods on antinutrients and *in vitro* digestibility of protein and starch in faba and kidney beans. *Food Chem* 2000;68:159–65.

61. Tharanathan RN, Mahadevamma S. A review: Grain legumes a boon to human nutrition. *Trends Food Sci Tech* 2003;14:507–18.

62. Arija I, Centeno C, Viveros A, Brenes A, Marzo F, Illera JC, et al. Nutritional evaluation of raw and extruded kidney bean (*Phaseolus vulgaris* L. var. *pinto*) in chicken diets. *Poultry Sci* 2006;85:635–44.

63. Drago SR, Velasco-González OH, Torres RL, González RJ, Valencia ME. Effect of the extrusion on functional properties and mineral dialyzability from *Phaseolus vulgaris* bean flour. *Plant Food Hum Nutr* 2007;62:43–8.

64. Anton AA, Ross KA, Beta T, Fulcher RG, Arntfield SD. Effect of predehulling treatments on some physical and nutritional properties of navy and pinto beans (*Phaseolus vulgaris* L.). *LWT-Food Sci Technol* 2008;41:771–8.

65. Anton AA, Fulcher RG, Arntfield SD. Physical and nutritional impact of fortification of corn starch-based extruded snacks with common bean (*Phaseolus vulgaris* L.) flour: Effects of bean addition and extrusion cooking. *Food Chem* 2009;113:989–96.

66. Nyombaire G, Siddiq M, Dolan KD. Physico-chemical and sensory quality of extruded light red kidney bean (*Phaseolus vulgaris* L.) porridge. *LWT-Food Sci Technol* 2011;44 1597–02.

67. Lambein F, Kuo YH. *Lathyrus sativus, a neolithic crop with a modern future? An overview of the present situation. Proc. Int. Symp. Lathyrus sativus – cultivation and nutritive value in animal and human*. Poland: Lublin-Radom; 1997.

68. Grela ER, Jensen SK, Jakobsen K. Fatty acid composition and content of tocopherols and carotenoids in raw and extruded grass pea (*Lathyrus sativus* L). *J Sci Food Agr* 1999;79:2075–8.

69. Kasprzak M, Rzedzicki Z. Effect of bath temperature and soaking time on the dynamics of water holding capacity of everlasting pea-wheat extrudates. *Int Agrophys* 2007;21:241–8.

70. Artz WE, Warren C, Villota R. Twin-screw extrusion modification of a corn fiber and corn starch extruded blend. *J Food Sci* 1990;55:746–50.

71. Arêas JAG. Extrusion of food proteins. *Crit Rev Food Sci* 1992;32:365–92.

72. Alonso R, Orúe E, Marzo F. Effects of extrusión and conventional processing methods on protein and antinutritional factor contents in pea seeds. *Food Chem* 1998;63:505–12.

73. Quintana RBR, Cánovas GVB, Morales JJZ, Morales AA, Ramos AQ. Functional and nutritional properties of extruded whole pinto bean meal (*Phaseolus vulgaris* L.). *J Food Sci* 1998;63(1):113–6.

74. Shimelis EA, Rakshit SK. Effect of processing on antinutrients and *in vitro* digestibility of kidney bean (*Phaseolus vulgaris* L.) varieties grown in East Africa. *Food Chem* 2007;103:161–72.

75. Robutti JL, Borras FS, González RJ, Torres RL, De Greef DM. Endosperm properties and extrusion cooking behaviour of maize cultivars. *LWT-Food Sci Technol* 2002;35:663–9.

76. González RJ, Torres RL, De Greef DM, Bonaldo AG. Effect of extrusion conditions and structural characteristics on melt viscosity of starchy materials. *J Food Engn* 2006;74:96–107.

77. Ruíz-Ruíz J, Martínez-Ayala A, Drago S, González R, Bentancur-Ancona D, Chel-Guerrero L. Extrusion of a hard-to-cook vean (*Phaseolus vulgaris* L.) and quality protein maize (*Zea mays* L.) flour blend. *LWT-Food Sci Technol* 2008;41:1799–07.

78. González RJ, Torres RL, De Greef DM, Drago SR, Cuggino MI, Chel Guerrero LA, et al. Extrusión-cocción de una mezcla maíz-vigna unguiculata: factores que afectan las propiedades físicas del extrudido y la viscosidad de las dispersiones de la harina precocida. In: Betancur DA, Chel Guerrero LA, Castellanos Ruelas AF, editors. *Utilización de recursos naturales tropicales para el desarrollo de alimentos, cap13*. Mérida, Mexico: UADY; 2010. p. 172–88.

79. Launay B, Lisch JM. Twin-screw extrusion cooking of starches: Flow behavior of starch pastes, expansion and mechanical properties of extrudates. *J Food Engn* 1983;**2**:259–80.

80. Wagner LR. Some like it hot … and some like it hotter. *Snack World* 1989;**46**:38–40.

81. Jamora JJ, Rhee KS, Rhee KC. Chemical and sensory properties of expanded extrudates from pork meat-defatted soy flour blends with onion, carrot and oat. *J Food Sci Nutr* 2002;**6**:158–62.

82. Díaz AL. *Food quality and properties of quality protein maize*. College Station, TX: MS Thesis. Texas A&M University; 2003.

83. Guy RC, Horne AW. Extrusion and co-extrusion of cereals. In: Blanshard JM, Litchell JV, editors. *Food structure – its creation and evaluation*. London, UK: Butterworths; 1988.

84. Padmanabhan M, Bhattacharya M. Extrudate expansion during extrusion cooking of foods. *Cereal Food World* 1989;**34**:945–9.

85. Arhaliass A, Bouvier JM, Legrand J. Melt growth and shrinkage at the exit of the die in the extrusion-cooking process. *J Food Engn* 2003;**60**:185–92.

86. Kokini JL, Moraru CI. Nucleation and Expansion During Extrusion and Microwave Heating of Cereal Foods. *Compr Rev Food Sci F* 2003;**2**:120–38.

87. Patil RT, Berrios JJ, Tang J, Swanson BG. Evaluation of methods for expansion properties of legume extrudates. *Am Soc Agri Biol Engn* 2007;**23**(6):777–83.

88. Shirani G, Ganesharanee R. Extruded products with Fenugreek (*Trigonella foenum-graecium*) chickpea and rice: Physical properties, sensory acceptability and glycaemic index. *J Food Engn* 2009;**90**:44–52.

89. Martinez-Serna M, Hawkes J, Villota R. Extrusion of natural and modified whey proteins in starch-based systems. In: Spiess WEL, Schubert H, editors. *Engineering and food: Advanced processes*. London, UK: Elsevier Applied Science; 1990. p. 346–65.

90. Onwulata CL, Konstance RP, Smith PW, Holsinger VH. Physical properties of extruded products as affected by cheese whey. *J Food Sci* 1998;**63**:814–8.

91. Pérez AA, Drago SR, Carrara CR, De Greef DM, Torres RL, González RJ. Extrusion cooking of maize-soybean mixture: Factors affecting expanded product characteristics and flour dispersion viscosity. *J Food Engn* 2008;**87**(3):333–40.

92. Suknark K, Philips RD, Chinnan MS. Physical properties of directly expanded extrudates formulated from partially defatted peanut flour and different types of starch. *Food Res Int* 1997;**30**:575–83.

93. Yagci S, Gögüs F. Response surface methodology for evaluation of physical and functional properties of extruded snack foods developed from food-by-products. *J Food Engn* 2008;**86**:122–32.

94. Kirby AR, Ollet AL, Parker R, Smith AC. An experimental study of screw configuration effects in the twin-screw extrusion cooking of maize grits. *J Food Engn* 1988;**8**:247–72.

95. Colonna P, Tayeb J, Mercier C. Extrusion cooking of starch and starchy products. In: Mercier C, Linko P, Harper JM, editors. *Extrusion cooking*. St Paul, MN: AACC; 1989. p. 247–19.

96. Frias J, Giacomino S, Peñas E, Pellegrino N, Ferreyra V, Apro N, et al. Assessment of the nutritional quality of raw and extruded *Pisum sativum* L. var. *laguna* seeds. *LWT-Food Sci Technol* 2011;**44**:1303–8.

97. Vasanthan T, Gaosong J, Yeung J, Li J. Dietary fibre profile of barley flour as affected by extrusion cooking. *Food Chem* 2002;**77**:35–40.

98. FAO/WHO/UNU. *Energy and protein requirements, report of the joint FAO/WHO/UNU expert consultation*. Geneva, Switzerland: Technical Report Series No. 724; 1985.

99. Singh S, Wakeling L, Gamlath S. Retention of essential amino acids during extrusion of protein and reducing sugars. *J Agr Food Chem* 2007;**55**:8779–86.

100. Ainsworth P, Fuller D, Plunkett A, Ibanoglu S. Influence of extrusion variables on the protein *in vitro* digestibility and protein solubility of extruded soy tarhana. *J Sci Food Agr* 1999;**79**:675–8.

101. Zamora NC. Efecto de la extrusión sobre la actividad de factores antinutricionales y digestibilidad *in vitro* de proteínas y almidón en harinas de Canavalia ensiformis. *Arch Latinoam Nutr* 2000;**53**:293–8.

102. Singh S, Gamlath S, Wakeling L. Nutritional aspects of food extrusion: a review. *Int J Food Sci Tech* 2007;**42**:916–29.

103. Van der Poel AFB, Gravendeel S, Boer H. Effect of different processing methods on tannin content and *in vitro* protein digestibility of faba bean (*Vicia faba* L.). *Anim Feed Sci Tech* 1991;**33**:49–58.

104. Pastor-Cavada E, Juan R, Pastor JE, Alaiz M, Vioque J. Antioxidant activity of seed polyphenols in fifteen wild Lathyrus species from South Spain. *LWT-Food Sci Technol* 2009;**42**:705–9.

105. Pastor-Cavada E, Juan R, Pastor JE, Alaiz M, Girón-Calle J, Vioque J. Antioxidative activity in the seeds of 28 *Vicia* species from southern Spain. *J Food Biochem* 2011;**35**:1373–80.

106. Viscidi KA, Dougherty MP, Briggs J, Camire ME. Complex phenolic compounds reduce lipid oxidation in extruded oat cereal. *Lebensm Wiss Technol* 2004;**37**:789–96.

107. Dlamini NR, Dykes L, Rooney LW, Waniska RD, Taylor JR. Condenses tannins in traditional wet-cooked and modern extrusion-cooked sorghum porridges. *Cereal Chem* 2009;**86**(2):191–6.

108. Repo-Carrasco-Valencia R, Peña J, Kallio H, Salminen S. Dietary fiber and other functional componets in two varieties of crude and extruded Kiwicha (*Amaranthus caudatus*). *J Cereal Sci* 2009;**49**:219–24.

109. Ziegler EE, Filer LJ. *Conocimientos Actuales sobre nutrición*, 7th edn. Washington, DC: OMS. ILSI Pub Cientif; 1990.

110. Hazell T, Johnson IT. Influence of food processing on iron availability *in vitro* from extruded maize-based snack foods. *J Sci Food Agr* 1989;**46**:365–74.

111. Lombardi-Boccia G, Dilullo G, Carnovale E. *In vitro* dialysability from legumes: influence of phytate and extrusión cooking. *J Sci Food Agr* 1991;**48** 599–05.

112. Fairweather-Tait SJ, Symss LL, Smith AC, Johnson IT. The effect of extrusion cooking on iron absorptions from maize and potato. *J Sci Food Agr* 1987;**39**:341–8.

113. Monsen ER, Hallberg L, Layrisse M, Hegsted DM, Cook JD, Mertz W, et al. Estimation of available dietary iron. *Am J Clin Nutr* 1978;**31**:134–41.

114. Martín de Portela ML. *Vitaminas y minerales en nutrición*, 1st edn. Buenos Aires, Argentina: Libreros López; 1993.

115. Hallberg L, Rossander L, Skanberg AB. Phytates and the inhibitory effect of bran on iron absorption in man. *Am J Clin Nutr* 1987;**45**:9888–996.

116. Brune M, Rossander-Hulten L, Hallberg L, Gleerup A, Sandberg AS. Iron absorption from bread in humans: inhibiting effects of cereal fiber, phytate and inositol phosphates with different numbers of phosphate group. *J Nutr* 1992;**122**:442–9.

117. Sandberg AS. Bioavailability of minerals in legumes. *Br J Nutr* 2002;**88**:S281–5.

118. Alonso R, Rubio LA, Muzquiz M, Marzo F. The effect of extrusion cooking on mineral bioavailability in pea and kidney bean seed meals. *Anim Feed Sci Tech* 2001;**94**:1–13.

Rice Bran Antioxidants in Health and Wellness

Md. Shafiqul Islam[*, †], *Naoki Matsuki*[**], *Reiko Nagasaka*[‡],
Kazuyuki Ohara[‡, ¶], *Takamitsu Hosoya*[§], *Hiroshi Ozaki*[*, §§],
Hideki Ushio[§§, ¶], *Masatoshi Hori*[*, §§]

[*]The University of Tokyo, Department of Veterinary Pharmacology, Graduate School of Agriculture and Life Sciences, Tokyo, Japan, [†]Bangladesh Agricultural University, Department of Pharmacology, Mymensingh, Bangladesh, [**]The University of Tokyo, Department of Veterinary Clinical Pathobiology, Graduate School of Agriculture and Life Sciences, Tokyo, Japan, [‡]Tokyo University of Marine Science and Technology, Department of Food Science and Technology, Tokyo, Japan, [§]Tokyo Medical and Dental University, Institute of Biomaterials and Bioengineering, Graduate School of Biomedical Science, Tokyo, Japan, [§§]The University of Tokyo, Development of Advanced Technology Laboratory Research Center for Food Safety, Tokyo, Japan, [¶]The University of Tokyo, Laboratory of Marine Biochemistry, Graduate School of Agriculture and Life Sciences, Tokyo, Japan

RICE BRAN ANTIOXIDANTS

Increased concern about the safety of synthetic antioxidants has led to an increased interest in the exploration of effective natural antioxidants. In a world where science merges with health, phytochemicals are the next big thing. Rice is one of the world's most important food crops, and more than half the people in the world eat rice as the main part of their diet. In some parts of the world, the word "to eat" literally means "to eat rice." Rice bran is a component of raw rice that is obtained when it is removed from the starchy endosperm in rice milling process (Fig. 34.1).[1] There is emerging interest in the use of naturally occurring antioxidants for the management of a number of pathophysiological conditions, most of which involve free radical damage.[2] Dietary antioxidants form one of the defense mechanisms that protects the body against the damaging effects of reactive oxygen species (ROS). Natural products have received great attention for disease prevention owing to their various health benefits, their noticeable lack of toxicity and side effects, and the limitations of chemotherapeutic agents. Some thousand chemical compounds can occur in food, but only few of them have nutritional significance. Various extraction methods have shown that rice bran phytochemicals contain a mixture of antioxidant components such as phenolic acids, anthocyanins, α-tocopherol and γ-oryzanol, and gallic, hydroxybenzoic, and protocatechuic acids.[3,4] Among these antioxidant components, rice bran oil is a rich source of oryzanols. The name oryzanol was derived from rice bran of *Orysae sativa L.*, because it was first purified from the unsaponifiable fraction of rice bran oil. Initially γ-oryzanol was considered to be a single compound, but since then it has been characterized as a mixture of ferulic acid esters of several sterols and triterpene alcohols called α-, β- and γ-oryzanol, of which γ-oryzanol has been the most commonly mentioned compound. γ-Oryzanol contains a number of phytosteryl ferulates, such as 24-methylenecycloartanyl ferulate, cycloartenyl ferulate, campesteryl ferulate, β-sitosteryl ferulate, and campestanyl ferulate; the mixture of these is referred to as γ-oryzanol.[5] Structurally all components of γ-oryzanol contain one unit of ferulic acid (i.e., a ferulic acid moiety) and a residual moiety that is triterpene alcohol or sterol (Fig. 34.2).[1,6] The ferulic acid moiety of rice bran's phytosteryl ferulates plays a pivotal role in free radical scavenging (DPPH free radical) and inhibition of cholesterol oxidation. On the other hand, *in vitro* studies on NIH 3T3 fibroblast cells under induced oxidative stress by H_2O_2 showed antioxidative effects both of ferulic acid and sterol moieties of phytosteryl ferulates.[7] γ-Oryzanol is a white or slightly yellowish tasteless powder with little or no odor, and contains only 1–3% rice bran oil.

(A)

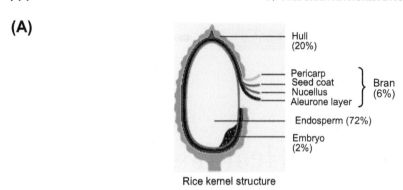

Rice kernel structure

(B)

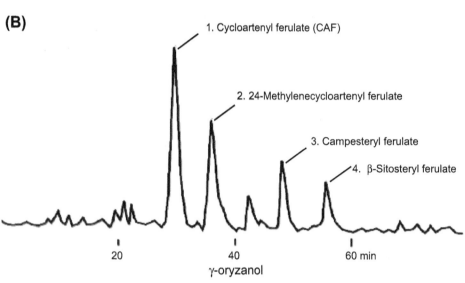

γ-oryzanol

FIGURE 34.1 (A) Rice kernel showing different parts of structure. (B) HPLC elution showing rice bran γ-oryzanol contains (1) cycloartenyl ferulate; (2) 24-methylenecycloartanyl ferulate; (3) campesteryl ferulate, and (4) β-sitosteryl ferulate. *Figure adapted from Islam* et al.[1]

BIOMEDICAL IMPORTANCE OF RICE BRAN ANTIOXIDANTS FOR OXIDATIVE STRESS

Over the past 30 years, the fields of free radical chemistry and biology have risen from relative obscurity to become mainstream elements of biomedical investigation and pharmaceutical development.[8] Antioxidants in rice bran have professed health benefits, as well as their antioxidant characteristic of improving the storage ability of food additives for further benefits to health. At the molecular level, cells produce many by-products of oxidative metabolic processes during pathophysiological states, called free radicals. These free radicals can cause damage to the cell wall, cell components, and genetic material. Among the molecules of a cell, mitochondria are an important source of ROS, and the uncontrolled and/or sustained increase in reactive oxygen species production by mitochondria causes oxidative damage to biological molecules, which could be implicated in the pathogenesis of cancer, diabetes mellitus, atherosclerosis, neurodegenerative diseases, rheumatoid arthritis, ischemia/reperfusion injury, obstructive sleep apnea, and other diseases.[9] Scientific evidence suggests that oxidative stress-oriented diseases can be managed

with rice bran antioxidant treatments, as the therapeutic effects of rice bran's extracts for antioxidative purposes and their ability to scavenge reactive oxygen species are well established. Various research findings have revealed that these antioxidant components, such as 24-methylenecycloartanyl ferulate, cycloartenyl ferulate, campesteryl ferulate, and β-sitosteryl ferulate, are able to inhibit lipid peroxidation and free radical production, and scavenge the free radicals from the body.[7] Therefore, natural antioxidants from rice bran could provide a potential means to treat conditions in which the formation of reactive oxygen species exceeds the capability of the natural protective mechanisms.[10] During the course of radical oxidation cholesterol may play an important role in lipid bilayer stabilization, as cholesterol-modified cell membrane provoked the effects on peroxidation, with corresponding increases in oxidative damage in the cell, possibly as a consequence of lipid bilayer destabilization.[11] The structure of γ-oryzanol components is similar to that of cholesterol, an important component in reducing oxidation stress and maintaining the functionality of cells. In accordance with the structural relationship theory, γ-oryzanol components such as cycloartenyl ferulae significantly inhibited oxidative stress in NIH 3T3 fibroblast cells stimulated with H_2O_2.[7] Besides the

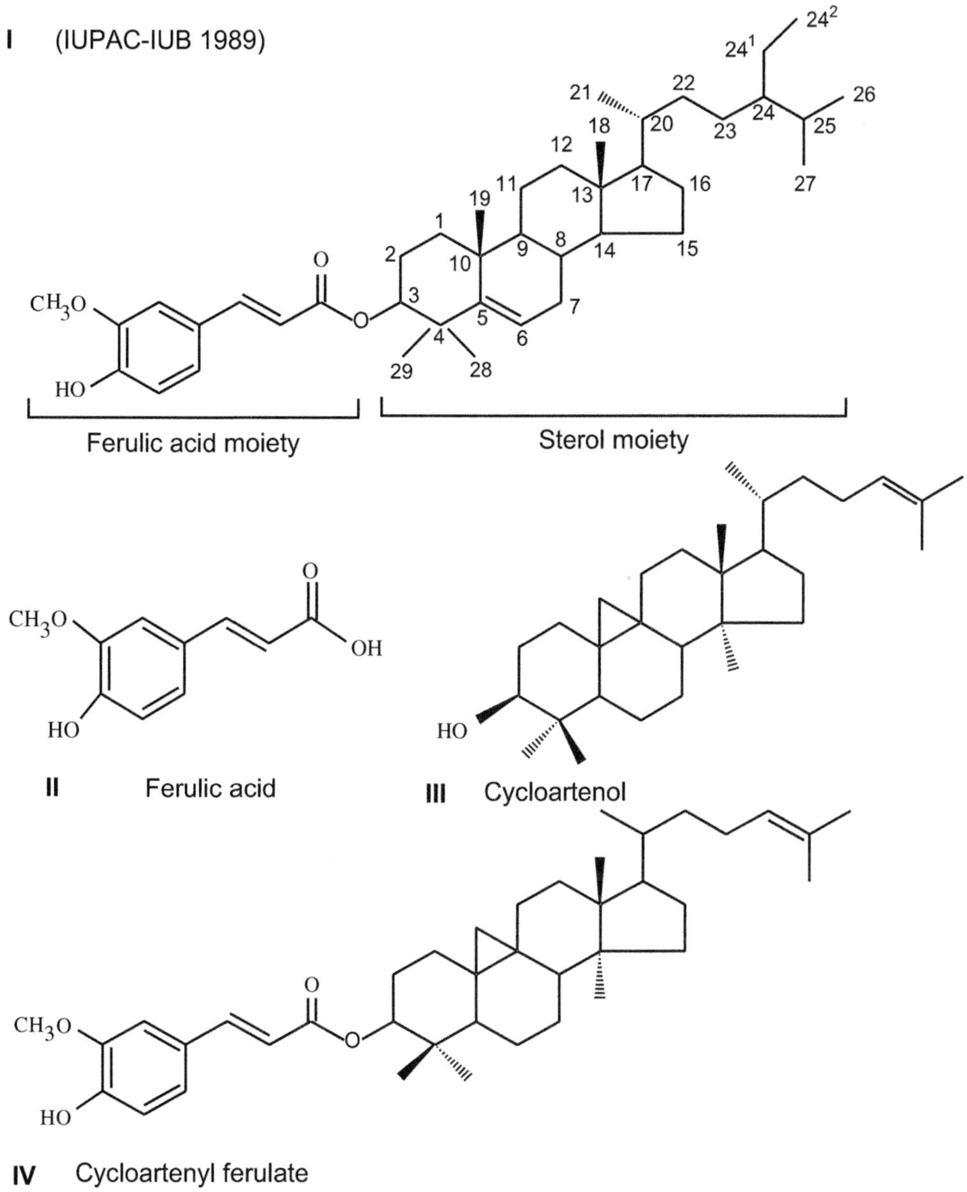

I (IUPAC-IUB 1989)

Ferulic acid moiety

Sterol moiety

II Ferulic acid

III Cycloartenol

IV Cycloartenyl ferulate

FIGURE 34.2 IUPAC-IUB 1989 showing ferulic acid and sterol moiety (I), ferulic acid structure (II), sterol moiety cycloartenol (III), and cycloartenyl ferulate, a combination of ferulic acid and sterol moiety cycloartenol (IV). *Figure adapted from Islam et al.*[1]

cholesterol theory, cycloartenyl ferulate significantly enhanced superoxide dismutase (SOD) activity in LPS-stimulated RAW 264.7 macrophages.[12] It is notable that the sterol moiety alone, cycloartenol (CA), is also able to inhibit significantly the intracellular ROS production.[7] In addition, CA showed chemopreventive potential on benzoyl peroxide- and UVB radiation-induced cutaneous tumor and oxidative stress in murine skin. Benzoyl peroxide (20 mg/animal/0.2 ml acetone) and UVB radiation (0.420 J/m^2 per second) treatment decreased the activities of cutaneous antioxidant enzymes, namely catalase, glutathione peroxidase, glutathione reductase, glucose-6-phosphate dehydrogenase, and phase II metabolizing enzymes such as glutathione-S-transferase and quinone reductase, and depleted the level of cutaneous glutathione. There was also enhancement

in cutaneous microsomal lipid peroxidation, xanthine oxidase activity, [14C]-ornithine decarboxylase activity and [3H]-thymidine incorporation into cutaneous DNA. Moreover, CA applied topically prior to the application of benzoyl peroxide at dose levels of 0.2 mg and 0.4 mg/kg body weight significantly inhibited epidermal ornithine decarboxylase activity, DNA synthesis, lipid peroxidation, and xanthine oxidase activity ($P < 0.001$). In addition, CA treatment recovered the inhibitory activity of benzoyl peroxide, such as depleted glutathione, antioxidant, and phase II metabolizing enzymes to a significant level ($P < 0.001$).[13]

Another major component of rice bran extract, ferulic acid, the possible metabolite of γ-oryzanol, potentially prevented decreases in reduced glutathione (GSH), SOD, catalase (CAT), and glutathione peroxidase (GPx) activities induced by gamma radiation.[8] The inherent quality of ferulic acid's ability to scavenge reactive oxygen species is similar to that of the body defense mechanism, SOD.

RICE BRAN ANTIOXIDANTS FOR GASTROINTESTINAL COMPLAINTS

Rice bran γ-oryzanol has therapeutic potency for many gastrointestinal diseases. Colorectal cancer is an important public health problem, and one of the most fearsome complications of inflammatory bowel diseases (IBDs) – mainly ulcerative colitis (UC) but also Crohn's colitis. Many basic medical scientific studies for gastrointestinal diseases have been reported since 1962. Rice bran γ-oryzanol has been reported to inhibit gastric secretion and experimental ulcers in rats.[14] The inhibitory effects of γ-oryzanol on gastric secretions were slightly effective for histamine-stimulated acid secretion, non-effective for carbachol-stimulated secretion, and significantly inhibited tetragastrin-stimulated secretion. It was further revealed that the effect of γ-oryzanol on acid secretion stimulated by tetragastrin was prevented by vagotomy but not by splanchnicotomy. Therefore, this scientific evidence suggests that the gastric antisecretory effect of γ-oryzanol is mediated by the vagus nerve, which plays a role in the action of gastrin.[14] In another study, pretreatment with γ-oryzanol (100 mg/kg, s.c., once daily × 5) depressed the gastric secretion stimulated by insulin or 2-deoxy-D-glucose, but the potency was less than that with atropine (10 mg/kg, s.c.). γ-Oryzanol had no effect on the decrease in the serum glucose level or on the increase in the gastrin level induced by insulin injection, while atropine enhanced these responses. Therefore, it is considered that the inhibitory action of γ-oryzanol on gastric secretion may be due to depression of the vagus system, but the mode of action is different from that of atropine.[15] Rice bran γ-oryzanol, cycloartenyl ferulate, and ferulic acid (the metabolite of γ-oryzanol) were extensively studied in dextran sulfate sodium (DSS)-induced colitis mice. γ-Oryzanol, cycloartenyl ferulate, and ferulic acid ameliorate colonic inflammation in DSS-induced colitis in mice.[16] This amelioration was associated with inhibition of myeloperoxidase (MPO) activity, decreased production of cytokines such IL-1β, TNF-α, and IL-6, and inhibition of COX-2 and NF-κB activity in colitis tissue. Still, the medical treatment of IBD relies on the use of aminosalicylates, corticosteroids, immunosuppressive drugs (azathioprine, 6-mercaptopurin, methotrexate, cyclosporin), and antibiotics. However, aminosalicilates (5-amino salicylic acid [5-ASA] derivatives) and/or glucocorticoids remain the principal means of therapy for IBD at different stages of the disease. 5-ASA-based agents are usually well tolerated but frequently induce side effects, such as acute pancreatitis, abdominal pain, diarrhea, nausea, headache, anemia, renal failure, and anaphylaxis. Therefore, rice bran γ-oryzanol and its components are prominent candidate seed compounds for treatment of gastrointestinal complaints.

RICE BRAN ANTIOXIDANTS FOR INFLAMMATION

It is well recognized that a secondary effect of ROS production is the induction of NF-κB activation, which mediates inflammation. Therefore, antioxidants can protect against inflammation through inhibition of the inflammatory signaling cascade NF-κB pathway. There is still controversy over whether γ-oryzanol and its antioxidant components inhibit NF-κB signaling directly, or indirectly through their antioxidant ability. The alteration or correction of undesired cellular functions caused by abnormal proinflammatory signal transmissions mediated by NF-κB is an important inherent quality of chemopreventive and chemoprotective phytochemicals and phytonutrients.[17] Rice bran's antioxidant components have diverse anti-inflammatory effects. In both *in vivo* colitis and *in vitro* RAW 264.7 macrophages, γ-oryzanol and antioxidant components significantly inhibit IκB-α degradation levels, resulting in the inhibition of NF-κB p65 nuclear translocation.[7,16] These components are also able to inhibit iNOS and NO production in activated 264.7 RAW macrophages by interfering with NF-κB activation.[12] In addition, *trans*-ferulic acid and γ-oryzanol also ameliorate ethanol-induced liver injury in mice.[18] Moreover, rice bran oil markedly prevents inflammatory activity against inflammation of mouse ear when evoked by 12-O-tetradecanoylphorbol-13-acetate (TPA).[19] On the other hand, free triterpene alcohol, CA, has been reported as a powerful anti-inflammatory compound and also inhibits leukocyte infiltration against carrageenan-induced peritonitis in mice.[20] CA also inhibits phospholipase A2 (PLA2) *in vitro*.[20] Pretreatment with γ-oryzanol, as well as its components (cycloartenyl ferulate, ferulic acid, or cycloartenol), dose-dependently inhibits LPS-mediated NF-κB activation in bovine aortic endothelial cells (BAECs).[21]

RICE BRAN ANTIOXIDANTS FOR HYPERCHOLESTEROLEMIC– HYPERLIPIDEMIC PATIENTS

Atherosclerosis is a chronic disease of large arteries due to accumulation of oxidized lipid on the vascular wall, neointima formation, fibrous cap formation, and migration of inflammatory cells onto the injured endothelium. The molecular mechanism of atherosclerosis begins when injured endothelial cells start to increase the expression of adhesion molecules such as E-selectin, vascular cell adhesion molecule-1 (VCAM-1), and intercellular adhesion molecule-1 (ICAM-1), which assist the progress of leukocyte adhesion to the endothelium and migration to the subendothelial area, ultimately producing atherosclerosis in the advanced stage. Recently, rice bran γ-oryzanol has been reported to potentially suppress lipopolysaccharide (LPS)-induced adhesion molecules such as vascular cell adhesion molecule-1, intercellular adhesion molecule-1, and E-selectin in bovine aortic endothelial cells.[21] In addition, pretreatment with γ-oryzanol dose dependently reduces U937 monocyte adhesion to bovine aortic endothelial cells. Dyslipidemia is one of the main risk factors for atherosclerosis, a major contributor to cardiovascular disease. One of the most important functions of rice bran oil is its potential cholesterol-lowering properties. Several reports suggest that rice bran oil and its major components (unsaturated fatty acids, triterpene alcohols, phytosterols, tocotrienols, and α-tocopherol) improve the plasma lipid profile of rodents, rabbits, nonhuman primates, and humans by reducing total plasma cholesterol and triglyceride concentration while increasing high density lipoprotein cholesterol (HDL-C).[22,23] A study in dyslipidemic rats that were on a diet containing 10% refined rice bran oil reported significantly lower total serum cholesterol levels, free esterified, and low and very low density lipoprotein cholesterol (LDL-C, VLDL-C).[24] Another study in monkeys also demonstrated that rice bran oil reduced serum total cholesterol and LDL-C, and that these reductions were not accompanied by a reduction in HDL-C.[25] Studies on human volunteers with dyslipidemia also showed that γ-oryzanol treatment significantly improved their lipid profile, and their inflammatory and oxidative stress levels.[26–30] In chronic schizophrenic patients with dyslipidemia treated with γ-oryzanol (100 mg, three times daily for 16 weeks) significantly decreased LDL-C and total cholesterol without changing HDL-C.[26] A study on human volunteers revealed that intake of rice bran oil (by using it as cooking oil) for 50 days significantly decreased lipid peroxides, triglycerides, LDL-C and VLDL-C in the blood.[28] Most interestingly, combined dietary supplementation of γ-oryzanol, vitamin E, and niacin to dyslipidemic volunteers dramatically improved the lipid profile, ROS and total antioxidant capacity. Thus, there is evidence that γ-oryzanol lowers plasma non-HDL-C levels and raises plasma HDL-C, possibly through increased fecal excretion of cholesterol and its metabolites.[23,29] Although the detailed mechanisms behind the cholesterol-lowering ability of γ-oryzanol are not fully understood, regular consumption of γ-oryzanol is recommended as part of a therapeutic lifestyle change in order to reduce LDLC in patients with hyperlipidemia. Rice bran's triterpene alcohols, such as cycloartenol (CA) and 24-methylene

cycloartanol, significantly reduce cholesterol and triglyceride levels in hypercholesterolemic rats.[31] Endogenous sterol excretion increases in animals given CA. The accumulation of CA in the liver inhibits cholesterol esterase activity, which in turn leads to a reduction in circulating cholesterol levels. On the other hand, rice bran's oil, which is rich in tocopherols and tocotrienols, may improve oxidative stability. Tocotrienols inhibit HMG CoA reductase, resulting in hypocholesterolemia.[31] The hypolipidemic effect of this oil has also been established in human subjects. Therefore, rice bran oil could be a suitable edible oil for patients with hyperlipidemia, and is a prominent candidate as preventive medicine for atherosclerosis and other chronic vascular diseases.

RICE BRAN ANTIOXIDANTS FOR NEOPLASIA

Rice is a staple diet in Asia, where the incidence of breast and colon cancer is markedly below that in the Western world. Rice bran's phytosteryl ferulate products have received a great deal of interest regarding their protective and/or preventative effects in relation to colon cancer. Several studies on rice bran phytosteryl ferulates have demonstrated their anticarcinogenic activity in the colon.[32] The inherent quality of rice bran is reported to reduce azoxymethane-induced colon tumor incidence, initiation of the tumor, and the size of the tumor in rats. Possible mechanisms of the anticolonic cancer effect of phytosterols have been analyzed in vitro. In human colorectal adenocarcinoma SW480 cell lines, the anticancer activity of CAF is mediated through the elevated death receptors DR4 and DR5, mitochondrial apoptosis pathways, depletion of anti-apoptotic Bcl-2, upregulation of pro-apoptotic Bak, dissipation of the mitochondrial membrane potential, and the release of cyto c and Smac/DIABLO (caspase-dependent death effectors) from mitochondria into the cytosol.[33] Besides all of this, CAF also sensitizes the metastatic and resistant colon cancer SW620 to TNF-related apoptosis-inducing ligand (TRAIL)-induced apoptosis and to the enhanced activation of caspase-8 and -3. It has also been reported that β-sitosterol inhibits the growth of HT-29 cells, a human colon cancer cell line, and this may be mediated through the influence of signal transduction pathways that involve membrane phospholipids.[34,35] It has been reported that dietary phytosteryl ferulates mitigate the growth and spread of breast cancer when the MDA-MB-231 cell line is xenografted into SCID mice.[35] Cycloartenyl trans-ferulate and 24-methylenecycloartenyl trans-ferulate also show moderate cytotoxicity against human breast adenocarcinoma MCF-7 cells.[36] A water-soluble component of rice bran extract exhibits antiproliferative effects on leukemia tumor cell growth *in vitro*. These studies strongly suggest that rice bran-derived antioxidant phytochemicals may ameliorate other types of carcinogenesis. Indeed, genetic mouse models of breast, prostate, and intestinal cancer reveal that a diet containing 30% rice bran greatly inhibits the number of adenomas in *ApcMin* mice.[37] Other related compounds of CAF, such as β-sitosterol, campesterol, and stigmasterol, also show anticancer activity in the colon, breast, and prostate.[38] It is reported that rice bran sitosterol ferulate, 24-methylcholesterol ferulate, cyclo-artenol ferulate, and 24-methylenecycloartanol ferulate are able to inhibit 12-O-tetradecanoylphorbol-13-acetate (TPA)-induced inflammation and markedly suppress the tumor-promoting effect of TPA in 7,12-dimethylbenz[*a*] anthracene-initiated mice.[39] However, it is still unclear whether these anticancer effects of phytosterols are related to antioxidant- and/or NF-κB-inhibited potency.

Ferulic acid inhibits the growth of colon cancer cells, and is also reported to inhibit 4-nitroquinoline-1-oxide (4NQO)-induced oral carcinogenesis in rats. The incidences of tongue carcinomas and preneoplastic lesions (severe dysplasia) in rats of the group given ferulic acid in the diet at a dose of 500 ppm, after exposure to 4NQO for 5 weeks in drinking water at a dose of 20 ppm, was significantly lower on termination of the experiment (32 weeks) in the group with the carcinogen alone ($P < 0.005$ and $P < 0.001$ respectively). In addition, the effects of rice germ on azoxymethane (AOM)-induced formation of aberrant crypt foci (ACF) also revealed similar effects in male F344 rats. Numbers of ACF/colon, ACF/cm^2, and aberrant crypts/colon in the group treated with AOM (15 mg/kg s.c. once a week for 3 weeks) and gamma-amino butyric acid (GABA)-enriched defatted rice germ (2.5% in diet), or the group with AOM and rice germ (2.5% in diet), were smaller than those of the group with AOM alone ($P < 0.005$). Exposure to defatted rice germ or rice germ during the initiation phase or the post-initiation phase also decreased incidences of AOM-induced large bowel neoplasms ($P < 0.05$).[40]

RICE BRAN ANTIOXIDANTS AMELIORATE TYPE 2 DIABETES VIA INCREASED ADIPONECTIN SECRETION

Oxidative stress is considered to be a key factor in the development of diabetes and its related complications. Although there are few studies on phytochemicals against diabetes mellitus, it is reported that rice trienol, a crude lipophilic rice bran extract that contains phytosterols, tocotrienols, tocopherols, squalene, and other compounds, greatly prevents oxidative damage in this disease.[41] Therefore, rice bran components might ameliorate diabetes mellitus through their antioxidative ability. However, the molecular mechanisms of these crude lipophilic rice bran extracts for diabetes mellitus have not been clarified. Adipose tissue has been recognized as an organ that not only stores excess energy but is also the source of a variety of bioactive substances, such as adipocytokines, including TNF-α and IL-6. Adipocytokines are known to induce inflammatory responses in various tissues such as vascular walls and muscles. Recently, a novel adipocytokine named adiponectin has been identified in adipose tissue and is positively correlated with insulin sensitivity.[42] In type 2 diabetes, circulating levels of adiponectin are lower compared to controls matched by body mass index, indicating that adiponectin is a new target molecule that ameliorates type 2 diabetes. It has been confirmed that proinflammatory cytokines dramatically reduce adiponectin secretion in adipocytes, and rice bran γ-oryzanol increases adiponectin secretion in adipocytes in mice. Moreover, γ-oryzanol upregulates adiponectin secretion by activating peroxisomal proliferator activated receptor γ (PPARγ) through the inhibition of NF-κB activity.[43] Interestingly, γ-oryzanol has the ability to increase adiponectin secretion, but only under the condition of activated NF-κB.[43] It has been documented that ferulic acid may lower blood sugar levels of type 1 and type 2 diabetic mice by enhancing insulin secretion. The hypoglycemic effects of a phenolic acid fraction (the ethyl acetate fraction, EAE) of rice bran and of ferulic acid in C57BL/KsJ db/db mice significantly decreased blood glucose levels and increased plasma insulin levels. EAE or ferulic acid groups had significantly elevated hepatic glycogen synthesis and glucokinase activity compared with the control group. Plasma total cholesterol and low density lipoprotein (LDL) cholesterol concentrations were significantly decreased by EAE and ferulic acid administration. These findings suggest that EAE and ferulic acid may be beneficial for treatment of type 2 diabetes because they regulate blood glucose levels by elevating glucokinase activity and production of glycogen in the liver.[44] Other findings include increased glycogen synthesis and glucokinase activity in the liver, while total cholesterol and LDL cholesterol were decreased. Therefore, ferulic acid may be beneficial in type 2 diabetes and for the management of diabetic complications.

RICE BRAN ANTIOXIDANTS FOR ALLERGY SYNDROME

It is well established that NF-κB-related inflammation has a pivotal role in the late phase of allergy. Therefore, γ-oryzanol may have a potent anti-allergic effect in the case of late phases of allergy by inhibiting NF-κB action. Moreover, there are no reports about the effects of γ-oryzanol on mast cell degranulation, which is a main event in type I allergy. It has been reported that rice bran oil modulates the immune system by enhancing B-lymphocyte proliferation and TH1-type cytokine levels such as IL-2 or TNF-α, and in reducing the Th2 cytokine IL-4 and IgE levels known for their anti-allergenic properties.[45] CAF and γ-oryzanol from rice bran oil were found to attenuate the dinitrophenyl–human serum albumin (DNP-HAS)-induced passive cutaneous anaphylaxis reaction in the dorsal skin of rats. CAF and γ-oryzanol also inhibit the degranulation of mouse monoclonal anti-DNP antibody (DNP-IgE)-sensitized RBL-2H3 mast cells stimulated with anti-DNP-HAS.[46] On the other hand, ferulic acid, which does not have the sterol chemical structure of cycloartenyl ferulate, did not alter mast cell degranulation, although ferulic acid did have a strong antioxidant property, suggesting that the anti-allergic potency of cycloartenyl ferulate is not related to antioxidant ability. The negative charge moiety of the sterol structure of cycloartenyl ferulate may capture IgE, which in turn inhibits mast cell degranulation.

RICE BRAN ANTIOXIDANTS FOR POST-MENOPAUSAL SYNDROME

Nowadays, γ-oryzanol is often used for treating the menopause, although it is unclear how it benefits the post-menopausal syndrome, and especially hot flushes. Some researchers suspect it might be helpful due to effects on luteinizing hormone. The United States National Cholesterol Education Panel (NCEP) evaluated the effect of rice bran oil compared with the effects of canola, corn, and olive oils on 15 middle-aged and elderly subjects (8 post-menopausal women and 7 men, age range 44–78 years) with elevated low density lipoprotein (LDL) cholesterol concentrations (range 133–219 mg/dL). Plasma cholesterol and LDL-C concentrations were similar and statistically indistinguishable when the subjects consumed the rice bran, canola, and corn oil-enriched diets, and lower than when they consumed the olive oil-enriched diet.[47]

RICE BRAN ANTIOXIDANTS IN REDUCING THYROID STIMULATING HORMONE

A single oral dose (300 mg) of rice bran derived γ-oryzanol produced a significant reductionion the elevated serum TSH levels in hypothyroid patients, while chronic treatment with γ-oryzanol resulted in decreased serum TSH levels in six of eight patients.[48] Moreover, there was no change in the serum levels of thyroxine-iodine and triiodothyronine, and no difference in the serum TSH response to TRH in hypothyroid patients and normal subjects. Therefore, γ-oryzanol inhibits serum TSH levels in patients with primary hypothyroidism, possibly by direct action at the hypothalamus rather than the pituitary.[48]

RICE BRAN ANTIOXIDANTS IN PRESERVATION OF FOOD AND SKIN COLOR

Ferulic acid has been reported to maintain the color tone of green peas, prevent discoloration of Green Tea, and prevent oxidation from turning banana black, thus reducing bacterial contamination. Ferulic acid (0.01–0.5%) as well as γ-oryzanol (0.05–0.5%) administered to Red Sea Bream (*Pagrus major*) for 98 days led to a brighter color in those treated than in the controls due to the preventive effects of ferulic acid and γ-oryzanol against photo-oxidation of lutein and astaxanthin.[49] Moreover, the structure of ferulic acid is similar to that of tyrosine and is believed to inhibit melanin formation through competitive inhibition with tyrosine. Ferulic acid (0.5%) is able to protect human skin from UV irradiation.[50] The ferulic acid ester also exhibited an inhibitory effect on melanin production, and is anticipated to become a potential pigmentation inhibitor. With these positive finding, ferulic acid has been widely used in cosmetics applications for absorbing the long UV wavelength, as sunscreen or as a whitening agent.

MISCELLANEOUS USES OF RICE BRAN PHYTOCHEMICALS

The structure of ferulic acid is similar to that of nor-metanephrine, the first metabolite of norepinephrine, hence mimicking a stimulatory effect on somatotrophin in the pituitary gland.[51] However, ferulic acid did not affect luteinizing hormone or thyroid hormones. Ferulic acid (9.5 mg/kg bw) decreased angiotensin-1-converting enzyme (ACE) activity in the plasma, corresponding well with the reduction of blood pressure (BP) in stroke-prone spontaneously hypertensive rats (SHRSP). Plasma total cholesterol and triglyceride levels were lower 2 hours after administration. The mRNA expression of genes involved in lipid and drug metabolism was downregulated in ferulic acid-treated rats.[52] Ferulic acid (100 mg/kg) provides neuroprotection against oxidative stress-related apoptosis following cerebral ischemia/reperfusion injury by inhibiting ICAM-1 mRNA expression in rats. Ferulic acid decreased the level of ICAM-1 mRNA and the number of microglia/macrophages, and subsequently downregulated inflammation-induced oxidative stress and oxidative stress-related apoptosis, suggesting that ferulic acid provides neuroprotection against oxidative stress-related apoptosis by inhibiting ICAM-1 mRNA expression after cerebral ischemia/reperfusion injury in rats.[53] Ferulic acid attenuated amyloid-β-peptide induced memory impairment in mice, indicating that this molecule enhances learning ability and memory function.[54] γ-Oryzanol is used as a supplement by body builders and athletes, as it is thought to increase testosterone levels, promote endorphins, and stimulate lean muscle tissue growth. However, there is still controversy regarding whether γ-oryzanol is an appropriate nutrient supplement for body builders and athletes.[55] Clinical studies have, however, revealed that γ-oryzanol is able to increases the brain chemical norepinephrine, and it has been administered to people suffering from mild anxiety.

References

1. Islam SM, Nagasaka R, Ohara K, Hosoya T, Ozaki H, et al. Biological abilities of rice bran-derived antioxidant phytochemicals for medical therapy. *Curr Top Med Chem* 2011;**11**:1847–53.

2. Soobrattee MA, Neergheen VS, Luximon-Ramma A, Aruoma OI, Bahorun T. Phenolics as potential antioxidant therapeutic agents: mechanism and actions. *Mutat Res* 2005;**579**(1–2):200–13.

3. Xu Z, Hua N, Godber JS. Antioxidant activity of tocopherols, tocotrienols, and gamma-oryzanol components from rice bran against cholesterol oxidation accelerated by 2,2'-azobis (2-methylpropionamidine) dihydrochloride. *J Agric Food Chem* 2001;**49**(4): 2077–81.

4. Laokuldilok T, Shoemaker CF, Jongkaewwattana S, Tulyathan V. Antioxidants and antioxidant activity of several pigmented rice brans. *J Agric Food Chem* 2011;**59**(1):193–9.

5. Xu Z, Godber JS. Purification and identification of components of gamma-oryzanol in rice bran Oil. *J Agric Food Chem* 1999;**47**(7):2724–8.

6. IUPAC-IUB Joint Commission on Biochemical Nomenclature (JCBN). The nomenclature of steroids. Recommendations 1989. *Eur J Biochem* 1989;**186**(3):429–58.

7. Islam MS, Yoshida H, Matsuki N, Ono K, Nagasaka R, Ushio H, et al. Antioxidant, free radical-scavenging, and NF-kappaB-inhibitory activities of phytosteryl ferulates: structure-activity studies. *J Pharmacol Sci* 2009;**111**(4):328–37.

8. Castro L, Freeman BA. Reactive oxygen species in human health and disease. *Nutrition* 2001;**17**(2):3–5, 161.

9. Droge W. Free radicals in the physiological control of cell function. *Physiol Rev* 2002;**82**(1):47–95.

10. Raha S, Robinson BH. Mitochondria, oxygen free radicals, disease and ageing. *Trends Biochem Sci* 2000;**25**(10):502–8.

11. Lopez-Revuelta A, Sanchez-Gallego JI, Hernandez-Hernandez A, Sanchez-Yague J, Llanillo M. Increase in vulnerability to oxidative damage in cholesterol-modified erythrocytes exposed to t-BuOOH. *Biochim Biophys Acta* 2005;**1734**(1):74–85.

12. Nagasaka R, Chotimarkorn C, Shafiqul IM, Hori M, Ozaki H, Ushio H. Anti-inflammatory effects of hydroxycinnamic acid derivatives. *Biochem Biophys Res Commun* 2007;**358**(2):615–9.

13. Sultana S, Alam A, Khan N, Sharma S. Inhibition of benzoyl peroxide and ultraviolet-B radiation induced oxidative stress and tumor promotion markers by cycloartenol in murine skin. *Redox Rep* 2003;**8**(2):105–12.

14. Mizuta K, Kaneta H, Itaya K. [Effects of gamma-oryzanol on gastric secretions in rats [authors' transl.]. *Nihon Yakurigaku Zasshi* 1978;**74**(2):285–95.

15. Mizuta K, Itaya K. Effects of gamma-oryzanol and atropine on gastric secretion stimulated by insulin or 2-deoxy-D-glucose [authors' transl]. *Nihon Yakurigaku Zasshi* 1978;**74**(4):517–24.

16. Islam MS, Murata T, Fujisawa M, Nagasaka R, Ushio H, Bari AM, et al. Anti-inflammatory effects of phytosteryl ferulates in colitis induced by dextran sulphate sodium in mice. *Br J Pharmacol* 2008;**154**(4):812–24.

17. Surh YJ. NF-kappa B and Nrf2 as potential chemopreventive targets of some anti-inflammatory and antioxidative phytonutrients with anti-inflammatory and antioxidative activities. *Asia Pac J Clin Nutr* 2008;**17**(Suppl. 1):269–72.

18. Chotimarkorn C, Ushio H. The effect of trans-ferulic acid and gamma-oryzanol on ethanol-induced liver injury in C57BL mouse. *Phytomedicine* 2008;**15**(11):951–8.

19. Akihisa T, Yasukawa K, Yamaura M, Ukiya M, Kimura Y, Shimizu N, et al. Triterpene alcohol and sterol ferulates from rice bran and their anti-inflammatory effects. *J Agric Food Chem* 2000;**48**(6): 2313–9.

20. Ahumada C, Saenz T, Garcia D, De La Puerta R, Fernandez A, Martinez E. The effects of a triterpene fraction isolated from Crataegus monogyna Jacq. on different acute inflammation models in rats and mice. Leucocyte migration and phospholipase A2 inhibition. *J Pharm Pharmacol* 1997;**49**(3):329–31.

21. Sakai S, Murata T, Tsubosaka Y, Ushio H, Hori M, Ozaki H. gamma-Oryzanol reduces adhesion molecule expression in vascular endothelial cells via suppression of nuclear factor-kappaB activation. *J Agric Food Chem* 2012;**60**(13):3367–72.

22. Cicero AF, Gaddi A. Rice bran oil and gamma-oryzanol in the treatment of hyperlipoproteinaemias and other conditions. *Phytother Res* 2001;**15**(4):277–89.

23. Wilson TA, Nicolosi RJ, Woolfrey B, Kritchevsky D. Rice bran oil and oryzanol reduce plasma lipid and lipoprotein cholesterol concentrations and aortic cholesterol ester accumulation to a greater extent than ferulic acid in hypercholesterolemic hamsters. *J Nutr Biochem* 2007;**18**(2):105–12.

24. Seetharamaiah GS, Chandrasekhara N. Studies on hypocholesterolemic activity of rice bran oil. *Atherosclerosis* 1989;**78**(2–3):219–23.

25. Wilson TA, Ausman LM, Lawton CW, Hegsted DM, Nicolosi RJ. Comparative cholesterol lowering properties of vegetable oils: beyond fatty acids. *J Am Coll Nutr* 2000;**19**(5):601–7.

26. Nicolosi RJ, Ausman LM, Hegsted DM. Rice bran oil lowers serum total and low density lipoprotein cholesterol and apo B levels in nonhuman primates. *Atherosclerosis* 1991;**88**(2–3):133–42.

27. Sharma RD, Rukmini C. Rice bran oil and hypocholesterolemia in rats. *Lipids* 1986;**21**(11):715–7.

28. Sasaki J, Takada Y, Handa K, Kusuda M, Tanabe Y, Matsunaga A, et al. Effects of gamma-oryzanol on serum lipids and apolipoproteins in dyslipidemic schizophrenics receiving major tranquilizers. *Clin Ther* 1990;**12**(3):263–8.

29. Rong N, Ausman LM, Nicolosi RJ. Oryzanol decreases cholesterol absorption and aortic fatty streaks in hamsters. *Lipids* 1997;**32**(3):303–9.

30. Rajnarayana K, Prabhakar MC, Krishna DR. Influence of rice bran oil on serum lipid peroxides and lipids in human subjects. *Indian J Physiol Pharmacol* 2001;**45**(4):442–4.

31. Rukmini C, Raghuram TC. Nutritional and biochemical aspects of the hypolipidemic action of rice bran oil: a review. *J Am Coll Nutr* 1991;**10**(6):593–601.

32. Raicht RF, Cohen BI, Fazzini EP, Sarwal AN, Takahashi M. Protective effect of plant sterols against chemically induced colon tumors in rats. *Cancer Res* 1980;**40**(2):403–5.

33. Kong CK, Lam WS, Chiu LC, Ooi VE, Sun SS, Wong YS. A rice bran polyphenol, cycloartenyl ferulate, elicits apoptosis in human colorectal adenocarcinoma SW480 and sensitizes metastatic SW620 cells to TRAIL-induced apoptosis. *Biochem Pharmacol* 2009;**77**(9):1487–96.

34. Awad AB, Chen YC, Fink CS, Hennessey T. Beta-sitosterol inhibits HT-29 human colon cancer cell growth and alters membrane lipids. *Anticancer Res* 1996;**16**(5A):2797–804.

35. Awad AB, Fink CS. Phytosterols as anticancer dietary components: evidence and mechanism of action. *J Nutr* 2000;**130**(9):2127–30.

36. Luo HF, Li Q, Yu S, Badger TM, Fang N. Cytotoxic hydroxylated triterpene alcohol ferulates from rice bran. *J Nat Prod* 2005;**68**(1):94–7.

37. Verschoyle RD, Greaves P, Cai H, Edwards RE, Steward WP, Gescher AJ. Evaluation of the cancer chemopreventive efficacy of rice bran in genetic mouse models of breast, prostate and intestinal carcinogenesis. *Br J Cancer* 2007;**96**(2):248–54.

38. Hudson EA, Dinh PA, Kokubun T, Simmonds MS, Gescher A. Characterization of potentially chemopreventive phenols in extracts of brown rice that inhibit the growth of human breast and colon cancer cells. *Cancer Epidemiol Biomarkers Prev* 2000;**9**(11):1163–70.

39. Yasukawa K, Akihisa T, Kimura Y, Tamura T, Takido M. Inhibitory effect of cycloartenol ferulate, a component of rice bran, on tumor promotion in two-stage carcinogenesis in mouse skin. *Biol Pharm Bull* 1998;**21**(10):1072–6.

40. Mori H, Kawabata K, Yoshimi N, Tanaka T, Murakami T, Okada T, et al. Chemopreventive effects of ferulic acid on oral and rice germ on large bowel carcinogenesis. *Anticancer Res* 1999 Sep-Oct;**1**9(5A):3775–8.

41. Kanaya Y, Doi T, Sasaki H, Fujita A, Matsuno S, Okamoto K, et al. Rice bran extract prevents the elevation of plasma peroxylipid in KKAy diabetic mice. *Diabetes Res Clin Pract* 2004;**66**(Suppl. 1):S157–60.

42. Kadowaki T, Yamauchi T, Kubota N, Hara K, Ueki K, Tobe K. Adiponectin and adiponectin receptors in insulin resistance, diabetes, and the metabolic syndrome. *J Clin Invest* 2006;**116**(7):1784–92.

43. Ohara K, Uchida A, Nagasaka R, Ushio H, Ohshima T. The effects of hydroxycinnamic acid derivatives on adiponectin secretion. *Phytomedicine* 2009;**16**(2–3):130–7.

44. Jung EH, Kim SR, Hwang IK, Ha TY. Hypoglycemic effects of a phenolic acid fraction of rice bran and ferulic acid in C57BL/KsJ-db/db mice. *J Agric Food Chem* 2007;**55**(24):9800–4.

45. Sierra S, Lara-Villoslada F, Olivares M, Jimenez J, Boza J, Xaus J. Increased immune response in mice consuming rice bran oil. *Eur J Nutr* 2005;**44**(8):509–16.

46. Oka T, Fujimoto M, Nagasaka R, Ushio H, Hori M, Ozaki H. Cycloartenyl ferulate, a component of rice bran oil-derived gamma-oryzanol, attenuates mast cell degranulation. *Phytomedicine* **17**(2): 152–156.

47. Lichtenstein AH, Ausman LM, Carrasco W, Gualtieri LJ, Jenner JL, Ordovas JM, et al. Rice bran oil consumption and plasma lipid levels in moderately hypercholesterolemic humans. *Arterioscler Thromb* 1994;**14**(4):549–56.

48. Shimomura Y, Kobayashi I, Maruto S, Ohshima K, Mori M, Kamio N, et al. Effect of gamma-oryzanol on serum TSH concentrations in primary hypothyroidism. *Endocrinol Jpn* 1980;**27**(1):83–6.

49. Maoka T, Tanimoto F, Sano M, Tsurukawa K, Tsuno T, Tsujiwaki S, et al. Effects of dietary supplementation of ferulic acid and gamma-oryzanol on integument color and suppression of oxidative stress in cultured red sea bream, *Pagrus major*. *J Oleo Sci* 2008;**57**(2):133–7.

50. Murray JC, Burch JA, Streilein RD, Iannacchione MA, Hall RP, Pinnell SR. A topical antioxidant solution containing vitamins C and E stabilized by ferulic acid provides protection for human skin against damage caused by ultraviolet irradiation. *J Am Acad Dermatol* 2008;**59**(3):418–25.

51. Gorewit RC. Pituitary and thyroid hormone responses of heifers after ferulic acid administration. *J Dairy Sci* 1983;**66**(3):624–9.

52. Ardiansyah Ohsaki Y, Shirakawa H, Koseki T, Komai M. Novel effects of a single administration of ferulic acid on the regulation of blood pressure and the hepatic lipid metabolic profile in stroke-prone spontaneously hypertensive rats. *J Agric Food Chem* 2008;**56**(8):2825–30.

53. Cheng CY, Su SY, Tang NY, Ho TY, Chiang SY, Hsieh CL. Ferulic acid provides neuroprotection against oxidative stress-related apoptosis after cerebral ischemia/reperfusion injury by inhibiting ICAM-1 mRNA expression in rats. *Brain Res* 2008;**1209**: 136–50.

54. Yan JJ, Cho JY, Kim HS, Kim KL, Jung JS, Huh SO, et al. Protection against beta-amyloid peptide toxicity in vivo with long-term administration of ferulic acid. *Br J Pharmacol* 2001;**133**(1):89–96.

55. Grunewald KK, Bailey RS. Commercially marketed supplements for bodybuilding athletes. *Sports Med* 1993;**15**(2):90–103.

Organic Rice Bran Oils in Health

Khongsak Srikaeo

Pibulsongkram Rajabhat University, Faculty of Food and Agricultural Technology, Muang Phitsanulok, Thailand

INTRODUCTION

Rice is the most important cereal crop in Asia, and is a staple food in most populations of this region. It is grown in more than 100 countries, and there are around 18,000 varieties accounting for about 25% of the world's food grain production. Milling of paddy yields approximately 70% of rice (endosperm) as the major product, and by-products consisting of 20% rice husk, 8% rice bran, and 2% rice germ.[1-6]

Rice bran constitutes about 10% of the weight of rough rice. It is comprised of pericarp, aleurone, sub-aleurone, seed coat, nucellus along with the germ, and a small portion of endosperm. The percentage and composition of rice bran vary according to the rice variety, pretreatment before milling, the type of milling system, and the degree of milling. Rice bran is light in color, sweet in taste, moderately oily, and has a slightly toasted nutty flavor. Texture varies from a fine, powder-like consistency to a flake, depending on the stabilization process.[7-11]

Rice bran contains 12–22% oil, 11–17% protein, 6–14% fiber, 10–15% moisture, and 8–17% ash. It is rich in vitamins, including vitamin E, thiamin, and niacin, and minerals such as aluminum, calcium, chlorine, iron, magnesium, manganese, phosphorus, potassium, sodium, and zinc.[7,12] It also contains a significant amount of nutraceutical compounds and approximately 4% unsaponifiables, mainly comprised of naturally occurring antioxidants such as tocopherols, tocotrienols, and oryzanol.[13]

It was earlier used primarily as animal feed, but is now finding major applications in the form of rice bran oil (RBO).[14,15]

RBO is traditionally consumed in Asian rice producing countries, with growing interest in Western markets.[16-19] It is in steady demand as "healthy oil" in Japan, where approximately 80,000 tonnes is consumed annually.[20] Traditionally RBO has been used for frying food, due to its oxidative stability and flavor; it is now considered to

be a good substitute for vegetable oils.[21,22] It is widely used in pharmaceutical, food, and allied industries due to its unique properties, high medicinal value, and therapeutic applications.[23,24]

Recently, interest in RBO has escalated with its identification as a healthy oil. It is well established that RBO is one of the most nutritious and health-beneficial edible oils, as it contains high level of physiologically active compounds. γ-Oryzanol and phytosterols have the capacity to lower blood cholesterol and decrease cholesterol absorption. Tocotrienols and γ-oryzanol are known as powerful antioxidants, which are associated with the prevention of cardiovascular diseases and some cancers.[25-30]

Organic production of RBO provides more nutraceuticals. However, most commercial productions of RBO involve the use of hazardous chemical extraction and various refining processes, which are not permitted in organic food production. Moreover, the extensive refining processes dramatically reduce the nutritional values of RBO.

This chapter reviews the health benefits of RBO, with special focus on organic RBO. Aspects on processing are also discussed.

CONVENTIONAL RBO PRODUCTION

Generally, RBO is difficult to process due to its high levels of free fatty acids (FFAs), waxes, bran fines, and pigment content. These factors lead to high refining losses when traditional refining processes are employed. However, with careful attention to processing techniques, beginning with the rice mill, RBO can be produced economically with reasonable yields and quality.[31]

The processing of RBO starts with stabilization of the rice bran. The stabilized rice bran is then extracted for crude RBO. The crude oil is then refined by a number of refining steps. These processes have been summarized and discussed by different authors.[8,22]

Various commercial efforts to extract the oil have been made for a very long time. RBO with low FFA content can be extracted with hexane from extrusion stabilized bran. Non-stabilized bran, although having a high FFA, can also be used for production of oil. Preprocessing of the bran through an extruder, expander, or expeller may be used to form either a flake or pellet, which results in improved solvent flow through an extraction bed.[32]

Earlier methods to recover the oil used hydraulic pressing.[22] In a Japanese system for pressing, the raw bran is cleaned by sifting and air classification to remove whole and broken grains and hulls, and, in some instances, to recover rice germ. The bran is then steam cooked, dried, pre-pressed, and finally expeller pressed. Hexane extraction may be by batch, battery, or continuous type. All three systems were recently operating in Japan. Continuous systems operate in Brazil, Burma, Egypt, India, Mexico, Taiwan, Thailand, and the United States. The bran in the most efficient systems is stabilized, pelletized, and, if required, dried. After the pretreated bran is placed in the extractor, hexane is pumped in and allowed to percolate through the bran to extract the oil. Countercurrent extraction is used.

The miscella (solvent plus oil) is passed through filters to remove the bran fines before evaporation for solvent and crude oil recovery. The production of fines from expander stabilized bran depends on the stabilization condition. The flake size is larger if expanded at 120°C, but the flakes are fragile and easily broken. Flakes with high moisture content are more resistant to breakage. Final bran moisture is about 6%.

Pelletizing of the bran improves percolation and minimizes fines in the miscella. Pellets are 6–8 mm in diameter. Moistening during pelletizing reduces the fines problem. Parboiled bran does not produce the hard pellets found for raw bran, possibly because of protein denaturation during parboiling. Binding of the fines in the pellet is assisted by starch gelatinization during heating of the bran. Parboiled bran also presents problems in sticking to dryer surfaces, resulting in self-ignition in the dryer. Prior mixing with raw bran alleviates the problem.

Extraction of RBO by supercritical fluid has been investigated.[33] Minor reductions in oil yield may occur. The oil yield is 17.98% with supercritical CO_2, 18.23% with CO_2–ethanol, and 20.21% with hexane.

Extraction yields crude RBO which then needs to go through many refining steps. The composition of crude RBO has a major effect on refining. The crude oil typically contains up to 0.5% bran fines and 0.5–5% wax. Agitated storage tanks are required, and heated tanks and lines also are necessary to prevent crystallization of waxes. Refining losses may be in excess of 10 times the amount of FFAs when the crude oil has a relatively low FFA (<10%) content. Lower refining losses of approximately twice the amount of FFAs have been reported.[32]

Refining of crude RBO involves dewaxing, degumming, neutralization of free fatty acids, bleaching to improve color, and steam deodorization.

Crude RBOs contain bran fines, and the removal of fines prior to degumming and refining gives better oil quality and yield.[34] Refined RBO is a light yellow color (Lovibond 3.0 R 30Y) with a mild background odor and flavor reminiscent of rice. Similar to peanut oil, the flavor and odor are complementary to the flavor of many fried foods, such as fish, chicken, and chips.

Dewaxing

Waxes can increase refining losses. The wax content of crude oil depends on the variety of rice used, milling technique, method of oil extraction, and extraction temperature. Extraction temperature affects both the type of wax present and its quantity – for example, extraction at 50°C yields two to three times more wax than extraction at 20°C.

Initial dewaxing may consist simply of gravity settling followed by decanting. The oil is gradually cooled to allow for wax crystallization, followed by filtration or centrifugation to recover the wax sludge. The foots recovered may be added back to the defatted bran, sold as an animal feed oil, or further processed for oil recovery and wax purification. Wax recovery involves acetone washing and fractionation with isopropanol.

Attempts have been made to recover the wax using cold and hot extraction. Wax yields of 1.29–1.82% of the crude oil are obtained. Continuous dewaxing of RBO by chilling the oil or miscella to less than 20°C followed by filtration through plate and frame filters is practiced. Sodium silicate has been used as an aid for dewaxing. The characteristics and physical properties of a purified rice bran wax are similar to those of carnauba wax. Additional dewaxing may be used during degumming and alkali refining. Dewaxing of refined, bleached oil by cooling to approximately 5°C followed by filtration is necessary for production of high-grade, chill-proof oil.[22]

Degumming and Deacidification

The phospholipids in rice oil are similar in composition to those in other oil sources. These may be recovered as rice lecithin.[22] Production of food-grade lecithin requires prior removal of bran fines and waxes. Regular water degumming may be used.

Temperatures above 80°C are required to prevent crystallization and removal of waxes with the gums. If food-grade lecithin is not being produced, filtration of bran fines is not required. Pretreatment with phosphoric or organic acid is necessary to remove non-hydratable phospholipids. Food-grade surfactants may be added to improve wax removal.[35] Degumming at less than 50°C actually assists in wax removal. Wet gums may be added to defatted bran as a method for disposal.[8]

Both alkali and physical refining have been used for FFA removal. With alkali refining, batch or continuous methods may be used. Oil may be pretreated with phosphoric or organic acid for phospholipid hydration. The oil is then treated with 16- to 30-baume caustics with 20–40% excess. The soaps settle and may be recovered as "soapstock" or foots.[36]

Continuous refining consists of in-line mixers, heaters, and centrifuges. The combined oils plus alkali are rapidly heated to 55–70°C to assist in breaking the emulsion of hydrated soap in oil. In instances where neutralization is combined with dewaxing, separation is performed at 28–32°C. Water washing or post-neutralization treatment with silicates to remove final traces of soaps and phospholipids is the same as for conventional oils. Miscella refining, or refining while still in solvent, may also be used. Higher refining yields and good-quality neutralized oil with less color are advantages of miscella refining. Losses are near the calculated amount based on titrated values. Rice oil miscella is often variable.[36]

Excessive losses may occur in refining of RBO. A 5% FFA crude oil has losses ranging from 12% to 40% by the cup method. The cause of high refining losses is unknown, although it is assumed the losses are caused by the presence of partial esters, oxidized components, and waxes, as well as high FFA acidity. Steam refining is practiced by various refineries in Japan and the United States. In calculating the amount of caustic required for caustic neutralization, the oil is titrated to a phenolphthalein endpoint. This titration endpoint includes not only the FFA, but also the oryzanol compounds. With the higher caustic addition, the oryzanol is transferred to the soapstock away from the oil, and the nutritional benefit of these compounds is lost. An alternative indicator for titration uses alkali blue;[22] this indicator reflects only the acidity contributed by the free fatty acids.

Bleaching, Hydrogenation, and Deodorization

Standard methods are used for bleaching, hydrogenation, and deodorization of RBO. Bleaching uses activated carbon or bleaching earth.[36] Activated carbon is seldom used because of the high costs and difficulties in handling. Bleach clay dosage depends on the characteristics of the rice bran oil as well as that of the bleaching earth, and dosages range from 2% to 10%. Newer silica bleaching earths are more effective in achieving satisfactory oil colors.

Deodorization or steam stripping is used to remove objectionable odors resulting from peroxides, aldehydes, and ketones, as well as characteristic RBO odors and flavors. The oil is heated to 220–250°C under 3–5 mmHg vacuum. Semicontinuous deodorizer units are the most common types used. Storage of deodorized RBO is the same as for other oils.

Physical refining, also called steam refining, combines deacidification with deodorization. Physical refining is more efficient for high FFA oils, giving better yields of neutralized oil than alkali refining.[22]

Winterization

In addition to wax, RBO contains sufficient saturated and high melting glycerides to require winterization to achieve a cold test of 5 hours. Without winterization, dewaxed rice oil is frequently cloudy or turbid even at room temperature or slightly lower. Winterization consists of cooling the oil under defined rates and to specific temperatures, followed by filtration. With rice oil, winterization consists of cooling 30–35°C oil slowly at a uniform rate to 15°C over a 12-hour period with slow agitation, then further cooling to 4–5°C without agitation followed by holding over a 24- to 48-hour period, allowing higher melting components to crystallize. The type of crystals formed depends on the cooling rate and the temperature differentials.

Large, stable crystals are desired for filterability. Filter aids may be added to assist separation of the crystals from the viscous oil. Cold tests of the winterized oil of 5–7 hours are near maximum.

Miscella winterization more effectively separates the high melting solids from RBO. Hexane, acetone, and isopropyl acetate are among the solvents used. The miscella is slowly cooled to 15°C over 12 hours with agitation, then to 4–5°C without agitation, and held for 24–48 hours before filtering.

More recently, membrane-based separation and purification technologies have been established as an efficient, cost-effective, and environmentally friendly process for solid–liquid, solute–solvent, and liquid–liquid separation applications.

Membrane separation is primarily a size-exclusion based pressure-driven process. Performance of membrane separation is affected by membrane composition, temperature, pressure, velocity of flow, and interaction between components of the feedstock and with the membrane surface.[31]

ORGANIC RBO PRODUCTION

The processing of organic foods must comply with national and international regulations, which may differ from region to region. In general, organic foods are produced using methods that do not involve modern synthetic inputs such as synthetic pesticides and chemical fertilizers. Organic foods must not be processed using irradiation, industrial solvents, or chemical food additives. Processed organic food usually contains only organic ingredients. If non-organic ingredients are present, at least a certain percentage of the food's total plant and animal ingredients must be organic (95% in the United States, Canada, and Australia), and any non-organically produced ingredients are subject to various agricultural requirements. Foods claiming to be organic must be free of artificial food additives, and are often processed with fewer artificial methods, materials, and conditions (such as chemical ripening, food irradiation, and genetically modified ingredients). Pesticides are allowed as long as they are not synthetic. To be certified organic, products must be grown and manufactured in a manner that adheres to standards set by the country they are sold in.

Organic RBO may be produced from cold-pressed rice bran. This produces crude RBO. Crude oils of vegetable origin contain impurities of varying types. These impurity levels are affected by storage and handling, as well as extraction processes. With increasing demand for healthy products, organic RBO is very appealing as a specialty oil in a niche market. Srikaeo and Pradit[37] mentioned that most organic RBOs in Thailand are produced by small-scale manufacturers using a single-screw compression press for oil extraction. This process is less capital-intensive and requires no sophisticated machinery, but results in very low production yields. Crude RBO produced by this method also contains high amount of impurities. The oil is usually high in FFAs, waxes, and bran fines. This causes problems such as dark color, haziness, a higher amount of unsaponifiables, and foaming during frying, consequently creating setbacks for its marketing as edible oil. As mentioned earlier, industrial processing of vegetable oils as well as RBO is generally obtained by solvent extraction and processed by degumming, alkali-refining, bleaching, winterizing, and deodorizing. Due to its physical and chemical characteristics, crude RBO is considered the most difficult oil to refine to meet edible oil specifications. Moreover, the industrial refining process requires the use of hazardous chemicals such as sodium hydroxide (alkali refining), which is not allowed for organic RBO processing.

Rice bran for production of organic RBO must have been farmed organically and processed via organic-certified facilities. Industrial solvent extraction and chemical refining processes must be avoided. Therefore, commercial large-scale production of organic RBO is currently not viable. Organic RBO is usually marketed as high-value food or dietary supplements, and not as an edible cooking oil. For example, commercial organic RBOs sold in Thailand are usually marketed as health food supplements. They can also come in the form of soft gels or capsules.

In the market for organic food consumer trust is a delicate issue, since consumers are not able to verify whether a product is an organic product, even after consumption. Organic products must be produced according to organic principles, which refer to the production process rather than to the endproduct.[38] Certified organic products can be identified by organic certification logos, which differ from country to country. In a single country, there may also be several organic labeling schemes.

EFFECTS OF PROCESSING ON RBO COMPONENTS

As discussed above, crude RBO needs careful refining due to the high content of impurities.

Chemical refining seems the most appropriate and straightforward process to obtain a refined oil with a bland taste, light color, and good (cold) stability. It consists of degumming, dewaxing, alkali neutralization, bleaching, and deodorization.[31] However, the operating costs of chemical refining are quite high due to oil losses during neutralization, and environmental problems caused by the production of large soapstock waste streams. Moreover, high percentages of the valuable minor compounds are lost.[39–42] Consumer interest in minimally processed oils of high nutritional value necessitates continuous research regarding appropriate refining processes.

The problems of soapstock disposal and of losses of oryzanol and neutral oil can be reduced by using a weak acid salt (such as sodium bicarbonate) to achieve a refined RBO with a high yield and with good oryzanol retention. Furthermore, this oil can be treated with small amounts of concentrated caustic to yield a refined RBO and a nutraceutical-rich concentrate. Other alternative methods to chemical refining are miscella refining, mixed solvent refining, and physical or steam refining.[31] The latter process is commonly used for high FFA feedstocks (palm oil, coconut oil), and has the advantages of producing no soapstock and yielding lower oil and micronutrient losses.[42] However, steam refining requires a rigorous pretreatment to remove interfering pigments, waxes, and phospholipids.[43] For this pretreatment, many different degumming and dewaxing methods are described, such as degumming with water or acid, super degumming, enzymatic degumming, combined degumming/dewaxing, miscella dewaxing, and solvent dewaxing.[31] Notably, most of these methods, which involve chemicals and extreme condition processes, are not allowed for organic RBO processing.

Furthermore, studies on the use of different types of membranes show that they have the potential for use in all stages of RBO refining,[44] and for increasing the retention of oryzanol in the RBO.[45] Despite these encouraging results, a major drawback of membrane processing, especially in an industrial environment, is the difficulty of preventing fouling and/or cleaning fouled membranes.[31] In industrial practice, rice bran is still mostly chemically refined. Earlier attempts to apply physical refining failed because it was not possible to produce refined oil with a sufficiently light color.

Recently, membrane technology has been applied to the oil industry. However, much work has yet to be done on membrane processing of RBO.[46]

Membrane processes seem to be a beneficial process for refining the oil as well as preserving the natural antioxidants in oil. Subramanian et al.[47] studied membrane permeation of TAG (>800 Da)–tocopherols (431 Da) model systems, where tocopherols did not permeate (−51 to −29% rejection) through non-porous membranes and consequently its concentration in the feed increased from 0.144 to 0.67%. However, the total permeate flux remained almost constant (0.098 and 0.104 kg/m² per hour) throughout the process, despite a large change in tocopherol concentration in the feed.

Oryzanol, which is the unique phytonutrient in RBO, was found to be reduced dramatically during the oil refining process. Degumming and dewaxing of crude RBO removed only 1.1% and 5.9% of oryzanol, respectively, while the alkali treatment removed 93.0–94.6% of oryzanol from the original crude oil. Oryzanol lost during the refining process is retained in the soapstock, which is not one of the edible oil products.

The oryzanol content in some commercial RBOs has been reported. Crude RBO contained 1.8–2.4%, degummed RBO contained 1.7–2.2%, chemically refined RBO contained 0.1–0.2%, physically refined RBO contained 1.0–1.7%, and soapstocks contained 2.2–6.7% of oryzanol. Attempts have been made to isolate ozyzanol from the soapstock by-products.

HEALTH BENEFITS OF RBO

RBO is an unconventional vegetable oil believed by some populations to be healthy due to its high levels of antioxidants and phytosterols. It is superior to other vegetable oils because it contains ω-3 and ω-6 fatty acids, particularly due to oryzanol and higher amounts of unsaponifiables.[48,49]

It seems that RBO and its components are able to improve the plasma lipid pattern of hypercholesterolemic patients safely. The available data in humans suggest that RBO is an edible oil of preference for improving plasma lipid and lipoprotein profiles.[20]

The hypolipidemic response of RBO was investigated in non-human primates fed on semi-purified diets containing blends of oils including RBO at 0–35% kcals as dietary fat. The study demonstrated that the degree of reduction of serum total cholesterol (TC) and low density lipoprotein cholesterol (LDL-C) was highly correlated with initial serum cholesterol levels in monkeys fed on a standard diet. Further, RBO supplementation in the diet significantly influenced serum TC and LDL-C, causing up to 40% reduction in LDL-C without affecting HDL-C levels when RBO was the sole dietary oil.[50]

Similar to animal studies, a range of human studies has shown that RBO is an edible oil of preference for improving serum cholesterol levels and lipoprotein profiles. The first scientific statement regarding RBO's antihyperlipidemic property in humans was published in 1970. RBO blended with corn, safflower, and sunflower oil was consumed by healthy young women for 7 days to evaluate the effect of blending different vegetable oils on serum cholesterol levels. It was observed that the hypocholesterolemic effect of RBO was comparable to that of other vegetable oils, such as corn, safflower, and sunflower oils. Furthermore, the blended oil still exerted hypocholesterolemic effects, even when 5 eggs were consumed daily for 7 consecutive days. In contrast, there was an increase in HDL-cholesterol after consumption of the blended oil, and consequently the atherogenic index was significantly improved.[51,52]

The hypocholesterolemic effects of RBO were evaluated in moderately non-obese hyperlipoproteinemic human subjects fed on RBO for a longer period. For comparison, the control group continued use of palm or groundnut oils. The RBO-treated patients showed a 16–25% decrease in plasma total cholesterol and 32–35% drop in triglycerides after 15–30 days of treatment as compared to the control group.[53]

The diets of healthy volunteers with normal cholesterol levels were supplemented with a margarine enriched with RBO sterols to assess the impact of sterols present in the unsaponifiable fraction of RBO on the lipid profile. The subjects were instructed to continue usual dietary and physical activities while supplementing their diets with control margarine containing traces of sterols, or margarine enriched with 2.1 g/day of the sterols from RBO for 3 weeks each. The enriched margarine significantly lowered total and LDL cholesterol compared to control.[54]

The roles of the RBO components that promote health benefits are discussed in more detail below.

Fatty Acids

Dietary fat is a crucial factor in the regulation of cholesterol levels, and there is overwhelming evidence to support the hypocholesterolemic effects of vegetable oils rich in polyunsaturated fatty acids, mainly linoleic acid. Growing interest in the health benefits of polyunsaturated fatty acids has focused on providing suitable sources of these constituents. Polyunsaturated fatty acids include linoleic acid (C18:2n6c), α-linolenic acid (ALA, C18:3n3), γ-linolenic acid (GLA, C18:3n6), arachidonic acid (AA, C20:4n6), eicosapentaenoic acid (EPA, C20:5n3), and docosahexaenoic acid (DHA, C22:6n3).

Polyunsaturated fatty acids are required in the body for normal functioning of the nervous, immune and inflammatory, cardiovascular, endocrine, respiratory, and reproductive systems. Their presence on membrane phospholipids can influence cellular activities. Fatty acids also alter membrane fluidity, consequently modulating changes in conformation or function of receptors, transporters and enzymes.[55,56]

Edible oils rich in polyunsaturated fatty acids have been reported to result in a decrease in total cholesterol, triglycerides, and low density lipoprotein cholesterol, as well as the beneficial HDL cholesterol. In RBO, the amount of linoleic acid is moderate and the proportion of oleic acid is relatively high. Studies have indicated that RBO has a significant hypocholesterolemic effect in both animals and humans when compared to other oils, in spite of containing only limited polyunsaturated fatty acids. The effect has been attributed to components such as tocotrienols, oryzanol, and mono-unsaturated fatty acid (the Mediterranean diet). The study with rats fed on a rice bran oil diet demonstrated a significant reduction in total serum cholesterol and LDL cholesterol, and an increase in fecal steroid excretion, compared with that of a peanut oil diet. Different research findings have proved that unsaponifiable fractions in RBO could compensate for its high saturated fats, and play a predominant role in decreasing cholesterol levels.[57–62]

Unsaponifiable Matter

Recently, RBO has received attention because of its unique health benefits,[63] attributed to its high level of unsaponifiable matter.[64] These are bioactive components with a nutraceutical value, and cannot be saponified by caustic treatment.[28] The unsaponifiables mainly comprise sterols (42–43%), triterpene alcohols (24–28%), and less polar components such as squalene or tocotrienols (19%), depending on the type of rice bran and the method used to extract and refine the lipids.[65,66] Crude RBO contains an unusually high content of unsaponifiables (3–5%), several times greater than most commonly used vegetable oils, whereas refined oil may contain 0.3–0.9% because the majority is removed during refining.[67] The content of the unsaponifiable material in refined RBO is regulated to be 0.5% under the Japan Agricultural Standard; this value is considerably higher than that of other vegetable oils.[20]

The unsaponifiable fraction in RBO also contains a unique complex of naturally occurring antioxidants, among which the tocopherols, tocotrienols, and oryzanol have received much attention.[68] The amount of α-tocopherol is relatively large (0.1% of the total oil) in RBO compared with other vegetable oils.[63]

There are several mechanisms by which unsaponifiables improve the serum biochemical profile, such as by interrupting the absorption of intestinal cholesterol rather than increasing the excretion of fat and neutral sterols, and increased fecal steroid excretion through interference with cholesterol absorption.[69–72]

Unsaponifiables prepared from RBO were evaluated in exogenously hypercholesterolemic rats. Animals were maintained for 2 weeks on a 0.5% cholesterol diet with 10% fat content (RBO, or a mixture of palm and safflower oils, or a mixture of palm and safflower oils plus 0.25% of unsaponifiable content prepared from RBO). Serum and liver total cholesterol concentrations were significantly lower and HDL levels significantly higher in both groups of rats consuming the unsaponifiables versus oil without added unsaponifiables.

Higher fecal excretion of cholesterol was noted in the two unsaponifiable groups as well. It was concluded that the unsaponifiable fraction of RBO acts to lower cholesterol by interrupting cholesterol absorption in the gut, and not by altering hepatic cholesterol metabolism.[70]

Monkeys were fed, in random order, a control diet or three experimental diets containing 20% energy content from RBO, canola oil, or corn oil, respectively. HDL levels were maintained on the RBO diet, while the rest of the diets showed a negative effect. The results suggest that the unsaponifiable fraction is critical for the oil's ability to decrease the risk of cardiovascular disease.[62]

Antioxidants

Any substance that delays or inhibits oxidation of the substrate, in spite of low concentrations, is called an antioxidant. The physiological role of antioxidants is to prevent damage to cellular components arising as a result of chemical reactions involving free radicals.[73] Several important nutraceutical compounds can be extracted from rice bran, which contains high levels of phytochemicals with antioxidant activities.[74] These phytochemicals include vitamin E, comprised of four homologues (α, β, γ, and δ) of tocopherol and tocotrienols,[75] and γ-oryzanol.[76] Vitamin E is considered to be the major chain-breaking antioxidant, especially in biological membranes.[77]

Rice bran is a rich natural source of vitamin E and γ-oryzanol.[78] It contains over 300 mg/kg vitamin E.[64] Vitamin E is a pale yellow, viscous oil.[7] It protects cell membranes by blocking oxidation of the unsaturated fatty acids and acting as a scavenger of free radicals. In addition to health benefits, antioxidants of rice bran and its oil have a potential use as additives to improve the storage stability and frying quality of foods.[79,80]

Oryzanol

The γ-oryzanol component in rice bran and RBO has the most potential as a nutraceutical, pharmaceutical, and cosmoceutical. This fraction contains ferulate

(4-hydroxo-3-methoxycinnamic acid) esters of sterols (campesterol, stigmasterol, and β-stigmasterol), and triterpene alcohols (cycloartenol, 24-methylene cycloartanol, cyclobranol).[81–83]

γ-Oryzanol was first isolated from RBO by Kaneko and Tsuchiya in 1954,[84] and was named because it was first discovered in RBO (*Oryza Sativa* L.). The most accessible natural source of γ-oryzanol is rice.[85] γ-Oryzanol is a white or slightly yellowish tasteless crystalline powder with little or no odor, and has a melting point of 137.5–138.5°C.[81] It is insoluble in water, slightly soluble in diethyl ether and n-heptane, and practically soluble in chloroform.[86] Initially it was reported to be a single component in rice bran,[103] but it is now known to be a mixture of at least 10 components.[87,88] Cycloartenyl ferulate, 24–methylene cycloartanyl ferulate, and campesteryl ferulate (Figure 35.1) are the three major components.

The concentration of γ-oryzanol in RBO ranges from 115 to 780 ppm, depending on the degree and method of processing.[89] γ-Oryzanol content in rice bran is 13–20 times (w/w) higher than that of total tocopherols and tocotrienols.[90] It has been observed that about 20% of the unsaponifiable fraction in RBO is oryzanol. Different extraction methods can result in different levels of these components, because some tocotrienols and

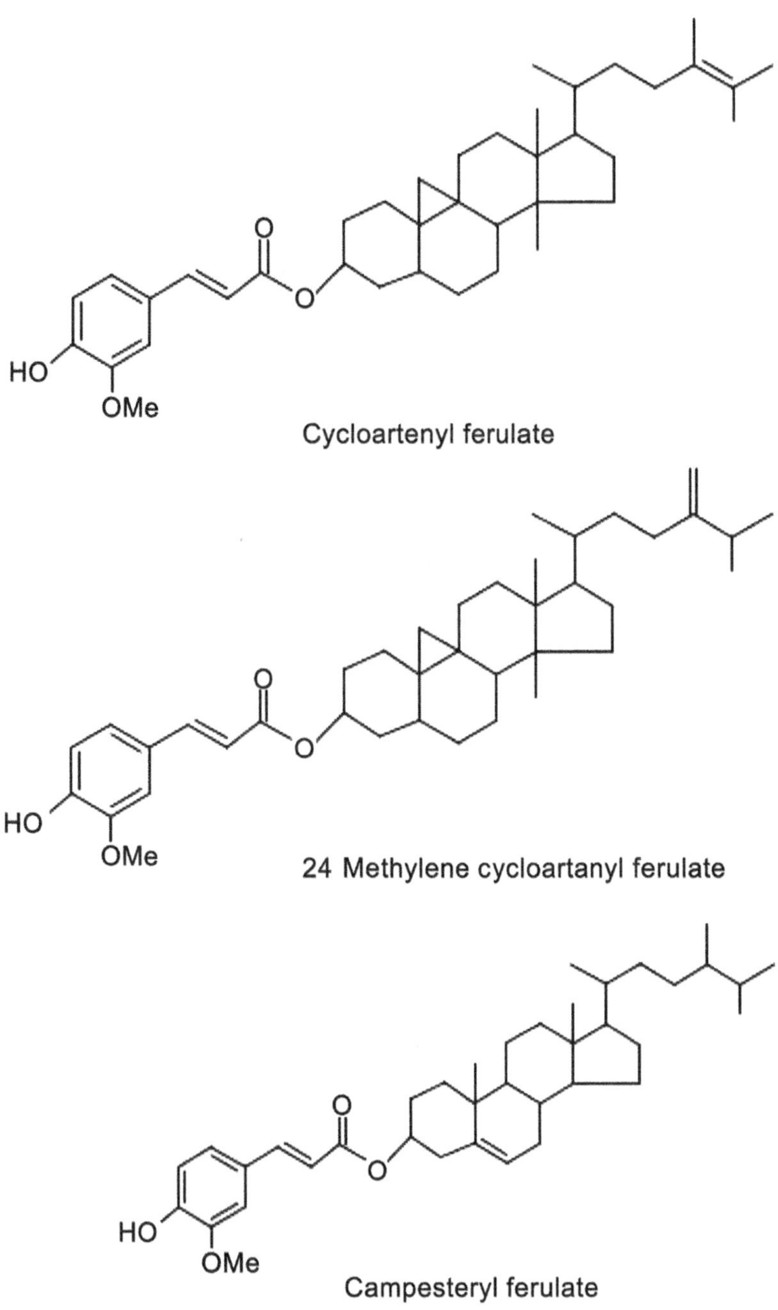

FIGURE 35.1 Three major components of γ-oryzanol.

Cycloartenyl ferulate

24 Methylene cycloartanyl ferulate

Campesteryl ferulate

A. OVERVIEW OF RICE AND HEALTH

tocotrienol-like compounds are bound to cellular components in the rice bran.[67,91]

The complete role of γ-oryzanol as a functional ingredient has not so far been thoroughly observed; on the other hand, health claims including antioxidant activity,[81] reduction of serum cholesterol,[92] reduction of cholesterol absorption,[65] increase of HDL cholesterol,[23] inhibition on platelet aggregation,[93] inhibition of tumor promotion,[94] and menopausal syndrome treatment[89] have been investigated.

For its antioxidant property, at the molecular and cellular levels, antioxidants serve to deactivate certain particles called free radicals. One *in vitro* study found that γ-oryzanol was more than four times as effective at stopping tissue oxidation as was vitamin E. The nutritional function of the γ-oryzanol components may be related to their antioxidant property because of the ferulic acid structure. Ferulic acid is a phenolic acid antioxidant.[95–99]

The antioxidant capacities of γ-oryzanol components were studied by using a linolenic acid model.[100] The three major components of γ-oryzanol (24-methylene cycloartanyl ferulate, cycloartenyl ferulate, and campesteryl ferulate) evidenced significant antioxidant activity when they were mixed with linoleic acid in a molar ratio of 1:100 and 1:250, but not in a molar ratio of 1:500. Antioxidant activities of tocopherols, tocotrienol, and γ-oryzanol oxidation were studied, and the highest antioxidant activity was found for 24-methylene cycloartanyl ferulate. All the three major γ-oryzanol componeents had activities higher than that of any of the four vitamin E components (α-tocopherol, α-tocotrinol, γ-tocopherol and γ-tocotrienol).[30] Inhibition of cholesterol autoxidation by the non-saponifiable fraction in rice bran was studied by Kim *et al.*[101] in an aqueous model system.

One of the most important properties of γ-oryzanol is its cholesterol-lowering property. There are several studies on humans and animals showing that the RBO has the property of lowering low density lipoprotein cholesterol and total serum cholesterol and increasing high density lipoprotein cholesterol to some extent either by influencing the absorption of dietary cholesterol or by enhancing the conversion of cholesterol to fecal bile acids and sterols. Further studies confirmed that the γ-oryzanol component of RBO is responsible for the hypocholesterolemia.[102–107]

The mechanism of the cholesterol-lowering action of γ-oryzanol was investigated.[67] Hamsters were rendered cholesterolemic by feeding them chow-based diets (containing coconut oil and 0.1% cholesterol with or without γ-oryzanol) for 7 weeks. Relative to control animals, oryzanol administration resulted in a significant reduction of plasma total cholesterol (28%) and non-high density lipoprotein cholesterol (non-HDL-C; 34%) levels, and a 25% reduction in cholesterol adsorption. Aortic fatty streak formation was reduced by 67% in the γ-oryzanol treated animals. It was concluded that γ-oryzanol was at least partly responsible for the cholesterol-lowering action of RBO, and is associated with the reduction in aortic fatty streak formation. It has been reported[108] that the serum total, LDL + VLDL cholesterol, and free esterified levels of rats maintained on a 10% RBO diet were lower than those of rats maintained on a 10% ground nut oil diet. Addition of 5% γ-oryzanol to the diet containing rice bran further reduced the serum cholesterol. These studies concluded that the cholesterol-lowering property of RBO might be due to γ-oryzanol and/or other non-saponifiable constituents present in RBO. Moreover, hypertriglyceridemia induced by fructose was lower in animals maintained on a 0.5% γ-oryzanol containing diet than in the corresponding controls. Blending of RBO with other vegetable oils in suitable proportions was reported to magnify the hypocholesterolemic activity, compared with the effect of each oil alone.[101] γ-Oryzanol may also lower the plasma cholesterol level. Although the mechanism underlying this effect is not known at present, the presence of γ-oryzanol and tocopherols in the rice bran is thought to be responsible for this favorable effect. The blending may have a practical significance. The effect of γ-oryzanol on atheroma formation in hypercholesterolemic rabbits has also been studied.[109] The effect of RBO and γ-oryzanol in the treatment of hyperlipoproteinemia has been investigated.[23] When added to a high cholesterol diet, it also inhibits platelet aggregation, preventing heart attacks and strokes. The nutritional and biochemical aspects of the hypolipidemic action of RBO have been reviewed, including the physiological, antioxidant, and hypocholesterolemic properties of γ-oryzanol.[110]

Regarding effects on serum TSH (thyroid stimulating hormone), a single oral dose (300 mg) of γ-oryzanol extracted from rice bran oil produced a significant reduction in the elevated serum TSH level in hypothyroid patients. Similarly, chronic treatment with γ-oryzanol resulted in a decreased serum TSH level in six of eight patients. There was no change in the serum level of thyroxine-iodine and triiodothyronine during the study. In addition, there was no difference in the serum TSH response to thyroid releasing hormone in hypothyroid patients and normal subjects. These observations suggest that γ-oryzanol inhibits serum TSH levels in patients with primary hypothyroidism, possibly by a direct action at the hypothalamus rather than the pituitary.[23]

Effects on muscle, γ-oryzanol/ferulic acid, inposine, chromium, and medium chain triacyl glycerol are used as ergogenic aids by strength/power athletes.[111] The effect of γ-oryzanol supplementation during resistance exercise training has been explained by Fry and colleagues.[112] These findings have created an interest in using γ-oryzanol as a sports supplement.

The carcinogenic potential of γ-oryzanol was studied in F344 rats[113] and B6C3F1 mice.[114] The findings indicate that, under the experimental conditions described, γ-oryzanol was not carcinogenic in F344 rats and B6C3F1 mice. The inhibitory effect of cycloartenol ferulate, a component of rice, on tumor promotion in two-stage carcinogenesis in mouse skin was studied.[94] According to this study, the active components of rice bran (sitosterol ferulate, 24-methylcholesterol ferulate, cycloartenol ferulate, and 24-methylenecycloartanol ferulate) markedly inhibited the TPA-induced inflammation in mice.

Cycloartenol ferulate, a component of γ-oryzanol in RBO, shows marked inhibition of the tumor promoting effect of TPA in 7,12-dimethylbenz[a]anthracene-initiated mice. The modifying effects of phytic acid and γ-oryzanol on the promotion stage of rat carcinogenesis, and RBO anticancer properties, were studied.[28,115]

In addition to γ-oryzanol, bioactive components from RBO have been shown to play a protective role against the alteration caused by a hypercholesterolemic diet. Male Sprague-Dawley rats were fed for 4 weeks with a normal diet, high-cholesterol diet, or high-cholesterol diet supplemented with the concentrated bioactive components from RBO. The high-cholesterol diet increased serum cholesterol in rats, compared with those fed on the normal diet. Serum HDL cholesterol was significantly increased in rats on the bioactive components from RBO group. Supplementation with bioactive compounds from RBO also lowered the activities of a biomarker of damage in liver function (aspartate transaminase). It was found that bioactive components from RBO have a significant practical value for protecting against the alterations caused by a hypercholesterolemic diet, and antioxidative ingredients which suppress lipid peroxidation.[102]

Tocols (Tocopherols and Tocotrienols)

Vitamin E consists of tocopherols and tocotrienols, collectively known as tocols. Humans and animals cannot synthesize this vitamin; they primarily acquire tocols from plants. Tocopherols and tocotrienols differ in the number and positions of methyl groups on the fused chromonol ring, and the absence or presence of three double bonds in the isoprenoid side chain. The structural differences between tocotrienols and tocopherols influence their biological activities.[116]

Tocotrienol has three double bonds within the main body of the molecule at the 3′, 7′, and 11′ positions of the hydrocarbon tail. Just like edible oils with a high level of polyunsaturated fatty acids, the presence of these double bonds give greater fluidity to tocotrienols and make it much easier for the body to incorporate them into cell membranes.[117] The major forms of tocotrienol are α-tocotrienol (5,7,8-trimethyltocotrienols), γ-tocotrienol (7,8-dimethyltocotrienol), and δ-tocotrienol (8-methyltocotrienol).[87]

RBO also contains high concentrations of the tocopherols compared with other oil seeds. Approximately 1% (v/v) of the unsaponifiable fraction of RBO is α-tocopherol. HPLC analysis of RBO showed that 1 g of RBO contains 3.02 mg of α-tocopherol.[118] Tocotrienols are present in vegetable oils like palm oil and RBO.[118,119] Barley, oat, palm, and rice brans contain more than 70% tocotrienols, known as the tocotrienols/tocotrienol rich fraction.[120] Two novel tocotrienols, d-P21-T3 (desmethyl tocotrienol) and d-P25-T3 (didesmethyl tocotrienol), have been identified and isolated from stabilized rice bran.[118] RBO is a rich source of tocotrienols, ranging from 72–1157 ppm depending upon different bran sources and commercial refining methods.

Approximately 1.7% (v/v) of the unsaponifiable fraction of RBO is tocotrienol. HPLC analysis of RBO showed that 1 g of RBO contains 0.5 mg of γ-tocotrienol.[118] It has been observed that human consumption of 240 mg/day of tocotrienols for up to 2 years caused no adverse effects, and they are safe at even much higher levels. The content and biological activities of tocotrienols are higher than those of tocopherols.[121]

MECHANISMS

The mechanism of action of rice bran and its oil on lipid metabolism is not yet clear. However, the most probable hypothesis for RBO's hypolipidemic action is its specific content of phytosterols, polyphenols (γ-oryzanol), and tocols (tocopherols and tocotrienols). The cholesterol-lowering effects of RBO are possibly attributable to its relatively high unsaponifiables, physiologically bioactive in controlling cholesterol levels in subjects. These compounds have been found to work synergistically to exhibit hypocholesterolemic effects.

In terms of phytosterols, there are several mechanisms through which plant sterols affect the cholesterol concentration in the body, such as formation of non-absorbable complexes with cholesterol, altering the size and/or stability of the micelles, interfering with cholesterol esterification in the mucosal cell, and interacting with protein receptors required in cholesterol absorption.[67] It is generally assumed that plant sterols inhibit intestinal absorption of dietary and biliary cholesterol, because of the structural similarities with cholesterol. Some studies have indicated that plant sterols contributed more hypocholesterolemic effects than unsaponifiables. In addition, some plant sterols may be more active than others.[62] Among the sterols, β-sitosterol has been recognized as the predominant cholesterol-lowering component.[54,122]

There are numerous mechanisms by which oryzanol lowers cholesterol levels, including:

1. Cholesterol-esterase inhibition by cycloartenol or by the inhibition of the accumulation of cholesterol esters within macrophages, or by the modulation of cholesterol acid esterase and acyl-CoA-cholesterol-acyltransferase[60]
2. The sterol moiety of γ-oryzanol being partly split off from the ferulic acid part in the small intestine by cholesterol esterase[20]
3. An effect on biliary secretion resulting in increased fecal excretion of cholesterol and bile acids[93]
4. Direct inhibition of lipid metabolism
5. Increased fecal excretion of cholesterol and its metabolites
6. Oryzanol exercising its effects on cholesterol metabolism at sites other than the intestine.[123]

In case of tocols, cholesterol-lowering mechanisms include:

1 Antioxidant activity that inhibits cholesterol oxidation
2. Inhibition of HMG-CoAR, a key enzyme in the endogenous synthesis of cholesterol, via increasing the controlled degradation of reductase protein and decreasing the efficiency of the translation of HMG-CoA-R messenger RNA.[124,125]
3. Inhibition of the activity of 3-hydroxy-3-methylglutaryl-coenzyme A (HMG-CoA) reductase, the liver enzyme that is critical to the rate at which cholesterol is synthesized.[126]
4. Inhibition of cholesterol synthesis by suppressing HMG-CoA reductase activity through a posttranscriptional mechanism in HepG2 cells.[127]
5. A decrease in serum total and LDL cholesterol by inhibition of the hepatic enzymic activity of β-hydroxy-β-methylglutaryl coenzyme A.[128]

CONCLUSIONS

It is well established that RBO is one of the most nutritious and health-beneficial edible oils as it contains high level of nutraceuticals. Organic RBO may be produced by cold-pressing of stabilized organic rice brans. This produces crude RBO, which usually contains some impurities such as FFA, wax, and bran fines. Most commercial productions of RBO apply several processes for refining of crude RBO, which may include degumming, dewaxing, alkali neutralization, bleaching, and deodorization. Refining processes involve the use of hazardous chemicals and extreme process conditions, and therefore dramatically reduce the nutritional value of RBO. For example, alkali treatment removes up to 95%

of γ-oryzanol from the original crude oils. RBO components that promote health benefits come mainly from its fatty acids, unsaponifiable matter, antioxidants, oryzanol, tocols, and other bioactive compounds. These components have the capacity to lower blood cholesterol and decrease cholesterol absorption. They are also known as antioxidants, which are associated with the prevention of cardiovascular disease.

References

1. Hoed VV, Depaemelaere G, Ayala JV, Santiwattana P, Verhé R, Greyt WD. Influence of chemical refining on the major and minor components of rice bran oil. *JAOCS* 2006;**83**:315–21.
2. Champagne ET. *Rice Chemistry and Technology*. 3rd ed. St Paul, MN: American Association of Cereal Chemists; 2004.
3. Hernandez N, Rodriguez-Alegría ME, Gonzalez F, Lopez-Munguia A. Enzymatic treatment of rice bran to improve processing. *JAOCS* 2000;**77**:177–80.
4. Champagne ET, Wood DF, Juliano BO, Bechtel DB. The Rice Grain and Its Gross Composition. In: Champagne ET, editor. *Rice Chemistry and Technology* 3rd ed. St Paul, MN: American Association of Cereal Chemists; 2004. p. 77–107.
5. Bond N. Rice Milling. In: Champagne ET, editor. *Rice Chemistry and Technology* 3rd edn St Paul, MN: American Association of Cereal Chemists; 2004. p. 283–300.
6. de Deckere EA, Korver O. Minor constituents of rice brain oil as functional foods. *Nutr Rev* 1996;**54**:S120–6.
7. Hu W, Wells JH, Shin TS, Godber JS. Comparison of isopropanol and hexane for extraction of vitamin E and oryzanols from stabilized rice bran. *JAOCS* 1996;**73**:1653–6.
8. Orthoefer FT, Eastman J. Rice Bran and Oil. In: Champagne ET, editor. *Rice Chemistry and Technology* 3rd ed. St Paul MN: American Association of Cereal Chemists; 2004. p. 569–93.
9. Saunders RM. Rice bran: Composition and potential food uses. *Food Rev Int* 1985;**3**:465–95.
10. Saunders RM. The properties of rice bran as a food stuff. *Cereal Foods World* 1990;**35**(632):634–6.
11. Luh DS. *Rice: Production and utilization*. Westport, CT: AVI Publishing; 1980.
12. Marshall WE, Wadsworth JI. *Rice science and technology*. New York, NY: Marcel Dekker; 1994.
13. Ju YH, Vali SR. Rice bran oil as a potential resource for biodiesel: A review. *J Sci Ind Res* 2005;**64**:866–82.
14. Shahidi F. *Bailey's Industrial Oil and Fat Products*. 6th ed. John Wiley & Sons; 2005. Volume 2 Edible Oil and Fat Products: Edible Oils.
15. Hammond N. Functional and nutritional characteristics of rice bran extracts. *Cereal Foods World* 1994;**39**:752–4.
16. Jariwalla RJ. Rice bran products: Phytonutrients with potential applications in preventive and clinical medicine. *Drugs under Exp Clin Res* 2001;**27**:17–26.
17. Kim JS, Godber JS. Oxidative stability and vitamin E levels increased in restructured beef roasts with added rice bran oil. *J Food Quality* 2001;**24**:17–26.
18. Nasirullah. Development of deep frying edible vegetable oils. *J Food Lipids* 2001;**8**:295–304.
19. Childs NW. Production and Utilization of Rice. In: Champagne ET, editor. *Rice Chemistry and Technology* 3rd ed. St. Paul, MN: American Association of Cereal Chemists; 2004. p. 1–23.
20. Sugano M, Tsuji E. Rice bran oil and cholesterol metabolism. *J Nutr* 1997;**127**:521–4.
21. Sayre RN, Nayyar DK, Saunders RM. Extraction and refining of edible oil from extrusion-stabilized rice bran. *JAOCS* 1985;**62**:1040–3.

22. Orthoefer FT. Rice bran oil. In: Shahidi F, editor. *Bailey's Industrial Oil and Fat Products. Volume 2 Edible Oil and Fat Products: Edible Oils*. John Wiley & Sons; 2005. p. 465–89.

23. Cicero AF, Gaddi A. Rice bran oil and γ-oryzanol in the treatment of hyperlipoproteinaemias and other conditions. *Phytotherapy Res* 2001;**15**:277–89.

24. Amarasinghe BMWPK, Gangodavilage NC. Rice bran oil extraction in Sri Lanka: Data for process equipment design. *Food Bioproducts Proc* 2004;**82**:54–9.

25. Nantiyakul N, Furse S, Fisk ID, Tucker G, Gray DA. Isolation and characterization of oil bodies from Oryza sativa bran and studies of their physical properties. *J Cereal Sci* 2013;**57**:141–5.

26. Most MM, Tully R, Morales S, Lefevre M. Rice bran oil, not fiber, lower cholesterol in humans. *Am J Clin Nutr* 2005;**81**:64–8.

27. Rong N, Ausman LM, Nicolosi RJ. Oryzanol decreases cholesterol absorption and aortic fatty streaks in hamsters. *Lipids* 1997;**32**:303–9.

28. Sugano M, Koba K, Tsuji E. Health benefits of rice bran oil. *Anticancer Res* 1999;**19**:3651–7.

29. Wester I. Cholesterol-lowering effect of plant sterols. *Eur J Lipid Sci Technol* 2000;**102**:37–44.

30. Xu Z, Hua N, Godber JS. Antioxidant activity of tocopherols, tocotrienols, and γ-oryzanol components from rice bran against cholesterol oxidation accelerated by 2,2′-azobis (2-methylpropionamidine) dihydrochloride. *J Agric Food Chem* 2001;**49**:2077–81.

31. Ghosh M. Review on recent trends in rice bran oil processing. *JAOCS* 2007;**84**:315–24.

32. Prabhakar JV, Venkatesh KVL. A simple chemical method for stabilization of rice bran. *JAOCS* 1986;**63**:644–6.

33. Kuk MS, Dowd MK. Supercritical CO_2 extraction of rice bran. *JAOCS* 1998;**75**:623–8.

34. Mishra A, Gopalakrishna AG, Prabhakar JV. Factors affecting refining losses in rice (*Oryza sativa* L.) bran oil. *JAOCS* 1988;**65**:1605–9.

35. Sah A, Agrawal BKD, Shukla LS. A new approach in dewaxing and refining rice bran oil. *JAOCS* 1983;**60**:466.

36. Bhattacharyya AC, Majumdar S, Bhattacharyya DK. Edible quality rice bran oil from high FFA rice bran oil by miscella refining. *JAOCS* 1986;**63**:1189–91.

37. Srikaeo K, Pradit M. Simple Techniques to Increase the Production Yield and Enhance the Quality of Organic Rice Bran Oils. *J Oleo Sci* 2011;**60**:1–5.

38. Jahn G, Schramm M, Spiller A. The reliability of certification: Quality labels as a consumer policy tool. *J Consum Policy* 2005;**28**:53–73.

39. De BK, Bhattacharyya DK. Physical refining of rice bran oil in relation to degumming and dewaxing. *JAOCS* 1998;**75**:1683–6.

40. Krishna AGG, Khatoon S, Shiela PM, Sarmandal CV, Indira TN, Mishra A. Effect of refining of crude rice bran oil on the retention of oryzanol in the refined oil. *JAOCS* 2001;**78**:127–31.

41. Tandy DC, McPherson WJ. Physical refining of edible oil. *JAOCS* 1984;**61**:1253–8.

42. Seetharamaiah GS, Prabhakar JV. Oryzanol content of Indian rice bran oil and its extraction from soapstock. *J Food Sci Technol* 1986;**23**:270–3.

43. Narayana T, Kaimal B, Vali SR, Surya BV, Rao K, Chakrabarti PP, et al. Origin of problems encountered in rice bran oil processing. *Eur J Lipid Sci Technol* 2002;**104**:203–11.

44. Manjula S, Subramanian R. Simultaneous degumming, dewaxing and decolorizing crude rice bran oil using nonporous membranes. *Sep Purif Technol* 2009;**66**:223–8.

45. Manjula S, Subramanian R. Enriching oryzanol in rice bran oil using membranes. *Appl Biochem Biotechnol* 2008;**151**:629–37.

46. De BK, Das R, Dutta BK, Bhattacharyya BK. Membrane degumming and dewaxing of rice bran oil and its refining. *Eur J Lipid Sci Technol* 1998;**100**:416–21.

47. Subramanian R, Nakajima M, Kimura T, Mackawa T. Membrane process for premium quality expeller-pressed vegetable oils. *Food Res Int* 1998;**31**:587–93.

48. Stöggl W, Huck C, Wongyai S, Scherz H, Bonn G. Simultaneous determination of carotenoids, tocopherols, and gamma-oryzanol in crude rice bran oil by liquid chromatography coupled to diode array and mass spectrometric detection employing silica C30 stationary phases. *J Sep Sci* 2005;**28**:1712–8.

49. Krishna AGG, Khatoon S, Babylatha R. Frying performance of processed rice bran oils. *J Food Lipids* 2005;**12**:1–11.

50. Nicolosi RJ, Ausman LM, Hegsted DM. Rice bran oil lowers serum total and low density lipoprotein cholesterol and Apo B levels in nonhuman primates. *Artherosclerosis* 1991;**88**:133–42.

51. Suzuki S, Oshima S. Influence of blending of edible fats and oils on human serum cholesterol level (Part 1). *Jpn J Nutr* 1970;**28**:3–6.

52. Suzuki S, Oshima S. Influence of blending of edible fats and oils on human serum cholesterol level (Part 2). *Jpn J Nutr* 1970;**28**:194–8.

53. Raghuram TC, Rao UB, Rukmini C. Studies on hypolipidemic effects of dietary rice bran oil in human subjects. *Nutr Rep Int* 1989;**39**:889–95.

54. Vissers MN, Zock PL, Meijer GW, Katan MB. Effect of plant sterols from rice bran oil and triterpene alcohols from sheanut oil on serum lipoprotein concentrations in humans. *Am J Clin Nutr* 2000;**72**:1510–5.

55. Certik M, Shimizu S. Biosynthesis and regulation of microbial polyunsaturated fatty acid production. *J Biosci Bioeng* 1999;**87**:1–14.

56. Calder PC. N-3 polyunsaturated fatty acids and inflammation: From molecular biology to the clinic. *Lipids* 2003;**38**:343–52.

57. Schaefer EJ, Levy RI, Ernst ND, Van Sant FD, Brewer Jr HB. The effect of low cholesterol, high polyunsaturated fat and low fat diets on plasma lipid and lipoprotein cholesterol levels in normal and hypocholesterolemic subjects. *Am J Clin Nutr* 1981;**34**:1758–63.

58. Mattson FH, Grundy SM. Comparison of effects of dietary saturated, monounsaturated and polyunsaturated fatty acids on plasma lipids and lipoproteins in man. *J Lipid Res* 1985;**26**:194–202.

59. Rukmini C. Chemical, nutritional and toxicological studies on rice bran oil. *Food Chem* 1988;**30**:257–68.

60. Rukmini C, Raghuram TC. Nutritional and biochemical aspects of the hypolipidemic action of rice bran oil: A review. *J Am Coll Nutr* 1991;**10**:593–601.

61. Nicolosi RJ, Ausman LM, Hegsted DM. Rice bran oil lowers serum total and low density lipoprotein cholesterol and apo B levels in nonhuman primates. *Atherosclerosis* 1991;**88**:133–42.

62. Wilson TA, Ausman LM, Lawton CW, Hegsted DM, Nicolosi RJ. Comparative cholesterol lowering properties of vegetable oils: Beyond fatty acids. *J Am Coll Nutr* 2000;**19**:601–7.

63. Nicolosi RJ, Rogers EJ, Ausman LM, Orthoefer FT. Rice bran oil and its health benefits. In: Marshall WE, Wordsworth JI, editors. *Rice science and technology*. New York: Marcel Dekker; 1994. p. 421–37.

64. Shin T, Godber JS, Martin DE, Wells JH. Hydrolytic stability and changes in E vitamers and oryzanol of extruded rice bran during storage. *J Food Sci* 1997;**62**:704–28.

65. Lloyd BJ, Siebenmorgen TJ, Beers KW. Effect of commercial processing on anti-oxidants in rice bran. *Cereal Chem* 2000;**77**:551–5.

66. Dunford NT, King JW. Thermal gradient deacidification of crude rice bran oil utilizing supercritical carbon dioxide. *JAOCS* 2001;**78**:121–5.

67. Rong N, Ausman LM, Nicolosi RJ. Oryzanol decreases cholesterol absorption and aortic fatty steaks in Hamsters. *Lipids* 1997;**32**:303–9.

68. Sayre RN, Earl L, Kratzer FH, Saunders RM. Effects of diets containing raw and extrusion cooked rice bran on growth and efficiency of feed utilization of broilers. *Br Poult Sci* 1988;**29**:815–23.

69. Kahlon TS, Chow FI, Chiu MM, Hudson CA, Sayre RN. Cholesterol lowering by rice bran and rice bran oil unsaponifiable matter in hamsters. *Cereal Chem* 1996;**73**:69–74.

A. OVERVIEW OF RICE AND HEALTH

70. Nagao K, Sato M, Takenaka M, Ando M, Iwamoto M, Imaizumi K. Feeding unsaponifiable compounds from rice bran oil does not alter hepatic mRNA abundance for cholesterol metabolism-related proteins in hypercholesterolemic rats. *Biosci Biotechnol Biochem* 2001;**65**:371–7.

71. Ikeda I, Nakashima YK, Sugano M. Effects of cycloartenol on absorption and serum levels of cholesterol in rats. *J Nutr Sci Vitaminol* 1985;**31**:375–84.

72. Sharma RD, Rukmini C. Rice bran oil and hypocholesterolemia in rats. *Lipids* 1986;**21**:715–7.

73. Halliwell B, Gutteridge JC. The definition and measurement of antioxidants in biological systems. *Free Radic Biol Med* 1995;**18**:125–6.

74. Chen MH, Bergman CJ. A rapid procedure for analyzing rice bran tocopherol, tocotrienol and γ-oryzanol contents. *J Food Composit Anal* 2005;**18**:319–31.

75. Birringer M, Pfluger P, Kluth D, Landes N, Brigelius-Flohe R. Identities and differences in the metabolism of tocotrienols and tocopherols in HepG2 Cells. *J Nutr* 2002;**132**:3113–8.

76. Akihisa T, Yasukawa K, Yamaura M, Ukiya M, Kimura Y, Shimizu N, et al. Triterpene alcohol and sterol ferulates from rice bran and their anti-inflammatory effects. *J Agric Food Chem* 2000;**48**:2313–9.

77. Ricciarelli R, Zingg JM, Azzi A, Vitamin E. protective role of a Janus molecule. *FASEB J* 2001;**15**:2314–25.

78. Yu S, Nehus ZT, Badger TM, Fang N. Quantification of vitamin E and gamma-oryzanol components in rice germ and bran. *J Agric Food Chem* 2007;**55**:7308–13.

79. Nesaretnam K, Stephen R, Dils R, Darbre P. Tocotrienols inhibit the growth of human breast cancer cells irrespective of estrogen receptor status. *Lipids* 1998;**33**:461–9.

80. Nanua JN, McGregor JU, Godber JS. Influence of high-oryzanol rice bran oil on the oxidative stability of whole milk powder. *J Dairy Sci* 2000;**83**:2426–31.

81. Xu Z, Godber JS. Comparison of supercritical fluid and solvent extraction methods in extracting γ-oryzanol from rice bran. *JAOCS* 2000;**77**:547–51.

82. Fang N, Yu S, Badger TM. Characterization of triterpene alcohol and sterol ferulates in rice bran using LC-MS/MS. *J Agric Food Chem* 2003;**51**:3260–7.

83. Miller A, Frenzel T, Schmarr HG, Engel KH. Coupled liquid chromatography–gas chromatography for the rapid analysis of γ-oryzanol in rice lipids. *J Chromatograpy A* 2003;**985**:403–10.

84. Kaneko R, Tsuchiya T. New compound in rice bran and germ oils. *J Chem Soc Jpn* 1954;**57**:526.

85. Seitz LM. Stanol and sterol esters of ferulic and p-coumaric acids in wheat, corn, rye, and triticale. *J Agric Food Chem* 1989;**37**:662–7.

86. Bucci R, Magrì AD, Magrì AL, Marini F. Comparison of three spectrophotometric methods for the determination of γ-oryzanol in rice bran oil. *Anal Bioanal Chem* 2003;**375**:1254–9.

87. Xu Z, Godber JS. Purification and identification of components of γ-oryzanol in rice bran oil. *J Agric Food Chem* 1999;**47**:2724–8.

88. Kim JS, Godber JS, King JM, Prinyawiwatkul W. Inhibition of cholesterol autoxidation by the nonsaponifiable fraction in rice bran in an aqueous model system. *JAOCS* 2001;**78**:685–9.

89. Rogers EJ, Rice SM, Nicolosi RJ, Carpenter DR, McClelland CA, Romanczyk LJ. Identification and quantitation of γ-oryzanol components and simultaneous assessment of tocols in rice bran oil. *JAOCS* 1993;**70**:301–7.

90. Bergman CJ, Xu Z. Genotype and environment effects on tocopherols, tocotrienols and γ-oryzanol contents of Southern US rice. *Cereal Chem* 2003;**80**:446–9.

91. Yu S, Nehus ZT, Badger TM, Fang N. Quantification of Vitamin E and γ-oryzanol Components in Rice Germ and Bran. *J Agric Food Chem* 2007;**55**:7308–13.

92. Akihisa T, Yasukawa K, Yamaura M, Ukiya M, Kimura Y, Shimizu N, et al. Triterpene alcohol and sterol ferulates from rice bran and their anti-inflammatory effects. *J Agric Food Chem* 2000;**48**:2313–9.

93. Seetharamaiah GS, Krishnakantha TP, Chandrasekhara N. Influence of oryzanol on platelet aggregation in rats. *J Nutrit Sci Vitaminol* 1990;**36**:291–7.

94. Yasukawa K, Akihisa T, Kimura Y, Tamura T, Takido M. Inhibitory effect of cycloartenol ferulate, a component of rice bran, on tumor promotion in two-stage carcinogenesis in mouse skin. *Biol Pharm Bull* 1998;**21**:1072–6.

95. Hiramitsu T, Armstrong D. Preventive effect of antioxidants on lipid peroxidation in the retina. *Ophthalmic Res* 1991;**23**:196–203.

96. Cuvelier ME, Richard H, Berset C. Comparison of the antioxidative activity of some acid-phenols: Structure activity relationship, Bioscience. *Biotechnol Biochem* 1992;**56**:324–30.

97. Marinova EM, Yanishlieva NV. Effect of Temperature on the antioxidative action of the inhibitors in lipid autoxidation. *J Sci Food Agric* 1992;**60**:313–8.

98. Marinova EM, Yanishlieva NV. Effect of lipid unsaturation on the antioxidative activity of some phenolic acids. *JAOCS* 1994;**71**:427–34.

99. Pratt DE. Water-soluble antioxidant activity in soybeans. *J Food Sci* 1972;**37**:322–3.

100. Xu Z, Godber JS. Antioxidant activities of major components of γ-oryzanol from rice bran using a linoleic acid model. *JAOCS* 2001;**78**:465–9.

101. Kim JS, Godber JS, King JM, Prinyawiwatkul W. Inhibition of cholesterol autoxidation by nonsaponifiable fraction fine rice bran in an aqueous model system. *JAOCS* 2000;**78**:685–9.

102. Ha TY, Han S, Kim SR, Kim IH, Lee HY, Kim HK. Bioactive components in rice bran oil improve lipid profiles in rats fed a high-cholesterol diet. *Nutr Res* 2005;**25**:597–606.

103. Rukmini C. Chemical nutritional and toxicological studies of rice bran oil. *Food Chem* 1988;**30**:257–68.

104. Nicolosi RJ, Ausman LM, Hegsted DM. Rice bran oil lowers serum total and low density lipoprotein cholesterol and Apo B levels in nonhuman primates. *Artherosclerosis* 1991;**88**:133–42.

105. Kahlon TS, Saunders RM, Sayre RN, Chow FI, Chiu MM, Betschart AA. Cholestrol-lowering effects of rice bran and rice bran oil fractions in hypercholestrolemic hamsters. *Cereal Chem* 1992;**69**:485–9.

106. Sasaki J, Takada Y, Handa K, Kusuda M, Tanabe Y, Matsunaga A, et al. Effects of gamma-oryzanol on serum lipids and apolipoproteins in dyslipidemic schizophrenics receiving major tranquilizers. *Clin Therapeutics* 1990;**12**:263–8.

107. Lichtenstein AH, Ausman LM, Carrasco W. Rice bran oil consumption and plasma lipid levels in moderately hypercholesterolemic humans. *Arteriosclerosis Thromb* 1994;**14**:549–56.

108. Seetharamaiah GS, Chandrasekhara N. Studies on hypocholesterolemic activity of rice bran oil. *Atherosclerosis* 1989;**78**:219–23.

109. Hiramatsu K, Tani T, Kimura Y, Izumi S, Nakane PK. Effect of gamma-oryzanol on atheroma formation in hypercholesterolemic rabbits. *Tokai J Exp Clin Med* 1990;**15**:299–305.

110. Rukmini C, Raghuram TC. Nutritional and biochemical aspects of the hypolipidemic action of rice bran oil: a review. *J Am Coll Nutr* 1991;**10**:593–601.

111. Rosenbloom C, Millard Stafford M, Lathrop J. Contemporary ergogenic aids used by strength/power athletes. *J Am Dietetic Associat* 1992;**92**:1264–6.

112. Fry AC, Bonner E, Lewis DL, Johnson RL, Stone MH, Kraemer WJ. The effects of gamma-oryzanol supplementation during resistance exercise training. *Int J Sport Nutr* 1997;**7**:318–29.

113. Tamagawa M, Shimizu Y, Takahashi T, Otaka T, Kimura S, Kadowaki H, et al. Carcinogenicity study of gamma-oryzanol in F344 rats. *Food Chem Toxicol* 1992;**30**:41–8.

114. Tamagawa M, Otaki Y, Takahashi T, Otaka T, Kimura S, Miwa T. Carcinogenicity study of gamma-oryzanol in B6C3F1 mice. *Food Chem Toxicol* 1992;**30**:49–56.

115. Hirose M, Fukushima S, Imaida K, Ito N, Shirai T. Modifying effects of phytic acid and gamma-oryzanol on the promotion stage of rat carcinogenesis. *Anticancer Res* 1999;**19**:3665–70.

116. Qureshi AA, Pearce BC, Nor RM, Gapor A, Peterson DM, Elson EC. Dietary alpha-tocopherol attenuates the impact of gamma-tocotrienol on hepatic 3-hydroxy-3-methylglutaryl coenzyme A reductase activity in chickens. *J Nutr* 1996;**126**:389–94.

117. Yap SP, Yuen KH, Wong JW. Pharmacokinetics and bioavailability of alpha-, gamma- and delta-tocotrienols under different food status. *J Pharm Pharmacol* 2001;**53**:67–71.

118. Qureshi AA, Mo H, Packer L, Peterson DM. Isolation and identification of novel tocotrienols from rice bran with hypocholesterolemic, antioxidant, and antitumor properties. *J Agric Food Chem* 2000;**48**:3130–40.

119. Stephens NG, Parsons A, Schofield PM, Kelly F, Cheeseman K, Mitchinson MJ. Randomised controlled trial of vitamin E in patients with coronary disease: Cambridge heart antioxidant study (CHAOS). *Lancet* 1996;**347**:781–6.

120. Patel M, Naik SN. Gamma-oryzanol from rice bran oil – a review. *J Sci Ind Res* 2004;**63**:569–78.

121. Qureshi AA, Sami SA, Salser WA, Khan FA. Synergistic effect of tocotrienol-rich fraction (TRF25) of rice bran and lovastatin on lipid parameters in hypercholesteroleic humans. *J Nutr Biochem* 2001;**12**:318–29.

122. Trautwein EA, Schulz C, Rieckhoff D, Rau AK, Erbersdobler HF, Groot WA, et al. Effect of esterified 4-desmethylsterols and-stanols or 4, 4′-dimethylsterols on cholesterol and bile acid metabolism in hamsters. *Br J Nutr* 2002;**87**:227–37.

123. Wilson TA, Nicolosia RJ, Woolfreya B, Kritchevsky D. Rice bran oil and oryzanol reduce plasma lipid and lipoprotein cholesterol concentrations and aortic cholesterol ester accumulation to a greater extent than ferulic acid in hypercholesterolemic hamsters. *J Nutr Biochem* 2007;**18**:105–12.

124. Parker RA, Pearce BC, Clark RW, Gordon DA, Wright JJ. Tocotrienols regulate cholesterol production in mammalian cells by post-transcriptional suppression of 3-hydroxy-3-methylglutaryl-coenzyme A reductase. *J Biol Chem* 1993;**268**:11230–8.

125. Khor HT, Chieng DY, Ong KK. Tocotrienols inhibit HMG-CoA reductase activity in the guinea pig. *Nutr Res* 1995;**15**:537–44.

126. Khor HT, Ng TT. Effects of administration of tocopherol and tocotrienols on serum lipids and liver HMG CoA reductase activity. *Int J Food Sci Nutr* 2000;**51**:S3–11.

127. Pearce BC, Parker RA, Deason ME, Qureshi AA, Wright JJK. Hypocholesterolemic activity of synthetic and natural tocotrienols. *J Med Chem* 1992;**35**:3595–606.

128. Qureshi AA, Sami SA, Salser WA, Khan FA. Dose dependent suppression of serum cholesterol by tocotrienol rich fraction (TRF25) of rice bran in hypercholesterolemic humans. *Atherosclerosis* 2002;**161**:199–207.

Fermented Rice Bran Attenuates Oxidative Stress

Dongyeop Kim[*†], *Gi Dong Han*[*]

[*]Yeungnam University, Department of Food Science and Technology, College of Natural Resources, Gyeongsan, Republic of Korea, [†]Hokkaido University, Division of Applied Bioscience, Graduate School of Agriculture, Sapporo, Japan

INTRODUCTION

An imbalance between oxidants and antioxidants in favor of oxidants is termed oxidative stress, which potentially leads to damage.[1] The current concept of oxidative stress involves metabolic stress-related pathways participating in cellular and extracellular metabolic events.[2] Oxidants are formed as normal products of aerobic metabolism, but can also be produced at elevated rates under pathophysiological conditions. Meanwhile, various biological oxidants have been shown to cover large ranges, and experimental studies have revealed that cells and organisms require oxidant defense mechanisms.[3] Oxidants can damage all types of molecules, including DNA, lipids, proteins, and carbohydrates.[4] Hence, oxidative stress is involved in processes such as mutagenesis, carcinogenesis, membrane damage, lipid peroxidation, protein oxidation, and fragmentation, as well as carbohydrate damage.[5–7] The first line of defense in cells and organs against oxidative stress is protection against reactive oxygen species (ROS)-induced damage.[8] In parallel with oxidative stress elicited by aerobic metabolism, animal and human cells have developed a ubiquitous antioxidant defense system consisting of superoxide dismutase (SOD), catalase (CAT), glutathione peroxidase (GPx), and glutathione reductase together with a number of low molecular-weight antioxidants such as ascorbate, α-tocopherol, glutathione, and vitamins, etc.[2,6,7]

Dietary antioxidants are obtained from functional foods or nutraceuticals, which are food products that provide medical or health benefits such as the prevention and treatment of diseases. They promote the concept of food as not only necessary for living but also a source of mental and physical wellbeing, contributing to the prevention and reduction of risk factors of several diseases as well as enhancing certain physiological functions.[9,10] To date, there has been a global trend toward using the natural substances present in medicinal and dietary plants as therapeutic antioxidants. The use of antioxidants in food, cosmetics, and the therapeutic industry offers a promising alternative to synthetic antioxidants, especially butylated hydroxytoluene (BHT) and butylated hydroxyanisole (BHA), due to their low cost, high compatibility with dietary intake, and lack of harmful effects to the human body.[6,11]

Whole foods represent the simplest example of functional foods. Among them, whole grain and whole grain-based products have the ability to enhance health beyond the simple provision of energy and nutrients. The chemical components in whole grains, including dietary fiber, insulin, β-glucan, phenolics, and tocopherols, possess health-enhancing properties, and whole grain seems to play a role in the prevention of diseases such as cardiovascular diseases and hypertension, type 2 diabetes mellitus, obesity, and cancer.[12,13] In particular, antioxidant components as secondary metabolites in plant foods have been highlighted and continue to be demonstrated as health components (Table 36.1).[14]

FERMENTED CEREAL FOODS AND PREVENTION OF OXIDATIVE DISORDERS

Fermentation

Fermentation has been used for almost 5000 years, and is an effective and low-cost technology for preserving foods as well as improving quality and safety. Further,

TABLE 36.1   Antioxidant Components in Plant Foods*

		Functional Components	
Class/Components	Source	Potential Benefit	Chemical Structure

CAROTENOIDS

β-Carotene	Carrots, various fruits	Neutralizes free radicals; antioxidant defenses	
Lutein, zeaxanthin	Kale, collards, spinach, corn, citrus	Maintains healthy vision	
Lycopene	Tomatoes and processed tomato products	Maintains prostate health	

FLAVONOIDS

Anthocyanidins	Berries, cherries, red grapes	Antioxidant defenses; maintains brain function	
Flavonols	Onions, apples, broccoli, tea, cocoa, chocolate, apples, grapes	Neutralize free radicals; antioxidant defenses, and maintains heart health	
Flavanones	Citrus foods	Neutralize free radicals; bolster cellular antioxidant defenses	
Proanthocyanidins	Cranberries, cocoa, apples, strawberries, grapes, wine, peanuts, cinnamon	Maintains urinary tract health and heart health	

TABLE 36.1 Antioxidant Components in Plant Foods*—cont'd

Functional Components			
ISOTHIOCYANATES			
Sulforaphane	Cauliflower, broccoli, Brussels sprouts, cabbage, kale, horseradish	Enhances detoxification of undesirable compounds and bolsters cellular antioxidant defenses	
PHENOLS			
Caffeic acid, ferulic acid	Apples, pears, citrus fruits, some vegetables	Bolster cellular antioxidant defense, maintains healthy vision and heart health	Hydroxycinnamic acid — R; Caffeic acid — OH; Ferulic acid — OCH₃
SULFIDES/THIOLS			
Diallyl sulfide, allyl methyl trisulfide	Garlic, onions, leeks, scallions	Enhances detoxification of undesirables	
Dithiolethiones	Cruciferous vegetables: broccoli, cabbage, bok choy, collards	Maintains healthy immune function	
WHOLE GRAINS			
Whole grains	Cereal grains	Reduces risk of coronary heart disease and cancer, contributes to reduced risk of diabetes	

Information obtained from the International Food Information Council Foundation.[14]

it adds value, enhances nutritional quality and digestibility, and provides dietary enrichment. All of these changes are coordinated by microorganisms that are present naturally or through inoculation in raw materials.[15,16] Common fermenting bacteria include species of *Leuconostoc*, *Lactobacillus*, *Streptococcus*, *Pediococcus*, *Micrococcus*, and *Bacillus*. The fungal genera most frequently found are *Aspergillus*, *Paeciloyces*, *Cladosporium*, *Fusarium*, *Penicillium*, and *Trichothecium*.[17] Among fermenting microbes, yeasts are common and important microorganisms in food, beverages, and medicine. Fermentation can be also applied to the design and manufacture of functional foods containing components that exert particular beneficial health effects.[15]

Fermented Cereal Foods

Cereal grains are considered to be one of the most pivotal sources of dietary proteins, carbohydrates, vitamins, minerals, and fiber. However, they contain lower protein content compared with dairy products, and they are deficient in certain essential amino acids such as lysine. Grains also have disadvantages due to the presence of antinutrients such as phytic acid, tannins, and polyphenols.[18]

In general, fermentation of cereals can reduce the levels of carbohydrates as well as some non-digestible poly- and oligosaccharides. Furthermore, certain amino acids may be synthesized, and the availability of vitamin B may be improved.[18,19] Fermentation also provides optimum pH conditions for enzymatic degradation of phytate, generally improving the shelf-life, texture, taste, and aroma of the resulting product. Hence, fermented cereals are very widely produced as food, including bread and beer, with improved shelf-life and overall acceptance.[15]

The major cereal sources for fermentation are maize, sorghum, millet, rice, and wheat.[19] During fermentation of cereal foods, nutrients such as protein and minerals are lost due to their conversion to metabolites or upon preparation of the grain as a fermentation substrate to avoid unexpected conversions. Therefore, the grain should be polished, or foreign matter removed, prior to fermentation. Intensive research on yeast is currently concerned with the conversion of carbohydrates into alcohol and other aromatic components, such as esters, organic acids, and carbonyls.[16]

Cereal Bran

Bran is high in fiber and contains a phytochemical-rich outer layer of cereal grains. To reduce the risk of obesity, diabetes, coronary problems, and cancer, high intake of whole grain foods having potential health benefits is strongly recommended owing to their abundance of indigestible fibers.[20] Hence, cereal bran is considered an important ingredient in functional food development, and various attempts have been made in parallel to determine which constituents in bran play crucial roles in the prevention of lifestyle diseases. In fact, polyphenolic compounds have been shown to ameliorate the effects of various lifestyle diseases due to their biological activities, which include antioxidative activity.[21] Bran contains phenolics bound in dietary fibers and β-glucan, which has a wide spectrum of biological activities. Most phenolic acids exist in bound form within cereal bran. Common phenolic acids in bran include ferulic acid, vanillin acid, caffeic acid, syringic acid, and p-coumaric acid.[22] Among these, ferulic acid is a component of lignocellulose cross-linked with lignin and polysaccharides, and it contributes to the rigidity and strength of plant cell wall structures.[23,24] Hence, ferulic acid is the most common phenolic acid found in cereal grains and is mostly present in the pericarp, aleurone, and embryo, but only minimally in the starchy endosperm.[25] Ferulic acid can be found in free, conjugated (soluble), or bound (insoluble) form in whole cereal grains.[26]

Fermentation as an Enzyme Reaction in Cereal Bran for Formation of Free Ferulic Acid

Ferulic acid is a very attractive natural antioxidant that is mainly present in whole cereal grains in the form of feruloylated oligosaccharides. The formation state of ferulic acid affects its bioavailability and resulting effectiveness as an antioxidant. For instance, although previous research has shown that feruloylated oligosaccharides more effectively inhibit lipid and low density lipoprotein (LDL) oxidation than free ferulic acid, free ferulic acid may effectively defend against various diseases due to its high bioavailability.[27,28] Ferulic acid was shown to be efficiently transported in its free form in an *in vitro* model of the colonic epithelium consisting of co-cultured Caco-2 and mucus-producing HT29-MTX cells.[29] Prior to absorption, phenolic acid esters are de-esterified from dietary fiber in the gastrointestinal tract due to the action of bacterial feruloyl esterase. Other works have revealed that free phenolic acids, including ferulic acid, are very easily absorbed into blood plasma and excreted in urine. In particular, structural changes may alter the absorption of phenolic compounds from the gastrointestinal tract as well as their antioxidant activity in blood plasma.[30]

Feruloyl esterase (EC 3.1.1.73) constitutes a subclass of carboxylic ester hydrolases (EC 3.1.1) that catalyzes the formation of ferulate ester groups between phenolic acid and polysaccharides involved in the cross-linking of hemicellulose and lignin in plant cell walls.[31,32] This enzyme is widely distributed in plants and microorganisms, and is utilized often in the food, feed, and pharmaceutical industries. Regarding function, feruloyl esterase can mediate the release of ferulic acid from agro-by-products, which can then be used as an antioxidant or transformed into other valuable molecules such as styrenes, polymers, epoxides, alkylbenzenes, vanillic acid derivatives, proteocatechuric acid-related catechols, guaiacol, catechol, and vanillin.[33]

FERMENTED RICE BRAN

What is Fermented Rice Bran?

Fermented rice bran (FRB), a new type of nutritional food adjunct, contains novel beneficial compounds possessing useful biological functions. For instance, it has been reported that FRB comprises various bioactivities; rice bran fermented with *Saccharomyces cerevisiae* has antistress and antifatigue effects, whereas polysaccharide extract of rice bran fermented with *Lentinus edodes* shows anticancer properties.[34,35] FRB extracts have inhibitory effects on melanogenesis mediated through the downregulation of MITF along with reduced cytotoxicity, as well as allergic and inflammatory reactivity through inhibition of degranulation, histamine release, and proinflammatory cytokine regulation.[36,37] Our group previously investigated whether or not FRB can ameliorate the oxidative stress induced by high glucose and hydrogen peroxide in adipocytes by analyzing ROS production. Rice bran extracts fermented by *Issatchenkia orientalis* showed higher free phenolic content compared to non-FRB. Further, FRB strongly inhibited ROS generation and upregulated the expression of PPAR-γ and adiponectin. This result was corroborated by another study in which FRB was shown to ameliorate oxidative stress-induced insulin resistance by neutralizing free radicals.[38]

Characteristics of Yeast, *Issatchenkia orientalis*, for Rice Bran Fermentation Using Solid-State Fermentation

Solid-State Fermentation (SSF)

Fermentation processes may be divided into two systems: submerged fermentation (SmF), which is based on microorganism cultivation in a liquid medium containing nutrients, and solid-state fermentation (SSF), which involves microbial growth, metabolism, and product formation on solid particles in a very small volume of water. In recent years, many researchers have demonstrated that SSF has a large impact on productivity, leading to higher yields and improved product characteristics compared to SmF.[39]

SSF has emerged as a potential technology for obtaining microbial products, including feed, fuel, food, industrial chemicals, and pharmaceutical products. SSF is defined as fermentation involving solids in the absence of free water, although the substrate must possess sufficient moisture to support microbial growth and metabolism. SSF offers numerous opportunities for the processing of agro-industrial residues, as solid-state processes have lower energy requirements, produce less wastewater, and are environmentally friendly due to efficient solid waste disposal.[40]

Although many bioactive compounds are still produced by SmF, there has been an increasing trend over recent decades towards utilization of SSF due to its greater overall efficiency.[41] SSF is often used to increase the amount of phenolic compounds in food products, thereby enhancing antioxidant activity. For example, bioprocessing of black beans for the preparation of koji containing various food-grade filamentous fungi, such as Aspergillus sp. and Rhizopus sp., has been shown to enhance antioxidant activity, possibly due to higher phenol and anthocyanin contents.[42] Further, fermented wheat grains are considered to be antioxidant-rich and more bioactive compared to non-fermented wheat grains. Two different filamentous fungi, Aspergillus oryzae and Aspergillus awamori, used in SSF are very effective in improving the phenolic content and antioxidant properties of wheat grains.[43] The chemical composition and bioactivity of stale rice can also be improved by SSF with Cordyceps sinensis.[44]

Besides increasing antioxidant activity, bioconversion of phenolic compounds by SSF can also alter food properties, with beneficial effects on human health.[39] According to Randhir and Shetty, SSF has been shown to significantly increase the phenolic content of mung beans, thereby enhancing antioxidant activity. This increase in antioxidant activity contributes to α-amylase inhibition, which is relevant to the control of diabetes, as well as the inhibition of Helicobacter pylori growth linked to peptic ulcer management.[45]

To develop bioprocesses using SSF, selection of a suitable microorganism substrate, and optimal conditions, including process, extraction, and purification parameters, should be carried out. For example, water activity and moisture content can critically influence microbial activity, which is why only fungi and yeast are typically suitable for SSF. Therefore, precise control of moisture content could be used to modify metabolic production or excretion in microorganisms. Further, the temperature of fermentation is very important as it ultimately affects microbial growth, spore formation and germination, and production formation. Heat transfer into and out of the SSF system is closely related with the level of aeration. However, a major problem encountered during SSF on a solid substrate is heat accumulation due to limited heat transfer.[40,46]

Yeast Fermentation in Food Processing

The claimed health benefits of fermented functional foods are either directly due to interactions between ingested live microorganisms, bacteria, or yeast with the host (probiotic effect) or indirectly due to ingestion of microbial metabolites produced during fermentation (biogenic effect). The biogenic properties of fermented functional foods are the result of microbial production of bioactive metabolites such as vitamins, bioactive peptides, organic acids, or fatty acids during fermentation.[47]

Fermentation plays at least five roles in food processing: (1) enrichment of the human diet through a wide diversity of flavors, aromas, and textures in foods; (2) preservation of substantial amounts of food through lactic acid, alcoholic, acetic acid, alkaline, and high salt fermentation; (3) biological enrichment of food substrates with vitamins, protein, essential amino acids, and essential fatty acids; (4) detoxification during food fermentation processing; and (5) reduction of cooking times and fuel requirements.[48]

Commonly used yeasts in food fermentation and processing are a part of the Saccharomyces family. Yeasts play a significant role in the food industry, as they produce enzymes that catalyze favorable desirable chemical reactions. Yeasts are a type of fungi in that they are unicellular organisms which reproduce asexually by budding. Similar to bacteria and molds, yeasts can have both beneficial and non-beneficial effects in food processing.

Yeasts are important fermentation agents in many food products and beverages. In yeast fermentation, basic ingredients such as grains, especially sugar or starch, are broken down by enzymes into dextrin and, subsequently, glucose, with the finished product depending on the production conditions and starting material. Other required molecules include usable nitrogen, trace oxygen, essential fatty acids and sterol, vitamins, and inorganic ions for efficient fermentation.[49] In line with this, metabolites from the yeast fermentation process have been studied in terms of their nutritional and ecological functions.[50] The main metabolites of yeast are ethanol and CO_2, and their production forms the basis of the alcoholic beverage and bread industries. Equally important to high final product quality is the contribution of yeast to aroma and flavor formation through the production of higher alcohols, esters, and organic acids.[51]

Fungi, yeast, and bacteria are used in SSF of rice bran for the production of functional food ingredients, feed, and ethanol. Among them, *Saccharomyces cerevisiae* var. *boulardii* (*S. boulardii*) has probiotic activity and is widely used as a dietary supplement for the prevention and treatment of intestinal disease. The wide spectrum of biomedical activities and food processing applications of *S. boulardii* has grown significantly over the past decade and includes, but is not limited to, protection against enteric pathogens, modification of lymphocyte proliferation, and differential release of plant secondary metabolites from foods such as wine, sourdough, and cheese. *Sacchromyces boulardii* has also been shown to be beneficial for the modification of food components, including breakdown of dietary phytate and biofortification of folate, to improve nutritional value and health properties.[52]

Issatchenkia orientalis, a multi-stress tolerant yeast, has been isolated from food, liquor, and soil. *I. orientalis* is widely used as a dietary supplement, protein source, and alternative candidate to improve wine quality and enzymatic production.[53–55]

Stress-tolerant microorganisms have certain advantages with respect to both cost and convenience. Thermotolerant microorganisms can reduce cooling costs and aid the simultaneous saccharification and fermentation process for converting biomass. Further, acid- and salt-tolerant microorganisms minimize the risk of bacterial contamination and reduce costs.[56] *I. orientalis* can withstand high temperature fluctuations, resulting in high biomass yields with great potential for improving the efficiency of fermentation.[46,57]

Future Prospects for Rice Bran Fermentation

Dietary rice bran intake and rice bran components have demonstrated protective effects against chronic diseases, including cardiovascular and certain oxidative stress-induced lifestyle diseases. Previous studies have shown that rice varieties are not equal in terms of levels of bioactive components. How these phytochemicals are altered by microbial fermentation and metabolism is an emerging area of research that merits careful investigation when assessing bioactivity and health benefits.[52]

OXIDATIVE STRESS AND ANTIOXIDANTS

Oxidative Stress and Antioxidant Defense

In the mid-1950s, Denham Harman articulated a free-radical theory of aging in which endogenous oxygen radicals are generated in cells, resulting in a pattern of cumulative damage.[58] This free-radical theory of aging originally implied that the targets of ROS were random, indiscriminate, and cumulative. However, although

oxidants may certainly function stochastically, accumulating evidence has implicated ROS as specific signaling molecules under both physiological and pathophysiological conditions. ROS generation is essential to the maintenance of homeostasis, within certain boundaries. Under certain situations of metabolic stress, even mitochondrial-derived oxidants seem to function as signaling molecules. Hence, elevated intracellular oxidant levels have two potential effects: damage to various cell components, and activation of specific signaling pathways.[59]

ROS encompass a variety of diverse chemical species, including superoxide anions, hydroxyl radicals, and hydrogen peroxide. These various radical species can be generated either exogenously or intracellularly from several different sources. Cytosolic enzyme systems contributing to oxidative stress include the expanding family of NADPH oxidases, which constitute a superoxide-generating system.[60,61] The effects of ROS are largely counteracted by an intricate antioxidant defense system consisting of antioxidant enzymes along with SOD, catalase, and glutathione peroxidase as enzymatic scavengers. SOD speeds up the conversion of superoxide to hydrogen peroxide, whereas catalase and glutathione peroxidase convert hydrogen peroxide to water. Various other non-enzymatic, low molecular mass molecules are important in ROS scavenging, including ascorbate, pyruvate, flavonoids, carotenoids, and glutathione.[62]

The balance between ROS production and antioxidant defense determines the overall degree of oxidative stress. Oxidative stress is considered to cause molecular and cellular damage in tissues. Many environmental stimuli, including cytokines, ultraviolet (UV) radiation, chemotherapeutic agents, hyperthermia, and even growth factors, generate high levels of ROS that can perturb the normal redox balance and shift cells into a state of oxidative stress.[59] Thus, ROS play a role in aging as well as the pathogenesis of numerous diseases, such as diabetes, cancer, neurodegenerative disease, and respiratory tract disorders.[63] Cell survival is dependent on adaptation or resistance to stress as well as repair or replacement of damaged molecules. A number of stress-response mechanisms have evolved to promote adaptation of cells and organisms to acute stress in either a cooperative or an antagonistic fashion.[59]

Diseases Related to Oxidative Stress and Antioxidant Therapy

Cancer

Chronic inflammation is induced by biological, chemical, and physical factors, and is associated with an increased risk of cancer. The link between inflammation and cancer has been supported by epidemiological and experimental data, and confirmed by anti-inflammatory therapies that show efficacy in cancer prevention and treatment.[64–67]

Sources of inflammation are widespread, and include microbial and viral infections; exposure to allergens, radiation, and toxic chemicals; autoimmune and chronic diseases; obesity; consumption of alcohol; tobacco use; and a high calorie diet. In general, a longer inflammation period is associated with a higher risk of cancer.[68,69] There are two stages of inflammation: acute and chronic. Acute inflammation, as the initial stage of inflammation, persists only for a short time and is usually beneficial to the host. However, if acute inflammation lasts for a long period of time, the second stage of inflammation, known as chronic inflammation, sets in, predisposing the host to various chronic illnesses such as cancer.[70] During inflammation, mast cells and leukocytes are recruited to sites of damage, leading to a "respiratory burst" caused by the elevated uptake of oxygen and, eventually, increased release and accumulation of ROS.[71,72]

In recent years, considerable evidence has demonstrated that ROS mediate the link between chronic inflammation and cancer. Cancer is a multistage process separated into at least three stages: initiation, promotion, and progression.[73–75] Oxidative stress is associated with all three of these stages. During the initiation stage, ROS may damage DNA by introducing gene mutations and structural alterations. In the promotion stage, ROS contribute to abnormal gene expression, blockage of cell-to-cell communications, and modification of second-messenger systems, thereby elevating proliferation of initiated cells or reducing apoptosis. Finally, oxidative stress may also participate in the progression stage of cancer by introducing DNA alterations to the initiated cell population.[76]

There is a variety of DNA repair enzymes that control the balance between production and removal of ROS, although antioxidants are more specific and efficient in protecting cells from radicals. This antioxidant system includes both endogenous and exogenous enzymatic and non-enzymatic antioxidants.[77]

Cardiovascular Diseases

Oxidative stress in cardiac and vascular myocytes describes injury caused to cells due to increased formation of ROS and/or reduced antioxidant reserve. Elevation of ROS generation seems to be due to impaired mitochondrial reduction of molecular oxygen, secretion of ROS by white blood cells, endothelial dysfunction, and auto-oxidation of catecholamines, as well as exposure to radiation or air pollution. On the other hand, reduction of the antioxidant reserve, which serves as a defense mechanism in cardiac and vascular myocytes, appears to be due to exhaustion and/or alteration of gene expression. The deleterious effects of ROS are mainly due to their ability to induce changes in subcellular organelles, resulting in intracellular Ca^{2+}-overload. Although a definite cause–effect relationship between oxidative stress and cardiovascular disease remains to be established, increased formation of ROS, indicating elevated oxidative stress, has been observed under a wide variety of experimental and clinical conditions. Furthermore, antioxidant therapy has been shown to exert beneficial effects on hypertension, atherosclerosis, ischemic heart disease, cardiomyopathies, and congestive heart failure. Antioxidants such as tocopherol (vitamin E) and ascorbic acid protect against lipid peroxidation as well as acting as cytosolic and extracellular antioxidants, respectively. Although both cardiac and vascular myocytes are protected by endogenous antioxidant defense mechanisms, they have no defense in situations of excessive oxidative stress. Therefore, antioxidant supplementation may be important. In addition to their therapeutic properties, cardiovascular drugs are considered as antioxidant supplements when given to patients suffering from cardiovascular disease.[78]

Neurodegenerative Diseases

Oxidative stress has long been recognized as important in the etiologies of numerous late-onset neurodegenerative diseases. In line with this, aging is an important risk factor for Alzheimer disease and Parkinson disease. Most theories regarding aging promote the idea that cumulative oxidative stress leads to mitochondrial mutation, mitochondrial dysfunction, and oxidative disease.[79]

However, a number of controversies have emerged as the roles of ROS in aging and age-related diseases become increasingly recognized. Based on the close association between oxidative stress and neurodegenerative disease, the rationale for antioxidant-based therapies is clear. The most widely studied antioxidant-based therapies are vitamin E (reduces lipid peroxidation in the brain), vitamin C (intracellular reducing molecule), and coenzyme Q10 (transfers electrons from complexes I and II to complex III in the respiratory chain). The role of vitamin E in the central nervous system is not fully understood, although it is a lipid-soluble molecule with antioxidant function that appears to neutralize the effects of peroxide and prevent lipid peroxidation in membranes.[80]

Insulin Resistance, Hyperglycemia, and Diabetes

Traditionally, the major function of adipose tissue is considered to be energy storage. However, there is increasing evidence that adipose tissue plays an important role in physiological processes, including an endocrine function. Adipocytes secrete proteins with a variety of functions, including glucose homeostasis, inflammation, energy balance, and lipid metabolism, all of which are regulated by insulin.[81] Further, adipose tissue secretes an adipocytokine related to insulin resistance.[82]

Insulin resistance is defined as a clinical state in which a normal or elevated level of insulin results in an attenuated biological response.[83] Insulin resistance is a key feature of non-insulin-dependent diabetes mellitus (NIDDM), and it occurs in such clinical settings as pregnancy, sepsis, cancer, cachexia, obesity, starvation, acromegaly, burn trauma, and metabolic syndrome.[84]

NIDDM is associated with accelerated production of oxygen-free radicals as well as reduced scavenging of oxidatively modified proteins.[85] Hyperglycemia is a symptom of insulin resistance that creates oxidative stress through the overproduction of free radicals.[86] Several reports have claimed that hydrogen peroxide as a free radical has insulin-mimetic effects. For example, a recent report observed reduced insulin activity in response to oxidative stress.[87–89]

Glucose is the primary fuel and regulator in pancreatic islet β-cell function. The primary function of insulin is to maintain blood glucose levels within a normal range. However, this homeostatic relationship is disrupted when glucose remains at supraphysiological levels for protracted periods of time – a consequence referred to as glucose toxicity.[90–92] Resultant defects in insulin content and secretion have been ascribed to the adverse effects of glucose on insulin gene expression, as evidenced by loss of insulin mRNA expression, insulin gene promoter activity, and DNA binding of transcription factors.[93,94] Although the toxic effects of glucose on β-cell function have been shown to be associated with alteration of insulin gene expression and insulin synthesis, no mechanism of action has yet been elucidated. Among potential mechanisms, chronic oxidative stress induced by glucose toxicity, resulting in ROS production, is considered to be potentially responsible for the progression of diabetes mellitus.[95]

In general, the development of type 2 diabetes is associated with pancreatic β-cell dysfunction along with insulin resistance. Normal β cells can compensate for insulin resistance by increasing insulin secretion, whereas insufficient compensation leads to the onset of glucose intolerance. Once hyperglycemia becomes apparent, β-cell function deteriorates progressively.[96–98]

Hyperglycemia as a direct cause of these phenomena, such as β-cell glucose toxicity, has been confirmed in various studies. Chronic hyperglycemia may impair β-cell function at the level of insulin synthesis as well as insulin secretion; when β-cell-derived cell lines are exposed to a high glucose concentration for a long time period, insulin gene transcription and insulin content are dramatically reduced.[94,99,100]

Under diabetic conditions, ROS are produced mainly through glycation reactions, which occur in various tissues and play a role in the development of diabetic complications. On the other hand, induction of glycation in diabetes was originally found in neural cells and the crystalline lens. Indeed, advanced glycation end products (AGEs) have been detected in β cells exposed to high glucose concentrations.[95,100–102]

ROS production is the primary initiation event of various pathogenic mechanisms, including oxidative stress linked with hyperglycemia and complications associated with diabetes mellitus.[103] ROS are generated in the mitochondria by the electron transport chain, and are scavenged by antioxidant enzymes such as mitochondrial manganese superoxide dismutase and glutathione peroxidase under normal conditions. However, excessive ROS production resulting in diabetes mellitus is mediated by the disruption of antioxidant enzymes.[104] Over the past century, the incidence of chronic metabolic diseases, particularly obesity and type 2 diabetes, has increased dramatically in developing countries.[105] Chronic metabolic diseases are associated with exposure to stress-induced defects in the regulation and coordination of homeostatic systems related to energy and nutrient management.[106] AGEs are considered to be molecular mediators of tissue damage in response to diabetic complications.[107] AGEs have been found at increasingly higher concentrations in renal glomeruli and tubules injured during diabetes mellitus.[108,109] Consequently, accumulation of AGEs can promote inflammation as well as metabolic and homeostasis failure via interactions with specific receptors and binding proteins. In fact, evidence supports interactions between AGEs and specific receptors involved in the pathogenesis of diabetic nephropathy.[110]

Since numerous studies have demonstrated that oxidative stress is mediated by hyperglycemia-induced generation of free radicals, antioxidants could be used to ameliorate oxidative stress.[111] Expression of antioxidant enzymes, such as superoxide dismutase, catalase, and glutathione peroxidase, is known to be very low in islet cells compared with other tissues and cells. Therefore, β cells exposed to oxidative stress may become rather sensitive, suggesting that glycation and subsequent oxidative stress are at least partially responsible for the toxic effects of hyperglycemia. Kaneto *et al.* and Matsuoka *et al.* previously revealed that glycation-mediated ROS production reduces insulin gene transcription and causes apoptosis in β cells.[102,112,113]

Organisms and animals possess their own intrinsic antioxidant defense systems that can be endogenously strengthened. This is especially true for the pancreas, as it has a relatively weak intrinsic defense system against oxidative stress. Such antioxidant supplements include *N*-acetyl-L-cysteine (NAC), which scavenges hydrogen peroxide, and vitamins C and E, which are well-known dietary antioxidants. Vitamin E is lipophilic and inhibits lipid peroxidation, scavenging lipid peroxyl radicals to yield lipid hydroperoxides and tocopheroxyl radical. Vitamin C, a water-soluble vitamin, functions cooperatively with vitamin E by regenerating tocopherol from tocopheroxyl radical. Kaneto *et al.* demonstrated that antioxidant treatment (NAC, vitamins C and E) was beneficial for treating diabetes and provided protection to β cells against glucose toxicity in D57BL/KsJ-*db*/*db* mice.[112,114]

ANTIOXIDANT EFFECTS OF FERMENTED RICE BRAN ON OXIDATIVE STRESS

Alternative Clinical Trials with Antioxidants

Biological antioxidants are natural molecules that prevent the uncontrolled formation of free radicals and activated oxygen species by mainly scavenging and reducing molecules. Redox recycling markedly increases the biological efficacy of antioxidants by reducing the need for *de novo* synthesis or large uptake of antioxidant nutrients.[115]

There has been an increasing interest in the therapeutic usage of naturally occurring antioxidants. In particular, phenolics are considered as potential therapeutic agents against a wide range of ailments, including neurodegenerative disease, cancer, diabetes, cardiovascular dysfunction, inflammatory diseases, and aging.[116] Phenolics are widely distributed in the plant kingdom and are thus an integral part of the human diet, with significant amounts reported in vegetables, fruits, and beverages.[117] Phenolics also exhibit a wide range of biological effects, including antibacterial, anti-inflammatory, anti-allergic, hepatoprotective, antithrombotic, antiviral, anticarcinogenic, and vasodilatory activities.[118] Dietary plant phenolic compounds have been reported to exert a variety of biological actions, such as free radical scavenging, metal chelation, modulation of enzymatic activity, signal transduction, and activation of transcription factors and gene expression.[118,119] They have received particular attention over the past decade due to their putative roles in the prevention of several human diseases, particularly atherosclerosis and cancer.[119]

Most epidemiological studies have shown that whole grains are protective against diabetes, obesity, cancer, and cardiovascular disease. There are many potential mechanisms responsible for the protective effects of whole grains due to their abundance of nutrients and phytochemicals, especially phenolic compounds.[120]

Rice bran contains many types of phenolic acids, the most abundant of which is ferulic acid, known as a strong antioxidant that may be responsible for most of the bioactivity of rice bran.[12]

Bioactive Ingredients of Fermented Rice Bran

Rice bran consists of a nutritious mixture of proteins, lipids, energy, and minerals. The bioactive food components in rice bran include γ-oryzanol, tocopherols, tocotrienols, polyphenols (ferulic acid and α-lipoic acid), phytosterols (β-sitosterol, campesterol, and stigmasterol), and carotenoids (α-carotene, β-carotene, lycopene, lutein, and zeazanthin). Rice bran also contains essential amino acids (tryptophan, histidine, methionine, cysteine, and arginine) as well as micronutrients (magnesium, calcium, phosphorous, manganese, and nine B vitamins).[121]

During fermentation, the amounts of phytochemicals are enhanced according to the variety of rice bran. In particular, the ferulic acid content was shown to be significantly elevated in Neptune rice bran upon *S. boulardii* fermentation.[53]

Ferulic Acid

Ferulic acid is a ubiquitous plant constituent produced by phenylalanine and tyrosine metabolism. It is present in seeds and leaves in both its free form as well as covalently linked to lignin and other biopolymers. The antioxidant potential of ferulic acid can be attributed to the structural characteristics of its electron-donating substituents.[122] Ferulic acid as a secondary metabolite is often found in seeds of plants such as rice, wheat, and oats, as well as coffee, apples, artichokes, peanuts, etc.[123] It is a naturally occurring antioxidant as well as being reactive toward free radical by-products of metabolic processes implicated in DNA damage, cancer, and cell aging.[6]

Phytochemicals can exert anticancer activities partially based on their ability to quench ROS, thereby protecting critical cellular molecules (DNA, proteins, and lipids) from oxidative damage.[124] Ferulic acid has been shown to exhibit anticarcinogenic effects against azoxymethane-induced colon carcinogenesis in F344 rats.[125] It has also been reported to repress skin tumorigenesis promoted by 12-O-tetradecanoylphorbol-acetate as well as inhibit pulmonary cancer in mice.[126,127]

Diabetes is a common endocrine disorder characterized by hyperglycemia, which causes excessive production of free radicals as well as oxidative stress. Ferulic acid directly neutralizes free radicals produced in response to streptozotocin treatment in the pancreas. This reduction of oxidative stress in the pancreas may also attenuate the risks associated with streptozotocin, which affects β-cell proliferation and insulin secretion. Thus, glucose utilization may be restored and blood glucose levels reduced as a result of the elevated insulin secretion induced by ferulic acid.[128] Nomura *et al.* reported that amide compounds from ferulic acid induce stimulation of insulin secretion in rat pancreatic RIN-5F cells.[129] Further, ferulic acid has been shown to suppress the blood glucose level in streptozotocin-induced diabetic mice and KK-Ay mice when administrated orally at levels ranging from 0.01% to 0.1%.[130]

Case Report: Improving the Effects of Fermented Rice Bran Extract and Ferulic Acid on Oxidative Stress

Inhibitory Effects of Fermented Rice Bran Extract and Ferulic Acid on ROS Generation

ROS generation was evaluated in 3T3-L1 adipocytes following induction of oxidative stress by hydrogen peroxide (100 μM) for 12 hours. Treatment with FRB

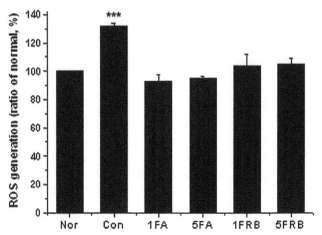

FIGURE 36.1 Inhibitory effects of ferulic acid and fermented rice bran extract on ROS generation in 3T3-L1 adipocytes treated with hydrogen peroxide. Measurement of cellular redox status with rates of dichlorofluorescein (DCF) oxidation. Two different concentrations of fermented rice bran extract (FRB) and ferulic acid (FA) were applied: 1FRB (10 μg/mL), 5FRB (50 μg/mL), 1FA (10 μM), and 5FA (50 μM). The results as mean values are shown with SD ($n=3$) (***$P<0.001$). ROS generation was assessed by DCFDA oxidation (carboxy-H_2DCFDA). Cells were plated onto 24-well plates at an initial density of 1×10^4 cells per well, followed by induction of differentiation. Cells were washed three times with 0.5 mL of HBSS per well. Following the addition of 20 μM DCFDA (final concentration), DCF fluorescence was followed continuously for 1 hour using a thermostatic plate reading spectrofluorometer (TECAN, infinite M200, Austria) at excitation and emission wavelengths of 495 and 525 nm, respectively. The amounts of cell proteins in each well were measured by bicinchoninic acid reaction, and DCF fluorescence levels were corrected for variations in total protein content between wells.

extract or ferulic acid significantly reduced ROS generation to 92.97–94.54% and 103.79–104.69%, respectively. However, there was no significant difference in ROS reduction between ferulic acid and FRB extract at all concentrations (Fig. 36.1).

NIDDM is associated with increased oxidative stress caused by accelerated production or reduced scavenging of ROS. Some studies have indicated that treatment with antioxidants such as cysteine or N-acetylcystein (NAC) protects β cells from ROS-mediated damage.[84] Other studies have found evidence that diabetes is associated with an antioxidant/pro-oxidant imbalance. In addition to impaired antioxidant defense, increased production of ROS has also been proposed.[131]

Improvement of Adipogenesis under Oxidative Stress by Fermented Rice Bran Extract and Ferulic Acid

3T3-L1 adipocytes were treated with FRB extract or ferulic acid for 12 hours before induction of oxidative stress. Oxidative stress caused a decrease in the triglyceride concentration in 3T3-L1 adipocytes by inhibiting adipogenesis (Fig. 36.2). However, treatment with FRB extract or ferulic acid increased the amount of

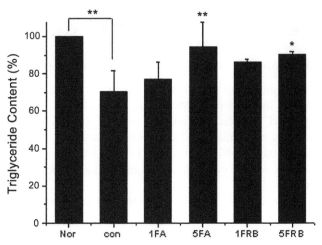

FIGURE 36.2 Inhibitory effects of ferulic acid and fermented rice bran extract on lipolysis of 3T3-L1 adipocytes treated with hydrogen peroxide. Lipid accumulation was assessed by quantification of A_{490}. Two different concentrations of fermented rice bran extract (FRB) and ferulic acid (FA) were applied: 1FRB (10 μg/mL), 5FRB (50 μg/mL), 1FA (10 μM), and 5FA (50 μM). The results as mean values are shown with SD ($n=3$) (*$P<0.05$, **$P<0.01$). After adipocyte differentiation, cells were stained with Oil Red O. Cells were washed twice with PBS and fixed with 10% formaldehyde in PBS for 1 hour. After the formaldehyde was discarded, Oil Red O staining was performed in isopropanol for 1 hour. Stained droplets were dissolved in isopropanol and then quantified by measuring the absorbance at 490 nm. The result is shown as relative triglyceride content.

triglycerides in a dose-dependent manner. A high volume of FRB extract (50 μg/mL) or ferulic acid (50 μM) resulted in significant improvement of adipogenesis. It was previously reported that normal insulin signaling in adipocytes is impaired during insulin resistance, leading to reduction of insulin-mediated glucose uptake and metabolism. During this period, free fatty acids are released from adipose triglyceride stores into the circulation, whereupon they are oxidized for fuel.[34,35]

Effects of Fermented Rice Bran Extract and Ferulic Acid on MRNA Expression of Molecules Related to Metabolic Homeostasis

The mRNA expression levels of glucose transporter 4 (GLUT4) and adiponectin, which are strongly related to homeostasis of adipocytes, were elevated at high concentrations of FRB extract and ferulic acid (Fig. 36.3). Higher doses of FRB extract or ferulic acid upregulated the expression of adiponectin and GLUT4, which is related to glucose transportation and insulin sensitivity. Ferulic acid at a concentration of 50 μM increased the expression of GLUT4 (135.13%) more so than other groups (Fig. 36.3A). In the glucose utilization assay, a higher dose of ferulic acid significantly increased glucose utilization in 3T3-L1 adipocytes. Adiponectin is a novel adipocytokine that regulates fat and insulin metabolism.[132] Secretion of adiponectin from adipocytes

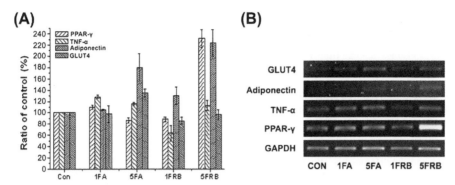

FIGURE 36.3 **Effects of ferulic acid and fermented rice bran extract on mRNA expression of molecules related to glucose utilization and adipogenesis in 3T3-L1 cells treated with hydrogen peroxide (100 μM).** (A) mRNA expression levels of PPAR-γ, TNF-α, adiponectin, and GLUT4 in 3T3-L1 cells were semi-quantified by RT-PCR. (B) Representative agarose gel electrophoretic patterns of PCR products are shown. Two different concentrations of fermented rice bran extract (FRB) and ferulic acid (FA) were applied: 1FRB (10 μg/mL), 5FRB (50 μg/mL), 1FA (10 μM), and 5FA (50 μM). Densitometric signal ratios of molecules to internal control (glyceraldehydes-3-phosphatedehydrogenase [GAPDH]) were analyzed.

may be disturbed during insulin resistance, with a recent study showing that disruption of adiponectin causes insulin resistance.[133,134] In addition, reduced plasma adiponectin levels have been described in patients with diabetes, presumably as a result of increased ROS.[135] Due to the functional consequences of ROS production in adipocytes that are associated with insulin resistance and alterations in serum levels of adiponectin, the increases of ROS induced an inflammatory response in adipocytes when they were exposed to hyperglycemia and its ROS production.[136]

In addition, catecholamine is thought to induce insulin resistance via the downregulation of adiponectin gene expression.[137] GLUT4 is a glucose transporter (GLUT) isoform located primarily in muscle cells and adipocytes that acts as the main insulin-responsive glucose transporter.[130] An *in vitro* study reported that 3T3-L1 adipocytes exposed to micromolar concentrations of hydrogen peroxide for induction of oxidative stress show decreased GLUT4 expression.[137] Further, various groups have shown that GLUT4 expression in adipose tissue is reduced in obese, non-diabetic, type 2 diabetes mellitus subjects.[138–140] Expression of tumor necrosis factor-alpha (TNF-α) as an inhibition factor of insulin signaling showed no drastic changes among the treatment groups (Fig. 36.3). However, expression of peroxisome proliferator-activated receptor gamma (PPAR-γ), a ligand-activated nuclear transcription factor, was dramatically elevated by FRB extract (50 μg/mL) treatment (Fig. 36.3). In a previous study, PPAR-γ was identified as a key transcription factor in adipogenesis.[34]

Thus, FRB extract ameliorated insulin resistance induced by oxidative stress by neutralizing free radicals and increasing glucose metabolism in adipocytes. This property could be attributed to ferulic acid as a potential antioxidant present in FRB extract.

CONCLUSION

Oxidative stress is caused by metabolic stress in response to a state of imbalance between oxidants and antioxidants, in favor of oxidants. For prevention of oxidant-induced damage, a ubiquitous antioxidant defense system together with antioxidants derived from plant foods was highlighted in this chapter. ROS play a role in aging as well as the pathogenesis of numerous diseases. Cereal grains are considered to be one of the most pivotal sources of dietary nutrients. Specifically, bran, which is high in fiber and contains a phytochemical-rich outer layer of cereal grains, is considered to be an important ingredient for reducing the risk of lifestyle-related diseases. Bran is composed of phenolics bound in dietary fibers and β-glucan, which has a wide spectrum of biological activities. To date, SSF has emerged as a potential technology for the development of bioactive products. It has also been employed to increase the content of phenolic compounds in certain foods. Thus, fermented cereal grains, especially bran with its abundance of bioactive molecules, are good ingredients as well as advanced sources of antioxidants.

References

1. Sies H. Oxidative stress: oxidants and antioxidants. *Exp Physiol* 1997;**82**:291–5.
2. Rahman T, Hosen I, Islam MMT, Shekhar HU. Oxidative stress and human health. *Adv Biosci Biotech* 2012;**3**:997–1019.
3. Sies H. Strategies of antioxidant defense. *Eur J Biochem* 1993;**15**:213–9.
4. Hawkins CL, Morgan PE, Davies MJ. Quantification of protein modification by oxidants. *Free Rad Biol Med* 2009;**45**:965–88.
5. Klaunig JE, Kamendulis LM, Hocevar BA. Oxidative stress and oxidative damage in carcinogenesis. *Toxicol Pathol* 2010;**38**:96–109.
6. Lobo V, Patil A, Phatak A, Chandra N. Free radicals, antioxidants and functional foods: Impact on human health. *Pharmacogn Rev* 2010;**4**:118–26.

7. Wei YH, Lee HC. Oxidative stress, mitochondrial DNA mutation, and impairment of antioxidant enzymes in aging. *Exp Bio med* 2002;**227**:671–82.

8. Yu BP. Cellular defenses against damage from reactive oxygen species. *Physiol Rev* 1994;**74**:139–62.

9. López-Varela S, González-Gross M, Marcos A. Functional foods and the immune system: A review. *Eur J Clin Nutr* 2002;**56**:S29–33.

10. Roberfroid MB. What is beneficial for health? The concept of functional food. *Food Chem Toxicol* 1999;**37**:1034–41.

11. Papas AM. Diet and antioxidant status. *Food Chem Toxicol* 1999; **37**:999–1007.

12. Gani A, Wani SM, Masoodi FA, Hameed G. Whole-grain cereal bioactive compounds and their health benefit: A review. *J Food Process Technol* 2012;**3**:146.

13. Jones JM, Engleson J. Whole Grains: Benefits and challenges. *Annu Rev Food Sci Technol* 2010;**1**:19–40.

14. International Food Information Council Foundation. *Media guide on food safety and nutrition: 2004–2006*. Washington: DC. International Food Information Council Foundation; 2006.

15. Fleet GH. The commercial and community significance of yeasts in food and beverage production. In: Querol A, Fleet GH, editors. *Yeast in food and beverages*. Heidelberg, Germany: Springer-Verlag; 2006. pp. 1–12.

16. Romano P, Capece A, Jespersen L. Taxonomic and ecological diversity of food and beverage yeasts. In: Querol A, Fleet GH, editors. *Yeast in food and beverages*. Heidelberg, Germany: Springer-Verlag; 2006. pp. 13–54.

17. Blandino A, Al-Aseeri Pandiella SS, Cantero D, Webb C. Cereal-based fermented foods and beverages. *Food Res Int* 2003;**36**:527–43.

18. Chavan JK, Kadam SS. Critical reviews in food science and nutrition. *Food Sci* 1989;**28**:348–400.

19. Haard NF, Odunfa SA, Lee CH. Quintero-Ramírez, Lorence-Quiñones A, Wacher-Radarte C. Fermented cereals: A global perspective. *FAO Agric Ser Bull* 1999;**138**.

20. Patel S. Cereal bran: the next super food with significant antioxidant and anticancer potential. *Mediterr J Nutr Metab* 2012;**5**:91–104.

21. Hasler CM. Functional foods: Their role in disease prevention and health promotion. *Food Tech* 1998;**52**:63–70.

22. Sosulski F, Krygier K, Hogge L. Free, esterified, and insoluble-bound phenolic acids. 3. Composition of phenolic acids in cereal and potato flours. *J Agric Food Chem* 1982;**30**:337–40.

23. Bondia-Pons I, Aura AM, Vuorela S, Kolehmainen M, Mykkänen H, Poutanen K. Rye phenolics in nutrition and health. *J Cereal Sci* 2009;**49**:323–36.

24. Liyama K, Lam TBT, Stone BA. Covalent cross-links in the cell wall. *Plant physiol* 1994;**104**:315–20.

25. Cyran MR, Saulnier L. Association and structural diversity of hemicelluloses in the cell walls of rye outer layers: comparison between two ryes with opposite breadmaking quality. *J Agric Food Chem* 2007;**55**:2329–41.

26. Adom KK, Liu RH. Antioxidant activity of grains. *J Agric Food Chem* 2002;**50**:6182–7.

27. Meyer AS, Donovan JL, Pearson DA, Waterhouse AL, Frankel EN. *J Agric Food Chem* 1998;**46**:1783–7.

28. Szwajgier D, Pielecki J, Targoński Z. The release of ferulic acid and feruloylated oligosaccharides during wort and beer production. *J I Brewing* 2005;**111**:372–9.

29. Poquet L, Clifford MN, Williamson G. Transport and metabolism of ferulic acid through the colonic epithelium. *Drug Metab Dispos* 2008;**36**:190–7.

30. Szwajgier D, Jakubczyk A. Biotransformation of ferulic acid by *Lactobacillus acidophilus* K1 and selected *Bifidobacterium* strains. *Acta Sci Pol Technol Aliment* 2010;**9**:45–59.

31. Fazary AE, Ju YH. Feruloyl esterases as biotechnological tools: current and future perspectives. *Acta Bioch Bioph Sin* 2007;**39**: 811–28.

32. Crepin VF, Faulds CB, Connerton IF. Functional classification of the microbial feruloyl esterases. *Appl Microbiol Biotechnol* 2004;**63**:647–52.

33. Ou S, Zhang J, Wang Y, Zhang N. Production of feruloyl esterase from *Aspergillus niger* by solid-state fermentation on different carbon sources. *Enzyme Res* 2011:848–939.

34. Kim KM, Yu KW, Kang DH, Suh HJ. Anti-stress and anti-fatigue effect of fermented rice bran. *Phytother Res* 2002;**16**:700–2.

35. Kim HY, Kim JH, Yang SB, Hong SG, Lee SA, Hwang SJ, et al. A polysaccharide extracted from rice bran fermented with *Lentinus edodes* enhances natural killer cell activity and exhibits anticancer effect. *J Med Food* 2007;**10**:25–31.

36. Chung SY, Seo YK, Park JM, Seo MJ, Park JK, Kim JW, et al. Fermented rice bran downregulates MITF expression and leads to inhibition of alpha-MSH-induced melanogenesis in B16F1 melanoma. *Biosci Biotechnol Biochem* 2009;**73**:1704–10.

37. Fan JP, Choi KM, Han GD. Inhibitory effects of water extracts of fermented rice bran on allergic response. *Food Sci Biotechnol* 2010;**19**:1573–8.

38. Kim D, Han GD. Ameliorating effects of fermented rice bran extract on oxidative stress induced by high glucose and hydrogen peroxide in 3T3-L1 adipocytes. *Plant Foods Hum Nutr* 2011;**66**:285–90.

39. Martins S, Mussatto SI, Martínez-Avila G, Montañez-Saenz J, Aguilar CN, Teixeira JA. Bioactive phenolic compounds: production and extraction by solid-state fermentation. A review. *Biotechnol Adv* 2011;**29**:365–73.

40. Pandey A. Solid-state fermentation. *Biochem Engin J* 2003;**13**:81–4.

41. nee'Nigam PS. Production of bioactive secondary metabolites. In: nee'Nigam PS, Pandey A, editors. *Biotechnology for agro-industrial residues utilization*. Dordrecht, The Netherlands: Springer; 2009. pp. 130–46.

42. Lee IH, Hung YH, Chou CC. Solid-state fermentation with fungi to enhance the antioxidative activity, total phenolic and anthocyanin contents of black bean. *Int J Food Microbiol* 2008;**121**:150–6.

43. Bhanja T, Kumari A, Banerjee R. Enrichment of phenolics and free radical scavenging property of wheat koji prepared with two filamentous fungi. *Bioresour Technol* 2009;**100**:2861–6.

44. Zhang A, Lei A, Lu Y, Lu Z, Chen Y. Chemical composition and bioactivity changes in stale rice after fermentation with. *Cordyceps sinensis J Biosci Bioeng* 2008;**106**:188–93.

45. Randhir R, Shetty K. Mung beans processed by solid-state bioconversion improves phenolic content and functionality relevant for diabetes and ulcer management. *Innovat Food Sci Emerg Tech* 2007;**8**:197–204.

46. Bryan WL. Solid-state fermentation of sugars in sweet sorghum. *Enzyme Microb Tech* 1990;**12**:437–42.

47. Stanton C, Ross RP, Fitzgerald GF, Van Sinderen D. Fermented functional foods based on probiotics and their biogenic metabolites. *Curr Opin Biotechnol* 2005;**16**:198–203.

48. Steinkraus KH. Fermentations in world food processing. *Compr Rev Food Sci Food Safe* 2002;**1**:23–32.

49. Snyder C, Ingledew M. Nutrition in fermentation. *Biofuels Business* 2009:55–6.

50. Carnevali P, Ciati R, Leporati A, Paese M. Liquid sourdough fermentation: Industrial application perspectives. *Food Microbiol* 2007;**24**:150–4.

51. Fredlund E. *Central carbon metabolism in the biocontrol yeast Pichia anomala*. PhD Thesis. Uppsala, Sweden: Department of Microbiology, Swedish University of Agricultural Sciences; 2004.

52. Ryan EP, Heuberger AL, Weir TL, Barnett B, Broeckling CD, Prenni JE. Rice bran fermented with *Saccharomyces* boulardii generates novel metabolite profiles with bioactivity. *J Agric Food Chem* 2011;**59**:1862–70.

53. Koh JH, Suh HJ. Biological activities of thermo-tolerant microbes from fermented rice bran as an alternative microbial feed additive. *Appl Biochem Biotechnol* 2009;**157**:420–30.

54. Hong SK, Lee HJ, Park HJ, Hong YA, Rhee IK, Lee WH, et al. Degradation of malic acid in wine by immobilized *Issatchenkia orientalis* cells with oriental oak charcoal and alginate. *Lett Appl Microbiol* 2010;**50**:522–9.

55. Quan CS, Fan SD, Ohta Y. Immobilization of *Candida krusei* cells producing phytase in alginate gel beads: an application of the preparation of *myo*-inositol phosphates. *Appl Microbiol Biotechnol* 2003;**62**:41–7.

56. Isono N, Hayakawa H, Usami A, Mishima T, Hisamatsu M. A comparative study of ethanol production by *Issatchenkia orientalis* strains under stress conditions. *J Biosci Bioeng* 2012;**113**:76–8.

57. Chinn MS, Nokes SE. Temperature control of a solid substrate cultivation deep-bed reactor using an internal heat exchanger. *Trans ASAE* 2003;**46**:1741–9.

58. Harman D. Aging: a theory based on free radical and radiation chemistry. *J Gerontol* 1957;**2**:298–300.

59. Finkel T, Holbrook NJ. Oxidants, oxidative stress and the biology of ageing. *Nature* 2000;**408**:239–47.

60. Suh YA, Arnold RS, Lassegue B, Shi J, Xu X, Sorescu D, et al. Cell transformation by the superoxide-generating oxidase Mox1. *Nature* 1999;**401**:79–82.

61. Geiszt M, Kopp JB, Várnai P, Leto TL. Identification of Renox, an NAD(P)H oxidase in kidney. *Proc Natl Acad Sci USA* 2000;**97**:8010–4.

62. Chae HZ, Kang SW, Rhee SG. Isoforms of mammalian peroxiredoxin that reduce peroxides in presence of thioredoxin. *Methods Enzymol* 1999;**300**:219–26.

63. Anderson D, Phillips BJ, Tian-Wei YU, Edwards AJ, Ayesh R, Butterworth KR. Effects of vitamin C supplementation in human volunteers with a range of cholesterol levels on biomarkers of oxygen radical-generated damage. *Pure Appl Chem* 2000;**72**:973–83.

64. Bartsch H, Nair J. Chronic inflammation and oxidative stress in the genesis and perpetuation of cancer: role of lipid peroxidation, DNA damage, and repair. *Langenbecks Arch Surg* 2006;**391**:499–510.

65. Grivennikov SI, Greten FR, Karin M. Immunity, inflammation, and cancer. *Cell* 2010;**140**:883–99.

66. Grivennikov SI, Karin M. Inflammation and oncogenesis: a vicious connection. *Curr Opin Genet Dev* 2010;**20**:65–71.

67. Gonda TA, Tu S, Wang TC. Chronic inflammation, the tumor microenvironment and carcinogenesis. *Cell Cycle* 2009;**8**:2005–13.

68. Schetter AJ, Heegaard NH, Harris CC. Inflammation and cancer: interweaving microRNA, free radical, cytokine and p53 pathways. *Carcinogenesis* 2010;**31**:37–49.

69. Aggarwal BB, Vijayalekshmi RV, Sung B. Targeting inflammatory pathways for prevention and therapy of cancer: short-term friend, long-term foe. *Clin Cancer Res* 2009;**15**:425–30.

70. Lin WW, Karin M. A cytokine-mediated link between innate immunity, inflammation, and cancer. *J Clin Invest* 2007;**117**:1175–83.

71. Hussain SP, Hofseth LJ, Harris CC. Radical causes of cancer. *Nat Rev Cancer* 2003;**3**:276–85.

72. Coussens LM, Werb Z. Inflammation and cancer. *Nature* 2002;**420**:860–7.

73. Ames BN, Gold LS. Animal cancer tests and cancer prevention. *J Natl Cancer Inst Monogr* 1992;**1992**:125–32.

74. Guyton KZ, Kensler TW. Oxidative mechanisms in carcinogenesis. *Br Med Bull* 1993;**49**:523–44.

75. Schulte-Hermann R, Timmermann-Trosiener I, Barthel G, Bursch W. DNA synthesis, apoptosis, and phenotypic expression as determinants of growth of altered foci in rat liver during phenobarbital promotion. *Cancer Res* 1990;**50**:5127–35.

76. Stevenson DE, Walborg Jr EF. The role of oxidative stress in chemical carcinogenesis. *Environ Health Perspect* 1998;**106**:289–95.

77. Reuter S, Gupta SC, Chaturvedi MM, Aggarwal BB. Oxidative stress, inflammation, and cancer: How are they linked? *Free Radic Bio Med* 2010;**49**:1603–16.

78. Dhalla NS, Temsah RM, Netticadan T. Role of oxidative stress in cardiovascular diseases. *J Hypertens* 2000;**18**:655–73.

79. Lin MT, Beal MF. Mitochondrial dysfunction and oxidative stress in neurodegenerative diseases. *Nature* 2006;**443**:787–95.

80. Gandhi S, Abramov AY. Mechanism of oxidative stress in neurodegeneration. *Oxid Med Cell Longev* 2012. 2012: 428010.

81. Trayhurn P, Beattie JH. Physiological role of adipose tissue: white adipose tissue as an endocrine and secretory organ. *Proc Nutr Soc* 2001;**60**:329–39.

82. Mlinar B, Marc J, Janez A, Pfeifer M. Molecular mechanisms of insulin resistance and associated diseases. *Clinica Chimica Acta* 2007;**375**:20–35.

83. Cefalu WT. Insulin resistance: cellular and clinical concepts. *Exp Biol Med* 2001;**226**:13–26.

84. Houstis N, Rosen ED, Lander ES. Reactive oxygen species have a causal role in multiple forms of insulin resistance. *Nature* 2006;**440**:944–8.

85. Cross CE, Halliwell B, Borish ET, Pryor WA, Ames BN, Saul RL, et al. Oxygen radicals and human disease. *Ann Intern Med* 1987;**107**:526–45.

86. Aragno M, Parola S, Tamagno E, Brignardello E, Manti R, Danni O, et al. Oxidative derangement in rat synaptosomes induced by hyperglycemia: restorative effect of dehydroepiandosterone treatment. *Biochem Pharmacol* 2000;**60**:389–95.

87. Heffetz D, Bushkin I, Dror R, Zick Y. The insulinomimetic agents H_2O_2 and vanadate stimulate protein tyrosine phosphorylation in intact cells. *J Biol Chem* 1990;**265**:2896–902.

88. Hayes GR, Lockwood DH. Role of insulin receptor phosphorylation in the insulinomimetic effects of hydrogen peroxide. *Proc Natl Acad Sci USA* 1987;**84**:8115–9.

89. Rudich A, Kozlovsky N, Potashnik R, Bashan N. Oxidant stress reduces insulin responsiveness in 3T3-L1 adipocyte. *Am J physiol* 1997;**272**:E935–40.

90. Unger RH, Grundy S. Hyperglycaemia as an inducer as well as a consequence of impaired islet cell function and insulin resistance: implications for the management of diabetes. *Diabetologia* 1985;**28**:119–21.

91. Rossetti L, Giaccari A, DeFronzo RA. Glucose toxicity. *Diabetes Care* 1990;**13**:610–30.

92. Robertson RP, Olson LK, Zhang HJ. Differentiating glucose toxicity from glucose desensitization: a new message from the insulin gene. *Diabetes* 1994;**43**:1085–9.

93. Robertson RP, Zhang HJ, Pyzdrowski KL, Walseth TF. Preservation of insulin mRNA levels and insulin secretion in HIT cells by avoidance of chronic exposure to high glucose concentrations. *J Clin Invest* 1992;**90**:320–5.

94. Olson LK, Redmon JB, Towle HC, Robertson RP. Chronic exposure of HIT cells to high glucose concentrations paradoxically decreases insulin gene transcription and alters binding of insulin gene regulatory protein. *J Clin Invest* 1993;**92**:514–9.

95. Baynes JW. Role of oxidative stress in development of complications in diabetes. *Diabetes* 1991;**40**:405–12.

96. Porte Jr D. Banting Lecture 1990. β-cells in type II diabetes mellitus. *Diabetes* 1991;**40**:166–80.

97. DeFronzo RA, Bonadonna RC, Ferrannini E. Pathogenesis of NIDDM: a balanced overview. *Diabetes Care* 1992;**15**:318–68.

98. Yki-Jarvinen H. Glucose toxicity. *Endocrine Rev* 1992;**13**:415–31.

99. Robertson RP, Zhang HJ, Pyzdrowski KL, Walseth TF. Preservation of insulin mRNA levels and insulin secretion in HIT cells by avoidance of chronic exposure to high glucose concentrations. *J Clin Invest* 1992;**90**:320–5.

100. Hunt JV, Smith CC, Wolff SP. Autoxidative glycosylation and possible involvement of peroxides and free radicals in LDL modification by glucose. *Diabetes* 1991;**39**:1420–4.

101. Kaneto H, Fujii J, Myint T, Miyazawa N, Islam KN, Kawasaki Y, et al. Reducing sugars trigger oxidative modification and

apoptosis in pancreatic b-cells by provoking oxidative stress through the glycation reaction. *Biochem J* 1996;**320**:855–63.

102. Tajiri Y, Moller C, Grill V. Long term effects of aminoguanidine on insulin release and biosynthesis: evidence that the formation of advanced glycosylation end products inhibits B cell function. *Endocrinology* 1997;**138**:273–80.

103. Baynes JW, Thorpe SR. Role of oxidative stress in diabetic complication: a new perspective on an old paradigm. *Diabetes* 1999;**48**:1–9.

104. Pitkänen S, Robinson BH. Mitochondrial complex I deficiency lead to increased production of superoxide radicals and induction of superoxide dismutase. *J Clin Invest* 1996;**98**:345–51.

105. Hossain P, Kawar B, Nahas ME. Obesity and diabetes in the developing world-a growing challenge. *N Engl J Med* 2007;**356**:213–5.

106. Hotamisligil GS. Inflammation and metabolic disorders. *Nature* 2006;**444**:860–7.

107. Miura J, Yamagishi S, Uchigata Y, Takeuchi M, Yamamoto H, Makita Z, et al. Serum levels of non-carboxymethyllysine advanced glycation endproducts are correlated to severity of microvascular complications in patients with type 1 diabetes. *J Diabetes Complications* 2003;**17**:16–21.

108. Horie K, Miyata T, Maeda K, Miyata S, Sugiyama S, Sakai H, et al. Immunohistochemical colocalization of glycoxidation products and lipid peroxidation products in diabetic renal glomerular lesions. Implication for glycoxidative stress in the pathogensis of diabetic nephropathy. *J Clin Invest* 1997;**100**:2995–3004.

109. Forbes JM, Cooper ME, Thallas V, Burns WC, Thomas MC, Brammar GC, et al. Reduction of the accumulation of advanced glycation end products by ACE inhibition in experimental diabetic nephropathy. *Diabetes* 2002;**51**:3274–82.

110. Vlassara H. The AGE-receptor in the pathogenesis of diabetic complications. *Diabetes Metab Res Rev* 2001;**17**:436–43.

111. Johansen JS, Harris AK, Rychly DJ, Ergul A. Oxidative stress and the use of antioxidants in diabetes: linking basic science to clinical practice. *Cardiovasc Diabetol* 2005;**29**:5–15.

112. Tiedge M, Lortz S, Drinkgern J, Lenzen S. Relation between antioxidant enzyme gene expression and antioxidative defense status of insulin-producing cells. *Diabetes* 1997;**46**:1733–42.

113. Matsuoka T, Kajimoto Y, Watada H, Kaneto H, Kishimoto M, Umayahara Y, et al. Glycation-dependent, reactive oxygen species-mediated suppression of the insulin gene promoter activity in HIT cells. *J Clin Invest* 1997;**99**:144–50.

114. Stahl W, Sies H. Antioxidant defense: vitamins E and C and carotenoids. *Diabetes* 1997;**46**:14–8.

115. Chaudière J, Ferrari-lliou R. Intracellular antioxidants: from chemical to biochemical mechanisms. *Food Chem Toxicol* 1999;**37**:949–62.

116. Soobrattee MA, Neergheen VS, Luximon-Ramma A, Aruoma OI, Bahorun T. Phenolics as potential antioxidant therapeutic agents: Mechanism and actions. *Mutat Res* 2005;**579**:200–13.

117. Luximon-Ramma A, Bahorun T, Crozier A, Zbarsky V, Datla KK, Dexter DT, et al. Characterization of the antioxidant functions of flavonoids and proanthocyanidins in Mauritian black teas. *Food Res Int* 2005;**38**:357–67.

118. Middleton E, Kandaswami C, Theoharides TC. The effects of plant flavonoids on mammalian cells: implications for inflammation, heart disease and cancer. *Pharmacol Rev* 2000;**52**:673–839.

119. Nardini M, Ghiselli A. Determination of free and bound phenolic acids in beer. *Anal Nutr Clin Methods* 2004;**84**:137–43.

120. Slavin J. Why whole grains are protective: biological mechanisms. *Proc Nutr Soc* 2003;**62**:129–34.

121. Ryan EP. Bioactive food components and health properties of rice bran. *J Am Vet Med Assoc* 2011;**238**:593–600.

122. Kanaski J, Aksenova M, Stoyanova A, Butterfield DA. Ferulic acid antioxidant protection against hydroxyl and peroxyl radical oxidation in synaptosomal and neuronal cell culture systems *in vitro*: structure activity studies. *J Nutr Biochem* 2002;**13**:273–81.

123. Parr AJ, Bolwell GP. Phenols in the plant and in man. The potential for possible nutritional enhancement of the diet by modifying the phenols content or profile. *J Sci Food Agric* 2000;**80**:985–1012.

124. Roy M, Chakrabarty S, Sinha D, Bhattacharya RK, Siddiqi M. Anticlastogenic, antigenotoxic and apoptotic activity of epigallocatechin gallate: a green tea polyphenol. *Mutat Res* 2003;**523**:33–41.

125. Kawabata K, Yamamoto T, Hara A, Shimizu M, Yamada Y, Matsunaga K, et al. Modifying effects of ferulic acid on azoxymethane-induced colon carcinogenesis in F344 rats. *Cancer Lett* 2000;**157**:15–21.

126. Asanoma M, Takahashi K, Miyabe M, Yamamoto K, Yoshimi N, Mori H, et al. Inhibitory effect of topical application of polymerized ferulic acid, a synthetic lignin, on tumor promotion in mouse skin two stage tumorigenesis. *Carcinogenesis* 1993;**14**:1321–5.

127. Lesca P. Protective effects of ellagic acid and other plant phenols benzo[a]pyrene- induced neoplasia in mice. *Carcinogenesis* 1983;**4**:1651–3.

128. Balasubashini MS, Rukkumani R, Viswanathan P. Ferulic acid alleviates lipid peroxidation in diabetic rats. *Phytother Res* 2004;**18**:310–4.

129. Noumura E, Kashiwada A, Hosoda A, Nakamura K, Morishita H, Tsuno T, et al. Synthesis of amide compounds of ferulic acid and their stimulatory effects on insulin secretion *in vitro*. *Bioorg Med Chem* 2003;**11**:3807–13.

130. Ohnishi M, Matuo T, Tsuno T, Hosoda A, Nomura E, Taniguchi H, et al. Antioxidant activity and hypoglycemic effect of ferulic acid in streptozotocin induced diabetic mice and KK-AY mice. *Biofactors* 2004;**21**:315–9.

131. Kahn BB, Flier JS. Obesity and insulin resistance. *J Clin Invest* 2000;**106**:473–81.

132. Kubota N, Terauchi Y, Yamauchi T, Kubota T, Moroi M, Matsui J, et al. Disruption of adiponectin causes insulin resistance and neointimal formation. *J Biol Chem* 2002;**277**:25863–6.

133. Maeda N, Shimomura I, Kishida K, Nishizawa H, Matsuda M, Nagaretani H, et al. Diet-induced insulin resistance in mice lacking adiponectin/ACRP30. *Nat Med* 2002;**6**:731–7.

134. Mlinar B, Marc J, Janez A, Pfeifer M. Molecular mechanisms of insulin resistance and associated diseases. *Clinica Chimica Acta* 2007;**375**:20–35.

135. Cao Y, Tao L, Yuan Y, Jiao X, Lau WB, Wang Y, et al. Endothelial dysfunction in adiponectin deficiency and its mechanisms involved. *J Mol Cell Cardiol* 2009;**46**:413–9.

136. Lin Y, Berg AH, Iyengar P, Lam TK, Giacca A, Combs TP, et al. The hyperglycemia-induced inflammatory response in adipocytes: the role of reactive oxygen species. *J Biol Chem* 2005;**280**:4617–26.

137. Most MM, Tulley R, Morales S, Lefevre M. Rice bran oil, not fiber, lowers cholesterol in human. *Am J Clin Nutr* 2005;**81**:64–78.

138. Olefsky JM. Treatment of insulin resistance with peroxisome proliferator-activated receptor γ agonists. *J Clin Invest* 2000;**106**:467–72.

139. Pessler D, Rudich A, Bashan N. Oxidative stress impairs nuclear proteins binding to the insulin responsive element in the GLUT4 promoter. *Diabetologia* 2001;**44**:2156–64.

140. Rhodes CJ, White MF. Molecular insights into insulin action and secretion. *Eur J Clin Invest* 2002;**32**:3–13.

141. Rudich A, Kozlovsky N, Potashnik R, Bashan N. Oxidant stress reduces insulin responsiveness in 3T3-L1 adipocyte. *Am J physiol* 1997;**272**:E935–40.

37

Rice Bran Oil's Role in Health and Cooking

Abdul Rohman[*,†]

Gadjah Mada University, Department of Pharmaceutical Chemistry, and Research Center of Halal Products, Yogyakarta, Indonesia, †Center of Research for Fiqh Science and Technology (Cirst) Universiti Teknologi Malaysia, Skudai, Malaysia

INTRODUCTION

Rice is the staple food for two-thirds of the world's population. The milling process of rice will remove the bran (10%) and the husk (20%) to release the starchy endosperm (70%). Rice bran is one of the abundant co-products produced during rice milling to obtain white rice.[1] The bran is the hard outer layer of rice, consisting of aleurone and pericarp.[2] Rice bran has been recognized as an excellent source of vitamins, minerals, and some phytochemicals, such as gamma-oryzanol, tocopherols, tocotrienols and phytosterols; however, it has been under-utilized in humans and used primarily in feed formulation. During the past two decades, some studies have shown that rice bran is a unique complex of naturally occurring antioxidant compounds.[3,4] It has been reported to contain an inherently high level of γ-oryzanol, a medicinally important antioxidant.[1] Moreover, rice bran is reported to possess health benefits for humans, including a hypolipidemic effect, the reduction of low density lipoprotein (LDL) cholesterol, an increase in the ratio of high density lipoprotein (HDL) cholesterol/LDL, growth promotion, development of lean muscles, and stimulation of the hypothalamus.[5,6] Rice bran has also been assessed as a potential source of edible oil to obtain rice bran oil (RBO).[7] It has been reported that rice bran contains 15–25% of oil, depending upon the degree of milling, the variety of rice, and other agro-climatic conditions.[8]

Rice bran is the source of rice bran oil (RBO). RBO, also known as rice oil, is used extensively in Asian countries such as Japan, Korea, China, Taiwan, Thailand, Indonesia, and Pakistan. In Japan, RBO is the preferred oil, for its subtle flavor and odor.[9] India, Japan, and China have been recognized as the most successful countries in RBO production.[10] Table 37.1 shows the production of RBO in some countries. Initially, the method used for recovering RBO from rice bran was the hydraulic pressing technique. In the fats and oils industry, RBO is obtained using solvent extraction with non-polar solvents such as hexane. With the advances in extraction techniques, some new extraction methods have been proposed for RBO production – for example, supercritical fluid extraction.[11]

Several phytochemical components present in RBO have potential significance for the diet and for health. Crude RBO is composed of 4% unsaponifiable fraction, 2–4% free fatty acids, and 88–89% neutral lipids. The unsaponifiable fraction is a complex mixture of naturally occurring antioxidant compounds such as tocotrienols, tocopherols, and γ-oryzanol, all of which demonstrate antioxidant properties.[12,13] γ-Oryzanol present in RBO has received great attention due to its high antioxidant activity, which is greater than that of tocopherols and tocotrienols;[14] therefore, RBO can be considered as a functional food oil.

Some biological activities related to RBO supplementation have been reported. RBO is capable of reducing harmful low density lipoprotein (LDL) cholesterol without reducing high density lipoprotein (HDL),[15–17] increasing antioxidant level in serum,[18] and preventing some types of cancer,[19] without causing any allergenic reactions when ingested.[20] Furthermore, RBO has a very good shelf-life compared to other cooking oils, such as palm oil and soybean oil, because of some of the antioxidant components present in it. RBO also has low viscosity, allowing less oil to be absorbed during cooking, and thus reducing overall calorie intake.[21]

RECOVERING RICE BRAN OIL

Rice bran is the source of rice bran oil; therefore, the quality of the RBO depends on the rice bran used for recovery of the oil. The quality of rice bran depends on the rice variety, treatment of the grain before milling,

TABLE 37.1 Production of Rice Bran Oil by Country*[9]

Country	Thousand Tonnes
Bangladesh	1.5
Brazil	1.5
Burma	17.6
Cambodia	4.6
China	90
India	472.7
Indonesia	0.15
Japan	65
Korea	11.7
Republic of Korea	9.2
Laos	2.6
Nepal	7.6
Pakistan	3.7
Sri Lanka	5.5
Thailand	7.8
Vietnam	7.6
Total	722.2

* *Does not include US production, which is 15.9–18.0 thousand tonnes.*

type of milling system, degree of milling, and fractionation occurring during milling.[1] The presence of contaminants in rice bran, such as broken rice and layers from the endosperm, will affect the oil content.[9]

Over the past 60 years, considerable efforts have been made to recover RBO from rice bran. Earlier methods were based on hydraulic pressing.[9] In a Japanese system for pressing, the raw bran is cleaned by sifting and air spraying to remove whole and broken grains and hulls, and, in some instances, to recover rice germ. The bran is then steam cooked, dried, pre-pressed, and pressed. For commercial purposes, RBO is obtained via extraction processes using non-polar solvent such as hexane. The process of oil extraction is shown in Figure 37.1.

Rice bran contains some active enzymes which are endogenously present or produced as a result of microbial activity activated during milling processes.[22] Such enzymes include α-amylase, β-amylase, ascorbic acid oxidase, catalase, dehydrogenase, cytochrome oxidase, esterase, deoxyribonuclease, flavin oxidase, α- and β-glycosidase, invertase, lecithinase, lipase, pectinase, lipoxygenase, peroxidase, phosphatase, phytase, proteinase, and succinate dehydrogenase. However, the most important ones affecting the destabilization of rice bran are lipase, lipoxygenase, and peroxidase.[9] Lipase will hydrolyze the oil into glycerol and free fatty acids, which give the product a rancid smell and bitter taste

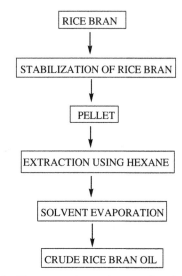

FIGURE 37.1 The process for production of crude rice bran oil.

that renders the bran unsuitable for human consumption, while lipoxygenase and peroxidase will affect the quality and shelf-life of rice bran. Therefore, rice bran needs to be stabilized in order to inactivate rice bran against those enzymes.

Rice bran can be stabilized by various methods, including dry heating, wet heating, and extrusion. Some chemical stabilizers, such as sodium meta-bisulfate, can also be used.[23] The most practical method is the extrusion or expansion method; here, excessive moisture is not added, hence eliminating the need of drying step. In the dry heating technique, simple hot air drying is applied. This can reduce the moisture content to approximately 3–4%. Wet heating (sometimes along with pH adjustment) is more effective than dry heating for rice bran stabilization. Steam cookers, autoclaves, blanchers, and screw extruders with injected steam and water can be used during wet heating.[9,24] Other methods used for rice bran stabilization include microwave heating,[25,26] stabilization using ohmic heating,[27] and dielectric heating.[28]

Hexane is a non-polar solvent with a boiling point of 68°C, and is therefore the solvent of choice for oil extraction from rice bran to yield rice bran oil (RBO). Hexane is directly blended with previously stabilized rice bran at 20°C at a solvent to bran ratio of 2:1 (wt/wt). Furthermore, hexane can be removed from the miscella (extracted oil and solvent mixture) by vacuum rotary evaporator to yield crude rice bran oil. However, hexane has some limitations, such as its high cost, easy flammability, and contribution to health and environmental hazards. Therefore, some short-chain alcohols such as ethanol and isopropyl alcohol have been proposed as alternatives for RBO extraction due to their safety and lower cost compared with hexane.[29] Short-chain alcoholic solvents can extract more non-glyceride materials than hexane, due to their greater polarity.[30] Ethanol has been preferred for the extraction of RBO rich in tocopherols, tocotrienols, and B vitamins, while isopropyl alcohol has been used for the extraction of rice bran oil rich in B vitamins alone.[31] Recently, some other extraction methods have been proposed for recovering RBO, such as supercritical fluid extraction (SFE). SFE can extract RBO more efficiently than conventional solvent extraction; however, the drawbacks of this technology include the high cost of equipment for extraction, and the involvement of solvents at their critical point. One of the solvents used is carbon dioxide in its critical state.[32–35]

Some researchers have used an enzymatic reaction prior to solvent extraction in order to recover more oil. The yields of RBO obtained were high when rice bran was treated with cellulase and pectinase enzymes and subsequently extracted with n-hexane. However, the application of enzymatic treatment alone did not result in high yields.[36,37] Hanmoungjai *et al.*[38] used Alcalase for extraction of RBO, giving a yield of 79%. RBO has also been extracted using enzyme-assisted aqueous extraction under optimized conditions using mixtures of protease (368 U), α-amylase (80 U), and cellulose (380 U), which gave a yield of 77%.[39]

To ensure its stability and fitness for human consumption, crude RBO must be refined. The color of crude RBO is dark greenish brown to light yellow, depending on the condition of the bran, the extraction method, and the composition of the bran. Pigments include carotene, chlorophyll, and Maillard browning products. The purpose of the refining process is to remove undesirable matter that interferes with the physical, chemical, and sensory characteristics of RBO. The refining process of crude RBO improves the quality of RBO, is economical, and yields by-products, such as γ-oryzanol, inositol, and phytosterols, which are of pharmaceutical and nutritional interest.[40,41] The important steps of RBO refining involve dewaxing, degumming, neutralization of free fatty acids, bleaching to improve color, and steam deodorization. Refined RBO is a light yellow color with a mild background odor and flavor reminiscent of rice.[9] Figure 37.2 illustrates the refining process,[41] which can be carried out either physically or chemically. Some stages in the refining processes of RBO can cause significant losses of or changes in the composition of valuable minor components such as γ-oryzanol and tocopherols.[42,43]

PHYSICOCHEMICAL PROPERTIES OF RICE BRAN OIL

Regarding the growing demand for and scientific awareness of the nutritional and functional properties of oils, including rice bran oil (RBO), the assessment of quality and details of the composition of RBO is of great

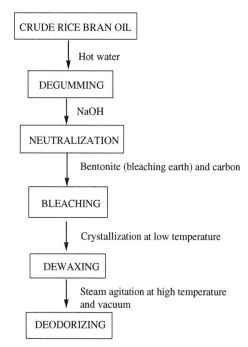

FIGURE 37.2 The steps in rice bran oil (RBO) refining.

interest for some researchers.[3,44–46] Edible oils, including RBO, are characterized by their major and minor components. Crude RBO is composed of 4% unsaponifiable matter, such as tocopherols and tocotrienols; 2–4% free fatty acids (FFAs) at the time of milling; and 88–89% triacylglycerols (neutral lipids). An FFA level of less than 5% is desirable when producing RBO, because a high level of FFAs requires a higher degree of refining. The unsaponifiable fraction is a complex mixture of naturally occurring antioxidant compounds, such as tocopherol, tocotrienols and oryzanol.[10] Furthermore, RBO is very stable at high temperatures and has a smoke point of 254°C; this is relatively high because of the high content of saturated fatty acid and waxes, making RBO suitable for cooking and frying. Table 37.2 shows the composition of crude RBO obtained by hexane extraction of stabilized bran.

Table 37.3 gives a typical specification for finished/refined RBO. This is similar to those for palm oil and peanut oil. RBO has a characteristic nutty and earthy flavor. The fatty acid composition of RBO is most similar to that of peanut or groundnut oil. Palmitic, oleic, and linoleic acids are the main fatty acids in RBO (>90%).[9,47] Palmitic–linolenic–oleic, palmitic–linoleic–linoleic, oleic–linoleic–palmitic, linolenic–linoleic–palmitic, and trioleic are the major triglycerides in RBO. RBO also contains 2.5–3.2% of unsaponifiable matter such as tocopherols (vitamin E), γ-oryzanol, and phytosterols. These are reported to have some beneficial effects for human health.

The components of RBO that are promising as nutraceutical and pharmaceutical compounds are tocopherols

TABLE 37.2   The Composition of Crude Rice Bran Oil[9]

Lipid Type		Percent
Saponifiable lipids		90–96
	Neutral lipids	88–89
	Triacylglycerols	83–86
	Diacylglycerols	3–4
	Monoacylglycerols	6–7
	Free fatty acids	2–4
	Waxes	6–7
	Glycolipids	6–7
	Phospholipids	4–5
Unsaponifiable lipids		4–2
	Phytosterols	43
	Sterol esters	10
	Triterpene alcohols	28
	Hydrocarbons	18
	Tocopherols	1

TABLE 37.3   Product Specification of Refined Rice Bran Oil[9]

Characteristic	Value
Iodine value (Wijs method, g/100g sample)	99–108
Peroxide value (meq/kg)	1.0 max
Moisture (%)	0.05 max
Color (5.25 – in Lovibond red)	5.0 max
Free fatty acid (% as oleic)	0.05 max
Flavor/odor	7 min.
Chlorophyll (ppb)	75 max.
Saponification value	180–190
Unsaponifiable matter	3–5
Smoke point	213°C
Refractive index	1470–1473
Specific gravity	0.916
AOM[a] (h)	17.5
Acid value	1.2
Iodine value	100
Saponification value	211.8
Unsaponifiable matter	4.2
Fatty acid composition	Percent
C14:0	0.6
C16:0	21.5
C18:0	2.9
C18:1	38.4
C18:2	34.4
C18:3	2.2
C20:0	–
C22:0	–

[a] *Oxidative stability as determined by the active oxygen method.*

and γ-oryzanol.[6,48,49] Chemically, γ-oryzanol found in RBO is a mixture of steryl and other triterpenyl esters of ferulic acids (cycloartenyl ferulate, 24-methylene cycloartenyl ferulate, and β-sitosterol ferulate and campesteryl ferulate) (Figure 37.3). Important rice bran ferulates are cycloartenyl ferulate, 24-methylene cyclo-artanyl ferulate, and campesteryl ferulate.[49] Various authors have reported on the level of γ-oryzanol in refined RBO. Pestana *et al.*[44] reported that the concentration of γ-oryzanol in refined RBO is 29mg/100g sample, while Rogers *et al.*[50] reported that γ-oryzanol was present in refined RBO in the range of 10–80mg per 100g oil. The difference could be due to the dissimilar processing conditions.

Refined RBO also contains tocopherols (Ts) and tocotrienols (T3s), namely α-, β-, γ- and δ-T and α-, β-, γ- and δ-T3. The chemical structures of tocopherols and tocotrienols are shown in Figure 37.4. Crude RBO contains 19–46mg of α-T/100g oil, 1–3mg of β-T/100g oil, 1–10mg of γ-T/100g oil, and 0.4–0.9mg of δ-T/100g oil; and 14–33mg of α-T3/100g oil, and 9–69mg of γ-T3 (Table 37.3). The mean content of total tocols (T and T3) was 93mg/100g for crude RBO and 50mg/100g for refined RBO.[9] Rice bran stabilization, storage, and the method of extraction affect the concentration of tocols in RBO.[51,52] Due to the high content of Ts and T3s, RBO showed better stability than the palm olein in deep frying of French fries, making RBO ideal for frying and cooking processes.[53,54]

During the refining process the composition of some components of RBO, such as fatty acids, γ-oryzanol and

tocopherols, can change. Pestana *et al.*[44] reported that α-T concentration increased slightly in the course of refining, particularly during the processes of degumming, neutralization, and bleaching. It can be deduced that α-T was stable throughout the entire refining process, even during deodorizing, where the temperature is 230°C, while levels of other tocopherols decreased slightly during refining. However, the total T contents were slightly increased during refining because of the increase in α-T. In addition, the fatty acid composition of RBO did not change during refining. Hoed *et al.*[43] also reported that, during the refining process of RBO, the concentration of α-T was increased while the level γ-T was slightly decreased. The authors also stated that there

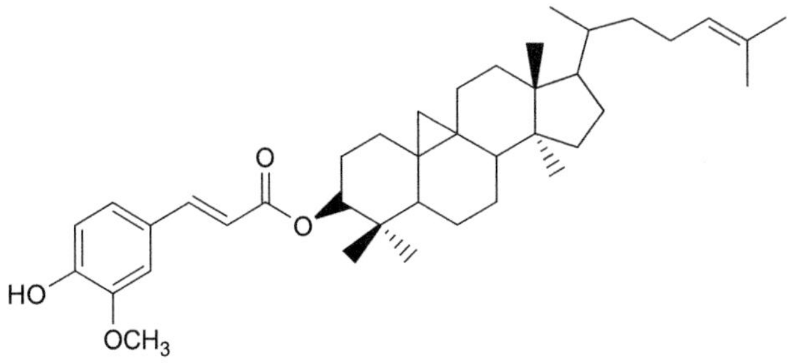

FIGURE 37.3 Some ferulates in oryzanol.

Cycloartenyl ferulate

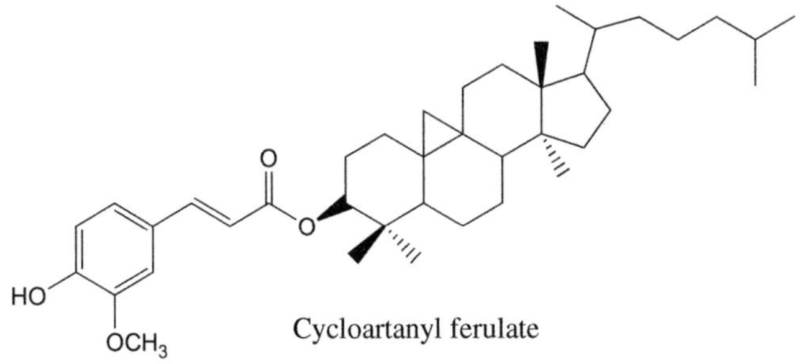

Cycloartanyl ferulate

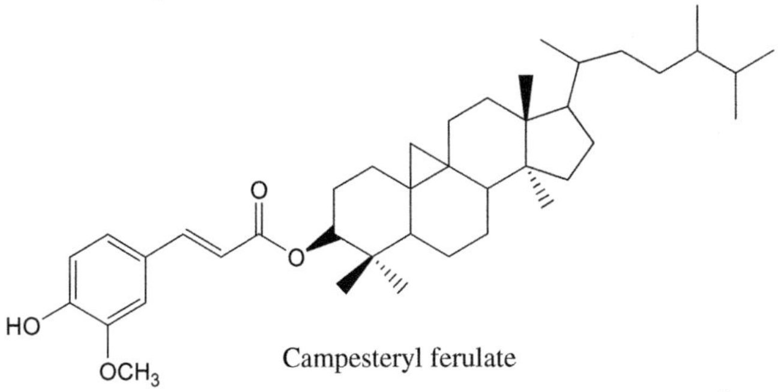

Campesteryl ferulate

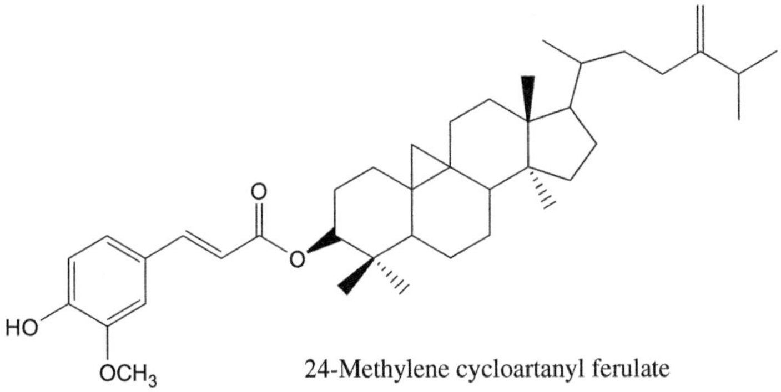

24-Methylene cycloartanyl ferulate

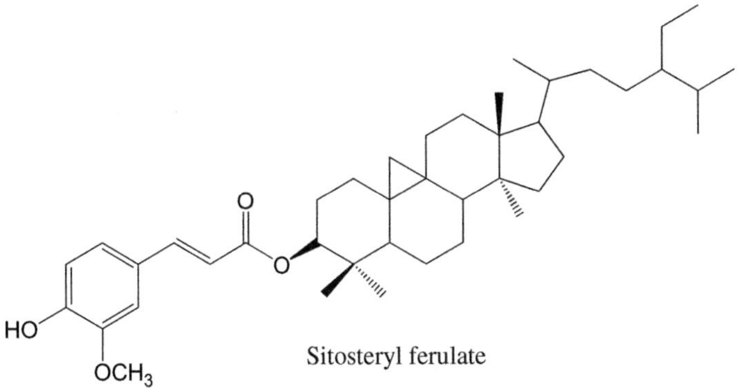

Sitosteryl ferulate

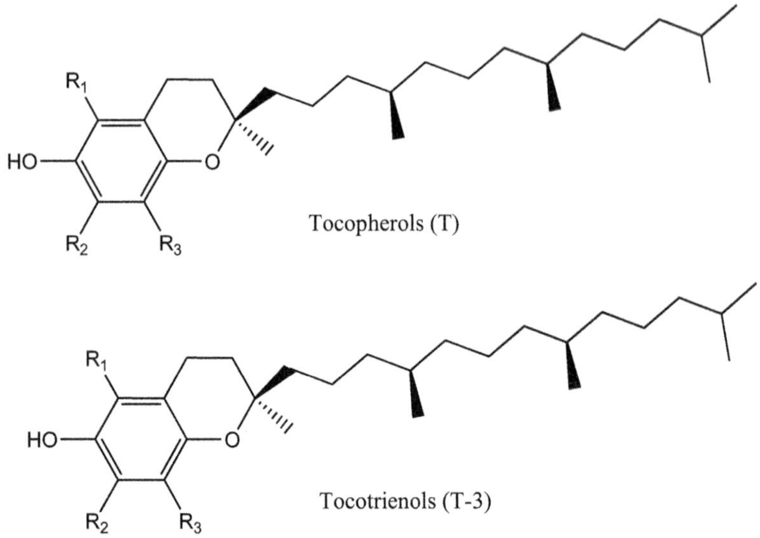

FIGURE 37.4 The chemical structures of tocopherols (T) and tocotrienols (T3).

Tocopherols (T)

Tocotrienols (T-3)

	R₁	R₂	R₃
α-T (T-3)	CH₃	CH₃	CH₃
β-T (T-3)	CH₃	H	CH₃
γ-T (T-3)	H	CH₃	CH₃
δ-T (T-3)	H	H	CH₃

was almost no change in the tocopherol concentration during deodorization at 238°C for 90 minutes.

Almost all of the γ-oryzanol components decreased in similar proportions during the several steps of refining. The concentrations of the main γ-oryzanol components did not decrease significantly during degumming; however, the neutralization process produced substantial losses of all the γ-oryzanol components.[44] Significant reductions in γ-oryzanol concentrations were produced during bleaching. A significant further reduction of the total γ-oryzanol concentration was produced during deodorizing, but not during dewaxing. The concentration of γ-oryzanol in refined RBO is just 2% of its initial value in crude RBO.[44,55] The loss of γ-oryzanol components during neutralization was also reported by Krishna and colleagues.[56] They explained that γ-oryzanol components are probably more soluble in an alkaline medium, or may react and precipitate during neutralization; as a consequence, the polar free ferulic acid is dragged along with the sediment. γ-Oryzanol components were also degraded during deep frying.[57,58]

NUTRITIONAL ASPECTS OF RICE BRAN OIL

Rice bran oil (RBO) is an ideal oil for cooking and frying, due to its high levels of tocopherols and tocotrienols, which offer good stability comparable to peanut oil, olive oil, and cottonseed oil. RBO is also preferred over other vegetable oils for its flavor. Potato chips fried with RBO showed flavor and odor stability at elevated temperatures. In some cases, RBO is blended with frying oils such as soybean oil and palm oil in order to reduce the increase in total polar materials.[9,10]

RBO has some unique properties which render it suitable for use in the food and pharmaceutical industries. One such feature is the presence of significant levels of minor elements that are beneficial to human health, such as tocopherols, tocotrienols, oryzanol, and phytosterols. RBO is reported to possess some biological activity, such as antioxidant and cholesterol-lowering effects. Due to its antioxidant action, RBO is attracting great interest in the research world as a functional food oil.

Antioxidant Activity

The antioxidants at cellular and molecular levels are capable of deactivating free radicals.[59] The phenolic compounds can scavenge free radicals by donating their hydrogen form.[60,61] The minor components of RBO, namely γ-oryzanol, phytosterols, and other phytosterol conjugates, are considered to have antioxidant properties against free radicals. Due to its phenolic property, the ferulic acid ester of γ-oryzanol is known to be a potent radical scavenger.[62,63] Studies have shown that one test-tube of γ-oryzanol is four times as effective as an equivalent amount of tocopherols in inhibiting cellular oxidation. When the four tocopherols (α-, β-, γ-, and δ-tocopherol) were compared, γ-oryzanol components exhibited higher antioxidant capacities. All these factors can be used to develop RBO as a functional food oil that is known to have antioxidant properties.[64,65]

Hypocholesterolemic Effect of Rice Bran Oil

The unsaponifiable matter and saturated fatty acids present in RBO are correlated with a hypocholesterolemic effect.[66] The significance of the unsaponifiable matter is supported by various studies, both non-clinical or clinical. It has been shown that the capacity of RBO to lower serum total cholesterol (TC) and low density lipoprotein cholesterol (LDL-C) is greater than predicted, based on its fatty acid composition.[67]

Suzuki et al.[68] observed that daily consumption of 60 g of a combination of 70% RBO and 30% safflower oil in healthy young women could lower plasma TC levels more effectively than the respective oils alone, or their combination in other proportions, even within 7 days. Moreover, Tsuji and her colleagues observed that the blended oil exerted a hypocholesterolemic effect on seven young female volunteers, even when five eggs were daily consumed for 7 consecutive days, associated with a significant increase of plasma HDL-C level.[69]

Raghuram et al.[70] reported, in humans, that those fed with RBO for a longer period showed a significant hypocholesterolemic effect compared to other studied oils. Nicolosi et al.[67] also reported that RBO has unique hypocholesterolemic effects in non-human primates, which are not attributed to the fatty acids present in RBO. Ausman et al.[71] compared the activity of RBO, canola, and coconut oils in reducing cholesterol plasma. Both plasma total cholesterol (TC) and low-density lipoprotein cholesterol (LDL-C) were significantly reduced with RBO but not with canola. RBO also showed a significant 15–17% reduction in cholesterol absorption with no effect on excretion of bile acid. The authors stated that these results suggest that the lipid lowering found in RBO is correlated with decreased cholesterol absorption, but not with hepatic cholesterol synthesis.

Since the 1950s, phytosterol components such as β-sitosterol and sitostanol have been reported to be cholesterol-lowering agents. Most studies undertaken have therefore focused on the action of phytosterols in reducing LDL-C and circulating cholesterol levels. These results indicate that these agents may be hypolipidemic agents in mild hypercholesterolemia by altering the lipid metabolism.[72,73,74]

Gamma-oryzanol was reported to possess similar hypocholesterolemic effects. Low and high consumption of (γ-oryzanol-containing) rice bran oil for 4 weeks reduced plasma total cholesterol (TC) to 6.3%, low density lipoprotein-cholesterol (LDL-C) to 10.5%, and the LDL-C/high density lipoprotein cholesterol (HDL-C) ratio to 18.9%.[75] Moreover, some unsaponifiable matter

contained in RBO was shown to significantly reduce liver cholesterol levels.[76] RBO blended with safflower oil at a definite proportion (7:3, wt/wt) magnified the hypocholesterolemic efficacy, compared with the effect of each oil alone.[77] Similar results were also reported regarding the hypocholesterolemic effect of γ-oryzanol. When hyperlipidemic subjects were administered 300 mg/day of γ-oryzanol for 3 months, a significant decrease in plasma TC and LDL-C was observed in both hypercholesterolemic and hypertriglyceridemic patients, while a relevant increase in HDL-C was caused only in the hypercholesterolemic group. In none of the above-mentioned studies were any side effects reported.[78,79] Seetharamaiah and Chandrasekhara[80] studied the effect of RBO on cholesterol level. The serum total, free, esterified and (LDL + VLDL)-cholesterol levels maintained on a 10% refined RBO diet were significantly lower than in those on a 10% groundnut oil diet; HDL-cholesterol showed a tendency to be higher. Addition of oryzanol, at a level of 0.5%, to the diet containing RBO revealed a further significant decrease in serum TC.[80]

Tocopherols and tocotrienols (α-, β-, γ-, and δ-) contained in RBO and other edible oils have been studied extensively as hypocholesterolemics in both human[81,82] and non-human[83,84] experiments. Ts and T3s administered intravenously are capable of inhibiting HMGCoA-R, an important enzyme involved in the endogenous synthesis of cholesterol, mainly through two post-transcriptional actions: increasing the controlled degradation of protein reductase, and decreasing the efficiency of the translation of HMGCoA-R messenger RNA.[85,86] In addition, α-T appears to induce HMGCoA-R activity.[87] However, not all clinical trials confirm the antihypercholesterolemic effects of T3 in humans, and some researchers suggest caution regarding this claim.[88,89]

Coronary Heart Disease

It is well recognized that the death rate due to coronary heart disease (CDC) is lower in Mediterranean countries than in Northern Europe and North America. Conclusions from these studies acclaimed the Mediterranean diet, which is very rich in complex carbohydrates, mono- and polyunsaturated fatty acids, fiber, and antioxidants (which can be present in certain oils, like RBO); and poor in cholesterol, and saturated and oxidized fatty acids.[90] An epidemiological study on distinct populations showed that there is a linear relationship between plasma lipid levels and CDC; this appears to hold true even if the elevated plasma cholesterol is only borderline.[91]

For the evaluation of CHD, the levels of individual circulating cholesterols have greater influence than total cholesterol. LDL is directly related to the development of CHD, while HDL has an inverse relationship with

CHD.[92,93] In human diets, supplementation with soluble sitostanol significantly reduced total circulating cholesterol and LDL levels by 7.5% and 10%, respectively.[94] Blending of 45% RBO with palm oil led to an increased antioxidant status and hence and improved CDC index.[95]

Non-Nutritional Uses of Rice Bran Oil

Some publications have reported the use of RBO in areas not associated with nutrition. Non-food uses of RBO include feed formulations, soaps, and glycerin. Waxes may be used as a carnauba wax replacement in confectionery, cosmetics, and polishing compound products. The use of RBO as a specialty ingredient in the cosmetic/personal care market, where the demand is for natural, value-added healthy ingredients, is growing.[9]

The presence of γ-oryzanol in RBO can function as a protective agent against UV light-induced lipid peroxidation, and as a consequence can be used as a potent sunscreen agent. The ferulic acid and its esters present in γ-oryzanol stimulate hair growth and prevent skin aging.[96,97]

RBO also contains approximately 500 ppm of tocotrienols. When applied to the skin, T3 penetrates and is absorbed rapidly. T3 accumulates in the skin and acts as the first defense layer with antioxidant properties. As a consequence, T3 stabilizes the free radicals generated in the skin when exposed to oxidative rays. T3 will thus protect against skin damage induced by ultraviolet rays.[98]

CONCLUSION

Rice bran is an under-used co-product of rice milling. The value is partially captured through extraction and refining of the rice bran oil (RBO). RBO contains microcomponents such as γ-oryzanols, phytosterols, tocopherols, tocotrienols, and dietary fibers like β-glucan, pectin, and gum. It has been reported to have several beneficial health effects, as an antioxidant, as an anticholesterolemic, and in reducing coronary heart disease. Moreover, RBO can be used in the cosmetics and pharmaceutical industries. Due to its stability, RBO is ideal for frying and cooking processes. Furthermore, RBO has good taste and performance which is ideal for salad, cooking, and frying applications.

References

1. Saunders RM. Rice bran composition and potential food uses. *Food Rev Int* 1986;**8**:415–98.
2. Hernandez N, Rodriguez-Alegría ME, Gonzalez F, Lopez-Munguia A. Enzymatic treatment of rice bran to improve processing. *J Am Oil Chem Soc* 2000;**77**:177–80.
3. Anwar F, Anwer T, Mahmood Z. Methodical characterization of rice (*Oryza sativa*) bran oil from Pakistan. *Grasas y Aceites* 2005;**56**(2):125–34.
4. Moldenhauer KA, Champagne ET, McCaskill DR, Guraya H. Functional products from rice. In: Mazza G, editor. *Functional Foods*. Lancaster, PA: Technomic Publishing Co., Inc; 2003. p. 71–89.
5. Seetharamiah GS, Chandrasekhra N. Studies on hypocholesterolemic activity of rice bran oil. *Atherosclerosis* 1989;**78**:219–23.
6. Rukmini C, Raghuram TC. Nutrional and biochemical aspects of the hypolipidemic action of rice bran oil: A review. *J Am Coll Nutr* 1991;**10**:593–601.
7. Rukmani C. Nutritional significane of rice bran oil. *Indian J Med Res* 1995;**102**:241–4.
8. Prasad RPN. Refining of rice bran oil. *Lipid Technol* 2006;**18**(12):275–9.
9. Orthoefer FT. Rice Bran Oil in Bailey's Industrial Oil and Fat Products. In: Shahidi F, editor. 6th ed. New York, NY. USA: John Wiley & Sons, Inc; 2005.
10. Nagendra Prasad MN, Sanjay KR, Shravya Khatokar M, Vismaya MN, Nanjunda Swamy S. Health Benefits of Rice Bran – A Review. *J Nutr Food Sci* 2011;**1**:108.
11. Dunford NT, Teel JA, King JW. A Continuous counter-current supercritical fluid deacidification process for phytosterol ester fortification in rice bran oil. *Food Res Int* 2003;**36**:175–9.
12. Sugano M, Suji ET. Rice bran oil and human health. *Biomed Environ Sci* 1996;**9**:242–6.
13. Westrate JA, Meiger GW. Plant sterol-enriched margarines and reduction of plasma total and LDL-cholesterol concentration in normocholestrolaemic and mildly hypercholesterolaemic subjects. *Eur J Clin Nutr* 1998;**52**:334–43.
14. De BK, Bhattacharyya DK. Physical refining of rice bran oil in relation to degumming and dewaxing. *J Am Oil Chem Soc* 1998;**75**:1683–6.
15. Nicolosi RJ, Austam LM, Hegsted DW. Rice bran oil lowers serum total and low density lipoprotein cholesterol and apo-B levels in nonhuman primates. *Atherosclerosis* 1991;**88**:133–9.
16. Sharma RD, Rukmini C. Rice bran oil and hypocholesterolemia in rats. *Lipids* 1986;**21**:715–20.
17. Wilson TA, Nicolosi RJ, Woolfrey B, Kritchevsky D. Rice bran oil and oryzanol reduce plasma lipid and lipoprotein cholesterol concentrations and aortic cholesterol ester accumulation to a greater extent than ferulic acid in hypercholesterolemic hamsters. *J Nutr Biochem* 2007;**18**:105–12.
18. Xu ZM, Hua N, Gobder JS. Antioxidant activity of tocopherols, tocotrienols, and c-oryzanol components from rice bran against cholesterol oxidation accelerated by 2-2'-azo-bis(2-methylpropionamidine) dihydrochloride. *J Agric Food Chem* 2001;**49**:2077–81.
19. Gosh M. Review on Recent Trends in Rice Bran Oil Processing. *J Am Oil Chem Soc* 2007;**84**:315–24.
20. Crevel RWR, Kerkhoff MAT, Konong MMG. Allergenicity of refined vegetable oils. *Food Chem Toxicol* 2000;**38**:385–7.
21. Chakrabarty MM. Rice bran: a new source for edible and industrial oil. In: Erickson David R, editor. *Proceedings of world conference on edible fats and oils processing*. Champaign: AOCS Press; 1989. p. 331–40.
22. Orthoefer FT, Eastman J. Chapter 19: Rice bran and oil. In: Champagne ET, editor. *Rice: Chemistry and Technology*. St Paul, MN: American Association of Cereal Chemists; 2004.
23. Yoon SH, Kim SK. Oxidative stability of high fatty acid rice bran oil at different stages of refining. *J Am Oil Chem Soc* 1994;**75**:227–9.
24. Hammond NA. *Method for stabilizing rice bran and rice bran products*. US Patent Number; 1994. 5292537 A.
25. Tao J, Rao R, Liuzzo J. Microwave heating for rice bran stabilization. *J Microwave Power and Electromagnetic Energy* 1993;**28**(3):156–64.
26. Ramezanzadeh FM, Rao RM, Prinyawiwatkul W, Marshall WE, Windhauser M. Effects of microwave heat, packaging, and storage temperature on fatty acid and proximate compositions in rice bran. *J Agric Food Chem* 2000;**48**(2):464–7.
27. Lakkakula RN, Lima M, Walker T. Rice bran stabilization and rice bran oil extraction using ohmic heating. *Bioresource Technol* 2004;**92**:157–61.

28. Sreenarayanan VV, Chattopadhyay PK. Rice bran stabilization by dielectric heating. *J Food Proc Preservation* 1986;**10**(2):89–98.

29. Meinke WW, Holland BR, Harris WD. Solvent extraction of rice bran, production of B-vitamin concentrate and oil by isopropanol extraction. *J Am Oil Chem Soc* 1949;**26**:532–4.

30. Lusas EW, Watkins LR, Koseoglu S. Isopropyl alcohol to be tested as solvent. *INFORM* 1991;**2**:970–6.

31. Seetharamaiah GS, Prabhakar JV. Oryzanol content of Indian rice bran oil & its extraction from soap stock. *J Food Sci Technol* 1986;**23**:270–3.

32. Kim H, Lee S, Park K, Hong I. Characterization of extraction and separation of rice bran oil rich in EFA using SFE process. *Separation and Purification Technol* 1999;**15**:1–8.

33. Ramsay ME, Hsu JT, Novak RA, Reightler WJ. Processing rice bran by supercritical fluid extraction. *Food Technol* 1991;**45**:98–104.

34. Kuk MS, Dowd MK. Supercritical CO2 extraction of rice bran. *J Am Oil Chem Soc* 1998;**75**:623–8.

35. Zhao W, Shishikura A, Fujimoto K, Ara K, Saito S. Fractional extraction of rice bran oil with supercritical CO_2. *Jpn Agric Biol Chem* 1987;**51**:1773–7.

36. Sengupta R, Bhattacharyya DK. Enzymatic Extraction of Mustard Seed and Rice Bran. *J Am Oil Chem Soc* 1996;**73**:687–92.

37. Hernandez N, Rodriguez-Alegria ME, Gonzalez F, Lopez-Munguia A. Enzymatic Treatment of Rice Bran to Improve Processing. *J Am Oil Chem Soc* 2000;**77**:177–80.

38. Hanmoungjai P, Pyle DL, Niranjan K. Enzymatic process for extracting oil & protein from rice bran. *J Am Oil Chem Soc* 2001;**78**:817–21.

39. Sharma A, Khare SK, Gupta MN. Enzyme-Assisted Aqueous Extraction of Rice Bran Oil. *J Am Oil Chem Soc* 2001;**78**(9):949–51.

40. Ferrari RA, Schulte E, Esteves W, Brühl L, Mukherjee KD. Minor constituents of vegetable oils during industrial processing. *J Am Oil Chem Soc* 1996;**73**:587–92.

41. Rodrigues CEC, Onoyama MM, Meirelles AJA. Optimization of the rice bran oil deacidification process by liquid–liquid extraction. *J Food Eng* 2006;**73**:370–8.

42. Patel M, Naik SN. Gamma-oryzanol from rice bran oil – A Review. *J Sci Ind Res* 2004;**63**:569–78.

43. Van Hoed V, Depaemelaere G, Villa Ayala J, Santiwattana P, Verhé R, De, et al. Influence of chemical refining on the major & minor components of rice bran oil. *J Am Oil Chem Soc* 2006;**83**:315–21.

44. Pestana VR, Zambiazi RC, Mendonc CRB, Bruscatto MH, Lerma-García MJ, Ramis-Ramos G. Quality Changes and Tocopherols and c-Oryzanol Concentrations in Rice Bran Oil During the Refining Process. *J Am Oil Chem Soc* 2008;**85**:1013–9.

45. Misra R, Sharma HK. Effect of frying conditions on the physico-chemical properties of rice bran oil and its blended oil. *J Food Sci Technol* 2011.

46. Choudhary M, Grover K. Effect of Deep-Fat Frying on Physico-chemical Properties of Rice Bran Oil Blends. *IOSR J Nursing and Health Sci* 2013;**1**(4):1–10.

47. Rohman A, Che Man YB. The chemometrics approach applied to FTIR spectral data for the analysis of rice bran oil in extra virgin olive oil. *Chemometrics and Intelligent Laboratory Systems* 2012;**110**:129–34.

48. Desai ID, Bhagavan H, Salkeld R, de Oliveira JED. Vitamin E content of crude and refined vegetable oils in Southern Brazil. *J Food Composit Anal* 1988;**3**:231–8.

49. Narayan AV, Barhate RS, Raghavarao KSMS. Extraction and Purification of Oryzanol from Rice Bran Oil and Rice Bran Oil Soapstock. *J Am Oil Chem Soc* 2006;**83**(8) 663–630.

50. Rogers EJ, Rice SM, Nicolosi RJ, Carpenter DRMC, Clelland CA, Romanczyk LJ. Identification and quantitation of γ-oryzanol components and simultaneous assessment of tocols in rice bran oil. *J Am Oil Chem Soc* 1993;**70**:301–7.

51. Gimeno E, de la Torre-Carbot K, Lamuela-Raventós RM, Castellote AI, Fitó M, de la Torre R, et al. Changes in the phenolic content of low density lipoprotein after olive oil consumption in men. A randomized crossover controlled trial. *Br J Nutr* 2008;**98**(6):1243–50.

52. Bruscatto MH, Zambiazi RC, Sganzerla M, Pestana VR, Otero D, Lima R, et al. Degradation of tocopherols in rice bran oil submitted to heating at different temperatures. *J Chromatography Sci* 2009;**47**(9):762–5.

53. Fan HY, Sharifudin MS, Hasmadi M, Chew HM. Frying stability of rice bran oil and palm olein. *Int Food Res J* 2013;**20**(1):403–7.

54. Naz A, Butt MS. Oxidative stability of wheat germ and rice bran oils in frying. *Int J Food Safety* 2011;**13**:232–6.

55. Pestana-Bauer VR, Zambiazi RC, Mendonça CRB, Beneito-Cambra M, Ramis-Ramos G. γ-Oryzanol and tocopherol contents in residues of rice bran oil refining. *Food Chem* 2012;**134**:1479–83.

56. Krishna AG, Kumar HGA, Khatoon S, Prabhakar DS. Effect of cooking of rice bran on the quality of extracted oil. *J Food Lipids* 2006;**13**:341–53.

57. Khuwijittjaru P, Yuenyong T, Pongsawatmanit R, Adachi S. Degradation kinetics of gamma-oryzanol in antioxidant-stripped rice bran oil during thermal oxidation. *J Oleo Sci* 2009;**58**(10):491–7.

58. Nasirullah, Rangaswamy BL. Oxidative stability of healthful frying oil medium and uptake of inherent nutraceuticals during deep frying. *J Am Oil Chem Soc* 2005;**82**(10):753–7.

59. Higash–Okai K, Kanbara K, Amano K, Hagiwara A, Sugita C, et al. Potent antioxidative and antigenotoxic activity in aqueous extract of Japanese rice bran - association with peroxidase activity. *Phytotherapy Res* 2004;**18** b: 628–633.

60. Ijana M, Djordjevic, Slavica S, Šiler-Marinkovic, Suzana I. Dimitrijevic-Brankovic Antioxidant Activity and Total Phenolic Content in Some Cereals and Legumes. *Int J Food Properties* 2011;**14**(1):175–84.

61. Cicerale S, Conlan XA, Sinclair AJ, Keast RSJ. Chemistry and Health of Olive Oil Phenolics. *Crit Rev Food Sci Nutr* 2008;**49**(3):218–36.

62. Wang T, Hicks KB, Moreau R. Antioxidant activity of phytosterols, oryzanol & other phytosterol conjugates. *J Am Oil Chem Soc* 2002;**79**:1201–6.

63. Zhimin Xu, Godber JS, Xu Z. Antioxidant activities of major components of gamma-oryzanol from rice bran using a linolenic acid model. *J Am Oil Chem Soc* 2001;**78**:465–9.

64. Xu Z, Hua N. Godber JS Antioxidant activity of tocopherols, tocotrienols & γ-oryzanol components from rice bran against cholesterol oxidation accelerated by 2,2′-Azo-bis (2-methylpropionamidin) Dihydrochloride. *J Agric Food Chem* 2001;**49**:2077–81.

65. Nakatani N, Tachibana Y, Kikuzaki H. Establishment of a model substrate oil for antioxidant activity assessment by oil stability index method. *J Am Oil Chem Soc* 2001;**78**:19–23.

66. Nagao K, Sato M, Takenaka M, Ando M, Iwamoto M, Imaizumi K. Feeding unsaponifiable compounds from rice bran oil does not alter hepatic mRNA abundance for cholesterol metabolism-related proteins in hypercholesterolemic rats. *Biosci Biotechnol Biochem* 2001;**65**:371–7.

67. Nicolosi RJ, Ausman LM, Hegsted DM. Rice bran oil lowers serum total and low density lipoprotein cholesterol and apo B levels in nonhuman primates. *Atherosclerosis* 1991;**88**:133–42.

68. Suzuki S, Oshima S. Influence of blending of edible fats and oils on human serum cholesterol level (Part 1). *Jpn J Nutr* 1970;**28**:3–9.

69. Tsuji E, Itoh H, Itakura H. Comparison of effects of dietary saturated and polyunsaturated fats on the serum lipids levels. *Clinical Therapeutics in Cardiovascular Disease* 1989;**8**:149–51.

70. Raghuram TC, Rao UB, Rukmini C. Studies on hypolipidemic effects of dietary rice bran oil in human subjects. *Nutr Rep Int* 1989;**39**:889–95.

71. Ausman LM, Ni Rong T, Nicolosi RJ. Hypocholesterolemic effect of physically refined rice bran oil: studies of cholesterol metabolism and early atherosclerosis in hypercholesterolemic hamsters. *J Nutr Biochem* 2005;**16**:521–9.

72. Kahlon TS, Saunders RM, Sayre RN, Chow FI, Chiu MM, et al. Cholesterol-lowering effects of rice bran & rice bran oil fractions in hypercholesterolemic hamsters. *Cereal Chem* 1992;**69**:485–9.

73. Ling WH, Jones PJH. Dietary Phytosterols: A review of metabolism, benefits and side effects. *Life Sci* 1995;**57**:195–206.

74. Frank N, Andrews FM, Elliott SB, Lew J, Boston RC. Glucose dynamics in mares Effects of rice bran oil on plasma lipid concentrations, lipoprotein composition, and glucose dynamics in mares. *J Anim Sci* 2005;**83**:2509–18.

75. Berger A, Rein D, Schäfer A, Monnard I, Gremaud G, Lambelet P, et al. Similar cholesterol-lowering properties of rice bran oil, with varied γ-oryzanol, in mildly hypercholesterolemic men. *Eur J Nutr* 2005;**44**:163–73.

76. Kahlon TS, Chow FI, Chiu MM, Hudson CA, Sayre RN. Cholesterol lowering by rice bran & rice bran oil unsaponifiable matter in hamsters. *Cereal Chem* 1996;**73**:69–74.

77. Sugano M, Tsuji E. Rice bran oil and cholesterol metabolism. *J Nutr* 1997;**127**(3):521S–4S.

78. Yoshino G, Kazumi T, Amano M, Takeiwa M, Yamasaki T, Takashima S, et al. Effects of gamma-oryzanol and probucol on hyperlipidemia. *Curr Therapy Res* 1989;**45**:975–82.

79. Yoshino G, Kazumi T, Amano M, Takeiwa M, Yamasaki T, Takashima S, et al. Effects of gamma-oryzanol on hyperlipidemic subjects. *Curr Therapy Res* 1989;**45**:543–52.

80. Seetharamaiah GS, Chandrasekhara N. Studies on hypocholesterolemic activity of rice bran oil. *Atherosclerosis* 1989;**78**(2):219–23.

81. Lichtenstein AH, Ausman LM, Carrasco W, Gualtieri LJ, Jenner JL, Ordovas JM, et al. Rice bran oil consumption and plasma lipid levels in moderately hypercholesterolemic humans. *Arteriosclerosis and Thrombosis* 1994;**14**:549–56.

82. Qureshi AA, Qureshi N, Wright JK. Lowering of serum cholesterol in hypercholesterolemic humans by tocotrienols (palmvitee). *Am J Clin Nutr* 1991;**S53**:1021–6.

83. Pearce BC, Parker RA, Deason ME, Quereshi AA, Wright JJK. Hypocholesterolemic activity of synthetic and natural tocotrienols. *J Med Chem* 1992;**35**:3595–606.

84. Hood RL, Sidhu GS. Effect of guar gum and tocotrienols on cholesterol metbolism in the Japanese quail. *Nutr Res* 1992;**S12**:116–27.

85. Khor HT, Chieng DY, Ong KK. Tocotrienols inhibit liver HMGCoA reductase activity in the Guinea pig. *Nutr Res* 1995;**15**:537–44.

86. Parker RA, Pearce BC, Clarck RW, Gordon DA, Wright JJK. Tocotrienols regulate cholesterol production in mammalian cells by posttrascriptional suppression f 3-Hydroxy-3-Methyl- Glutaryl-Coenzyme A reductase. *J Biol Chem* 1993;**268**:11230–8.

87. Qureshi AA, Pearce BC, Nor RM, Gapor A, Peterson DM, Elson CE. Dietary γ-tocopherol attenuates the impact of α-tocotrienol on hepatic 3-hydroxy-3-methyl-glutaryl coenzymeA reductase activity in chickens. *J Nutr* 1996;**126**:389–94.

88. Kerckhoffs DA, Brouns F, Hornstra G, Mensink RP. Effects on the human serum lipoprotein profile of beta-glucan, soy protein and isoflavones, plant sterols and stanols, garlic and tocotrienols. *J Nutr* 2002;**132**:2494–505.

89. Mustad VA, Smith CA, Ruey PP, Edens NK, De Michele SJ. Supplementation with 3 compositionally different tocotrienol supplements does not improve cardiovascular disease risk factors in men and women with hypercholesterolemia. *Am J Clin Nutr* 2002;**76**:1237–43.

90. Cicero AFG, Derosa G. Rice bran and its main components: potential role in the management of coronary risk factors. *Curr Topics in Nutr Res* 2005;**3**(1):29–46.

91. Durrington PN, Prais H, Bathanagar D. Indications for cholesterol lowering medication, comparison of risk-assessment methods. *Lancet* 1999;**353**:278–81.

92. Sayre B, Saunders R. Rice bran & rice bran oil. *Lipid Technol* 1990:272–6.

93. Margolis S, Dobs AS. Nutritional management of plasma lipid disorders. *J Am Coll Nutr* 1989;**8**:33S–45S.

94. Vanhanen HT, Blomqvist S, Ehnholm C, Hyvönen M, Jauhiainen M, Torstila I, et al. Serum cholesterol, cholesterol precursors, and plant sterols in hypercholesterolemic subjects with different apoE phenotypes during dietary sitostanol ester treatment. *J Lipid Res* 1993;**34**:1535–44.

95. Azrina A. *The Effects of Rice Bran and Blended Race Bran Oils On Indices of Coronary Heart Disease*. Malaysia: PhD Thesis, Universiti Putra Malaysia; 2005.

96. Noboru K, Yusho T. Oryzanol Containing Cosmetics. *Jpn Patent* 1970;**70**:32078.

97. Shugo M. Anti-dandruff and anti-itching shampoo. *Jpn Patent* 1979;**79**:36306.

98. Eitenmiller RR. Vitamin E Content of fats and oils: nutritional implications. *Food Technol* 1997;**51**:78–81.

NOVEL APPROACHES TO BRAN AND WHOLE GRAINS

Amino Acid Production from Rice Straw Hydrolyzates

Christian Matano, Tobias M. Meiswinkel, Volker F. Wendisch

Bielefeld University, Faculty of Biology & CeBiTec, Bielefeld, Germany

INTRODUCTION

Rice is one of the largest food crops in the world, with around 380 million tonnes of production by the three major producing countries: China, India, and Indonesia.[1] Rice straw is the main by-product generated during the process of edible rice culture. Currently, a great amount of straw is burned *in situ*, piled or spread in the field, incorporated into the soil, or used as mulch for the subsequent crop. Some of the rice straw is gathered in the form of bales and utilized for many purposes.[2] Traditional uses of straw are for livestock bedding and fodder, craft arts (such as basket or hat manufacture), and as a construction material (as in bricks or cobs, made from a mixture of clay and straw). More recently, new uses of this agro-waste have been proposed – for example, as biomass for fuel or energy production, or feedstock for production of chemicals. The burning of straw *in situ* is very common in some of the higher-production countries (such as Thailand, China, and northern India), but it raises environmental and health concerns; although this practice, compared to the removal of straw for further use, reduces the losses of sulfur, phosphorus, and potassium from the soil, it releases air pollutants, leading to respiratory problems among the local population.[3,4] A disadvantage of the utilization of straw bales in animal feeding is straw's low digestible energy and nutrient content. Traditional usage in crafts cannot make use of all the straw produced worldwide: in China alone around 200 million tonnes of rice are produced every year, and up to half the yield is straw.[1]

The use of rice straw as renewable resource for direct energy production through combustion or liquid biofuel production via torrefaction has been recently reviewed and presented as a promising, although immature, technology for agro-waste disposal.[5,6] Another option for the valorization of this carbon-neutral renewable source is its utilization as a substrate in industrial fermentation plants for the production of biofuels or other high-value products.

Through appropriate pretreatments, lignocellulosic biomass is transformed into nutrients (mainly fermentable sugars) suitable as a substrate for microbial fermentations. Several lines of research have shown advances in ethanol production by engineered microorganisms from rice straw hydrolyzates.[7–9]

The use of microorganisms in the manufacture of food, pharmaceutical, or industrial products is already established in large-scale biotechnological processes of immense economic importance. Most of these production processes, however, currently rely on media based on starch and molasses, which are relatively expensive and have competing uses in nutrition. A desirable advance, in the perspective of environmental sustainability, would be to broaden the spectrum of substrates usable by the microorganisms, developing producing strains able to utilize or co-utilize wastes from the agro- and food industries as carbon sources. Increasingly, lignocellulosic biomass hydrolyzates are used as a feedstock for industrial fermentations. These biomass hydrolyzates consist of complex mixtures of different fermentable sugars, but also contain inhibitors and salts that affect the performance of the product-generating microorganisms.[10]

This chapter is intended to provide the reader a glimpse into the potential for utilization of underexploited agro-waste such as rice straw as a substrate for industrial biotechnological processes involving *Corynebacterium glutamicum*, one of the most important microorganisms for producing bulk amino acids and organic acids at the multi-million tonne scale.[11,12]

Amino acids are fundamental to human and animal life, as they are the building blocks of proteins and precursors of other important molecules such as neurotransmitters.

Depending on the particular mammalian species, 8–10 of the so-called essential amino acids cannot be produced by the organism and must therefore be supplied in food or feed. Improving food and feed by adding essential amino acids that are underrepresented in natural feedstuffs reduces feed costs, improves feed efficiency, enhances animal growth, and reduces excretion of excess nitrogen (e.g., in manure). At least to some extent, the addition of amino acids to animal feed compensates for environmental problems caused by excrement-related nitrogen pollution in the soil, and helps in responding to the steady increase in meat consumption in Asia and Central and South America. The practice of feeding amino acids as a means of improving the growth of livestock has been in use since the 1960s,[13] and there is a history of more than five decades of safe use of corynebacterial fermentation products.

The market volume for feed amino acids (L-lysine, DL-methionine, L-threonine, and L-tryptophan) and for food amino acids (L-glutamic, L-aspartic acid, and L-phenylalanine) has been constantly growing over the past 20 years.[12] Glutamic acid is used as flavor enhancer, in the form of monosodium glutamate (MSG), while aspartic acid and phenylalanine are starting materials for the peptide sweetener aspartame, used, for example, in "lite" sodas. Other amino acids find applications in the pharmaceuticals, cosmetics, and agriculture sectors.[12] From the perspective of biotechnology, rice agro-waste is relevant mostly for the production of bulk amino acids, as in the million-tonne scale production of L-glutamate and L-lysine. In this respect, rice agro-waste constitutes a potential carbon source for fermentation, disregarding the presence of other high-value products that may be extracted and purified from these heterogeneous matrices. Treatments necessary to decompose lignocellulosic agro-wastes should be cheap in order to compete with molasses or starch hydrolyzates.

LIGNOCELLULOSIC BIOMASS AS WASTES FROM AGRO-INDUSTRY

Lignocellulosic biomass and agricultural wastes are currently underutilized, and their proper recycling may even be an ecological problem – for example, field burning of remains such as rice straw causes increased air pollution and health problems.[14] For the large-scale biotechnological production of commodity chemicals, substrates must also be available at large-scale level; therefore, abundant agro-wastes represent viable candidates as alternate carbon sources. Lignocellulose is composed mainly of cellulose (40–50%), hemicellulose (25–30%), and lignin (10–20%).[15] Hemicellulose is a heteropolymer of various hexose (glucose, galactose, and mannose) and pentose (xylose and arabinose) sugars.

Thus, lignocellulosic hydrolyzates contain not only glucose as a major component, but also significant fractions of xylose (5–20%) and arabinose (1–5%).[16] Unfortunately, relatively few native strains of industrial microorganisms can utilize pentose sugars as fermentable substrates.[17] The lack of pentose-utilizing, industrially relevant microorganisms often hampers the implementation of successful industrial processes based on lignocellulosic biomass, although successful examples of metabolic engineering (e.g., of *Saccharomyces cerevisiae* for ethanol production from pentoses) have been described.[16,18–21] Notably, lignocellulosic hydrolyzates contain mixtures of a number of carbon sources, and fermentation processes based on them are difficult if the microorganisms employed are characterized by sequential carbon source utilization. It is an inherent advantage of *Corynebacterium glutamicum* that it simultaneously utilizes carbon sources present in blends.[22–25] Considerable efforts have been made to utilize hemicellulose for the production of organic acids like lactic acid or succinic acid, and of alcohols like ethanol.[19,26] Amino acid fermentation using hemicellulosic biomasses only came into the focus recently.[27,28] Lignocellulosic hydrolyzates often present a challenge to industrial microorganisms as they contain growth inhibitors. A wide variety of methods for pretreatment of lignocellulosic biomass has been developed, the most common are steam explosion, ammonia fiber explosion, acid hydrolysis, or alkaline hydrolysis;[29–33] these pretreatment methods are suitable for releasing monomeric sugars, but also release inhibitory substances. Inhibitors can be divided into three categories: furan derivatives such as 5-hydroxymethyl-2-furaldehyde (HMF); a wide variety of phenolics; and weak acids such as acetic, formic, or levulinic acid.[34–36] Therefore, it is highly desirable that a robust biotechnological system is used, which can at least tolerate or even preferably utilize these inhibitors; for example, *Corynebacterium glutamicum* is able to utilize acetic acid, which acts as a fermentation inhibitor to many microorganisms, as a carbon source.[37]

Rice Straw

In biotechnological applications, rice straw hydrolyzates have been studied regarding their use in ethanol production by engineered microorganisms,[7–9] and also for the production of amino acids such as L-glutamate and L-lysine.[27,28,38] Interesting for fermentation are the relatively high contents of cellulose and hemicellulose (32–47%, 19–27%) in rice straw, which have to be processed to allow access to the monomeric sugars.[39,40] In terms of hemicellulose these are mainly pentoses, among which xylose is dominant.[41] Therefore, biotechnological applications must consider the need for an organism able to utilize as much as possible of the available carbon sources.

Rice Husks

Rice husks are the outer shells of rice grains, and are separated from the grains during milling. Rice husks have been heavily researched, but with a different focus – not so much on utilization as a carbon source,[42,43] but rather as a filtering agent used in waste water treatment for removal of heavy metal ions such as Cr(VI) or Cd(II),[44–49] or for the production of activated carbon[50,51] or nano-filter and nano-pore materials.[52–55]

Wheat Bran

Wheat bran is usually created during milling for white flour production. During whole grain production, only the husks are removed and the grain and bran are processed further.[56] A great deal of research has been undertaken regarding wheat bran, the majority concentrating on dietary factors, but biotechnological usage of wheat bran has also received attention. In this respect, ethanol production with *Saccharomyces cerevisiae*,[57,58] production of various enzymes (e.g., cellulases) using mainly *Aspergillus* species[59–62] on wheat bran, and production of acids like L-lactic acid using *Lactobacilli* and *Lactococci* species on whole wheat flour, have been developed.[63]

Silage Juice

Ensiling is the process of preserving wet plant material by applying anaerobic conditions, either in storage silos or by wrapping in plastic. The green plant material is left to wither to a dry mass content of one-third, and anaerobic conditions are ensured by compression. The anaerobic conditions and the low pH, due to the conversion of most of the water-soluble carbohydrates into lactic acid by lactic acid bacteria, preserve the silage from spoiling coliform bacteria and clostridia.[64] The dominating compounds in sugar beet and corn silages are sucrose and starch, respectively, whereas grass silage does not have a major component.[65] Lactic acid itself is a valuable intermediate for the manufacture of biodegradable polymers,[66] but recovery costs from silage are very high.[67]

Other Residues

Besides the previously described lignocellulosic wastes, there are other wastes that can be used as feedstock for industrial fermentation either alone or together with the conventional substrates for fermentation. Here, only three examples are given: lactose in whey, formed during the manufacture of cheese and casein; glycerol from the biodiesel production process; and amino sugars that can be derived from shrimp-shell wastes.

Lactose

Whey streams, a major by-product of dairy industries, could be used as an abundant and renewable raw material for microbial fermentations, with lactose providing the carbon source. The lactose can constitute as much as $50\,g/L$. Whey disposal is an environmental problem, since it is highly polluting and generated in large quantities. The utilization of lactose from whey as a substrate for industrial fermentation is problematic, because most of the relevant microorganisms lack the capacity for lactose uptake and/or degradation pathways.[68] Moreover, whey is typically too dilute for the task.

Glycerol

Glycerol is a good source of carbon and energy for the growth of several microorganisms, and may be suitable for biotechnological production of a number of chemicals in fermentative processes. It arises in the biodiesel production process as a major by-product of plant-seed oil transesterification with methanol, with a stoichiometric yield of 10% (w/w) with respect to the biodiesel produced. In 2010, around 1.6 million tonnes of glycerol were produced as a necessary by-product during biodiesel production, and the trend for biodiesel production, and thus for glycerol production, is growing.[69]

Amino Sugars

Amino sugars, such as glucosamine and N-acetyl glucosamine (GlcNac), have undisputed potential because they could serve both as a carbon and as a nitrogen source for fermentation processes. GlcNac is part of the bacterial cell wall, a peptidoglycan, together with units of N-acetylmuramic acid, cross-linked with oligopeptides. GlcNac is the monomeric unit of chitin, the main component of cell walls of fungi, the radulas of mollusks, the beaks of cephalopods, and the exoskeleton of arthropods and insects. It occurs in nature together with its deacetylated form, glucosamine. The chitin fractions of arthropods contribute up to 12% of the organic nitrogen in soil.[70–72] Although chitin is the second most abundant natural polysaccharide on Earth, with a global annual turnover of 100 billion tonnes, it has yet to find a use in large quantities. The glucosamine fraction of shellfish waste could represent an example of an alternative, renewable source for industrial fermentations.[73]

CORYNEBACTERIUM GLUTAMICUM AS A WORKHORSE FOR BIOTECHNOLOGY

C. glutamicum is a rod-shaped Gram-positive soil bacterium, isolated in Japan in the 1950s for its ability to produce glutamate.[74] This finding opened the way to intensive exploitation of the organism in industrial biotechnology from the 1960s onward. The taste-enhancing power of monosodium glutamate was in fact discovered at the beginning of the 20th century by Kikunae Ikeda, and production based on bacterial fermentation of this flavor additive rapidly replaced previous production methods, which were based on vegetable protein hydrolysis or direct synthesis with acrylonitrile.[75] Currently, more than 2.6 million tonnes of L-glutamate are produced every year.[76] Another relevant product from *C. glutamicum* fermentation is L-lysine, of which more than 1.4 million tonnes is produced per year.[13]

However, glutamate and lysine are not the only products obtainable via *C. glutamicum* fermentations. Strains for the fermentative production of other L-amino acids, such as L-arginine, L-ornithine, L-threonine, L-valine, L-isoleucine, L-serine, or L-methionine, have been developed.[77,78] Moreover, *C. glutamicum* has been engineered for the production of a variety of L-amino acids and other products, such as organic acids, alcohols, and diamines.

Similarly, use of alternative carbon sources that (unlike the traditional sugars sucrose, glucose, and fructose) do not have competing applications in the food industry has become possible by metabolic engineering.[78] Interestingly, *C. glutamicum* is resistant to the various growth inhibitors, such as furans, phenols, and acids, that are formed during lignocellulose pretreatment under the chosen conditions, thereby opening up the prospect of production processes from agro-wastes.[78]

Natural Carbon Sources for *C. glutamicum*

C. glutamicum is able to use a variety of carbohydrates, alcohols, and organic acids as single or combined sources of carbon and energy for growth and production – for example, the sugars glucose, fructose, and sucrose, or the organic acids gluconate, acetate, propionate, pyruvate, and lactate.[22,79–85]

Industrial production processes using *C. glutamicum*, however, currently rely only on glucose, sucrose, and fructose, derived from starch hydrolyzates (mainly in North America) or molasses (dominating in Europe, South America, and Asian production plants).[86] In *C. glutamicum* these sugars are substrates of the phosphotransferase system (PTS), which phosphorylates its substrate by utilizing phosphoenolpyruvate[87] concomitantly to allow uptake into the cell. However, PTS-independent uptake of glucose has been discovered and characterized in *C. glutamicum*.[88–90]

A relevant aspect of *C. glutamicum* in the perspective of the use of rice hydrolyzates as (co-)substrate is that the growth of the organism is not much affected by the presence of acetate and alcohols that usually act as inhibitors for many other organisms. Some of these chemicals can already be utilized as a carbon source by the wild type, but engineering of the organism in order to achieve full exploitation of the heterogeneous variety of carbon sources present in the hydrolyzates has also been followed successfully.

Another important feature of *C. glutamicum* is its ability to co-utilize different carbon sources, when supplemented as mixtures. For example, co-utilization can be observed during monophasic growth of *C. glutamicum* on glucose with organic acids such as lactate, pyruvate, acetate, and propionate plus acetate.[22] Diauxic growth and sequential utilization of carbon sources with preferential utilization of glucose occurs only rarely – for example, with mixtures of glucose and ethanol.[79] Thus, adaptation of the *C. glutamicum* metabolism to the presence of various carbon sources is clearly different from that in other well-studied bacteria, such as *Escherichia coli* or *Bacillus subtilis*, in which catabolite repression enables consumption of the additional carbon source only when the preferred one is exhausted.[37]

Acetate

Acetate can serve as a carbon source for *C. glutamicum*.[22] The growth rate and biomass yield on acetate are lower than on glucose or acetate–glucose mixtures, indicating an increased energy metabolism. The carbon consumption rate in media with acetate–glucose mixtures resulted from the simultaneous consumption of acetate and glucose, and was comparable to carbon consumption rates with either acetate or glucose alone.[22] Only at initial concentrations higher than 180 mM was a concentration-dependent lag phase (up to 2 days at 400 mM) observed, and the growth rate decreased significantly.[22] This effect might be due to a detrimental effect of acetate functioning as an uncoupler of the transmembrane pH gradient,[91] or, as shown for *E. coli*, to the interference of acetate with methionine biosynthesis.[92]

Cellobiose

Although present in cellulosic hydrolyzates, the disaccharide cellobiose is not fermented by most of the industrial microorganisms.[93] A *C. glutamicum* R mutant gained the ability to consume D-cellobiose, due to mutations in a phosphotransferase permease subunit (*bglF* gene), specific for the transport of the β-glucosides arbutin and salicin.[94] For utilization of cellobiose, the phospho-β-glucosidase gene (*bglA*) is also necessary. Both these genes are present in *C. glutamicum* R., but are absent from other strains. Under oxygen-deprived conditions, the simultaneous utilization of cellobiose, glucose, and xylose for the production of lactic and succinic acid could be demonstrated.[93]

Aromatics

It is known that lignin-derived phenolic compounds (vanillin, ferulic acid, benzoate, 4-hydroxybenzoate, vanillate, and phenol) are the main growth inhibitors in lignocellulosic hydrolyzates for microbial fermentation.[95,96] Surprisingly, at least for acid production under oxygen deprivation conditions, *C. glutamicum* is not affected by these substances, displaying a high tolerance to several phenolic inhibitors.[97] In addition, it has an impressive ability to utilize aromatic compounds, making it particularly interesting in the perspective of a bioprocess based on agro-wastes hydrolyzates, such as rice straw.

C. glutamicum wild type can grow on benzoate, phenol,[98] 3-hydrobenzoate, gentisate,[99] protocatechuate, vanillate, 4-hydroxybenzoate, 4-cresol,[100,101] resorcinol,[102] benzyl alcohol, 2,4-dihydroxybenzoate, 3,5-dihydroxytoluene,[101] naphthalene,[103] vanillin, and ferulic acid.[84] The robust ability of *C. glutamicum* to grow with these aromatic compounds partially relies on its multiple transporters for their uptake. Although aromatic compounds can enter the cells by passive diffusion when present at high concentrations, active transport increases the efficiency and rate of substrate acquisition in natural environments where these compounds are present at low concentrations.[101] The peripheral pathways leading to aromatic-ring cleavage in *C. glutamicum* have recently been reviewed, and will not be described here.[104]

Engineering of *C. glutamicum* for Access to Alternative Carbon Sources

C. glutamicum has been engineered for efficient utilization of substances serving as poor growth substrates – for example, rapid growth with intermediates of the tricarboxylic acid cycle, including malate, fumarate, and succinate, was achieved.[105,106] Moreover, *C. glutamicum* strain development was focused on the utilization of carbon sources inaccessible to the wild-type strain, with particular attention paid to those available from the agro- and fisheries industries.

One of the main objectives of industrial biotechnology is to offer the possibility to complement and, in the long term, replace the petro-based economy. Therefore, research on metabolic engineering of *C. glutamicum* is increasingly oriented towards access to alternative carbon sources that are economically viable and do not find competing applications in nutrition. Examples of this trend are illustrated in this section, such as engineering access to arabinose, xylose, and cellobiose present in lignocellulosic hydrolyzates from agro-industrial wastes,[27,28,107] glycerol from the biodiesel industry, and the chitin component glucosamine.[69,108,109]

Arabinose

The aldopentose monosaccharide arabinose is one of the most abundant sugars in lignocellulosic hydrolyzates derived from agricultural or forestry production.

In bacteria, arabinose typically enters the pentose phosphate pathway as xylulose-5-phosphate, following a three-step enzymatic conversion process: in the first step, arabinose isomerase (AraA) converts arabinose to ribulose; second, ribulokinase (AraB) phosphorylates ribulose to ribulose-5-phosphate; and finally this is converted to xylulose-5-phosphate by ribulose-5-phosphate 4-epimerase (AraD).[110] *C. glutamicum* ATCC 31831 was able to utilize low concentrations of arabinose upon expression of the arabinose transporter gene *araE*.[111] Arabinose has been used as a carbon source for the production of organic acids,[111] as well as for the production of the amino acids L-glutamate, L-lysine, L-ornithine, and L-arginine,[107] and the diamine putrescine.[112]

Xylose

Like arabinose, the aldopentose xylose is also present in lignocellulosic hydrolyzates and is typically utilized in bacteria via the pentose phosphate pathway after isomerization to xylulose and phosporylation to xylulose-5-phosphate. The genome of *C. glutamicum* does not encode xylose isomerase XylA, but possesses a xylulokinase gene (*xylB*) encoding the enzyme responsible for phosphorylation of xylulose. Heterologous expression of *xylA* from *E. coli* was sufficient to enable growth with xylose as the sole carbon source. Additional expression of *E. coli xylB* increased the growth rate of the recombinant *C. glutamicum* strain.[26] In order to achieve simultaneous utilization of mixed sugars, *C. glutamicum* ATCC 31831 has been equipped with the transporter gene *araE* in addition to the xylose utilization genes, resulting in fast consumption of xylose.[111] To prove its biotechnological usability, anaerobic production of succinic and lactic acid,[26] as well as aerobic production of cadaverine[113] and of the amino acids L-glutamate and L-lysine, from xylose was demonstrated.[27,28]

Lactose

C. glutamicum wild type is unable to metabolize lactose or galactose. Engineering of the organism has been attempted in order to achieve production of lysine in dairy-based substrates, such as whey. Heterologous expression of the *lac* genes from *E. coli* allows growth on lactose.[114] Nevertheless, only the glucose liberated by decomposition of lactose is utilized in this way.

Combined heterologous expression of the lactose permease and β-galactosidase genes from *Lactobacillus delbrueckii*, and the aldose-1-epimerase, galactokinase, UDP-glucose-1-P-uridylyltransferase, and UDP-galactose-4-epimerase from *Lactococcus lactis* subsp. *cremoris* MG1363, allowed the use of both the glucose and galactose components of lactose. Whey-based L-lysine production was possible, although growth in the whey-based medium was slower as compared to that with glucose.[115]

Glycerol

Glycerol occurs as a waste product in the biodiesel industry. In the transesterfication reactions of plant oils and fats with methanol or ethanol, fatty acids react to fatty acid methyl/ethyl esters (FAME, FAEE) whereas the glycerol backbone of the lipids accumulates as the major by-product, with a stoichiometric share of 10% (w/w). As 16 million tonnes of biodiesel were produced in 2009,[116] waste glycerol of 1.6 million tonnes accumulated. In the biorefinery concept, glycerol and additional side-streams of the biodiesel process, such as residues from plants used as source of oil or fat (e.g., residues from rape seeds) are to be valorized. To enable glycerol utilization in *C. glutamicum*, plasmid borne expression of *E. coli* genes encoding for glycerol kinase and glycerol-3-phosphate dehydrogenase was shown to be sufficient.[108] To further increase growth performance, the *E. coli* glycerol facilitator gene was expressed in addition.[108] When carrying this plasmid, *C. glutamicum* was able to efficiently utilize glycerol as the sole source of carbon. Moreover, this strain co-utilized glycerol with glucose. Recombinants carrying this plasmid were also used for succinate production.[117] The functions of homologues encoded in the *C. glutamicum* genome (cg3198 and cg1853) have not been reported;[108] however, their ectopic overexpression was shown to support growth of *C. glutamicum* with glycerol as the sole carbon source.[118]

Glucosamine

Recently, the PTS[Glc] transport system, whose major substrate is glucose, has been identified as also being responsible for glucosamine uptake in *C. glutamicum*.[119] Overproduction of the endogenous glucosamine-6-phosphate deaminase NagB entailed fast growth on glucosamine. Various recombinant strains overexpressing endogenous *nagB* were shown to utilize glucosamine as a substrate for production of the amino acid L-lysine and of the diamine putrescine.[109]

Typical Products from C. glutamicum

Glutamate

As mentioned above, *C. glutamicum* was isolated from nature in 1956, and revolutionized monosodium glutamate (MSG) production. The accumulation of glutamate in the supernatant occurred under particular conditions, such as biotin limitation[120] or after addition of certain detergents.[121] The initial explanation for glutamate overproduction was the leak model, which focuses on fatty acid synthesis and membrane alteration: under biotin limitation the cell membrane permeability for glutamate is enhanced, due to decreased fatty acid and phospholipid contents.[86] Later evidences disagreed with this model: it was shown that glutamate secretion is not a passive process and the membrane permeability is not changed, since other amino acids, as well as acetate and ions such as H[+], K[+], and Cl[−], do not leak from the cell during glutamate overproduction.

Furthermore, it was confirmed that membrane fluidity does not change under biotin-limited conditions.[122] Export of L-glutamate by a carrier has been described,[123] and attributed to a homologue of the mechanosensitive channel of small conductance (mscCG) of *E. coli* in the glutamate secretion.[124] NCgl1221 is a mechanosensitive channel gated by membrane tension, and functions not only for glutamate secretion but also as an osmotic safety valve.[125–127]

L-glutamate production involves metabolic changes,[86] and may occur via glutamate dehydrogenase or the GS-GOGAT system.[128] Precursor supply requires anaplerosis by PEP carboxylase and/or pyruvate carboxylase.[129–131] Flux of 2-oxoglutarate to L-glutamate is switched at the level of the 2-oxoglutarate dehydrogenase (ODHC) activity. In its unphosphorylated form, the small soluble protein OdhI binds to and inhibits ODHC, thus funneling 2-oxoglutarate flux towards L-glutamate and resulting in L-glutamate excretion. ODHC is not inhibited and is fully active when OdhI is phosphorylated by one of the serine protein kinases PknG, PknA, PknB, and PknL.[132–135] Consequently, engineering strategies resulting in unphosphorylated OdhI improved L-glutamate production.

Lysine

Large-scale production of L-lysine with *C. glutamicum* started as early as 1958 at Kyowa Hakko's plant in Japan. Other companies joined the business, and since then the biotechnological manufacturing of L-lysine has undergone continuous improvement by strain improvement and process engineering.[136] In short, the flux through the split lysine biosynthesis pathway[137] was increased by overexpression of the gene for the key enzyme aspartokinase, *lysC*, or by introduction of *lysC* alleles coding for versions of aspartokinase that are not feedback-inhibited by lysine.[138,139] Introducing *hom* mutations that cause a restricted homoserine dehydrogenase flux[140] reduced the formation of by-products. The carbon precursor supply for lysine biosynthesis was improved in *C. glutamicum*, which possesses the two anaplerotic C3-carboxylating enzymes PEP carboxylase[141] and pyruvate carboxylase,[129,142] as well as the C4-decarboxylating enzymes PEP carboxykinase[143] and malic enzyme,[144] and oxaloacetate decarboxylase.[145] Overexpression of the pyruvate carboxylase gene, as well as deletion of the PEP carboxykinase gene, improved lysine production.[130,131,146] Regeneration of the co-factor NADPH occurs primarily in the pentose phosphate pathway,[147–149] and flux into the pentose phosphate pathway was increased by deletion of the phosphoglucoisomerase gene *pgi*, precluding utilization of glucose-6-phosphate in glycolysis,[150] or by expression of mutant alleles of the glucose-6-phosphate dehydrogenase gene *zwf* or of the 6-phosphogluconate dehydrogenase gene *gnd*.[150–152] Increased pentose phosphate pathway flux and L-lysine production was achieved on sucrose[153] and, in some strains, on fructose[154] by overexpression of *fbp*, which encodes fructose-1,6-bisphosphatase.[155]

Engineering of *C. glutamicum* for New Products

Development of genetic engineering tools in recent decades, sequencing of the genome of the organism, and the rapid evolution of "*-omics*" technologies have allowed tremendous expansion of the spectrum of products obtainable from *C. glutamicum*.[78]

Great advances have been made in the understanding of its key regulatory features for access to new products via metabolic engineering. Nowadays, *C. glutamicum* can be considered as a versatile platform for the production of several other chemicals.[156] This section summarizes the wide range of products that can be obtained from the organism.

Diamines

Due to their reactivity, basicity, and surface activity, polyamines have found a wide variety of commercial applications, mainly as intermediates in the synthesis of functional products (e.g., polyamides/epoxy curing, fungicides, anthelmintic/pharmaceuticals, petroleum production, oil and fuel additives, paper resins, chelating agents, fabric softeners/surfactants, bleach activators, and asphalt chemicals).[157] Diamines can be synthesized by bacteria and used as monomers for the production of polyamides. Thus, the main commercial interest in biogenic polyamines is their use in the polymer industry.[158] Nylon-4,6 is an example of an industrial polyamide containing a biogenic diamine that can also be synthesized by bacteria. This polyamide is produced from putrescine and adipic acid (hexanedioic acid), and is now on the market – for example, as Stanyl™ (DSM, The Netherlands). The total market for plastics has grown over the past six decades, at an average of 9% per year, and the polyamide fraction has also grown, at 4.5% per year in recent years, reaching a production volume of 2.4 million tonnes per year in 2007.[159] The market share of specialty polyamides is about 2% of this market. At present, the production of monomers for use in the polyamide industry is mainly based on chemical routes, with few exceptions, such as 1,10-decamethylenediamine, which is isolated from castor oil and used for the production of PA-10,10 (e.g., Vestamid® TerraDS; Evonik Degussa, Germany). More recently, a drive towards a low-carbon footprint of materials and applications and towards the development of sustainable processes is expected

to further biotechnological polyamine production. In bacteria, the pathways of polyamine biosynthesis start with the amino acids L-lysine, L-ornithine, L-arginine, or L-aspartic acid. Since a million-tonne scale industry for the fermentative production of amino acid is thriving and strains overproducing L-lysine, L-ornithine, and L-arginine are available, it is reasonable to engineer these amino acid-producing corynebacteria for polyamine production.[158]

PUTRESCINE (1,4-DIAMINOBUTANE)

C. glutamicum can be engineered for the overproduction of putrescine, via the arginine- or ornithine decarboxylase pathways. The latter pathway is preferable, as it comprises one rather than two or three reactions in the arginine decarboxylase pathway.[158] Putrescine production by *C. glutamicum* was optimized to the highest yield published to date by fine-tuning OTC activity and by expressing the ornithine decarboxylase gene *speC* from *E. coli* from an anabolism-based *argF* addiction plasmid, ensuring stable putrescine production by the engineered *C. glutamicum* strain.[160] In a recent study, putrescine production has also been achieved using glucosamine as the sole carbon source or as co-substrate together with glucose in a production strain harboring an overexpression plasmid for the glucosamine-6-phosphate deaminase gene. Product formation with glucosamine was comparable to that with glucose with respect to concentrations, yields, and rates.[109]

CADAVERINE (1,5-DIAMINOPENTANE)

Like putrescine, cadaverine is a biogenic diamine which can be used as precursor of polyamides.[78] L-lysine producing *C. glutamicum* strains can easily be engineered to produce cadaverine, as only a single enzymatic reaction has to be added; namely, lysine decarboxylase.[113] Later, cadaverine production with enzymatic hydrolyzates of hemicellulose particles from oat spelts[113] and starch-based cadaverine production[161] were developed.

Organic Acids

In the past few years the research interest in the production of organic acids by *C. glutamicum* fermentations has grown constantly. The organism has been engineered to produce a wide range of such molecules, finding application in many fields, including the food, cosmetics, and pharmaceuticals industries. Studies have been published regarding the production of pyruvic, lactic, 2-oxoglutaric, 2-ketoisovaleric, and pantothenic acids. Due to its importance, the engineering of *C. glutamicum* for the production of succinic acid will be presented as example.

SUCCINIC ACID

Succinic acid is a bulk chemical with a global production of 16,000–30,000 tonnes, and an annual growth of

10%.[162] It can be used as a de-icer, in the food and beverage industry, or as a building block for various commodity chemicals as well as biodegradable polymers such as polybutylene succinate and polybutylene succinate adipate.[163] It is currently mainly produced from fossil fuels by a chemical process, but biological processes for succinic acid production may become more economically competitive with increases in fossil fuel prices. Succinic acid occurs in living organisms as an intermediate of the tricarboxylic acid cycle, and may be excreted as an end product during anaerobic fermentation by some anaerobic and facultative anaerobic organisms.[164,165] In *C. glutamicum*, deletion of the lactate dehydrogenase gene (*ldhA*) and overexpression of the anaplerotic pyruvate carboxylase gene (*pyc*) led to production of 146 g/L succinic acid, with productivity of 3.2 g/L per hour under anaerobic conditions.[163] Redox-balanced anaerobic succinate production from glucose and formate was achieved by heterologous expression of a formate dehydrogenase gene.[166] Under aerobic conditions, combined overexpression of phosphoenolpyruvate carboxylase (*ppc*) and pyruvate carboxylase (*pyc*) genes to impel anaplerosis and deletion of acetic acid-forming genes and of succinic acid-oxidizing genes (*sdhCAB*) resulted in a strain producing 10.6 g/L succinic acid in a growth-independent manner. Subsequent overexpression of *E. coli* glycerol utilization genes *glpFKD* allowed this strain to produce almost the same amount of succinic acid from glycerol.[78]

Alcohols

ETHANOL

Ethanol production was achieved in *C. glutamicum* by heterologous expression of the *Zymomonas mobilis* pyruvate decarboxylase gene (*pdc*) and overexpression of an alcohol dehydrogenase gene (*adhB*). The former enzyme catalyzes decarboxylation of pyruvic acid to acetaldehyde, which is eventually reduced by the latter enzyme to ethanol. With these modifications, lactic and succinic acid were produced as by-products. In order to avoid this problem, the lactate dehydrogenase (*ldh*) and phosphoenolpyruvate carboxylase (*ppc*) genes were disrupted. The resulting strain produced about 10 g/L ethanol under oxygen-deprivation conditions.[167]

ISOBUTANOL

Higher alcohols are gaining interest as biofuels due to a higher energy density and lower corrosivity and hygroscopicity compared to ethanol. Moreover, they are compatible with existing infrastructure. Isobutanol is a higher alcohol that can be produced in two steps from 2-ketoisovalerate, the immediate precursor of L-valine. Since *C. glutamicum* has been successfully engineered for production of L-valine[168,169] and 2-ketoisovalerate,[170] it appeared to be a suitable organism for isobutanol production. A 2-ketoisovalerate-producing strain has been engineered with heterologous expression of a 2-ketoacid decarboxylase gene (*kivd*) from *Lactococcus lactis* and overexpression of the native alcohol dehydrogenase gene (*adhA*), in order to convert 2-KIV to isobutanol. The pyruvate carboxylase *pyc* and lactate dehydrogenase *ldh* genes were deleted to channeling more carbon through the isobutanol pathway. The resultant strain produced 4.9 g/L isobutanol in 120 hours.[171] Blombach *et al.* achieved more than two-fold higher titers of butanol after re-engineering their 2-ketoisovalerate-producing strain, with deletions of *ldh* and a number of other genes to further increase pyruvic acid, 2-ketoisovalerate, and co-factor availability: *aceE* and *pqo* deletions served the first purpose, *ilvE* deletion the second, and *mdh* deletion the third. Upon additional expression of the *E. coli pntAB* operon encoding transhydrogenase, 13 g/L isobutanol could be attained under oxygen deprivation conditions.[172]

PROPANDIOL

1,2-Propanediol is used in the food, cosmetics, and pharmaceuticals industries, and has a worldwide market of more than half a million tonnes per year. It can be produced by *C. glutamicum* upon heterologous expression of *E. coli* methylglyoxal synthase gene (*mgs*) and overexpression of a putative aldo-keto reductase gene (cgR_2242). The former enzyme catalyzes the conversion of the glycolytic intermediate dihydroxyacetone phosphate (DHAP) to methylglyoxal, which is reduced to 1,2-propanediol by the latter enzyme. The resulting strain has a production capability of 1.8 g/L in 90 hours via fed-batch fermentation.[173]

CAROTENOIDS

C. glutamicum contains the glycosylated C50 carotenoid decaprenoxanthin as yellow pigment, which is synthesized starting from isopentenyl pyrophosphate.[174,175] *C. glutamicum* possesses a certain degree of redundancy in carotenoid biosynthesis, as two functional phytoene synthases exist.[176] Recently, its potential for carotenoid overproduction could be demonstrated, as metabolic engineering of only the terminal reactions leading to lycopene resulted in considerable lycopene production.[176]

OUTLOOK

Broadening of the substrate spectrum for industrial microbial fermentations, and here in particular for *C. glutamicum* fermentations, is an ongoing trend, and it will not concentrate only on biomass-derived monomeric sugars. Rather, research also needs to be directed towards the utilization of polymers of differing complexity, such as starch, glucan, or chitin. The initial successes of amino acid production based on rice straw hydrolyzates and similar depolymerized biomass substrates have been obtained largely at the laboratory scale. Thus, future biotechnological research needs to address transfer to the technical scale, and process intensification and integration.

References

1. FAO. *FAO Rice Market Monitor, November*; 2012. Volume XV, Issue No. 4 Available at: www.fao.org/docrep/017/ap772e/ap772e.pdf. [accessed 18.02.13].

2. Dobbermann BA, Fairhust TH. Rice Straw Management. *Better Crops Int* 2002;**16**:7–11.

3. Lemieux PM, Lutes CC, Santoianni DA. Emissions of organic air toxics from open burning: a comprehensive review. *Prog Energ Combust* 2004;**30**(1):1–32.

4. Zheng YG, Chen XL, Wang Z. Microbial biomass production from rice straw hydrolysate in airlift bioreactors. *J Biotechnol* 2005;**118**(4):413–20.

5. Matsumura Y, Minowa T, Yamamoto H. Amount, availability, and potential use of rice straw (agricultural residue) biomass as an energy resource in Japan. *Biomass Bioenerg* 2005;**29**(5):347–54.

6. Nigam PS, Singh A. Production of liquid biofuels from renewable resources. *Prog Energ Combust* 2011;**37**(1):52–68.

7. Chen WH, Lin TS, Guo GL, Huang WS. Ethanol production from rice straw hydrolysates by *Pichia stipitis*. *Enrgy Proced* 2012;**14**:1261–6.

8. Lin TH, Huang CF, Guo GL, Hwang WS, Huang SL. Pilot-scale ethanol production from rice straw hydrolysates using xylose-fermenting *Pichia stipitis*. *Bioresource Technol* 2012;**116**:314–9.

9. Sakamoto T, Hasunuma T, Hori Y, Yamada R, Kondo A. Direct ethanol production from hemicellulosic materials of rice straw by use of an engineered yeast strain codisplaying three types of hemicellulolytic enzymes on the surface of xylose-utilizing *Saccharomyces cerevisiae* cells. *J Biotechnol* 2012;**158**(4):203–10.

10. Rumbold K, van Buijsen HJ, Gray VM, et al. Microbial renewable feedstock utilization: a substrate-oriented approach. *Bioengineered bugs* 2010;**1**(5):359–66.

11. Wendisch VF, editor. *Amino Acid Biosynthesis – Pathways, Regulation and Metabolic Engineering*. Heidelberg, Germany: Springer; 2007.

12. Leuchtenberger W, Huthmacher K, Drauz K. Biotechnological production of amino acids and derivatives: current status and prospects. *Appl Microbiol Biotechnol* 2005;**69**(1):1–8.

13. Ajinomoto. *Feed-Use Amino Acids Business*. Available at: www.ajinomoto.com/ir/pdf/Feed-useAA-Oct2011.pdf; 2011 [accessed 20.04.12].

14. Mussatto SI, Roberto IC. Optimal experimental condition for hemicellulosic hydrolyzate treatment with activated charcoal for xylitol production. *Biotechnol Prog* 2004;**20**(1):134–9.

15. Wyman CE. Production of low cost sugars from biomass: progress, opportunities, and challenges. In: Overend RP, Chornet E, editors. *Biomass: a growth opportunity in green energy and value added products*. Oxford, UK: Pergamon Press; 1999. p. 867–72.

16. Aristidou A, Penttila M. Metabolic engineering applications to renewable resource utilization. *Curr Opin Biotechnol* 2000;**11**(2):187–98.

17. Jeffries TW, Jin YS. Ethanol and thermotolerance in the bioconversion of xylose by yeasts. *Adv Appl Microbiol* 2000;**47**:221–68.

18. Becker J, Boles E. A modified *Saccharomyces cerevisiae* strain that consumes L-arabinose and produces ethanol. *Appl Environ Microbiol* 2003;**69**(7):4144–50.

19. Hahn-Hagerdal B, Karhumaa K, Fonseca C, Spencer-Martins I, Gorwa-Grauslund MF. Towards industrial pentose-fermenting yeast strains. *Appl Microbiol Biotechnol* 2007;**74**(5):937–53.

20. Hahn-Hagerdal B, Karhumaa K, Jeppsson M, Gorwa-Grauslund MF. Metabolic engineering for pentose utilization in *Saccharomyces cerevisiae*. *Adv Biochem Eng Biotechnol* 2007;**108**:147–77.

21. Karhumaa K, Wiedemann B, Hahn-Hagerdal B, Boles E, Gorwa-Grauslund MF. Co-utilization of L-arabinose and D-xylose by laboratory and industrial *Saccharomyces cerevisiae* strains. *Microb Cell Fact* 2006;**5**:18.

22. Wendisch VF, de Graaf AA, Sahm H, Eikmanns BJ. Quantitative determination of metabolic fluxes during coutilization of two carbon sources: comparative analyses with *Corynebacterium glutamicum* during growth on acetate and/or glucose. *J Bacteriol* 2000;**182**(11):3088–96.

23. Wendisch VF. Genetic regulation of *Corynebacterium glutamicum* metabolism. *J Microbiol Biotechnol* 2006;**16**(7):999.

24. Netzer R, Krause M, Rittmann D, et al. Roles of pyruvate kinase and malic enzyme in *Corynebacterium glutamicum* for growth on carbon sources requiring gluconeogenesis. *Arch Microbiol* 2004;**182**(5):354–63.

25. Blombach B, Seibold GM. Carbohydrate metabolism in *Corynebacterium glutamicum* and applications for the metabolic engineering of L-lysine production strains. *Appl Microbiol Biotechnol* 2010;**86**(5):1313–22.

26. Kawaguchi H, Vertes AA, Okino S, Inui M, Yukawa H. Engineering of a xylose metabolic pathway in *Corynebacterium glutamicum*. *Appl Environ Microbiol* 2006;**72**(5):3418–28.

27. Gopinath V, Meiswinkel TM, Wendisch VF, Nampoothiri KM. Amino acid production from rice straw and wheat bran hydrolysates by recombinant pentose-utilizing *Corynebacterium glutamicum*. *Appl Microbiol Biotechnol* 2011;**92**(5):985–96.

28. Meiswinkel TM, Gopinath V, Lindner SN, Nampoothiri KM, Wendisch VF. Accelerated pentose utilization by *Corynebacterium glutamicum* for accelerated production of lysine, glutamate, ornithine and putrescine. *Microbial biotechnology* 2012.

29. Esteghlalian A, Hashimoto AG, Fenske JJ, Penner MH. Modeling and optimization of the dilute-sulfuric-acid pretreatment of corn stover, poplar and switchgrass. *Bioresource Technol* 1997;**59**(2-3):129–36.

30. Fan LT, Gharpuray MM, Lee YH. *Cellulose hydrolysis*. Berlin, New York: Springer-Verlag; 1987.

31. McMillan JD. Pretreatment of lignocellulosic biomass. In: Himmel ME, Baker JO, Overend RP, editors. *Enzymatic conversion of biomass for fuels production*. Washington, DC: American Chemical Society; 1994. p. 292–324.

32. Meshartree M, Dale BE, Craig WK. Comparison of Steam and Ammonia Pretreatment for Enzymatic-Hydrolysis of Cellulose. *Appl Microbiol Biotechnol* 1988;**29**(5):462–8.

33. Sun Y, Cheng JY. Hydrolysis of lignocellulosic materials for ethanol production: a review. *Bioresource Technol* 2002;**83**(1):1–11.

34. Almeida JRM, Modig T, Petersson A, Hahn-Hagerdal B, Liden G, Gorwa-Grauslund MF. Increased tolerance and conversion of inhibitors in lignocellulosic hydrolysates by *Saccharomyces cerevisiae*. *J Chem Technol Biot* 2007;**82**(4):340–9.

35. Dunlop AP. Furfural formation and behavior. *Ind Eng Chem* 1948;**40**(2):204–9.

36. Palmqvist E, Hahn-Hagerdal B. Fermentation of lignocellulosic hydrolysates. II: inhibitors and mechanisms of inhibition. *Bioresource Technol* 2000;**74**(1):25–33.

37. Gerstmeir R, Wendisch VF, Schnicke S, et al. Acetate metabolism and its regulation in Corynebacterium glutamicum. *J Biotechnol* 2003;**104**(1-3):99–122.

38. Gopinath V, Murali A, Dhar KS, Nampoothiri KM. *Corynebacterium glutamicum* as a potent biocatalyst for the bioconversion of pentose sugars to value-added products. *Appl Microbiol Biotechnol* 2012;**93**(1):95–106.

39. Saha BC. Hemicellulose bioconversion. *J Ind Microbiol Biotechnol* 2003;**30**(5):279–91.

40. Zamora R, Sanchez Crispin JA. Production of an acid extract of rice straw. *Acta Cient Venez* 1995;**46**(2):135–9.

41. Roberto IC, Mussatto SI, Rodrigues RCLB. Dilute-acid hydrolysis for optimization of xylose recovery from rice straw in a semi-pilot reactor. *Ind Crop Prod* 2003;**17**(3):171–6.

42. Gullon P, Moura P, Esteves MP, Girio FM, Dominguez H, Parajo JC. Assessment on the fermentability of xylooligosaccharides from rice husks by probiotic bacteria. *J Agric Food Chem* 2008;**56**(16):7482–7.

43. Sankh SN, Deshpande PS, Arvindekar AU. Improvement of Ethanol Production Using *Saccharomyces cerevisiae* by Enhancement of Biomass and Nutrient Supplementation. *Appl Biochem Biotech* 2011;**164**(8):1237–45.

44. Ajmal M, Rao RAK, Anwar S, Ahmad J, Ahmad R. Adsorption studies on rice husk: removal and recovery of Cd(II) from wastewater. *Bioresource Technol* 2003;**86**(2):147–9.

45. Kumar U, Bandyopadhyay M. Fixed bed column study for Cd(II) removal from wastewater using treated rice husk. *J Hazardous Materials* 2006;**129**(1-3):253–9.

46. Kumar U, Bandyopadhyay M. Sorption of cadmium from aqueous solution using pretreated rice husk. *Bioresource Technol* 2006;**97**(1):104–9.

47. Sobhanardakani S, Parvizimosaed H, Olyaie E. Heavy metals removal from wastewaters using organic solid waste-rice husk. *Environ Sci Pollut Res Int* 2013.

48. Thakur AK, Gupta AK. Water absorption characteristics of paddy, brown rice and husk during soaking. *J Food Eng* 2006;**75**(2):252–7.

49. Zulkali MMD, Ahmad AL, Norulakmal NH. *Oryza sativa* L. husk as heavy metal adsorbent: Optimization with lead as model solution. *Bioresource Technol* 2006;**97**(1):21–5.

50. Chen Y, Zhu Y, Wang Z, et al. Application studies of activated carbon derived from rice husks produced by chemical-thermal process – a review. *Adv Colloid Interface Sci* 2011;**163**(1):39–52.

51. Kalderis D, Bethanis S, Paraskeva P, Diamadopoulos E. Production of activated carbon from bagasse and rice husk by a single-stage chemical activation method at low retention times. *Bioresour Technol* 2008;**99**(15):6809–16.

52. Bansal V, Ahmad A, Sastry M. Fungus-mediated biotransformation of amorphous silica in rice husk to nanocrystalline silica. *J Am Chem Soc* 2006;**128**(43):14059–66.

53. Hwang MJ, Lee SY, Han CS. A study on electric conductivity of phosphoric acid supported on nano-pore rice husk silica in H2/Pt/H3PO4 / RHS/Pt/O2 fuel cells. *J Nanosci Nanotechnol* 2006;**6**(11):3491–3.

54. Kim HJ, So SJ, Han CS. A study on modification of nanoporous rice husk silica for hydrophobic nano filter. *J Nanosci Nanotechnol* 2010;**10**(5):3705–8.

55. Lee SY, Han CS. Nano filter from sintered rice husk silica membrane. *J Nanosci Nanotechnol* 2006;**6**(11):3384–7.

56. Hemery Y, Rouau X, Lullien-Pellerin V, Barron C, Abecassis J. Dry processes to develop wheat fractions and products with enhanced nutritional quality. *J Cereal Sci* 2007;**46**(3):327–47.

57. Favaro L, Basaglia M, Casella S. Processing wheat bran into ethanol using mild treatments and highly fermentative yeasts. *Biomass Bioenerg* 2012;**46**:605–17.

58. Gomathi D, Muthulakshmi C, Kumar DG, Ravikumar G, Kalaiselvi M, Uma C. Production of Bio-Ethanol from Pretreated Agricultural Byproduct Using Enzymatic Hydrolysis and Simultaneous Saccharification. *Microbiology* 2012;**81**(2):201–7.

59. Kang SW, Park YS, Lee JS, Hong SI, Kim SW. Production of cellulases and hemicellulases by Aspergillus niger KK2 from lignocellulosic biomass. *Bioresource Technol* 2004;**91**(2):153–6.

60. Kumar NSM, Ramasamy R, Manonmani HK. Production and optimization of L-asparaginase from *Cladosporium* sp. using agricultural residues in solid state fermentation. *Ind Crop Prod* 2013;**43**:150–8.

61. Mahadik ND, Puntambekar US, Bastawde KB, Khire JM, Gokhale DV. Production of acidic lipase by *Aspergillus niger* in solid state fermentation. *Proc Biochem* 2002;**38**(5):715–21.

62. Sukumaran RK, Singhania RR, Mathew GM, Pandey A. Cellulase production using biomass feed stock and its application in lignocellulose saccharification for bio-ethanol production. *Renew Energ* 2009;**34**(2):421–4.

63. Hofvendahl K, HahnHagerdal B. L-lactic acid production from whole wheat flour hydrolysate using strains of *Lactobacilli* and. *Lactococci. Enzyme and Microbial Technol* 1997;**20**(4):301–7.

64. McDonald P, Henderson AR, Heron SJ. Microorganisms. In: McDonald P, Henderson AR, Heron SJ, editors. *The Biochemistry of Silage*. Aberystwyth, UK: Chalcombe Publications; 1991. p. 81–152.

65. Neuner A, Wagner I, Sieker T, et al. Production of l-lysine on different silage juices using genetically engineered *Corynebacterium glutamicum*. *J Biotechnol* 2013;**163**(2):217–24.

66. Sodergard A, Stolt M. Properties of lactic acid based polymers and their correlation with composition. *Prog Polym Sci* 2002;**27**(6):1123–63.

67. Datta R, Tsai SP, Bonsignore P, Moon SH, Frank JR. Technological and economic potential of poly (lactic acid) and lactic acid derivatives. *FEMS Microbiol Rev* 1995;**16**:221–31.

68. Domingues L, Guimaraes PM, Oliveira C. Metabolic engineering of *Saccharomyces cerevisiae* for lactose/whey fermentation. *Bioengineered Bugs* 2010;**1**(3):164–71.

69. Wendisch VF, Meiswinkel TM, Lindner SN. Use of glycerol in biotechnological applications. In: Montero G, Stoytcheva M, editors. *Biodiesel – Quality, Emissions and Byproducts*. Rijeka, Croatia: InTech - Open Access Publisher; 2011. p. 305–40.

70. Appuhn A, Joergensen RG, Raubuch M, Scheller E, Wilke B. The automated determination of glucosamine, galactosamine, muramic acid, and mannosamine in soil and root hydrolysates by HPLC. *J Plant Nutr Soil Sc* 2004;**167**(1):17–21.

71. Stevenson FJ. Organic forms of soil nitrogen. In: Stevenson FJ, editor. *Nitrogen in agricultural soils Madison, Wis.* American Society of Agronomy; 1982. p. 101–4.

72. Parsons JW. Chemistry and distribution of amino sugars in soils and soils organisms. In: Paul EA, Ladd JN, editors. *Soil biochemistry*. New York, NY: Marcel Dekker; 1981. p. 197–227.

73. Tharanathan RN, Kittur FS. Chitin – the undisputed biomolecule of great potential. *Crit Rev Food Sci Nutr* 2003;**43**(1):61–87.

74. Kinoshita S, Udaka S, Shimono M. Studies on the amino acid fermentation. Production of L-glutamic acid by various microorganisms. *J Gen Appl Microbiol* 1957;**3**:193–205.

75. Lindemann B, Ogiwara Y, Ninomiya Y. The discovery of umami. *Chem Senses* 2002;**27**(9):843–4.

76. Ajinomoto. *Food Products Business*. Available at: www.ajinomoto. com/ir/pdf/Food-Oct2010.pdf; 2010 [accessed 20.04.12].

77. Kinoshita SA. Short History of the Birth of the Amino Acid Industry in Japan. In: Eggeling L, Bott M, editors. *Handbook of Corynebacterium glutamicum*. Boca Raton, FL: CRC Press; 2005. p. 1–5.

78. Zahoor A, Lindner SN, Wendisch VF. Metabolic engineering of *Corynebacterium glutamicum* aimed at alternative carbon sources and new products. *Computational and Structural Biotechnol J* 2012;**3**(4). http://dx.doi.org/10.5936/csbj.201210004.

79. Arndt A, Eikmanns BJ. The alcohol dehydrogenase gene *adhA* in *Corynebacterium glutamicum* is subject to carbon catabolite repression. *J Bacteriol* 2007;**189**(20):7408–16.

80. Chaudhry MT, Huang Y, Shen XH, Poetsch A, Jiang CY, Liu SJ. Genome-wide investigation of aromatic acid transporters in. *Corynebacterium glutamicum. Microbiology* 2007;**153**(Pt 3):857–65.

81. Claes WA, Puhler A, Kalinowski J. Identification of two *prpDBC* gene clusters in *Corynebacterium glutamicum* and their involvement in propionate degradation via the 2-methylcitrate cycle. *J Bacteriol* 2002;**184**(10):2728–39.

82. Cocaign M, Monnet C, Lindley ND. Batch kinetics of *Corynebacterium glutamicum* during growth on various carbon sources: use of substrate mixtures to localise metabolic bottlenecks. *Appl Microbiol Biotechnol* 1993;**40**:526–30.

83. Frunzke J, Bott M. Regulation of iron homeostasis in *Corynebacterium glutamicum*. In: Burkovski A, editor. *Corynebacteria – genomics and molecular biology*. Caister, UK: Caister Academic Press; 2008. p. 241–66.

84. Merkens H, Beckers G, Wirtz A, Burkovski A. Vanillate Metabolism in *Corynebacterium glutamicum*. *Curr Microbiol* 2005;**51**:59–65.

85. Netzer R, Peters-Wendisch P, Eggeling L, Sahm H. Cometabolism of a nongrowth substrate: L-serine utilization by Corynebacterium glutamicum. *Appl Environ Microbiol* 2004;**70**(12):7148–55.

86. Kimura E. L-Glutamate Production. In: Eggeling L, Bott M, editors. *Handbook of Corynebacterium glutamicum*. Boca Raton, FL: CRC Press; 2005. p. 439–64.

87. Parche S, Burkovski A, Sprenger GA, Weil B, Kramer R, Titgemeyer F. *Corynebacterium glutamicum*: a dissection of the PTS. *J Mol Microbiol Biotechnol* 2001;**3**(3):423–8.

88. Lindner SN, Seibold GM, Henrich A, Kramer R, Wendisch VF. Phosphotransferase system-independent glucose utilization in *Corynebacterium glutamicum* by inositol permeases and glucokinases. *Appl Environ Microbiol* 2011;**77**(11):3571–81.

89. Lindner SN, Seibold GM, Kramer R, Wendisch VF. Impact of a new glucose utilization pathway in amino acid-producing *Corynebacterium glutamicum*. *Bioengineered bugs* 2011;**2**(5).

90. Lindner SN, Petrov DP, Hagmann CT, et al. Phosphotransferase system- (PTS-) mediated glucose uptake is repressed in phosphoglucoisomerase-deficient *Corynebacterium glutamicum* strains. *Appl Environ Microbiol* 2013.

91. Baronofsky JJ, Schreurs WJ, Kashket ER. Uncoupling by Acetic Acid Limits Growth of and Acetogenesis by *Clostridium thermoaceticum*. *Appl Environ Microbiol* 1984;**48**(6):1134–9.

92. Roe AJ, O'Byrne C, McLaggan D, Booth IR. Inhibition of *Escherichia coli* growth by acetic acid: a problem with methionine biosynthesis and homocysteine toxicity. *Microbiology* 2002;**148**(Pt 7):2215–22.

93. Sasaki M, Jojima T, Inui M, Yukawa H. Simultaneous utilization of D-cellobiose, D-glucose, and D-xylose by recombinant *Corynebacterium glutamicum* under oxygen-deprived conditions. *Appl Microbiol Biotechnol* 2008;**81**(4):691–9.

94. Kotrba P, Inui M, Yukawa H. A single V317A or V317M substitution in Enzyme II of a newly identified beta-glucoside phosphotransferase and utilization system of *Corynebacterium glutamicum* R extends its specificity towards cellobiose. *Microbiology* 2003;**149**(Pt 6):1569–80.

95. Klinke HB, Thomsen AB, Ahring BK. Inhibition of ethanol-producing yeast and bacteria by degradation products produced during pre-treatment of biomass. *Appl Microbiol Biotechnol* 2004;**66**(1):10–26.

96. Parawira W, Tekere M. Biotechnological strategies to overcome inhibitors in lignocellulose hydrolysates for ethanol production: review. *Crit Rev Biotechnol* 2011;**31**(1):20–31.

97. Sakai S, Tsuchida Y, Nakamoto H, et al. Effect of lignocellulose-derived inhibitors on growth of and ethanol production by growth-arrested *Corynebacterium glutamicum* R. *Appl Environ Microbiol* 2007;**73**(7):2349–53.

98. Shen XH, Liu ZP, Liu SJ. Functional identification of the gene locus NCgl2319 and characterization of catechol 1,2-dioxygenase in *Corynebacterium glutamicum*. *Biotechnol Lett* 2004;**26**(7):575–80.

99. Shen XH, Jiang CY, Huang Y, Liu ZP, Liu SJ. Functional identification of novel genes involved in the glutathione-independent gentisate pathway in *Corynebacterium glutamicum*. *Appl Environ Microbiol* 2005;**71**(7):3442–52.

100. Qi SW, Chaudhry MT, Zhang Y, et al. Comparative proteomes of *Corynebacterium glutamicum* grown on aromatic compounds revealed novel proteins involved in aromatic degradation and a clear link between aromatic catabolism and gluconeogenesis via fructose-1,6-bisphosphatase. *Proteomics* 2007;**7**(20):3775–87.

101. Shen XH, Liu SJ. Key enzymes of the protocatechuate branch of the beta-ketoadipate pathway for aromatic degradation in *Corynebacterium glutamicum*. *Sci China Ser C* 2005;**48**(3):241–9.

102. Huang Y, Zhao KX, Shen XH, Chaudhry MT, Jiang CY, Liu SJ. Genetic characterization of the resorcinol catabolic pathway in *Corynebacterium glutamicum*. *Appl Environ Microbiol* 2006;**72**(11):7238–45.

103. Lee SY, Le TH, Chang ST, Park JS, Kim YH, Min J. Utilization of phenol and naphthalene affects synthesis of various amino acids in *Corynebacterium glutamicum*. *Curr Microbiol* 2010;**61**(6):596–600.

104. Shen XH, Zhou NY, Liu SJ. Degradation and assimilation of aromatic compounds by *Corynebacterium glutamicum*: another potential for applications for this bacterium? *Appl Microbiol Biotechnol* 2012;**95**(1):77–89.

105. Youn JW, Jolkver E, Kramer R, Marin K, Wendisch VF. Identification and characterization of the dicarboxylate uptake system DccT in *Corynebacterium glutamicum*. *J Bacteriol* 2008;**190**(19):6458–66.

106. Youn JW, Jolkver E, Kramer R, Marin K, Wendisch VF. Characterization of the dicarboxylate transporter DctA in *Corynebacterium glutamicum*. *J Bacteriol* 2009;**191**(17):5480–8.

107. Schneider J, Niermann K, Wendisch VF. Production of the amino acids L-glutamate, L-lysine, L-ornithine and L-arginine from arabinose by recombinant *Corynebacterium glutamicum*. *J Biotechnol* 2011;**154**(2-3):191–8.

108. Rittmann D, Lindner SN, Wendisch VF. Engineering of a glycerol utilization pathway for amino acid production by *Corynebacterium glutamicum*. *Appl Environ Microbiol* 2008;**74**(20):6216–22.

109. Uhde A, Youn JW, Maeda T, et al. Glucosamine as carbon source for amino acid-producing *Corynebacterium glutamicum*. *Appl Microbiol Biotechnol* 2013;**97**(4):1679–87.

110. Kawaguchi H, Sasaki M, Vertes AA, Inui M, Yukawa H. Engineering of an L-arabinose metabolic pathway in *Corynebacterium glutamicum*. *Appl Microbiol Biotechnol* 2008;**77**(5):1053–62.

111. Sasaki M, Jojima T, Kawaguchi H, Inui M, Yukawa H. Engineering of pentose transport in *Corynebacterium glutamicum* to improve simultaneous utilization of mixed sugars. *Appl Microbiol Biotechnol* 2009;**85**(1):105–15.

112. Meiswinkel TM, Gopinath V, Lindner SN, Nampoothiri KM, Wendisch VF. Accelerated pentose utilization by *Corynebacterium glutamicum* for accelerated production of lysine, glutamate, ornithine and putrescine. *Microbial Biotechnology* 2013;**6**(2):131–40.

113. Buschke N, Schroder H, Wittmann C. Metabolic engineering of *Corynebacterium glutamicum* for production of 1,5-diaminopentane from hemicellulose. *Biotechnol J* 2011;**6**(3):306–17.

114. Brabetz W, Liebl W, Schleifer KH. Studies on the utilization of lactose by *Corynebacterium glutamicum*, bearing the lactose operon of. *Escherichia coli. Arch Microbiol* 1991;**155**(6):607–12.

115. Barrett E, Stanton C, Zelder O, Fitzgerald G, Ross RP. Heterologous expression of lactose- and galactose-utilizing pathways from lactic acid bacteria in *Corynebacterium glutamicum* for production of lysine in whey. *Appl Environ Microbiol* 2004;**70**(5):2861–6.

116. Licht FO. *World Ethanol and Biofuels Report* 2010;**8**(13):265.

117. Litsanov B, Brocker M, Bott M. Glycerol as a substrate for aerobic succinate production in minimal medium with *Corynebacterium glutamicum*. *Microbial biotechnology* 2013;**6**(2):189–95.

118. Meiswinkel TM, Rittmann D, Lindner SN, Wendisch VF. Crude glycerol-based production of amino acids and putrescine by *Corynebacterium glutamicum*. *Biores Technol* 2013 http://dx.doi.org/10.1016/ j. biortech. 2013.02.053 (in press).

119. Postma PW, Lengeler JW, Jacobson GR. Phosphoenolpyruvate:carbohydrate phosphotransferase systems of bacteria. *Microbiol Rev* 1993;**57**(3):543–94.

120. Shiio I, Otsuka SI, Takahashi M. Effect of biotin on the bacterial formation of glutamic acid. I. Glutamate formation and cellular premeability of amino acids. *J Biochem* 1962;**51**:56–62.

121. Duperray F, Jezequel D, Ghazi A, Letellier L, Shechter E. Excretion of glutamate from *Corynebacterium glutamicum* triggered by amine surfactants. *Biochim Biophys Acta* 1992;**1103**(2):250–8.

122. Neubeck M, Prenner E, Horvat P, Bona R, Hermetter A, Moser A. Membrane Fluidity in Glutamic Acid-Producing Bacteria *Brevibacterium* sp ATCC13869. *Archives of Microbiology* 1993;**160**(2):101–7.

123. Gutmann M, Hoischen C, Kramer R. Carrier-mediated glutamate secretion by *Corynebacterium glutamicum* under biotin limitation. *Biochim Biophys Acta* 1992;**1112**(1):115–23.

124. Nakamura J, Hirano S, Ito H, Wachi M. Mutations of the *Corynebacterium glutamicum* NCgl1221 gene, encoding a mechanosensitive channel homolog, induce L-glutamic acid production. *Appl Environ Microbiol* 2007;**73**(14):4491–8.

125. Becker M, Borngen K, Nomura T, et al. Glutamate efflux mediated by *Corynebacterium glutamicum* MscCG, *Escherichia coli* MscS, and their derivatives. *Biochim Biophys Acta* 2013;**1828**(4):1230–40.

126. Hashimoto K, Murata J, Konishi T, Yabe I, Nakamatsu T, Kawasaki H. Glutamate is excreted across the cytoplasmic membrane through the NCgl1221 channel of *Corynebacterium glutamicum* by passive diffusion. *Biosci Biotechnol Biochem* 2012;**76**(7):1422–4.

127. Nakayama Y, Yoshimura K, Iida H. A gain-of-function mutation in gating of *Corynebacterium glutamicum* NCgl1221 causes constitutive glutamate secretion. *Appl Environ Microbiol* 2012;**78**(15):5432–4.

128. Kholy ER, Eikmanns BJ, Gutmann M, Sahm H. Glutamate Dehydrogenase Is Not Essential for Glutamate Formation by *Corynebacterium glutamicum*. *Appl Environ Microbiol* 1993;**59**(7):2329–31.

129. Peters-Wendisch PG, Wendisch VF, de Graaf AA, Eikmanns BJ, Sahm H. C3-carboxylation as an anaplerotic reaction in phosphoenolpyruvate carboxylase-deficient *Corynebacterium glutamicum*. *Arch Microbiol* 1996;**165**(6):387–96.

130. Peters-Wendisch PG, Kreutzer C, Kalinowski J, Patek M, Sahm H, Eikmanns BJ. Pyruvate carboxylase from *Corynebacterium glutamicum*: characterization, expression and inactivation of the *pyc* gene. *Microbiology* 1998;**144**(Pt 4):915–27.

131. Peters-Wendisch PG, Schiel B, Wendisch VF, et al. Pyruvate carboxylase is a major bottleneck for glutamate and lysine production by *Corynebacterium glutamicum*. *J Mol Microbiol Biotechnol* 2001;**3**(2):295–300.

132. Niebisch A, Kabus A, Schultz C, Weil B, Bott M. Corynebacterial protein kinase G controls 2-oxoglutarate dehydrogenase activity via the phosphorylation status of the OdhI protein. *J Biol Chem* 2006;**281**(18):12300–7.

133. Schultz C, Niebisch A, Gebel L, Bott M. Glutamate production by *Corynebacterium glutamicum*: dependence on the oxoglutarate dehydrogenase inhibitor protein OdhI and protein kinase PknG. *Appl Microbiol Biotechnol* 2007;**76**(3):691–700.

134. Bott M. Offering surprises: TCA cycle regulation in *Corynebacterium glutamicum*. *Trends Microbiol* 2007;**15**(9):417–25.

135. Schultz C, Niebisch A, Schwaiger A, et al. Genetic and biochemical analysis of the serine/threonine protein kinases PknA, PknB, PknG and PknL of *Corynebacterium glutamicum*: evidence for non-essentiality and for phosphorylation of OdhI and FtsZ by multiple kinases. *Mol Microbiol* 2009;**74**(3):724–41.

136. Kelle R, Hermann T, Bathe B. L-Lysine production. In: Eggeling L, Bott M, editors. *Handbook of Corynebacterium glutamicum*. Boca Raton, FL: CRC Press; 2005. p. 465–88.

137. Schrumpf B, Schwarzer A, Kalinowski J, Puhler A, Eggeling L, Sahm H. A functionally split pathway for lysine synthesis in *Corynebacterium glutamicum*. *J Bacteriol* 1991;**173**(14):4510–6.

138. Schrumpf B, Eggeling L, Sahm H. Isolation and prominent characteristics of an L-lysine hyperproducing strain of *Corynebacterium glutamicum*. *Appl Microbiol Biotechnol* 1992;**37**:566–71.

139. Thierbach G, Kalinowski J, Bachmann B, Pühler A. Cloning of a DNA fragment from *Corynebacterium glutamicum* conferring aminoethyl cysteine resistance and feedback resistance to aspartokinase. *Appl Microbiol Biotechnol* 1990;**32**(4):443–8.

140. Ohnishi J, Hayashi M, Mitsuhashi S, Ikeda M. Efficient 40 degrees C fermentation of L-lysine by a new *Corynebacterium glutamicum* mutant developed by genome breeding. *Appl Microbiol Biotechnol* 2003;**62**(1):69–75.

141. Eikmanns BJ, Follettie MT, Griot MU, Sinskey AJ. The phosphoenolpyruvate carboxylase gene of *Corynebacterium glutamicum*: molecular cloning, nucleotide sequence, and expression. *Mol Gen Genet* 1989;**218**(2):330–9.

142. Peters-Wendisch PG, Wendisch VF, Paul S, Eikmanns BJ, Sahm H. Pyruvate carboxylase as an anaplerotic enzyme in *Corynebacterium glutamicum*. *Microbiology* 1997;**143**:1095–103.

143. Jetten MS, Sinskey AJ. Characterization of phosphoenolpyruvate carboxykinase from *Corynebacterium glutamicum*. *FEMS Microbiol Lett* 1993;**111**:183–8.

144. Gourdon P, Baucher MF, Lindley ND, Guyonvarch A. Cloning of the malic enzyme gene from *Corynebacterium glutamicum* and role of the enzyme in lactate metabolism. *Appl Environ Microbiol* 2000;**66**(7):2981–7.

145. Klaffl S, Eikmanns BJ. Genetic and functional analysis of the soluble oxaloacetate decarboxylase from *Corynebacterium glutamicum*. *J Bacteriol* 2010;**192**(10):2604–12.

146. Riedel C, Rittmann D, Dangel P, et al. Characterization of the phosphoenolpyruvate carboxykinase gene from *Corynebacterium glutamicum* and significance of the enzyme for growth and amino acid production. *J Mol Microbiol Biotechnol* 2001;**3**(4):573–83.

147. Marx A, de Graaf AA, Wiechert W, Eggeling L, Sahm H. Determination of the fluxes in the central metabolism of *Corynebacterium glutamicum* by nuclear magnetic resonance spetroscopy combined with metabolite balancing. *Biotechnol Bioeng* 1996;**49**:111–29.

148. Marx A, Eikmanns BJ, Sahm H, de Graaf AA, Eggeling L. Response of the Central Metabolism in Corynebacterium glutamicum to the use of an NADH-Dependent Glutamate Dehydrogenase. *Metabolic Engineering* 1999;**1**(1):35–48.

149. Marx A, Striegel K, de Graaf AA, Sahm H, Eggeling L. Response of the central metabolism of *Corynebacterium glutamicum* to different flux burdens. *Biotechnol Bioeng* 1997;**56**:168–80.

150. Marx A, Hans S, Mockel B, Bathe B, de Graaf AA. Metabolic phenotype of phosphoglucose isomerase mutants of *Corynebacterium glutamicum*. *J Biotechnol* 2003;**104**(1-3):185–97.

151. Ohnishi J, Katahira R, Mitsuhashi S, Kakita S, Ikeda M. A novel gnd mutation leading to increased L-lysine production in *Corynebacterium glutamicum*. *FEMS Microbiol Lett* 2005;**242**(2):265–74.

152. Ando S, Ochiai K, Yokoi H, Hashimoto S, Yonetani Y. Novel glucose-6-phosphate dehydrogenase. *Patent WO0198472* 2002; (2002-01-02).

153. Georgi T, Rittmann D, Wendisch VF. Lysine and glutamate production by *Corynebacterium glutamicum* on glucose, fructose and sucrose: Roles of malic enzyme and fructose-1,6-bisphosphatase. *Metab Eng* 2005;**7**(4):291–301.

154. Becker J, Klopprogge C, Zelder O, Heinzle E, Wittmann C. Amplified expression of fructose 1,6-bisphosphatase in *Corynebacterium glutamicum* increases in vivo flux through the pentose phosphate pathway and lysine production on different carbon sources. *Appl Environ Microbiol* 2005;**71**(12):8587–96.

155. Rittmann D, Schaffer S, Wendisch VF, Sahm H. Fructose-1,6-bisphosphatase from *Corynebacterium glutamicum*: expression and deletion of the *fbp* gene and biochemical characterization of the enzyme. *Arch Microbiol* 2003;**180**(4):285–92.

156. Wendisch VF. Synthetic biology approaches to carbon utilization of *Corynebacterium glutamicum*. *J Biotechnol* 2010;**150** S548–S54S.

157. Kroschwitz JI, Seidel A. *Kirk-Othmer encyclopedia of chemical technology*. 5th ed. Hoboken, NJ: Wiley-Interscience; 2004.

158. Schneider J, Wendisch VF. Putrescine production by engineered *Corynebacterium glutamicum*. *Appl Microbiol Biotechnol* 2010;**88**(4):859–68.

159. Platt DK. *Rapra Technology Limited. Engineering and high performance plastics market report: a Rapra market report.* Shrewsbury, UK: Rapra Technology Ltd; 2003.

160. Schneider J, Eberhardt D, Wendisch VF. Improving putrescine production by *Corynebacterium glutamicum* by fine-tuning ornithine transcarbamoylase activity using a plasmid addiction system. *Appl Microbiol Biotechnol* 2012;**95**(1):169–78.

161. Tateno T, Okada Y, Tsuchidate T, Tanaka T, Fukuda H, Kondo A. Direct production of cadaverine from soluble starch using *Corynebacterium glutamicum* coexpressing alpha-amylase and lysine decarboxylase. *Appl Microbiol Biotechnol* 2009;**82**(1):115–21.

162. NNFCC. *NNFCC Renewable Chemicals Factsheet: Succinic Acid.* Available at: www.nnfcc.co.uk/publications/nnfcc-renewable-chemicals-factsheet-succinic-acid; 2010 [accessed 18.02.13].

163. Okino S, Noburyu R, Suda M, Jojima T, Inui M, Yukawa H. An efficient succinic acid production process in a metabolically engineered *Corynebacterium glutamicum* strain. *Appl Microbiol Biotechnol* 2008;**81**(3):459–64.

164. Glassner DA, Datta R. inventors; Process for the production and purification of succinic acid. USA; 1992.

165. Guettler MV, Jain MK, Rumler D. *inventors; Method for making succinic acid, bacterial variants for use in the process, and methods for obtaining variants.* USA; 1996.

166. Litsanov B, Brocker M, Bott M. Toward Homosuccinate Fermentation: Metabolic Engineering of *Corynebacterium glutamicum* for Anaerobic Production of Succinate from Glucose and Formate. *Appl Environ Microbiol* 2012;**78**(9):3325–37.

167. Inui M, Kawaguchi H, Murakami S, Vertes AA, Yukawa H. Metabolic Engineering of *Corynebacterium glutamicum* for Fuel Ethanol Production under Oxygen-Deprivation Conditions. *J Mol Microbiol Biotechnol* 2004;**8**(4):243–54.

168. Blombach B, Schreiner ME, Bartek T, Oldiges M, Eikmanns BJ. *Corynebacterium glutamicum* tailored for high-yield L-valine production. *Appl Microbiol Biotechnol* 2008;**79**(3):471–9.

169. Blombach B, Arndt A, Auchter M, Eikmanns BJ. L-Valine production during growth of pyruvate dehydrogenase complex-deficient *Corynebacterium glutamicum* in the presence of ethanol or by inactivation of the transcriptional regulator SugR. *Appl Environ Microbiol* 2009;**75**(4):1197–200.

170. Krause FS, Blombach B, Eikmanns BJ. Metabolic engineering of *Corynebacterium glutamicum* for 2-ketoisovalerate production. *Appl Environ Microbiol* 2010;**76**(24):8053–61.

171. Smith KM, Cho KM, Liao JC. Engineering *Corynebacterium glutamicum* for isobutanol production. *Appl Microbiol Biotechnol* 2010;**87**(3):1045–55.

172. Blombach B, Riester T, Wieschalka S, et al. *Corynebacterium glutamicum* tailored for efficient isobutanol production. *Appl Environ Microbiol* 2011;**77**(10):3300–10.

173. Niimi S, Suzuki N, Inui M, Yukawa H. Metabolic engineering of 1,2-propanediol pathways in *Corynebacterium glutamicum*. *Appl Microbiol Biotechnol* 2011;**90**(5):1721–9.

174. Krubasik P, Kobayashi M, Sandmann G. Expression and functional analysis of a gene cluster involved in the synthesis of decaprenoxanthin reveals the mechanisms for C-50 carotenoid formation. *Eur J Biochem* 2001;**268**(13):3702–8.

175. Krubasik P, Sandmann G. A carotenogenic gene cluster from *Brevibacterium linens* with novel lycopene cyclase genes involved in the synthesis of aromatic carotenoids. *Molecular and General Genetics* 2000;**263**(3):423–32.

176. Heider SA, Peters-Wendisch P, Wendisch VF. Carotenoid biosynthesis and overproduction in *Corynebacterium glutamicum*. *BMC Microbiol* 2012;**12**(1):198.

Germinated Barley Foodstuff Dampens Inflammatory Bowel Disease

Osamu Kanauchi*, Keiichi Mitsuyama†, Akira Andoh**

*Kirin Holdings Co., Ltd, Strategic Research and Development Department, Chuo-ku, Tokyo, Japan, and Shiga University of Medical Science, Otzu, Japan, †Kurume University School of Medicine, Inflammatory Bowel Disease Center, Division of Gastroenterology, Kurume, Japan, **Shiga University of Medical Science, Division of Mucosal Immunology, Graduate School of Medicine, Otsu, Shiga, Japan

INTRODUCTION

Barley and its Utility Value

Barley is a short-season, early maturing crop with less sensitivity to dryness or poor land than wheat. It is used commercially for animal feed, malt production (barley is one of the most important ingredients in beer production), and human consumption. In 2007, world barley production reached 136 million tonnes. Barley is the second most important coarse grain after maize (785 million tonnes in 2007), and far outweighs sorghum (65 million tonnes). The main production sites are in the European Union (Spain, Germany, and France), in Russia, and in Canada.[1]

The main use of barley is for feeding livestock, with only 13% being processed into malt. Beer is an ancient beverage dating back more than 5000 years, as illustrated in Mesopotamian clay tablets. Over time, different types of starchy plants have been used for brewing, including maize (in South America), soy (in India and Persia), millet and sorghum (in Africa), and rice (in the Far East). Nowadays, beer production from barley malt is the most common brewing process adopted worldwide.[1]

Barley is reported to have health-beneficial effects[2] and is usually (after removing the inedible, fibrous outer hull) eaten as barley meal (porridge or gruel) in Scotland or *sawiq* in the Arab world, or soups and stews in Eastern Europe. In non-alcoholic drink categories, it is used as a barley tea called *mugicha* in Japan, or a coffee substitute called *caffè d'orzo* (coffee of barley) in Italy. However, its consumption volume is not significant.

Germinated Barley Foodstuff (GBF) and the Beer Brewing Process

Beer is the fifth most consumed beverage in the world, with its production estimated at more than 1.3 billion hectoliters in 2002.[3] Beer is made in three steps: (1) immersing malted barley in hot water and separating the barley extract from the residue; (2) boiling this extract with hops; and (3) cooling the extract and fermenting it using yeast. Brewer's spent grain (BSG) is a by-product of the first step. The endosperm of the malted barley is transferred to the beer, and BSG remains, containing the husk, scutellum (mainly aleurone), pericarp, testa, and so on.[4] Over the years, BSG has been used as feed for livestocks and its safety considered to be very high.

Germinated barley foodstuff (GBF) is obtained by separating the aleurone and scutellum from BSG. This food preparation method is very safe, as it physically separates GBF from BSG and does not use any chemical process. GBF contains glutamine-rich protein and ample dietary fiber sources.[4] There are many types of commercial dietary fibers, which may be divided into two types: water-soluble fiber and water-insoluble fiber.[5] Certainly some types of dietary fiber could assist in defecation, but feeding certain kinds of dietary fiber may cause diarrhea or constipation in some people, due to the indigestibility of such fiber. If a new dietary fiber could be produced with a low risk of causing diarrhea or constipation, these symptoms in patients who have trouble with elimination may be alleviated.[6,7] The aim of this series of researches is to establish a new prebiotic treatment for improving bowel movements in several diseases without adverse effects.

Gut Microbial Ecology and Inflammatory Bowel Disease

A comprehensive culture-independent phylogenetic analysis of microbes has shown that at least 2000 bacterial species live in the gastrointestinal tract of a single individual.[8,9] There is a gradual increase in the bacterial population along the small bowel, from approximately 10^4 cfu/g of luminal content in the jejunum to 10^7 cfu/g in the distal ileum, with a predominance of Gram-negative aerobes and some obligate anaerobes.[10] Bacterial concentrations increase sharply from the distal to the ileocecal valve. The colon is heavily populated with anaerobes, with bacterial counts of 10^{14} cfu/g of luminal content. Around 80% of gut bacteria represent uncultured organisms.[11] It is now well established that inflammatory bowel disease (IBD), including Crohn's disease and ulcerative colitis (UC), is caused by an overwhelming immune response to luminal commensal bacteria in the mucosal tissue, which are a characteristic feature of the gastrointestinal system. Interaction between commensal bacteria and the mucosal immune system plays an important role in maintaining health and preventing development of this disease. Identification of the link between intestinal microbiota and IBD has led to numerous studies investigating the therapeutic potential of bacterial modification of the luminal environment using probiotics and prebiotics. Although complementary studies employing molecular techniques to identify specific bacterial groups have also been applied to the study of intestinal microbiota in IBD,[12–14] these studies do not support the presence of specific pathogenic bacteria in IBD. However, it was reported that the diversity of mucosal microbiota in CD and UC were significantly reduced, in comparison with healthy control subjects. This reduced diversity in IBD was due to a loss of such normal anaerobic bacteria as *Bacteroides* species, *Eubacterium* species, and *Lactobacillus* species.[15]

PREPARATION OF GBF AND ITS PROPERTIES

The BSG is pressed three times using a roll-mill (AS26 Künzel Bayern; roll rotating rate 1000 rpm : 350–450 rpm; roll gap, 0.02–0.06 mm) to grind the particles and isolate the husk fraction. Subsequently, milled BSG is suspended in about 10 times the volume of water, mixed well, and strained using a 50-mesh (300-μm) sieve to obtain the protein and dietary fiber-rich fraction (GBF). The wet GBF is then centrifuged in a high-speed decanter (ZSL-V Tanabe Co., Tokyo, Japan) and dried in a dry chamber at 70–80° or lyophylized. Figure 39.1 illustrates this process. The recovery rate is about 25% (dry matter basis to BSG). The chemical compositions of GBF and BSG are shown in Table 39.1. The amino acid compositions of GBF, casein

as the standard protein, and gluten as glutamine (Gln)-rich protein are shown in Table 39.2.[4] The settling volume (SV) of the dietary fibers plays an important role in their physiological effects in the gastrointestinal tract. The SV of GBF was 8.2 mL/g in artificial digestive conditions and 15.8 ml/g in alkaline conditions (1.0-N NaOH solution).[4] Interestingly, the aleurone layer of GBF contains, arabinoxylan in the cell wall, which emits fluorescence under excitation by ultraviolet light.[16,17] During the germination process, the barley and rice seeds change dramatically in their chemical composition due to the synthesis of low-lignified hemicellulose for stretching of their roots and germ (Table 39.3, Figure 39.1)

GBF AS A PREBIOTIC IN HEALTHY HUMAN SUBJECTS AND ANIMALS

In a Normal Animal Model (Change in Bowel Movement)

Male Sprague-Dawley rats or Balb/C mice were used, and individually housed in metabolic cages in a conventional animal experiment facility. After an acclimatization period, animals were divided into experimental groups on the basis of body weight. Subsequently, each group was fed an experimental diet. The basic experimental diet composition is shown in Table 39.4, and animals were allowed free access to their diet and drinking water. The feces excreted during the final 3 days of the respective experiments were collected, counted, and their dry weight weighed after lyophilization. On the final day, the animals were anesthetized with urethane, and their small intestines and cecal content were collected. Detailed experimental and analytical procedures were described in respective papers with reference numbers.

In normal (healthy) animal models, GBF significantly increased the fecal output compared with the control group (Fig. 39.2). To determine the active ingredients of GBF, we confirmed the effects of Gln or Gln-rich protein, representative water-soluble or insoluble fibers, on fecal output. Sequentially, we isolated the main components of GBF, dietary fiber, and the protein fraction, and estimated the active ingredients of GBF for improving bowel movement. Gln-rich protein or Gln itself could not improve defecation, and the three main dietary fiber components (cellulose as control, hemicellulose, and lignin, all purchased as reagents) and their mixture also could not reproduce the GBF effect. On the contrary, hemicellulose induced mild diarrhea, then fecal output was dramatically reduced. Water-soluble fibers could not increase normal fecal output but induced diarrhea; in particular, polydextrose caused severe diarrhea and prevented us from collecting fecal pellets. The reason behind these secretory motor effects is still unknown. The raw material BSG attenuated fecal

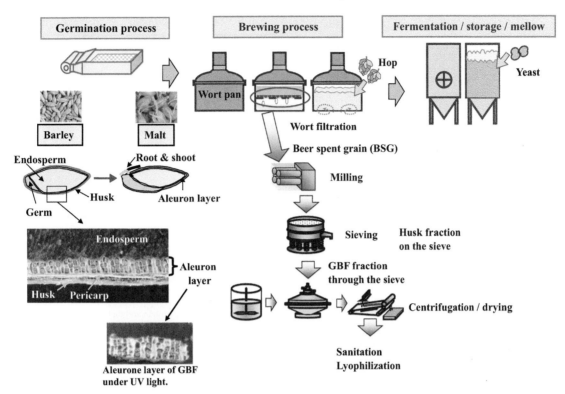

FIGURE 39.1 Schematic production of beer and germinated barley foodstuffs. Beer is made in three steps: (1) immersing malted barley in hot water and separating the barley extract from the residue; (2) boiling this extract with hops; and (3) cooling the extract and fermenting it using yeast. Brewer's spent grain (BSG) is a by-product of this first step. Germinated barley foodstuff (GBF) was obtained by separating the aleurone and scutellum from BSG by physical means only, not by any chemical process. For plants, the newly synthesized low-lignified hemicellulose, which is accumulated in the scutellum and aleurone fractions, is utilized for the stretching of their roots and germ. The aleurone layer of GBF contains arabinoxylan in the cell wall, which emits fluorescence under excitation by ultraviolet light. Please see color plate at the back of the book.

TABLE 39.1 Chemical Composition and Dietary Fiber Component of Germinated Barley Foodstuff and Beer Spent Grains

	Chemical Composition (% Weight)	
	GBF	BSG
Water	7.8	4.0
Protein	46.0	24.0
Lipids	10.2	10.6
Ash	2.0	2.4
Dietary fiber*	34.0	59.0
	Composition of Dietary Fiber (% Dietary Fiber)	
	GBF	BSG
Cellulose	26.0	43.0
Hemicellulose	49.9	36.9
Lignin	24.1	20.1

As natural detergent fiber.[4]

output significantly, and other water-insoluble fibers could not improve defecation. In addition, GBF potently increased the cecal short-chain fatty acid (SCFA) production induced by microbiota.[4,18]

Healthy Human Subjects (Change in Microbiota, SCFA, and Bowel Movement)

Fecal weight was monitored to evaluate the effect of GBF on defecation in healthy volunteers (Fig. 39.3A). First, 9 g of cellulose daily was administered to volunteers for 3 days, and feces were collected for the last 2 days as a control period. Next, 30 g of GBF was administered to volunteers for 28 days and feces were collected for the last 2 days. GBF significantly increased fecal output.[19] The effect of GBF on microflora in healthy volunteers was determined: 9 g of GBF was administered to volunteers (3 g of GBF each time, three times a day after a meal) for 14 days. Feces were collected from all subjects on days 0 and 14. Figure 39.3B summarizes the anaerobic microbes, *Bifidobacterium* and *Eubacterium limosum*, in the feces before (control) and after GBF administration. GBF administration had no significant effect on the growth of the aerobic strains (data not shown). The anaerobic microbiota, *Bifidobacterium* and *Eubacterium*, were significantly increased by GBF administration. Although the fecal contents of acetate, propionate, and butyrate were increased by GBF administration, only the butyrate content was significantly increased (Fig. 39.3C).[20] It was speculated that GBF lowered fecal pH mainly via the

TABLE 39.2 Amino Acid Composition of Casein, Germinated Barley Foodstuff, and Gluten

	Casein	GBF	Gluten
	(% of Total Amino Acids)		
Arg	3.65	4.83	1.50
Lys	7.12	3.19	1.96
His	2.60	2.29	2.15
Phe	5.03	5.77	5.88
Tyr	5.47	3.35	3.49
Leu	8.77	8.95	6.49
Ile	5.73	4.12	2.99
Met	2.86	2.07	1.64
Val	6.42	5.44	2.94
Ala	2.69	4.87	1.98
Gly	1.82	3.57	2.67
Pro	10.68	10.52	12.99
Gln	9.23	22.21	40.16
Glu	12.96	0.45	1.67
Ser	5.47	4.73	4.93
Thr	3.91	3.67	2.46
Asp	5.64	6.56	2.59
Trp	1.30	1.26	0.24
Cys	0.35	2.15	1.27

TABLE 39.3 Chemical Composition and its Dietary Fiber Component of Germinated Barley Foodstuff and Beer Spent Grains

	Chemical Composition (% Weight)				
	GBF	Barley		Rice	
		Raw	Germinated	Raw	Germinated
Water	7.8	6.5	8.0	8.0	7.6
Protein	46.0	18.0	11.5	16.3	17.6
Lipids	10.2	6.6	5.9	19.4	9.4
Ash	2.0	5.8	5.5	5.4	4.5
Dietary fiber*	34.0	32.1	30.7	28.8	31.6
	Composition of Dietary Fiber (% of Dietary Fiber)				
	GBF	Barley		Rice	
		Raw	Germinated	Raw	Germinated
Cellulose	26.0	36.7	21.6	34.3	21.8
Hemicellulose	54.1	55.3	73.6	46.1	70.9
Lignin	19.9	8.0	4.7	19.4	7.2

* As natural detergent fiber.[38]

TABLE 39.4 Composition of Experimental Diets

	Control (g/kg diet)	GBF (g/kg diet)
Casein	146.0	100.0
Vitamin mixture[a]	10.0	10.0
Mineral mixture[b]	35.0	35.0
Choline chloride	2.0	2.0
Cellulose	30.0	
GBF		100.0
DSS[c]	According to the experimental condition (0.5–3.0%)	
Corn oil	50.0	50.0
Corn starch	To make 1 kg	

GBF, germinated barley foodstuff; DSS, dextran sodium sulfate.
In experimental diets, the protein and dietary fiber contents of all groups were compensated to same level with casein and cellulose, respectively.
[a,b] Vitamin and mineral mixtures were prepared according to the AIN 93 formula.
[c] When DSS is added, the volume of corn starch is adjusted.

increase in *Bifidobacterium*. Reducing the pH in the lumen has been reported to keep the microflora in a preferred condition and to prevent abnormal fermentation in the lower intestine.[21] In addition to *Bifidobacterium*, *Eubacterium*, which is one kind of butyrate-producing bacteria, was also increased by GBF administration in humans.

THE EFFECTS OF GBF ON DYSFUNCTION OF THE GASTROINTESTINAL TRACT IN ANIMAL MODELS

Improvement of Constipation

Oral loperamide administration is known to cause mild constipation in rats.[22,23] To evaluate the improving effect of GBF on constipation, Sprague-Dawley rats with constipation induced by loperamide received GBF in their diet (2 mg/kg body weight). Bowel movements were higher in the GBF-fed rats than in the control (cellulose-fed) group, and fecal water content was also higher in the GBF-fed rats. The concentration of SCFAs in cecal content, especially butyrate, was significantly higher in the GBF group than in the control group. These findings suggest that GBF helps to normalize defecation not only in diarrhea but also in constipation, due to its high water-holding capacity and utilization by microbiota (as prebiotics).[24]

Alleviation of Enteritis

Methotrexate (MTX), an antimetabolite used for neoplastic treatment, inhibits the enzyme dihydrofolate

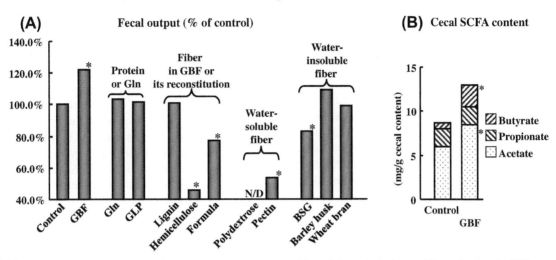

FIGURE 39.2 Change in fecal output by GBF and related component (A), and short-chain fatty acids production in GBF treatment (B). In fecal output, data was shown as % value of control treated group. Short-chain fatty acid content is expressed as the mean ($n=6~9$). GLP, glutamine peptide (purchased from DMV Japan Co. Tokyo, Japan); Lignin (purchased from Tokyo Kasei Kogyo Co. Tokyo, Japan); Hemicellulose, water-soluble hemicellulose; Formula, a mixture of cellulose, hemicellulose and lignin similar in composition to GBF's dietary fiber; PD, polydextrose, and PC, pectin from apple (PD and PC were used as representative water-soluble fibers); BSG, beer spent grain; Barley husk, husk-rich fraction by milling and sieving of BSG. Wheat bran is used as a representative water-insoluble fiber. Data are expressed as the mean changes±SD; * represents a significant difference compared with Cont ($P<0.05$). *Data are modified from original data in previous studies.*[4,18] Please see color plate at the back of the book.

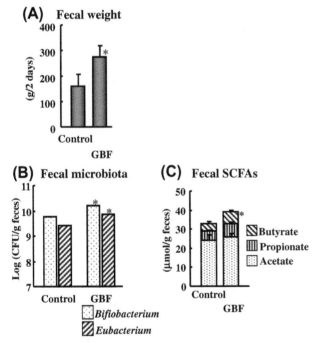

FIGURE 39.3 Change in fecal weight (A), fecal microbiota analysis (B), and fecal short-chain fatty acid content (C) in healthy volunteers. In (A), 9 g daily of cellulose was administered to volunteers ($n=10/$ group) for 3 days and feces were collected the last 2 days as a control period; sequentially, 30 g of GBF was administered to volunteers for 28 days and feces were collected the last 2 days. GBF significantly increased fecal output. (B) Summary of the anaerobic microbes *Bifidobacterium* and *Eubacterium limosum* in the feces and short-chain fatty acid content before (control) and after GBF administration ($n=9/$group). Data are expressed as the mean changes±SEM; * represents a significant difference between the Cont and GBF ($P<0.05$). *Data are modified from original data in previous studies.*[19] Please see color plate at the back of the book.

reductase and is used as enteritis model. MTX-induced enteritis is characterized histologically by crypt loss, villus fusion and atrophy, capillary dilatation, and a mixed inflammatory cellular infiltrate, and shows symptoms resembling the side effects (body weight loss, severe diarrhea, mucosal damage) of patients undergoing chemotherapy.[25] GBF contains Gln as a relatively stable and insoluble protein fraction. Gln is considered to be a trophic factor for small intestinal epithelia, which is important during severe illness; however, its clinical use, including parenteral nutrition, is precluded by its instability.[26] In addition, it has recently been shown that Gln may modulate mucosal immune function, including decrease of TLR-4, MyD88, and TRAF6 mRNA expression.[27]

Based on the presence of Gln in GBF, its potency in alleviating mucosal damage in the MTX-enteritis model was examined. After consumption of GBF, Gln, or a glutamine-rich (gluten) diet, GBF more effectively prevented diarrhea and mucosal damage, compared with the control, Gln-, or gluten-fed groups. Furthermore, GBF increased mucosal protein content and sucrase activity compared to the Gln- or gluten-fed group. The bacterial translocation and elevation of MPO activity induced by MTX were depressed by the consumption of GBF. GBF also dramatically attenuated small intestinal mucosal damage by histological observation. GBF has a potential as therapeutic diet to decrease the adverse effects of neoplastic chemotherapy.[28]

Improvement of Fecal Formation in Ceco-Colectomized Model

Colectomy is known to cause severe diarrhea due to malfunction of water and electrolyte absorption and the decrease of fecal forming ability. The human colon absorbs more than 90% of the fluid passing across the ileocecal valve, and has a huge capacity to collect sodium and electrolytes against the osmotic pressure or electrochemical gradient.[29,30] After colectomy, the main site of water or electrolyte absorption is lost; furthermore, extirpation of the ileocecal valve, which largely contributes to bowel function, results in a marked decrease in quality of life for the patients.[30]

In a ceco-colectomy model in rats, GBF significantly decreased the incidence of diarrhea. This effect was linked to its high water-holding capacity and the modulation of osmotic pressure in the lower intestine of GBF. In addition, Gln in GBF may have contributed to the early recovery of mucosal integrity due to an improving epithelium as a trophic effect.

Preventive and Therapeutic Effects in IBD Models

After having investigated the efficacy of GBF in several bowel movement dysfunction models, we tested its effects on IBD models. IBD, which comprises CD and UC, is considered to be one of the most important and serious dysfunctions of bowel movement. Childhood-onset UC is typically extensive throughout the intestine, whereas adults are equally likely to develop UC confined to the distal colon. There is evidence that commensal or pathogenic bacteria play a significant role as an environmental trigger.[31] Recent data from experimental colitis using animal models indicates that disruption of the mucosal barrier function may induce pathologic immune responses to luminal bacteria, resulting in acute and chronic inflammation.[32] Furthermore, it is speculated that improving the mucosal integrity of the intestinal barrier function may help to reduce intestinal inflammation. Identification of the link between intestinal microbiota and IBD has led to many studies investigating the therapeutic potential of bacterial modification of the luminal environment using probiotics and prebiotics.[33,34] It is on this basis that we carried out an evaluation of the efficacy of GBF and prebiotics in experimental IBD.

Dextran sodium sulfate (DSS)-induced colitis

More than 60 different kinds of animal models have been established to study IBD. They are classified primarily into chemically induced, cell-transfer, congenial mutant, and genetically engineered models.[35] In the first step, we chose the chemically induced DSS colitis model, since it is one of the most commonly used due to its high reproducibility and convenience. DSS colitis induces diarrhea, bloody feces, mucosal ulceration, shortening of the colon, and weight loss, which are some of the representative symptoms in human IBD.[36]

In this model, the preventive effects of GBF on colitis were determined and compared with those of sulfasalazine (SASP), a drug used to treat inflammatory bowel disease. As shown in Figure 39.4,[37] after GBF administration the clinical symptoms of colitis, including body weight loss and mucosal damage, were significantly attenuated compared with the control group. GBF more effectively prevented bloody diarrhea and mucosal damage in colitis compared with controls and SASP. GBF increased mucosal integrity and barrier function, and ameliorated serological inflammatory parameters (IL-8 and α_1-acid glycolprotein), while significantly increasing SCFA production, compared with the control group. SCFA production including butyrate induced by microbiota significantly inhibited transcriptional factors and proinflammatory cytokine production, including nuclear factor kappa B (NF-κB) and the signal transducer and activator of transcription 3 (STAT3). In addition, GBF had a significantly high absorption ability for bile acids, which reduced the inflammatory response.[37]

Both germinated and non-germinated samples of gramineous seeds (barley and rice) were prepared to unveil whether germination had any role in GBF effects. Interestingly, the germinated rice and barley fraction had the same effects as GBF, while the non-germinated sample had no effect, suggesting a key role of germination in the protective influence of GBF in the DSS model.[38] During germination, low-lignified hemicellulose is accumulated in the germ and aleurone fraction, and this synthesized hemicellulose is utilized by plants to extend the roots or shoots. The synthesized dietary fiber fraction has high water-holding capacity and is easily degraded by the microbiota, and may therefore contribute to the high butyrate production by microbiota.[38] In our previous study, the dietary fiber fraction and protein fraction were prepared from GBF, and we compared the preventive effect of these samples on colitis with that of GBF. The dietary fiber fraction attenuated the bloody diarrhea, serum inflammatory parameters and increased SCFA content, while the protein fraction had no effect.[39]

Subsequently, we investigated the role of SCFAs, which are mainly by-products of microbiota in the lower gastrointestinal tract. It is well known that SCFAs have pleiotrophic effects towards epithelial cells, namely by providing an important energy source for the mucosa, and increasing vascular flow, motility, and sodium absorption.[40] In addition, butyrate, via rectal administration, was reported to be effective in reducing colonic

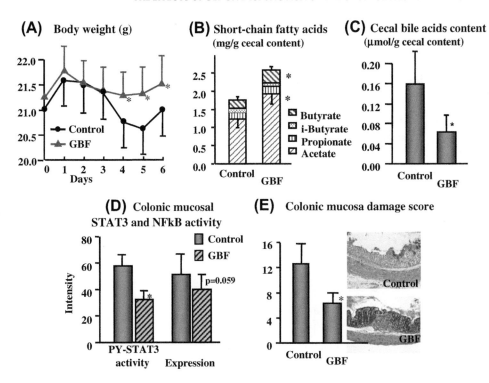

FIGURE 39.4 Change in body weight (A), fecal short-chain fatty acid (SCFA) content (B), cecal bile acids content (C), colonic mucosal signal transducer and activator of transcription 3 (STAT3), and nuclear factor kappa B (NF-κB) activity (D), and colonic mucosal damage score and representative histology (E) in dextran sulfate sodium colitis mouse model. Data are expressed as the mean changes±SEM (n = 10/group); * represents a significant difference between the Cont and GBF (P < 0.05). *Data are modified from original data in a previous study.[37]* Please see color plate at the back of the book.

mucosal damage in colitis patients.[41,42] Interestingly, the utilization of SCFAs, including butyrate, in mitochondria without glucose oxidation is inhibited by ibuprofen, a non-steroidal anti-inflammatory drug, and ibuprofen itself is known to induce colitis.[43] The preventive effects of GBF on DSS-induced colitis were abolished by ibuprofen, and the severity of the colitis enhanced, compared to control animals. We therefore concluded that one of the active ingredients of GBF was likely to be microbiota-induced butyrate. Since oral butyrate had no therapeutic effects and intrarectal butyrate showed preventative effects on colitis, locally administered butyrate appears to play an important role in pathogenesis of colitis.[44]

Gene-Manipulated Spontaneous Colitis Models – (CD4+CD45RB^high T-Cell Transferred SCID Mouse [CD45RB model], HLAB27 Transgenic Rats)

The colitis induced by CD4 + CD45RB^high T cells transferred to the SCID mouse (CD45RB model) is mediated by Th1 responses associated with interferon-γ (IFN-γ and tumor necrosis factor-α(TNF-α) productions. TNF-α is derived primarily from non-lymphoid cells in the recipient.[35] In the CD45RB^high transferred model, GBF had the same preventive effects on colitis as seen in the DSS-induced model. Figure 39.5 shows that GBF clearly suppressed body weight loss, incidence of occult blood (Fig. 39.5A), and colonic mucosal damage (Fig. 39.5B). Although SCFAs did not increase in this experiment, GBF itself attenuated IL-6 production (Fig. 39.5C) and IFN-γ mRNA expression

(Fig. 39.5D). This might represent another relevant mechanism by which GBF prevents colitis, independently of SCFA increase.[45]

The HLA-B27 transgenic rat is also a well-characterized IBD model. These rats, which overexpress the human HLA-B27/b2 microglobulin gene, spontaneously develop an inflammatory disease mainly located in the lower gastrointestinal tract. The HLA-B27 gene is associated with inflammatory disorders, including IBD. HLA-B27-expressing innate immune cells and the presence of enteric bacteria are essential in the development of intestinal inflammation in this model.[46] GBF significantly reduced bleeding and colonic mucosal hyperplastic changes, as well as the level of serum inflammatory chemokine interleukin-8.[47] In conclusion, as described above, GBF exerted preventive and therapeutic effects on the development of colitis in three completely different colitis rodent models.

Colon Cancer Model and Chronic Colitis

It is known that the risk of contracting colorectal cancer (CRC) is higher in patients with IBD than in the general population.[48,49] A greater risk is observed in IBD patients who have experienced extensive colorectal inflammation which continues for longer periods of time.[50] The risks of contracting colitic cancer with chronic inflammation are several times higher than in the general population. GBF has potential anti-inflammatory effects because it contains microbiotic

(A) Change in body weight and occult blood score

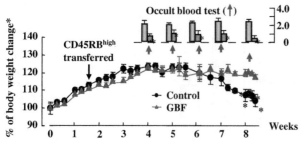

(B) Mucosal damage score   **(C)** Mucosal IL-6   **(D)** IFN-γ m RNA level

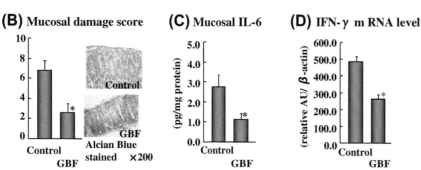

FIGURE 39.5 Change in body weight and occult blood score (A), mucosal damage score and representative histology (B), mucosal interleukin-6 (IL-6) (C), and expression of interferon gamma (IFN-γ) (D) in CD45RB[high] transferred model. Data are expressed as mean changes ± SEM ($n = 10$); * represents significant different between control and GBF groups ($P < 0.05$). *Data are modified from original data in a previous study.[45] Please see color plate at the back of the book.*

metabolites, SCFAs.[51,52] Thus, the use of prebiotics is considered to be a rational strategy to prolong the remission period in IBD, with limited adverse effects and a reduced risk of colorectal cancer, in comparison to the administration of steroids or immune suppressive agents, which show severe adverse effects. GBF was found to attenuate the incidence of sporadic colorectal cancer in an azoxymethane (AOM) rodent model. GBF increased the anticarcinogenic factor slc5a8, the mucosa protecting factor heat shock protein 25, and cecal SCFAs.[53] In addition, GBF downregulated toll-like receptor 4 (TLR4) and cyclooxygenase-2 (COX-2) mRNA in the colonic mucosa, and prevented the incidence of aberrant crypt foci (Fig. 39.6A–C).[54] It has been previously reported that TLR4 is upregulated in inflammatory intestinal mucosa and carcinogenic regions.[55,56]

In the repeated and intermittent DSS administration animal model (chronic colitis model), the incidence of adenomatous dysplasia and of high-grade dysplasia were greatly decreased by GBF concomitantly with a reduction in the stratified squamous epithelium area, when compared to control (Fig. 39.6D).[57] In the GBF group, the proliferative rate (proliferating cell nuclear antigen PCNA-labeling index) in the colonic epithelium damaged by chronic inflammation was significantly lower than that of the control group. Interestingly, in the subacute inflammatory phase, GBF significantly attenuated the mucosal damage score while the PCNA labeling index of the colonic mucosa was significantly higher than that of the control group.[57]

GBF AS A BENEFICAL FOOD FOR ULCERATIVE COLITIS PATIENTS

Adjunctive Therapeutic Usage in the Active Period

The first GBF trial enrolled 10 patients with mild to moderately active UC who had been unresponsive to or intolerant of standard treatment. The patients consumed 30 g of GBF every day for 4 weeks in a non-randomized, open-label fashion. After 4 weeks, it was discovered that treatment with GBF resulted in clinical and endoscopic improvements (Fig. 39.7A, B), with an increase in fecal butyrate. Despite continued treatment with standard drugs, the patients had an exacerbation of the disease within 4 weeks after discontinuing GBF treatment.[58]

To confirm the above result, we continued with the multicenter open control trial. Eighteen patients with mild to moderately active UC were divided into a GBF-treated group and a control group, using a random allocation protocol. The control group was given standard anti-inflammatory therapy for UC, and the GBF group received standard UC therapy with 20–30 g GBF administered daily for 4 weeks. The efficacy of GBF was determined by clinical score. In some patients, fecal microbiota analysis and endoscopic examination were performed. By 4 weeks of GBF treatment, a significant improvement in the clinical score of the GBF group was confirmed; however, serum inflammatory parameters had not changed. No adverse effects were observed with GBF treatment. Endoscopic examination confirmed that

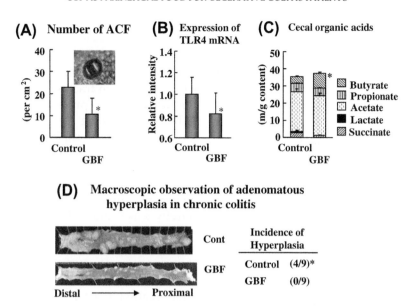

FIGURE 39.6 Change in the incidence of aberrant crypt foci (ACF) (A) and the expression of mRNA of toll-like receptor 4 (TLR4 mRNA) and cyclooxygenase-2 (COX-2) (B) in colonic mucosa, and cecal organic acids content (C) in the azoxymethane-induced colon cancer model. (D) shows representative hyperplastic adenoma in control rats and the incidence of hyperplastic adenoma in the cyclic administered DSS chronic colitis model. Aberrant crypt foci (ACF) were counted under a light microscope per 1 cm² of the distal colon at 100× magnification. Aberrant crypts appeared larger and had a thicker epithelial lining compared to normal crypts, and were gathered into a focus consisting of several crypts. (A) ACF in the germinated barley foodstuff (GBF) group were significantly lower than in the control (Cont) group. (B) The expression levels of toll-like receptor 4 (TLR4) in the colonic mucosa were normalized to the expression levels of the housekeeping gene glyceraldehyde-3-phosphate dehydrogenase. (C) Cecal short-chain fatty acid content. (D) Representative macroscopic observation of the entire colon in both groups and incidence of hyperplasia are shown. Data are expressed as mean changes±SD; $P < 0.05$ for the differences between the Cont and the GBF. *Data modified from original data in previous studies: (A–C)[54], (D)[57].* Please see color plate at the back of the book.

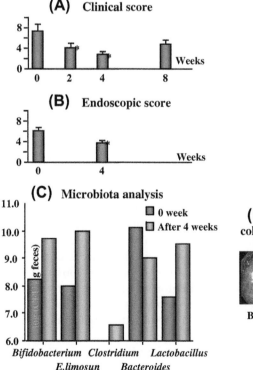

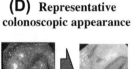

FIGURE 39.7 Change in the clinical score (A) and endoscopic score (B) in mild to moderately active ulcerative colitis patients who consumed 30g GBF every day for 4 weeks. Representative change in microbiota analysis (C) and endoscopic observation (D) in active moderate ulcerative colitis patient with daily administration of 20–30g of GBF for 4 weeks. Mild to moderately active ulcerative colitis patients who had been unresponsive to or intolerant of standard treatment consumed 30g of GBF every day for 4 weeks in a non-randomized, open-label fashion. After 4 weeks of treatment with GBF, clinical and endoscopic improvements were observed (A, B).[58] Data are expressed as mean changes±SEM ($n = 10$); * represents significant different between 0 week and 2 or 4 weeks after GBF treatment ($P < 0.05$). Microbiota analysis showed increases of *Bifidobacterium* and *Eubacterium limosum* (butyrate producer), and a decrease in *Bacteroides* (C). (D) Representative colonic mucosal appearance at baseline and after GBF treatment. *Data are modified from original data in a previous study.[59]* Please see color plate at the back of the book.

mucosal damage was reduced, and microbiota analysis showed an increase in *Bifidobacterium* and *Eubacterium limosum* (butyrate producer) and a decrease in *Bacteroides* (Figure 39.7C, D).[59] Today, GBF is sold as medical food for UC patients with the approval of the Ministry of Health, Labor and Welfare in Japan.

Prophylactic Usage to Prolong the Remission Period

Although the prebiotic GBF alone is insufficient to ameliorate completely an acute colonic inflammation and displays a relatively long latency before showing efficacy, it is considered that GBF would be useful for maintaining remission without causing serious adverse effects. In other words, maintaining remission by modulating the colonic luminal environment should be a major treatment strategy[31,60] that can minimize the risk of developing colitic cancer. Medical therapy of UC has two main goals: one is rapidly to suppress the inflammation in active disease, and the other is to prolong remission by improving the intestinal condition. In line with the latter strategy, in the present study we assessed the efficacy of GBF in patients with UC during remission. To investigate the efficacy of GBF as a maintenance therapy in patients with UC in remission, 59 such patients were enrolled in double-blind placebo control study. They were divided into a control group ($n = 37$) and a GBF group ($n = 22$). Patients in the control group were given a standard treatment for 12 months, while patients in the GBF group received a standard treatment plus 20 g of GBF daily. The patients in the GBF group showed significantly better clinical activity indexes at 3, 6, and 12 months compared with the patients in the control group. The cumulative recurrence rate in the GBF group with steroid tapering treatment was significantly lower compared with the rate in the control group. In this study, no adverse effects except for some bloating (as seen in the ingestion of dietary fiber) were observed.

FURTHER PROSPECTS FOR GBF AS A NEUTRACEUTICAL

GBF is a by-product of BSG, and was initially developed as dietary fiber. However, we were able to reveal the hidden benefits of GBF as functional foods for UC patients, and GBF has been available in Japan as a medical food approved by the Ministry of Health, Labour and Welfare since 2000. Prebiotics are non-digestible food constituents given to benefit the host by selectively stimulating the growth or activity of one or a limited number of bacterial species already resident in the colon.[61–63] The prebiotic GBF is thought to have unique characteristics,

such as a partly degraded lattice-like structure and increase in Gln-rich protein synthesis due to germination process. The fiber fraction of GBF can enhance the fecal forming ability and is easily utilized by microbiota, while the protein fraction of GBF is a stable trophic carrier for Gln to the epithelium.

Before describing further the prospects of GBF as a nutraceutical, we recapitulate here the effects of other prebiotics on IBD. Fructooligosaccharides (FOS) have been shown to stimulate *Lactobacilli* and *Bifidobacteria*,[64,65] and increase SCFAs in the colon.[66] Lindsay *et al.*[67] investigated the efficacy of FOS in IBD patients, and disease activity was decreased with increase of fecal *Bifidobacteria* and the proportion of dendritic cells expressing TLR2 and TLR4. Psyllium (Ispaghula husk), long used by clinicians to maintain stool consistency in both constipation and diarrhea, ameliorated the development of colonic inflammation in a colitis model.[68,69] Hallert *et al.*[70] studied the efficiency of psyllium in relieving gastrointestinal symptoms for 4 months in a placebo-controlled trial of 29 patients with UC who were in remission, and the symptoms score in psyllium groups was significantly superior than that of control.

Bran, the hard outer layer of cereal grains consisting of combined aleurone and pericarp, is particularly rich in dietary fiber, and contains significant quantities of starch, protein, fat, vitamins, and dietary minerals. Bran is present in, and may be milled from, any cereal grain, including oats, rice, and wheat. In inactive UC patients, bran increased the fecal butyrate level without any signs of disease relapse or increasing gastrointestinal complaints in these patients.[71]

Another option to modulate the intestinal environment is to administer probiotics. The intestinal tract contains a complex ecosystem in which a subtle balance exists between the gut microflora and the host epithelium. In IBD this delicate balance is broken down, and as a result a harmful immune response is driven.[72] However, the changes in microbiotic composition may be transient; if so, implantation of exogenous bacteria will have a limited applicability.[73] Potential mechanisms of probiotic action include competitive interactions, production of antimicrobial metabolites, influences on the epithelium, and immune modulation.[74] Prebiotics alter the composition or balance of intestinal microbiota in the host such that *Bifidobacteria* and *Lactobacilli* reach greater prominence without having to add exogenous microbiota. This so-called healthier microbiota should provide increased resistance to gut infections and may also have immunomodulatory properties. In many cases prebiotics cannot be absorbed by the epithelium and are converted into other metabolites, including SCFAs. Therefore, we suggest that prebiotic treatment in gastrointestinal dysfunction including IBD is the most rational way to proceed.

There is evidence that disruption of mucosal barrier function may induce pathologic immune responses to luminal bacteria, resulting in acute and chronic inflammation.[75–79] Therefore, it is speculated that improving the mucosal integrity of the intestinal barrier function may help to reduce the onset of colorectal cancer, as well as chronic inflammation in IBD. Interestingly, murine models of intestinal inflammation are attenuated in germ-free conditions[80] and intestinal tumorigenesis is intimately linked to intestinal inflammation, and, by extension, to microbial sensing by pattern recognition receptors (PRRs), which signals may modulate the neoplastic and infiltrating immune cells. GBF is not a medicine but a food that is recognized as safe and suitable for ingestion over long periods of time. Additional investigations are warranted to characterize the exact underlying mechanisms of GBF properties as an inhibitor of chronic inflammation and a reducer of colorectal cancer incidence.

CONCLUSIONS

Although more detailed basic and clinical studies are required, the use of nutraceutical preventive treatments such as prebiotics, including GBF, for IBD and colorectal cancer may prove useful without causing the adverse effects observed in treatments with anti-inflammatory drugs or anticancer drugs. In the near future, the benefits of GBF and its use as a cutting-edge therapy compared to other probiotics or prebiotics on the market will be confirmed. This novel therapy approach in patients with IBD may help to extend the remission periods and reduce the risk of contracting colonic cancer. It may also be helpful in modulating the colonic environment in healthy humans.

Acknowledgements

This chapter is dedicated to Dr Shuhachi Kiriyama, Osamu Kanauchi's tutor at university and Professor Emeritus in Hokkaido University, who passed away in October 2011. The authors also thank Dr Muriel Larauche and Professor Yvette Taché (University of California, Los Angeles) for critical reviewing.

References

1. *FAO/EBRD: Barley, malt, beer.* Agribusiness handbook. Available at: ftp://ftp.fao.org/docrep/fao/012/i1003e/i1003e00.pdf; 2009.
2. Harris KA, Kris-Etherton PM. Effects of whole grains on coronary heart disease risk. *Curr atheroscler Rep* 2010;**12**:368–76.
3. Aliyu S, Bala M. Brewer's spent grain: A review of its potentials and applications. *African J Biotechnol* 2011;**10**:324–31.
4. Kanauchi O, Agata K. Protein, and dietary fiber-rich new foodstuff from brewer's spent grain increased excretion of feces and jejunum mucosal protein content in rats. *Biosci Biotechnol Biochem* 1997;**61**:29–33.
5. Anderson JW, Smith BM, Gustafson NJ. Health benefits and practical aspects of high-fiber diets. *Am J Clin Nutr* 1994;**59**: 1242S–7S.
6. Scarlett Y. Medical management of fecal incontinence. *Gastroenterology* 2004;**126**:S55–63.
7. Pattee PL, Thompson WG. Drug treatment of the irritable bowel syndrome. *Drugs* 1992;**44**:200–6.
8. Neish AS. Microbes in gastrointestinal health and disease. *Gastroenterology* 2009;**136**:65–80.
9. Guarner F. The intestinal flora in inflammatory bowel disease: normal or abnormal? *Curr Opin Gastroenterol* 2005;**21**:414–8.
10. Guarner F, Malagelada JR. Gut flora in health and disease. *Lancet* 2003;**361**:512–9.
11. Eckburg PB, Bik EM, Bernstein CN, Purdom E, Dethlefsen L, Sargent M, et al. Diversity of the human intestinal microbial flora. *Science* 2005;**308**:1635–8.
12. Bibiloni R, Mangold M, Madsen KL, Fedorak RN, Tannock GW. The bacteriology of biopsies differs between newly diagnosed, untreated, Crohn's disease and ulcerative colitis patients. *J Med Microbiol* 2006;**55**:1141–9.
13. Prindiville T, Cantrell M, Wilson KH. Ribosomal DNA sequence analysis of mucosa-associated bacteria in Crohn's disease. *Inflamm Bowel Dis* 2004;**10**:824–33.
14. Seksik P, Sokol H, Lepage P, Vasquez N, Manichanh C, Mangin I, et al. Review article: the role of bacteria in onset and perpetuation of inflammatory bowel disease. *Aliment Pharmacol Ther* 2006;**24**(Suppl. 3):11–8.
15. Ott SJ, Musfeldt M, Wenderoth DF, Hampe J, Brant O, Folsch UR, et al. Reduction in diversity of the colonic mucosa associated bacterial microflora in patients with active inflammatory bowel disease. *Gut* 2004;**53**:685–93.
16. Kanauchi O, Mitsuyama K, Saiki T, Nakamura T, Hitomi Y, Bamba T, et al. Germinated barley foodstuff increases fecal volume and butyrate production at relatively low doses and relieves constipation in humans. *Int J Mol Med* 1998;**2**:445–50.
17. Hartley RD, Harris PJ. Biochemical Systematics and Ecology. *Biochem Syst Ecol* 1981;**9**:189–203.
18. Kanauchi O, Agata K, Fushiki T. Mechanism for the increased defecation and jejunum mucosal protein content in rats by feeding germinated barley foodstuff. *Biosci Biotechnol Biochem* 1997;**61**: 443–8.
19. Kanauchi O, Mitsuyama K, Saiki T, Fushikia T, Iwanaga T. Germinated barley foodstuff increases fecal volume and butyrate production in humans. *Int J Mol Med* 1998;**1**:937–41.
20. Kanauchi O, Fujiyama Y, Mitsuyama K, Araki Y, Ishii T, Nakamura T, et al. Increased growth of Bifidobacterium and Eubacterium by germinated barley foodstuff, accompanied by enhanced butyrate production in healthy volunteers. *Int J Mol Med* 1999; **3**:175–9.
21. Aoe S, Ohta F, Ayano Y. Effect of water-soluble dietary fiber on intestinal microflora in rats. *J Jpn Soc Nutr Food Sci* 1988;**41**: 203–11.
22. Sandhu BK, Milla PJ, Harries JT. Mechanisms of action of loperamide. *Scand J Gastroenterol Suppl* 1983;**84**:85–92.
23. Sandhu BK, Tripp JH, Candy DC, Harries JT. Loperamide: studies on its mechanism of action. *Gut* 1981;**22**:658–62.
24. Kanauchi O, Hitomi Y, Agata K, Nakamura T, Fushiki T. Germinated barley foodstuff improves constipation induced by loperamide in rats. *Biosci Biotechnol Biochem* 1998;**62**:1788–90.
25. de Koning BA, Sluis M, Lindenbergh-Kortleve DJ, Velcich A, Pieters R, Buller HA, et al. Methotrexate-induced mucositis in mucin 2-deficient mice. *J Cell Physiol* 2007;**210**:144–52.
26. Scheppach W, Loges C, Bartram P, Christl SU, Richter F, Dusel G, et al. Effect of free glutamine and alanyl-glutamine dipeptide on mucosal proliferation of the human ileum and colon. *Gastroenterology* 1994;**107**:429–34.

27. Kessel A, Toubi E, Pavlotzky E, Mogilner J, Coran AG, Lurie M, et al. Treatment with glutamine is associated with down-regulation of Toll-like receptor-4 and myeloid differentiation factor 88 expression and decrease in intestinal mucosal injury caused by lipopolysaccharide endotoxaemia in a rat. Clin Exp Immunol 2008;151:341–7.

28. Kanauchi O, Mitsuyama K, Saiki T, Agata K, Nakamura T, Iwanaga T. Preventive effects of germinated barley foodstuff on methotrexate-induced enteritis in rats. Int J Mol Med 1998;1:961–6.

29. Ohigashi S, Hoshino Y, Ohde S, Onodera H. Functional outcome, quality of life, and efficacy of probiotics in postoperative patients with colorectal cancer. Surg Today 2011;41:1200–6.

30. Luboshits J, Goldberg G, Chubadi R, Achiron A, Atsmon J, Hayslett JP, et al. Functional adaptation of rat remnant colon after proximal hemicolectomy. Dig Dis Sci 1992;37:175–8.

31. Nagalingam NA, Lynch SV. Role of the microbiota in inflammatory bowel diseases. Inflamm Bowel Dis 2012;18:968–84.

32. Petersson J, Schreiber O, Hansson GC, Gendler SJ, Velcich A, Lundberg JO, et al. Importance and regulation of the colonic mucus barrier in a mouse model of colitis. Am J Physiol Gastrointest Liver Physiol 2011;300:G327–33.

33. Jonkers D, Penders J, Masclee A, Pierik M. Probiotics in the management of inflammatory bowel disease: a systematic review of intervention studies in adult patients. Drugs 2012;72:803–23.

34. Nanau RM, Neuman MG. Nutritional and probiotic supplementation in colitis models. Dig Dis Sci 2012;57:2786–810.

35. Mizoguchi A. Animal models of inflammatory bowel disease. Prog Mol Biol Translational Sci 2012;105:263–320.

36. Smith P, Mangan NE, Walsh CM, Fallon RE, McKenzie AN, van Rooijen N, et al. Infection with a helminth parasite prevents experimental colitis via a macrophage-mediated mechanism. J Immunol 2007;178:4557–66.

37. Kanauchi O, Serizawa I, Araki Y, Suzuki A, Andoh A, Fujiyama Y, et al. Germinated barley foodstuff, a prebiotic product, ameliorates inflammation of colitis through modulation of the enteric environment. J Gastroenterol 2003;38:134–41.

38. Kanauchi O, Nakamura T, Agata K, Mitsuyama K, Iwanaga T. Effects of germinated barley foodstuff on dextran sulfate sodium-induced colitis in rats. J Gastroenterol 1998;33:179–88.

39. Kanauchi O, Iwanaga T, Andoh A, Araki Y, Nakamura T, Mitsuyama K, et al. Dietary fiber fraction of germinated barley foodstuff attenuated mucosal damage and diarrhea, and accelerated the repair of the colonic mucosa in an experimental colitis. J Gastroenterol Hepatol 2001;16:160–8.

40. Kles KA, Chang EB. Short-chain fatty acids impact on intestinal adaptation, inflammation, carcinoma, and failure. Gastroenterology 2006;130:S100–5.

41. Andoh A, Bamba T, Sasaki M. Physiological and anti-inflammatory roles of dietary fiber and butyrate in intestinal functions. jpen 1999;23:S70–3.

42. Scheppach W, Christl SU, Bartram HP, Richter F, Kasper H. Effects of short-chain fatty acids on the inflamed colonic mucosa. Scand J Gastroenterol Suppl 1997;222:53–7.

43. Roediger WE, Millard S. Selective inhibition of fatty acid oxidation in colonocytes by ibuprofen: a cause of colitis? Gut 1995;36:55–9.

44. Kanauchi O, Iwanaga T, Mitsuyama K, Saiki T, Tsuruta O, Noguchi K, et al. Butyrate from bacterial fermentation of germinated barley foodstuff preserves intestinal barrier function in experimental colitis in the rat model. J Gastroenterol Hepatol 1999;14:880–8.

45. Kanauchi O, Oshima T, Andoh A, Shioya M, Mitsuyama K. Germinated barley foodstuff ameliorates inflammation in mice with colitis through modulation of mucosal immune system. Scand J Gastroenterol 2008;43:1346–52.

46. Schepens MA, Schonewille AJ, Vink C, van Schothorst EM, Kramer E, Hendriks T, et al. Supplemental calcium attenuates the colitis-related increase in diarrhea, intestinal permeability, and extracellular matrix breakdown in HLA-B27 transgenic rats. J Nutr 2009;139:1525–33.

47. Kanauchi O, Andoh A, Iwanaga T, Fujiyama Y, Mitsuyama K, Toyonaga A, et al. Germinated barley foodstuffs attenuate colonic mucosal damage and mucosal nuclear factor kappa B activity in a spontaneous colitis model. J Gastroenterol Hepatol 1999;14:1173–9.

48. Eaden JA, Abrams KR, Mayberry JF. The risk of colorectal cancer in ulcerative colitis: a meta-analysis. Gut 2001;48:526–35.

49. Rutter MD, Saunders BP, Wilkinson KH, Rumbles S, Schofield G, Kamm MA, et al. Cancer surveillance in longstanding ulcerative colitis: endoscopic appearances help predict cancer risk. Gut 2004;53:1813–6.

50. Lukas M. Inflammatory bowel disease as a risk factor for colorectal cancer. Dig Dis 2010;28:619–24.

51. Kanauchi O, Mitsuyama K, Andoh A. The therapeutic impact of manipulating microbiota in inflammatory bowel disease. Curr Pharm Des 2009;15:2074–86.

52. Koh SJ, Kim JS. Prebiotics: germinated barley foodstuff for the prevention of colitis-associated colon cancer? J Gastroenterol Hepatol 2011;26:1219–20.

53. Kanauchi O, Mitsuyama K, Andoh A, Iwanaga T. Modulation of intestinal environment by prebiotic germinated barley foodstuff prevents chemo-induced colonic carcinogenesis in rats. Oncol Rep 2008;20:793–801.

54. Fukuda M, Komiyama Y, Mitsuyama K, Andoh A, Aoyama T, Matsumoto Y, et al. Prebiotic treatment reduced preneoplastic lesions through the downregulation of toll like receptor 4 in a chemo-induced carcinogenic model. J Clin Biochem Nutr 2011;49:57–61.

55. Fukata M, Chen A, Vamadevan AS, Cohen J, Breglio K, Krishnareddy S, et al. Toll-like receptor-4 promotes the development of colitis-associated colorectal tumors. Gastroenterology 2007;133:1869–81.

56. Fukata M, Hernandez Y, Conduah D, Cohen J, Chen A, Breglio K, et al. Innate immune signaling by Toll-like receptor-4 (TLR4) shapes the inflammatory microenvironment in colitis-associated tumors. Inflamm Bowel Dis 2009;15:997–1006.

57. Komiyama Y, Mitsuyama K, Masuda J, Yamasaki H, Takedatsu H, Andoh A, et al. Prebiotic treatment in experimental colitis reduces the risk of colitic cancer. J Gastroenterol Hepatol 2011;26:1298–308.

58. Mitsuyama K, Saiki T, Kanauchi O, Iwanaga T, Tomiyasu N, Nishiyama T, et al. Treatment of ulcerative colitis with germinated barley foodstuff feeding: a pilot study. Aliment Pharmacol Ther 1998;12:1225–30.

59. Kanauchi O, Suga T, Tochihara M, Hibi T, Naganuma M, Homma T, et al. Treatment of ulcerative colitis by feeding with germinated barley foodstuff: first report of a multicenter open control trial. J Gastroenterol 2002;37(Suppl. 14):67–72.

60. Sartor RB. Current concepts of the etiology and pathogenesis of ulcerative colitis and Crohn's disease. Gastroenterol Clin North Am 1995;24:475–507.

61. Gibson GR, Roberfroid MB. Dietary modulation of the human colonic microbiota: introducing the concept of prebiotics. J Nutr 1995;125:1401–12.

62. Macfarlane S, Macfarlane GT, Cummings JH. Review article: prebiotics in the gastrointestinal tract. Aliment Pharmacol Ther 2006;24:701–14.

63. Galvez J, Rodriguez-Cabezas ME, Zarzuelo A. Effects of dietary fiber on inflammatory bowel disease. Mol Nutr Food Res 2005;49:601–8.

64. Kleessen B, Hartmann L, Blaut M. Oligofructose and long-chain inulin: influence on the gut microbial ecology of rats associated with a human faecal flora. Br J Nutr 2001;86:291–300.

65. Bovee-Oudenhoven IM, ten Bruggencate SJ, Lettink-Wissink ML, van der Meer R. Dietary fructo-oligosaccharides and lactulose inhibit intestinal colonisation but stimulate translocation of salmonella in rats. Gut 2003;52:1572–8.

66. Campbell JM, Fahey Jr GC, Wolf BW. Selected indigestible oligo-saccharides affect large bowel mass, cecal and fecal short-chain fatty acids, pH and microflora in rats. *J Nutr* 1997;**127**:130–6.

67. Lindsay JO, Whelan K, Stagg AJ, Gobin P, Al-Hassi HO, Rayment N, et al. Clinical, microbiological, and immunological effects of fructo-oligosaccharide in patients with Crohn's disease. *Gut* 2006;**55**:348–55.

68. Marteau P, Flourie B, Cherbut C, Correze JL, Pellier P, Seylaz J, et al. Digestibility and bulking effect of ispaghula husks in healthy humans. *Gut* 1994;**35**:1747–52.

69. Rodriguez-Cabezas ME, Galvez J, Camuesco D, Lorente MD, Concha A, Martinez-Augustin O, et al. Intestinal anti-inflammatory activity of dietary fiber (Plantago ovata seeds) in HLA-B27 transgenic rats. *Clin Nutr* 2003;**22**:463–71.

70. Hallert C, Kaldma M, Petersson BG. Ispaghula husk may relieve gastrointestinal symptoms in ulcerative colitis in remission. *Scand J Gastroenterol* 1991;**26**:747–50.

71. Hallert C, Bjorck I, Nyman M, Pousette A, Granno C, Svensson H. Increasing fecal butyrate in ulcerative colitis patients by diet: controlled pilot study. *Inflamm Bowel Dis* 2003;**9**:116–21.

72. Kanauchi O, Mitsuyama K, Araki Y, Andoh A. Modification of intestinal flora in the treatment of inflammatory bowel disease. *Curr Pharm Des* 2003;**9**:333–46.

73. Bouhnik Y, Pochart P, Marteau P, Arlet G, Goderel I, Rambaud JC. Fecal recovery in humans of viable Bifidobacterium sp ingested in fermented milk. *Gastroenterology* 1992;**102**:875–8.

74. Collins MD, Gibson GR. Probiotics, prebiotics, and synbiotics: approaches for modulating the microbial ecology of the gut. *Am J Clin Nutr* 1999;**69**:1052S–7S.

75. Schultz M, Scholmerich J, Rath HC. Rationale for probiotic and antibiotic treatment strategies in inflammatory bowel diseases. *Dig dis* 2003;**21**:105–28.

76. Subramanian S, Campbell BJ, Rhodes JM. Bacteria in the pathogenesis of inflammatory bowel disease. *Curr Opin Infect Dis* 2006;**19**:475–84.

77. Podolsky DK. Inflammatory bowel disease. *N Engl J Med* 2002;**347**:417–29.

78. Mizoguchi A, Mizoguchi E. Inflammatory bowel disease, past, present and future: lessons from animal models. *J Gastroenterol* 2008;**43**:1–17.

79. Sansonetti PJ, Di Santo JP. Debugging how bacteria manipulate the immune response. *Immunity* 2007;**26**:149–61.

80. Asquith M, Powrie F. An innately dangerous balancing act: intestinal homeostasis, inflammation, and colitis-associated cancer. *J Exp Med* 2010;**207**:1573–7.

B. NOVEL APPROACHES TO BRAN AND WHOLE GRAINS

40

Development of Functional Foods (Enzyme-Treated Rice Fiber) from Rice By-products

Osamu Kanauchi*, Muriel Larauche[†], Yvette Taché[†]

*Kirin Holdings Co., Ltd, Strategic Research and Development Department, Chuo-ku, Tokyo, Japan, and Shiga University of Medical Science, Otzu, Japan, [†]CURE: Digestive Diseases Research Center and Oppenheimer Family Center for Neurobiology of Stress, Digestive Diseases Division at the University of California Los Angeles, VA Greater Los Angeles Healthcare System, Los Angeles, California, USA

INTRODUCTION

Rice and its Utility Values

Rice is one of the most important cereal products worldwide, and is grown in more than 100 countries. Milling of paddy rice (or rough rice) yields 70% white rice (endosperm) as the major product as well as by-products comprising 20% rice husk, 8% rice bran, and 2% rice germ. During this whitening process, the husk and bran have to be removed from the grain to produce white rice; rice is then utilized after the appropriate degree of polishing to obtain the desired whiteness.[1] Utilization of rice and its derivatives is shown in Figure 40.1. White rice is a major staple grain, especially in Asia, and represents more than 25% of the world's grain production. Husk is utilized as a soil fertilizer or a source of silicon-based materials under proper production controls.[2] The rice bran is the hard outer layer of the rice, consisting of the aleurone, pericarp, and germ. Rice bran contains protein, fat, fiber, minerals, residual starch, and many kinds of functional micronutrients. Although rice bran was originally used mainly for cattle feed, it is now a major source of rice oil because rice bran can be stabilized by a variety of methods such as thermal control or cold storage.[3] During the oil extraction process, rice bran is separated into two fractions: fat-soluble and fat-insoluble. Subsequently, the fat-soluble fraction is degraded into four fractions (gum, wax, oil, and residue) and the fat-insoluble fraction is divided into four major components (protein, dietary fiber, phytate, and γ-aminobutyrate or GABA). Although rice production in Japan is not very large, Japan is now considered as a promising producer of nutraceuticals or the high-value fraction from rice bran. In this chapter, we focus on the effects of rice bran and its derivatives.[4]

In addition to the rancidity due to lypolysis caused by endogenous lipase or microbiota activity or denaturation of the fat fraction, there is the disadvantage that rice bran also contains unfavorable compounds, including trypsin inhibitor and hemagglutinin; however, the rice oil extracting procedure (thermal process denaturation and solvent extraction) can destroy these antinutritional fractions. Presently, rice bran is a major source of fat and used as an important by-product of rice in the world. Defatted rice bran contains 10–20% protein, 1–4% fat, 40–60% dietary fiber and residual starch, and 8–15% ash. It is also rich in unsaponifiables (vitamins and sterol compounds).

Rice Bran and its Physiological and Functional Properties

Dietary Fiber of Rice Bran

Using thermal processing techniques, rice bran can be stabilized to prevent the development of rancidity, and incorporated into breads and other products.[5] Rice bran itself has some nutritional and physiological functions, including hypolipidemic effects.[6] According to reports, full-fat rice bran reduced plasma total cholesterol or low density lipoprotein cholesterol due to the residual fat-soluble fraction (phytosterols or γ-oryzanol).[6,7] The fecal bulking property of rice bran was also described as being the same as that of wheat bran in the rat.[8] However, in clinical trials it was shown that rice bran was more effective than wheat bran as a means of increasing the output of stool and decreasing the fecal transit time.[5,9,10] In addition, the dietary fiber fraction of rice bran was also reported to reduce the risk of coronary heart disease mortality by reducing blood pressure or improving insulin resistance.[1]

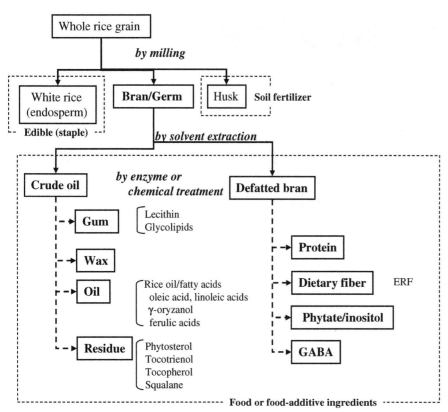

FIGURE 40.1 The utilization of rice grain and its derivatives.

Protein or Amino Acid Isolated from Rice Bran

In addition to the fiber fraction of rice bran, the protein fraction or isolate is also available for use as a functional food. The nutritional and pharmaceutical potential of the protein fraction of rice bran has long been recognized; however, it was difficult to use it as a supplement or functional food for three reasons. First, the protein fraction was a composite of albumin, globulin, glutelin, and prolamin. Secondly, rice bran protein showed strong aggregation and poor solubility. Finally, rice bran has a high phytate and dietary fiber content, and these two components could bind with proteins, making the protein bodies very hard to separate from other components.[11] However, application of the new technique with alkaline or phytase and xylanase utilization made the use of rice bran protein isolate possible. This isolate has an amino acid profile similar to those of casein or soybean protein isolates, except for the lysine content.[11] Recently, alcalase-treated rice bran was reported to show a poor digestive rate in the gastrointestinal tract and to have an inhibitory effect on colon and hepatic cancer cell proliferation.[12] Interestingly, in Japan rice bran was used for the substrate of GABA, which was produced by *Lactobacillus–Saccharomyces*, and GABA was utilized as a functional food for reducing the risk of hypertension or neural dysfunction.[4]

Fat-Soluble Fraction Including Unsaponifiables of Rice Bran

Rice bran is also an important vegetable oil source because it contains relatively high levels of oleic acid, which has hypocholesterolomic and anti-inflammatory effects[13] and is recognized as the best source of phytosterols. In addition, rice bran oil contains minor components, such as γ-oryzanol and tocopherols,[14,15] and considerable amounts of cycloartenol and 24-methylene cycloartanol, which have been reported to have anti-inflammatory effects or inhibitory effects on anti-human immunodeficiency virus-1 reverse transcriptase.[16,17]

Miscellaneous (Phytate)

Phytate is a complex form of both phosphate and inositol in rice grains. Although it forms a heterogeneous mixture with dietary minerals (zinc, iron, etc.) and can induce mineral-related deficiency, its consumption also provides protection against a variety of cancers via its antioxidant properties. Supplementation with phytase or phytase treatment can reverse the adverse effects of phytate in rice bran.[18] Conversely, in the case of hypercalciuric stones, phytate is reported to be one of the most effective substances to reduce the intestinal absorption of calcium, and rice bran treatment should be effective in the prevention of recurrences of hypercalciuric stones.[19]

TABLE 40.1 Chemical Composition of Rice Bran and Enzyme-Treated Rice Fiber (ERF)

	Rice bran	ERF
Protein	17.6	14.9
Lipids	3.5	12.9
Dietary fiber[a]	28.2	74.5
Cellulose[b]	(30.2 %)	(32.8 %)
Hemicellulose[b]	(48.2 %)	(42.8 %)
Lignin[b]	(21.5 %)	(24.4 %)
Carbohydrate[c]	33.0	
Ash	11.6	2.1
Water	11.5	3.6

Original data appeared in Komiyama et al.[36]

[a] Data obtained by the method of Southgate.[20a]

[b] Data within parentheses indicate % of dietary fiber.

[c] Carbohydrate data were calculated by the formula 100 − Protein − Lipids − Dietary Fiber − Ash

PREPARATION OF ENZYME-TREATED RICE FIBER (ERF) AND ITS CHARACTERISTICS

Preparation of ERF and its Properties

Enzyme-treated rice bran fiber (ERF) is a newly developed prebiotic which contains hemicellulose-rich dietary fiber made from rice bran. Since the detailed preparation of ERF was previously reported, we only briefly describe the method in this section.[20] Approximately 25% of defatted and stabilized rice bran is suspended in water (80°C) and heat-resistant amylase is subsequently added and maintained at 80°C for 60 minutes in order to remove the residual starch fraction. Sequentially, the insoluble fraction is isolated using a #200 meshed sieve (aperture size 75 μm) and then hydrolyzed using hemicellulase and protease at 50°C (pH 5.0, adjusting by lactic acid) for 12 hours. After hydrolysis, this insoluble fraction is heated at 80°C for 20 minutes to halt enzyme activity and subsequently sterilized and dried in hot air to obtain ERF. The recovery rate is approximately 20%.

The chemical composition of ERF is shown in Table 40.1.[21] It contains roughly 70% hemicellulose rich dietary fiber and about 15% protein by weight. The physiological function of this dietary fiber seems to be related to its physical properties. The settling volume (SV) in water of dietary fiber is a physical parameter that can be conveniently measured and contributes to the bulk-forming activity of the dietary fiber studied.[22] The SV of ERF was determined to be 30.1 mL, which is an important value in assessing the bulking effect in the lower intestinal tract.[23] In addition, the SV of ERF

TABLE 40.2 Settling Volume of Insoluble Dietary Fiber

Fiber Source	Settling Volume (mL)
Cellulose	3.5
ERF	30.1
Rice bran	4.5

is considerably higher than those of cellulose and raw material, rice bran (Table 40.2).

Utilization of ERF by Microbiota

Enzyme-treated rice bran fiber is considered to be a prebiotic; therefore, it is very important to evaluate the assimilation rate of ERF by the intestinal microbiota. This evaluation was carried out by representative anaerobic human intestinal bacterial strains, including two *Bifidobacterium* strains (*B. breve*, JCM 1192; and *B. longum*, JCM 1217) and two lactobacilli strains (*L. acidophilus*, JCM 1132; and *L. casei*, JCM 1134) as probiotics; two *Bacteroides* strains (*B. distasonis*, JCM 5825; and *B. ovatus*, JCM 5824) as opportunistic microbiota; and the butyrate-producing microbiota *Eubacterium limosum* (*E. limosum*, JCM 6421). A detailed experimental procedure has been published.[24] Briefly, ERF was added to the peptone–yeast (PY) medium (sole carbon source) at a rate of 0.5% (PY–ERF medium) under anaerobic condition at 37°C. After incubation, the pH and concentrations of organic acids (acetate, propionate, butyrate, iso-butyrate, succinate, lactate) were determined.

In addition, six of the above mentioned strains (excluding *E. limosum*) were used to investigate the mechanism of bacterial butyrate production. Respective strains were inoculated with or without *E. limosum*. ERF was efficiently utilized by *B. longum* and *L. acidophilus*, which showed that microbiota could convert ERF to organic acids. *B. breve*, *L. casei*, the two bacteroides strains, and *E. limosum* could not utilize ERF directly, as evidenced by the fact that no major increases in organic acid production were observed in the PY–ERF medium as compared with the PY medium. The total organic acid contents increased and the organic acid production profiles changed dramatically for all strains incubated together with *E. limosum*. Among the two probiotic strains (*L. acidophilus* and *L. casei*), the butyrate content was higher than that for *E. limosum* alone. Furthermore, there was a dramatic decrease in lactate production and a marked increase in acetate production among both of the lactobacillus strains. With regard to the two *Bacteroides* strains, there was an increase in total organic acid content and a decrease in succinate content, although there was no change in butyrate content, as compared with *E. limosum* alone (Table 40.3).[20]

TABLE 40.3   Change in Organic Acid Production Profiles of Representative Intestinal Microbiota (μmol/L)

	Succinate		Lactate		Acetate		Propionate		Butyrate	
		+E[a]		+E		+E		+E		+E
B. breve	0.05	0.15	1.58	0.00	11.93	15.09	0.10	0.25	0.00	2.08
B. longum	1.44	1.17	0.00	0.00	5.57	12.20	10.62	3.15	0.00	1.92
L. acidophilus	0.35	0.45	13.84	0.00	0.43	12.72	0.16	0.33	0.00	5.09
L. casei	0.00	0.07	13.10	0.00	1.22	8.80	0.40	0.72	0.00	6.20
B. distasonis	2.59	0.30	3.29	0.00	3.85	12.42	2.85	7.68	0.00	1.29
B. ovatus	2.68	1.25	6.53	0.00	2.80	10.48	0.34	3.64	0.00	2.50
E. limosum (E)	0.04		0.00		9.74		0.13		2.58	2.63

In this experiment, ERF was added to peptone yeast medium as the sole carbon source at 0.5%. Data are the means of triplicate samples.

We used seven representative microbiota: two *Bifidobacterium* strains (*B. breve*, JCM 1192 and *B. longum*, JCM 1217) and two *Lactobacillus* strains (*L. acidophilus*, JCM 1132 and *L. casei*, JCM 1134) as probiotics, two *Bacteroides* strains (*B. distasonis*, JCM 5825 and *B. ovatus*, JCM 5824) as opportunitistic microbiota, and the butyrate-producing microbiota, *Eubacterium limosum* (*E. limosum*, JCM 6421).

In regard to *L. acidophilus* and *L. casei*, the butyrate content was greater than that for *E. limosum* alone. For both lactobacillus strains, there was a dramatic decrease in lactate production and a marked increase in acetate and butyrate production. In the case of the two *Bacteroides* strains, there was an increase in the total organic acid content and a decrease in the succinate content, although there was no increase in butyrate content, as compared with *E. limosum* alone.

[a] *E. limosum (E) was co-cultured with six respective strains.*

THE EFFECTS OF ERF ON DYSFUNCTION OF GASTROINTESTINAL TRACT IN ANIMAL MODELS

Improving Manifestations of Inflammatory Bowel Disease

As described in Chapter 39, the resident luminal bacteria seem to be an important factor in the development of inflammatory bowel disease (IBD), which is characterized by an intractable and chronic relapsing inflammation of the colon.[25–30] Interaction between commensal bacteria and the mucosal immune system plays an important role in maintaining health and preventing the development of IBD. Recent data on experimental colitis using animal models indicate that the disruption of the mucosal barrier function may induce pathologic immune responses to luminal bacteria, thus resulting in acute and chronic inflammation.[31] Therefore, it is speculated that improving the mucosal integrity of the intestinal barrier function may help to reduce intestinal inflammation. Prebiotics, which are safe, indigestible food constituents given to benefit the host by selectively stimulating the growth or activity of beneficial microbiota already resident in the gastrointestinal tract, have been used as IBD therapy.[32,33] Recently, stabilized rice bran has been reported to have some beneficial ingredients (e.g., dietary fiber, antioxidant product, etc. ...).[34] In addition, some fat-soluble fractions of food have also been shown to have an immune modulatory effect.[35] Therefore, it is speculated that food stuffs rich in dietary fiber, which are derived from rice bran, might have a beneficial effect on IBD patients. The ERF is a newly developed prebiotic that contains dietary fiber and a fat-soluble fraction. As

mentioned above, maintaining the composition of beneficial microbiota by prebiotics is considered to be one of the appropriate ways to treat IBD.

Chemically-Induced Colitis Model (Dextran Sodium Sulfate)

Animal treatment and experimental conditions are described in Chapter 39, and the detailed experimental procedure was previously described.[36] Briefly, 9-week-old female BALB/c mice were divided into three groups: control group; 4% of rice bran (as raw material of ERF) diet group; and 4% of ERF diet group. Dietary protein and dietary fiber levels were adjusted to the same level among groups. After 1 week of pre-feeding with the respective diets, colitis was induced by adding 2.5% dextran sulfate sodium (DSS) to the diets. Body weights were monitored throughout the experimental period. Animals were sacrificed at day 6 after the initiation of colitis, and the serum, colon, spleen, and cecal content were collected. The weight of the spleen and cecal contents and the length of the entire colon were measured. Serum interleukin-6 (IL-6) levels were also determined.

Rice bran itself had a slightly preventive effect on DSS-induced colitis, and this action was significantly reinforced by the enzyme treatment (ERF). ERF significantly attenuated body weight loss, compared with the control group, while rice bran did not show significant difference compared with the control group (Fig. 40.2A). In addition, shortening of the colon length (Fig. 40.2B), one of representative clinical inflammatory manifestation in the colitic mouse, was significantly prevented by ERF. Moreover, ERF significantly suppressed the increase of spleen weight, compared with that of control and rice bran (Fig. 40.2C). Although detailed data are not

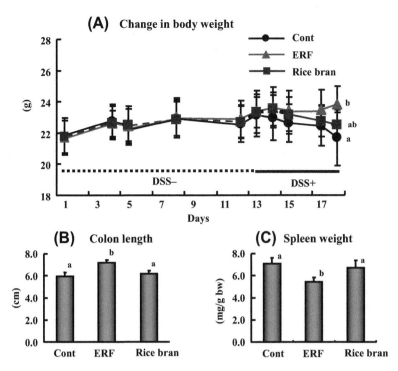

FIGURE 40.2 Change in body weight (A), colon length (B), and weight of spleen per body weight (C) in mice with DSS colitis fed control (Cont), enzyme-treated rice fiber (ERF), or its raw material rice bran diet. Data are expressed as mean ± SD. Each group contains 10 mice. a,b: Values not sharing a common letter represent differences among the three groups.[36] Please see color plate at the back of the book.

shown, ERF significantly increased cecal acetate, propionate, and butyrate in this colitis model; furthermore, the *Clostridium* genus was significantly decreased compared with control group. Hata *et al.* reported that HLA-B27 transgenic rats showed a dramatic increase in the number of *Clostridium* and *Eubacterium*, in parallel with the progression of colitis.[37] Another study, by Kleessen *et al.*,[38] also indicates that bacterial invasion of the mucosa was evident in 83.3% of colonic biopsy specimens from the of UC patients. Although the precise mechanism of such alterations of the gut microbiota remains controversial, ERF certainly excluded the two detrimental genera and therefore is considered to maintain a preferable intestinal microbiota, while also preventing dysbiosis, thereby decreasing the effect of a detrimental immune response.

Immune-Dysfunction Colitis Model (CD4+CD45RB*high* T-Cell Transferred)

To prevent interaction between DSS and ERF, we used a different colitis model: the CD45RB[high] transferred mode. This colitis is only caused by immune dysfunction and not by chemical irritation. The effects of ERF were evaluated by inducing colitis through the transfer of CD4+ CD45RB[high] T cells to female CB17/Icr SCID mice.[39] The recipient SCID mice were started on the respective diets 2 weeks prior to the transfer. After 7 weeks of transfer, the SCID mice were sacrificed. In the second set of adoptive transfer experiments, the CD4+ T cells derived from the spleen of first transferred mice were immediately isolated, and then pooled for two groups (control, and germinated barley foodstuff [GBF]), respectively.

Sequentially, the CD4+ T cells (a mixture of naïve and memory or effector CD4+ T cells) of the spleen from control and ERF mice were re-transferred to other SCID mice fed the same AIN93G diet. Both groups were maintained for an additional 10 weeks and then sacrificed after the T cell re-transfer, and colitis was evaluated.[36]

ERF treatment effectively attenuated body weight loss, as shown by the significantly higher body weight in ERF mice than controls in the first transfer period (Fig. 40.3A) At the end of the first transfer experiment, CD4+CD69+ gated T-cells populations (parameter of activation of T cells) were significantly attenuated compared with those of the control group (Fig. 40.3B). Peripheral serum IL-6 (representative of inflammatory parameters) was also significantly suppressed by ERF (Fig. 40.3C). In the secondary transfer model, mice with CD4+ T cells derived from ERF treatment had a significantly attenuated body weight loss (Fig. 40.3D). Although the same diet was fed to both groups, once it was acquired the T cell character remained thereafter. In Figure 40.3E, the mucosal damage score in mice that received CD4+ T cells derived from ERF treatment group is lower than that of the control group, although it did not reach statistical significance ($P = 0.089$).

Overview of the Preventive Effects of ERF on Colitis

Prebiotics and their metabolites have been reported to have pleiotropic beneficial effects on the colonic mucosa, including metabolic (immune modulator – i.e., regulator of transcriptional factor), trophic (energy source for epithelium; short-chain fatty acids, SCFAs produced by commensal microbiota), and protective (absorbing bile acids) functions in IBD.[40–43] It was also reported that rice bran oil reinforced the Th1-dominant immune response in an *in vitro* study.[44] Since ERF contains both insoluble fiber and fat fractions, we tried to evaluate the preventive effects of ERF on colitis models.

ERF, which includes large amounts of partially dismantled cell wall structure, possibly increasing its prebiotic ability, was shown to prevent the major symptoms of colitis, including wasting, shortening of colon length, megalosplenia, and a decrease of inflammatory cytokine production (detailed data not shown). Although the cellular mechanisms of ERF anti-inflammatory effects on colitis remain to be fully elucidated, some of these effects were thought to be derived from modulating the microbiota and increasing SCFA production. Indeed, it is well known that butyrate[45] and acetate[42] ameliorate epithelial inflammation in IBD. In particular, butyrate has a unique ability to downregulate the activation of NF-κB or phosphorylate, the signaling transducer and activator of transcription 3.[46] Interestingly, recent reports show that colonic mucosal inflammation can increase the number of enterochromaffin cells and the production of 5-HT in a rodent IBD model, and that this change might contribute to the dysmotility seen in IBD.[47,48]

Since ERF contains fat and dietary fiber fractions, the fat-soluble fraction of ERF might also be considered to contribute to the observed anti-inflammatory effects. The relative hydrophilic fraction (methanol-soluble fraction) was indeed found to have a potent ability to inhibit the induction of dendritic cells (DCs) and to stimulate cell growth, in comparison to that of the control (detailed data not shown). This methanol-soluble fraction contained a mixture of ferulic acids and its esters of either triterpene alcohols or phytosterols (oryzanol), free fatty acids (n-3 or n-6).[36] Interestingly, oryzanol itself did not have any stimulation of cell growth and differentiation effects (detailed data not shown). Although further detailed studies will be needed, as described above, ERF might contain anti-inflammatory molecules that alter the differentiation of the immune cells involved in inflammation.

Alleviation of Irritable Bowel Syndrome by ERF

Irritable bowel syndrome (IBS) is a common functional bowel disorder of unclear etiology, characterized by recurrent abdominal pain and altered bowel habits without structural abnormalities, affecting up to 15% of adults in the US[49] and 5–10% in Asia.[50] Stress is an important factor in the onset, maintenance, and exacerbation of IBS symptoms.[51,52] Recently, interactions between intestinal microbiota, mucosal barrier function, and immune system have been identified as playing a role in IBS pathogenesis.[53,54] An imbalance in the gastrointestinal microbial population induced by

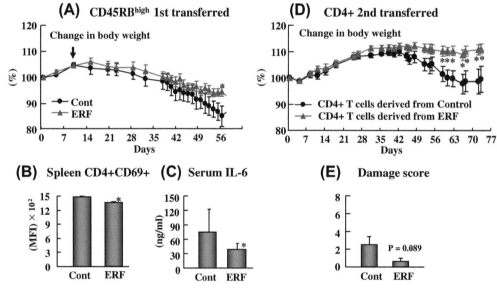

FIGURE 40.3 Change in body weight (A) in mice with colitis due to transfer of CD4+CD45RB[high] T cells fed either control (Cont; *n* = 10) or enzyme-treated rice fiber (ERF; *n* = 10) diet. Data are expressed as the mean ± SD. The body weights of the Cont and ERF groups on day 0 were 16.3 ± 0.2 and 16.4 ± 0.2, respectively. The downward arrow represents the day of CD4+CD45RB[high] T cell transfer. (B) Mean fluorescent intensity (MFI) of CD4+CD69+ T cells in the mesenteric lymph nodes. (C) Serum interleukin-6 concentration. (D) Change in body weight in mice with colitis due to 2nd transfer of CD4+ T cells which were derived from 1st transferred colitis mice fed either Cont or ERF diet. (E) Colonic mucosal damage score and final spleen weight per g body weight. Data are expressed as the mean changes ± SD; * represents a significant difference between the Cont and ERF groups (*P* < 0.05).[36] Please see color plate at the back of the book.

infection, dietary changes, or antibiotics can produce low-grade inflammation, as observed in a subset of IBS patients.[55] Conversely, alterations in gut transit, which can be related to dietary factors, stress, or antibiotics, may also contribute to the abnormalities observed in enteric microbiota metabolic activity, including fermentation processes.[56] Furthermore, visceral hypersensitivity, a key feature of IBS,[57] can be associated with low-grade colonic mucosal inflammation in a subset of patients.[58]

The microbiota of the gastrointestinal tract forms a complex ecosystem, and the use of probiotics and antibiotics has been reported to change the diversity and quantity of microbiota in IBS patients.[59,60] Probiotics such as VSL#3 and prebiotics such as bran have shown efficacy in the clinical or preclinical treatment of IBS.[61,62] While the underlying mechanisms remain unclear, it has been reported that probiotics change the microbiota in IBS patients and improve mucosal immune, motor, and mucosal barrier function. These effects subsequently result in positive changes in fermentation and visceral sensitivity. However, probiotic therapy is of short duration, as the administered probiotics are excreted in the feces within several days after the termination of administration. Prebiotics have also been reported to alleviate IBS symptoms mainly through the modulation of the microbiota and the increase of SCFA production.[61,62] Although prebiotics generally must be present in relatively high-dose volumes to show efficacy in IBS patients, prebiotics have been reported to increase selectively beneficial endogenous microbiota without the administration of exogenous microbiota (probiotics). Indeed, prebiotics as indigestible food constituents provide specific substrates ready to be metabolized by the beneficial gut microbiota, thereby stimulating their growth or activity.[36,53] Prebiotics are also a source of SCFAs that provide energy to the epithelium and exhibit anti-inflammatory properties.[33]

Here we report the effects of chronic feeding of 4% ERF prebiotic in two rodent models of stress-related modulation of visceral pain induced by repeated restraint stress and water avoidance.

Restraint Stress-Induced Visceral Hypersensitivity

Experimental details have been published previously.[20] Briefly, male Sprague-Dawley rats were divided into three groups: a control diet group, an ERF (4%) diet group, and a Polycarbophil-Ca (PC, 500 mg/kg) diet group (used as positive control), which were fed the respective diets *ad libitum* for 14 days. They were then subjected to restraint stress (4h per day) or no stress during the latter 3 days of this period. Defecation and the abdominal withdrawal reflex (AWR) to colorectal distension (CRD) were monitored and, following euthanasia, the 5-HT content, 5-HT positive cells, proinflammatory markers, cytokine-induced

neutrophils chemoattractant (CINC)-1, and tumor necrosis factor (TNF)-α content in the distal colonic mucosa were measured, along with organic analysis of the cecal content.

In the control diet and PC diet groups, repeated restraint stress significantly decreased the pain threshold; however, ERF diet prevented reduction in the pain threshold due to restraint stress (Table 40.4). In the control diet group, restraint stress produced a significant increase in colonic mucosal 5-HT content. This response did not occur in the ERF and PC diet groups exposed, or not, to restraint stress (Table 40.4). However, the number of 5-HT positive cells (primarily enterochromaffin cells and mast cells) was similar among the six groups and no inflammatory damage was observed. No significant differences were observed in the levels of CINC-1 and TNF-α. Restraint-stressed rats showed a significant decrease in food intake, but no change in body weight compared to non-stressed rats. This was associated with an increase in defecation, except for rats treated with ERF. In the absence of stress, the butyrate cecal content in the ERF group and the succinate content in the PC group were significantly higher than those in the control diet rats. Restraint stress significantly decreased acetate and butyrate production in the ERF diet group; however, the butyrate content was higher in the restraint-stress ERF group than in the stress-negative control diet group.

TABLE 40.4 Change in the Perception of Pain Threshold to Colorectal Distension Induced by the Barostat Method

Treatment	Diet Group		
	Control	ERF	Polycarbophyl-Ca
PERCEPTION OF PAIN THRESHOLD BY CRD (mmHG)			
Stress −	30.4 ± 2.9	27.4 ± 2.0	34.24.4
Stress +	20.2 ± 2.8*	26.8 ± 3.7	20.8 ± 2.2*
COLONIC MUCOSAL 5-HT CONTENT (NG/MG PROTEIN)			
Stress −	88.3 ± 8.0	89.9 ± 24.6	74.3 ± 30.9
Stress +	133.7 ± 14.2*	100.5 ± 8.1	94.5 ± 10.6

CRD, colorectal distension.
Behavioral responses to CRD were evaluated in all groups by measuring abdominal withdrawal reflex (AWR) scores. A score of 3 was set as the threshold intensity, which was taken as visceral hypersensitivity. A balloon was distended with air to exert a pressure of 5 mmHg for 1 minute and the baseline colonic contraction was confirmed. After this baseline evaluation, rats were allowed to calm and their baseline CRD reached a steady state. Thereafter, CRD was performed in a stepwise fashion. This process involved 30 sec of distention followed by 20 sec of rest from 10 to 52 mmHg with 3 mmHg increases in pressure. In the control and Polycarbophyl-Ca groups, restraint stress significantly decreased the pain threshold; however, ERF prevented any reduction in the pain threshold due to restraint stress. In the control group, restraint stress produced a significant increase in colonic mucosal serotonin content; however, there were no significant differences in the serotonin content between stress-positive and stress-negative rats in the ERF and PC groups.
Data are shown as the mean ± SE; * indicates a significant difference between stress-positive and -negative rats in the same dietary group (P < 0.05).

Repeated Water Avoidance Stress-Induced Visceral Analgesia

As recently reported,[63] male Wistar rats were fed the 4% ERF diet (two groups) or standard control diet (two groups) for 37 days starting at the weaning period and continuing until they reached adulthood (6–6.5 weeks). After monitoring their baseline visceromotor response (VMR) to colorectal distension (CRD) on day 0 using a non-invasive method relying on intraluminal pressure measurements,[63,64] rats were either exposed to water avoidance stress (WAS) or not for 10 consecutive days. Body weight and defecation were monitored daily. On days 1 (acute WAS) and 10 (rWAS), 45–50 min after the end of the stress session, and on day 11, 24 h after the last rWAS session, rats were subjected to CRD protocol and VMR was monitored in all groups. Immediately after the last CRD, animals were euthanized and cecum and distal colon collected to measure organic acid content and histological assessment, respectively (Table 40.5).

Repeated WAS induced an immediate analgesia compared to baseline in standard diet fed rats. The ERF diet potentiated the immediate and induced a delayed visceral analgesia to rWAS compared to baseline (Fig. 40.4). In rats fed the standard diet, 86%, 67%, and 86% of animals developed visceral analgesia in response to rWAS when tested at day 1, 10, or 11, respectively, while 100% exhibited visceral analgesia in rats fed ERF diet consistently over the 3 days of testing. The ERF diet compared with control diet decreased the percentage of rats developing hyperalgesia in response to rWAS at 60 mmHg CRD over the 10 days of stress. While there were no differences in the percentage of rats developing hyperalgesia in non-stressed rats at days 1, 10, and 11 in rWAS groups, 14.3%, 33.3%, and 14.3% fed the standard diet developed hyperalgesia at days 1, 10, and 11 ($n=6–8$/ group) respectively, but none did so in the ERF diet fed group ($n=8–9$/group) ($P=0.0478$, Fisher's exact test). Interestingly, lower concentrations in the cecal content of isobutyrate and total butyrate (isobutyrate+butyrate), but not butyrate alone, were correlated with a lower visceral pain response (overall AUC during CRD on day 11) (Rp=0.41, $P=0.0368$, and Rp=0.42, $P=0.0335$, respectively) in stressed and non-stressed animals fed either ERF or standard diet. In animals fed the standard diet, rWAS evoked slight colonic inflammation with mild invasion of inflammatory cells and submucosal edema that was rarely observed in non-stressed animals or in rWAS stressed animals fed ERF. Defecation was higher in the ERF-treated group than in the standard diet group. Lastly, animals on the standard diet still maintained a 1.3-fold higher body weight gain than rats on the ERF diet over the 10 days of rWAS or no stress.

Overview of the Modulating Effects of ERF on Visceral Sensitivity

The use of both models showed that ERF is able to prevent the development of repeated 4-h restraint stress-related visceral hypersensitivity, and to potentiate repeated

TABLE 40.5 Visceromotor Response after Water Avoidance Stress (WAS) or No Stress in Rats Fed Standard or Enzyme-Treated Rice Fiber Diet

Time Post WAS[a]	CRD Pressure (mmHg)	Standard Diet[a]		ERF Diet[a]	
		No stress	WAS	No stress	WAS
		Analgesia (%)[b]	Analgesia (%)[b]	Analgesia (%)[b]	Analgesia (%)[b]
45 min day 1	40	15.8 ± 17.6	-32.4 ± 15.2[c]	26.0 ± 23	-29.5 ± 12.3[d]
	60	1.0 ± 9.7	-30.0 ± 10.8[c]	12.9 ± 13.8	-28.7 ± 6.0[de]
		($n=7$)	($n=7$)	($n=8$)	($n=8$)
45 min day 10	40	-26.4 ± 11.7	-36.2 ± 17.8[d]	3.7 ± 21.3	-49.3 ± 11.6[de]
	60	-23.7 ± 18.6	-20.6 ± 12.2	21.6 ± 23.5	-38.9 ± 7.3[d]
		($n=7$)	($n=7$)	($n=8$)	($n=9$)
45 min day 11	40	7.5 ± 38.7	-28.2 ± 15.0	-4.1 ± 21.5	-49.8 ± 12.6[d]
	60	30.4 ± 15.4	-24.3 ± 9.6[d]	5.8 ± 15.1	-34.3 ± 10.8[d]
		($n=5$)	($n=7$)	($n=6$)	($n=8$)

[a] Rats were fed 4% ERF diet or standard control diet starting at the weaning period for 37 days, then tested for baseline visceromotor response (VMR) to colorectal distention (CRD) response (day 0) and thereafter exposed daily to 1 h WAS for 10 consecutive days or no stress (days 1–10), while still maintained on a standard or 4% ERF diet. Non-stressed animals were kept in their home cages. On days 1 (acute WAS) and 10 (rWAS), 45–50 min after the end of the stress session, and on day 11, 24 h after the last rWAS session, rats were subjected to CRD protocol and VMR was monitored in all groups.

[b] Each value represents the mean ± SE of % VMR changes from baseline (day 0) in number of animal indicated by n in columns). Minus values represent analgesia.

[c] P < 0.05

[d] P < 0.01 vs baseline

[e] P < 0.05 vs respective diet non-stressed group, two-way ANOVA, Bonferroni post hoc test.

1-h WAS-induced visceral analgesia, in rats. There is growing evidence that stress exposure alters the structures of the intestinal microbiota.[65] The mechanisms involved in the modulation of visceral pain by chronic ERF feeding to reduce stress-related hypersensitivity and to enhance stress-induced analgesia are most likely quite different, even though they may share some underlying connections. It appears that in the repeated 4-h restraint-stress model, the main effect of ERF was on the serotonergic system, while in the rWAS model ERF may have enhanced visceral analgesia by preventing rWAS-induced subtle immune and structural histological changes in colonic mucosa, as demonstrated by the reduction in the percentage of rats exhibiting histological alterations. However, it may also be speculated that the prevention of stress-related dysbiosis by chronic ERF feeding may contribute to dampen the mechanisms involved in hypersensitivity while enhancing analgesic mechanisms through a local action, along with the communication of the gut microbiota to the brain being increasingly recognized.[66] Further studies are warranted to gain better insight into these mechanisms.

MODULATION OF COLONIC ENVIRONMENT BY RICE BRAN AND ITS HEALTH BENEFITS

It is reported that diet, intestinal microbes, and/or Western lifestyle contribute to the abnormal immunological response of the digestive tract. As Japanese economic growth began to develop around 1960, Japanese people began to incorporate more animal proteins and fats, and breads, which are universally present in Western lifestyle food, into their diet. This change in dietary pattern has been positively associated with the incidence rate of IBD.[67] Interestingly, it is reported that dietary habit (ingestion of brown rice containing rice bran) or residential area significantly changed fecal microbiota.[68,69]

Rice bran is known for its unique preventive effects on pathogenic bacterial colonization due to the increase of the phylum *Firmicutes* involving *Lactobacillus*. In addition, it is reported that phytochemicals in rice bran may inhibit pathogen entry and intracellular replication of pathogenic bacteria by modulating the epithelial microenvironment.[70] Rice bran needs to be stabilized to prevent the development of rancidity, therefore the added starch may be easily utilized by microbiota, compared with wheat bran. Furthermore, rice bran is more abundant in water-soluble fiber than wheat bran.[8–10] Thus, it is speculated that rice bran has higher potency of bowel movement and stimulation of mucosal growth than other brans. Generally, the benefits of dietary fiber derive from its physical properties, water-holding capacity, and bile acid binding capacity,[71] in addition to being a substrate for probiotics (prebiotics) and the action of short-chain fatty acid produced by microbiota.[72] Verschoyle *et al.* reported the cancer chemopreventive effects of rice bran in a unique paper.[73] In this report, the prophylactic effect of rice bran was evaluated on the genetic model of mammary, prostate (TRAMP), and intestinal carcinogenesis

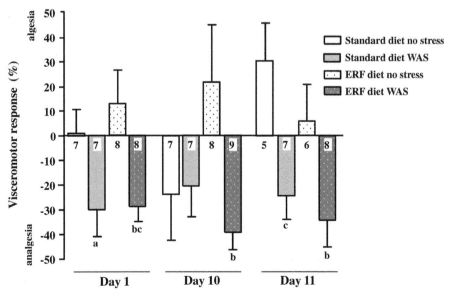

FIGURE 40.4 Change in visceromotor response after water avoidance stress or no stress in rats fed standard or enzyme-treated rice fiber diet. Rats were fed 4% ERF diet or standard control diet starting at the weaning period for 37 days, then tested for baseline visceromotor response (VMR) to colorectal distension (CRD at 60 mmHg) response (day 0) and thereafter exposed daily to 1 h WAS for 10 consecutive days or no stress (days 1–10), while still maintained on standard or 4% ERF diet. Non-stressed animals were kept in their home cages. On days 1 (acute WAS) and 10 (rWAS), 45–50 min after the end of the stress session, and on day 11, 24 h after the last rWAS session, rats were subjected to CRD protocol and VMR was monitored in all groups. Each value represents the mean±SE of % VMR changes from baseline (day 0) in number of animals (indicated in columns). Minus values represent analgesia. [a]$P < 0.05$ vs baseline, [b]$P < 0.01$ vs baseline; [c]$P < 0.05$ vs respective diet non-stressed group, two-way ANOVA, Bonferroni *post hoc* test.

(Apc[min]) mice. Interestingly, rice bran did not affect carcinoma development in the mammary prostate carcinogenic model; however, consumption of rice bran significantly reduced the numbers of colonic adenomas and bleeding, compared with control. This means that the anticarcinogenic component of rice bran cannot be transported to a remote organ from the gastrointestinal tract. Although the detailed reason is still not clear, it is a very important point in the understanding of rice bran anticarcinogenic effects.

Finally, we introduce other important health benefits of rice bran in the major metabolic syndrome (diabetes and hyperlipidemia). Rice bran has a blood glucose-lowering effect, which is thought to derive from its high content of dietary fiber and from the potential benefit of rice bran intake in the prevention of diabetic vascular complications.[71] This latter effect seems to be linked to an increase in the viscosity of the digests in the intestinal tract, and inhibition of the glucose diffusion or attenuation of α-amylase activity.[71] It was reported that full-fat rice bran has an ameliorating effect on hypercholesterolemia in humans. The relatively high content of water-soluble fiber and rice oil fraction including oryzanol were considered to be active ingredients.[7]

CONCLUSIONS

In recent years, there have been reports that the consumption of unpolished rice is beneficial due to some of the nutrients contained. Some fat-soluble fractions of rice bran have also been reported to have an immune modulatory effect.[44] Therefore, it was considered that foodstuffs rich in dietary fiber, which is derived from rice bran, might have a beneficial effect on gastrointestinal dysfunction. ERF is a newly developed prebiotic which contains dietary fiber and a fat-soluble fraction.[36] Although the mechanisms underlying IBD and IBS are quite different, both diseases have a common pathogenesis: overwhelming immune response in some subtypes.[74,75] In addition, IBS has a heterogeneous clinical presentation that includes abnormal bowel movements and abdominal pain, which are also symptoms of IBD.[76] It is known that modulation of microbiota plays an important role in the mechanism of both IBS and IBD.[77,78] Therefore, we evaluated the efficacy of prebiotic ERF in preclinical models of these two gastrointestinal conditions. ERF had potent anti-inflammatory effects on chemical and genetic IBD models[36] and prevented the development of stress-induced visceral hypersensitivity in IBS models while enhancing stress-induced visceral analgesia[63,79] due to the modulation of microbiota and increase of SCFA production. In addition to our results, many researchers have published the beneficial effects of rice bran and its related products for health promotion

or disease prevention. Although further detailed studies are required to gain a deeper insight into the cellular mechanisms, our data support the benefits of ERF utilization for gastrointestinal conditions such as IBS and IBD in a clinical setting in the near future. This nutraceutical product may also be helpful in modulating the colonic environment in healthy humans as well as patients.

Acknowledgements

Research was supported by Central Labs for Frontier Technology Kirin Holdings Co. Ltd Japan, and National Institute of Health grants, P50 DK-64539 (to Y. Taché and M. Larauche), Center Grant DK-41301 (Animal Core, to Y. Taché), and Veterans Administration Research Career Scientist Award (to Y. Taché).

References

1. Nagendra Prasad M, Sanjay K, Shravya Khatokar M, Vismaya M, Nanjunda Swamy S. Health Benefits of Rice Bran - A Review. *J Nutr Food Sci* 2011;1. http://dx.doi.org/10.4172/2155-9600.1000108.
2. Chandrasekhar S, Satyanarayana KG, Pramada PN, Raghavan P, Gupta TN. Review Processing, properties and applications of reactive silica from rice husk—an overview. *J Mater Sci* 2003;38:3159–68.
3. Khan SH, Butt MS, Anjum FM, Jamil A. Antinutritional appraisal and protein extraction from differently stabilized rice bran. *Pak J Nutr* 2009;8:1281–6.
4. Arai S. Global view on functional foods: Asian perspectives. *Br J Nutr* 2002;88(Suppl. 2):S139–43.
5. James C, Sloan S. Functional Properties of Edible Rice Bran in Model Systems. *J Food Sci* 1984;49:310–1.
6. Truswell AS. Cereal grains and coronary heart disease. *Eur J Clin Nutr* 2002;56:1–14.
7. Gerhardt AL, Gallo NB. Full-fat rice bran and oat bran similarly reduce hypercholesterolemia in humans. *J Nutr* 1998;128:865–9.
8. Gestel G, Besancon P, Rouanet JM. Comparative evaluation of the effects of two different forms of dietary fibre (rice bran vs. wheat bran) on rat colonic mucosa and faecal microflora. *Ann Nutr Metab* 1994;38:249–56.
9. Tomlin J, Read NW. Comparison of the effects on colonic function caused by feeding rice bran and wheat bran. *Eur J Clin Nutr* 1988;42:857–61.
10. Johnson IT. Fibre source for the food industry. *Proc Nutr Soc* 1990;49:31–8.
11. Wang M, Hettiarachchy NS, Qi M, Burks W, Siebenmorgen T. Preparation and functional properties of rice bran protein isolate. *J Agric food Chem* 1999;47:411–6.
12. Kannan A, Hettiarachchy N, Johnson MG, Nannapaneni R. Human colon and liver cancer cell proliferation inhibition by peptide hydrolysates derived from heat-stabilized defatted rice bran. *J Agric Food Chem* 2008;56:11643–7.
13. van Dijk SJ, Feskens EJ, Bos MB, Hoelen DW, Heijligenberg R, Bromhaar MG, et al. A saturated fatty acid-rich diet induces an obesity-linked proinflammatory gene expression profile in adipose tissue of subjects at risk of metabolic syndrome. *Am J Clin Nutr* 2009;90:1656–64.
14. Jiang Y, Wang T. Phytosterols in cereal by-products. *J Am Oil Chem Soc* 2005;82:439–44.
15. Hoed VV, Depaemelaere G, Ayala JV, Santiwattana P, Verhe R, De Greyt W. Influence of chemical refining on the major and minor components of rice brain oil. *J Am Oil Chem Soc* 2006;83:315–21.

16. Akihisa T, Ogihara J, Kato J, Yasukawa K, Ukiya M, Yamanouchi S, et al. Inhibitory effects of triterpenoids and sterols on human immunodeficiency virus-1 reverse transcriptase. *Lipids* 2001;**36**:507–12.

17. Akihisa T, Yasukawa K, Yamaura M, Ukiya M, Kimura Y, Shimizu N, et al. Triterpene alcohol and sterol ferulates from rice bran and their anti-inflammatory effects. *J Agric Food Chem* 2000;**48**:2313–9.

18. Kumara V, Sinhab AK, Makkara HPS, Beckera K. Dietary roles of phytate and phytase in human nutrition: A review. *Food Chem* 2010;**120**:945–59.

19. Ohkawa T, Ebisuno S, Kitagawa M, Morimoto S, Miyazaki Y, Yasukawa S. Rice bran treatment for patients with hypercalciuric stones: experimental and clinical studies. *J Urol* 1984;**132**:1140–5.

20. Kanauchi O, Mitsuyama K, Komiyama Y, Yagi M, Andoh A, Sata M. Preventive effects of enzyme-treated rice fiber in a restraint stress-induced irritable bowel syndrome model. *Int J Mol Med* 2010;**25**:547–55.

21. Southgate DAT. Determination of Carbohydrates in Foods. II. Unavailable Carbohydrates. *J Sci Food Agric* 1969;**20**:331–5.

22. Tanabe H, Sugiyama K, Matsuda T, Kiriyama S, Morita T. Small intestinal mucins are secreted in proportion to the settling volume in water of dietary indigestible components in rats. *J Nutr* 2005;**135**:2431–7.

23. Hayashi K, Hara H, Asvarujanon P, Aoyama Y, Luangpituksa P. Ingestion of insoluble dietary fibre increased zinc and iron absorption and restored growth rate and zinc absorption suppressed by dietary phytate in rats. *Br J Nutr* 2001;**86**:443–51.

24. Kanauchi O, Fujiyama Y, Mitsuyama K, Araki Y, Ishii T, Nakamura T, et al. Increased growth of Bifidobacterium and Eubacterium by germinated barley foodstuff, accompanied by enhanced butyrate production in healthy volunteers. *Int J Mol Med* 1999;**3**:175–9.

25. Kanauchi O, Mitsuyama K, Andoh A. The therapeutic impact of manipulating microbiota in inflammatory bowel disease. *Curr Pharm Des* 2009;**15**:2074–86.

26. Sandborn WJ. Current directions in IBD therapy: what goals are feasible with biological modifiers? *Gastroenterology* 2008;**135**: 1442–7.

27. Sansonetti PJ, Di Santo JP. Debugging how bacteria manipulate the immune response. *Immunity* 2007;**26**:149–61.

28. Subramanian S, Campbell BJ, Rhodes JM. Bacteria in the pathogenesis of inflammatory bowel disease. *Curr Opin Infect Dis* 2006;**19**:475–84.

29. Maynard CL, Weaver CT. Intestinal effector T cells in health and disease. *Immunity* 2009;**31**:389–400.

30. Maynard CL, Weaver CT. Immunology: Context is key in the gut. *Nature* 2012;**471**:169–70.

31. Mizoguchi A, Mizoguchi E. Inflammatory bowel disease, past, present and future: lessons from animal models. *J Gastroenterol* 2008;**43**:1–17.

32. Looijer-van Langen MA, Dieleman LA. Prebiotics in chronic intestinal inflammation. *Inflamm Bowel Dis* 2009;**15**:454–62.

33. Szilagyi A. Use of prebiotics for inflammatory bowel disease. *Can J Gastroenterol* 2005;**19**:505–10.

34. Henderson AJ, Kumar A, Barnett B, Dow SW, Ryan EP. Consumption of rice bran increases mucosal immunoglobulin A concentrations and numbers of intestinal Lactobacillus spp. *J Med Food* 2012;**15**:469–75.

35. Islam MS, Murata T, Fujisawa M, Nagasaka R, Ushio H, Bari AM, et al. Anti-inflammatory effects of phytosteryl ferulates in colitis induced by dextran sulphate sodium in mice. *Br J Pharmacol* 2008;**154**:812–24.

36. Komiyama Y, Andoh A, Fujiwara D, Ohmae H, Araki Y, Fujiyama Y, et al. New prebiotics from rice bran ameliorate inflammation in murine colitis models through the modulation of intestinal homeostasis and the mucosal immune system. *Scand J Gastroenterol* 2011;**46**:40–52.

37. Hata K, Andoh A, Sato H, Araki Y, Tanaka M, Tsujikawa T, et al. Sequential changes in luminal microflora and mucosal cytokine expression during developing of colitis in HLA-B27/beta2-microglobulin transgenic rats. *Scand J Gastroenterol* 2001;**36**:1185–92.

38. Kleessen B, Kroesen AJ, Buhr HJ, Blaut M. Mucosal and invading bacteria in patients with inflammatory bowel disease compared with controls. *Scand J Gastroenterol* 2002;**37**:1034–41.

39. Kanauchi O, Oshima T, Andoh A, Shioya M, Mitsuyama K. Germinated barley foodstuff ameliorates inflammation in mice with colitis through modulation of mucosal immune system. *Scand J Gastroenterol* 2008;**43**:1346–52.

40. Araki Y, Andoh A, Fujiyama Y, Kanauchi O, Takenaka K, Higuchi A, et al. Germinated barley foodstuff exhibits different adsorption properties for hydrophilic versus hydrophobic bile acids. *Digestion* 2001;**64**:248–54.

41. Guarner F, Malagelada JR. Gut flora in health and disease. *Lancet* 2003;**361**:512–9.

42. Maslowski KM, Vieira AT, Ng A, Kranich J, Sierro F, Yu D, et al. Regulation of inflammatory responses by gut microbiota and chemoattractant receptor GPR43. *Nature* 2009;**461**:1282–6.

43. Thibault R, De Coppet P, Daly K, Bourreille A, Cuff M, Bonnet C, et al. Down-regulation of the monocarboxylate transporter 1 is involved in butyrate deficiency during intestinal inflammation. *Gastroenterology* 2007;**133**:1916–27.

44. Sierra S, Lara-Villoslada F, Olivares M, Jimenez J, Boza J, Xaus J. Increased immune response in mice consuming rice bran oil. *Eur J Nutr* 2005;**44**:509–16.

45. Kanauchi O, Iwanaga T, Mitsuyama K, Saiki T, Tsuruta O, Noguchi K, et al. Butyrate from bacterial fermentation of germinated barley foodstuff preserves intestinal barrier function in experimental colitis in the rat model. *J Gastroenterol Hepatol* 1999;**14**:880–8.

46. Kanauchi O, Serizawa I, Araki Y, Suzuki A, Andoh A, Fujiyama Y, et al. Germinated barley foodstuff, a prebiotic product, ameliorates inflammation of colitis through modulation of the enteric environment. *J Gastroenterol* 2003;**38**:134–41.

47. Chin A, Svejda B, Gustafsson BI, Granlund AB, Sandvik AK, Timberlake A, et al. The role of mechanical forces and adenosine in the regulation of intestinal enterochromaffin cell serotonin secretion. *Am J Physiol Gastrointest Liver Physiol* 2012;**302**:G397–405.

48. Coates MD, Johnson AC, Greenwood-Van Meerveld B, Mawe GM. Effects of serotonin transporter inhibition on gastrointestinal motility and colonic sensitivity in the mouse. *Neurogastroenterol Motil* 2006;**18**:464–71.

49. Longstreth GF, Thompson WG, Chey WD, Houghton LA, Mearin F, Spiller RC. Functional bowel disorders. *Gastroenterology* 2006;**130**:1480–91.

50. Chang FY, Lu CL, Chen TS. The current prevalence of irritable bowel syndrome in Asia. *J Neurogastroenterol Motil* 2010;**16**: 389–400.

51. Dickhaus B, Mayer EA, Firooz N, Stains J, Conde F, Olivas TI, et al. Irritable bowel syndrome patients show enhanced modulation of visceral perception by auditory stress. *Am J Gastroenterol* 2003;**98**:135–43.

52. Posserud I, Agerforz P, Ekman R, Bjornsson ES, Abrahamsson H, Simren M. Altered visceral perceptual and neuroendocrine response in patients with irritable bowel syndrome during mental stress. *Gut* 2004;**53**:1102–8.

53. Spiller R. Review article: probiotics and prebiotics in irritable bowel syndrome. *Aliment Pharmacol Ther* 2008;**28**:385–96.

54. Tana C, Umesaki Y, Imaoka A, Handa T, Kanazawa M, Fukudo S. Altered profiles of intestinal microbiota and organic acids may be the origin of symptoms in irritable bowel syndrome. *Neurogastroenterol Motil* 2010;**22**(512–519): e114–515.

55. Collins SM, Denou E, Verdu EF, Bercik P. The putative role of the intestinal microbiota in the irritable bowel syndrome. *Dig Liver Dis* 2009;**41**:850–3.

56. Oufir LE, Barry JL, Flourie B, Cherbut C, Cloarec D, Bornet F, et al. Relationships between transit time in man and in vitro fermentation of dietary fiber by fecal bacteria. *Eur J Clin Nutr* 2000;**54**:603–9.

57. Bouin M, Plourde V, Boivin M, Riberdy M, Lupien F, Laganiere M, et al. Rectal distention testing in patients with irritable bowel syndrome: sensitivity, specificity, and predictive values of pain sensory thresholds. *Gastroenterology* 2002;**122**:1771–7.

58. Ohman L, Simren M. Pathogenesis of IBS: role of inflammation, immunity and neuroimmune interactions. *Nature Rev* 2010;**7**:163–73.

59. Kassinen A, Krogius-Kurikka L, Makivuokko H, Rinttila T, Paulin L, Corander J, et al. The fecal microbiota of irritable bowel syndrome patients differs significantly from that of healthy subjects. *Gastroenterology* 2007;**133**:24–33.

60. Madden JA, Hunter JO. A review of the role of the gut microflora in irritable bowel syndrome and the effects of probiotics. *Br J Nutr* 2002;**88**(Suppl. 1):S67–72.

61. Camilleri M. Probiotics and irritable bowel syndrome: rationale, mechanisms, and efficacy. *J Clin Gastroenterol* 2008;**42**(Suppl. 3 Pt 1): S123–5.

62. Saulnier DM, Ringel Y, Heyman MB, Foster JA, Bercik P, Shulman RJ, et al. The intestinal microbiome, probiotics and prebiotics in neurogastroenterology. *Gut Microbes* 2012;**4**.

63. Larauche M, Mulak A, Yuan PQ, Kanauchi O, Tache Y. Stress-induced visceral analgesia assessed non-invasively in rats is enhanced by prebiotic diet. *World J Gastroenterol* 2012;**18**:225–36.

64. Larauche M, Mulak A, Kim YS, Million M, Taché Y. Sex differences in visceral sensitivity induced by repeated psychological stress in rats: differential role of opioid pathway. *Gut* 2010;**59**(Suppl. III) A104(abs).

65. Bailey MT, Dowd SE, Galley JD, Hufnagle AR, Allen RG, Lyte M. Exposure to a social stressor alters the structure of the intestinal microbiota: implications for stressor-induced immunomodulation. *Brain Behav Immun* 2011;**25**:397–407.

66. Forsythe P, Kunze WA, Bienenstock J. On communication between gut microbes and the brain. *Curr Opin Gastroenterol* 2012;**28**:557–62.

67. Asakura H, Suzuki K, Kitahora T, Morizane T. Is there a link between food and intestinal microbes and the occurrence of Crohn's disease and ulcerative colitis? *J Gastroenterol Hepatol* 2008; **23**:1794–801.

68. Benno Y, Endo K, Miyoshi H, Okuda T, Koishi H, Mitsuoka T. Effect of rice fiber on human fecal microflora. *Microbiol immunol* 1989;**33**:435–40.

69. Benno Y, Endo K, Mizutani T, Namba Y, Komori T, Mitsuoka T. Comparison of fecal microflora of elderly persons in rural and urban areas of Japan. *Appl Environ Microbiol* 1989;**55**:1100–5.

70. Kumar A, Henderson A, Forster GM, Goodyear AW, Weir TL, Leach JE, et al. Dietary rice bran promotes resistance to Salmonella enterica serovar Typhimurium colonization in mice. *BMC Microbiol* 2012;**12**:71.

71. Seki T, Nagase R, Torimitsu M, Yanagi M, Ito Y, Kise M, et al. Insoluble fiber is a major constituent responsible for lowering the post-prandial blood glucose concentration in the pre-germinated brown rice. *Biol Pharm Bull* 2005;**28**:1539–41.

72. Wong JM, de Souza R, Kendall CW, Emam A, Jenkins DJ. Colonic health: fermentation and short chain fatty acids. *J Clin Gastroenterol* 2006;**40**:235–43.

73. Verschoyle RD, Greaves P, Cai H, Edwards RE, Steward WP, Gescher AJ. Evaluation of the cancer chemopreventive efficacy of rice bran in genetic mouse models of breast, prostate and intestinal carcinogenesis. *Br J Cancer* 2007;**96**:248–54.

74. Langhorst J, Junge A, Rueffer A, Wehkamp J, Foell D, Michalsen A, et al. Elevated human beta-defensin-2 levels indicate an activation of the innate immune system in patients with irritable bowel syndrome. *Am J Gastroenterol* 2009;**104**:404–10.

75. Ohman L, Isaksson S, Lundgren A, Simren M, Sjovall H. A controlled study of colonic immune activity and beta7+ blood T lymphocytes in patients with irritable bowel syndrome. *Clin Gastroenterol Hepatol* 2005;**3**:980–6.

76. Bercik P, Verdu EF, Collins SM. Is irritable bowel syndrome a low-grade inflammatory bowel disease? *Gastroenterol Clin North Am* 2005;**34**:235–45, vi-vii.

77. Borody TJ, Khoruts A. Fecal microbiota transplantation and emerging applications. *Nature Rev* 2011;**9**:88–96.

78. Spiller R, Lam C. The shifting interface between IBS and IBD. *Curr Opin Pharmacol* 2011;**11**:586–92.

79. Kanauchi O, Nakamura T, Agata K, Mitsuyama K, Iwanaga T. Effects of germinated barley foodstuff on dextran sulfate sodium-induced colitis in rats. *J Gastroenterol* 1998;**33**:179–88.

Chickpea (*Cicer arietinum* L.) Fortification of Cereal-Based Foods to Increase Fiber and Phytochemical Content

Clara Fares, Valeria Menga

Consiglio per la Ricerca e la Sperimentazione in Agricoltura, Cereal Research Centre, Foggia, Italy

INTRODUCTION

Legumes are recognized as the second most important plant source for human and animal foods.[1] They are also the third largest family among the flowering plants, consisting of approximately 650 genera and 20,000 species.[2] Among all of these species only a few are widely cultivated, such as lentils, chickpeas, dry beans, and peas, which are among the most important crops in the world because of their nutritional quality.[3] Legumes are a rich source of complex carbohydrates, proteins, vitamins, and minerals.[4,5] On this basis, some studies are focusing their attention on unexplored or underused legumes, or on those that are concentrated in particular regions of the world, with a view to their potential for the alleviation of hunger in developing countries, and especially for children and pregnant women.[6] Indeed, among the most serious problems in developing countries, protein–energy malnutrition has become critical, and this can be attributed to both an increasing population and an enhanced dependence on a cereal-based diet, due to a reduction in fertile land.[7]

Chickpea (*Cicer arietinum* L.) has great relevance for human nutrition and in livestock industries, where it represents an alternative source of energy and protein.[8] This is a popular crop that grows in tropical, subtropical, and temperate regions around the world. The 2010 world production was 10,918,081 tonnes, with 11,982,140 Ha under harvest. Chickpea is grown mainly in Asia, which has 89% of the total harvested area and 85% of the total world production of chickpea. In particular, the most important grower and the main consumer is India, with 8,210,000 Ha dedicated to its production, which can amount to 7,480,000 tonnes of chickpeas per year (FAOSTAT, http://faostat.fao.org/default.aspx).

Chickpea seeds vary in size, shape, and color.[9] Based on this variation, the chickpea can be classified into two types: "kabuli" and "desi."[10] The kabuli type of chickpea has a thin seed coat that can range in color from white to cream, with a 100-seed weight of 28–70 g. Desi chickpea seeds have a thicker skin and an irregularly shaped seed coat that can range in color from cream, to black, brown, yellow, and green, and contains anthocyanin. Kabuli chickpeas are grown in temperate regions, whereas desi chickpeas are grown in the semi-arid tropics.[11]

The chickpea is an excellent source of nutrients. Kabuli chickpeas contain about 21.3% protein, 5.7% fat, and 60.4 % carbohydrate (75% of which is starch), while desi chickpeas contain about 30% protein, 4.6% fat, and 62.6% carbohydrate (61% of which is starch).[5] Chickpea protein is rich in lysine and arginine, but particularly deficient in sulfur-containing amino acids (i.e., methionine and cysteine).[11] This legume is also a good source of absorbable calcium, phosphorus, magnesium, iron, and potassium.[12] Like all legumes that grow in rotation with other crops, chickpea represents a valuable source of nitrogen for the soil due to its ability to fix nitrogen from the atmosphere. Aslam *et al.*[13] have reported the total nitrogen fixed by a chickpea crop as 74 kg/Ha.

Like all legumes, chickpea turns out to be an excellent source of fiber too. The fiber content of kabuli chickpeas is about 15.4%, while there is much more fiber in the desi chickpeas, at about 24.6%.[5] Chickpea contains both soluble dietary fiber (SDF) and insoluble dietary fiber (IDF), based on its solubility during extraction and isolation.[14] The IDF includes lignin, cellulose, and hemicelluloses, while the SDF includes pectins, β-glucans, galactomanan gums, and a set of non-digestible substances that include inulin and resistant starch.[15] The insoluble fraction of the fiber is related to intestinal regulation, whereas the SDF is associated with a decrease in cholesterol levels and adsorption of glucose in the intestine.[16] A significant component of carbohydrate that acts like SDF is seen in a group of low molecular weight soluble sugars, the α-galactosides. Rincon et al.[17] reported that desi chickpeas have a significantly higher total dietary fiber and IDF than kabuli chickpeas due to the thicker hulls of the desi cultivars. Different domestic processing methods, such as decortication, soaking, fermentation, toasting, and industrial hydrothermal treatments, can remove antinutritional factors and promote the digestibility of chickpea.

The phytochemicals in chickpea are mainly related to the dietary fiber. These compounds are a heterogeneous group of substances that include glucosinolates, a wide group of polyphenols (e.g., flavonoids, phenolic acids, stilbenes, and lignans), and carotenoids. In chickpea, the main phenolic compounds include phenolic acids, flavonols, flavones, isoflavones, anthocyanins, and condensed tannins.[18,19] These phenolics have diverse biological activities, such as antioxidation, apoptosis, anti-aging, anticancer, anti-inflammation, anti-atherosclerosis, and cardiovascular protection. According to Segev et al.,[20] the colored chickpea cultivars (desi) are richer in antioxidant compounds than the cream-colored kabuli chickpeas. The biological functions of the antioxidant compounds arise through their protection of the organism against molecules that are reactive oxygen species (ROS). The production and subsequent protection system against ROS is common to all living species. Under normal conditions, ROS appear as by-products formed as a result of successive single-electron reductions of molecular oxygen (O_2), and include superoxide, hydrogen peroxide, and hydroxyl radicals. The levels of ROS inside a cell are kept low by the relevant protective mechanisms, which include catalase, superoxide dismutase, and peroxidase. However, under certain stress conditions cells can no longer react by producing high amounts of ROS.[21]

Despite all of these relevant characteristics, the chickpea whole seed market has a low commercial value, and therefore any attempt to isolate and or increase the use of these individually components (such as dietary fiber, phytochemicals) in the production of foods will expand the use of this crop. In this context, several studies have focused on how to separate the functional ingredients of chickpea seeds. Xiaoli et al.[22] investigated 19 cultivars of chickpea to evaluate the optimal conditions (solvent, solvent/seed ratio, temperature) for the extraction of the oligosaccharides, which represent a selected substrate for the growth and health of the human gut microflora. In this study, they reported that the optimum conditions to extract these substances were 50% ethanol–water as solvent and a ratio of 10:1 of solvent to defatted flour of the chickpea, at 50°C for 30 minutes. Under these conditions, one of the cultivars among those they examined showed the highest α-galactoside content and a low sucrose content, which represents the most limiting condition in the preparation of high-purity, sucrose-free α-galacto-oligosaccharides (α-GOS). However, to date, the food product applications proposed for chickpea are all related to its use for fiber enrichment of bread and pasta, and for changing the texture of some low-fat pork bologna, and for this reason most of the studies being carried out on this legume are desirable, to take full advantage of its potential.[23]

CARBOHYDRATE AND ANTIOXIDANT PROFILE OF CHICKPEA SEEDS

The chickpea grain is a noted source of carbohydrate, which is represented by starch, the main constituent, and dietary fiber and α-GOS. Starch is the most relevant storage polysaccharide in plants, and it occurs as granules in the chloroplast of green leaves and in the amyloplast of seeds, pulses, and tubers. At the molecular level, starch consists of two main structural components: amylose, in which the linear glucose polymers are linked together by α-D-(1–4) linkages; and amylopectin, which is a branched molecule with α-D-(1–4) linkages and α-D-(1–6) linkages. Amylopectin is more abundant than amylose in starch granules. In particular, starch represents the most relevant fraction in chickpea cotyledons, varing in the range of 30.8% to 37.9% dry matter, in which can be noted trace amounts of protein, ash, and lipid (Table 41.1)[24–27] Differences in the amounts and characteristics of starch have been found in relation to the kabuli and desi chickpea types. The starch granules of chickpea are mostly oval and smooth, and do not have fissures on the surface.[24,25] As reported by Miao et al.,[25] kabuli starch differs from desi starch in several parameters: a higher granule size, a higher yield, a lower amylose content, higher gelatinization parameters, and

TABLE 41.1 Chemical Composition of Chickpea Starch (Kabuli Type)

	Content (g/100 g)	References
Starch	30.8–37.9	Hoover and Ratnayake[24], Singh et al.[27], Miao et al.[25]
Ash	0.05–0.07	Hoover and Ratnayake[24], Singh et al.[27], Miao et al.[25]
Protein	0.1–0.89	Hoover and Ratnayake[24], Singh et al.[27], Miao et al.[25], Huang et al.[26]
Lipid	0.09–0.50	Hoover and Ratnayake[24], Singh et al.[27], Miao et al.[25], Huang et al.[26]
Amylose	23.2–31.8	Hoover and Ratnayake[24], Singh et al.[27], Miao et al.[25]; Huang et al.[26]

higher crystallinity, which in turn might be responsible for the higher value of *in vitro* digestibility of kabuli starch in comparison to desi starch. In any case, both chickpea starches represent foods with a low glycemic index (GI).

According to Englyst et al.,[28] starch can be classified into rapidly digestible starch (RDS), slowly digestible starch (SDS), and resistant starch (RS), based on the rate of glucose released during starch hydrolysis by digestive enzymes. Both SDS and resistant starch have a positive impact on human health. SDS stabilizes glucose metabolism and has a medium to low GI, and thus all of the foods that contain SDS are indicated for people with type 2 diabetes, as it does not produce hyperglycemia followed by hypoglycemia.[29] The GI defines the rate at which the blood glucose increases after an intake of 50 g carbohydrate.[30] The higher the GI, the faster the absorption of carbohydrates, and foods with low GIs are recommended (GI < 55).[31] The resistant starch has been defined as the sum of starches and their degradation products that escape absorption in the small intestine and reach the colon, to be fermented by the microbial flora.[32] The positive effects of these starch fractions on human health will be discussed extensively later.

The α-GOS are low molecular weight, non-reducing sugars that are widespread in the plant kingdom, and they are soluble in water and water–alcohol solutions. These mostly accumulate in the storage organs of plants,[33] where they have protective physiological functions that are associated with drought tolerance and frost resistance,[34] and with germination inhibition under drought conditions.[35] The most abundant α-GOS in chickpea seeds are, in decreasing order: ciceritol, stachyose, raffinose, and verbascose, and their amounts vary from 4.18% to 8.53% (Table 41.2). According to the investigation of 19 chickpea varieties by Xiaoli et al.,[22] there

can be considerable variations in the levels of α-GOS and sucrose, and especially for verbascose, which was only detected in seven varieties. In the various chickpea varieties, the range of variability for α-GOS that has been quoted in the literature is particularly wide: Alajaji and Adawy[36] reported raffinose contents five-fold higher than those reported by Aguilera et al.,[37] while Xiaoli et al.[22] reported double the content of ciceritol with respect to that reported by De Berrios and colleagues.[38] Despite this documented variability, almost all studies have agreed that ciceritol is the most representative α-GOS in chickpea and lentil.[22,39]

These sugars are interesting for the growth of the intestinal bifidobacteria, and as they are not digested they reach the colon intact, where they are substrates for luminal fermentation, which increases the bifidobacteria population in the colon.[40] This occurs due to the lack of the α-galactosidase enzyme in the upper human intestinal tract. This characteristic allows α-GOS to be considered as prebiotics, like resistant starch, and therefore they are considered beneficial for the health of the colon lumen.[41] The positive actions of bifidobacteria in limiting the growth of pathogenic microbes and of other indigenous harmful microflora are due to the production of short-chain fatty acids (SCFAs), seen as mainly acetic acid and lactic acid in a 3:2 molar ratio, and to their production of some antibiotics.[42] The SCFAs are involved in colon physiology through their several actions: attenuation of inflammation processes, proliferation of enterocytes, colorectal carcinogenesis, production of nitrogenous metabolites, and, as indicated above, colonization by pathogens.[43] Moreover, the acidification of the colon lumen as a result of the production of these SCFAs is involved in mineral availability, mainly for Ca and Mg.[44] Interesting, the effects that the SCFAs have on lipid metabolism also result in lower low-density lipoprotein (LDL) cholesterol.[45]

When the α-GOS levels are very high, such as with an intake of >3 g/day,[46] negative factors can prevail over these positive ones in the overall assessment of advantages/disadvantages arising from this consumption of legumes. Indeed, because of the microbial fermentation in the lower intestinal tract, the α-GOS are metabolized with the production of large amounts of carbon dioxide, hydrogen, methane, and SCFAs, which in turn lower the pH.[47] The α-GOS that are most involved in flatus production are raffinose, stachiose, and verbascose. The presence of high levels of these flatus α-GOS in the intestinal tract can result in disorders such as diarrhea and abdominal cramp; moreover, they can decrease the dietary energy and interfere with other nutrients. Among these disorders, flatus production is considered the most important factor that discourages people from eating chickpeas and other pulses. Chickpeas and lentils have lower levels of these α-GOS that are involved in flatus

TABLE 41.2 α-GOS Content in Chickpea Seeds

Component	Content (g/100 g)	References
Sucrose	0.79–3.21	Alajaji-Adawy[36]; Xiaoli et al.[22], Aguilera et al.[37], De J. Berrios et al.[38], Wang et al.[5]
α-GOS:		
Ciceritol	2.69–4.04	Xiaoli et al.[22], Aguilera et al.[37], De J. Berrios et al.[38]
Stachyose	1.14–2.56	Alajaji-Adawy[36], Xiaoli et al.[22], Aguilera et al.[37], De J. Berrios et al.[38], Wang et al.[5]
Raffinose	0.32–1.45	Alajaji-Adawy[36], Xiaoli et al.[22], Aguilera et al.[37], De J. Berrios et al.[38], Wang et al.[5]
Verbascose	0.03–0.48	Alajaji-Adawy[36], Xiaoli et al.[22], Wang et al.[5]

production, as these pulses have the highest levels of cic-eritol,[46] whereas Peterbauer and Richter[48] demonstrated that this is more slowly hydrolyzable by α-galactosidase than the other α-GOS.

Processing of the chickpea is considered to be a standard way to decrease these flatulence-causing factors, and can be summarized as the following methods: soaking, cooking, germination, fermentation, and addition of the α-galactosidase enzyme. As the α-GOS are water soluble, it is relatively easy to remove a large amount of these sugars by soaking the chickpeas and discarding this water. This process is standard in domestic preparation of chickpeas and other legume seeds. The effectiveness of soaking depends on several factors, such as the water:seed ratio, length of time,[49] temperature, addition of salt to the water, and also legume species and variety.[50] According to studies by Vidal-Valverde et al.,[51] about 1–10% of the release of these water-soluble sugars can be ascribed to the leaching process, while the remaining loss can be attributed to the metabolic processes that are triggered in the soaking seeds. The effects of soaking on the mineral content of legume and cereal seeds have been investigated, and, according to the report of Lestienne et al.,[49] this treatment is not a good method for improving mineral bioavaibility. Alajaji and El-Adawy[37] observed that both traditional and microwave cooking are effective in reducing α-GOS. Indeed, in their study there was a loss of 35% of the sucrose, 47% of the raffinose, 41% of the stachiose, and all of the verbascose, compared to their levels in raw chickpea. They thus hypothesized that the loss occurred through diffusion and leaching into the boiling water.

Germination has also been shown to be effective in reducing the levels of α-GOS by up to 100%, through the release of α-galactosidase.[52] Fermentation is also a domestic way to reduce the α-GOS, which are hydrolyzed by the bacterial α-galactosidase. A study conducted by Zamora and Fields[53] showed that with the natural fermentation of chickpea seeds, the prevalence of lactic bacteria was responsible for the reduction in α-GOS levels, as these bacteria only use oligosaccharides for their growth. Naturally, depending on the Lactobacillus strains adopted, it is possible to modulate the quality and quantity of this α-GOS reduction, although it was indicated that natural fermentation is more effective compared to controlled fermentation by selected bacterial strains.[54,55] The removal of α-GOS through the addition of α-galactosidase from different sources (e.g., Aspergillus spp.) has been reported as a good tool for the food industry to obtain complete hydrolysis of all of the sugars involved in flatulence production.[56,57]

Genetic manipulation of α-GOS levels has also been reported as an effective method for their removal, and Kerr et al.[58] patented the inhibition of galactinol synthase activity. However, due to the physiological importance

of the α-GOS during seed development and storage, Griga et al.[59] suggested the activation of α-galactosidase to degrade α-GOS after harvesting, or by the transfer of α-galactosidase from a thermophilic bacterium in the grain legumes (e.g., Thermotoga neapolitana). This bacterium has its optimum temperature near to 100°C, and can be activated during food processing. An alternative way suggested by Frías et al.[60] was a reduction in the α-GOS levels through promotion of the synthesis of related compounds, such as the galactosyl cyclitols, and in this way maintaining the protective nature of these compounds while decreasing their flatus potential, as ciceritol is more slowly hydrolyzed by α-galactosidase than the other α-GOS.

Dietary Fiber

Dietary fiber encompasses a mixture of indigestible polysaccharides (e.g., cellulose, hemicelluloses, oligosaccharides, pectins, gums), lignin, and waxes. Recently, the American Association of Cereal Chemists provided a definition of dietary fiber that perhaps best describes its physiological role. According to this definition, dietary fiber is:[61]

> the edible parts of plants of analogous carbohydrates that are resistant to digestion and absorption in the human intestine with complete or partial fermentation in the large intestine. Dietary fiber includes polysaccharides, oligosaccharides, lignin, and associated plant substances. Dietary fiber promotes beneficial physiological effects, including laxation, and/or cholesterol attenuation, and/or blood glucose attenuation.

Dietary fiber is classified into IDF and SDF, according to their different physiological roles. IDF primarily promotes the transit of fecal bulk, improves laxation, and promotes colon health by enhancing the growth of the gut microflora (acting as prebiotics). SDF is involved in the control of glucose and lipids.[62]

Strong epidemiological and experimental data have shown that an increased consumption of SDF has a strong effect on the lowering of multiple risk factors for cardiovascular disease (CVD). Under the term of syndrome X, several risk factors have been clustered together – dyslipidemia, hypertension, and hyperglycemia – and Reaven[63] postulated that insulin resistance underlies the increase in this disease, which was later defined as metabolic syndrome.[64] In this context, the effects of the SDF of legumes, cereals, and vegetables have been studied, and the potential synergies between SDF and other phytochemicals for lowering the risk of the metabolic syndrome have been widely reviewed.[65]

The total dietary fiber content of chickpea varies from about 15% to 23%, although large differences have been reported for the ratio between IDF and SDF. Between the studies of Martin-Cabrejas et al.[66] and Wang et al.,[67] this ratio was very similar (13:1 and 11:1, respectively), while the greatest differences were seen between the studies of Fares and Menga[19] and Aguilera et al.[37] (3:1 and 21:1, respectively). This range of variability might be attributable to the kernel size, as the major difference between the cotyledon fibers and the hulls is in the concentration of cellulose, lignin, and hemicellulose, which are typically of the cell wall.[68] Similar observations were reported by Wang et al.,[67] who stated that large-sized seeds have a lower proportion of hull to cotyledon in the ratio between the surface to the volume, and therefore larger chickpea seeds show less IDF than small-sized seeds. Several processing conditions can also alter this ratio, and will be treated extensively in the next sections.

Phytochemicals

Legume seeds contain a large variety of phytochemicals, which are molecules that are involved in several biological functions, and in which great interest has arisen over the past few years for their use as a natural source of these compounds.[69,70] Phenolic compounds are the most typical phytochemicals, and in legumes they are represented by the specific chemical structures of the isoflavonoids and 5-deoxyisoflavonoids.[71] In plants, these compounds have pivotal roles both in the defense against pathogens and as chemical signals in symbiotic nitrogen fixation. Antioxidants can be classified into three main categories according to their origin and their structural characteristics: endogenous antioxidants present in enzymatic systems (e.g., isozymes of catalase, superoxide dismutase, peroxidise); non-enzymatic antioxidants that can be endogenous (e.g., selenoprotein, glutathione) or exogenous (e.g., vitamins, carotenoids, polyphenols); and exogenous non-enzymatic antioxidants, which are secondary antioxidants of the chain-breaking type, as they block free radicals from becoming less reactive radicals.

There are numerous methodologies for the extraction and quantification of antioxidants in foods. Different solvent systems have been tested for the extraction of antioxidants from legumes, including water; aqueous mixtures of ethanol, methanol, and acetone;[72,73] absolute methanol and ethanol;[74] and 80% acidified methanol.[19,75] However, according to Xu and Chang,[76] who carried out a comparative study on the phenolic profiles and antioxidant activities of various legumes using six solvent systems, the best extraction solvents for the total phenolic compounds, total flavonoids content, and antioxidant activities from chickpea are 50% acetone, 80% acetone, and 70% ethanol, respectively. The extraction methods also greatly influence subsequent analyses. Table 41.3 shows data from recent studies on the total phenolic compounds, phenolic acids, flavonoids, and proanthocyanidins. Here, comparison among these data can cause problems, as the concentrations are often very different.

According to Pirisi et al.,[78] who studied the phenolic compounds in olive oil, these discrepancies depended on the various analytical methods and on the use of different standard equivalent units chosen for the calibration curves. Indeed, various different standards are used to quantify the results from colorimetric measurements, and as these standards can have different numbers of active hydroxyl groups, the responses will be different – and this, in turn, will provide different results.[79]

For the total phenolics, the variability ranges from 0.2 mg catechins eq/g[20] to 3.04 mg/g.[75] This variability was previously noted by Bravo,[80] who reported a total phenolic content in chickpea of 0.78–2.3 mg/g. The study by Segev et al.[20] reported that more than 95% of the total phenolic content and total flavonoid content is concentrated in the seed coat, and that the colored desi chickpea seeds contain more antioxidants than the kabuli chickpea. The levels of these compounds in the colored seeds, with respect to the cream-colored kabuli seeds, showed up to 13-fold, 11-fold, and 31-fold greater total phenolic content, total flavonoid content, and antioxidant activity, respectively.

Some studies have also highlighted differences between the free phenolic compounds that are more readily available, and the bound phenolic compounds that are acid esterified to the cell walls, showing that the free fraction is more represented in the chickpea compared to other legumes.[19,81] As reported by Han and Baik,[81] both the free and the bound fractions of the phytochemicals are located in the cotyledons, as removing the coats does not significantly change the antioxidant activities detected in decorticated seeds, in comparison to raw seeds. Specific phenolic compounds have been described for the chickpea too, as shown in Table 41.3: the phenolic acids, flavonoids, and proanthocyanidins. The phenolic acids (or phenolcarboxylic acids) are organic compounds that contain at least one phenolic hydroxyl group and a carboxyl group. These are divided into two groups, the benzoic acid derivatives and cinnamic acid derivatives, both of which act as antioxidants. According to Fares and Menga,[19] the phenolic acid content in chickpea seed is 43.06 μg/g.

Flavonoids, including the flavones, flavanols, and condensed tannins, are recognized for their ability to counteract oxidative stress. In particular, the condensed tannins (or proanthocyanidins) have an important role in seed defense systems.[82] The mean total flavonoid content in chickpea seeds is lower compared to soybean, lentil, and the common bean.[18] Also, for the proanthocyanidins, the amounts detected are strongly influenced both by the extraction system and by the cultivar. This is indicated by the range of data reported in Table 41.3, which for the catechins covers from 0.05 mg CAE/g to 1.85 mg CAE/g, as reported by Xu and Chang,[76] who tested six solvents in their investigation. According to

TABLE 41.3   Total Phenolics, Phenolic Acids, Flavonoids, Proanthocyanidins and Antioxidant Activity of Raw Chickpea

Compound	Content	Unit	Method	Reference(s)
Total phenolics				
	2.2	mg/g		Han and Baik[81]
	0.2–6.8	mg catechins eq/g		Segev et al.[20]
	1.41–1.67	mg gallic acid eq/g		Xu and Chang[76,89]
	0.87	mg ferulic acid eq/g		Fares and Menga[19]
	2.79–3.04	mg/g		Martin-Cabrejas et al.[75]
Phenolic acids				
	43.06	µg/g		Fares and Menga[19]
Flavonoid				
	0.1–1.08	mg catechins eq/g		Segev et al.[20]
	0.18–3.16	mg catechins eq/g		Xu and Chang[76]
Proanthocyanidins				
	0.05–1.85	mg catechins eq/g		Xu and Chang[76]
	1.96–2.19	mg/g		Martin-Cabrejas et al.[75]
Antioxidant activity				
	1.23	µmol trolox equivalent/g	LDL	Xu et al.[18]
	0.73–1.13	µmol trolox equivalent/g	FRAP	Xu and Chang[76]
	16.48	µmol trolox equivalent/g	ABTS	Fares and Menga[19]
	18.66	µmol trolox equivalent/g	ORAC	Halvorsen et al., 2002[77]
	5.13–34.66	µmol trolox equivalent/g	ORAC	Xu and Chang[76,89]
	0.30–3.68	µmol trolox equivalent/g	DPPH	Xu and Chang[75,89]

Martin-Cabrejas,[75] who tested two Spanish chickpea varieties, Castellano and Sinlao, the range was from 1.96 mg/g to 2.19 mg/g.

Existing methods for the identification of the antioxidant properties in vitro are numerous, and, again, each method has its own specificity. These can largely be divided into two types, depending on their scavenging of ROS or of non-biological stable radicals. The ROS scavengers more closely reflect what actually happens in a biological system (i.e., oxygen radical absorbance capacity, LDL), while use of the second type of scavenger is easier and faster as a laboratory routine (2,2′-azinobis[3-ethylbenzothiazoline-6-sulphonic acid] [ABTS], 2,2-diphenyl-1-picrylhydrazyl [DPPH], ferric-reducing antioxidant power [FRAP]). In any case, all of these assays assess the activity of a scavenger against radicals in the foods tested. Table 41.3 shows the results of studies on antioxidants that were performed using several analytical methods, and, as can clearly be seen, different methods with different reaction mechanisms can lead to different results.[76] For this reason, as these measurements are antioxidant system-dependent, the simultaneous use of several methodologies is preferable to provide a more complete picture of the antioxidant properties of the system tested. However, all of these studies are in agreement, in terms that the chickpea can be considered a "functional" food due to its high antioxidant activity. Indeed, in a comparative study among legumes, Xu et al.[18] showed that a cream chickpea variety has an antioxidant activity (as measured using DPPH) that is comparable to those of soybean and green pea varieties.

In terms of human health, these compounds can have protective effects when their dietary intake is consistent.[83] They have several biological properties, acting as an antioxidant, modulating enzyme detoxification, stimulating the immune system, decreasing platelet aggregation, and modulating hormone metabolism.[84] In general, antioxidants are defined as "any substance that is present in low concentrations compared to an oxidizable substrate, and is able to slow or inhibit the oxidation of the substrate."[85] In this way, oxidizable substrates, such as lipids, proteins, and DNA, are protected from oxidation, and thus remain stable. Several reports have indicated that these molecules are involved in the prevention of several degenerative diseases, through the protection of the tissues against oxidative stress.[86]

Recently, Henry-Vitrac et al.[87] reported that the soybean isoflavones (daidzein, daidzin, genistein, genistin, equol) can have potent anti-amyloidogenic activities *in vitro* in Alzheimer disease. They showed that the aglycones and equol (the major metabolite of daidzein) can inhibit fibril formation by up to 30%, which demonstrates that soy isoflavone might have a nutritional value for the prevention of the pathophysiology of Alzheimer disease.

TECHNOLOGICAL PROCESSES TO IMPROVE THE CHICKPEA NUTRITIONAL PROFILE

Technological food processes are useful tools to improve the flavor and palatability of legumes. In this way, starch gelatinization and protein denaturation occurs, which is accompanied by seed softening.[9] Such treatments are important for the reduction of some antinutritional substances, too, such as the condensed tannins that inhibit the digestibility of protein and phytic acid, which reduce the bioavailability of some essential minerals,[88] and also to modify the starch and fiber content, including the α-GOS.

Cooking encompass the traditional boiling process, pressure cooking, and microwave cooking, and this is the widest way to process legumes, with the promotion of several changes in the physical characteristics and chemical compositions of the dry legumes.[89] However, a lot of other thermal processes can be used to enhance the nutritional characteristics of legumes, such as toasting,[19,90] extrusion cooking technology,[38] dehydration,[66] and new technology to extract or reduce the α-GOS.[46,91] Pre-cooking processes (e.g., dehulling/abrading, soaking) can also be useful for the reduction of some antinutritional factors and improvement of the organoleptic characteristics of chickpea.

The effectiveness of the cooking process will depend on the size, composition, and structure of the legume seed,[92] and therefore pretreatments such as dehulling or abrading affect the cooking properties, as reported by Otto and colleagues.[93] This technology changes the composition and structure of the seed due to the different distributions of the various substances within the seed itself. According to Klamczynska et al.,[92] who investigated the chemical composition of legume cotyledons of chickpea, with wrinkled peas and smooth peas, the largest change in seed composition was as a result of progressive abrasion, and these chemical changes differed among the species and among the cultivars of the same species due to their different proportions of seed coat. A general decrease in protein content and an increase in starch suggested that this legume has a higher protein content in the outer layer, while the higher starch content is in the inner portion of the seed. However, no relevant changes were observed by Han and Baik[81] for the antioxidant properties of chickpea after removing the coat of the raw seed, both in the free and bound fractions, which suggests that the hull of chickpea is not a good source of phytochemicals.

Prior to cooking, soaking is the preliminary step that helps to increase the tissue texture, shorten the cooking time, and further reduce the hardness of the seed.[89] During soaking there is a significant decrease in the content of all of the soluble sugars, with a decrease in the α-GOS highlighted of about 25% by Martin-Cabrejas et al.[66] and of about 27% by Frías et al.[94] This has been attributed to both leaching and activation of metabolic processes in the soaking seeds. According to Frías et al.,[94] the starch content also decreases with soaking, in relation to the solution used and the type of legume considered; in particular, they noted that in chickpea the decrease in the starch content was about 20–21%. Martin-Cabrejas et al.[66] reported an increase of about 10% in the IDF after the soaking process. Finally, a decrease in the phenolic compounds in legumes such as beans, peas, lentils, and chickpea has been reported,[95] although Xu and Chang[89] showed that only in chickpea and peas does the loss observed in the total phenolic content decrease with increases in the hydration rate. This finding was hypothesized to be due to the longer soaking time, which allows the cotyledons to absorb a lot of the phenolics that are lost into the soaking water. According to Han and Baik,[81] in chickpea there is no change in the antioxidant activity of the bound fraction, while the free fraction is increased.

An alternative technological process to improve the nutritional quality and obtain edible products with good sensorial characteristics is fermentation. Reyes-Moreno et al.[96] tested a solid-state fermentation process for producing chickpea "tempeh" flour, a traditional fermented food that is usually produced with different strains of the fungus *Rhizopus* spp. for fermenting boiled and dehulled soybean. This treatment increased the protein content of chickpea, and simultaneously decreased the lipids and ash. Reyes-Moreno et al.[96] thus argued that, in a first step, the protein increase was due to the dehulling and leaching of the solid material during this treatment, as previously reported in other studies.[97] After the fermentation, this was related to an increase in the fungus biomass, with the fat reduction attributed to the use of the fatty acids as an energy source by the fungus. In addition, the phytic acid content decreased in parallel with an increase in fermentation time, due to the phytase activity of the *Rhizopus*.

Seed germination also finds applications in the production of novel foods that are thereby more digestible for people who prefer to eat only vegetables. The germination process is widely used to enhance the nutritive value of legumes, by inducing the formation of enzymes that eliminate or reduce the antinutritional and indigestible factors, like trypsin inhibitor, phytic acid, tannins, and α-GOS.[98] Indeed, during germination, a multitude of chemical changes occurs that mobilizes the stored carbohydrates, free amino acids, and essential nutrients, which results in more useful forms for human metabolism.[99] El-Adaway[100] studied the effects of germination on chickpea seed and reported an increase in the crude protein, non-protein nitrogen, and crude fiber due to the degradation of the seed components to simple peptides, while a decrease in the fat and total carbohydrate content was attributed to their use as an energy source during germination. Moreover, according to El-Adawy,[100] germination is more effective for a reduction in α-GOS, and especially raffinose and stachyose, and is more efficient in the retention of minerals and B vitamins, when compared with cooking. Ghavidel and Prakash[101] also reported a significant effect of germination on the bioavailability of chickpea nutrients, antinutrients, and minerals. A positive effect was seen for protein content, thiamine, bioavailable iron, and calcium, while there was a reduction in the SDF and in phytic acid and tannins.

The cooking and thermal processing of chickpea results in improved protein quality and overall nutritional quality. The traditional cooking after soaking of chickpea leads to a reduction in the total soluble sugars of 36%, and in particular in sucrose and ciceritol.[66] Similarly, Frías et al.[94] showed a minimal decrease in the starch after cooking, with respect to the soaked seed, with a much larger reduction in the available sugars and α-GOS, the reduction of which ranged from 45% to 58%. According to the literature, the elimination of these sugars is connected with the removal of the soaking and cooking solutions.[36] Wang et al.[67] reported a significant increase in both the SDF and IDF in boiled cooked chickpea, compared to raw samples, which was probably due to the protein–fiber complexes formed after all of the chemical modifications caused by the cooking process. Changes in the structure of the cell wall and the storage polysaccharides also occurred, which, in turn, reduces the solubility of the dietary fiber. The increase in the resistant starch content that is seen results from retrogradation of starch after gelatinization.[4] Boiling is generally regarded as a destructive process for antioxidant compounds, and Xu and Chang[89] reported a reduction of 85–95% in free radical scavenging (with DPPH) of cooked seeds, a reduction of 56–69% in the oxygen radical absorbance capacity, and a reduction in the total phenolic compounds too; these losses showed an increasing tendency with the extension of the cooking time. Han and Baik[81] showed a reduction in free radical scavenging using DPPH for free phytochemicals, while they saw no significant changes in antioxidant activity for bound

phytochemicals. This decrease in the antioxidant activity of the free phytocheminals was attributed to a loss of the soluble antioxidant compounds during the cooking.

An alternative cooking method to the traditional one is pressure boiling, and, according to Xu and Chang,[89] there are significant differences between standard and pressure boiling of chickpea in terms of its antioxidant properties. They showed that when measured as the oxygen radical absorbance capacity, the antioxidant properties were significantly increased in the case of pressure boiling, as compared to the respective original unprocessed chickpea. This finding might be due to the formation of novel compounds, such as Maillard reaction products, which have antioxidant activity.[102] De Almeida Costa et al.[103] reported that the combination of pressure boiling with freeze-drying leads to a small increase in the nutrient levels (about 10% for the IDF), with the exception of the resistant starch, which was probably due to their method of analysis, as this was not designed to estimate the changes in the resistant starch. Daur et al.[90] instead studied the nutritional quality of pressure cooked chickpea, and highlighted a general deterioration of all of its nutritional characteristics, compared to the raw seed.

Among the hydrothermal processes used to obtain a more tender product, there is also microwave cooking, a method that can replace traditional cooking. Esmat et al.[3] showed that microwave cooking decreases the protein, fat, and ash, with respect to the raw chickpea, similar to traditional cooking, but it also led to an increase in the crude fiber of about 51.9%, with respect to the 40% with traditional cooking. In addition, microwave cooking was useful to reduce the α-GOS and antinutritional factors, similar to conventional cooking. Alajaji and El-Adawy[36] observed a smaller loss of riboflavin, thiamine, niacin, and pyridoxine with microwave cooking compared to standard boiling, and the same was seen for the mineral content, which retained to a greater degree by microwave cooking with respect to traditional cooking. It is therefore quite clear that microwave cooking is useful not only for saving time and energy, but also for obtaining a nutritionally better product.

Toasting or roasting represents another way to change the chemical composition and texture of chickpea, and this consists of heating a substance to a high temperature, of over 100°C, for a specific period of time. Fares and Menga[19] adopted this method to evaluate the carbohydrate and antioxidant modifications that can occur in chickpea flour, and they evaluated the effects of partial replacement of semolina with toasted chickpea flour on the nutritional and cooking quality of pasta. Here, the protein content increased from 23.4% in the raw chickpea to 26.5% in the toasted chickpea, with increases also in the resistant starch and IDF. The increase in IDF might also be attributable to Maillard reaction products. These products, in turn, result in an increase in the phenolics and antioxidant activity of toasted chickpea, which are always higher for the free fraction, as compared to the bound fraction. In addition, it is very interesting to note that with toasting there was a reduction in the starch, with a lowering of the GI of this novel chickpea flour. These data indicate that chickpea toasting induces significant changes in the carbohydrate and antioxidant profiles of the resulting flours, enhancing the overall nutritional profile, and that it is possible to use this flour to improve the nutritional characteristics of pasta.

Toasted chickpea is used as an ingredient in the preparation of ethnic foods, such as "leblebi," as studied by Koksel and colleagues.[104] In leblebi production, chickpea seeds are subjected to three sequential heat treatments that are performed at around 75°C for several minutes. After the first and second heat treatments the chickpeas are allowed to rest in 3-cm thick layers for 5 days, and after the third heat treatment they are left for 1 month. Following these heat treatments, water is added slowly to increase the moisture content by 10%, and after a rest period of several hours the husks become detached from the cotyledons. The dehulled chickpeas are reheated to approximately 50°C for 5 minutes, rested for 2 days, and then roasted for 3 minutes at 130°C. This process substantially increased the porosity of the chickpeas and decreased the stiffness, in comparison to raw seeds. Koksel et al.[104] also highlighted that the physical properties induced by the roasting process improved the organoleptic and nutritional goodness of the new product.

More recently, a new technology has been spreading that provides added value for new legume-based foods: extrusion cooking. This represents an ideal method for manufacturing a number of food products, ranging from snacks and breakfast cereals to baby food. However, as this is a complex multivariate process, it requires careful control if the product quality is to be maintained. Extrusion cooking can be described as a process whereby moistened starchy and/or proteinaceous material is cooked and worked into a viscous, plastic-like dough. This physical treatment combines heating of the food products with the extrusion process, which can be described as the shaping of a material by forcing it through a specially designed opening (die). These processes are designed to increase the beneficial effects of the heating and to reduce its detrimental effects, to create fully cooked, shelf-stable food products with enhanced textural attributes and flavor.[38] According to De Berrios et al.,[38] extruded chickpea has lower concentrations of total available carbohydrate with respect to the raw flour, and this is believed to be due to the transformation of the starch and other polysaccharides into lower molecular weight compounds that can, in turn, form Amadori compounds (derivatives of aminodeoxysugars formed as part of the Maillard reaction) and other compounds. As a consequence of the temperature used, the oligosaccharide content decreased, probably because the $2 \rightarrow 1$-furanosidic bonds in sucrose and raffinose can be broken during extrusion cooking and the formation of lower molecular weight sugars.[105]

Industrial dehydration has been tested as a feasible method for the processing of chickpea, which improves the nutritional characteristics of chickpea and makes the seeds ready-to-use in special foods for specific consumers. According to Martin-Cabrejas et al.,[66] who tested soaking, traditional cooking, and dehydration, this treatment produces the greatest reductions in the SDF of chickpea, of about 53%, and in particular of about 56% for stachiose and raffinose, the sugars that are primarily responsible for the associated flatulence. This process thus transforms the chickpea into a food that can be used by people with digestive problems. Finally, it is important to note that, according to Martin-Cabrejas et al.,[66] positive effects are also observed for the fiber content, which is increased in both the SDF and IDF.

Chickpea is nourishing, and has excellent nutritional value, with the use of domestic and/or industrial processes enhancing these features. For example, discarding the water solutions after the soaking and cooking of chickpea represents an excellent technique to greatly decrease the concentrations of α-GOS and almost all of the antinutritional factors. It is also clear that each process used modifies the organoleptic and chemical compositions of chickpea in a different way. In this regard, the choice of one technique rather than another can be very useful to preserve all of the nutritional substances – for example, the use of microwaves instead of traditional cooking to retain more of the vitamins and minerals.

However, new technologies, such as toasting, industrial dehydration, and cooking extrusion, are perhaps the most effective for the overall improvement of the organoleptic and nutritional value of the chickpea, thus turning it into a functional food too, which is much more useful for human health.

CHICKPEA FLOUR IN CEREAL-BASED PRODUCTS

Through the increase in medical and scientific knowledge, consumers are becoming strongly interested in understanding the relationships between diet and disease and have become more interested in the composition of their foods. In this context, research on functional foods has focused on the possibility of fortifying cereal-based products, such as durum wheat pasta and bakery products, through the addition of raw materials of vegetable origin in order to increase the protein nutritional value, dietary fiber, and mineral content.[106,107] Bearing in mind that pasta and bakery products are staple and cheap foods that have key roles in the human diet, the dietary intake of substances beneficial to health through the consumption of these products should help to reduce the incidence of diseases typical of developed countries, such as metabolic syndrome and cancer. This would thus significantly reduce the national health costs for the treatment of these widespread diseases in a population that is growing both in terms of a longer life and a less healthy lifestyle (e.g., excessive consumption of food, sedentary lifestyle).

Pasta itself is recognized as a healthy food with a low fat content, no cholesterol, and a low GI,[108] with the capability of carrying "nutraceutical" substances[104] with antioxidant activities.[109] According to the study of Goni and Valentin-Gamazo,[110] pasta with the addition of 25% raw chickpea flour results in increased protein, fat, and mineral content, and a significantly lower GI, than pasta made with only durum wheat semolina. Interestingly, the GI of the pasta with chickpea and the pasta control were in the normal ranges for slowly digestible carbohydrate, but the GI was significantly lower in the case of the pasta with added chickpea flour. Both types of pasta showed lower starch hydrolysis with respect to bread. The use of chickpea flour, both toasted and raw, in the production of durum wheat pasta was evaluated in the study of Fares and Menga:[19] with 20% toasted chickpea as a flour replacement, the protein content, resistant starch, and total dietary fiber increased proportionally with the percentage of chickpea flour added, and by the greatest amounts with the addition of toasted chickpea flour. An increase in the phenolic acids was also seen, and this was attributed to the positive effects due to the inclusion of the chickpea flour, which had a good supply of free phenolic acids. Therefore, Fares and Menga[19] hypothesized that the toasting process can further reduce the caloric intake of chickpea flour, as indicated by the resistant starch and IDF increase, and the reduction in the available sugars. These in turn might be responsible for reduced effects on the postprandial blood glucose response, while providing a wider range of low-GI foods for consumers.

On the other hand, in Brazil and India, chickpea-based food snacks have been developed to help prevent malnutrition in young children.[111] Thus, for all of the favorable properties described above, chickpea is considered an ideal complement to cereals in a healthy diet, for both developed and developing countries.

Despite the broad consensus in the scientific community about the positive effects on nutritional enhancement of cereal-based products through the inclusion of chickpea flour (raw or processed), the data concerning the effects of chickpea flour addition on the organoleptic properties of pasta and bakery products are controversial. Among the favorable characteristics, among the legumes, chickpea has few "beany" flavors, and also for this reason it is the preferred ingredient for improvement of cereal-based products. Apart from the flavor, any negative effects on the organoleptic properties of pasta will certainly be related to the form of the addition, such as if the chickpea flour is produced from dehulled or whole seeds. The dehulling process of chickpea seeds is effective in increasing the cooking quality of chickpea-enriched pasta, as shown in the study by Wood,[112] while the inclusion of whole seed flour decreases the cooking behavior due to dilution of the gluten network by the non-gluten flour.[19,113] Wood[112] showed that chickpea-fortified spaghetti has a lower cooking loss and less stickiness than durum wheat control spaghetti. This behavior was shown to be related to both the increased protein content and the non-starch polysaccharides due to the fortification with dehulled chickpea. Thus, the reduced cooking loss was associated with the increase in the protein–polysaccharide matrix, which prevented the loss of amylose during cooking, while the reduced stickiness of the fortified spaghetti was attributed to the high amylose content of the chickpea flour. Another relevant finding relates to the industrial application of pre-cooked foods, as spaghetti fortified with dehulled chickpea retains its firmness after refrigeration much better than with just durum wheat. This opens up a new market if this food is subjected to canning and microwave re-heating.

Sabanis and colleagues[113] studied the effects of the inclusion of up to 50% raw chickpea flour in durum wheat lasagna, and showed that the nutritional value of the pasta increased with the level of fortification, but the cooking characteristics deteriorated with higher levels of substitution. Fares and Menga[19] studied four levels of replacement with raw and toasted whole seed chickpea flour (5%, 10%, 15%, and 20%), and stated that while the protein and total dietary fiber increased according to the chickpea substitution, the total organic matter, which is a measure of the overall cooking behavior, worsened. Therefore, for the overall acceptability of chickpea-fortified durum wheat pasta, the threshold levels of replacement with chickpea flour appear to be acceptable up to 20% if the flour is obtained from coated seeds,[19,113,114] or up to 50% with dehulled seeds.[112] Similarly, Gomez et al.[115] studied the effects of chickpea flours (with and without their coats) and the varietal influence on cake quality. Here, they showed that it is feasible to use chickpea flours to totally or partially replace wheat flour in the preparation of layer and sponge cakes. In this study, they also showed that dehulled chickpea flour produced higher and softer cakes than those produced with whole chickpea flour, and a varietal influence was also observed.

The impact of chickpea inclusion in the formulation of bread has also been studied. Two recent studies have been carried out by Yamsaengsun et al.[116] and Hefnawy and colleagues.[117] The first of these studies[116] stated that the addition of whole seed chickpea flour increased crumb firmness and slightly decreased the bread volume, for both white and whole wheat breads. Moreover, they investigated the effects of this inclusion on the bread color parameters, and found that chickpea substitution increased the yellowness and darkness of white bread, while the color parameters of whole wheat bread were not affected. The second of these two studies[117] investigated the impact of partial and total replacement of wheat flour by whole seed chickpea flour on the quality characteristics of toasted bread. They found that the addition of 15% and 30% chickpea flour decreased the volume of the bread, but that the toasted bread produced had acceptable characteristics in terms of weight, volume, texture, and crumb structure, comparable to those of the bread control. Chickpea flour obtained from dehulled seeds has been tested in the preparation of chapattis, a steam leavened flat bread that is popular in India. Here, Kadam et al.[118] evaluated the use of different sources of commodities to make good-quality chapattis, and they reported that wheat flour with 20% dehulled chickpea flour was the best blend to obtain chapattis with the same taste as the control.

Chickpea flour has also been used in the preparation of extruded foods, such as snacks. In the first studies that were carried out by Battistuti et al.,[119] it was confirmed that the most acceptable chickpea snack was actually rated higher than a commercial corn snack. Chavez-Jauregui et al.[111] added bovine lung to chickpea flour and stated that these new snacks had improved nutritional quality and the same acceptability as commercial brands. Similar results were obtained in a prior study by Cardoso-Santiago and Arêas,[120] who also stated that a 30-g pack of a snack with a 10% blend of chickpea and bovine lung can provide up to 30% of the recommended daily allowance for iron.

The use of composite flours containing wheat or other cereal sources and pulses is increasing in several countries throughout the world, with the production of a wide range of products with excellent organoleptic and enhanced nutritional properties. In the current literature, there is evidence concerning the formulation of functional cereal products through the addition of raw chickpea flour and/or chickpea flour modified by treatments aimed at increasing its nutritional compounds (e.g., fiber, antioxidants). Among all of these, pasta and bakery products have attracted the attention of a number of studies, as this now appears to be an appropriate way to produce high-quality and inexpensive foods, and to increase the market supply of new foods for consumers.

CONCLUSIONS

According to a wide study conducted by Kalogeropoulos et al.[70] on the most widely consumed legumes, the dietary intake of macronutrients and micronutrients by the consumption of one serving of cooked dry legume (125 g) was particularly impressive. For cooked chickpea, Kalogeropoulos et al.[70] reported that this provides about 11.6% protein, 3.7% carbohydrate, 5.8% fat, 9.8% phytosterols, and over 100% dietary fiber (the daily intake recommended by the USDA Food Guide is 31 g dietary fiber, and this chickpea serving supplies 40.7 g dietary fiber). Therefore, without loading consumers with calories, chickpea represents a notable source of dietary fiber and phytochemicals. Another factor that has an important role in this food choice is seen in its preparation. Social changes have significantly modified the timing and methods of meal preparation, so much so that today people prefer products that are ready and quick to cook. Therefore, the idea of cereal-based products that include processed chickpea represents an attempt to optimize the development of a unique meal that can be guaranteed to support a healthy and balanced diet.

References

1. Vietmeyer ND. Lesser-known plants of potential use in agriculture and forestry. *Science* 1986;**232**:1379–84.
2. Doyle JJ. Phylogeny of the legume family: an approach to understanding the origins of nodulation. *Ann Rev Ecol Syst* 1994;**25**:325–49.
3. Esmat AAA, Helmy IMF, Barch GF. Nutritional Evaluation and functional Properties of Chickpea (*Cicer arietinum* L.) Flour and the improvement of Spaghetti Produced from its. *J Am Sci* 2010;**6**:1055–72.
4. Costa GE, Queiroz-Monici K, Reis S, Oliveira AC. Chemical composition, dietary fiber and resistant starch contents of raw and coke pea, common bean, chickpea and lentil legumes. *Food Chem* 2006;**84**:48–55.
5. Wang X, Gao W, Zhang J, Zhang H, Li J, He X, et al. Subunit, amino acid composition and *in vitro* digestibility of protein isolates from Chinese kabuli and desi chickpea (*Cicer arietinum* L.) cultivars. *Food Res Int* 2010;**43**:567–72.
6. Arinathan V, Mohan VR, De Britto AJ. Chemical composition of certain tribal pulses. *Int J Food Sci Nutr* 2003;**54**:209–17.
7. FAO. *Food Insecurity: when people live with hunger and fear starvation.* Rome, Italy: FAO; 2000.
8. Bampidisa VA, Christodouloub V. Chickpeas (*Cicer arietinum* L.) in animal nutrition: A review. *Anim Feed Sci and Tech* 2011;**168**:1–20.
9. Singh U, Rao PV, Seetha R. Effect of dehulling on nutrient losses in chickpea (*Cicer arietinum* L.). *J Food Compos Anal* 1992;**5**:69–76.
10. Nizakat B, Amal BK, Gul SSK, Zahid M, Ihsanullah I. Quality and consumers acceptability studies and their inter-relationship of newly evolved desi type chickpea genotypes. Quality evolution of new chickpea genotypes. *Int J of Food Sci Tech* 2007;**42**(5):528–34.
11. Iqbal A, Ateeq N, Khalil IA, Perveen S, Saleemullah S. Physicochemical characteristics and amino acid profile of chickpea cultivars grown in Pakistan. *J Food Service* 2006;**17**:94–101.
12. Christodoulou V, Bampidis VA, Hucko B, Ploumi K, Iliadis C, Robinson PH, et al. Nutritional value of chickpeas in rations of lactating ewes and growing lambs. *Anim Feed Sci Technol* 2005;**118**:229–41.
13. Aslam M, Mahmood IA, Herridge DF. Contribution of chickpea fixed N2 in increasing rain-fed wheat production in Potohar. *Pakistan. Soil Sci. Soc. Pak* Nov. 13-16, 2000:26.

14. Tungland B, Meyer D. Non-digestible oligo- and polysaccharides (dietary fiber): Their physiology and role in human health and food. *Compr Rev Food Sci F* 2002;**1**(3):90–109.

15. Rodríguez R, Jiménez A, Fernández-Bolaños J, Guillén R, Heredia A. Dietary fibre from vegetable products as a source of functional ingredients. *Trends Food Sci Tech* 2006;**17**:3–15.

16. Scheneeman BO. Soluble vs insoluble fibre-different physiological responses. *Food Tech* 1987;**41**:81–2.

17. Rincon F, Martinez B, Ibanez MV. Proximate composition and antinutritive substances in chickpea (*Cicer arietinum* L.) as affected by the biotype factor. *J Sci Food Agric* 1998;**78**:382–388.

18. Xu BJ, Yuan SH, Chang SKC. Comparative analyses of phenolic composition, antioxidant capacity, and color of cool season legumes and other selected food legumes. *J Food Sci* 2007;**72**:S167–77.

19. Fares C, Menga V. Effects of toasting on the carbohydrate profile and antioxidant properties of chickpea (*Cicer arietinum* L.) flour added to durum wheat pasta. *Food Chem* 2012;**131**:1140–8.

20. Segev A, Badani H, Kapulnik Y, Shomer I, Oren-Shamir M, Galili S. Determination of Polyphenols, Flavonoids, and antioxidant capacity in colored chickpea. *J Food Sci* 2010;**75**(2):115–9 S.

21. Jacks TJ, Davidonis GH. Superoxide, hydrogen peroxide, and the respiratory burst of fungally infected plant cells. *Mol Cell Biochem* 1996;**158**:77–9.

22. Xiaoli X, Liyi Y, Shuang H, Wei L, Yi S, Hao M, et al. Determination of oligosaccharide content in 19 cultivars of chickpea (*Cicer arietinum* L) seeds by high performance liquid chromatography. *Food Chem* 2008;**111**:215–9.

23. Tosh SM, Yada S. Dietary fibres in pulse seed and fractions: characterization, functional attributes, and applications. *Food Res Int* 2010;**43**:450–60.

24. Hoover R, Ratnayake WS. Starch characteristics of black bean, chickpea lentil, navy bean and pinto bean cultivars grown in Canada. *Food Chem* 2002;**78**:489–98.

25. Miao M, Zhang T, Jiang B. Characterizations of kabuli and desi chickpea starches cultivated in China. *Food Chem* 2009;**113**:1025–32.

26. Huang J, Schols HA, van Soest JJG, Jin Z, Sulmann E, Voragen AGJ. Physicochemical properties and amylopectin chain profiles of cowpea, chickpea and yellow pea starches. *Food Chem* 2007;**101**:1338–45.

27. Singh N, Sandhu KS, Kaur M. Characterization of starches separated from Indian chickpea (*Cicer arietinum* L.) cultivars. *J Food Sci* 2004;**47**:441–9.

28. Englyst HN, Kingman SM, Cummings JH. Classification and measurement of nutritionally important starch fractions. *Eur J Clin Nutr* 1992;**46**:S33–50.

29. Han J, BeMiller JN. Preparation and physical characteristics of slowly digesting modified food starches. *Carbohyd Polym* 2007;**67**:366–74.

30. Jenkis AL. The glycemic index: Looking back 25 years. *Cereal foods world* 2007;**52**:50–3.

31. Rizkalla SW, Bellisle F, Slama G. Health benefits of low glycemix index foods, such as pulses, in diabetic patients and health individuals. *Brit J Nut* 2002;**88**:S255–62.

32. *Euresta, European Flair Action Concerted on Resistant Starch. Department of human nutrition.* Wageningen, The Netherlands: Wageningen Agricultural University Newsletter III; 1992 7.

33. Frías J, Vidal-Verde C, Kozlowska H, Gorecki R, Honke J, Hedley CL. Evolution of soluble carbohydrates during the development of pea, faba bean, and lupin seeds. *Z Lebensm Unters Forsch* 1996;**203**:27–32.

34. Larsson S, Johansson LA, Svenningsson M. Soluble sugars and membrane lipids in winter wheats (*Triticum Aestivum* L.) during cold acclimatation. *Eur J Agron* 1993;**1**:85–90.

35. Horbowicz M, Obendorf RL. Seed dessication tolerance and storability: Dependence on flatulence-producing oligosaccharids and cyclitols – review and survey. *Seed Sci Res* 1994;**4**:385–405.

36. Alajaji SA, El-Adawy TA. Nutritional composition of chickpea (*Cicer arietinum* L.) as affected by microwave cooking and other traditional cooking methods. *J Food Compos Anal* 2006;**19**:806–12.

37. Aguilera Y, Martin-Cabrejas MA, Benìtez V, Mollà E, Lopez-Andréu F, Esteban RM. Changes in carbohydrate fraction during dehydration process of common legumes. *J Food Compos Anal* 2009;**22**:678–83.

38. De J, Berrios J, Morales P, Cámara M, Sánchez-Mata MC. Carbohydrate composition of raw and estrude pulse flours. *Food Res Int* 2010;**43**:531–6.

39. Quemener B, Brillouet JM. Ciceritol, a pinitol diga-lactoside from seeds of chickpea, lentil and with lupin. *Phytochemistry* 1983;**22**:1745–51.

40. Alles MS, Hartemink R, Meyboom S, Harryvan JL, Van Laere KM, Nagengast FM, et al. Effect of transgalactoolisaccharides on the composition of the human intestinal microflora and on putative risk markers for colon cancer. *Am J Clin Nutr* 1999;**69**:980–91.

41. Bouhnik Y, Raskine L, Simoneau G, Vicaut E, Neut C, Flouriè B, et al. The capacity of nondigestible carbohydrates to stimulate fecal bifidobacteria in healthy humans: a double-blind randomized, placebocontrolled, parallel-group, dose–response relation study. *Am J Clin Nutr* 2004;**80**:1658–64.

42. Roberfroid M. Functional food concept and its application to prebiotics. *Dig. Liver Dis* 2002;**34**:S105–10.

43. Topping DL, Clifton PM. Short chain fatty acids and human colonic function: roles of resistant starch and non resistant starch polysaccharides. *Physiology Rev* 2001;**81**:1031–64.

44. Scholz-Ahrens KE, Schaafsma G, van den Heuvel EGHM, Schrezenméir J. Effects of prebiotics on mineral absorption. *Am J Clin Nutr* 2001;**73**:459S–64S.

45. Bazzano LA, Tees CH, Nguyen MT. Effect of non-soy legume consumption on cholesterol levels: a meta-analysis of randomized controlled trials. *Circulation* 2008;**118**:1122.

46. Martinez-Villaluenga C, Frías J, Vidal-Verde C. Alpha-Galactosides: antinutritional factors or functional ingredients? *Crit Rev Food Sci Nutr* 2008;**48**:301–16.

47. Naczk M, Amarowicz R, Shahidi F. α-Galactosides of sucrose in foods: composition, flatulence-causing effects, and removal. *ACS Symposium Series* 1997;**662**:127–51.

48. Peterbauer T, Richter A. Biochemistry and physiology of raffinose family oligosaccharides and galactosyl cyclitol in seeds. *Seed Sci Res* 2001;**11**:185–97.

49. Lestienne I, Icard-Vernière C, Mouquet C, Picq C, Trèche S. Effect of soaking whole cereal and legume seeds on iron, zinc and phytate contents. *Food Chem* 2005;**89**:421–5.

50. Sat IG, Keles F. The effect of soaking and cooking on the oligosaccharide content of seker a dry bean variety (*P. vulgaris*, L) grown in Turkey. *Pakistan J Nutr* 2002;**1**(5):206–8.

51. Vidal-Valverde C, Sierra I, Frías J, Prodanov M, Sotomayor C, Hedley CL, et al. Nutritional evaluation of lentil flours obtained after short time soaking processes. *Eur Food Res Technol* 2002;**214**:220–6.

52. Aranda P, Dostalova J, Frías J, Lopez-Jurado M, Kozlowska H, Pokorny J, et al. Nutrition. In: Hedley CL, editor. *Carbohydrates in Grain Legume Seeds. Improving Nutritional Quality and Agronomic Characteristics.* Wallingford, UK: International; 2001. p. 61–87.

53. Zamora FA, Fields ML. Nutritive quality of fermented cowpea (*Vigna sinensis*) and chickpea (*Cicer arietinum*). *J Food Sci* 1979;**44**:234–6.

54. Doblado R, Frías J, Muñoz R, Vidal-Verde C. Fermentation of vigna sinensis var. carilla flours by natural microflora and Lactobacillus species. *J Food Protein* 2003;**66**:2313–20.

55. Granito M, Torres A, Frías J, Guerra M, Vidal-Verde C. Effect of natural and controlled fermentation on flatus-producing compounds of beans (*P. vulgaris*). *J Sci Food Agric* 2003;**83**:1004–9.

56. Viana SF, Guimaraes VM, José IC, Oliveira MGA, Costa NMB, Barros EG, et al. Hydrolysis of oligosaccharides in soybean flour by α-galactosidase. *Food Chem* 2005;**93**:665–70.

57. Song D, Chang SK. Enzymatic degradation of oligosaccharides in pinto bean flour. *J Agric Food Chem* 2006;**54**:1296–301.

58. Kerr PS, Pearlstein RW, Schweiger BJ, Becker-Manley MF, Pierce JW. Nucleotide sequences of galactinol synthase from zucchini and soybeans. U.S. *Patent* 1998 5773699.

59. Griga M, Kosturkova G, Kuchuk N, Ilieva-Stoilova M. Biotechnology. In: Hedley CL, editor. *Carbohydrates in Grain Legume Seeds*. Wallingford, UK: Improving Nutritional Quality and Agronomic Characteristics. International; 2001. p. 145–207.

60. Frías J, Bakhash A, Jones DA, Arthur AE, Vidal-Valverde C, Rhodes MJC, et al. Genetic analysis of raffinose oligosaccharide pathway in lentil seeds. *J exp Bot* 1999;**50**:469–76.

61. American Association of Cereal Chemists (AACC 2001). The definition of dietary fibre. (Report of the Dietary Fibre Definition Committee to the Board of Directors of the AACC) Cereal Food World 46(3): 112–126.

62. Jenkis DJA, Kendall CWC, Axelsen M, Augustin LSA, Vuksan V. Viscous and nonviscous fibres, nonabsorbable a low glycemix index carbohydrates, blood lipids and coronary hearth disease. *Curr Opin Lipidol* 2000;**11**:49–56.

63. Reaven GM. Banting lecture 1988: role of insulin resistance in human desease. *Diabetes* 1988;**37**:1595–607.

64. Ford ES, Giles WH, Dietz WH. Prevalence of the metabolic syndrome among Us adults: findings from the Third National Health and Nutrition Examination Survey. *JAMA* 2002;**287**:356–9.

65. Hertog MGL, Kromhout D, Aravanis C. Flavonoid intake and long term risk of coronary heart disese and cancer in seven countries study. *Arch Int Med* 1995;**155**:381–6.

66. Martin-Cabrejas M, Aguilera Y, Benitez V, Mollá E, Lòpez-Anréu F, Esteban RM. Effect of industrial dehydration on the soluble carbohydrates and dietary fiber fractions in legumes. *J Agric Food Chem* 2006;**54**:7652–7.

67. Wang N, Hatcher DW, Tyler RT, Toews R, Gawalko EJ. Effect of cooking on the composition of beans (*Phaseolus vulgaris* L.) and chickpea (*Cicer arietinum* L.). *Food Res Int* 2010;**43**:589–94.

68. Dalgetty DD, Baik BK. Isolation and characterization of cotyledon fibres from peas lentils and chickpeas. *Cereal Chem* 2003;**80**(3):310–5.

69. Amarowicz R, Pegg RB. Legumes as a source of natural antioxidants. *Eur J Lipid Sci Tech* 2008;**110**:865–78.

70. Kalogeropoulos N, Chiou A, Ioannou M, Karathanos V, Hassapidou M, Andrikopoulos N. Nutritional evaluation and bioactive microconstituents (phytosterols, tocopherols, polyphenols, triterpenic acid in cooked dry legumes usually consumed in the Mediterranean countries. *Food Chem* 2010;**121**:682–90.

71. Aoki T, Tomoyoshi A, Shin-ichi A. Flavonoids of leguminous plants: structure, biological activity and biosynthesis. *J Plant Res* 2000;**113**:475–88.

72. Zielinski H, Kozlowska H. Antioxidant activity and total phenolics in selected cereal grains and their different morphological fraction. *J Agri Food Chem* 2000;**48**:2008–16.

73. Yu LL, Perret J, Harris M, Wilson J, Qian M. Free radical scavenging properties of wheat extracts. *J Agri Food Chem* 2002;**50**:1619–24.

74. Zhou KQ, Yu LL. Effects of extraction solvent on wheat bran antioxidant activity estimation. *Lebensm-Wiss Technol* 2004;**37**:717–21.

75. Martin-Cabrejas MA, Aguilera Y, Pedrosa MM, Cuadrado C, Hernández T, Díaz S, et al. The impact of dehydratation process on antinutrients and protein digestibility of some legume flours. *Food Chem* 2009;**114**:1063–8.

76. Xu BJ, Chang SKC. Comparative analyses of phenolic composition, antioxidant capacity, and color of cool season legumes as affected by extraction solvents. *J Food Sci* 2007;**72** S159–S156.

77. Halvorsen BL, Holte K, Myhrstad MC, Barikmo I, Hvattum E, Remberg SF, et al. A systematic screening of total antioxidants in dietary plants. *J. Nutr* 2002;**132**:461–71.

78. Pirisi FMP, Cabras C, Falqui C, Migliorini M, Muggelli M. Phenolic compounds in virgin olive oil. 2. Reappraisal of the extraction, HPLC separation and quantification procedures. *J. Agric Food Chem* 2000;**48**:1191–6.

79. Hrncirik K, Fritsche S. Comparability and reliability of different techniques for the determination of phenolic compounds in virgin olive oil. *Eur J Lipid Sci Technol* 2004;**106**:540–9.

80. Bravo L. Polyphenols: chemistry, dietary sources, metabolism and nutritional significance. *Nutr Rev* 1998;**56**:317–33.

81. Han H, Baik BK. Antioxidant activity and phenolic content of lentils (*Lens culinaris*), chickpea (*Cicer arietinum* L.), peas (*Pisum sativum* L.) and soybeans (*Glycine max*) and their quantitative changes during processing. *Int J Food Sci Tech* 2008;**43**:1971–8.

82. Troszynska A, Ciska E. Phenolic compounds of seed coats of white and coloured varieties of pea (*Pisum sativum* L) and their total antioxidant activity. *Czech J Food Sci* 2002;**20**:15–22.

83. Kasum CM, Jacobs Jr DR, Nicodemus K, Folsom AR. Dietary risk factors for upper aerodigestive tract cancers. *Int J Cancer* 2002;**99**(2):267–72.

84. Thompson LU. Antioxidant and hormone-mediated health benefits of whole grains. *Crit Rev Food Sci Nutr* 1994;**34**:473–97.

85. Antolovich M, Prenzler PD, Patsalides E, McDonald S, Robards K. Methods for testing antioxidant activity. *Analyst* 2002;**127**:183–98.

86. Crozier A, Jaganath IB, Clifford MN. Dietary phenolics: Chemistry, bioavailability and effects on health. *Nat Prod Rep* 2009;**26**:1001–43.

87. Henry-Vitrac C, Berbille H, Mérillon JM, Vitrac X. Soy isoflavones and potential inhibitors of Alzheimer β-amyloid fibril aggregation *in vitro*. *Food Res Int* 2010;**43**:2176–8.

88. Wang N, Hatcher DW, Gawalko EJ. Effect of variety and processing on nutrients and certain anti-nutrients in field peas (*Pisum sativum*). *Food Chem* 2008;**111**:132–8.

89. Xu BJ, Chang SKC. Effect of soaking, boiling and steaming on total phenolic content and antioxidant activities of cool season food legumes. *Food Chem* 2008;**110**:1–13.

90. Daur I, Khan IA, Jahangir M. Nutritional Quality of roasted and pressure- cooked chickpea compared to raw. *Sarhad J Agric* 2008:24117–22.

91. Torres A, Frías J, Vidal-Verde C. Changes in chemical composition of lupin seeds (*Lupinus angusifolius* L.) after selective α-galactoside extraction. *J Sci Food Agric* 2005;**85**:2468–74.

92. Klameczynska B, Czuchajowska Z, Baik BK. Composition, soaking, cooking properties and thermal characteristics of starch of chickpeas, wrinkled peas and smooth peas. *Int J Food Sci Tech* 2001;**36**:563–72.

93. Otto T, Baik BK, Czuchajowska Z. Microstructure of seeds, flours and starch of legumes. *Cereal Chem* 1997;**74**:445–51.

94. Frías J, Vidal-Verde C, Sotomayor C, Diaz-Pollan C, Urbano G. Influence of processing on available carbohydrate content and antinutritional factors of chickpeas. *Eur Food Res Technol* 2000;**210**:340–5.

95. López-Amorós ML, Hernández T, Estrela I. Effect of germination on legume phenolic compounds and their antioxidant activity. *J Food Comp Anal* 2006;**19**:277–83.

96. Reyes-Moreno C, Cuevas-Rodriguez EO, Milan-Carrilo J, Ardenas-Valenzuela OG, Barron-Hoyos J. Solid state fermentation process for producing chickpea (*Cicer arietinum* L) tempeh flour: physiochemical and nutritional characteristics of the product. *J Sci Food Agric* 2004;**84**:271–8.

97. Paredes-Lopez O, Gonzáles-Castañeda J, Cárabez-Trejo A. Influence of solid substrate fermentation on the chemical composition of chickpea. *J Ferm Bioeng* 1991;**71**:58–62.

98. Bau HM, Villanme C, Nicolas JP, Méjean L. Effect of germination on chemical composition, biochemical constitutes and antinutritional factors of soy bean (*Glycine max*) seeds. *J Sci Food Agric* 1997;**73**:1–9.

99. Fernandez-Orozco R, Piskula MK, Zielinski H, Kozlowska H, Frías J, Vidal-Valverde C. Germination as a process to improve the antioxidant capacity of *Lupinus angustifolius* L. var. *Zapaton*. *Eur Food Res Technol* 2006;**223**:495–502.

100. El-Adawy T. Nutritional composition and antinutritional factors of chickpeas (*Cicer arietinum* L.) undergoing different cooking methods and germination. *Plant Food Hum Nutr* 2002;**57**:83–97.

101. Ghavidel RA, Prakash J. The impact of germination and dehullingon nutrients, antinutrients, in vitro iron and calciun bioavailability and *in vitro* starch and protein digestibility of some legume seeds. *LWT-Food Sci Tech* 2007;**40**:1292–9.

102. Manzocco L, Calligaris S, Mastrocola D, Vicoli MC, Lerici CR. Review of non-enzymatic browning and antioxidant capacity in processed foods. *Trends Food Sci Tech* 2001;**11**:340–6.

103. de Almeida Costa GE, da Silva Queiroz-Monici K. Pissini Machado Reis SM, Costa de Oliveira A. Chemical composition, dietary fibre and resistant starch contents of raw and cooked pea, common bean, chickpea and lentil legumes. *Food Chem* 2006;**94**:327–30.

104. Koksel H, Sivri D, Scanlon MG, Bushuk W. Comparison of physical properties of raw and roasted chickpea (leblebi). *Food Res Int* 1999;**31**:659–65.

105. Chiang BY, Johnson JA. Gelatinization of starch in extruded products. *Cereal Chem* 1977;**54**:436–43.

106. Tudorica CM, Kuri V, Brennan CS. Nutritional and physicochemical characteristics of dietary fibre enriched pasta. *J Agri Food Chem* 2002;**50**:347–56.

107. Chillo S, Laverse J, Falcone PM, Protopapa A, Del Nobile MA. Influence of the addition of buckwheat flour and durum wheat bran on spaghetti quality. *J Cereal Sci* 2008;**47**:144–52.

108. Fares C, Platani C, Baiano A, Menga V. Effect of processing and cooking on phenolic acid profile and antioxidant capacity of durum wheat pasta enriched with debranning fractions of wheat. *Food Chem* 2010;**119**:1023–9.

109. Cleary LJ, Brennan CS. Effect of beta-glucan on pasta quality. *Int J Food Sci Tec* 2006;**41**:910–8.

110. Goni I, Valentın-Gamazo C. Chickpea flour ingredient slows glycemic response to pasta in healthy volunteers. *Food Chem* 2003;**81**:511–5.

111. Chavez-Jàuregui RN, Cardoso-Santiago RA. Pinto e Silva MEM, Arêas JAG. Acceptability of snaks produced by the extrusion of amaranth and blend of chickpea and bovine lung. *Int J Food Sci Tech* 2003;**38**:795–8.

112. Wood A. Texture, processing and organoleptic properties of chickpea-fortified spaghetti with insights to the underlying mechanisms of traditional durum pasta quality. *J Cereal Sci* 2009;**49**:128–33.

113. Sabanis D, Makri E, Doxastakis G. Effect of durum flour enrichment with chickpea flour on the characteristic of dough and lasagne. *J Sci Food Agri* 2006;**86**:1938–44.

114. Zhao YH, Manthey FA, Chang SKC, Hou H-J, Yuan SH. Quality Characteristics of spaghetti as affected by green and yellow pea, lentil, and chickpea flours. *J Food Sci* 2005;**70**:371–6.

115. Gomez M, Oliete B, Rosell CM, Pando V, Fernández E. Studies on cake quality of wheat-chickpea flour blends. *LTW-Food Sci Tech* 2008;**41**:1701–9.

116. Yamsaengsun R, Schoenlechner R, Berghofer E. The effect of chickpea on the functional properties of white and whole wheat bread. *Int J Food Sci Tech* 2010;**45**:610–20.

117. Hefnawy TMH, El-Shourbagy GA, Ramadan MF. Impact of adding chickpea (*Cicer arietinum* L.), flour on the rheological properties of toast bread. *Int Food Res J* 2012;**19**(2):521–5.

118. Kadam ML, Salve RV, Mehrajfatema ZM, More SG. Development and evaluation of composite flour for Missi roti/chapatti. *J Food Process Tech (ISSN:2157-7110 JFPT, an open access journal)* 2012;**3**(1):1–7.

119. Battistuti JP, Barros RMC, Arêas JAG. Optimization of extrusion cooking process for chickpea (*Cicer arietinum* L.) defatted flour by response surface methodology. *J Food Sci* 1991;**56**(6):1695–8.

120. Cardoso-Santiago RA, Arêas JAV. Nutritional evaluation of snacks obtained from chickpea and bovine lung blends. *Food Chem* 2001;**74**:35–40.

Index

Note: Page numbers followed by "f" denote figures; "t" tables.

Color Plates

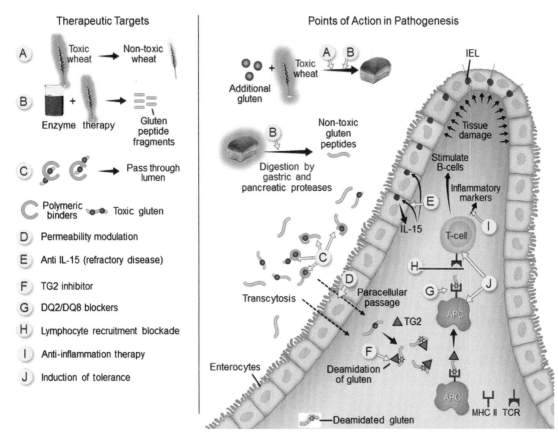

FIGURE 12.1 (A) Non-toxic wheat: generation of wheat species that lack the immunogenic gluten peptides. (B) Enzyme therapy: detoxification of the gluten peptides by enzymatic supplementation or treatment of the wheat flour with microbial proteases. (C) Polymeric binders: polymeric binders limit toxicity of gluten by preventing degradation and absorption. (D) Permeability modulation: zonulin antagonists (larazotide) inhibit gliadin-induced increased permeability by inhibition of zonulin release via receptor blockade. (E) Anti IL-15: gluten peptides evoke the innate immune response by inducing IL-15 expression and interaction between epithelial MIC and NKG2D receptor on surface of intraepithelial lymphocytes. This ligand–receptor interaction induces epithelial apoptosis by stimulation of the cytotoxic T lymphocytes. (F) TG2 inhibitors: gliadin peptides are deamidated by TG2 in the lamina propria. TG2 blockade can inhibit the adaptive immune response. (G) HLA blockade: Prevents binding of the gliadin peptides to HLA DQ2 or DQ8 on the surface of the antigen presenting cells. (H) Inhibition of T-lymphocyte recruitment blocks migration of immune cells to the intestinal tissues. (I) Anti-cytokine therapy: antibodies against IFN-γ and TNF-α produced in response to T-cell activation reduce mucosal injury in celiac disease. (J) Induction of immune tolerance: vaccine with immunogenic gluten peptides. Abbreviations: IL-15, interleukin; NKG2D, natural killer cell receptor D; MIC, major histocompatibility complex class I related chains; TG2, transglutaminase 2; IFN, interferon; TNF, tumor necrosis factor.

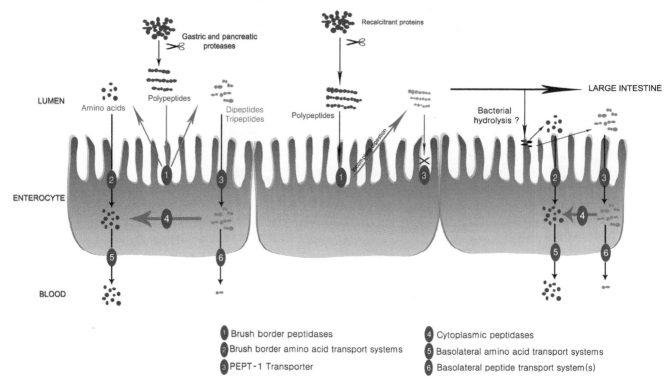

FIGURE 13.1 Model of protein digestion and absorption in the small intestine. Proteins are hydrolyzed to amino acids, dipeptides, and tripeptides by pancreatic and brush border membrane proteases. These products are transported into the enterocytes via specific transport systems in the brush border membrane. Once inside the cells, small peptides are subjected to hydrolysis by cytoplasmic peptidases to release free amino acids which are transported into the blood. The transport of small peptides across the basolateral membrane is a minor pathway. Recalcitrant proteins such as gluten prolamins are relatively resistant to proteolysis in the small intestine. As a result of the partial digestion, high molecular weight oligopeptides persist in the lumen of the small intestine because they are not transported by PEPT-1. These peptides could be hydrolyzed by bacterial proteases to easily absorbable compounds that would be used by the host.

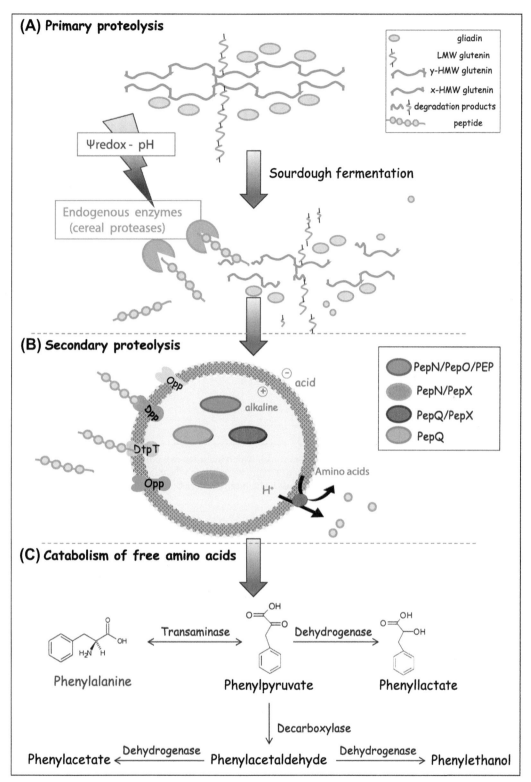

FIGURE 14.1 Schematic representation of the proteolysis during sourdough fermentation. (A) Primary proteolysis triggered by the acidification and reduction of disulfide bonds of gluten by hetero-fermentative lactobacilli, which in turn promote the primary activity of cereal proteases, which leads to the liberation of various sized polypeptides. (B) Secondary proteolysis by intracellular peptidases of sourdough lactic acid bacteria, which complete the proteolysis and liberate free amino acids. PepN, general aminopeptidase type N (EC3.4.11.11); PepO, endopeptidase (EC 3.4.23); PEP prolyl endopeptidyl peptidase (EC 3.4.21.26); PepX, X-prolyl dipeptidyl aminopeptidase (EC 3.4.14.5); PepQ, prolidase (EC 3.4.13.9). (C) Catabolism of free amino acids by sourdough lactic acid bacteria: example of catabolic reaction involving phenylalanine. *Figure adapted from Gobbetti et al.*[45]

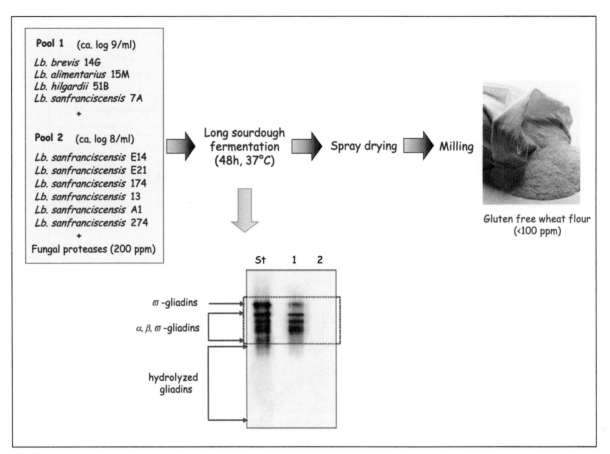

FIGURE 14.2 **Schematic representation of the biotechnology protocol, which includes two pools (1 and 2) of 10 selected sourdough lactobacilli, fungal proteases (200 ppm), and long fermentation time (48 h, 37°C).** The resulting wheat flour contains hydrolyzed gluten at less than 100 ppm, as shown by R5-Western blot gel. St, European gliadin standard; 1, chemically acidified dough; 2, dough fermented with selected lactobacilli and proteases. Lb, *Lactobacillus*.

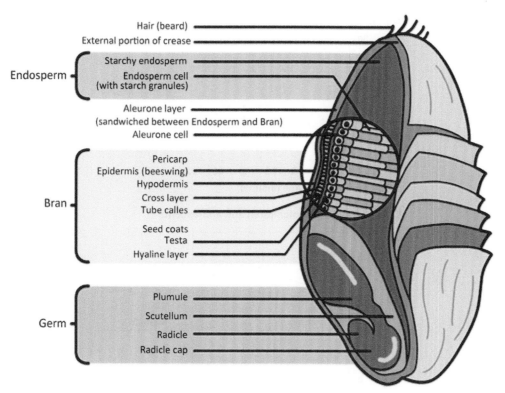

FIGURE 17.1 Structure of a wheat grain. http://www. g r a i n c h a i n . c o m / 1 4 - t o - 16/technology/images/seed.gif.

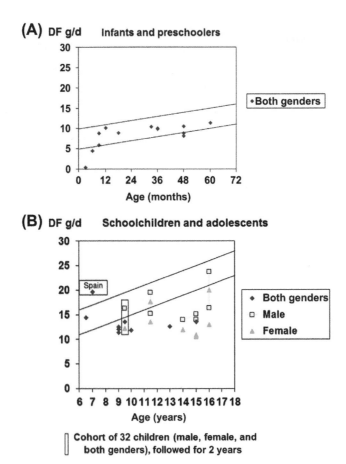

FIGURE 18.1 Mean dietary fiber intake according to mean age groups: (A) infants and preschoolers; (B) school children and adolescents. Means of age groups are approximate, since mean ages are not available from the literature; for instance, the calculated mean for age group 2–5 years is 48 months. Oblique lines represent the limits of the recommended DF intake according to the American Health Foundation: age (years) + 5–10 g/day.[47] *Information from a compilation of literature data*[49, 81–89]

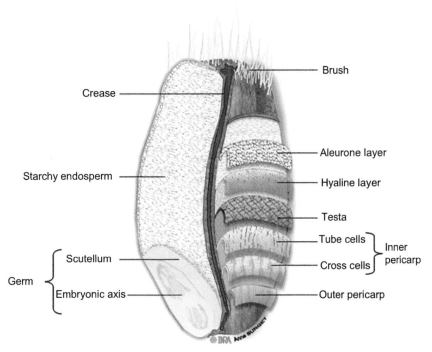

FIGURE 19.2 A histological representation of the wheat grain. *From Surget and Barron,[39] translated and reproduced with permission from the editor.*

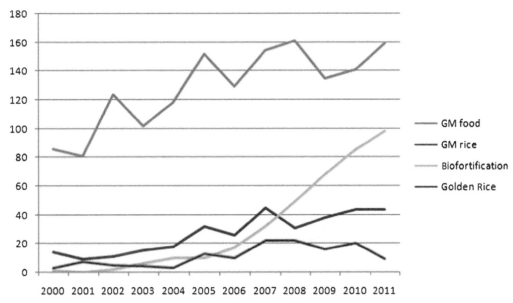

FIGURE 21.1 Number of articles on GM food, GM rice, biofortification and Golden Rice, as derived from the Web of Knowledge literature database (2000–2011). Note: Recent figures (2012) were not included as they were incomplete at the time of the study. *Source: own compilation, based on Web of Knowledge (2011).*

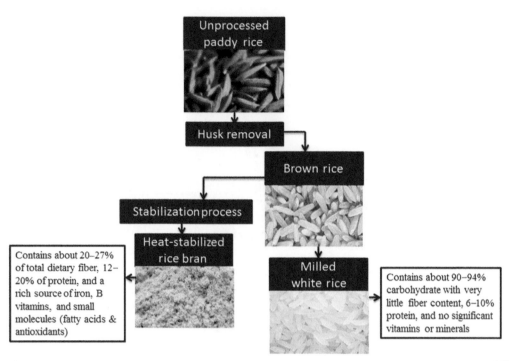

FIGURE 22.1 Whole grain rice processing and a summary of nutrient variations of white rice and rice bran end products.[10,57]

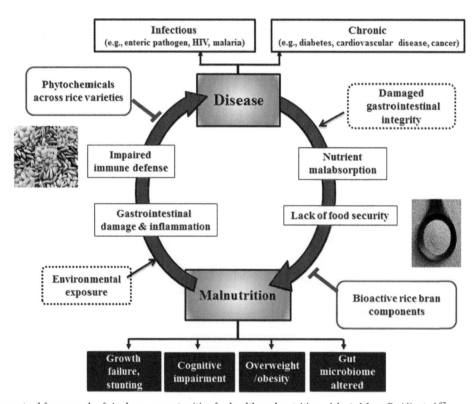

FIGURE 22.2 Conceptual framework of rice bran opportunities for health and nutrition. *Adapted from Preidis et al.*[87]

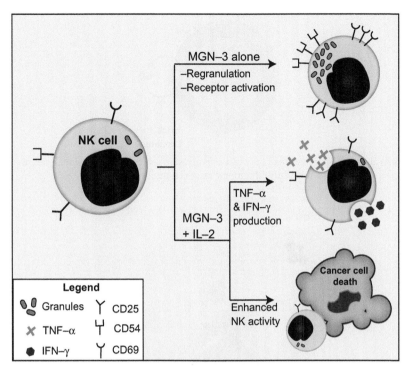

FIGURE 31.3 Natural killer augmentory effects by MGN-3/BioBran alone and its synergy with IL-2. Treatment with MGN-3/BioBran alone resulted in regranulation and receptor activation of NK cells. In addition, treatment of NK cells with MGN-3/BioBran and IL-2 increased TNF-α and IFN-γ secretions and enhanced NK cell activity.

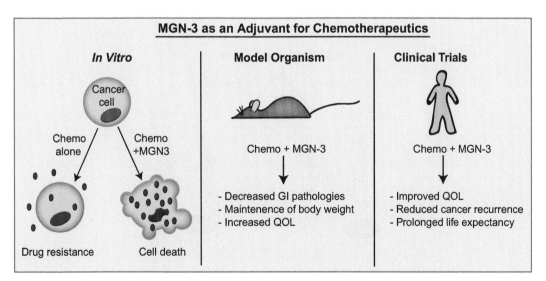

FIGURE 31.4 MGN-3/BioBran acts as an adjuvant for chemotherapeutic drugs in three different models; in vitro, and in animal and cancer patients. For *in vitro* studies, treatment with MGN-3/BioBran increased the accumulation of chemotherapy drugs (red ovals) in cancer cells, which ultimately induced apoptosis. In animal studies, MGN-3/BioBran improved QOL and maintained body weight, and in cancer patients it reduced cancer recurrence and prolonged life expectancy.

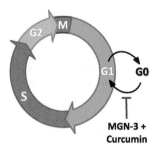

FIGURE 31.5 MGN-3/BioBran and curcumin treatment may cause an arrest in cell cycle progression. Evidence suggests that this combination of therapies arrests the cell cycle in G0–G1 transition, thus inhibiting cancer cell proliferation and growth.

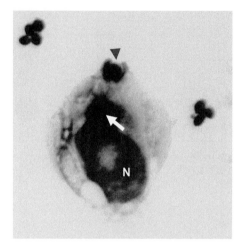

FIGURE 31.6 Breast cancer cells phagocytize baker's yeast. This image shows a Giemsa-stained cytospin preparation of MCF-7 cells at two different stages of yeast phagocytosis. One yeast is in the process of phagocytosis (red arrowhead), while the other has already been phagocytosed into the cancer cell (white arrow). Notice that the nucleus (N) is condensing and the nucleus to cytoplasm ratio is increasing.

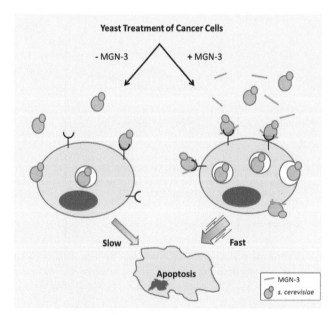

FIGURE 31.7 The co-culture of cancer cells with yeast in the presence of MGN-3/BioBran. MGN-3/BioBran enhances binding of yeast, leading to an increase in phagocytosis of yeast and subsequent increase in cancer cell apoptosis.

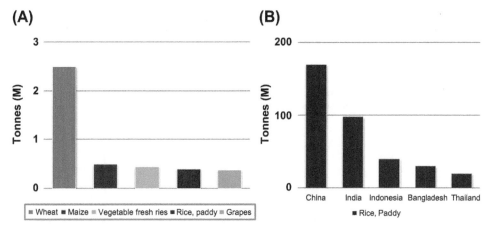

FIGURE 32.1 (A) Whole world production: proportion of rice amongst other grains (average 1961–2010). (B) Production of top five producers of rice (average 1961–2010). *Food and Agriculture Organization of the United Nations* (http://faostat3.fao.org/home/index.html#VISUALIZE).

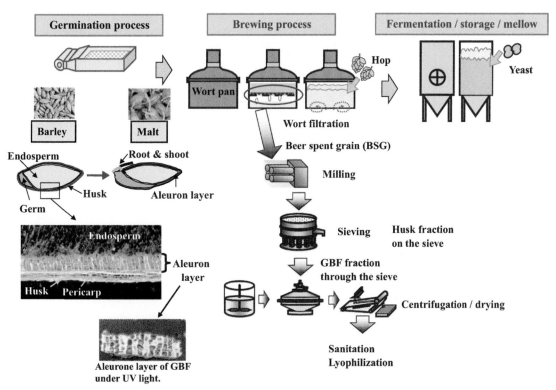

FIGURE 39.1 Schematic production of beer and germinated barley foodstuffs. Beer is made in three steps: (1) immersing malted barley in hot water and separating the barley extract from the residue; (2) boiling this extract with hops; and (3) cooling the extract and fermenting it using yeast. Brewer's spent grain (BSG) is a by-product of this first step. Germinated barley foodstuff (GBF) was obtained by separating the aleurone and scutellum from BSG by physical means only, not by any chemical process. For plants, the newly synthesized low-lignified hemicellulose, which is accumulated in the scutellum and aleurone fractions, is utilized for the stretching of their roots and germ. The aleurone layer of GBF contains arabinoxylan in the cell wall, which emits fluorescence under excitation by ultraviolet light.

Effects of GBF on fecal output and SCFA content

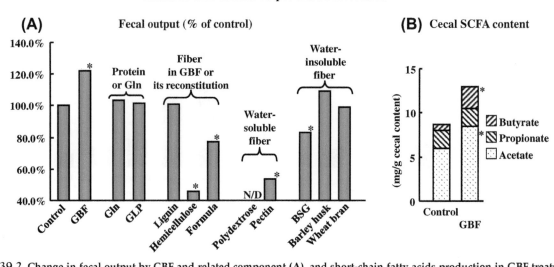

FIGURE 39.2 Change in fecal output by GBF and related component (A), and short-chain fatty acids production in GBF treatment (B). In fecal output, data was shown as % value of control treated group. Short-chain fatty acid content is expressed as the mean ($n = 6$~9). GLP, glutamine peptide (purchased from DMV Japan Co. Tokyo, Japan); Lignin (purchased from Tokyo Kasei Kogyo Co. Tokyo, Japan); Hemicellulose, water-soluble hemicellulose; Formula, a mixture of cellulose, hemicellulose and lignin similar in composition to GBF's dietary fiber; PD, polydextrose, and PC, pectin from apple (PD and PC were used as representative water-soluble fibers); BSG, beer spent grain; Barley husk, husk-rich fraction by milling and sieving of BSG. Wheat bran is used as a representative water-insoluble fiber. Data are expressed as the mean changes ± SD; * represents a significant difference compared with Cont ($P < 0.05$). *Data are modified from original data in previous studies.*[4,18]

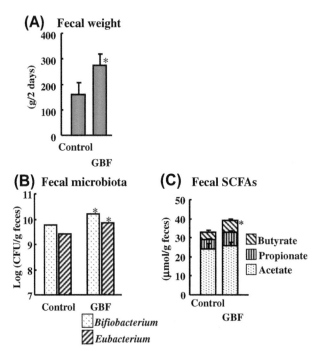

FIGURE 39.3 Change in fecal weight (A), fecal microbiota analysis (B), and fecal short-chain fatty acid content (C) in healthy volunteers. In (A), 9 g daily of cellulose was administered to volunteers ($n = 10$/group) for 3 days and feces were collected the last 2 days as a control period; sequentially, 30 g of GBF was administered to volunteers for 28 days and feces were collected the last 2 days. GBF significantly increased fecal output. (B) Summary of the anaerobic microbes *Bifidobacterium* and *Eubacterium limosum* in the feces and short-chain fatty acid content before (control) and after GBF administration ($n = 9$/group). Data are expressed as the mean changes ± SEM; * represents a significant difference between the Cont and GBF ($P < 0.05$). *Data are modified from original data in previous studies.*[19]

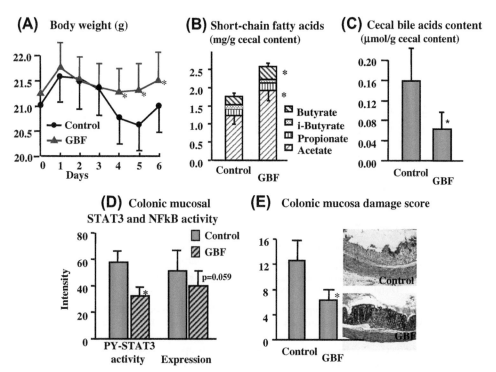

FIGURE 39.4 Change in body weight (A), fecal short-chain fatty acid (SCFA) content (B), cecal bile acids content (C), colonic mucosal signal transducer and activator of transcription 3 (STAT3), and nuclear factor kappa B (NF-κB) activity (D), and colonic mucosal damage score and representative histology (E) in dextran sulfate sodium colitis mouse model. Data are expressed as the mean changes ± SEM (n = 10/group); * represents a significant difference between the Cont and GBF (P < 0.05). *Data are modified from original data in a previous study.*[37]

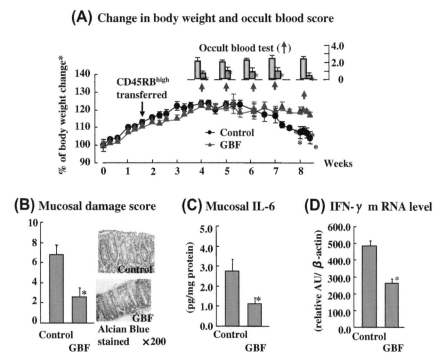

FIGURE 39.5 Change in body weight and occult blood score (A), mucosal damage score and representative histology (B), mucosal interleukin-6 (IL-6) (C), and expression of interferon gamma (IFN-γ) (D) in CD45RB[high] transferred model. Data are expressed as mean changes ± SEM (n = 10); * represents significant different between control and GBF groups (P < 0.05). *Data are modified from original data in a previous study.*[45]

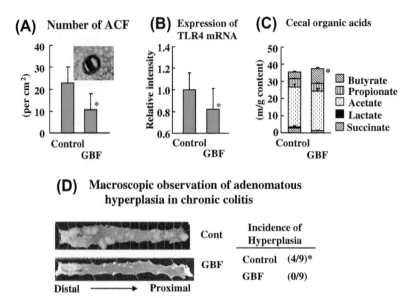

FIGURE 39.6 Change in the incidence of aberrant crypt foci (ACF) (A) and the expression of mRNA of toll-like receptor 4 (TLR4 mRNA) and cyclooxygenase-2 (COX-2) (B) in colonic mucosa, and cecal organic acids content (C) in the azoxymethane-induced colon cancer model. (D) shows representative hyperplastic adenoma in control rats and the incidence of hyperplastic adenoma in the cyclic administered DSS chronic colitis model. Aberrant crypt foci (ACF) were counted under a light microscope per 1 cm2 of the distal colon at 100× magnification. Aberrant crypts appeared larger and had a thicker epithelial lining compared to normal crypts, and were gathered into a focus consisting of several crypts. (A) ACF in the germinated barley foodstuff (GBF) group were significantly lower than in the control (Cont) group. (B) The expression levels of toll-like receptor 4 (TLR4) in the colonic mucosa were normalized to the expression levels of the housekeeping gene glyceraldehyde-3-phosphate dehydrogenase. (C) Cecal short-chain fatty acid content. (D) Representative macroscopic observation of the entire colon in both groups and incidence of hyperplasia are shown. Data are expressed as mean changes ± SD; $P < 0.05$ for the differences between the Cont and the GBF. *Data modified from original data in previous studies: (A–C)[54], (D)[57].*

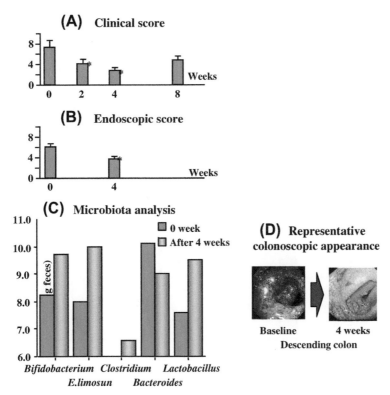

FIGURE 39.7 Change in the clinical score (A) and endoscopic score (B) in mild to moderately active ulcerative colitis patients who consumed 30 g GBF every day for 4 weeks. Representative change in microbiota analysis (C) and endoscopic observation (D) in active moderate ulcerative colitis patient with daily administration of 20–30 g of GBF for 4 weeks. Mild to moderately active ulcerative colitis patients who had been unresponsive to or intolerant of standard treatment consumed 30 g of GBF every day for 4 weeks in a non-randomized, open-label fashion. After 4 weeks of treatment with GBF, clinical and endoscopic improvements were observed (A, B).[58] Data are expressed as mean changes ± SEM ($n = 10$); * represents significant different between 0 week and 2 or 4 weeks after GBF treatment ($P < 0.05$). Microbiota analysis showed increases of *Bifidobacterium* and *Eubacterium limosum* (butyrate producer), and a decrease in *Bacteroides* (C). (D) Representative colonic mucosal appearance at baseline and after GBF treatment. *Data are modified from original data in a previous study.*[59]

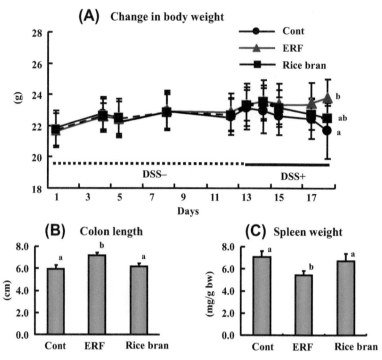

FIGURE 40.2 Change in body weight (A), colon length (B), and weight of spleen per body weight (C) in mice with DSS colitis fed control (Cont), enzyme-treated rice fiber (ERF), or its raw material rice bran diet. Data are expressed as mean ± SD. Each group contains 10 mice. a,b: Values not sharing a common letter represent differences among the three groups.[36]

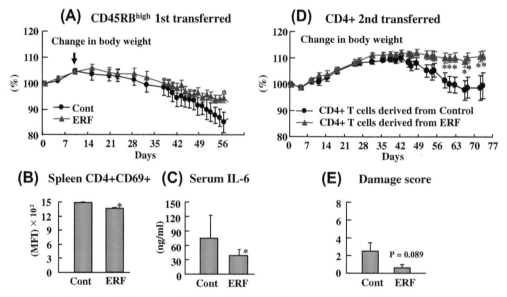

FIGURE 40.3 Change in body weight (A) in mice with colitis due to transfer of CD4+CD45RB^high T cells fed either control (Cont; $n = 10$) or enzyme-treated rice fiber (ERF; $n = 10$) diet. Data are expressed as the mean ± SD. The body weights of the Cont and ERF groups on day 0 were 16.3 ± 0.2 and 16.4 ± 0.2, respectively. The downward arrow represents the day of CD4+CD45RB^high T cell transfer. (B) Mean fluorescent intensity (MFI) of CD4+CD69+ T cells in the mesenteric lymph nodes. (C) Serum interleukine-6 concentration. (D) Change in body weight in mice with colitis due to 2nd transfer of CD4+ T cells which were derived from 1st transferred colitis mice fed either Cont or ERF diet. (E) Colonic mucosal damage score and final spleen weight per g body weight. Data are expressed as the mean changes ± SD; * represents a significant difference between the Cont and ERF groups ($P < 0.05$).[36]

Printed and bound by CPI Group (UK) Ltd, Croydon, CR0 4YY

08/05/2025

01864938-0002